Minimally Invasive Bariatric Surgery

Minimally Invasive Bariatric Surgery

Second Edition

Editors

Stacy A. Brethauer, MD
Assistant Professor of Surgery
  Cleveland Clinic Lerner College of Medicine
Bariatric and Metabolic Institute
Cleveland Clinic
Cleveland, OH, USA

Philip R. Schauer, MD
Professor of Surgery
  Cleveland Clinic Lerner College of Medicine
Director, Bariatric and Metabolic Institute
Cleveland Clinic
Cleveland, OH, USA

Bruce D. Schirmer, MD
Stephen H. Watts Professor of Surgery
Department of Surgery Health Sciences Center
University of Virginia Health System
Charlottesville, VA, USA

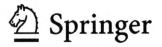 Springer

Editors

Stacy A. Brethauer, MD
Assistant Professor of Surgery
  Cleveland Clinic Lerner College of Medicine
Bariatric and Metabolic Institute
Cleveland Clinic
Cleveland, OH, USA

Philip R. Schauer, MD
Professor of Surgery
  Cleveland Clinic Lerner College of Medicine
Director, Bariatric and Metabolic Institute
Cleveland Clinic
Cleveland, OH, USA

Bruce D. Schirmer, MD
Stephen H. Watts Professor of Surgery
Department of Surgery
Health Sciences Center
University of Virginia Health System
Charlottesville, VA, USA

Videos to this book can be accessed at http://www.springerimages.com/videos/978-1-4939-1636-8

ISBN 978-1-4939-1636-8   ISBN 978-1-4939-1637-5 (eBook)
DOI 10.1007/978-1-4939-1637-5
Springer New York Heidelberg Dordrecht London

Library of Congress Control Number: 2014956872

Preface

It is truly amazing how rapidly the field of bariatric surgery has changed over the last two decades. As we proudly present our second edition of this text, it is clear that much has changed in our field even since the first edition was published. The obesity and diabetes epidemic that is upon us has spurred a sense of urgency among bariatric surgeons to provide safe and effective treatment to as many patients as possible and to educate our referring physicians about the benefits of these metabolic procedures. There is still much work to be done to provide even better access to patients and to ensure high quality care at a national level, but there are few, if any, disciplines in surgery that have come so far in such a short time as bariatric surgery. The morbidity and mortality rates after laparoscopic bariatric surgery are now equivalent to many other commonly performed elective operations such as hysterectomy, hip replacement, and cholecystectomy. That is a remarkable accomplishment that reflects the impact of laparoscopic techniques, advanced training programs, and an emphasis on quality patient care that have been the hallmarks of bariatric surgery since the 1990s.

This new edition highlights many of the advances in our field over the last 7 years with regard to the multidisciplinary management of the obese patients and surgical outcomes. Updated chapters on the medical and perioperative management of these patients provide state-of-the-art management pathways to guide practicing bariatric physicians and surgeons. Quality improvement, value-based care, and outcome reporting have entered the lexicon of every practicing surgeon now, and we have also added an important chapter on patient safety and quality improvement for the bariatric surgery program.

A major shift that has occurred in bariatric surgery over the last decade has been the acceptance of sleeve gastrectomy as a primary bariatric procedure. As sleeve gastrectomy surpasses gastric bypass in the United States as the most commonly performed procedure, there is still much debate about the long-term role of this relative newcomer to our field. This updated text incorporates current updates on techniques, outcomes, and management of complications after sleeve gastrectomy to address the successes and challenges of this operation. New investigative techniques and procedures, both surgical and endoscopic, comprise a small proportion of clinical activity currently, but are discussed in this update as these concepts may hold promise for less-invasive and more widely accepted interventions in the future.

This second edition provides surgical technique chapters written by leaders in the field accompanied by updated illustrations and videos to inform the resident or fellow preparing for the next day's case. Outcome chapters for each procedure reflect the current state of the evidence and the text also provides practical management strategies for complications that occur after each procedure accompanied by figures and images that illustrate these clinical challenges.

As the emphasis on weight loss after these operations has been overtaken by the discussion regarding metabolic benefits, we have added new chapters and authors to provide clear evidence-based updates focusing on the long-term effects of bariatric surgery on mortality, cancer, and the full spectrum of obesity-related comorbidities.

While it seems that change is the only certainty in the field of bariatric surgery, this updated textbook provides the most current snapshot of this exciting and evolving field. We hope you find the second edition of *Minimally Invasive Bariatric Surgery* a useful tool in your practice and a practical guide to educating residents and fellows.

Cleveland, OH, USA   Stacy A. Brethauer, M.D.
Cleveland, OH, USA   Philip R. Schauer, M.D.
Charlottesville, VA, USA   Bruce D. Schirmer, M.D.

Contents

Contributors

Ted D. Adams, Ph.D., M.P.H
Division of Cardiovascular Genetics, University of Utah School of Medicine, Salt Lake City, UT, USA
Health & Fitness Institute, Intermountain Healthcare, University of Utah School of Medicine, Salt Lake City, UT, USA

Cheguevara Afaneh, M.D.
Department of Surgery, New York Presbyterian Hospital, Weill Cornell Medical Center, New York, NY, USA

Eric P. Ahnfeldt, D.O.
Cleveland Clinic Foundation, Bariatric and Metabolic Institute, Cleveland, OH, USA

Abdulrahim AlAwashez, M.D., M.B.B.S., F.R.C.S.C.
Department of Surgery, Dalhousie University, St. Marha's Hospital, Antigonish, NS, Canada

Mohamed R. Ali, M.D.
Minimally Invasive and Bariatric Surgery, University of California, Davis Medical Center, Sacramento, CA, USA

Maria Altieri, M.D.
Department of General Surgery, Stony Brook University Hospital, Stony Brook, NY, USA

Luigi Angrisani, M.D.
Surgical Endoscopy, S. Giovanni Bosco Hospital, Naples, Italy

Dan E. Azagury, M.D.
Section of Bariatric and Minimally Invasive Surgery, Stanford University School of Medicine, Stanford, CA, USA

Sean J. Barnett
Cincinatti Children's Hospital Medical Center, Pediatric and General Thoracic Surgery, Cincinatti, OH, USA

Esam S. Batayyah, M.D., F.A.C.S.
Bariatric and Metabolic Institute, Cleveland Clinic, Digestive Disease Institute, Cleveland, OH, USA

Simon Biron, M.D., M.Sc.
Department of Surgery, IUCPQ (Hospital Laval), Quebec, QC, Canada

Stacy A. Brethauer, M.D.
Bariatric and Metabolic Institute, Cleveland Clinic, Digestive Disease Institute, Cleveland, OH, USA

Wendy A. Brown, M.B.B.S. (Hons), Ph.D., F.A.C.S., F.R.A.C.S.
Monash University Centre for Obesity Research and Education, Melbourne, VIC, Australia

Bartolome Burguera, M.D., Ph.D.
Research Unit, Division of Endocrinology, IUNICS, Hospital Universitario Son Espases, Palma de Mallorca, Spain

Guy-Bernard Cadière, M.D., Ph.D.
Department of Gastrointestinal Surgery, European School of Laparoscopic Surgery, Saint-Pierre University Hospital, Brussels, Belgium

Josemberg Marins Campos, M.D., Ph.D.
Department of General Surgery, Universidade Federal de Pernambuco, Recife, PE, Brazil

Pedro Paulo Caravatto, M.D.
The Center of Obesity and Diabetes, Hospital Oswaldo Cruz, São Paulo, Brazil

Aaron D. Carr, M.D.
Minimally Invasive and Bariatric Surgery, University of California, Davis Medical Center, Sacramento, CA, USA

Derrick Cetin, M.D.
Department of Bariatric Medicine, Cleveland Clinic Foundation, Bariatric Metabolic Institute, Cleveland, OH, USA

Bipan Chand
Department of Surgery, Stritch School of Medicine, Loyola University Chicago, Chicago, IL, USA

Ricardo Cohen, M.D.
The Center of Obesity and Diabetes, Hospital Oswaldo Cruz, São Paulo, Brazil

Janelle W. Coughlin, Ph.D.
Johns Hopkins University School of Medicine, Baltimore, MD, USA

Christopher R. Daigle, M.D.
Bariatric and Metabolic Institute, Cleveland Clinic, Cleveland, OH, USA

Adrian G. Dan, M.D. F.A.C.S.
Department of General Surgery, Akron City Hospital Summa Health System, Akron, OH, USA

Giovanni Dapri, M.D., Ph.D., F.A.C.S., F.A.S.M.B.S.
Department of Gastrointestinal Surgery, European School of Laparoscopic Surgery, Saint-Pierre University Hospital, Brussels, Belgium

Lance E. Davidson, Ph.D.
Division of Cardiovascular Genetics, University of Utah School of Medicine, Salt Lake City, UT, USA

John B. Dixon, M.B.S.B., Ph.D., F.R.A.C.G.P., F.R.C.P. (Edin)
Baker IDI Heart & Diabetes Institute, Clinical Obesity Research, Melbourne, VIC, Australia

Monica Dua, M.D.
Cleveland Clinic Foundation, Bariatric and Metabolic Institute, Cleveland, OH, USA

George M. Eid
Allegheny Health Network, Pittsburgh, PA, USA

Bamdad Farhad, D.O.
Department of Bariatric and Minimally Invasive Surgery, South Eastern Medical Center, Lumberton, NC, USA

George Fielding, M.D., M.B.B.S., F.R.A.C.S., F.R.C.S. (Glasgow)
Department of Surgery, New York University, New York, NY, USA

Christine Ren Fielding, M.D. F.A.C.S.
NYU Langone Medical Center, New York, NY, USA

Brandon T. Grover, D.O., F.A.C.S.
Department of General & Vascular Surgery, Gundersen Lutheran Health System, La Crosse, WI, USA

Giselle G. Hamad
Department of Surgery, University Pittsburgh Medical Center, Pittsburgh, PA, USA

Mia Hashibe, Ph.D., M.P.H.
Department of Family and Preventive Medicine, University of Utah School of Medicine, Salt Lake City, UT, USA

Leslie J. Heinberg, Ph.D.
Cleveland Clinic Lerner College of Medicine, Bariatric and Metabolic Institute, Cleveland Clinic, Cleveland, OH, USA

Daniel M. Herron, M.D., F.A.C.S.
Department of Surgery, Mount Sinai School of Medicine, New York, NY, USA

Kelvin D. Higa, M.D.
Minimally Invasive Bariatric Surgery, Fresno Heart and Surgical Hospital, Fresno, CA, USA

Jacques Himpens, M.D., Ph.D.
Department of Gastrointestinal Surgery, European School of Laparoscopic Surgery, Saint-Pierre University Hospital, Brussels, Belgium

Elizabeth A. Hooper, M.D.
General and Bariatric Surgery, Mercy Clinic and Hospital, Oklahoma City, OK, USA

Frédéric-Simon Hould, M.D., F.R.C.S.C.
Department of Surgery, Advanced Laparoscopy, Bariatric and Metabolic Surgery, Institut Universitaire de Cardiologie et de Pneumologie de Québec (IUCPQ), Laval University, Québec City, QC, Canada

Kelli C. Hughes, R.D., C.D.E.
University of Virginia Health System, Charlottesville, VA, USA

Steven C. Hunt, Ph.D.
Division of Cardiovascular Genetics, University of Utah School of Medicine, Salt Lake City, UT, USA

Dennis Hurwitz
UPMC Magee Women's Hospital—Plastic Surgery, University of Pittsburgh, Pittsburgh, PA, USA

Thomas H. Inge
Department of Pediatric and General Thoracic Surgery, Cincinatti Children's Hospital Medical Center, Cincinatti, OH, USA

Mohammad H. Jamal, M.B.Ch.B. (Hons), M.Ed., F.R.C.S.C.
Department of Surgery, Mubarak Teaching Hospital, Kuwait University, Kuwait City, Kuwait

Daniel B. Jones, M.D., M.S., F.A.C.S.
Department of General Surgery, Beth Israel Deaconess Medical Center, Boston, MA, USA

Stephanie B. Jones, M.D.
Department of Anesthesia, Critical Care and Pain Medicine, Beth Israel Deaconess Medical Center and Harvard Medical School, Boston, MA, USA

Julie J. Kim, M.D.
Department of Surgery, Tufts Medical Center, Boston, MA, USA

Shanu N. Kothari, M.D., F.A.C.S.
Department of General & Vascular Surgery, Gundersen Lutheran Health System, La Crosse, WI, USA

Matthew Kroh, M.D.
Digestive Disease Institute, Cleveland Clinic, Cleveland, OH, USA

Cindy M. Ku, M.D.
Department of Anesthesia, Critical Care, and Pain Medicine, Beth Israel Deaconess Medical Center, Boston, MA, USA

Nitin Kumar, M.D.
Division of Gastroenterology, Brigham and Women's Hospital/Harvard Medical School, Boston, MA, USA

Michele Lorenzo, M.D., Ph.D.
UOML Distretto 56, ASL—NA3 Sud, Torre Annunziata, Italy

Rebecca Lynch, M.D.
General Surgery, Summa Akron City Hospital, Akron, OH, USA

Simon Marceau, M.D., F.R.C.S.C.
Department of Surgery, IUCPQ (Hospital Laval), Quebec, QC, Canada

Karina A. McArthur
Kaiser Permanente Mid Atlantic, Holy Cross Hospital, Pittsburgh, PA, USA

Kathleen M. McCauley
Goodman Allen & Filetti, PLLC, Glen Allen, VA, USA

Emanuele Lo Menzo, M.D.
Department of General Surgery, Cleveland Clinic Florida, The Bariatric and Metabolic Institute, Weston, FL, USA

Marc P. Michalsky
Nationwide Children's Hospital, Columbus, OH, USA

Cyrus Moon, MD
Minimally Invasive Bariatric Surgery, Fresno Heart and Surgical Hospital, Fresno, CA, USA

John M. Morton, M.D., M.P.H.
Section of Bariatric and Minimally Invasive Surgery, Stanford University School of Medicine, Stanford, CA, USA

Fady Moustarah, M.D., M.P.H., F.R.C.S.C.
Department of Surgery, IUCPQ (Hospital Laval), Quebec, QC, Canada

Manoel Galvao Neto, M.D.
Department of Bariatric Endoscopy, Gastro Obeso Center, São Paulo, Brazil

Paul O'Brien, M.D.
Centre for Obesity Research and Education (CORE), Monash Medical School, Monash University, Melbourne, VIC, Australia

Jaisa Olasky, M.D.
Department of Surgery, Beth Israel Deaconess Medical Center, Boston, MA, USA

Debbie Pasini, R.N., B.S.N., C.B.N.
Bariatric Care Center, Summa Health System, Akron, OH, USA

Tarissa Petry, M.D.
The Center of Obesity and Diabetes, Hospital Oswaldo Cruz, São Paulo, Brazil

Alfons Pomp, M.D., F.A.C.S., F.R.C.S.C.
Department of Surgery, New York Presbyterian Hospital, Weill Cornell Medical Center, New York, NY, USA

Jaime Ponce, M.D., F.A.C.S., F.A.S.M.B.S.
Hamilton Medical Center—Dalton Surgery Group, Dalton, GA, USA

Pornthep Prathanvanich
Department of Surgery, Stritch School of Medicine, Loyola University Chicago, Chicago, IL, USA

Aurora Pryor, M.D.
Department of General Surgery, Stony Brook University Hospital, Stony Brook, NY, USA

Rebecca N. Puffer, M.P.H., R.D.
University of Virginia Health System, Charlottesville, VA, USA

Almino Cardoso Ramos
Department of Bariatric Surgery, Gastro Obeso Center, São Paulo, Brazil

M. Logan Rawlins, M.D.
Minimally Invasive & Bariatric Surgery, Department of Surgery, University of Virginia, Charlottesville, VA, USA

Hector Romero-Talamas, M.D.
Bariatric and Metabolic Institute, Cleveland Clinic, Cleveland, OH, USA

Raul J. Rosenthal, M.D.
Bariatric and Metabolic Institute, Cleveland Clinic, Weston, FL, USA

Mitchell S. Roslin, M.D.
Department of Surgery, Lenox Hill Hospital, New York, NY, USA

Francesco Rubino, M.D.
Section of Gastrointestinal Metabolic Surgery, Department of Surgery, Weill Cornell Medical College and New York Presbyterian Hospital, New York, NY, USA
Catholic University, Rome, Italy

Bruce D. Schirmer, M.D.
Department of Surgery, University of Virginia Health Systems, Charlottesville, VA, USA

Sajani Shah, M.D.
Department of Surgery, Tufts Medical Center, Boston, MA, USA

Scott A. Shikora, M.D.
Department of Surgery, Center of Metabolic & Bariatric Surgery, Brigham & Women's Hospital, Boston, MA, USA

Alpana Shukla, M.D., M.R.C.P.
Section of Gastrointestinal Metabolic Surgery, Department of Surgery, Weill Cornell Medical College and New York Presbyterian Hospital, New York, NY, USA
Catholic University, Rome, Italy

Lyz Bezerra Silva, M.D.
Department of General Surgery, Hospital Agamenon Magalhães, Recife, PE, Brazil

Mary B. Simmons, R.D.
Rockingham Memorial Hospital, Harrisonburg, VA, USA

Manish Singh, M.D.
Bariatric and Metabolic Institute in Affiliation with Cleveland Clinic Bariatric and Metabolic Institute, Doctors Hospital at Renaissance, Edinburg, TX, USA

Ashwin Soni, M.D., B. Sc.
Section of Gastrointestinal Metabolic Surgery, Department of Surgery, Weill Cornell Medical College and New York Presbyterian Hospital, New York, NY, USA
Catholic University, Rome, Italy

Harvey J. Sugerman, M.D.
Department of Surgery, Virginia Commonwealth University, Sanibel, FL, USA

Robert Sung, M.D.
Department of Surgery, Lenox Hill Hospital, New York, NY, USA
General SurgeryLenox Hill Hospital, New York, NY, USA

Samuel Szomstein, M.D.
Department of General and Vascular Surgery, Cleveland Clinic Florida, Weston, FL, USA

Christopher C. Thompson, M.D., M.Sc., F.A.C.G., F.A.S.G.E.
Division of Gastroenterology, Brigham and Women's Hospital/Harvard Medical School, Boston, MA, USA

Joan Tur, B.S., M.H.S., Ph.D.
Research Unit, Division of Endocrinology, IUNICS, Hospital Universitario Son Espases, Palma de Mallorca, Spain

Amanda R. Vest, M.B.B.S., M.R.C.P.
Heart and Vascular Institute, Cleveland Clinic, Cleveland, OH, USA

Krzysztof J. Wikiel
Department of Surgery, Magee-Women's Hospital of UPMC, Pittsburgh, PA, USA

Andrew S. Wu, M.D.
Department of Metabolic, Endocrine, and Minimally Invasive Surgery, Mount Sinai School of Medicine, New York, NY, USA

James B. Young, M.D., F.A.C.C.
Heart and Vascular Institute, Cleveland Clinic, Cleveland, OH, USA

Andrea Zelisko, M.D.
Cleveland Clinic Lerner College of Medicine, Digestive Disease Institute, Cleveland, OH, USA

1

The Global Burden of Obesity and Diabetes

John B. Dixon

One could only wonder what aliens who visited Earth briefly 40 years ago and returned today would think of the changes seen in the dominant intelligent life form inhabiting the planet. Large numbers of humans have become quite bloated, sluggish, and many have difficulty getting around. This would appear the most obvious change in the human condition during that period. What has happened? What has gone wrong? What will things be like should our visitors return in another 40 years?

The obesity-diabetes epidemic has rolled out progressively and inexorably since the 1970s, and little has been done globally to prevent it. The causes are poorly understood, and any attempts to change the trends appear piecemeal, tokenistic, and ineffective. Regions of the developing world that appeared to be protected with their economic and lifestyle characteristics are surpassing all expectations, and even those in rural areas of developing countries are running head first into the diabesity epidemic.

Obesity a Global Issue: The global age-standardized prevalence of obesity nearly doubled from 6.4 % in 1980 to 12.0 % in 2008. Half of this rise occurred in the 20 years between 1980 and 2000 and half occurred in the 8 years between 2000 and 2008 [1]. The magnitude of rise has varied with region, country, and gender; however, stabilization of the obesity prevalence is rare, and of great concern, the rise has accelerated globally over the last decade. In 1980, half of the 572 million adults with a BMI >25 kg/m^2 lived in just five countries headed by China 72 million and the USA 70 million. In 2008, countries with the most overweight people were China (241 million) and the USA (158 million). The largest absolute rise in obesity (BMI >30 kg/m^2) occurred in the USA (56 million) and China (42 million), followed by Brazil (20 million) and Mexico (18 million). The region with the highest global prevalence of obesity includes small islands in the Western Pacific such as Nauru, Samoa, Tonga, and the Cook Islands where obesity rates exceed 50 % and for some subgroups 70 % [1].

Of the high-income nations, there were divergent trends for both men and women with greater rises in obesity prevalence in Australasia and North America compared with Western Europe and high-income areas of Asia. Women had greater increases in obesity prevalence than men in sub-Saharan Africa and Latin America and the Caribbean. Men had greater a increase in prevalence throughout Europe and the high-income regions of the Asia-Pacific region [1]. "If the rates of weight gain (in Australia) observed in the first 5 years of this decade are maintained, our findings suggest that normal-weight adults will constitute less than a third of the population by 2025, and the obesity prevalence will have increased by 65 %" [2].

With increasing levels of obesity, we see an exponential rise in class III obesity (BMI >40 kg/m^2). In the USA between 2000 and 2005, the prevalence of obesity increased by 24 %, class III obesity by 50 %, and BMI >50 kg/m^2 by 75 %, two and three times faster, respectively [3]. Similar trends are reported in Australia [4]. The resultant exponential increase in class III obesity and super obesity is an expected trend as the mean BMI for a community steadily increases. There is also an important gender trend with increasing levels of obesity with women more likely to have the more severe forms of obesity Table 1. Scattered reports of a leveling off of obesity prevalence in small subsections of the community, for example, in adolescent and young adult women, should be treated cautiously as levels are still high, and we need to reflect about the weight trajectories of their mothers and grandmothers who at an equivalent age were generally more petite.

For years we have watched as the US CDC state by state obesity levels have risen year by year and reassured ourselves that either our state was not the worst or, better still, we lived outside the USA and were immune to the catastrophe within. But alas, we can now watch similar changes in the Canadian provinces and UK counties, and thanks to the International Association for the Study of Obesity (IASO), we have a global atlas of the emerging trends. Sadly no global area is or will remain immune.

S.A. Brethauer et al. (eds.), *Minimally Invasive Bariatric Surgery*,
DOI 10.1007/978-1-4939-1637-5_1, © Springer Science+Business Media New York 2015

TABLE 1. Estimates of the proportion of the US adult population with a BMI > 40 kg/m^2

	1960 (%)	1980 (%)	2000 (%)	2010 (%)
Women (USA)	1.4	2.8	6.1	7.4
Men (USA)	0.4	0.8	2.9	4.3

Adapted from the IASO website [5]

Ethnic Differences Risk: Ethnic-Based Action Points

Diabetes as a Global Issue: While it can be often assumed that the emerging epidemic of type 2 diabetes parallels the obesity epidemic, there are a range of other important considerations that influence the global and regional incidence, prevalence, and total burden of type 2 diabetes.

The International Diabetes Federation "World Diabetes Atlas" updated in 2012 provides an excellent overview of the global situation, and there are very important regional considerations. *Globally it is estimated that 371 million live with diabetes, an overall adult prevalence is 8.3 %, and half of these cases are undiagnosed*:

- Countries with the highest prevalence of diabetes are in two regions the Western Pacific Island nations and in the Middle East. Examples of the highest prevalence rates in adults include Federation of Micronesia (37 %), Nauru (31 %), and Marshall Islands (27 %) in the Western Pacific and Kuwait (24 %), Saudi Arabia (23 %), and Qatar (23 %) in the Middle East.
- Countries with the highest absolute numbers in descending order are China (92 million), India (63 million), the USA (24 million), and Brazil (14 million). And the region with the highest numbers is the Western Pacific with 132 million.
- Sub-Saharan Africa is the region with the highest level of undiagnosed diabetes (80 %).

It is the Asian area that now contributes to more than 60 % of the world's population with diabetes where some of the most dramatic increases in diabetes prevalence have occurred over recent decades. All Asian countries have seen major rises as the rapid socioeconomic growth and industrialization interact with populations that have a strong genetic and ethnic risk of diabetes. Asians develop diabetes at a lower threshold of environmental and anthropometric risk (BMI and waist circumference) [6]. Another striking characteristic of diabetes in the Asian region is the striking narrowing of the urban–rural divide in diabetes prevalence. While urbanization and industrialization were thought to drive increased risk of diabetes, it is now clear that the rural areas are following very closely behind. In the Shanghai region of China, urban diabetes prevalence rose from 11.5 to 14.1 % between 2002–2003 and 2009, while the rural diabetes prevalence rose from 6.1 to 9.8 % during the same period [7]. The rapid rise in diabetes numbers in China indicates a major public health problem that has occurred in parallel with the massive changes in development and gross domestic product [8].

A recent review of diabetes prevalence in the rural areas of low- and middle-income countries revealed a quadrupling of prevalence over the last 25 years. Diabetes prevalence increased over time, from 1.8 % in 1985–1989, 5.0 % in 1990–1994, 5.2 % in 1995–1999, 6.4 % in 2000–2004, to 8.6 % for 2005–2010 [9]. However, this is only part of the story as it is estimated that between 2010 and 2013, the number of adults with diabetes will increase by 69 % in developing countries, while the expected increase in developed countries is 20 % [10]. The diabetes burden in developing countries is also troubling as the increase in diabetes prevalence is dominated by the 40–59 age group, a time of productivity and employment, rather than being driven by aging as is the case developed countries (Fig. 1) [10].

Factors influencing the number of people with diabetes also vary considerable between developed and developing countries. If the incidence of diabetes exceeds mortality, then the prevalence rises. The absolute number of people with diabetes will be influenced by a range of factors, and the relative contributions of these factors vary considerably (Fig. 2). An increased prevalence of diabetes is not simply related to an increase incidence. In the period between 1999 and 2004 in Taiwan, the prevalence of diabetes increased 38 % and 24 % in men and women, respectively, but during the same period, incidence dropped 4 % and 13 %, respectively. An increased incidence in younger adults and a reduced incidence in the elderly increased prevalence substantially [11].

Diabetes incident and prevalence data from Ontario Canada between 1995 and 2005 provides another example of the interactions that lead to prevalence. During this period, the age- and sex-adjusted prevalence of diabetes in the province increased 69 %, from 5.2 % in 1995 to 8.8 % in 2005. The rate of increase in prevalence was greater in a younger population and the mortality of those with diabetes fell by 25 %. Thus, the increased prevalence in diabetes is attributed to both an increased incidence and improved survival [12].

The prevalence of diabetes in the USA is also greatly influenced by an increased survival of those with diabetes. During the period 1997 to 2004, the National Health Interview Survey found that age-adjusted excessive death rates for those with diabetes (compared with those without diabetes) declined by 60 %, from 5.8 additional deaths/1000 to 2.3 additional deaths/1000, for cardiovascular disease, and

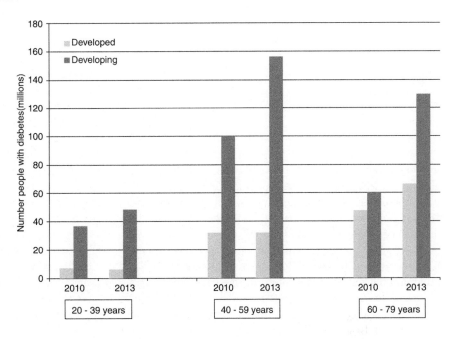

Fig. 1. The predicted number of people with diabetes in 2030 in comparison with 2010 (adapted from: Shaw, J.E. et al., Diabetes Res Clin Pract, (2010). **87**(1): p. 4–14).

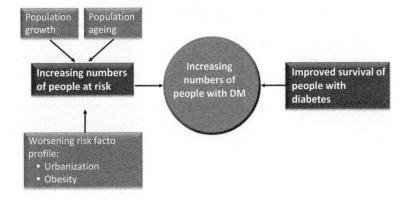

Fig. 2. The reasons associated with an increase in the numbers with diabetes. The relative impact of these population characteristic varies considerably between developed and developing countries.

for all-cause age-adjusted mortality a decline of 44 % from 10.8 to 6.1 deaths/1000. The declines were similar in both men and women [13]. Similar declines in mortality have been reported in other developed countries including Canada, Norway, and Finland. These encouraging findings have been attributed to a range of advances including systematic improvements in the quality and organization of care, improved models of chronic disease management, and the active promotion of self-care behaviors. More intensive pharmacotherapy targeting optimal levels of blood pressure [14] and cholesterol [15] has been shown to reduce morbidity and mortality, while the targets for glucose control remain more controversial [16]. There have also been reductions in smoking, limb amputations, and visual loss associated with retinopathy.

It becomes clear that while increasing levels of obesity play a major role in the increasing global population with diabetes, there are other major contributing determinants. The contrast in these determinants in developing compared with developed nations is presented in Table 2.

Causes Are Complex: The global biological determinants for the obesity-diabetes epidemic appear complex and poorly understood. They extend well beyond the global marketing of Westernized energy dense foods and the obligatory reduction in human movement that a developed society delivers. The interaction with the environment is far more complex, and a large number of additional conditions also appear to contribute to the evolving catastrophe. This complexity may partly explain the impotence of current preventative measures. Early life and metabolic programming appear to be very

TABLE 2. The differing determinants of the increasing population with diabetes in developing compared with developed countries

	Developed	Developing
Population growth	+	++
Population aging	+	+++
Increasing high-risk ethnicities	++	–
Increased incidence	+	++
Falling mortality	++	–

important factors contributing to obesity and may include genetics, maternal age, assertive mating, childhood infections, the pattern of established gut microbiota, and epigenetic programming changes to the ovum, the fetus, and the infant during the early years of life [17, 18]. The most important 4 years that influence a person's weight throughout the life cycle may well occur before the 3rd birthday. Early life programming sets an organism up for the environment that the organism is likely to encounter for living. To be programmed for a lean nutritional environment and being born into the "land of plenty" is aberrant representing a clear programming-environmental mismatch. One only has to look at the obesity and metabolic plight of indigenous populations globally when confronted with Western living conditions. It may not surprise that people of European origin fare best in "a land of plenty" and indeed may be the global exceptions in their resistance to developing diabetes and other metabolic disturbance associated with obesity.

Other environmental conditions are also likely to contribute to the obesity emidemic: sleep time over the decades has been reduced and is partly replaced with screen time; temperature-controlled environments reduce our energy expenditure in both heating and cooling our bodies; endocrine disrupters are widely dispersed within our environment and some contribute to weight gain; antibiotics and other factors have been designed to grow our food supply rapidly and efficiently may also change or gut microbiome to encourage weight gain; and iatrogenic contributions to weight gain through medications to treat mental illness, epilepsy, chronic autoimmune and inflammatory disease, and diabetes [17].

Obesity and Its Influence on Diabetes

The risk of developing type 2 diabetes at any given BMI is strongly related to ethnicity, and the World Health Organization and the International Diabetes Federation recommend modified action points for interventions based on ethnicity (Table 3).

Obesity also has additional influences on the number of people with diabetes for reasons beyond increased incidence.

Obesity is leading to an onset of type 2 diabetes in younger age groups. There is a negative relationship between BMI and the age of onset of type 2 diabetes [19, 20], and this is clearly associated with a longer period living with diabetes. Life expectancy for diabetes diagnosed at 30 years is quite different to that of 70 years.

In those with diabetes, overweight and obesity appears to be associated with lower age-adjusted mortality. A series of recent population assessments raise a very relevant issue with respect to diabetes, BMI, and mortality. All are different populations, but there are consistent findings and all would raise substantive questions about the value of weight loss in the overweight and class I obese BMI ranges.

Data from 5 pooled analyses of 5 large US longitudinal cohort studies were examined for incident diabetes in men and women over the age of 40 years and subsequent cardiovascular and all-cause mortality. After adjusting for demographics and established cardiovascular risk factors, those who were overweight and obese had a reduced all-cause and cardiovascular mortality [21].

Similar and very confronting data has been reported from Taiwan where a national diabetes registry is active [22]. Almost 90,000 diabetic patients were recruited after 1995 and the national death registry examined at the end of 2006 when 30 % had died. The adjusted analysis found that increasing body mass index was associated with progressive reduction in all-cause mortality. The effect was statistically significant for all causes of mortality other than cancer deaths. Those with a BMI >30 (which is uncommon in Taiwan) had the lowest mortality. This is one example of the obesity survival paradox.

A third study in Scotland examined BMI at the time of diabetes diagnosis in over 100,000 patients and mortality. There were 9,631 deaths between 2001 and 2007. BMI at the time of diagnosis was associated in a U-shaped mortality with the lowest index mortality in the overweight group. The authors question if weight loss interventions reduce mortality [23].

Black and Caucasian men followed by the USA VA medical centers also demonstrate an inverse relationship between BMI and diabetes mortality. The obese men, even those with a BMI > 35, have a lower mortality than normal-weight men [24].

These data add important contributions to the metabolic surgery—type 2 diabetes debate and raise issues about intentional weight loss in those not in the BMI > 35 category. This emerging data, combined with the issues with the large Sibutramine SCOUT study [25] and the premature cessation of the Look Ahead study for lack of hard end-point efficacy, all raise questions about any value in intentional weight loss in the overweight and class I obese BMI range in those with diabetes. It is becoming clear that bariatric-metabolic surgery will need to provide hard all-cause mortality, cardiovascular mortality, and suicide outcomes [26] data before it could be a broadly acceptable therapy for overweight and class I obese individual with diabetes. The same pattern has emerged for the approval of pharmacotherapy for weight loss and diabetes although it is easier to stop drug therapy than reverse bariatric procedures.

In summary, diabetes and obesity prevalence continues to rise, especially in the young and in developing countries.

TABLE 3. The classification of weight category by BMI

Classification	BMI (kg/m^2)	
	Principal cutoff points	Cutoff points for Asians
Normal range	18.5–24.9	18.5–22.9
		23.0–24.9
Pre-obese	25.0–29.9	25.0–27.4
		27.5–29.9
Obese class I	30.0–34.9	30.0–32.4
		32.5–34.9
Obese class II	35.0–39.9	35.0–37.4
		37.5–39.9
Obese class III	≥40.0	≥40.0

For Asian populations, classifications remain the same as the international classification, but public health action points for interventions are set at 23, 27.5, 32.5, and 37.5 [27]
We address eligibility and prioritization for bariatric surgery within the colored zones above
Source: Adapted from WHO 2004 [28]

Increasing obesity and its associated increase in incident diabetes do not explain all the increase in diabetes prevalence, and the determinants of prevalence vary considerably in developing countries when compared with developed. The morbidity and mortality associated with diabetes has decreased substantially in developed countries where the major increase in diabetes is likely to occur in those over 60 years. In contrast in developing countries, the obesity-diabetes epidemic burden will impact those of working age. Longitudinal epidemiological data indicates that overweight and obesity may be associated with improved survival in those with diabetes and that the benefits of intentional weight loss are unclear.

The burden of obesity and diabetes remains high globally, and national and regional obesity-diabetes prevention and management strategies are essential.

Acknowledgment: I would like to thank Professor Jonathan Shaw, at the Baker IDI Heart and Diabetes Institute, Melbourne, for sharing figures and data that I have used in the preparation of this chapter.

Review Questions and Answers

Question 1

What is the expected change in the proportion of people with severe obesity (class II, III, and BMI > 50) as the prevalence of obesity rises in a community?

(a) The rise in the prevalence of obesity leads to the same proportional rise in higher levels of obesity.
(b) The proportional rise in severe forms of obesity is less than expected because limited numbers have the propensity to become severely and super obese.
(c) The proportional (or percentage) rises far more rapid and becomes more so with higher BMI. The proportion of super obese (BMI >50) is rising rapidly.

(d) There is insufficient data to know how many in our communities have the more severe forms of obesity.

The answer is C.

Question 2

The increasing prevalence of diabetes in developed countries such as the USA is related to:
(a) Increased aging
(b) Increased overweight and obesity rates
(c) Increased survival of those with diabetes
(d) Increased proportion within the population with a high ethnic risk
(e) All of the above

The answer is E.

Question 3

Which of the following is true about diabetes prevalence in developing countries?
(a) Diabetes rates are much lower than in developed countries.
(b) Diabetes rates are only rising in urban regions.
(c) The expected increase in diabetes will have its greatest impact in the working years of middle age rather than the elderly.
(d) The expected increase in diabetes will have its greatest impact in elderly.
(e) Diabetes is not a major health issue in developing countries as it is in the developed.

The answer is C.

References

1. Stevens GA, Singh GM, Lu Y, Danaei G, Lin JK, Finucane MM, Bahalim AN, McIntire RK, Gutierrez HR, Cowan M, Paciorek CJ, Farzadfar F, Riley L, Ezzati M. National, regional, and global trends in adult overweight and obesity prevalences. Popul Health Metr. 2012;10:22.
2. Walls HL, Magliano DJ, Stevenson CE, Backholer K, Mannan HR, Shaw JE, Peeters A. Projected progression of the prevalence of obesity in Australia. Obesity (Silver Spring). 2012;20:872–8.
3. Sturm R. Increases in morbid obesity in the USA: 2000-2005. Public Health. 2007;121:492–6.
4. Walls HL, Wolfe R, Haby MM, Magliano DJ, de Courten M, Reid CM, McNeil JJ, Shaw J, Peeters A. Trends in BMI of urban Australian adults. Public Health Nutr. 1980–2000;2009:1–8.
5. IASO. USA prevalence of morbid obesity—adapted from the IASO website; 2013.
6. Ramachandran A, Snehalatha C, Shetty AS, Nanditha A. Trends in prevalence of diabetes in Asian countries. World J Diabetes. 2012;3:110–7.
7. Li R, Lu W, Jiang QW, Li YY, Zhao GM, Shi L, Yang QD, Ruan Y, Jiang J, Zhang SN, Xu WH, Zhong WJ. Increasing prevalence of type 2 diabetes in Chinese adults in Shanghai. Diabetes Care. 2012;35:1028–30.
8. Yang W, Lu J, Weng J, Jia W, Ji L, Xiao J, Shan Z, Liu J, Tian H, Ji Q, Zhu D, Ge J, Lin L, Chen L, Guo X, Zhao Z, Li Q, Zhou Z, Shan

G, He J. Prevalence of diabetes among men and women in China. N Engl J Med. 2010;362:1090–101.

9. Hwang CK, Han PV, Zabetian A, Ali MK, Narayan KM. Rural diabetes prevalence quintuples over twenty-five years in low- and middle-income countries: a systematic review and meta-analysis. Diabetes Res Clin Pract. 2012;96:271–85.

10. Shaw JE, Sicree RA, Zimmet PZ. Global estimates of the prevalence of diabetes for 2010 and 2030. Diabetes Res Clin Pract. 2010;87:4–14.

11. Chang CH, Shau WY, Jiang YD, Li HY, Chang TJ, Sheu WH, Kwok CF, Ho LT, Chuang LM. Type 2 diabetes prevalence and incidence among adults in Taiwan during 1999-2004: a national health insurance data set study. Diabet Med. 2010;27:636–43.

12. Lipscombe LL, Hux JE. Trends in diabetes prevalence, incidence, and mortality in Ontario, Canada 1995-2005: a population-based study. Lancet. 2007;369:750–6.

13. Gregg EW, Cheng YJ, Saydah S, Cowie C, Garfield S, Geiss L, Barker L. Trends in death rates among U.S. adults with and without diabetes between 1997 and 2006: findings from the national health interview survey. Diabetes Care. 2012;35:1252–7.

14. UK Prospective Diabetes Study Group. Tight blood pressure control and risk of macrovascular and microvascular complications in type 2 diabetes: UKPDS 38. BMJ. 1998;317:703–13 [see comments] [published erratum appears in BMJ 1999 Jan 2;318(7175):29].

15. Colhoun HM, Betteridge DJ, Durrington PN, Hitman GA, Neil HA, Livingstone SJ, Thomason MJ, Mackness MI, Charlton-Menys V, Fuller JH. Primary prevention of cardiovascular disease with atorvastatin in type 2 diabetes in the collaborative atorvastatin diabetes study (cards): multicentre randomised placebo-controlled trial. Lancet. 2004;364:685–96.

16. Currie CJ, Peters JR, Tynan A, Evans M, Heine RJ, Bracco OL, Zagar T, Poole CD. Survival as a function of HbA(1c) in people with type 2 diabetes: a retrospective cohort study. Lancet. 2010;375:481–9.

17. McAllister EJ, Dhurandhar NV, Keith SW, Aronne LJ, Barger J, Baskin M, Benca RM, Biggio J, Boggiano MM, Eisenmann JC, Elobeid M, Fontaine KR, Gluckman P, Hanlon EC, Katzmarzyk P, Pietrobelli A, Redden DT, Ruden DM, Wang C, Waterland RA, Wright SM, Allison DB. Ten putative contributors to the obesity epidemic. Crit Rev Food Sci Nutr. 2009;49:868–913.

18. Gluckman PD, Hanson MA. Developmental and epigenetic pathways to obesity: an evolutionary-developmental perspective. Int J Obes (Lond). 2008;32 Suppl 7:S62–71.

19. Hillier TA, Pedula KL. Characteristics of an adult population with newly diagnosed type 2 diabetes: the relation of obesity and age of onset. Diabetes Care. 2001;24:1522–7.

20. Durand ZW. Age of onset of obesity, diabetes and hypertension in Yap State, Federated States of Micronesia. Pac Health Dialog. 2007;14:165–9.

21. Carnethon MR, De Chavez PJ, Biggs ML, Lewis CE, Pankow JS, Bertoni AG, Golden SH, Liu K, Mukamal KJ, Campbell-Jenkins B, Dyer AR. Association of weight status with mortality in adults with incident diabetes. JAMA. 2012;308:581–90.

22. Tseng CH. Obesity paradox: differential effects on cancer and non-cancer mortality in patients with type 2 diabetes mellitus. Atherosclerosis. 2013;226:186–92.

23. Logue J, Walker JJ, Leese G, Lindsay R, McKnight J, Morris A, Philip S, Wild S, Sattar N. The association between BMI measured within a year after diagnosis of type 2 diabetes and mortality. Diabetes Care. 2013;36(4):887–93.

24. Kokkinos P, Myers J, Faselis C, Doumas M, Kheirbek R, Nylen E. BMI-mortality paradox and fitness in African American and Caucasian men with type 2 diabetes. Diabetes Care. 2012;35:1021–7.

25. James WP, Caterson ID, Coutinho W, Finer N, Van Gaal LF, Maggioni AP, Torp-Pedersen C, Sharma AM, Shepherd GM, Rode RA, Renz CL. Effect of sibutramine on cardiovascular outcomes in overweight and obese subjects. N Engl J Med. 2010;363:905–17.

26. Adams TD, Gress RE, Smith SC, Halverson RC, Simper SC, Rosamond WD, Lamonte MJ, Stroup AM, Hunt SC. Long-term mortality after gastric bypass surgery. N Engl J Med. 2007;357:753–61.

27. WHO. Appropriate body-mass index for Asian populations and its implications for policy and intervention strategies. Lancet. 2004;363:157–63.

28. WHO. Obesity: preventing and managing the global epidemic. Report of a who consultation. World Health Organ Tech Rep Ser. 2000;894:1–253.

2

Pathophysiology of Obesity Comorbidity: The Effects of Chronically Increased Intra-abdominal Pressure

Harvey J. Sugerman

Severe obesity is associated with multiple comorbidities that reduce the life expectancy and markedly impair the quality of life. Morbidly obese patients can suffer from central (android) obesity or peripheral (gynoid) obesity or a combination of the two. Gynoid obesity is associated with degenerative joint disease and venous stasis in the lower extremities. Android obesity is associated with the highest risk of mortality related to problems due to the metabolic syndrome or syndrome X, as well as increased intra-abdominal pressure (IAP). The metabolic syndrome is associated with insulin resistance, hyperglycemia, and type 2 diabetes mellitus (DM), which in turn are associated with nonalcoholic liver disease (NALD), polycystic ovary syndrome, and systemic hypertension [1–7]. Increased IAP is probably responsible in part or totally for obesity hypoventilation, venous stasis disease, pseudotumor cerebri, gastroesophageal reflux disease (GERD), stress urinary incontinence, and systemic hypertension. Central obesity is also associated with increased neck circumference and sleep apnea. Other comorbidities are not specifically associated with either the metabolic syndrome or an increased IAP, such as degenerative joint or disc disease.

A previous clinical study of patients with obesity hypoventilation syndrome noted extremely high cardiac filling (pulmonary artery and pulmonary capillary wedge) pressures, as high as or higher than in patients with congestive heart failure (CHF), but most of these patients were not in heart failure. It was initially hypothesized that this could have been secondary to hypoxemic pulmonary artery vasoconstriction; however, the pressures remained elevated immediately following gastric surgery for obesity despite postoperative mechanical ventilation and correction of both hypoxemia and hypercarbia. This pressure returned to normal within 6 to 9 months after surgically induced weight loss [8]. High lumbar cerebrospinal fluid (CSF) pressures were noted in obese women with pseudotumor cerebri (also known as idiopathic intracranial hypertension). Resolution of headache and marked decreases in CSF pressures were noted when restudied 34 ± 8 months following gastric bypass (GBP) surgery (Fig. 1) [9]. The cause(s) of these phenomena remained unexplained until women with stress overflow urinary incontinence, in whom resolution of the problem occurred within months following GBP surgery, underwent measurement of urinary bladder pressures (UBPs) in the gynecologic urodynamic laboratory before and 1 year following obesity surgery [10]. These women were noted to have extremely high UBPs that normalized following surgically induced weight loss. Their pressures were as high as, or even higher than, UBPs noted in critically ill patients with an acute abdominal compartment syndrome where treatment is urgent surgical decompression [11–13]. It was hypothesized that severely obese patients with central obesity have a chronic abdominal compartment syndrome with high UBPs, as an estimate of an increased IAP, and this would be related to a number of obesity comorbidity problems [14].

Animal Studies

Several studies were performed to evaluate the effects of acutely elevated IAP in a porcine model, using either an infusion of iso-osmotic polyethylene glycol normally used for bowel cleansing (Go-Lytely®), on the cardiovascular, pulmonary, and central nervous systems. Polyethylene glycol was chosen, as it is not osmotically active nor absorbed into the central circulation in significant amounts to cause significant changes in intravascular volume. UBPs correlated well ($r = 0.98$, $p < 0.0001$) with directly measured IAP in this model. Acutely elevated IAP produced a significant increase in the pulmonary wedge pressure (Fig. 2) and hemodynamic changes characterized by decreased cardiac output, increased filling pressures, and increased systemic vascular resistance. Pulmonary effects were hypoxia, hypercarbia, increased inspiratory pressure, and elevated pleural pressure [15]. These changes were consistent with the pulmonary pathology characteristic of obesity hypoventilation syndrome.

S.A. Brethauer et al. (eds.), *Minimally Invasive Bariatric Surgery*,
DOI 10.1007/978-1-4939-1637-5_2, © Springer Science+Business Media New York 2015

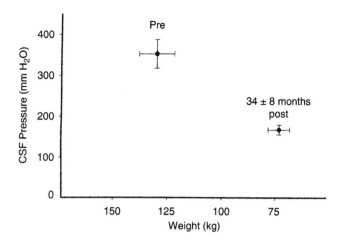

FIG. 1. Elevated cerebrospinal fluid (CSF) pressure prior to, and significant ($p < 0.001$) decrease 34 ± 8 months following, gastric surgery for severe obesity associated with pseudotumor cerebri (Sugerman et al. [9], with permission).

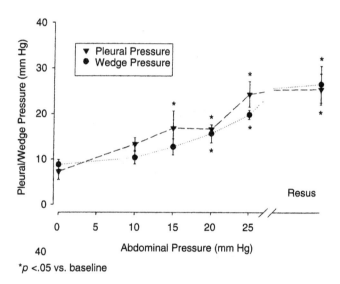

*$p < .05$ vs. baseline

FIG. 2. Progressive increase in pleural pressure and pulmonary artery wedge (occlusion) pressure with increasing intra-abdominal pressure associated with the intra-abdominal instillation of iso-osmotic polyethylene glycol in an acute porcine model. Resus, resuscitation (Ridings et al. [15], with permission).

As IAP increased, pleural pressure, central venous pressure, and intracranial pressure also increased (Fig. 3). When pleural pressure was prevented from rising by midline sternotomy and incision of the pleura and pericardium, the effects of rising IAP on the cardiovascular, pulmonary, and central nervous systems were all negated, except for the decrease in cardiac output [16]. Acute elevation of IAP caused increases (Figs. 4 and 5) in both plasma renin activity (PRA) and aldosterone levels [17].

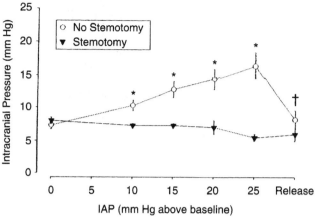

FIG. 3. Progressive increase in directly measured intracranial pressure with increasing intra-abdominal pressure associated with the intra-abdominal instillation of iso-osmotic polyethylene glycol in an acute porcine model and prevention of this increase in animals that had undergone a median sternotomy and pleuropericardiotomy (Bloomfield et al. [16], with permission).

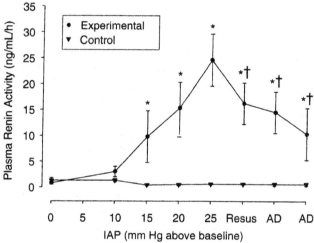

FIG. 4. Progressive increase in plasma renin activity with increasing intra-abdominal pressure (IAP) associated with the intra-abdominal instillation of iso-osmotic polyethylene glycol in an acute porcine model as compared to control animals that did not have their IAP increased; effect of volume expansion (resuscitation) and 30 and 60 min after abdominal decompression (AD). *$p < 0.05$ versus baseline and control animals; †$p < 0.05$ versus pre-resuscitation value (Bloomfield et al. [17], with permission).

Clinical Studies

During the course of this research, it was noted that conditions known to increase IAP such as pregnancy, laparoscopic pneumoperitoneum, and ascites are associated with pathologic consequences also encountered in the morbidly

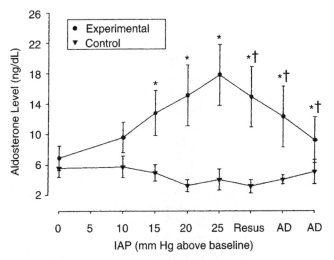

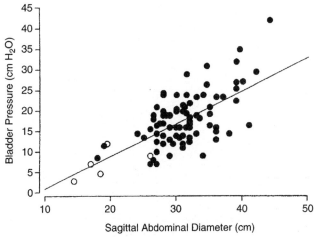

FIG. 5. Progressive increase in serum aldosterone levels with increasing IAP associated with the intra-abdominal instillation of iso-osmotic polyethylene glycol in an acute porcine model as compared to control animals that did not have their IAP increased; effect of volume expansion (resuscitation) and 30 and 60 min after abdominal decompression (AD). $*p < 0.05$ versus baseline and control animals; $\dagger p < 0.05$ versus pre-resuscitation value (Bloomfield et al. [17], with permission).

obese, such as gastroesophageal reflux, abdominal herniation, stress overflow urinary incontinence, and lower limb venous stasis [18–20]. Furthermore, it was noted that these comorbidities significantly improved in conjunction with the marked decrease in IAP [21]. Thus, the comorbidities that are presumed to be secondary to increased IAP in obese patients include CHF, hypoventilation, venous stasis ulcers, GERD, urinary stress incontinence, incisional hernia, pseudotumor cerebri, proteinuria, and systemic hypertension [9, 10, 21–25]. In recent years, there have been a number of other confirmatory studies regarding the pulmonary and hemodynamic effects of an increased IAP [26–31]. There have also been several studies documenting the effects of a high IAP in relation to pelvic floor dysfunction [32–35], as well as studies regarding the relationship between a high IAP and GERD, pseudotumor cerebri, venous stasis disease, and systemic hypertension [36–42].

In a study of 84 patients with severe obesity prior to GBP surgery and five nonobese patients prior to colectomy for ulcerative colitis, it was found that obese patients had a significantly higher UBP (18 ± 0.7 versus 7 ± 1.6 cmH$_2$O, $p < 0.001$) which correlated with the sagittal abdominal diameter (SAD, $r = 0.67$, $p > 0.001$, Fig. 6) and was greater ($p > 0.05$) in patients with (compared to those without) morbidity presumed due to increased IAP (Fig. 7) [14]. The waist/hip ratio (WHR) correlated with UBP in men ($r = 0.6$, $p > 0.05$) but not in women ($r = -0.3$), supporting the concept that the SAD is a better reflection of central obesity than the WHR. In 15 patients studied before and 1 year after GBP, there were

FIG. 6. Correlation between urinary bladder pressure and sagittal abdominal diameter in 84 morbidly obese patients (*filled circle*) and five control nonobese patients (0) with ulcerative colitis, $r = 0.67$, $p < 0.0001$) (Sugerman et al. [14], with permission).

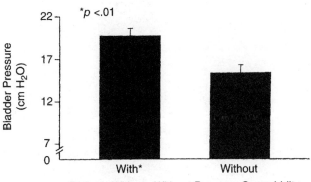

FIG. 7. Increased urinary bladder pressure in 67 patients with IAP-related morbidity and in 17 patients without IAP-related morbidity (Sugerman et al. [14], with permission).

significant ($p > 0.001$) decreases in weight (140 ± 8 to 87 ± 6 kg), body mass index (BMI) (52 ± 3 to 33 ± 2 kg/m^2), SAD (32 ± 1 to 20 ± 2 cm, Fig. 8), UBP (17 ± 2 to 10 ± 1 cmH$_2$O, Fig. 9), and obesity comorbidity with the loss of 69 ± 4 % of excess weight [15].

Discussion

The relationship of central obesity to the constellation of health problems known collectively as the metabolic syndrome appears well established [3, 7].

This has been presumed to be due to increased visceral fat metabolism. Increased UBP and its relationship to increased IAP have been used in postoperative patients as an indication for emergent re-exploration and abdominal decompression

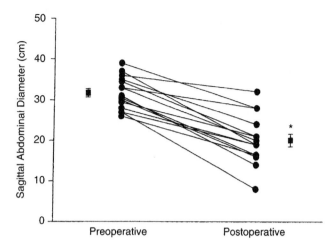

FIG. 8. Sagittal abdominal diameter before and 1 year after surgically induced weight loss. *Filled circle* = individual patient, *filled square* = mean ± standard error of the mean. *$p < 0.0001$ (Sugerman et al. [11], with permission).

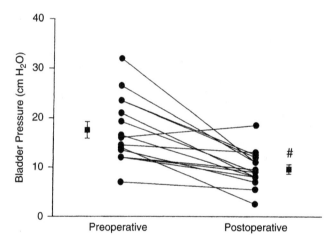

FIG. 9. Urinary bladder pressure before and 1 year after surgically induced weight loss. *Filled circle* = individual patient, *filled square* = mean ± standard error of the mean. *$p < 0.0001$ (Sugerman et al. [11], with permission).

for an acute abdominal compartment syndrome to correct oliguria and increased peak inspiratory pressures with mechanical ventilation [11–13]. The decision to perform emergency abdominal decompression is usually taken when the UBP is ≥ 25 cmH$_2$O. In the study of obese patients prior to GBP surgery, 11 patients had UBPs ≥ 25, four ≥ 30, and one ≥ 40 cmH$_2$O [14]. It became apparent after our previous study where we found very high UBPs in severely obese women with stress overflow urinary incontinence [10] that centrally obese patients may have a chronic abdominal compartment syndrome. We have also found a significantly higher ($p < 0.001$) risk of incisional hernia following open surgery for obesity (20 %) than after colectomy in mostly nonobese patients with ulcerative colitis (4 %) where two-thirds of the colitis patients were taking prednisone and had a much larger incision [23]. Four of the seven incisional

hernias in the colitis group occurred in patients with a BMI ≥ 30. Presumably, this increased risk of incisional hernia was due to an increased IAP in the obese patients.

UBPs were significantly higher in patients with comorbid factors mechanistically presumed to be associated with an elevated IAP than in patients with obesity-related problems that are not considered to be secondary to an increased IAP. The abdominal pressure-related morbidity factors chosen have been documented in pregnancy and cirrhotics with ascites, as well as obese patients, and included hypoventilation, venous stasis disease, GERD, urinary incontinence, pseudotumor cerebri, and incisional hernia. In another report we have found that obese women with pseudotumor cerebri have increased SAD, thoracic pressures as measured transesophageally, and cardiac filling pressures [24]. In addition, hypertension was considered to be probably related to IAP through one or more of the following mechanisms: (1) increased renal venous pressure, (2) direct renal compression [24], and (3) an increased intrathoracic pressure leading to a decreased venous return and decreased cardiac output. Each of these may lead to activation of the renin-angiotensin-aldosterone system, leading to sodium and water retention and vasoconstriction. The increased renal venous pressure could lead to a glomerulopathy with proteinuria. It is currently hypothesized that the hypertension seen in the morbidly obese is secondary to insulin-induced sodium reabsorption. However, systemic hypertension in the morbidly obese may not be associated with hyperinsulinemia, and these patients have been noted to have a decreased renal blood flow (RBF), glomerular filtration rate (GFR), and proteinuria [39]. This was confirmed in a porcine model where a cinch was placed around the right renal vein after left nephrectomy which was associated with a decreased GFR, increased aldosterone and renin, as well as proteinuria [43]. In another study, we found that chronically elevated IAP in a canine model led to the progressive development of systemic hypertension which resolved with restoration of a normal IAP [44]. Others have suggested that the increased ICP with central obesity and increased IAP is responsible for hypertension via the central nervous system [42]. Regardless of cause, surgically induced weight loss is associated with significant decreases in systemic arterial pressure [45].

Although the UBPs were measured supine in anesthetized, paralyzed patients and these pressures could be altered by the upright position, we believe the data to be clinically relevant. First, in the stress incontinence study, the pressures rose even further when the patient assumed a sitting or standing position [10]. Second, these pressures likely would be even higher in the absence of muscle paralysis. Third, most individuals spend 6–8 h sleeping in a supine or lateral decubitus position. Many severely obese patients, especially those with sleep apnea and hypoventilation, have found that they must sleep in the sitting position, presumably to lower the effect of the increased IAP on their thoracic cavity. It is also for this reason that patients with pseudotumor cerebri have more severe headaches in the morning upon awakening.

Although an increased WHR is a recognized measurement of central obesity and metabolic complications, we found a poor correlation between the WHR and UBPs in women but a good correlation in men. This is probably the result of the diluting effect of peripheral obesity, commonly present in women, on the estimate of central obesity. The greater problem of central obesity in men was reinforced by the finding of a greater SAD and UBP in men compared to women despite an equal BMI [14]. Unlike the WHR, the SAD provided good positive correlations with UBP in both men and women, corroborating the computed tomography (CT) scan data reported by Kvist et al. [46, 47] that the SAD is a better reflection of central obesity than the WHR.

In the study of UBP in patients following GBP surgery, significant weight loss was associated with a marked reduction in both pressure-related and non-pressure-related comorbidity, except for incisional hernias and the need for cholecystectomy. Several studies have documented improvement following surgically induced weight loss in conditions presumed to be caused by an abnormally high IAP, such as urinary incontinence [10, 32–35], respiratory insufficiency including sleep apnea and hypoventilation [8, 22–30], GERD [31, 48, 49], pseudotumor cerebri [9, 24, 41, 42], hypertension [45], and cardiac dysfunction [8, 45].

These possible pathophysiologic consequences of an increased IAP (hypertension, peripheral edema, proteinuria, increased CSF pressures, increased cardiac filling pressures, and increased hepatic venous pressures) suggest that the chronic abdominal compartment syndrome could be responsible for toxemia of pregnancy. This hypothesis is supported by the increased association of preeclampsia in primiparas (where the abdomen has never been stretched before), twin pregnancies, morbid obesity where an increased IAP is predictable, and its correction with parturition. Furthermore, there is no clinical animal model of preeclampsia, presumably because animals carry their fetuses in the prone position. The hypothesis is that an increased IAP compresses and reduces blood flow in the abdominal venous system which leads to fetal/placental ischemia, systemic hypertension, proteinuria, hepatic ischemia, platelet consumption in the spleen and liver, pulmonary insufficiency, and intracranial hypertension [50]. The placental/fetal ischemia is thought to cause an increased release of sFlt-1, endoglin, placental growth factor and a decreased VEGF.

Review Questions and Answers

Questions

1. Increased intra-arterial pressure is related primarily to the:
   (a) Hip circumference
   (b) Waist circumference
   (c) Waist:hip ratio
   (d) All of the above

2. Animal studies have shown that pseudotumor cerebri is a result of:
   (a) An increased thoracic pressure
   (b) An increased intra-abdominal pressure
   (c) An increased intracranial pressure
   (d) All of the above

3. Increased intra-abdominal pressure is associated with:
   (a) Urinary incontinence
   (b) Pseudotumor cerebri
   (c) Venous stasis disease
   (d) Obesity hypoventilation
   (e) All of the above

4. Roux-en-Y gastric bypass for severe obesity is associated with:
   (a) A significant decrease in body weight
   (b) A significant decrease in spinal fluid pressure
   (c) A significant improvement in arterial blood gases
   (d) All of the above

Answers

1. (b)
   The increased intra-abdominal pressure is secondary to an increased fat mass within the abdomen (i.e., central obesity). This is best measured by either the waist circumference or the sagittal abdominal diameter. Large lower abdominal obesity produces a large hip circumference; this reduces the waist:hip ratio, and therefore makes this ratio misleadingly low.

2. (d)
   The increased intra-abdominal pressure pushes the diaphragm cephalad and increases intrathoracic pressure. This decreases venous return from the brain, which leads to vascular engorgement and an increased intracranial pressure and severe headaches. It is called pseudotumor cerebri because there is no mass within the brain. It is also called "idiopathic intracranial hypertension."

3. (e)
   All of these obesity-related comorbidities are a result of an increased intra-abdominal pressure and all improve significantly after surgically induced weight loss.

4. (e)
   Surgically induced weight loss is associated with significant weight loss, decreased spinal fluid pressure and relief of severe headache associated with pseudotumor cerebri, improved respiratory function with a decreased $PaCO_2$ and increased PaO_2, and healing of venous stasis ulcers.

References

1. Eckel RH, Grundy SM, Zimmet PZ. The metabolic syndrome. Lancet. 2005;365(9468):1415–28.

2. Grundy SM, Brewer Jr HB, Cleeman JI, et al. Definition of metabolic syndrome: report of the National Heart, Lung, and Blood Institute/American Heart Association conference on scientific issues related to definition. Circulation. 2004;109(3):433–8.

3. National Cholesterol Education Program (NCEP) Expert Panel on Detection, Evaluation, and Treatment of High Blood Cholesterol in Adults (Adult Treatment Panel III). Third Report of the National Cholesterol Education Program (NCEP) Expert Panel on Detection, Evaluation, and Treatment of High Blood Cholesterol in Adults (Adult Treatment Panel III) final report. Circulation. 2002; 106(25):3143–421.

4. Ong JP, Elariny H, Collantes R, et al. Predictors of nonalcoholic steatohepatitis and advanced fibrosis in morbidly obese patients. Obes Surg. 2005;15(3):310–5.

5. Mattar SG, Velcu LM, Rabinovitz M, et al. Surgically induced weight loss significantly improves nonalcoholic fatty liver disease and the metabolic syndrome. Ann Surg. 2005;242(4):610–7; discussion 618–620.

6. Escobar-Morreale HF, Botella-Carretero JI, Alvarez Blasco F, et al. The polycystic ovary syndrome associated with morbid obesity may resolve after weight loss induced by bariatric surgery. J Clin Endocrinol Metab. 2005;90(12):6364–9.

7. Johnson D, Prud'homme D, Despres JP, et al. Relation of abdominal obesity to hyperinsulinemia and high blood pressure in men. Int J Obes Relat Metab Disord. 1992;16(11):881–90.

8. Sugerman HJ, Baron PL, Fairman RP, et al. Hemodynamic dysfunction in obesity hypoventilation syndrome and the effects of treatment with surgically induced weight loss. Ann Surg. 1988; 207(5):604–13.

9. Sugerman HJ, Felton III WL, Salvant Jr JB, et al. Effects of surgically induced weight loss on idiopathic intracranial hypertension in morbid obesity. Neurology. 1995;45(9):1655–9.

10. Bump RC, Sugerman HJ, Fantl JA, McClish DK. Obesity and lower urinary tract function in women: effect of surgically induced weight loss. Am J Obstet Gynecol. 1992;167(2):392–7; discussion 397–399.

11. Harman PK, Kron IL, McLachlan HD, et al. Elevated intra-abdominal pressure and renal function. Ann Surg. 1982;196(5):594–7.

12. Kron IL, Harman PK, Nolan SP. The measurement of intraabdominal pressure as a criterion for abdominal re-exploration. Ann Surg. 1984;199(1):28–30.

13. Ertel W, Oberholzer A, Platz A, et al. Incidence and clinical pattern of the abdominal compartment syndrome after "damage-control" laparotomy in 311 patients with severe abdominal and/or pelvic trauma. Crit Care Med. 2000;28(6):1747–53.

14. Sugerman H, Windsor A, Bessos M, Wolfe L. Intraabdominal pressure, sagittal abdominal diameter and obesity comorbidity. J Intern Med. 1997;241(1):71–9.

15. Ridings PC, Bloomfield GL, Blocher CR, Sugerman HI. Cardiopulmonary effects of raised intra-abdominal pressure before and after intravascular volume expansion. J Trauma. 1995;39(6): 1071–5.

16. Bloomfield GL, Ridings PC, Blocher CR, et al. A proposed relationship between increased intra-abdominal, intrathoracic, and intracranial pressure. Crit Care Med. 1997;25(3):496–503.

17. Bloomfield GL, Blocher CR, Fakhry IF, et al. Elevated intra-abdominal pressure increases plasma renin activity and aldosterone levels. J Trauma. 1997;42(6):997–1004; discussion 1004–1005.

18. Dent J, Dodds WJ, Hogan WJ, Toouli I. Factors that influence induction of gastroesophageal reflux in normal human subjects. Dig Dis Sci. 1988;33(3):270–5.

19. Nagler R, Spiro HM. Heartburn in late pregnancy. Manometric studies of esophageal motor function. J Clin Invest. 1961;40: 954–70.

20. Skudder PA, Farrington DT. Venous conditions associated with pregnancy. Semin Dermatol. 1993;12(2):72–7.

21. Sugerman H, Windsor A, Bessos M, et al. Effects of surgically induced weight loss on urinary bladder pressure, sagittal abdominal diameter and obesity co-morbidity. Int J Obes Relat Metab Disord. 1998;22(3):230–5.

22. Sugerman HJ, Fairman RP, Sood RK, et al. Long-term effects of gastric surgery for treating respiratory insufficiency of obesity. Am J Clin Nutr. 1992;55(2 Suppl):597S–601S.

23. Sugerman HJ, Kellum Jr JM, Reines HD. Greater risk of incisional hernia with morbidly obese than steroid-dependent patients and low recurrence with prefascial polypropylene mesh. Am J Surg. 1996;171(1):80–4.

24. Sugerman HJ, DeMaria EJ, Felton III WL, et al. Increased intra-abdominal pressure and cardiac filling pressures in obesity-associated pseudotumor cerebri. Neurology. 1997;49(2):507–11.

25. Sugerman HJ, Sugerman EL, Wolfe L, et al. Risks/benefits of gastric bypass in morbidly obese patients with severe venous stasis disease. Ann Surg. 2001;234:41–6.

26. Lambert DM, Marceau S, Forse RA. Intra-abdominal pressure in the morbidly obese. Obes Surg. 2005;15(9):1225–32.

27. Pelosi P, Quintel M, Malbrain ML. Effect of intra-abdominal pressure on respiratory mechanics. Acta Clin Belg Suppl. 2007;1:78–88.

28. Lumachi F, Marzano B, Fantl G, et al. Hypoxemia and hypoventilation syndrome improvement after laparoscopic bariatric surgery in patients with morbid obesity. In Vivo. 2010;24(3):329–31.

29. Wei YF, Tseng WK, Huang CK, et al. Surgically induced weight loss, including reduction in waist circumference, is associated with improved pulmonary function in obese patients. Surg Obes Relat Dis. 2011;7(5):599–604.

30. Gaszyriski TM. The effect of abdominal opening on respiratory mechanics during general anesthesia for open bariatric surgery in morbidly obese patients. Anestezjol Intens Ter. 2010;42(4):172–4.

31. El-Serag HB, Tran T, Richardson P, Ergun G. Anthropometric correlates of intragastric pressure. Scand J Gastroenterol. 2006;41(8): 887891.

32. Fantl JA. Genuine stress incontinence: pathophysiology and rationale for its medical management. Obstet Gynecol Clin North Am. 1989;16(4):827–40.

33. Laungani RG, Seleno N, Carlin AM. Effect of laparoscopic gastric bypass on urinary incontinence in morbidly obese women. Surg Obes Relat Dis. 2009;5(3):334–8.

34. Krause MP, Albert SM, Elsangedy HM, et al. Urinary incontinence and waist circumference in older women. Age Ageing. 2010;39(1): 69–73.

35. Lee RK, Chung S, Chughtai B, Te AE, Kaplan SA. Central obesity as measured by waist circumference is predictive of severity of lower urinary tract symptoms. BJU Int. 2012;110(4):540–5.

36. Van Rij AM, DeAlwis CS, Jiang P, et al. Obesity and impaired venous function. Eur J Vasc Endovasc Surg. 2008;35(6):739–44.

37. Arfvidsson B, Eklof B, Balfour J. Iliofemoral venous pressure correlates with intraabdominal pressure in morbidly obese patients. Vasc Endovascular Surg. 2005;39(6):505–9.

38. Varela JE, Hinojosa M, Nguyen N. Correlations between intra-abdominal pressure and obesity-related co-morbidities. Surg Obes Relat Dis. 2009;5(5):524–8.

39. Scaglione R, Ganguzza A, Corrao S, et al. Central obesity and hypertension: pathophysiologic role of renal haemodynamics and function. Int J Obes Relat Metab Disord. 1995;19(6):403–9.

40. Ben-Haim M, Mandell J, Friedman RL, Rosenthal RJ. Mechanisms of systemic hypertension during acute elevation of intraabdominal pressure. J Surg Res. 2000;91(2):101–5.

41. Hamdalla IN, Shamseddeen HN, Getty JL, et al. Greater than expected prevalence of pseudotumor cerebri: a prospective study. Surg Obes Relat Dis. 2013;9(1):77–82.

42. Rosenthal RJ, Hiatt JR, Phillips EH, et al. Intracranial pressure: effects of pneumoperitoneum in a large-animal model. Surg Endosc. 1997;11(4):376–80.

43. Doty J, Saggi BH, Sugerman HJ, et al. Effect of increased renal venous pressure on renal function. J Trauma. 1999;47(6): 1000–5.

44. Bloomfield GL, Sugerman HJ, Blocher CH, et al. Chronically increased intra-abdominal pressure produces systemic hypertension in dogs. Int J Obes Relat Metab Disord. 2000;24:819–24.

45. Vest AR, Heneghan HM, Agarwal S, Schauer PR, Young JB. Bariatric surgery and cardiovascular outcomes: a systematic review. Heart. 2012;98(24):1763–77.

46. Kvist H, Chowdhury B, Grangard U, et al. Total and visceral adipose-tissue volumes derived from measurements with computed tomography in adult men and women: predictive equations. Am J Clin Nutr. 1988;48(6):1351–61.

47. Kvist H, Chowdhury B, Sjostrom L, et al. Adipose tissue volume determination in males by computed tomography and 40K. Int J Obes. 1988;12(3):249–66.

48. Braghatto I, Korn O, Gutierrez L, et al. Laparoscopic treatment of obese patients with gastroesophageal reflux disease and Barrett's esophagus: a prospective study. Obes Surg. 2012;22(5):764–72.

49. Varela JE, Hinojosa MW, Nguyen NT. Laparoscopic fundoplication compared with laparoscopic gastric bypass in morbidly obese patients with gastroesophageal reflux disease. Surg Obes Relat Dis. 2009;5(2):139–43.

50. Sugerman HJ. Hypothesis: preeclampsia is a venous disease secondary to an increased intra-abdominal pressure. Med Hypotheses. 2011;77:841–9.

3

Medical Management of Obesity

Bartolome Burguera and Joan Tur

Scientific Evidence Supporting the Potential Efficacy of Medical Treatment of Obesity

It is generally believed in the scientific community that medical (nonsurgical) treatments alone have not been effective in achieving a significant long-term weight loss in obese adults. The situation is even less optimistic in regard to patients with obesity class II (moderate) and III (morbid obesity). However, very few studies have specifically examined the effects of nonsurgical treatment in these morbidly obese patients, so conclusions about nonsurgical therapy in this population are based on inference. In studies of class I (minimal) and class II obesity, medical therapy can achieve about 10 % body weight loss in 10–40 % of patients depending on study design, use of medications, and duration of the intervention. Duration of the weight loss response increases with duration of treatment and with use of medications and behavior modification.

Some studies have demonstrated the beneficial effect that dietary plans, behavior therapy programs, and physical activity have in helping to lose weight and to improve the comorbidities associated to obesity [19, 20]. Also, some clinical trials have shown the beneficial effect that drugs such as sibutramine and orlistat have had in reducing weight and improving the glycemic and lipid profiles in obese patients. The subjects participating in these clinical trials also received dietary advice. Their BMI was between 30 and 35 kg/m^2 and the average duration of these studies was only 1 year [20, 21].

It is very important to set realistic expectations before starting medical treatments of obesity. Both physician and the patient should be aware that a weight loss of 5–15 % reduces obesity-related health risks significantly. There are a substantial number of patients who respond to weight loss interventions with important changes in their lifestyle, which translates in long-term weight loss. Identifying the patients who will respond to nonsurgical interventions would be very important to maximize resources and avoid unnecessary surgeries. We need to keep in mind that bariatric surgery treats less than 1 % of the eligible morbid obese population, and that already implies waiting lists averaging more than 1 year. Should all the obese patients with the current indications ask for surgery, we simply would not have either the economical and infrastructure resources or the health professionals necessary to operate on 3–5 % of the Western population. Therefore, it is important to count with effective comprehensive interdisciplinary medical therapies alternative (and complementary) to bariatric surgery.

Setting unrealistic goals concerning the weight loss is frequently associated with weight management failure. Recent studies have shown the short efficacy of lifestyle interventions for the treatment of severe obesity and related comorbidities [22, 23].

Dietary Modifications

The macronutrient composition of different weight loss diets is a topic of great interest, and several clinical trials have attempted to compare their effectiveness [24–34] (Table 1). Most studies have indicated that hypocaloric diets, low in calories from carbohydrates, help patients to achieve a greater weight loss in the short term than low-fat diets [24–29]. In line with these observations, a Cochrane review confirmed that low-carbohydrate diets are associated with a greater weight loss than others [35]. Below are presented some of latest evidence and recommendations available [36].

Changes in Total Calorie Intake

The Balanced Hypocaloric Diet

Evidence:

A caloric restriction between 500 and 1,000 kcal daily induces weight loss ranging between 0.5 and 1.0 kg/week, equivalent to a weight loss of 8 % for an average period of 6 months (evidence level 1+).

S.A. Brethauer et al. (eds.), *Minimally Invasive Bariatric Surgery*,
DOI 10.1007/978-1-4939-1637-5_3, © Springer Science+Business Media New York 2015

TABLE 1. Some common diets

Type	Description	Average weight loss, kg (95 % CI)
Mediterranean diet	Fruits, nuts, red wine, fiber, whole grains, fish, and vegetable fat (extra virgin olive oil)	−4.4 kg (−5,9 to −2,9 kg)
Weight watchers	Moderate energy deficit Portion control	−2.8 kg (−5.9 to −0.7 kg)
LEARN	Moderate energy deficit (lifestyle, exercise, attitude, intensive lifestyle, relationships, nutrition) modification	−2.6 kg (−3.8 to −1.3 kg)
Ornish	Vegetarian based Fat restricted (<10 % of total calories)	−2.2 kg (−3.6 to −0.8 kg)
Zone	Low carbohydrate Carbohydrate/protein/fat 40/30/30	−1.6 kg (−2.8 to −0.4 kg)
Atkins	Very low carbohydrate Minimal fat restriction	−4.7 kg (−6.3 to −3.1 kg)

- Measures such as reducing portion sizes or reducing the energy density of the diet can facilitate compliance with a reduced-calorie diet and weight loss in obese patients (evidence level 3).

Recommendations:

- In obese adults, a caloric deficit of 500–1,000 kcal/day vs. caloric requirements is enough to induce a weight loss of 8 % in the first 6 months of therapy (grade A recommendation).
- The reduction on the portion sizes of serving and the energy density of the diet are effective measures to reduce the weight via dietary management (grade D recommendation).

Dietary Modifications Based on Different Combinations of Macronutrients

Modified-Fat Diets Versus Modified-Carbohydrate Diets

Evidence:

- Short term (6 months): a low-carbohydrate diet allows people to achieve greater weight loss than a low-fat diet (evidence level 1++).
- Long term (12 months or more): a low-carbohydrate diet allows people to achieve similar weight loss than a low-fat diet (evidence level 1+).
- Long term (12 months or more): a low-carbohydrate diet can help patients to achieve a further increase in the concentration of high-density cholesterol (HDL-Cl) and a greater reduction in the concentration of triglycerides than a low saturated fat diet (evidence level 1+).

- Long term (12 months or more): a low saturated fat diet can help patients to achieve a further decrease in the concentration of low-density cholesterol (LDL-Cl) than a low-carbohydrate diet (evidence level 2+).
- Low-carb diets cause more adverse effects than low-fat diets (evidence level 2++).
- Low-carb diets can increase long-time mortality if the fat contained is, mostly, from animal origin.

Recommendations:

- The reduction in the proportion of carbohydrates, with an increase in fats, is not helpful to enhance the effects of diet on weight loss (grade A recommendation).
- In an obese patient, a low-fat diet is useful to control the levels of LDL cholesterol, whereas a low-carb diet allows to achieve better triglyceride and HDL cholesterol control (grade B recommendation).
- Low-carb diets may not contain a high proportion of animal fats (grade D recommendation).

Modified-Carbohydrate Diets

Fiber-Enriched Diets

Evidence:

- There are not enough data to establish evidence on the role of a diet enriched with dietary fiber or whole grains on weight loss.
- Glucomannan supplements added to the diet may have a modest (satiating) effect, which encourages weight loss (level of evidence 1+).
- Fiber supplements (different than glucomannan) added to the diet can contribute minimally to weight loss (level of evidence 2+).
- The treatment of obesity with a diet enriched or supplemented with glucomannan, plantago ovata, and β-glucan lowers LDL cholesterol levels of obese patients (evidence level 1+).

Recommendations:

- In the treatment of obesity, fiber supplements (mainly glucomannan) may increase the effectiveness of the diet on weight loss (grade C recommendation).
- The prescription of diets enriched with fiber or fiber supplements (mainly glucomannan) may benefit obese people with lipid abnormalities (grade B recommendation).

Low Glycemic Index Diets

- The glycemic index (GI) is a system for quantifying the glycemic response of a food containing the same amount of carbohydrates with that of a reference food [37]. The glycemic load (GL) is the product of the GI and the amount of ingested carbohydrates and provides an indication of the amount of glucose available to metabolize or store after ingestion of food containing carbohydrates [38].

Evidence:

- In the treatment of obesity, dietary modifications in GI or GL have no persistent effect on weight loss (evidence level 1+).
- There are not enough data to establish evidence on the role of low-GI diets or low GL on maintenance of weight loss after a low-calorie diet.

Recommendations:

- As a specific strategy for the dietary management of obesity, the decrease in GL and GI, can't be recommended (grade A recommendation).

High-Protein Diets

Evidence:

- A high-protein diet can induce greater weight loss in the short term (less than 6 months) than a conventional diet, rich in carbohydrates (evidence level 2+).
- A high-protein diet does not induce greater weight loss in the long term (over 12 months) than conventional diet, rich in carbohydrates (evidence level 1+).
- There are insufficient data to establish the effectiveness of high-protein diets in the maintenance of weight loss after an initial phase of weight loss with other diets.
- A high-protein diet helps to preserve lean mass, better than a diet rich in carbohydrates (evidence level 2+).
- A high-protein diet can increase (in the long term) the risk of total mortality and cardiovascular mortality, mainly when the protein is of animal origin (evidence level 2+).

Recommendations:

- In the treatment of obesity, it is not recommended to induce changes in the proportion of dietary protein (grade A recommendation).
- To ensure the maintenance or the increase of the lean mass during a low-calorie diet, it is effective to increase the protein content of the diet above 1.05 g/kg (grade B recommendation).
- When a high protein is prescribed, the intake of animal protein in the diet should be limited, to prevent an increased risk of mortality in the very long term (grade C recommendation).

Meal Replacement Diets

Evidence:

- The use of commercial meal replacements for one or more meals a day may facilitate the monitoring of a hypocaloric diet more effectively, promoting, in this case, both weight loss and maintenance of weight loss (evidence level 1−).
- This benefit is greater when those meal replacements are used in the context of structured treatments that include physical activity, education, and food behavior modification (evidence level 3).
- There have not been clinically significant adverse effects associated with the use of meal replacements in the context of low-calorie diets (evidence level 3).

Recommendations:

- In obese or overweight adults, replacing some meals for meal replacements (in the context of low-calorie diets) can be useful for weight loss and its maintenance (grade D recommendation).

Very-Low-Calorie Diets

Evidence:

- In the short term (less than 3 months), very-low-calorie diets (VLCD) (400–800 kcal/day) result in a greater weight loss than low-calorie diets (>800 to <1,200 kcal/day) (evidence level 1+).
- In the long term (over 1 year), these diets do not result in a greater weight loss than low-calorie diets (evidence level 1+).
- The use of a VLCD before bariatric surgery, in patients with hepatic steatosis and increased surgical risk, can reduce surgical risk (evidence level 1+).
- At the moment, there are no data available to establish whether VLCD with commercial products help patients to reach an adequate protein intake.
- The VLCD presents a higher risk of adverse effects than the low-calorie diet (evidence level 1−).
- The evidence available does not support that the VLCD are associated with a greater lean mass loss in relation to fat mass loss, compared to less restrictive calorie diets.

Recommendations:

- The VLCD can be used in the treatment of obese patients, following a specific clinical indication and a close medical monitoring (grade D recommendation).
- The VLCD can't be used in patients who don't meet the guidelines, requirements, and criteria (grade A recommendation).
- Under medical supervision, and considering the possible adverse effects that can be observed, the use of VLCD can be justified in the preoperative bariatric surgery in patients with hepatic steatosis and increased surgical risk (grade B recommendation).
- Using VLCD with commercial products could be justified in the immediate postoperative of bariatric surgery to help the patient reach an adequate protein intake (grade D recommendation).

Mediterranean Diet (MedDiet)

Evidence:

- Studies point to a possible role of MedDiet in the prevention of overweight and obesity, although there are inconsistent results (evidence level 2−).
- The available evidence suggests that greater adherence to the MedDiet could prevent the increase of the abdominal circumference (evidence level 2+).

Recommendations:

- Increased adherence to the MedDiet could prevent overweight and obesity and prevent the increase of the abdominal circumference (grade C recommendation).

Benefits of the Mediterranean Diet:

Most prospective studies researching the association between dietary quality and risk of obesity found that an overall dietary pattern based on the traditional Mediterranean diet was inversely associated with the risk of obesity or weight gain [39–42]. The inverse association between the MedDiet and adiposity indices has also been reported in some studies [43–47]. Some clinical trials have added support for this association [48–50].

Nutrigenetic studies [51–53] have analyzed the biological and statistical interactions between the Mediterranean diet and its components and variations in key genes in lipid metabolism, inflammation, adipocytokines, obesity, diabetes, and cardiovascular disease (APOA1, APOA2, ABCA1, LIPC, COX-2, FTO, TCF7L2, PRKAG3, PRKAA2, ADIPOQ, CD36, NR1H3, etc.). There have been many statistically significant interactions in which greater adherence to the MedDiet, or some of its typical foods, is able to reverse the adverse effects that have risk allelic variants in these genes on their specific phenotypes, being able to modulate the adverse effects of certain genetic variants, dyslipidemia, hyperglycemia, and/or obesity.

This evidence suggests that the typical MedDiet pattern, based on whole foods, minimally processed, which includes fruits, nuts (walnuts), vegetables, legumes, whole grains, red wine, fiber, fish, vegetable protein, and vegetable fat (from extra virgin olive oil), has qualitative elements that promote weight loss and glycemic control and enhances the management of the metabolic syndrome [54]. It has recently been demonstrated a further reduction in the incidence of cardiovascular events in people at high risk who consumed a Mediterranean diet supplemented with extra virgin olive oil or nuts [55].

Physical Activity

Increased physical activity is an important component in the medical treatment of obesity; it represents an increase in energy expenditure. A class A evidence indicates that, with or without diet associated, the impact of physical activity has

good results for weight loss and its maintenance [56, 57]. However, subsequent recommendations of the American College of Sports Medicine indicate that physical activity in itself has a limited effect on weight loss [58].

Since the publication in 1999 of the report "A one year follow-up to Physical Activity and Health: A report of the Surgeon General" [59] in the USA, a large amount of evidence-based knowledge has been accumulated on the benefits of physical activity in overweight and obese individuals, although not so much in the morbidly obese.

In order to update the scientific knowledge, an Experts Committee reviewed new research and classified the degree of evidence of the benefits of physical activity on health. The results of this review were published in the report Physical Activity Advisory Committee Report, 2008 [60]. These guidelines suggest that the health benefits of physical activity include the prevention of disease and the reduction of multiple risk factors associated with many diseases and chronic conditions, becoming part of the treatment recommendations of some of these, as in the case of obesity.

Benefits of Physical Activity

The benefits of physical activity include reduced risk of premature death of any cause, CVD, T2DM, some cancers (breast cancer and colon cancer), depression, prevention of weight gain, weight loss (in combination with caloric restriction), and improvement of physical fitness and musculoskeletal fitness [61, 62]. Inactivity and low cardiorespiratory fitness are as important as overweight and obesity as mortality predictors [63].

In elderly people there is strong evidence supporting the improvement of cognitive function in people who are physically active and moderate evidence in regard to overall improvement in well-being [64] and functional health, reduction of abdominal obesity, reduced risk of developing hip fracture, risk reduction of lung cancer, and weight loss maintenance. In a recent systematic review and meta-analysis, Hobbs et al. [65] found that interventions in adults aged 55–70 years led to long-term improvements in physical fitness at 12 months; however, maintenance beyond this is unclear. Interventions which involved individually tailoring with personalized activity goals or provision of information about local physical activity opportunities in the community may be more effective in this population [65], and the benefits associated with regular exercise and physical activity contribute to a more healthy, independent lifestyle, greatly improving the functional capacity and quality of life in this population [66].

Recommendations for Physical Activity

Best practices:

1. All adults should avoid inactivity and all those who participate in physical activity should obtain some health benefits.

2. In order to obtain significant benefits of physical activity in adults, its duration should be at least 2.5 h/week (150 min) of moderate-intensity activity or 75 min of vigorous activity or a combination of both (category: "active").

3. To obtain additional benefits, adults should increase their aerobic activity to 300 min of moderate activity, or 150 of vigorous activity, or a combination of both (considered as "highly active") [60, 67].

The guidelines also recommend that adults should get involved in physical activity, increasing gradually its duration, frequency, and intensity, with the aim of minimizing the risk of injury.

As for the type of exercise recommended, muscle-strengthening activities involve all muscle groups 2 or more days a week. The elderly at risk of falling should also practice exercises to maintain and/or improve their balance.

There appears to be a linear relation between physical activity and health status, such that a further increase in physical activity and fitness will lead to additional improvements in health status. In addition to the recommendations from the guidelines, different studies provided data underlying the importance of avoiding a sedentary lifestyle as a key tool in health promotion [68, 69]. These recommendations are mainly addressed to obese people who are fairly inactive, encouraging them to reach gradually higher levels of physical activity in order to obtain the maximum benefit from its protective effects.

Some studies have focused attention on the sedentary profile of patients, in order to observe the benefit that certain dose of physical activity (in intensity and duration) would produce greater benefit in terms of weight loss and cardiovascular function. These studies concluded that the duration of exercise (150 min) is more important than the intensity (moderate vs. vigorous), but these studies did not include patients with BMI > 40 kg/m^2 [70].

The rise of new technologies on the development and marketing of instruments to measure the amount of physical activity (pedometers, accelerometers) will undoubtedly help to better determine the amount of physical activity needed to optimize the dose–response results on physical activity-based interventions [71].

There are few randomized controlled clinical trials evaluating the impact of physical activity in a lifestyle intervention in morbidly obese patients. Goodpaster et al. [22] conducted a trial designed specifically to evaluate the effects of an intensive lifestyle intervention on weight loss, abdominal fat, hepatic steatosis, and other cardiovascular risk factors in people with obesity (degrees II and III, BMI > 35 and > 40 kg/m^2, respectively) without T2DM. They concluded that, among patients with severe obesity, a lifestyle intervention involving diet combined with initial or delayed initiation of physical activity resulted in clinically significant weight loss and favorable changes in cardiometabolic risk factors.

In summary, the available evidence suggests that physically active people live longer than sedentary people and do so with a greater quality of life by improving their rest, reducing the risk of cardiovascular disease, type 2 diabetes, hypertension, dyslipidemia, and colon cancer. In relation to obesity, physical activity appears to help weight loss (although not induce weight loss by itself) and, in a dose sufficient, help in the maintenance of weight loss [57, 72–74].

Behavioral Therapy

Behavioral therapy is a key tool to help overweight and obese patients make long-term changes in their behavior by modifying and monitoring their food intake, increasing their physical activity, and controlling cues and environmental stimuli that trigger overeating [56, 57, 75–78].

Different eligibility criteria, target population, and inclusion criteria (T2DM and BMI) have been used in the most important clinical trials (Table 2). Two of the most cited studies involving behavioral therapy in the context of a lifestyle modification targeted diabetic and/or nondiabetic persons with elevated fasting and post-load plasma glucose concentrations: the Diabetes Prevention Program (DPP) [79] and the Action for Health in Diabetes (Look AHEAD) [80–82]. DPP participants (overweight, sedentary, and nondiabetic persons with elevated fasting and post-load plasma glucose concentrations) were randomly assigned to a metformin group, a lifestyle modification group, and a placebo group. The research team hypothesized that modifying these risk factors with a lifestyle intervention program or the administration of metformin would prevent or delay the development of diabetes. This program was based on 16 individual education sessions during the first 24 weeks and bimonthly the rest of the period. A low-fat, hypocaloric diet was prescribed (1,200–2,000 kcal/day depending on the degree of overweight), composed of conventional foods, and 150 min/week of physical activity (generally brisk walking), with a goal of losing 7 % of their initial body weight.

In the Look AHEAD study, more than 5,100 overweight participants with DM2 were randomized to a Diabetes Support and Education group (DSE) or an Intensive Lifestyle Intervention (ILI) with a weight loss goal of 7 % of their baseline weight and an increase of the time spent in physical activity to an average of 175 min a week. In the first 6 months, the patients attended to three group sessions and one individual visit. They used two meal replacement products a day, with a 1,200–1,800 kcal/day caloric intake goal. Between months 7–12, patients had a single and a group session per month, using one meal replacement product every day. From years 2–4, participants attended a single visit to the hospital and received a telephone call or an e-mail every month, with regular group sessions to help maintain a 7 % initial weight loss and/or neutralize possible weight regain.

TABLE 2. Eligibility criteria, population targeted, and inclusion criteria (T2DM and BMI) in the clinical trials Look AHEAD, DPP, LOSS, and TRAMOMTANA

	Ages eligible for study	Ethnically diverse population	Inclusion criteria: T2DM	Inclusion criteria: BMI
Look AHEAD	45–74	Yes	Yes	25 or higher (27 or higher if on insulin)
DPP	25 at least	Yes	No (ADA 1997 criteria) Impaired glucose tolerance (WHO 1985 criteria)	24 or higher (22 or higher in Asians)
LOSS	20–60	Yes	No	40 or higher
TRAMOMTANA	18–65	No	No	40 or higher

These two examples illustrate the wide range of approaches (Table 3) in regard to the number and configuration of individual visits, group sessions, dietary changes, exercise programs as well as patterns in weight loss and weight loss maintenance through these changes in lifestyle. The literature suggests that the current weight loss programs usually achieve a reduction of 7–10 % of the initial body weight [75, 83] after 6–9 months of intervention, and the combination of diet, physical activity, and behavioral changes can obtain even better results if anti-obesity agents are added to the therapy [84].

One of the biggest challenges is to maintain this weight loss over the medium- and long-term periods [77]. It is important to make these changes durable enough to allow a significant improvement in their comorbidities, quality of life [85, 86], and body composition [87].

One of the few clinical trials focused on the treatment of morbid obesity was the Louisiana Obese Subjects Study (LOSS Study) [23] (Table 4). The main objective of the study was to test whether, with brief training, primary care physicians could effectively implement weight loss for individuals with a BMI of 40–60 kg/m². In this 2-year randomized, controlled, clinical trial, the recommendations for patients in the Intensive Medical Intervention (IMI) group included a 900 kcal liquid diet for 12 weeks or less, group behavioral counseling, structured diet, and choice of pharmacotherapy (sibutramine hydrochloride, orlistat, or diethylpropion hydrochloride) during months 3–7 and continued use of medications and maintenance strategies for months 8–24.

Ryan et al. [23] obtained data indicating that severely obese patients randomized to an intensive weight loss program in primary care lost a significant amount of weight, compared to those receiving usual care (21 % of patients lost 10 % or more of the initial weight). The authors reported a weight loss of 5 % or higher in 31 % of the analyzed patients and a 10 % weight loss in 21 % of cases, with a significant improvement in many metabolic parameters. These results suggest that, with minimal training, primary care professionals could treat, successfully, a high percentage of morbidly obese patients. However, retention (retention rate in IMI group=51 %) and weight loss maintenance were two key points to improve, according with the researchers.

In a 1-year non-randomized controlled trial, Johnson et al. [88] compared changes in the dietary patterns of morbidly obese patients undergoing either laparoscopic gastric bypass surgery or a comprehensive lifestyle intervention program. Lifestyle intervention was associated with more favorable dietary 1-year changes than gastric bypass surgery in morbidly obese patients, as measured by intake of vegetables, whole grains, dietary fiber, and saturated fat.

A Spanish randomized clinical trial, performed in Mallorca (multidisciplinary treatment of morbid obesity—TRAMOMTANA) [89, 90], was designed to examine the effects of an Intensive Lifestyle Intervention (ILI) on the therapy of morbid obesity in comparison with a conventional obesity therapy group (COT) and with a third group consisting of patients already included in the bariatric surgery waiting list (SOG). The ILI group received behavioral therapy and nutritional/physical activity counseling. These morbidly obese patients attended weekly group meetings from weeks 1 through to 12 and biweekly from weeks 13 to 52. Meetings included 10–12 subjects, lasted 90 min, and were led by a registered nurse, who mastered in nutrition. The group sessions were focused on the qualitative aspects of the dietary habits, such as the distribution of energy intake, frequency of consumption, and food choices. The research team provided information on the benefits of the Mediterranean diet and encouraged the patients to follow this diet. There were no restrictions in calorie intake. A sport medicine physician prescribed daily home-based exercise (led by a physiotherapist), with gradual progression toward a goal of 175 min of moderate-intensity physical activity per week. Patients could receive treatment with weight loss medicines, such as orlistat or antidepressants at the endocrinologist discretion. Forty percent of the patients included in this group received treatment with sibutramine for a period of 1–2 months until it was withdrawn from the market in January of 2010.

The COT group received the standard medical treatment available for these patients (one visit with the endocrinologist every 6 months). Patients who received ILI achieved a significant weight loss compared with COT group (Fig. 1). The weight loss effect was already obtained after 6 months of ILI intervention. These results seriously question the efficacy of the COT approach to morbid obesity. Furthermore, they underscore the use of ILI programs to effectively treat morbidly obese patients which might help to reduce the number of candidate patients for

Table 3. Comparison of different lifestyle interventions: (1) Look AHEAD vs. DPP

	Frequency of sessions/visits	Format	Weight loss goal	Physical activity goal	Special features	Weight loss drugs	Meal replacements
Look AHEAD phase 1.1 (months 1–6)	Weekly	Three groups, one individual	Lose 7 % of initial weight	Exercise #175 min/week by month 6	Treatment toolbox	No	Two meal replacement products, one portion-controlled snack, and a self-selected meal each day
Look AHEAD phase 1.2 (months 7–12)	Three per month	Two groups, one individual		Increase minutes per week of activity; 10,000 steps/day goal			One meal replacement per day and two meals of self-selected foods are allowed
Look AHEAD phase 2 (months 13–48)	Two per month	One on site, one by mail or telephone. Additional: refresher groups are offered three times a year	Continued weight loss or weight maintenance		Advanced treatment toolbox orlistat		One meal replacement per day
Look AHEAD phase 3 (month 49+)	Two per year	On site. Additional phone calls and/or e-mail contacts. Participants may also join refresher groups			Additional support through newsletters, phone, or e-mail contact		
Diabetes Prevention Program (DPP), initial structured core curriculum (months 1–6)	16 in 24 weeks + 4 supervised phisic physical activity. Supervised sessions	Individual and group sessions	Lose 7 % of initial weight	150 min/week	Toolbox: adherence strategies, local and national network of training, feedback, and clinical support	No	Structured meal plans and meal replacement products were provided as an option for participants
Diabetes Prevention Program (DPP), maintenance program (months 7–12)	Face to face at least once every 2 months and by phone at least once between visits				Motivational campaigns. Small incentives (T-shirts, magnets, weight graphs. newsletters		

TABLE 4. Comparison of different lifestyle interventions: (2) LOSS vs. TRAMOMTANA

	Frequency of sessions/visits	Format	Weight loss goal	Physical activity goal	Special features	Weight loss drugs	Meal replacements
LOSS phase 1 (12 weeks or less)	No	No	Lose 10 % of initial weight	Exercise 150 min/week	Flexibility		Low-calorie liquid diet (900 kcal/day), 5 shakes per day
LOSS phase 2 (months 3–7)	4 weekly, then every 2 weeks Monthly physician visit	Group sessions + individual monthly physician visit			Individualized treatment strategies	Sibutramine Orlistat	Two daily meal replacements
LOSS phase 3 (months 8–24)	Monthly	Group sessions			$100 gift card rewarded attendance at month 24	Diethylpropion	One daily meal replacement, low-calorie liquid diet in 4- to 12-week episodes
TRAMOMTANA phase 1 (months 1–3)	Weekly	Four group sessions + 1 individual visit with specialist every 3 months	Lose 10 % of initial weight	Exercise 150 min/week by month 12	Social toolbox Rockport test Healthy cooking show Small incentives (umbrellas, magnets)	Sibutramine until withdrawal (40 % patients during 1–2 months)	No
TRAMOMTANA phase 2 (months 4–24)	Two per month	Two group sessions + 1 individual visit with specialist every 3 months			Social toolbox Rockport test Workshop: eat slowly and chew	No	

Fɪɢ. 1. One-year weight loss
in the TRAMOMTANA study.

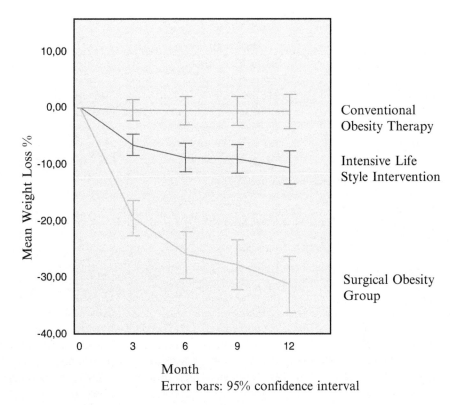

Fɪɢ. 1. One-year weight loss in the TRAMOMTANA study.

Error bars: 95% confidence interval

bariatric surgery, at a lower cost (evaluating medical visits, surgery, sessions, and meds).

Non-pharmacological strategies for weight reduction have reported 10 % losses that have been difficult to maintain [91]. Changes in dietary behavior, the stimulation of physical activity, and emotional support continue to be the mainstays for the management of obesity in adults, children, and adolescents.

Sustained caloric restriction (to 1,500 kcal/day for women and 1,800 for men), regardless of dietary macronutrient composition or regimen [19], has fairly similar effects on weight loss, ranging from 3 to 5 kg over 2 years [20]. The addition of physical exercise facilitates weight loss by increasing energy expenditure and increasing basal metabolic rate through an increase in muscle mass.

Unfortunately, lifestyle interventions alone rarely result in long-term weight loss and the majority of dieters return to baseline weight within 3–5 years. This even holds true for participants in weight loss trials who are offered education and intensive support to help prevent weight regain [21, 22].

The improvements described in morbidly obese patients using behavioral therapy as an element of an intensive lifestyle intervention could benefit a huge number of people: those who will undergo bariatric surgery and those who are not interested in surgery and just need to lose 5–10 % of the bodyweight. These interventions must be provided by multidisciplinary, academic, or clinical groups and can be provided at the hospital or primary care setting, to groups of 10–15 patients with an optimal duration of 20–26 weeks and a follow-up period of monitoring and maintenance (also 20–26 weeks) [57].

Overview of Current Obesity Medications

Lifestyle measures are the cornerstone of prevention and treatment of obesity. However, there is general agreement in the scientific community that the use of anti-obesity drugs should also be considered (after careful considerations of the pros and cons), in patients who did not have an optimal response to lifestyle interventions. Weight loss medications could also be considered in some cases as "jump-start" intervention, acting as coadjutant therapy to lifestyle interventions. In many circumstances adding medications to behavioral interventions helps to accomplish the recommended 10 % weight loss and also reinforces adherence to these lifestyle/behavioral interventions.

FDA guidance for the approval of new weight loss therapies intended for long-term use recommends a 5 % placebo-corrected weight reduction that should be maintained for at least 12 months after treatment initiation. Small, sustained reductions in weight can significantly improve CVR factors, particularly glycemia and BP, in overweight and obese individuals. The target adult population for drug therapy is set at BMI > 30 (or a BMI >27 plus a comorbidity such as HTA or T2DM). This opens up a potentially huge market for the development of new weight loss drugs. Despite the great strides in the understanding of the mechanisms involved in the hypothalamic regulation of appetite and energy balance, we still have a very limited armamentarium of drugs useful for the treatment of obesity.

TABLE 5. Drugs approved for treatment of obesity

Drug	Mechanism of action	Effect	Daily dosage	Average weight loss (kg)
Phentermine[a] (Adipex)	Augments central NE release	Decreases appetite	5–37.5 mg QD[b]	3.6 kg (12 weeks)
Diethylpropion[a] (Tenuate)	Augments central NE release	Decreases appetite	25 mg TID[c]	10 kg (12 weeks)
Orlistat[d] (Xenical)	Pancreatic and gastric	Decreases fat	120 mg TID	6 kg (1 year)
Orlistat[d,e] (Alli)[b]	Lipase inhibitor	Absorption	60 mg TID	
Lorcaserin (Belviq)	Agonist serotonin receptor 5-HT2C	Decreases appetite	10 mg BID	3.6 kg (1 year)
Phentermine and	Augments central NE and GABA release	7.5 mg/46 mg	8.1 kg (56 weeks)	
Topiramate CR (Qsymia®)	15 mg/92 mg	10.2 kg (56 weeks)		

[a]Approved only for short-term use (a few weeks)
[b]Usually taken mid-morning
[c]Taken 1 h before meals
[d]Taken with fatty meals or up to 1 h later; omit dose if meal is skipped; approved for up to 2 years' use. Diet should contain <30 % fat
[e]Available OTC

Given the previous history of several obesity medications that have been removed from the market due to significant side effects (HTA, depression, cardiac valvular abnormalities) and the current obesity-related health crisis, the need to identify safe and efficacious weight loss drugs is more than evident. Unfortunately, the medications currently available for obesity therapy are limited in number and efficacy (Table 5).

Sympathomimetic Amines

The oldest weight loss drugs still approved by the US FDA as weight loss adjuncts are sympathomimetic (amphetamine-like drugs) such as methamphetamine, phentermine, and diethylpropion. These medications act centrally as adrenergic stimulants, reducing appetite and increasing energy expenditure through generalized sympathetic activation.

Phentermine (Adipex®)

Phentermine (a central norepinephrine-releasing drug) is an approved anti-obesity agent, indicated as an adjunct to appropriate nutrition and physical exercise for short-term (up to 12 weeks) treatment of obesity. In the 1970s, phentermine hydrochloride was developed, with doses ranging from 8 to 37.5 mg [92].

Phentermine remains as the most widely prescribed weight loss drug in the USA. The phentermine hydrochloride salt easily dissociates in the GI tract, resulting in immediate release of the phentermine drug causing a significant appetite suppressant effect. Phentermine is classified by the FDA as a Schedule IV drug. It carries a risk for addiction and/or habituation, though its abuse potential is considered very low [93]. Short-term use of phentermine was associated with a mean weight loss of about 3 kg more than with placebo. No long-term (>1 year) randomized controlled trials of phentermine have been reported. Phentermine was widely used in combination with fenfluramine ("phen-fen"). Unfortunately, dexfenfluramine, a related drug, was found to cause valvular heart abnormalities and primary pulmonary hypertension and was removed from the market in 1997 [94].

Data on adverse events in weight loss trials that used sympathomimetic amines are limited but include increases in HR and BP, dry mouth, nervousness, insomnia, and constipation. Phentermine is contraindicated in patients with CAD, congestive heart failure (CHF), stroke, and uncontrolled HTA. There are no long-term data suggesting that treatment with this agent reduces CVD. Given the fact that phentermine is just approved for short-term use, this medication has very limited use in the management of obesity, as a chronic disease. However, as previously mentioned, it could be a helpful tool to use as a jump start to get patients motivated to participate in a lifestyle intervention program and start making small improvements in their daily habits, which could translate in long-term weight loss.

Diethylpropion (Tenuate®)

Diethylpropion is another amphetamine-like analogue, with fewer stimulant side effects, which has been approved by the US FDA for treatment of obesity since 1959. Diethylpropion is used as part of a short-term plan, along with a low-calorie diet, for weight reduction. Although most studies evaluating the efficacy of diethylpropion for weight loss were short term (less than 20 weeks), obese patients treated with diethylpropion lost an average of 3.0 kg of additional weight compared to placebo [95].

A report evaluated the efficacy of diethylpropion 50 mg BID or placebo for 6 months. After this period, all participants received diethylpropion in an open-label extension for an additional 6 months [96]. The study included 69 obese healthy adults who received a hypocaloric diet. After the initial 6 months, the diethylpropion group lost an average of 9.8 % of initial body weight vs. 3.2 % in the placebo group (Fig. 2). From baseline to month 12, the mean weight loss produced by diethylpropion was 10.6 %. Participants in the

FıG. 2. Effects of diethylpropion
in body weight change.

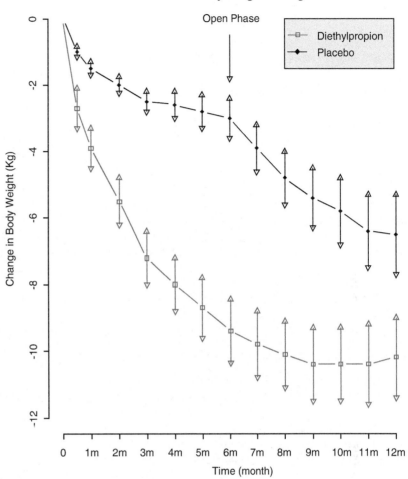

**Effects of Diethylpropion
in Body Weight Change**

placebo group who were switched to diethylpropion after 6 months lost an average of 7.0 % of their initial body weight. No differences in BP, pulse rate, EKG, and psychiatric evaluation were observed. As with phentermine, common side effects of diethylpropion included insomnia, dry mouth, dizziness, headache, mild increases in BP, and palpitations. Very few studies have evaluated the long-term use of diethylpropion.

Orlistat (Xenical®)

Orlistat is currently the only medication approved by the European Medicine Agency (EMEA) for the treatment of obesity [97]. Xenical acts by inhibiting the intestinal lipase, which translates into a reduction up to 30 % of ingested fat absorption. The recommended dosage is 1 capsule TID with meals. It has a dose-dependent effect: 120 mg decreases up to 30 % fat intake, whereas a dose of 60 mg decreases up to 25 %. In 2007, GlaxoSmithKline, under license from Roche, launched a low dose of orlistat (Alli®) which is not a necessary prescription.

The XENDOS study (XENical in the prevention of Diabetes in Obese Subjects) assessed the effect of the treatment with orlistat in 3,300 obese patients with impaired glucose tolerance [21], a 4-year, prospective, randomized, double-blind, placebo-controlled study; it demonstrated that orlistat (plus lifestyle modification) significantly reduced the incidence of T2DM and improved weight loss, when compared with placebo plus lifestyle changes. Mean weight loss after 4 years was significantly greater with orlistat (5.8 vs. 3.0 kg with placebo). The 3.0 kg weight loss achieved by the placebo plus lifestyle changes group over 4 years was comparable with that in the intensive lifestyle intervention arms of the DPS (3.5 kg) and DPP (3.5 kg). XENDOS was the first study to show that a weight loss agent such as orlistat in combination with lifestyle changes was more powerful than lifestyle changes alone helping patients to obtain long-term weight loss and improvements in their CVR factors. After 4 years' treatment, the cumulative incidence of diabetes was 9.0 % with placebo and 6.2 % with orlistat, corresponding to a risk reduction of 37.3 %. A meta-analysis of studies with orlistat [98] showed a drop of average weight of 2,39 kg.

Other benefits of orlistat include a reduction of LDL cholesterol more than expected by the drop in body weight.

Fat-soluble vitamin supplements should be taken 2 h before or after taking orlistat. The most common adverse effects included flatulence with discharge and fecal urgency, which occurred especially after high-fat dietary indiscretions, and were responsible for a significant rate of drug discontinuation. Serious, but very uncommon (only 12 cases), adverse effects have been reported such as liver damage, which were thought to be cases of individual hypersensitivity. Liver function should be monitored while doing Xenical therapy.

A study [99] warned of a possible link between reported cases of acute renal damage in orlistat users (incidence of 2 %). The authors hypothesized that the nonabsorbed dietary fat binds enteric calcium and reduces their ability to bind and sequestrate oxalate in the intestine that leads to excessive absorption of free oxalate with the consequent deposit in the renal parenchyma.

Xenical continues to be a useful therapy which could help obese patients to modified their dietary habits and lose weight.

Sibutramine (Meridia®, Reductil®)

Sibutramine was approved on November 1997 for weight loss and maintenance of weight loss in obese people, as well as in certain overweight people with other risks for CAD. Sibutramine induces weight loss by selectively inhibiting the neuronal reuptake of serotonin and norepinephrine within the hypothalamus. To a smaller degree, it also inhibits the reuptake of dopamine. Treatment with sibutramine resulted in an increase in satiety and a reduction in appetite [100, 101].

In a meta-analysis of randomized placebo-controlled trials of at least 1 year in duration (10 studies with 2,623 patients), sibutramine reduced body weight 4.3 kg more than placebo [102]. There was also a greater reduction in BMI in the sibutramine group and a 4 cm decrease in waist circumference with sibutramine therapy.

Sibutramine also prevented weight regain when administered after a dietary intervention. In the Sibutramine Trial of Obesity Reduction and Maintenance (STORM) study [103], 605 obese patients were treated with sibutramine (10 mg QD) and followed a low-energy diet for 6 months. Patients achieving >5 % weight loss after 6 months (n=467) were randomly allocated to continue sibutramine (10 mg QD uptitrated to 20 mg QD if weight regain occurred, or placebo for 18 months. The sibutramine group had less weight regain than the placebo group. In a subgroup of patients in STORM study, computed tomography showed a preferential reduction in visceral fat.

Sibutramine therapy was associated with an increase in BP and heart rate in some patients. As expected with any therapy for a chronic disease, significant weight regain was frequently observed after sibutramine therapy was discontinued. In the year 2010 both the EMA and FDA requested market withdrawal of sibutramine after reviewing data from the Sibutramine Cardiovascular Outcomes Trial (SCOUT) [104]. SCOUT was part of a post market requirement to look at cardiovascular safety of sibutramine after the European approval of the drug. It is important to emphasize that in this study patients participated for over 55 years with high CVR and that, in the vast majority of cases, they did not correspond with the type of patients for which this drug was originally approved for. After 6 years of treatment, the individuals who took sibutramine showed an increased risk of serious heart events, including nonfatal heart attack, nonfatal stroke, and death of 11.4 %, compared to 10.0 % in a placebo control group.

The results of the SCOUT were not surprising, if we take into account that most of the patients included in the SCOUT did not meet criteria for treatment with sibutramine. The odds were against sibutramine, because CVR is embedded in its mechanism of action and the study sample consisted of older obese patients, deliberately selected for high CVR, and exposed to sibutramine for 5 years (five times the maximum licensed duration of treatment) [105]. A large number of investigators and Scientific Societies felt that the SCOUT study was flawed as it only covered high-risk patients and did not consider obese patients who did not have cardiovascular complications or similar contraindications, especially considering that those were the patients who could really benefit from this medication.

Recently Approved Drugs for the Treatment of Obesity

Lorcaserin (Belviq®)

Lorcaserin is a new agonist of the 5-hydroxytryptamine (5-HT, or serotonin) receptor 5-HT2C. It binds selectively to the central 5-HT2C receptors, with poor affinity for 5-HT2A and 5-HT2B, respectively. Nonselective serotonergic agents, including fenfluramine and dexfenfluramine, were withdrawn from the market in 1997, after they were reported to be associated with valvular heart abnormalities [106]. Due to its selective agonist effect on 5-HT2C receptors, lorcaserin theoretically should not have similar cardiac adverse effects as fenfluramine.

Lorcaserin was approved by the FDA in June 2012, and it marked the end of a long era without any new drugs to treat obesity. The indication for lorcaserin is an addition to a reduced-calorie diet and exercise for patients who are obese or overweight with at least one medical comorbidity, such as T2DM, HTA, high cholesterol, or OSA. The mechanism by which lorcaserin results in weight loss appears to be by reducing appetite, which in turn reduces total energy intake. Three important phase 3 randomized clinical trials have evaluated the efficacy of lorcaserin helping obese patients to lose weight [107].

The BLOOM (Behavioral Modification and Lorcaserin for Overweight and Obesity Management) was a 104-week, clinical trial to assess the safety and efficacy of lorcaserin in obese patients. The primary outcome measure at year 1 was the proportion of patients achieving >5 % weight loss from baseline. At year 2 the primary outcome measure was the proportion of patients maintaining >5 % weight loss at week 104. In this study 3,182 obese adults (BMI >36 kg/m^2) were randomly assigned to lorcaserin (10 mg) or placebo BID for 1 year, followed by a 1-year extension period. All subjects participated in a behavioral modification program which included dietary and physical activity counseling. Obese patients treated with lorcaserin lost 3.6 kg more than controls at the end of the first year. Approximately 50 % of participants remained in the trial during year 2. Additionally, the weight reduction was maintained in more patients who continued to receive lorcaserin during the second year (68 %) than in patients who received a placebo (50.3 %) [108].

A second phase 3 Lorcaserin clinical trial was the BLOSSOM (Behavioral Modification and Lorcaserin Second Study for Obesity Management) [109]. In this 52-week clinical trial, 4,008 patients were treated with lorcaserin 10 mg QD or BID compared to placebo. The study was designed to assess the efficacy and safety of a dose range of lorcaserin when administered in conjunction with a nutritional and physical exercise program to promote weight loss, in obese patients and at-risk overweight patients. The primary outcome measure was again the proportion of patients achieving >5 % weight loss from baseline to week 52. Significantly more patients treated with lorcaserin 10 mg BID and QD lost at least 5 % of baseline body weight (47.2 % and 40.2 %, respectively) as compared with placebo (25.0 %). Weight loss of at least 10 % was achieved by 22.6 and 17.4 % of patients receiving lorcaserin 10 mg BID and QD, respectively, and 9.7 % of patients in the placebo group. Thus, the weight losses seen with lorcaserin were slightly greater than that seen in the orlistat studies, which provided 2–3 kg of placebo-subtracted weight loss. Headache, nausea, and dizziness were the most common lorcaserin-related adverse events.

A third lorcaserin trial BLOOM-DM (Behavioral Modification and lorcaserin for Overweight and Obesity Management in Diabetes Mellitus) [110] was carried out in 604 T2DM obese and overweight patients. The BLOOM-DM's purpose was to assess the weight loss effect of lorcaserin during and at the end of 1 year of treatment in patients treated with metformin, sulfonylurea (SFU), or either agent in combination with other oral hypoglycemic agents. Patients were randomized to lorcaserin 10 mg BID ($n=256$), lorcaserin 10 mg dosed QD ($n=95$), or placebo ($n=253$). Lorcaserin 10 mg BID met the three primary efficacy endpoints by producing statistically significant weight loss compared to placebo. At week 52, the data showed that weight loss was 4.5 % of total body weight with lorcaserin BID and 5 % with

lorcaserin QD vs. 1.5 % with placebo. Also 37.5 % of patients treated with lorcaserin 10 mg twice daily achieved at least 5 % weight loss, more than double the 16.1 % of patients taking a placebo. Additionally, 16.3 % of lorcaserin 10 mg BID patients achieved at least 10 % weight loss compared to 4.4 % of patients taking a placebo. HgA1C decreased by 0.9 % with lorcaserin BID, 1.0 % with lorcaserin QD, and 0.4 % with placebo. Symptomatic hypoglycemia occurred in 7.4 % of patients on lorcaserin BID, 10.5 % on lorcaserin QD, and 6.3 % on placebo.

Lorcaserin produced side effects in human clinical trials, but at rates not significantly different than placebo and mostly with mild and transient severity. The most common side effect was headache, experienced by about 18 % of drug arm participants compared to 11 % of placebo participants. Other reported side effects and their rates for lorcaserin and placebo patients, respectively, were as follows: upper respiratory tract infection (14.8 % vs. 11.9 %), nasopharyngitis (13.4 % vs. 12.0 %), sinusitis (7.2 % vs. 8.2 %), and nausea (7.5 % vs. 5.4 %). Lorcaserin has been associated with perceptual disturbances, and because lorcaserin has the potential to bind 5-HT2A receptors, it has been evaluated and found to have low abuse potential. Adverse events of depression, anxiety and suicidal ideation were infrequent and were reported at a similar rate in each treatment group. In agreement with the FDA, Arena conducted regular echocardiograms of the phase III participants. At the 3-, 6-, and 12-month intervals, the echocardiograms of participants of the BLOOM trial did not show any significant increase in valvulopathy over baseline.

Thus, lorcaserin is a new therapeutic tool to treat obesity and is a well-needed addition to an area where therapeutic agents are sparse. Lorcaserin has also been shown to improve glycemic control and it has modestly beneficial effects on lipids and BP as well. This data justifies the proposed indications for the use of lorcaserin as an adjunct to diet and physical activity for weight management, including weight loss and maintenance of weight loss in obese patients and overweight patients with at least 1 weight-related comorbidity.

Phentermine and Topiramate Controlled Release (Qsymia®)

The scientific literature and clinical experience tell us that anti-obesity drugs that specifically target just one area within the brain may have a limited effect inducing weight loss in obese patients; consequently the idea of targeting more than one circuit in the regulatory pathways of energy balance has become a popular and potentially efficient strategy to treat patients with obesity.

The FDA recently approved a combination of low doses of controlled-release (CR) phentermine and the anticonvulsant agent topiramate (in one capsule) for adults with a BMI ≥30 kg/m^2 or with a BMI ≥27 kg/m^2 and at least one weight-related comorbidity such as HTA, T2DM, and dyslipidemia

(July 2012). Several trials had evaluated the efficacy of this combination inducing weight loss in obese patients [111–115].

In the CONQUER clinical trial [111], 2,487 overweight and obese patients with HTA, high cholesterol or T2DM participated. Patients received a combination of phentermine-topiramate CR (7.5/46 or 15/92 mg) compared with placebo over 56 weeks [49]. At 56 weeks, change in body weight was −1.4, −8.1, and −10.2 kg in the patients assigned to placebo, phentermine-topiramate 7.5/46 mg, and phentermine-topiramate CR 15/92 mg, respectively. 21 % of the patients achieved at least 5 % weight loss with placebo, 62 % with phentermine-topiramate CR 7.5/46 mg, and 70 % with phentermine-topiramate CR 15/92 mg; for ≥10 % weight loss, the corresponding numbers were 7, 37, and 48 %.

In an extension of the CONQUER (the SEQUEL study) [112], investigators addressed the longer-term efficacy and safety of lifestyle intervention and two doses of phentermine-topiramate CR for an additional 52 weeks (total treatment duration of 108 weeks) in overweight and obese subjects with cardiometabolic disease. Overall, 84 % of subjects completed the study, with similar completion rates between treatment groups. At week 108, phentermine and topiramate CR was associated with significant, sustained weight loss compared with placebo. Mean percentage changes from baseline in body weight were −1.8, −9.3, and −10.5 % for placebo, 7.5/46, and 15/92, respectively. Phentermine-topiramate CR improved cardiovascular and metabolic variables and decreased rates of incident T2DM in comparison with placebo. Phentermine-topiramate CR was well tolerated over 108 weeks. Of note, phentermine-topiramate CR was less effective causing weight loss in the second year of use, although most individuals were able to maintain the weight they lost achieved in year 1.

In a third clinical trial (EQUIP) [113], 1,267 morbidly obese patients (BMI >35 kg/m^2) were included into three arms: placebo, phentermine-topiramate CR 3.75/23 mg, and phentermine-topiramate CR 15/92 mg with a total treatment duration of 56 weeks. Both doses of phentermine-topiramate CR yielded significantly greater 1-year weight loss compared with placebo, with a greater proportion of patients losing more than 5, 10, or 15 % of baseline body weight. Patients treated with phentermine-topiramate CR 15/92 and 3.75/23 lost 10.9 % and 5.1 % of body weight, respectively, when analyzed as ITT-LOCF, compared with 1.6 % weight loss on placebo and 14.4 and 6.7 % weight loss in completers-only analyses compared with 2.1 % weight loss with placebo. Of importance was that weight loss induced by phentermine-topiramate CR was accompanied by improvements in several cardiovascular and metabolic risk factors, such as waist circumference, systolic BP, and total cholesterol/HDL cholesterol ratio in both doses. As previously shown Phentermine-topiramate CR 15/92 treatment was also associated with significant improvements in diastolic BP, fasting glucose, LDL cholesterol, HDL cholesterol, and total cholesterol.

The most common adverse events were dry mouth (2, 13, and 21 %) in the groups assigned to placebo, phentermine-topiramate CR 7.5/46 mg, and phentermine-topiramate CR 15/92 mg, respectively, paraesthesia (2 %, 14 %, and 21 %, respectively) and constipation (6 %, 15 %, and 17 %, respectively) none of these events caused study discontinuation in more than 1 % of patients [116]. There was a dose-related increase in the incidence of psychiatric (e.g., depression, anxiety) and cognitive (e.g., disturbance in attention) adverse events in the active treatment group. Although BP improved slightly with active therapy, there was an increase in heart rate (0.6–1.6 beats/min) compared with placebo.

The FDA does not recommend the use of this drug combination in patients with recent stroke, unstable heart disease, HTA or CAD, glaucoma, hyperthyroidism or in patients who have taken monoamine oxidase inhibitors within 14 days. Women of child-bearing age should have a pregnancy test before starting this therapy and monthly thereafter. Because topiramate can produce renal stones, this combination preparation should be used cautiously in patients with a history of kidney stones.

A recommendation for the use of phentermine-topiramate CR was recently presented [115]. This algorithm titrates the dose starting with a phase-in dose of phentermine-topiramate CR 3.75/23 mg QD for 2 weeks. The dose then is increased to a half dose of 7.5/46 mg QD for 12 weeks. Patients are evaluated at that point for weight loss, and "responders" (patients with weight loss >3 %) are maintained on that dose. "Nonresponders" (those with weight loss <3 %) are either discontinued or receive increased doses. Those receiving increased doses are stepped up to an intermediate dose of 11.25/69 mg QD for 2 weeks, then the treatment is increased to a final full dose of 15/92 mg QD for 12 weeks. At the end of the full-dose period, responders with weight loss of 5 % or more are maintained on their doses. If an individual does not lose 5 % of body weight after 12 weeks on the highest dose, phentermine-topiramate CR should be discontinued gradually, as abrupt withdrawal of topiramate could cause seizures.

Phentermine-topiramate CR may be considered for obese postmenopausal women and men without CVD, particularly those who do not tolerate orlistat or lorcaserin [116]. The possibility of adding this combination therapy to orlistat should also be considered. Clinicians who prescribe and pharmacists who dispense the drug must be enrolled in a Risk Evaluation and Mitigation Strategy, which includes a medication guide, a patient brochure, and a formal training program for prescribers, detailing safety information [114].

In Europe, the combination of phentermine-topiramate CR has not been approved yet. The EMA's Committee for Medicinal Products for Human Use first rejected the product in October of 2012. In February of 2013 the EMA refused again to grant approval for this drug combination in the European Union.

TABLE 6. Effect of GLP-1 analogues on body weight compared to other T2DM therapies

Drug	Mechanism of action/effect	Daily dosage	Average weight change (kg)
Liraglutide (Victoza)	GLP-1 receptor agonist. Decreases appetite	1.8 mg (3 mg)	−4.8 to −7.2 kg (dose dependent; 20 weeks)
Exenatide (Byetta)	GLP-1 receptor agonist. Decreases appetite	5–10 µg	−2.8 to −4.4 kg (dose dependent, 30–82 weeks)
Exenatide ER (Bydureon)	GLP-1 receptor agonist. Decreases appetite	0.8–2 mg	−2.8 to −4.0 kg (dose dependent, 15–30 weeks)
Metformin (Glucophage)	Increases FA oxidation Decreases glucose absorption	2,000 mg	1–2 kg
DpP-4 inhibitors	(sitagliptin) Increase incretin (GLP-1 and GIP) levels (Vildagliptin, Saxagliptin, Linagliptin, Alogliptin)	VBF[a]	Weight neutral
Alpha-glucosidase	(acarbose, miglitol) Inhibit the breakdown and inhibitors Absorption of carbohydrates in the GI tract	25, 50, 100 mg	Weight neutral
Sulfonylurea	Stimulate insulin secretion	VBF[a]	+ 1 to +5 kg
Non-sulfonylurea	(meglitinides) Stimulate insulin secretion Secretagogues	0.5–1–2 mg	+0.7 to +2.4 kg
Thiazolidinediones	Enhancing of muscle/adipose tissue insulin sensitivity	15–30–45 mg	+ 1 to +5 kg
Insulin	Glucose uptake. Decreases appetite by inhibiting NPY/AgRP-secreting neurons	VBF[a]	+ 1 to +5 kg

[a]Varies by formulation (VBF)

Incretins as Potential Anti-obesity Drugs: GLP-1 Analogues

Glucagon-like peptide 1 (GLP-1) is an incretin hormone secreted from the L-cells in the lower gut in response to meal ingestion, which stimulates endogenous insulin secretion in a glucose-dependent manner. GLP-1 reduces appetite in lean and normal-weight individuals, as well as in obese individuals [117], and it has been shown to reduce body weight in overweight individuals with T2DM [118, 119] (Table 6). The underlying mechanism mediating the weight reducing effects of GLP-1 is most likely a combination of effects on the gastrointestinal tract and the central nervous system. GLP-1 also decreases blood glucagon levels and has been shown to promote B-cell growth and proliferation in animal models [120].

The combination of these mechanisms makes GLP-1 receptor stimulation, an interesting target to investigate for obesity therapy. However, a major drawback with endogenous GLP-1 with regard to administration as medical treatment is the short elimination half-life of <1.5 min after IV administration, due to rapid degradation by dipeptidyl peptidase (DPP-4) present on the capillary endothelium [121]. Hence, GLP-1 treatment has limited clinical value, and alternative therapeutic strategies have already been developed. A successful approach that has been employed to prolong the in vivo half-life of GLP-1 is to protect the peptide from cleavage by DPP-4 by exchanging amino acids at the second and third N-terminal positions of the peptide; cleavage by this enzyme is reduced [122].

Liraglutide (Victoza®)

Liraglutide is a long-acting GLP-1 analogue, with a 97 % structural homology to human GLP-1 and recently approved for the treatment of T2DM in the USA, EU, Japan, and other countries worldwide under the brand name Victoza® (Novo Nordisk) (1.2 or 1.8 mg QD) [123, 124]. Because GLP-1 decreases appetite and causes a dose-dependent weight loss in obese individuals [125], it could be an attractive treatment option for both T2DM and obesity. To explore the mechanism behind the observed weight loss with liraglutide, the effect of this drug on various body weight-related parameters known to be affected by native GLP-1 has been investigated. Results from various trials have shown that liraglutide 1.8 mg seems to exert a mild suppression of hunger ratings and increase postprandial fullness, as indicated by appetite rating endpoints [126].

More than 50 clinical trials with liraglutide have been completed (with doses up to 3.0 mg). Out of 10,000 subjects included, more than 7,000 subjects were exposed to liraglutide. A total of 986 obese subjects without T2DM (<9 % of all subjects) have been included to date in the obesity clinical development program for liraglutide. The first of three confirmatory phase 3 trials within the liraglutide obesity development program (NN8022-1923, o SCALE-Maintenance) was recently completed. Reporting is ongoing. The trial was a 56-week randomized, double-blind, placebo-controlled trial investigating treatment of liraglutide 3.0 mg vs. placebo as an adjunct to diet and exercise in overweight/obese subjects with comorbidities who had already lost at least 5 % of their body weight during a 4- to 12-week run-in period on a low-calorie diet. The mean weight loss for subjects in the run-in period was approximately 6 kg. From a body weight of approximately 100 kg at randomization, treatment with liraglutide for 56 weeks provided an additional estimated mean weight loss of 5.7 kg, compared to weight neutrality or maintenance in the placebo group (+0.16 kg vs. baseline). Treatment with liraglutide maintained and in some instances further improved beneficial effects on markers of glycemic control and CVR.

An important study including obese patient (BMI 30–40 kg/m²) without T2DM was conducted by Astrup et al. [125]. This placebo-controlled 20-week clinical trial included 564 obese individuals. They used one of four liraglutide doses (1.2, 1.8, 2.4, or 3.0 mg) compared to placebo-administered QD s.c. or to orlistat (120 mg) p.o. TID. Weight change analyzed by intention to treat was the primary endpoint. An 84-week open-label extension followed. Patients on liraglutide lost significantly more weight than did those on placebo or orlistat. Mean weight loss with liraglutide 1.2–3.0 mg was 4.8, 5.5, 6.3 g, and 7.2 kg compared with 2.8 kg with placebo and 4.1 kg with orlistat [127].

Treatment with liraglutide was generally well tolerated, with high completion rates in groups (75 % in liraglutide group, 70 % in placebo group). Serious adverse events were relatively uncommon, but were more frequent in liraglutide-treated subjects (4.2 %) compared to placebo (2.4 %). There were no events of pancreatitis or medullary thyroid cancer, and no treatment-related increases in blood calcitonin levels. The most commonly reported adverse events were from the gastrointestinal system, with nausea reported by 47 % of subjects in the liraglutide group compared to 17 % in the placebo groups and vomiting by 17 % vs. 2 %, respectively. It will be important to see the results from the studies currently conducted evaluating the efficacy and safety of liraglutide for the treatment of obesity and its impact on CVD disease.

Exenatide (Synthetic Exendin-4) (Byetta®)

Exenatide, an exendin-based GLP-1 receptor agonist, is a synthetic 39-amino acid peptide which was discovered in a search for biologically active peptides in venom from the Gila monster (Heloderma suspectum). It is currently available in the USA and EU (Eli Lilly). This reptilian protein shares 53 % amino acid homology to human GLP-1 [128] and is resistant to DPP4-mediated degradation.

Exenatide 5 or 10 µg administered twice daily s.c. was associated with a dose-dependent mean weight loss of up to 2.8 kg at 30 weeks, which increased to 4.4 kg at week 82 in an open-label trial extension [127, 129, 130]. Weight reductions were greatest in persons with the highest baseline BMI and in those taking metformin, with lesser reductions occurring in those patients taking an SU or a combination of metformin and SU.

At a dose of 10 µg BID, exenatide reduced HbA1c concentrations by 0.8–1.5 % [128–130]. In particular, exenatide lowered postprandial glucose levels after breakfast and dinner to a much greater degree than after lunch. A pooled analysis of three trials of adjunctive treatment with exenatide 5 or 10 µg BID showed a mean decrease in SBP and DBP of 2.6 and 1.9 mmHg, respectively, at week 104, suggesting sustained improvement in BP. Changes in lipid parameters at 82 weeks included decreased triglyceride (−38.6 mg/dL), LDLC (−1.6 mg/dL), and apolipoprotein B (−1.1 mg/dL) levels and an increase in HDL-C (+4.6 mg/dL). The most frequently reported adverse effects of exenatide were nausea and vomiting, which occurred in 40–60 % and ≤10 % of patients, respectively. Antibodies against exenatide were detected in 40–60 % of patients treated with the drug [128–130]. The clinical relevance of these antibodies cannot be known with certainty, but in the majority of patients, their presence does not seem to impair the efficacy of exenatide. Several additional GLP-1 agonists, including lixisenatide, albiglutide, and taspoglutide, are in various stages of clinical trials and have been modified to increase their half-lives.

Exenatide Long-Acting Release (Bydureon®)

The long-acting formulation exenatide LAR was developed to maintain a constant plasma level of the drug with once-weekly (QW) administration. Exenatide is incorporated into a matrix of poly(d,l-lactide-co-glycolide) (PLG), which previously has been used as a biomaterial in sutures and in extended release preparations. Once injected subcutaneously the compound breaks down over time and allows a controlled rate of drug delivery resulting in the longer duration of exenatide release [131]. Once released, exenatide is eliminated via the kidneys. Exenatide LAR exhibits a median half-life of 2 weeks and reaches steady-state plasma concentrations in approximately 6–10 weeks. Absorption is similar when given subcutaneously in the abdomen, thigh, or upper arm. When exenatide LAR 2 mg was given once weekly by injection, the concentration reached 50 pg/mL by end of week 2. This level has been associated with reduced fasting and postprandial plasma glucose in previous studies using continuous infusion of exenatide. Exenatide LAR was approved for marketing in the USA in 2011 and in Europe in 2013.

A small randomized, placebo-controlled, double-blinded phase 2 study compared exenatide LAR (0.8 or 2 mg) administered subcutaneously QW [132] in patients with T2DM during 15 weeks. From baseline to week 15, exenatide LAR reduced mean HbA_{1c} by −1.4 % (0.8 mg) and −1.7 % (2 mg) compared to +0.4 % with placebo. In the exenatide LAR 2 mg treatment arm, body weight reductions of 3.8 kg were seen, while no change was noted in either the 0.8 mg exenatide LAR and placebo arms. All results were clinically significant. No participants receiving exenatide withdrew from the study; adverse events reported included mild to moderate nausea, gastroenteritis, and hypoglycemia.

Several clinical trials including the DURATION Program (*D*iabetes therapy *U*tilization: *R*esearching changes in Hb*A*1c, weight and other factors *T*hough *I*ntervention with exenatide *ON*ce weekly) have evaluated the efficacy of exenatide LAR, compared to placebo and other antidiabetic drugs to improve body weight and metabolic parameters [133–136].

The clinical trial DURATION-1 studied the effect of exenatide QW in a head to head comparison against BID exenatide, over 30 weeks, in 295 patients with T2DM.

Treatment with exenatide LAR resulted in significantly greater improvements in HgA1C compared to exenatide BID (HgA1C changed from baseline, −1.9 %±0.08 vs. 1.5 %±.0.08). The weight loss did not differ between the two groups by 30 weeks (−3.7 kg for QW vs. −3.6 kg for BID), and about 75 % of the patients lost weight. Both treatments were associated with reduction in triglycerides and blood pressure. As previously seen, nausea was predominantly mild and transient and occurred less frequently with exenatide LAR. The size of the needle required for subcutaneous injection of exenatide LAR is bigger than that required for administration of exenatide (23 gauge [0.64 mm] vs. 29–32 gauge [0.24–0.34 mm]). Injection site reactions, such as erythema, nodules, or pruritus, are more common with exenatide LAR and have been reported in 10–15 % of patients [133]. By contrast, injection site reactions have been found in less than 2 % of patients treated with exenatide. The DURATION-1 study illustrates that exenatide QW is more effective in reducing HbA1c and fasting plasma glucose than BID, while the reduction in weight did not differ.

Most patients with T2DM often begin pharmacotherapy with metformin but eventually need additional treatment. In DURATION-2, exenatide QW (2 mg) was compared with pioglitazone (45 mg) and sitagliptin (100 mg) to assess the potential differences between these antidiabetic drugs as add-on therapy to metformin during a period of 26 weeks. In this study exenatide LAR produced superior HbA1c reduction (1.5 %) and weight loss (2.3 kg) compared to results obtained with sitagliptin (−0.9 % HgA1C, −1.5 kg weight loss) or pioglitazone (−1.2 % HgA1C, +2.8 kg weight gain) in a head to head study of patients with T2DM not achieving adequate glycemic control (starting HgA1C of 8.5 %) on metformin therapy [134]. The reduction in SBP was significantly greater with exenatide (−4 mmHg) compared with sitagliptin, but not pioglitazone. About 24 and 10 % registered nausea with exenatide and sitagliptin, while diarrhea was observed in 18 % and 10 %, respectively. Fewer patients withdrew from treatment with sitagliptin (13 %) than with exenatide (21 %) or pioglitazone (21 %). No major hypoglycemia occurred in any group.

In the open-label DURATION-3 trial [135], exenatide QW (2 mg) was compared with insulin glargine QD. Exenatide QW treatment resulted in greater HbA1c reduction (−1.5 %) after 26 weeks than insulin glargine (−1.3 %). Insulin glargine produced greater reduction in fasting glucose than did exenatide, while significantly greater reductions in postprandial glucose excursions were obtained with exenatide LAR.

Mean weight changes were −2.6 kg in the exenatide group and +1.4 kg in the insulin glargine-treated patients. Mean heart rate at week 26 was raised compared with baseline in the exenatide but not in the insulin glargine group. No other CVR factors including lipid concentrations differed between the groups. Risk of hypoglycemia was reduced with exenatide. One patient taking exenatide developed pancreatitis.

The number of patients who discontinued treatment because of adverse effects was 5 % (exenatide group) vs. 1 % (insulin glargine group). More patients discontinued exenatide QW than insulin glargine due to nausea and inject reactions.

The DURATION-4 study [136] assessed the relative efficacy of exenatide LAR head to head with metformin (2.5 g QD), pioglitazone (45 mg QD), or sitagliptin (100 mg QD). After 26 weeks of treatment, exenatide LAR produced an average weight loss of 2 kg, which was statistically significantly greater than the average 0.8 kg that patients lost with sitagliptin and the average 1.5 kg patients gained with Actos. Patients receiving metformin experienced an average weight loss of 2 kg. Patients randomized to exenatide LAR experienced a reduction in HgA1C of 1.5 % from baseline, which was significantly greater than the reduction of 1.2 % for sitagliptin in drug-naive subjects with T2DM. The most frequently reported adverse events among exenatide LAR users were nausea (11.3 %) and diarrhea (10.9 %) [136].

A recent article by Visboll et al. [137] presented a systematic review with meta-analyses of all randomized controlled trials of adult participants with a BMI of 25 or higher, with or without T2DM, and who received exenatide BID, exenatide QW, or liraglutide QD at clinically relevant doses for at least 20 weeks. They showed that GLP-1R agonist groups achieved a greater weight loss than control groups (weighted mean difference −2.9 kg). They recorded weight loss in the GLP-1R agonist groups for patients without T2DM (−3.2 kg) as well as patients with T2DM (−2.8 kg). In the overall analysis, GLP-1R agonists had beneficial effects on systolic and diastolic BP, plasma concentrations of cholesterol, and glycemic control. GLP-1R agonists were associated with nausea, diarrhea, and vomiting, but not with hypoglycemia.

Anti-obesity Medications in the Late Phase of Development

Naltrexone-Bupropion Extended Release (Tentatively Named Contrave)

This combination of naltrexone-bupropion extended release (SR) is not yet approved for marketing in the USA. Naltrexone is an opioid receptor antagonist that is approved for the treatment of alcohol and opioid dependence [138]. Bupropion is a dopamine and norepinephrine reuptake inhibitor that was first approved for the treatment of depression [139] and later for smoking cessation [140].

The safety and efficacy of this combination were studied by the Contrave Obesity Research (COR) program which consists of four randomized, double-blind, placebo-controlled, phase III clinical studies of 56-week duration (COR-I [141], COR-II [142], COR-BMOD (COR-Behavior MODification) [143], and COR-Diabetes), assessing the efficacy, safety, and tolerability of naltrexone SR-bupropion SR combination therapy in obese patients with or without T2DM.

In *COR-I trial* 1,742 obese patients were randomly assigned in a 1:1:1 ratio to a fixed oral (p.o.) of naltrexone-bupropion 32/360 mg SR (8+90 mg in each tablet, two tablets taken BID), naltrexone-bupropion 16/360 mg SR (4+90 mg in each tablet, two tablets taken BID), or matching placebo for 56 weeks [141]. Weight loss was significantly greater in the combination treatment groups compared with placebo. In the study population that completed 56 weeks of treatment, weight loss was −8.1 %, −6.7 %, and −1.8 % in the naltrexone-bupropion 32/360 SR, naltrexone-bupropion 16/360 SR, and placebo groups, respectively. Waist circumference, TG, CRP, and HOMA-IR were significantly reduced, and HDL-C levels were significantly increased in the combination treatment groups compared with placebo. COR-I investigators also reported greater improvements in the quality of life, eating behavior, and food craving in participants on naltrexone-bupropion SR compared with placebo.

The percentage of participants achieving weight loss of ≥10 % in the COR-II trial was also significantly higher in the naltrexone-bupropion 32/360 mg SR group compared with the placebo group (32.9 % vs. 5.7 %, respectively) as was the proportion of those achieving weight loss of ≥15 % (15.7 % vs. 2.4 % in the naltrexone-bupropion 32/360 mg SR group vs. placebo. The most frequently reported side effects were nausea, constipation, and headache.

In the COR-BMOD trial, 793 obese patients were randomly assigned in a 3:1 ratio to a fixed p.o. dose of naltrexone-bupropion 32/360 mg SR or placebo. All participants were on an energy-reduced diet and attended group behavioral modification sessions. At week 56 a significantly greater weight loss was observed in the naltrexone-bupropion SR group compared with placebo (−11.5 % vs. −7.3 %, respectively). Participants in both groups attended a similar number of BMOD sessions; the more sessions attended, the higher the percentage of weight reduction. The data showed that reductions in mean SBP and DBP were greater in the placebo group compared with the combination treatment group. Pulse rate was slightly increased in patients treated with naltrexone-bupropion SR, whereas it remained unchanged in the placebo group. This finding suggests that naltrexone-bupropion SR may attenuate the favorable effects of weight loss on BP. The smaller reduction in BP (as well as the small increase in pulse) in the naltrexone-bupropion SR group is consistent with the pharmacological properties of bupropion [144]. As previously shown, quality of life, as assessed by the IWQOL-Lite total score and subscales, was improved significantly more in the naltrexone-bupropion SR group compared with placebo.

Significantly more participants in the combination treatment group reported adverse events compared with placebo (nausea, 34.1 % vs. 10.5 %; constipation, 24.1 % vs. 14 %; dizziness, 14.6 % vs. 4.5 %; dry mouth, 8 % vs. 3 %; tremor, 5.8 % vs. 1 %; upper abdominal pain, 5.5 % vs. 1.5 %; and tinnitus, 5.3 % vs. 0.5 %, respectively) [143]. These adverse events were mostly mild to moderate in severity and occurred during the first weeks of the study. There were two serious cases of cholecystitis (followed by successful surgery) in patients on naltrexone-bupropion SR who had achieved weight loss >15 kg.

In the COR-Diabetes trial, 505 overweight or obese T2DM patients with a mean HbA1c = 8.0 % and on several oral hypoglycemic drugs were randomized in a 2:1 ratio to either naltrexone-bupropion 32/360 mg SR or placebo [145]. More patients on combination treatment lost >5 % of their initial weight compared with the placebo group (44.5 % vs. 18.9 %, respectively). Furthermore, reductions in mean HbA1c values were greater in the naltrexone-bupropion SR group compared with placebo (−0.6 % vs. −0.1 %, respectively), leading to a higher proportion of T2DM patients achieving HbA1c target levels of <7 % in the combination treatment group compared with placebo (44 % vs. 26 %, respectively).

Diabetic patients on naltrexone-bupropion SR showed significantly greater improvements in various cardiometabolic risk factors compared with placebo (waist circumference, −5 vs. 2.9 cm; TG, −11.2 % vs. −0.8 %; HDL-C, −3 % vs. −0.3 %). Mean reductions in LDL-C, fasting glucose, insulin, HOMA IR, and CRP levels were also greater in the combination group compared with placebo, although they did not reach significance. As previously shown the most frequently reported adverse events were nausea, vomiting, constipation, and dizziness. Discontinuation usually occurred due to nausea.

Even though the mechanisms by which the naltrexone-bupropion induces weight loss are not entirely understood, this combination deserves further evaluation because it can be an important new tool in the therapy of obesity. The combination of bupropion and naltrexone was favorably reviewed by an FDA Advisory Panel in 2012. The FDA has required a pre-marketing study of the combination drug with assessment of cardiovascular outcomes. There will be an interim analysis of the trial and the FDA may allow the marketing of the combination as Contrave as early as 2014, provided the cardiovascular outcomes are acceptable [146].

Cetilistat

Cetilistat (Norgine, Amsterdam, the Netherlands) is a lipase inhibitor and, while similar to the currently FDA-approved Roche's anti-obesity drug orlistat, may have a more tolerable side-effect profile due to a different molecular structure.

To determine the efficacy, safety, and tolerability of cetilistat in obese patients, a phase II, multicenter [147], randomized, placebo-controlled, parallel group study was developed. The 442 enrolled patients were advised a hypocaloric diet for a 2-week run-in period before they were randomized to either placebo or one of three different doses of cetilistat (60 mg TID, 120 mg TID, and 240 mg TID) for 12 weeks. Treatment with cetilistat reduced mean body weight to similar extents at all doses, which were statistically significant compared with placebo (60 mg TID 3.3 kg, 120 mg TID 3.5 kg, 240 mg TID 4.1 kg). Total serum and LDL cholesterol levels were likewise significantly reduced by 3–11 % at all doses of cetilistat. Cetilistat was well tolerated. The frequency of withdrawal owing to treatment-emergent adverse events was similar between cetilistat-treated groups (5.3–7.6 %) and placebo (7.6 %).

The incidence of GI adverse events was increased in the cetilistat-treated groups compared to placebo. However, those GI adverse events, such as flatus with discharge and oily spotting, only occurred in 1.8–2.8 % of subjects in the cetilistat-treated groups. Cetilistat produced a clinically and statistically significant weight loss in obese patients in this short-term 12-week study. This was accompanied by significant improvements in other obesity-related parameters.

Kopelman et al. [148] carried out a clinical trial to determine the efficacy and safety of cetilistat and orlistat relative to placebo in obese patients with T2DM, on metformin. Patients were randomized to placebo, cetilistat (40, 80, or 120 mg TID), or orlistat 120 mg TID, for 12 weeks. Similar reductions in body weight were observed in patients receiving cetilistat 80 or 120 mg TID or 120 mg TID orlistat (3.85, 4.32, 3.78 kg, respectively); and these reductions were significant vs. placebo. Statistically significant reductions in glycosylated hemoglobin were also noted. Discontinuation in the orlistat group was significantly worse than in the 120 mg cetilistat and placebo groups and was entirely due to gastrointestinal AEs.

Since successful management of obesity is likely to require long-term compliance with prescribed medication, cetilistat may have benefits over currently marketed anti-obesity drugs such as orlistat, with respect to better toleration. Takeda submitted a New Drug Application (NDA) to the Ministry of Health for cetilistat for the treatment of obesity with complications, based on data obtained from three phase III clinical trials in Japan in October of 2012. The three studies included a 52-week placebo-controlled study that evaluated the efficacy and safety of cetilistat and 24- and 52-week open-label safety studies that were conducted on obese patients with T2DM and dyslipidemia.

Conclusions

Obesity is a very serious global public health problem responsible for diseases such as CVD, T2DM, and hypertension, and it should be tackled by health-care providers as well as by health policy authorities. Obesity treatment should be individually tailored and the health risks and metabolic and psycho-behavioral characteristics of each patient should be taken into account before deciding what medical therapy could be more appropriate. Drugs must be prescribed over the long term for chronic weight management; they do not produce permanent weight loss. It is also very important to set up realistic expectations before starting the treatment of

obesity. Both physician and the patient should know that a weight loss of 5–10 % reduces obesity-related health risks significantly.

There are emerging data in the literature suggesting the possible effectiveness of medical, intensive, and interdisciplinary weight loss programs in subjects with morbid obesity. Behavioral therapy especially in the context of group therapy can be effective helping an important number of obese and morbidly obese patients to lose weight and to keep it off. The use of medications should be seriously considered as adjuvant therapy early in the course of the therapy. The current armamentarium to combat the obesity epidemic is very limited, and what is more worrisome, the list of new medications to treat this condition is also slim.

Unfortunately the history of significant side effects of some of these medications, and the fact that many healthcare legislators still feel that obesity is not a disease, has limited the effort of many governments to develop effective obesity prevention as well as obesity therapeutic programs. Also both socialized medicine and private insurance have put very limited effort in financing behavioral or pharmacological obesity therapies. These circumstances have also impacted in the general interest of pharmaceutical companies to develop new weight loss medications, which usually suffer exaggerated scrutiny by health regulatory agencies. In consequence, a large part of the drug development efforts have been switched to identify new T2DM treatments which interestingly cause weight loss as a side effect.

It is important to keep in mind that in addition to phentermine, diethylpropion, and orlistat, we have two new drugs, lorcaserin and the combination of phentermine and topiramate, approved for the treatment of the obesity, which could be useful tools to help treat our obese patients. Interesting new anti-obesity drugs are in the pipeline and hopefully some will reach the market in the near future. Meanwhile we should also take advance of the new GLP-1 analogues, which in some circumstances can be helpful to treat obese patients with T2DM.

New studies combining these medications and the ones to come in the context of lifestyle interventions will hopefully help to develop successful weight loss programs which bring some optimism to the field of obesity in the near future.

Review Questions and Answers

1. It is very important to set realistic expectations before starting medical treatments of obesity. What would be a realistic weight loss goal known to reduce the cardiovascular risk of patients?
   (a) 5–15 %
   (b) 3–10 %
   (c) 5–7 %
   (d) None of the above

CORRECT ANSWER (A): A −5 to −15% weight loss reduces obesity-related health risks significantly. There are a substantial number of patients who respond to weight loss interventions with important changes in their lifestyle, which translates in long-term weight loss.

2. Which of the following sentences would be false when we speak of the benefits of physical activity?
   (a) Reduced risk of premature death of any cause.
   (b) Reduced risk of diabetes mellitus.
   (c) Weight loss (without caloric restriction).
   (d) In elderly people there is strong evidence supporting the improvement of cognitive function in people who are physically active.

CORRECT ANSWER (A): The benefits of physical activity include reduced risk of premature death of any cause, cerebrovascular disease, diabetes mellitus, some cancers (breast cancer and colon cancer), depression, prevention of weight gain, weight loss (in combination with caloric restriction), improvement of physical fitness, and musculoskeletal fitness. Inactivity and low cardiorespiratory fitness are as important as overweight and obesity as mortality predictors.

In elderly people there is strong evidence supporting the improvement of cognitive function in people who are physically active and moderate evidence in regard to overall improvement in well-being, functional health, reduction of abdominal obesity, reduced risk of developing hip fracture, risk reduction of lung cancer, and weight loss maintenance.

3. Which of the following sentences is false when we speak of lifestyle modifications?
   (a) Changes in dietary behavior, the stimulation of physical activity, and emotional support continue to be the mainstays for the management of obesity in adults, children, and adolescents.
   (b) Lifestyle interventions alone result in long-term weight loss and the majority of dieters do not return to baseline weight within 3–5 years.
   (c) The improvements described in morbidly obese patients using behavioral therapy as an element of an intensive lifestyle intervention could benefit a huge number of people.
   (d) Lifestyle interventions can be provided at the hospital or primary care setting

CORRECT ANSWER (B): Lifestyle interventions alone rarely result in long-term weight loss and the majority of dieters return to baseline weight within 3–5 years.

4. Which of the following sentences is correct?
   (a) Phentermine is an approved anti-obesity drug for short-term therapy.
   (b) GLP-1 analogues are effective weight loss drugs.
   (c) Topiramate is an antiepileptic drug with a weight loss side effect.
   (d) Lorcaserin, in addition to a reduced-calorie diet and exercise, could be a potential useful drug to treat obesity.
   (e) All of the above.

CORRECT ANSWER (E).

5. Which of the following sentences is correct?
   (a) Bydureon is an exenatide long-acting release without weight loss effect.
   (b) Naltrexone is a dopamine reuptake inhibitor with weight loss effect.
   (c) Topiramate in combination with bupropion extended release is effective in causing weight loss.
   (d) Bupropion is an effective smoking cessation tool.
   (e) Cetilistat has central as well as gastrointestinal weight loss mechanism.

CORRECT ANSWER (D). Bupropion is a dopamine and norepinephrine reuptake inhibitor that was first approved for the treatment of depression [139] and later for smoking cessation [140].

References

1. Ogden CL, Carroll MD, Kit BK, Flegal KM. Prevalence of obesity in the United States, 2009–2010. NCHS Data Brief. 2012;(82):1–8.
2. The surgeon general's vision for a healthy and fit nation—2010—TOC.pdf [Internet]; cited 4/10/2013. Available from: http://www.ncbi.nlm.nih.gov/books/NBK44660/pdf/TOC.pdf
3. Berghofer A, Pischon T, Reinhold T, Apovian CM, Sharma AM, Willich SN. Obesity prevalence from a European perspective: a systematic review. BMC Public Health. 2008;8:200.
4. HSE 04/SUM BKLT—HSE2011-sum-bklet.pdf [Internet]; cited 4/16/2013. Available from: https://catalogue.ic.nhs.uk/publications/public-health/surveys/heal-surv-eng-2011/HSE2011-Sum-bklet.pdf
5. Gutierrez-Fisac JL, Guallar-Castillon P, Leon-Munoz LM, Graciani A, Banegas JR, Rodriguez-Artalejo F. Prevalence of general and abdominal obesity in the adult population of Spain, 2008–2010: the ENRICA study. Obes Rev. 2012;13(4):388–92.
6. Calle EE, Thun MJ, Petrelli JM, Rodriguez C, Heath Jr CW. Body-mass index and mortality in a prospective cohort of U.S. adults. N Engl J Med. 1999;341(15):1097–105.
7. Field AE. Impact of overweight on the risk of developing common chronic diseases during a 10-year period. Arch Intern Med. 2001;161(13):1581.
8. Strazzullo P, D'Elia L, Cairella G, Garbagnati F, Cappuccio FP, Scalfi L. Excess body weight and incidence of stroke: meta-analysis of prospective studies with 2 million participants. Stroke. 2010;41(5):e418–26.
9. Bogers RP, Bemelmans WJ, Hoogenveen RT, Boshuizen HC, Woodward M, Knekt P, et al. Association of overweight with increased risk of coronary heart disease partly independent of blood pressure and cholesterol levels: a meta-analysis of 21 cohort studies including more than 300 000 persons. Arch Intern Med. 2007;167(16):1720–8.

10. Alexander CM, Landsman PB, Teutsch SM, Haffner SM, Third National Health and Nutrition Examination Survey (NHANES III), National Cholesterol Education Program (NCEP). NCEP-defined metabolic syndrome, diabetes, and prevalence of coronary heart disease among NHANES III participants age 50 years and older. Diabetes. 2003;52(5):1210–4.

11. Renehan AG, Tyson M, Egger M, Heller RF, Zwahlen M. Body-mass index and incidence of cancer: a systematic review and meta-analysis of prospective observational studies. Lancet. 2008;371(9612):569–78.

12. Despres JP, Moorjani S, Lupien PJ, Tremblay A, Nadeau A, Bouchard C. Regional distribution of body fat, plasma lipoproteins, and cardiovascular disease. Arteriosclerosis. 1990;10(4):497–511.

13. Hubert HB, Feinleib M, McNamara PM, Castelli WP. Obesity as an independent risk factor for cardiovascular disease: a 26-year follow-up of participants in the Framingham heart study. Circulation. 1983;67(5):968–77.

14. Whaley-Connell A, Sowers JR. Indices of obesity and cardiometabolic risk. Hypertension. 2011;58:991–3.

15. Manson JE, Willett WC, Stampfer MJ, Colditz GA, Hunter DJ, Hankinson SE, et al. Body weight and mortality among women. N Engl J Med. 1995;333(11):677–85.

16. National diabetes fact sheet, 2007—ndfs_2007.pdf [Internet]; cited 5/3/2013. Available from: http://www.cdc.gov/diabetes/pubs/pdf/ndfs_2007.pdf

17. Finkelstein EA, Trogdon JG, Cohen JW, Dietz W. Annual medical spending attributable to obesity: payer-and service-specific estimates. Health Aff. 2009;28(5):w822–31.

18. Kaminsky J, Gadaleta D. A study of discrimination within the medical community as viewed by obese patients. Obes Surg. 2002;12(1):14–8.

19. Wing RR, Blair E, Marcus M, Epstein LH, Harvey J. Year-long weight loss treatment for obese patients with type II diabetes: does including an intermittent very-low-calorie diet improve outcome? Am J Med. 1994;97(4):354–62.

20. Arterburn DE, Crane PK, Veenstra DL. The efficacy and safety of sibutramine for weight loss: a systematic review. Arch Intern Med. 2004;164(9):994–1003.

21. Torgerson JS, Hauptman J, Boldrin MN, Sjostrom L. XENical in the prevention of diabetes in obese subjects (XENDOS) study: a randomized study of orlistat as an adjunct to lifestyle changes for the prevention of type 2 diabetes in obese patients. Diabetes Care. 2004;27(1):155–61.

22. Goodpaster BH, Delany JP, Otto AD, Kuller L, Vockley J, South-Paul JE, et al. Effects of diet and physical activity interventions on weight loss and cardiometabolic risk factors in severely obese adults: a randomized trial. JAMA. 2010;304(16):1795–802.

23. Ryan DH, Johnson WD, Myers VH, Prather TL, McGlone MM, Rood J, et al. Nonsurgical weight loss for extreme obesity in primary care settings: results of the Louisiana obese subjects study. Arch Intern Med. 2010;170(2):146–54.

24. Shai I, Schwarzfuchs D, Henkin Y, Shahar DR, Witkow S, Greenberg I, et al. Weight loss with a low-carbohydrate, Mediterranean, or low-fat diet. N Engl J Med. 2008;359(3):229–41.

25. Foster GD, Wyatt HR, Hill JO, McGuckin BG, Brill C, Mohammed BS, et al. A randomized trial of a low-carbohydrate diet for obesity. N Engl J Med. 2003;348(21):2082–90.

26. Stern L, Iqbal N, Seshadri P, Chicano KL, Daily DA, McGrory J, et al. The effects of low-carbohydrate versus conventional weight loss diets in severely obese adults: one-year follow-up of a randomized trial. Ann Intern Med. 2004;140(10):778–85.

27. Gardner CD, Kiazand A, Alhassan S, Kim S, Stafford RS, Balise RR, et al. Comparison of the Atkins, Zone, Ornish, and LEARN diets for change in weight and related risk factors among overweight premenopausal women: the A TO Z weight loss study: a randomized trial. JAMA. 2007;297(9):969–77.

28. Yancy Jr WS, Olsen MK, Guyton JR, Bakst RP, Westman EC. A low-carbohydrate, ketogenic diet versus a low-fat diet to treat obesity and hyperlipidemia: a randomized, controlled trial. Ann Intern Med. 2004;140(10):769–77.

29. Brehm BJ, Seeley RJ, Daniels SR, D'Alessio DA. A randomized trial comparing a very low carbohydrate diet and a calorie-restricted low fat diet on body weight and cardiovascular risk factors in healthy women. J Clin Endocrinol Metab. 2003;88(4):1617–23.

30. Samaha FF, Iqbal N, Seshadri P, Chicano KL, Daily DA, McGrory J, et al. A low-carbohydrate as compared with a low-fat diet in severe obesity. N Engl J Med. 2003;348(21):2074–81.

31. Yancy Jr WS, Westman EC, McDuffie JR, Grambow SC, Jeffreys AS, Bolton J, et al. A randomized trial of a low-carbohydrate diet vs orlistat plus a low-fat diet for weight loss. Arch Intern Med. 2010;170(2):136–45.

32. Astrup A, Meinert Larsen T, Harper A. Atkins and other low-carbohydrate diets: hoax or an effective tool for weight loss? Lancet. 2004;364(9437):897–9.

33. Foster GD, Wyatt HR, Hill JO, Makris AP, Rosenbaum DL, Brill C, et al. Weight and metabolic outcomes after 2 years on a low-carbohydrate versus low-fat diet: a randomized trial. Ann Intern Med. 2010;153(3):147–57.

34. Sacks FM, Bray GA, Carey VJ, Smith SR, Ryan DH, Anton SD, et al. Comparison of weight-loss diets with different compositions of fat, protein, and carbohydrates. N Engl J Med. 2009;360(9):859–73.

35. Thomas DE, Elliott EJ, Baur L. Low glycaemic index or low glycaemic load diets for overweight and obesity. Cochrane Database Syst Rev. 2007;(3):CD005105.

36. Gargallo Fernandez M, Marset JB, Lesmes IB, Izquierdo JQ, Sala XF, Salas-Salvado J, et al. FESNAD-SEEDO consensus summary: evidence-based nutritional recommendations for the prevention and treatment of overweight and obesity in adults. Endocrinol Nutr. 2012;59(7):429–37.

37. Jenkins DJ, Kendall CW, Augustin LS, Franceschi S, Hamidi M, Marchie A, et al. Glycemic index: overview of implications in health and disease. Am J Clin Nutr. 2002;76(1):266S–73.

38. Venn BJ, Green TJ. Glycemic index and glycemic load: measurement issues and their effect on diet-disease relationships. Eur J Clin Nutr. 2007;61 Suppl 1:S122–31.

39. Lassale C, Fezeu L, Andreeva VA, Hercberg S, Kengne AP, Czernichow S, et al. Association between dietary scores and 13-year weight change and obesity risk in a french prospective cohort. Int J Obes (Lond). 2012;36(11):1455–62.

40. Sanchez-Villegas A, Bes-Rastrollo M, Martinez-Gonzalez MA, Serra-Majem L. Adherence to a Mediterranean dietary pattern and weight gain in a follow-up study: the SUN cohort. Int J Obes (Lond). 2006;30(2):350–8.

41. Mendez MA, Popkin BM, Jakszyn P, Berenguer A, Tormo MJ, Sanchez MJ, et al. Adherence to a Mediterranean diet is associated with reduced 3-year incidence of obesity. J Nutr. 2006;136(11):2934–8.

42. Romaguera D, Norat T, Vergnaud AC, Mouw T, May AM, Agudo A, et al. Mediterranean dietary patterns and prospective weight change in participants of the EPIC-PANACEA project. Am J Clin Nutr. 2010;92(4):912–21.

43. Schroder H, Marrugat J, Vila J, Covas MI, Elosua R. Adherence to the traditional mediterranean diet is inversely associated with body mass index and obesity in a spanish population. J Nutr. 2004;134(12):3355–61.

44. Panagiotakos DB, Chrysohoou C, Pitsavos C, Stefanadis C. Association between the prevalence of obesity and adherence to the mediterranean diet: the ATTICA study. Nutrition. 2006;22(5):449–56.

45. Schroder H, Mendez MA, Ribas-Barba L, Covas MI, Serra-Majem L. Mediterranean diet and waist circumference in a representative national sample of young Spaniards. Int J Pediatr Obes. 2010;5(6):516–9.

46. Buckland G, Bach A, Serra-Majem L. Obesity and the Mediterranean diet: a systematic review of observational and intervention studies. Obes Rev. 2008;9(6):582–93.

47. Romaguera D, Norat T, Mouw T, May AM, Bamia C, Slimani N, et al. Adherence to the Mediterranean diet is associated with lower abdominal adiposity in European men and women. J Nutr. 2009;139(9):1728–37.

48. Cheskin LJ, Kahan S. Low-carbohydrate and Mediterranean diets led to greater weight loss than a low-fat diet in moderately obese adults. Evid Based Med. 2008;13(6):176.

49. McManus K, Antinoro L, Sacks F. A randomized controlled trial of a moderate-fat, low-energy diet compared with a low fat, low-energy diet for weight loss in overweight adults. Int J Obes Relat Metab Disord. 2001;25(10):1503–11.

50. Nordmann AJ, Suter-Zimmermann K, Bucher HC, Shai I, Tuttle KR, Estruch R, et al. Meta-analysis comparing Mediterranean to low-fat diets for modification of cardiovascular risk factors. Am J Med. 2011;124(9):841–51.e2.

51. Corella D, Ordovas JM. Nutrigenomics in cardiovascular medicine. Circ Cardiovasc Genet. 2009;2(6):637–51.

52. Corella D, Gonzalez JI, Bullo M, Carrasco P, Portoles O, Diez-Espino J, et al. Polymorphisms cyclooxygenase-2–765G>C and interleukin-6–174G>C are associated with serum inflammation markers in a high cardiovascular risk population and do not modify the response to a Mediterranean diet supplemented with virgin olive oil or nuts. J Nutr. 2009;139(1):128–34.

53. Corella D, Tai ES, Sorli JV, Chew SK, Coltell O, Sotos-Prieto M, et al. Association between the APOA2 promoter polymorphism and body weight in Mediterranean and Asian populations: replication of a gene-saturated fat interaction. Int J Obes (Lond). 2011;35(5):666–75.

54. Salas-Salvado J, Fernandez-Ballart J, Ros E, Martinez-Gonzalez MA, Fito M, Estruch R, et al. Effect of a Mediterranean diet supplemented with nuts on metabolic syndrome status: one-year results of the PREDIMED randomized trial. Arch Intern Med. 2008;168(22):2449–58.

55. Estruch R, Ros E, Salas-Salvado J, Covas MI, Corella D, et al. Primary prevention of cardiovascular disease with a Mediterranean diet. N Engl J Med. 2013;368:1279–90.

56. Clinical guidelines on the identification, evaluation, and treatment of overweight and obesity in adults—NCBI bookshelf [Internet]; cited 3/12/2013. Available from: http://www.ncbi.nlm.nih.gov/books/NBK2003/

57. Wadden TA, Webb VL, Moran CH, Bailer BA. Lifestyle modification for obesity: new developments in diet, physical activity, and behavior therapy. Circulation. 2012;125(9):1157–70.

58. Garber CE, Blissmer B, Deschenes MR, Franklin BA, Lamonte MJ, Lee IM, et al. American College of Sports Medicine position stand. quantity and quality of exercise for developing and maintaining cardiorespiratory, musculoskeletal, and neuromotor fitness in apparently healthy adults: guidance for prescribing exercise. Med Sci Sports Exerc. 2011;43(7):1334–59.

59. Morrow Jr JR, Jackson AW, Bazzarre TL, Milne D, Blair SN. A one-year follow-up to physical activity and health. A report of the surgeon general. Am J Prev Med. 1999;17(1):24–30.

60. Physical Activity Guidelines Advisory Committee report, 2008. To the Secretary of Health and Human Services. Part A: executive summary. Nutr Rev. 2009;67(2):114–20.

61. Shaw K, Gennat H, O'Rourke P, Del Mar C. Exercise for overweight or obesity. Cochrane Database Syst Rev. 2006;(4):CD003817.

62. Colberg SR, Sigal RJ, Fernhall B, Regensteiner JG, Blissmer BJ, Rubin RR, et al. Exercise and type 2 diabetes: The American College of Sports Medicine and the American Diabetes Association: joint position statement executive summary. Diabetes Care. 2010;33(12):2692–6.

63. Blair SN, Brodney S. Effects of physical inactivity and obesity on morbidity and mortality: current evidence and research issues. Med Sci Sports Exerc. 1999;31(11 Suppl):S646–62.

64. Netz Y, Wu MJ, Becker BJ, Tenenbaum G. Physical activity and psychological well-being in advanced age: a meta-analysis of intervention studies. Psychol Aging. 2005;20(2):272–84.

65. Hobbs N, Godfrey A, Lara J, Errington L, Meyer TD, Rochester L, et al. Are behavioral interventions effective in increasing physical activity at 12 to 36 months in adults aged 55 to 70 years? A systematic review and meta-analysis. BMC Med. 2013;11(1):75.

66. American College of Sports Medicine position stand. Exercise and physical activity for older adults. Med Sci Sports Exerc. 1998;30(6):992–1008.

67. Ekelund U, Brage S, Griffin SJ, Wareham NJ, ProActive UK Research Group. Objectively measured moderate- and vigorous-intensity physical activity but not sedentary time predicts insulin resistance in high-risk individuals. Diabetes Care. 2009;32(6):1081–6.

68. Healy GN, Dunstan DW, Salmon J, Cerin E, Shaw JE, Zimmet PZ, et al. Breaks in sedentary time: beneficial associations with metabolic risk. Diabetes Care. 2008;31(4):661–6.

69. Healy GN, Matthews CE, Dunstan DW, Winkler EA, Owen N. Sedentary time and cardio-metabolic biomarkers in US adults: NHANES 2003–06. Eur Heart J. 2011;32(5):590–7.

70. Chambliss HO. Exercise duration and intensity in a weight-loss program. Clin J Sport Med. 2005;15(2):113–5.

71. Bonomi AG, Westerterp KR. Advances in physical activity monitoring and lifestyle interventions in obesity: a review. Int J Obes (Lond). 2012;36(2):167–77.

72. Mekary RA, Feskanich D, Hu FB, Willett WC, Field AE. Physical activity in relation to long-term weight maintenance after intentional weight loss in premenopausal women. Obesity (Silver Spring). 2010;18(1):167–74.

73. Casazza K, Fontaine KR, Astrup A, Birch LL, Brown AW, Bohan Brown MM, et al. Myths, presumptions, and facts about obesity. N Engl J Med. 2013;368(5):446–54.

74. Wu T, Gao X, Chen M, van Dam RM. Long-term effectiveness of diet-plus-exercise interventions vs diet-only interventions for weight loss: a meta-analysis. Obes Rev. 2009;10(3):313–23.

75. Jeffery RW, Drewnowski A, Epstein LH, Stunkard AJ, Wilson GT, Wing RR, et al. Long-term maintenance of weight loss: current status. Health Psychol. 2000;19(1 Suppl):5–16.

76. Foster GD, Makris AP, Bailer BA. Behavioral treatment of obesity. Am J Clin Nutr. 2005;82(1 Suppl):230S–5.

77. Wing RR, Hill JO. Successful weight loss maintenance. Annu Rev Nutr. 2001;21:323–41.

78. Behavioral strategies in the treatment of obesity [Internet]; cited 4/3/2013. Available from: http://www-uptodate-com.proxy1.athensams.net/contents/behavioral-strategies-in-the-treatment-of-obesity?source=search_result&search=bahavioral+strategies,+obesity&selectedTitle=5~150

79. Diabetes Prevention Program (DPP) Research Group. The diabetes prevention program (DPP): description of lifestyle intervention. Diabetes Care. 2002;25(12):2165–71.

80. Look AHEAD Research Group, Pi-Sunyer X, Blackburn G, Brancati FL, Bray GA, Bright R, et al. Reduction in weight and cardiovascular disease risk factors in individuals with type 2 diabetes: one-year results of the look AHEAD trial. Diabetes Care. 2007;30(6):1374–83.

81. Wadden TA, Neiberg RH, Wing RR, Clark JM, Delahanty LM, Hill JO, et al. Four-year weight losses in the look AHEAD study: factors associated with long-term success. Obesity (Silver Spring). 2011;19(10):1987–98.

82. Ryan DH, Espeland MA, Foster GD, Haffner SM, Hubbard VS, Johnson KC, et al. Look AHEAD (action for health in diabetes):

design and methods for a clinical trial of weight loss for the prevention of cardiovascular disease in type 2 diabetes. Control Clin Trials. 2003;24(5):610–28.

83. Knowler WC, Barrett-Connor E, Fowler SE, Hamman RF, Lachin JM, Walker EA, et al. Reduction in the incidence of type 2 diabetes with lifestyle intervention or metformin. N Engl J Med. 2002;346(6):393–403.

84. Wadden TA, Berkowitz RI, Sarwer DB, Prus-Wisniewski R, Steinberg C. Benefits of lifestyle modification in the pharmacologic treatment of obesity: a randomized trial. Arch Intern Med. 2001;161(2):218–27.

85. Sovik TT, Aasheim ET, Taha O, Engstrom M, Fagerland MW, Bjorkman S, et al. Weight loss, cardiovascular risk factors, and quality of life after gastric bypass and duodenal switch: a randomized trial. Ann Intern Med. 2011;155(5):281–91.

86. Wyatt SB, Winters KP, Dubbert PM. Overweight and obesity: prevalence, consequences, and causes of a growing public health problem. Am J Med Sci. 2006;331(4):166–74.

87. Johannsen DL, Knuth ND, Huizenga R, Rood JC, Ravussin E, Hall KD. Metabolic slowing with massive weight loss despite preservation of fat-free mass. J Clin Endocrinol Metab. 2012; 97(7):2489–96.

88. Johnson LK, Andersen LF, Hofso D, Aasheim ET, Holven KB, Sandbu R, et al. Dietary changes in obese patients undergoing gastric bypass or lifestyle intervention: a clinical trial. Br J Nutr. 2012;30:1–8.

89. Tur J, Alos M, Iglesias L, Luque L, Colom A, Escudero A, et al. TRAMOMTANA (multidisciplinary treatment of morbid obesity: medication, behavioral therapy, nutritional support, and physical activity). From question to reality in an investigator-initiated clinical trial (II). Endocrinol Nutr. 2011;58(6):299–307.

90. Tur JJ, Escudero AJ, Alos MM, Salinas R, Teres E, Soriano JB, et al. One year weight loss in the TRAMOMTANA study. A randomized controlled trial. Clin Endocrinol (Oxf). 2013;79:791–9.

91. Butryn ML, Webb V, Wadden TA. Behavioral treatment of obesity. Psychiatr Clin North Am. 2011;34(4):841–59.

92. Colman E. Anorectics on trial: a half century of federal regulation of prescription appetite suppressants. Ann Intern Med. 2005;143(5):380–5.

93. Coyne TC. Phentermine–resin or salt–there are differences. Arch Intern Med. 1997;157(20):2381–2.

94. Jick H. Heart valve disorders and appetite-suppressant drugs. JAMA. 2000;283(13):1738–40.

95. Bray GA, Ryan DH. Medical therapy for the patient with obesity. Circulation. 2012;125(13):1695–703.

96. Cercato C, Roizenblatt VA, Leança CC, Segal A, Lopes Filho AP, Mancini MC, et al. A randomized double-blind placebo-controlled study of the long-term efficacy and safety of diethylpropion in the treatment of obese subjects. Int J Obes. 2009;33(8):857–65.

97. Orlistat for obesity. Med Lett Drugs Ther. 1999;41(1055):55–6.

98. Zhou YH, Ma XQ, Wu C, Lu J, Zhang SS, Guo J, et al. Effect of anti-obesity drug on cardiovascular risk factors: a systematic review and meta-analysis of randomized controlled trials. PLoS One. 2012;7(6):e39062.

99. Weir MA, Beyea MM, Gomes T, Juurlink DN, Mamdani M, Blake PG, et al. Orlistat and acute kidney injury: an analysis of 953 patients. Arch Intern Med. 2011;171(7):703–4.

100. Barkeling B, Elfhag K, Rooth P, Rossner S. Short-term effects of sibutramine (reductil) on appetite and eating behaviour and the long-term therapeutic outcome. Int J Obes Relat Metab Disord. 2003;27(6):693–700.

101. Berkowitz RI, Wadden TA, Tershakovec AM, Cronquist JL. Behavior therapy and sibutramine for the treatment of adolescent obesity: a randomized controlled trial. JAMA. 2003;289(14):1805–12.

102. Padwal R, Li SK, Lau DC. Long-term pharmacotherapy for obesity and overweight. Cochrane Database Syst Rev. 2004;(3): CD004094.

103. Hansen D, Astrup A, Toubro S, Finer N, Kopelman P, Hilsted J, et al. Predictors of weight loss and maintenance during 2 years of treatment by sibutramine in obesity. results from the European multi-centre STORM trial. Sibutramine trial of obesity reduction and maintenance. Int J Obes Relat Metab Disord. 2001;25(4): 496–501.

104. Caterson I, Coutinho W, Finer N, Van Gaal L, Maggioni A, Torp-Pedersen C, et al. Early response to sibutramine in patients not meeting current label criteria: preliminary analysis of SCOUT lead-in period. Obesity (Silver Spring). 2010;18(5):987–94.

105. Williams G. Withdrawal of sibutramine in Europe. BMJ. 2010;340:c824.

106. Gardin JM, Schumacher D, Constantine G, Davis KD, Leung C, Reid CL. Valvular abnormalities and cardiovascular status following exposure to dexfenfluramine or phentermine/fenfluramine. JAMA. 2000;283(13):1703–9.

107. BELVIQ—022529lbl.pdf [Internet]; cited 4/10/2013. Available from: http://www.accessdata.fda.gov/drugsatfda_docs/label/2012/022529lbl.pdf

108. Smith SR, Weissman NJ, Anderson CM, Sanchez M, Chuang E, Stubbe S, et al. Multicenter, placebo-controlled trial of lorcaserin for weight management. N Engl J Med. 2010;363(3):245–56.

109. BLOSSOM: behavioral modification and lorcaserin second study for obesity management—full text view—ClinicalTrials.gov [Internet]; cited 5/4/2013. Available from: http://clinicaltrials.gov/ct2/show/NCT00603902?term=Behavioral+Modification+and+Lorcaserin+Second+Study+for+Obesity+Management&rank=1

110. O'Neil PM, Smith SR, Weissman NJ, Fidler MC, Sanchez M, Zhang J, et al. Randomized placebo-controlled clinical trial of lorcaserin for weight loss in type 2 diabetes mellitus: the BLOOM-DM study. Obesity (Silver Spring). 2012;20(7):1426–36.

111. Gadde KM, Allison DB, Ryan DH, Peterson CA, Troupin B, Schwiers ML, et al. Effects of low-dose, controlled-release, phentermine plus topiramate combination on weight and associated comorbidities in overweight and obese adults (CONQUER): a randomised, placebo-controlled, phase 3 trial. Lancet. 2011; 377(9774):1341–52.

112. Garvey WT, Ryan DH, Look M, Gadde KM, Allison DB, Peterson CA, et al. Two-year sustained weight loss and metabolic benefits with controlled-release phentermine/topiramate in obese and overweight adults (SEQUEL): a randomized, placebo-controlled, phase 3 extension study. Am J Clin Nutr. 2012;95(2):297–308.

113. Allison DB, Gadde KM, Garvey WT, Peterson CA, Schwiers ML, Najarian T, et al. Controlled-release phentermine/topiramate in severely obese adults: a randomized controlled trial (EQUIP). Obesity (Silver Spring). 2012;20(2):330–42.

114. Qsymia REMS—UCM312598.pdf [Internet]; cited 4/10/2013. Available from: http://www.fda.gov/downloads/Drugs/DrugSafety/PostmarketDrugSafetyInformationforPatientsandProviders/UCM312598.pdf

115. VIVUS, inc.—VIVUS to present new data on qsymia™. In 30th annual scientific meeting of the obesity society [Internet]; cited 5/4/2013. Available from: http://ir.vivus.com/releasedetail.cfm?ReleaseID=708249

116. Johnson AM. Two new drugs approved for obesity. S D Med. 2012;65(9):356–7.

117. Doyle ME, Egan JM. Mechanisms of action of glucagon-like peptide 1 in the pancreas. Pharmacol Ther. 2007;113(3):546–93.

118. Gallwitz B. Glucagon-like peptide-1 analogues for type 2 diabetes mellitus: current and emerging agents. Drugs. 2011;71(13): 1675–88.

119. Hayes MR, De Jonghe BC, Kanoski SE. Role of the glucagon-like-peptide-1 receptor in the control of energy balance. Physiol Behav. 2010;100(5):503–10.

120. Buteau J, Foisy S, Joly E, Prentki M. Glucagon-like peptide 1 induces pancreatic beta-cell proliferation via transactivation of the epidermal growth factor receptor. Diabetes. 2003;52(1):124–32.

121. Mentlein R, Gallwitz B, Schmidt WE. Dipeptidyl-peptidase IV hydrolyses gastric inhibitory polypeptide, glucagon-like peptide-1(7–36)amide, peptide histidine methionine and is responsible for their degradation in human serum. Eur J Biochem. 1993;214(3):829–35.

122. Gallwitz B, Ropeter T, Morys-Wortmann C, Mentlein R, Siegel EG, Schmidt WE. GLP-1-analogues resistant to degradation by dipeptidyl-peptidase IV in vitro. Regul Pept. 2000;86(1–3):103–11.

123. Agerso H, Jensen LB, Elbrond B, Rolan P, Zdravkovic M. The pharmacokinetics, pharmacodynamics, safety and tolerability of NN2211, a new long-acting GLP-1 derivative, in healthy men. Diabetologia. 2002;45(2):195–202.

124. Degn KB, Juhl CB, Sturis J, Jakobsen G, Brock B, Chandramouli V, et al. One week's treatment with the long-acting glucagon-like peptide 1 derivative liraglutide (NN2211) markedly improves 24-h glycemia and alpha- and beta-cell function and reduces endogenous glucose release in patients with type 2 diabetes. Diabetes. 2004;53(5):1187–94.

125. Astrup A, Rossner S, Van Gaal L, Rissanen A, Niskanen L, Al Hakim M, et al. Effects of liraglutide in the treatment of obesity: a randomised, double-blind, placebo-controlled study. Lancet. 2009;374(9701):1606–16.

126. Flint A, Raben A, Astrup A, Holst JJ. Glucagon-like peptide 1 promotes satiety and suppresses energy intake in humans. J Clin Invest. 1998;101(3):515–20.

127. DeFronzo RA, Ratner RE, Han J, Kim DD, Fineman MS, Baron AD. Effects of exenatide (exendin-4) on glycemic control and weight over 30 weeks in metformin-treated patients with type 2 diabetes. Diabetes Care. 2005;28(5):1092–100.

128. Eng J, Kleinman WA, Singh L, Singh G, Raufman JP. Isolation and characterization of exendin-4, an exendin-3 analogue, from heloderma suspectum venom. Further evidence for an exendin receptor on dispersed acini from guinea pig pancreas. J Biol Chem. 1992;267(11):7402–5.

129. Buse JB, Henry RR, Han J, Kim DD, Fineman MS, Baron AD, et al. Effects of exenatide (exendin-4) on glycemic control over 30 weeks in sulfonylurea-treated patients with type 2 diabetes. Diabetes Care. 2004;27(11):2628–35.

130. Kendall DM, Riddle MC, Rosenstock J, Zhuang D, Kim DD, Fineman MS, et al. Effects of exenatide (exendin-4) on glycemic control over 30 weeks in patients with type 2 diabetes treated with metformin and a sulfonylurea. Diabetes Care. 2005;28(5):1083–91.

131. Tracy MA, Ward KL, Firouzabadian L, Wang Y, Dong N, Qian R, et al. Factors affecting the degradation rate of poly(lactide-co-glycolide) microspheres in vivo and in vitro. Biomaterials. 1999;20(11):1057–62.

132. Kim D, MacConell L, Zhuang D, Kothare PA, Trautmann M, Fineman M, et al. Effects of once-weekly dosing of a long-acting release formulation of exenatide on glucose control and body weight in subjects with type 2 diabetes. Diabetes Care. 2007;30(6):1487–93.

133. Drucker DJ, Buse JB, Taylor K, Kendall DM, Trautmann M, Zhuang D, et al. Exenatide once weekly versus twice daily for the treatment of type 2 diabetes: a randomised, open-label, non-inferiority study. Lancet. 2008;372(9645):1240–50.

134. Bergenstal RM, Wysham C, Macconell L, Malloy J, Walsh B, Yan P, et al. Efficacy and safety of exenatide once weekly versus sitagliptin or pioglitazone as an adjunct to metformin for treatment of type 2 diabetes (DURATION-2): a randomised trial. Lancet. 2010;376(9739):431–9.

135. Diamant M, Van Gaal L, Stranks S, Northrup J, Cao D, Taylor K, et al. Once weekly exenatide compared with insulin glargine titrated to target in patients with type 2 diabetes (DURATION-3): an open-label randomised trial. Lancet. 2010;375(9733):2234–43.

136. Russell-Jones D, Cuddihy RM, Hanefeld M, Kumar A, Gonzalez JG, Chan M, et al. Efficacy and safety of exenatide once weekly versus metformin, pioglitazone, and sitagliptin used as monotherapy in drug-naive patients with type 2 diabetes (DURATION-4): a 26-week double-blind study. Diabetes Care. 2012;35(2):252–8.

137. Vilsboll T, Christensen M, Junker AE, Knop FK, Gluud LL. Effects of glucagon-like peptide-1 receptor agonists on weight loss: systematic review and meta-analyses of randomised controlled trials. BMJ. 2012;344:d7771.

138. Lobmaier P, Kornor H, Kunoe N, Bjorndal A. Sustained-release naltrexone for opioid dependence. Cochrane Database Syst Rev. 2008;(2):CD006140.

139. Dhillon S, Yang LP, Curran MP. Bupropion: a review of its use in the management of major depressive disorder. Drugs. 2008;68(5):653–89.

140. Tong EK, Carmody TP, Simon JA. Bupropion for smoking cessation: a review. Compr Ther. 2006;32(1):26–33.

141. Greenway FL, Fujioka K, Plodkowski RA, Mudaliar S, Guttadauria M, Erickson J, et al. Effect of naltrexone plus bupropion on weight loss in overweight and obese adults (COR-I): a multicentre, randomised, double-blind, placebo-controlled, phase 3 trial. Lancet. 2010;376:595–605.

142. Apovian C, Aronne L, Rubino D, Still C, Wyatt H, Burns C, et al. A randomized, phase 3 trial of naltrexone SR/bupropion SR on weight and obesity-related risk factors (COR-II). Obesity (Silver Spring). 2013;21:935–43.

143. Wadden TA, Foreyt JP, Foster GD, Hill JO, Klein S, O'Neil PM, et al. Weight loss with naltrexone SR/bupropion SR combination therapy as an adjunct to behavior modification: the COR-BMOD trial. Obesity (Silver Spring). 2011;19(1):110–20.

144. Wellbutrin sr sustained-release tablets—us_wellbutrinSR.pdf [Internet]; cited 5/6/2013. Available from: http://us.gsk.com/products/assets/us_wellbutrinSR.pdf

145. Orexigen therapeutics announces data from COR Diabetes trial for contrave [Internet]; cited 5/6/2013. Available from: http://www.news-medical.net/news/20100628/Orexigen-Therapeutics-announces-data-from-CORDiabetes-trial-for-Contrave.aspx

146. Ryan DH, Bray GA. Pharmacologic treatment options for obesity: what is old is new again. Curr Hypertens Rep. 2013;15:182–9.

147. Bryson A, de la Motte S, Dunk C. Reduction of dietary fat absorption by the novel gastrointestinal lipase inhibitor cetilistat in healthy volunteers. Br J Clin Pharmacol. 2009;67(3):309–15.

148. Kopelman P, Bryson A, Hickling R, Rissanen A, Rossner S, Toubro S, et al. Cetilistat (ATL-962), a novel lipase inhibitor: a 12-week randomized, placebo-controlled study of weight reduction in obese patients. Int J Obes (Lond). 2007;31(3):494–9.

4
History of Bariatric and Metabolic Surgery

Adrian G. Dan and Rebecca Lynch

Abbreviations

ASBS   American Society for Bariatric Surgery
ASMBS American Society for Metabolic and Bariatric Surgery
JIB   Jejunoileal bypass
LRYGB Laparoscopic Roux-en-Y gastric bypass
LSG   Laparoscopic sleeve gastrectomy
VBG   Vertical banded gastroplasty

Introduction

Bariatric and metabolic surgery has evolved from humble beginnings as experimental surgery to become one of the most scientifically rooted and technically challenging surgical subspecialties used to battle the detrimental effects of the worldwide obesity epidemic. This evolution, now spanning more than six decades, has been driven by the efforts of visionaries who have trailblazed the concept of surgery for obesity, often in the face of controversy and prejudice. They have built upon the initiatives of those before them to achieve the fund of knowledge and the surgical methods that patients can be offered today. This thread of innovation was additionally impacted by the growth of the discipline of gastrointestinal surgery, the advent of the worldwide obesity epidemic, and the revolution of minimally invasive laparoscopic surgery at the turn of the twenty-first century.

This chapter and the historical timeline (Table 1) of bariatric and metabolic surgery are roughly subdivided into three periodical sections. The first 20 years are considered the *foundation* (1950s and 1960s) and witnessed the birth of the concept of gastrointestinal surgery for the achievement of weight loss. The next two decades (1970s and 1980s) saw the development and *evolution* of various procedures as well as the organization and expansion of the subspecialty. The last 20 years (1990s and 2000s) were marked by the application and refinement of *advanced minimally invasive surgery*

techniques, the explosion of research in metabolic and physiologic mechanisms, and the dawn of a new era of recognition and patient advocacy.

The Foundation

Although complex minimally invasive operations are commonplace today, the story of bariatric and metabolic surgery began as experimental surgery in the mid-twentieth century. In 1952, a Swedish surgeon by the name of Dr. Viktor Henrikson of Göteborg, Sweden, theorized that removal of a generous segment of the small intestine would lead to weight loss and improvement in overall health [1]. He based this theory upon learning of "favorable side effects" reported in patients undergoing small and large bowel resections for other disease processes. Henrikson selected, as his first patient, an obese 32-year-old female with complaints of constipation who had failed to lose weight despite following a strict weight loss program. He resected 105 cm of the small bowel to surgically assist in her weight loss and to improve her overall health and gastrointestinal function. Although this patient ultimately gained 2 kg over a 14-month period postoperatively, she subjectively reported better health, improved energy, and improved bowel function. This first bariatric surgical procedure led Henrikson to recommend further exploration of the potential benefits of bowel resection in obese patients via animal experimentation.

Around the same period of time, anecdotal clinical reports of humans surviving extensive small bowel resections were being reported in the literature. One such report by Dr. Herbert Meyer of New York described the outcome of a World War II veteran who lost the majority of his small bowel from acute mesenteric thrombosis during the Battle of the Bulge and went on to live a relatively normal life [2]. In 1954, Drs. Kremen and Linner of the University of Minnesota published an eloquent study evaluating the nutritional importance of the small intestine in canines [3]. They concluded that sacrificing a significant amount of distal small bowel

S.A. Brethauer et al. (eds.), *Minimally Invasive Bariatric Surgery*,
DOI 10.1007/978-1-4939-1637-5_4, © Springer Science+Business Media New York 2015

interferes with fat absorption and results in weight loss. This finding led them to proceed with the first documented human jejuno-intestinal bypass performed in 1954 at the Mount Sinai Hospital in Minneapolis, Minnesota. The interest in

TABLE 1. Major events in bariatric and metabolic surgery

Timeline of major events in the history of bariatric and metabolic surgery
1952 *First gastrointestinal operation to reduce weight by Henrikson in Sweden*
1954 *First gastrointestinal bypass procedure by Kremen and Linner in Minnesota*
1963 *First series of bariatric surgery patients reported by Payne*
1967 *Mason and Ito devise the loop gastric bypass*
1977 *Griffen publishes results of modification to a Roux-en-Y gastric bypass*
1978 *Scopinaro introduces the biliopancreatic diversion*
1980 *Vertical banded gastroplasty*
1983 *American Society of Bariatric Surgery (ASBS) founded in Iowa City*
1985 *First adjustable gastric bypass reported*
1988 *Biliopancreatic diversion with duodenal switch devised by Hess*
1991 *NIH consensus conference held on bariatric surgery*
1992 *First minimally invasive bariatric procedure (nonadjustable band)*
1993 *First laparoscopic Roux-en-Y gastric bypass performed by Wittgrove*
1995 *International Federation of Societies for Obesity (IFSO) founded in Stockholm*
1998 *First laparoscopic BPD with DS performed by Gagner*
2005 *ASBS accredits first bariatric Center of Excellence*
2007 *Diabetes Summit held in Rome, Italy*
2013 *AMA recognizes obesity as a disease*

such surgical intervention for obesity continued to grow, and in 1963, Payne and colleagues of the University of Southern California reported the results of 10 patients undergoing various types of intestinal bypass operations including jejunoileal (JIB) and jejunocolic shunts with end-to-side anastamoses (see Fig. 1) [4]. This represented the very first publication of a case series of patients undergoing gastrointestinal surgery, specifically with the intent of treating morbid obesity.

Multiple other variations on the jejunoileal and jejunocolic bypass followed. Each attempted to alleviate the complications of the preceding operations and determine the optimal amount of bowel to bypass. Dr. William Scott and colleagues at the Vanderbilt University Medical Center attempted an end-to-end anastomosis instead of an end-to-side anastomosis and varied the length of bypassed bowel showing improved weight loss in patients with more extensive bypass procedures, but worsened side effects [5].

The JIB became the most commonly utilized procedure for weight loss in the 1960s and 1970s. Although weight loss was commonly achieved and appealing, these procedures did not come without complications. As the popularity of the procedure increased, series of patients were studied, and the undesirable side effects became more evident. Malabsorption not only caused weight loss but also led to multiple nutritional deficiencies [6] and anaerobic bacterial overgrowth in the long blind loop of the small bowel [7]. This led to abdominal distention and absorption of bacterial products into the bloodstream resulting in distal manifestations. Patients often presented with a broad spectrum of complications including severe diarrhea, protein malnutrition, vitamin deficiencies, electrolyte imbalance, perianal irritation, polyarthralgias, calcium oxalate stones, nephropathy, and severe liver

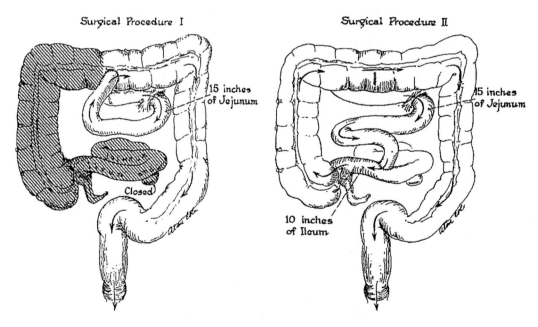

FIG. 1. Jejunoileal (*left*) and jejunocolic (*right*) bypass (by permission from AJS).

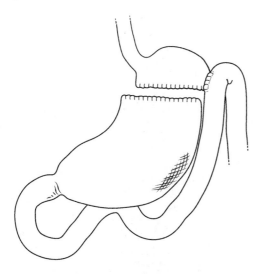

FIG. 2. The Mason-Ito gastric bypass procedure (Getch), with permission.

disease [7–9]. This often required surgeons to reverse such procedures and led to the eventual abandonment of the JIB procedure by the early 1980s [8, 10].

In an attempt to lessen the unfavorable side effects encountered with JIB, Mason and Ito at the University of Iowa developed the gastric bypass procedure. Dr. Edward Mason, commonly referred to as the father of bariatric surgery, worked within the department of surgery at the University of Iowa and met Dr. Chikashi Ito in September of 1965 in Edmonton, Canada, while attending a gastric physiology course. Dr. Robert Tidrick, chief of surgery at the University of Iowa, later hired Dr. Ito as a research collaborator. Mason and Ito ultimately collaborated on developing and studying a gastric bypass procedure based upon the Billroth II procedure which Mason had grown familiar with at the University of Minnesota under his mentor Dr. Owen H. Wangensteen. The main modification was that, unlike the antrectomy in the Billroth II reconstruction used by Wangensteen for peptic ulcer disease, the newer technique left the gastric antrum in place (see Fig. 2) [11].

Following animal experimentation in dogs, Mason and Ito performed the first gastric bypass procedure on May 10, 1966, on a 50-year-old woman with a BMI of 43 kg/m^2, whose morbid obesity was believed to play a major role in the failure of numerous ventral hernia repairs. This was the first report of a restrictive component to a bariatric operation [11].

The Evolution

While Mason and Ito's bypass procedure offered attractive results without the complications related to bacterial overgrowth, problems inherent to the Billroth II reconstruction affected patients postoperatively [11, 12]. These included bile reflux and afferent limb syndrome. In the 1970s,

Dr. Ward Griffen modified the drainage of the stomach from a short loop retrocolic gastrojejunostomy to a Roux-en-Y configuration [13]. Following Griffen's landmark publication in 1977, the Roux-en-Y configuration became the preferred method of reconstruction. The procedure continued to gain acceptance as the outcomes were compared to other obesity operations and superior results were noted. In 1987, Sugerman and colleagues reported that gastric bypass had significantly increased weight loss over VBG, and its apparent superiority led to cessation of randomization after only 9 months [14].

In a similar attempt to improve upon the detrimental effects of JIB, Scopinaro and colleagues from Genoa, Italy, introduced the idea of biliopancreatic diversion to allow for selective malabsorption without a blind loop of the small intestine. In 1979, after an experimental study on canines showed several advantages over JIB [15], they reported a series of 18 patients status post biliopancreatic diversion followed up to more than 1 year [16]. This procedure consisted of a hemigastrectomy with closure of the duodenal stump and a Roux-en-Y gastrojejunostomy. The jejunum was divided 20 cm distal to the ligament of Treitz resulting in a biliopancreatic limb which was anastomosed to the distal ileum leaving just 50 cm of common channel. The remaining 200 cm of the small bowel was brought up as a Roux limb to drain the stomach. Scopinaro's group reported excellent results in weight loss without the negative hepatic side effects observed with JIB, as well as biopsy-proven improvement in liver pathology. Longitudinal studies at 18 and 21 years showed excellent permanent weight loss results, although the authors warned about potential dangers if the operation was not performed as intended [17]. This radical malabsorptive procedure was complicated by anemia, bone demineralization, protein malabsorption, and marginal stomal ulceration [18, 19]. To this day, however, this procedure remains one of the most effective for long-term weight loss results.

In an effort to decrease the complications associated with Scopinaro's procedure, particularly the marginal ulceration observed with hemigastrectomy and gastrojejunal anastomosis, Dr. Douglas Hess devised and performed the first biliopancreatic diversion with duodenal switch procedure in Bowling Green, Ohio, on March 22, 1988 (Fig. 3) [20]. This operation consisted of creation of a gastric pouch along the lesser curvature of the stomach without disrupting the continuity of the pylorus to the duodenum and a Roux-en-Y duodenojejunostomy. The long tubular pouch in the shape of a sleeve led to the designation of the name "sleeve gastrectomy." His idea for creating a tubular gastrectomy as the gastric pouch instead of performing a hemigastrectomy was adapted from the duodenal switch procedure for anti-reflux described by DeMeester [21]. Studies showed that the addition of the duodenal switch improved marginal ulceration and dumping syndrome [21]. Despite these improvements, and the excellent weight loss results, this procedure still had its own set of drawbacks leading to reoperations and revisions [22].

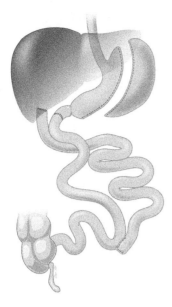

FIG. 3 Hess biliopancreatic diversion with duodenal switch (Getch), with permission.

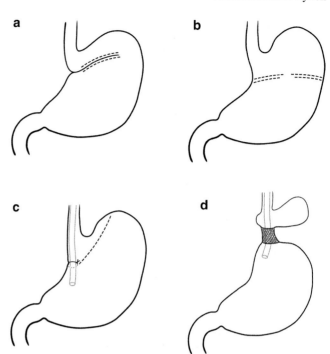

FIG. 4 Panel of gastroplasties (Getch), with permission.

Due to the significant complications encountered with malabsorptive procedures, numerous attempts were also made during the 1970s and 1980s to find a successful, purely restrictive procedure to decrease the stomach reservoir and limit caloric intake without interfering with small intestine anatomy. Printen and Mason introduced a horizontal gastroplasty involving a single staple line along the superior portion of the stomach starting from the lesser curvature [23] (Fig. 4). This formed a small gastric pouch connected to the remainder of the stomach through a channel at the end of the staple line along the greater curvature. Since the stomach reservoir was still able to dilate, adequate weight loss was not achieved, and other attempts with different stapling configurations followed. Gomez added a double-staple technique with mesh reinforcement that often failed due to mesh erosion and obstruction [24]. Pace also attempted to partition the stomach with a horizontal staple, but placed the channel between the upper and lower pouch in the center of the stomach [25]. Nonetheless, this allowed upper pouch dilation due to the thinner nature of the stomach wall near the greater curvature, and such procedures did not lead to lasting weight loss. Surgeons hypothesized that the fixed, thicker lesser curvature may be less likely to dilate. Long and Collins applied this theory by reorienting the staple line adjacent to the greater curvature by the angle of His obliquely toward the lesser curvature [26]. Despite this reorientation and efforts to stabilize the stoma with permanent suture, these procedures had limited success [27].

The gastroplasty variations ultimately led to the vertical banded gastroplasty (VBG) (Fig. 5) performed by Mason in 1980 which involved vertically partitioning the stomach at the angle of His through a window created near to the lesser curvature at the base of the pouch [28]. Polypropylene mesh

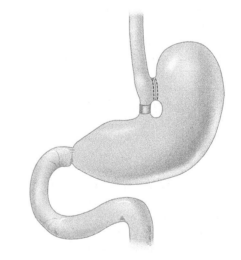

FIG. 5 Vertical banded gastroplasty (Getch), with permission.

was then placed around this window to secure the narrow, tubularized stomach reservoir. The VBG eventually was abandoned in favor of other operations such as the Roux-en-Y gastric bypass and adjustable gastric banding. Its drawbacks included stenosis of the pouch outlet due to excessive scarring and reaction to the foreign material, mesh erosion, and subsequent breakdown of the vertical staple line leading to loss of the intended restriction [29, 30].

Wilkinson and Peloso placed the first gastric band in 1978 in New Mexico. This consisted of a 2 cm-wide piece of polypropylene mesh placed around the superior portion of the fundus, restricting the channel for food passage [31].

Many other materials were then used for restriction including: Dacron used by Molina and Oria in Texas, silicone and Marlex mesh used by Näslund in Sweden, and a long 10.5 cm polypropylene clip with steel used by Bashour and Hill in the United States [32]. Although these methods were intended to be less invasive, several complications arose. Specifically, band migration, band erosion, and severe vomiting became significant early problems requiring interventions ranging from endoscopy with dilation to reoperation and revision. Late complications involved pouch dilation similar to that encountered with the earlier gastroplasties. On reoperation, surgeons found that many bands caused significant scarring, and the stoma size could not easily be altered after the first operation. Since the various gastroplasties attempted to this point incorporated staple lines and permanent alterations in gastric anatomy, surgeons across the world attempted to devise less invasive and potentially adjustable gastric restrictive options.

Silicone became the mainstay material for banding in 1983 given findings that it caused less tissue reaction and scarring [33]. Szinicz and Schnapka of Austria made novel modifications to the idea of banding and experimented with adjustable silicone bands in rabbits. Each band contained an inner balloon linked to a subcutaneous port allowing the balloon to be inflated or deflated with saline [34].

In 1985, Hallberg and Forsell of Sweden created an adjustable band to be utilized in humans, ultimately known as the *Swedish Adjustable Gastric Band* (SAGB) (Ethicon Endo-Surgery, Inc., Cincinnati, OH) [35]. During this same time, Kuzmak of the United States was developing an adjustable gastric band made from inflatable silastic silicone which became the *American Band* or *Lap-Band* (Allergan Inc, Irvine, CA)[36]. In 1986, Kuzmak reported the first case of an adjustable gastric band placement. These adjustable bands reduced the trouble of finding the perfect stomal size, since the aperture could now be adjusted through saline injections into a subcutaneous port. This feature made the purely restrictive banding operations much more tolerable by reducing emesis and pressure erosions when band pressures were properly adjusted. Similar weight loss rates were seen early on when compared with the vertical banded gastroplasty [36, 37].

The American Society for Metabolic and Bariatric Surgery

The creation of the American Society for Bariatric Surgery (ASBS) in 1983 had a major impact upon the development of the subspecialty. It provided a venue for the exchange of ideas and encouraged the application of scientific rigors to research methods.

In the late 1970s, Dr. Edward Mason, regarded as the father of bariatric and metabolic surgery, began hosting a yearly postgraduate course on obesity and obesity surgery. In 1983, Dr. Mason was invited as an honorary guest in Tokyo, Japan, to observe the creation of a Japanese obesity society as the problem had become more conspicuous in that country. Dr. Mason felt that if Japan had a need for an obesity society, then surely one should be created in the United States. Thus, he converted his 7th annual postgraduate course in bariatric surgery to the first meeting of what would become the ASBS. Dr. Mason became the first president of the society, and the first meeting hosted approximately 60 physicians and scientists in Iowa City, IA.

At that time, the overwhelming consensus within the surgical establishment remained that obesity was a result of gluttony and overindulgence. Prejudice existed not only within medicine against patients suffering from obesity but also within academic departments and societies against surgeons who held interest in weight loss surgery. Bariatric research studies were often not accepted at national meetings, unless they pointed out the potential complications and shortcomings of the current bariatric procedures. The ASBS meeting served as a setting where such research could be presented and critiqued without such bias. The society grew dramatically and advocated not only for research related to obesity surgery but also in other areas of the field such as access to care and establishment of quality standards. Dr. Mason's early efforts entailed forming a database first of his patients and those of his close circle of friends. Eventually, the database grew to include patients of other members of the society. Over time, several standardized databases were formed, including the Bariatric Ongoing Longitudinal Database (BOLD). Surgeons taking part in the ASBS Center of Excellence program were required to enter their patients into this database, providing a wealth of data for future bariatric research.

Armed with scientific evidence that bariatric surgery leads not only to weight loss but also extensive metabolic changes and resolution of numerous other metabolic comorbidities, the society voted to reflect this important aspect in 2007 and ratified the name change to the American Society for *Metabolic* and Bariatric Surgery (ASMBS). This concept was brought to the forefront and strongly endorsed by doctors Buchwald and Pories whose vision is credited with bringing about the dialogue to begin consideration of the name change. Through its evolution, the ASMBS became a force, championing significant endeavors in the areas of access to care, patient advocacy, research, data collection, and public relations among many others. In 2013, the ASMBS celebrated its 30-year anniversary and stands as one of the most respected and accomplished surgical societies in the world.

The International Federation of Societies for Obesity (IFSO)

In addition to the ASMBS, numerous societies across the world have sprung up to organize, support, and represent bariatric and metabolic surgeons and their patients. Societies exist in over 50 countries and are too numerous to mention in the scope of this chapter. In 1995, under the guidance and leadership of Dr. Nicola Scopinaro, many of the societies joined together to create the International Federation of Societies for Obesity and Metabolic Surgery (IFSO). This society holds meetings, where ideas can be exchanged between societies from different countries to help promote bariatric and metabolic surgery on a global basis.

The Minimally Invasive Era

The first minimally invasive weight loss procedure was the laparoscopic placement of a nonadjustable gastric band by Dr. Russell Broadbent in Australia performed on September 10, 1992 [38]. The work of Belachew, Cadiere, O'Brien, and Favretti assisted Inamed in engineering an improved adjustable gastric band. Belachew then placed the first laparoscopic adjustable gastric band on September 1, 1993 [39]. Complications mirrored that of the open gastric banding procedures, including band slippage, pouch dilation, and weight loss failure. Refinements such as the pars flaccid technique helped to decrease the complication [40–42]. This technique involved creation of a smaller stomach pouch and strategic posterior dissection along the diaphragmatic crura. The laparoscopic technique combined with the capability to adjust gastric restriction made this procedure more tolerable for patients than the rigid VBG and yielded a dramatic increase in its popularity. The *Lap-Band System* (Allergan Inc., Irvine, CA) gained FDA approval in the United States in 2001, and the *Realize* band (Ethicon Endo-Surgery, Inc., Cincinnati, OH) was introduced in the US market later in the decade. However, the past few years have witnessed a drop in the use of prosthetic restrictive devices due to the high rate of long-term complications, reoperations, and modest weight loss success when compared to other surgical options [43]. The laparoscopic sleeve gastrectomy has largely replaced banding as the preferred restrictive weight loss operation.

In October of 1993, Dr. Alan Wittgrove (Fig. 6) performed the first laparoscopic Roux-en-Y gastric bypass (LRYGB) [44]. Dr. Wittgrove's innovation was a landmark achievement not only for bariatric surgery but for the entire discipline of minimally invasive surgery. He was a visionary who attempted what few could imagine was even possible. In the late 1990s, other pioneers trailblazed the application of minimally invasive principles to the LRYGB. In doing so, the techniques became refined, and postoperative morbidity and mortality were decreased dramatically [45, 46]. With this decrease in morbidity, studies began to show improved quality of life with comparable weight loss in patients undergoing LRYGB versus open gastric bypass [47]. At the same time, reports boasting significant resolution of obesity and associated comorbid conditions were revealed by other prominent surgeons including Higa and Schauer, showing excellent results in sizable series of patients [48, 49]. The LRYGB became the most commonly performed bariatric operation in the 2000s.

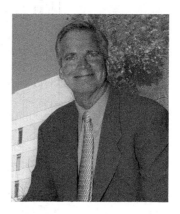

Fig. 6 Dr. Alan Wittgrove, with permission.

On July 25, 1999, Dr. Michel Gagner performed the first laparoscopic biliopancreatic diversion with duodenal switch procedure at the Mount Sinai Hospital in New York, NY [50]. This represented another landmark accomplishment with regard to the technical aspect of weight loss surgery. Long-term data also became available when Scopinaro and colleagues reported excellent results of the biliopancreatic diversion with studies following patients out as far as 20 years [19, 51]. The excellent weight loss results and resolution of metabolic comorbidities made this procedure particularly well suited for patients with super-morbid obesity. The minimally invasive approach was invaluable in this patient population where open surgery was difficult and wound-related complications could become catastrophic. Even with this approach, however, the potential to complete the operation was often hindered by massive intra-abdominal obesity, difficulty maintaining visualization, and occasional general physiologic instability. The procedure was sometimes aborted after completion of the sleeve gastrectomy, and such patients often exhibited a substantial amount of weight loss. This introduced the concept of the laparoscopic sleeve gastrectomy (LSG) which was initially shown to be useful as a first-step procedure for super-morbidly obese or high-surgical-risk individuals [52], a discovery also credited to Dr. Gagner.

Although the LSG was at first considered investigational, further research suggested its potential utility as a stand-alone operation [53]. In this setting when the LSG was intended to be the sole treatment of obesity, surgeons utilized smaller bougies to calibrate a narrow tubular sleeve for added restriction. The LSG was found to be useful beyond its restrictive capabilities with physiologic alterations that affected metabolic processes and decreased hunger [54]. These particular features and the lack of a need for a prosthetic restrictive device led to an increase of the popularity of the LSG in the late 2000s, and it rapidly replaced the LAGB as the preferred restrictive weight loss operation.

At the end of the decade, laparoscopic gastric plication, reported by Brethauer and colleagues as well as other international groups, received increasing attention [55]. The idea was to provide restriction without staple lines or prosthetic devices. In addition, other experimental modalities aimed at achieving weight loss without the risk of surgery include endoluminal gastric partitioning, the gastric balloon, endoscopically placed gastric sleeves, and neurostimulation.

A New Golden Era

The turn of the century ushered a new beginning for the subspecialty. The increased prevalence of obesity along with the laparoscopic surgical advancements caused a dramatic rise in the number of procedures performed. With this increase came new hurdles and political issues that needed to be addressed on behalf of bariatric patients and professionals. Efforts were undertaken on the part of the surgical societies to improve access to care and promote the public awareness of the efficacy and safety of surgical weight loss options.

In 2001, the catastrophic events which occurred in New York City on September 11 did not pass without a profound impact upon bariatric surgeons. This incident caused numerous insurance companies to close their medical malpractice business sections leaving many surgeons without coverage. In addition, the number of claims resulting from surgeons with inadequate training in complex minimally invasive procedures erupted, leading to apprehension to cover by malpractice insurance carriers. According to Dr. Kenneth Jones, who presided over the ASBS at the time, that combination was a "perfect storm" which produced a "near disaster for our subspecialty." The integration of bariatric surgery in the advanced laparoscopic fellowship training was instrumental as bariatric procedures became the "bread and butter" of advanced minimally invasive surgery. Appropriately trained surgeons began setting up comprehensive bariatric programs throughout the country and delivered quality of care which turned the tide and furthered the results of these new operations from the dubious problem-ridden procedures of the early days.

Aspects of bariatric care began enjoying positive portrayals and representation in the press. However, this was tarnished to some degree by surgeons who attempted advanced laparoscopic procedures after minimal proctoring instead of formal training. The development of bariatric-focused surgical fellowship programs overseen by the Minimally Invasive Surgery Fellowship Council provided a formal match for candidates and bariatric fellowship training programs. This enabled surgeons to appropriately learn and develop the advanced skills necessary to complete such procedures safely.

Several consensus conferences also served as a means to educate practitioners and to standardize bariatric and metabolic surgery. The first consensus conference on the role of bariatric surgery to treat obesity was chaired by Dr. Henry Buchwald in 1978. The guidelines were based upon a small body of literature that was available at that time, and it finally discouraged the use of the JIB. Throughout the next decade, the use of surgery for weight loss became more frequent with the advent of the RYGB and the VBG. In 1991, the NIH published a consensus statement on "gastrointestinal surgery for severe obesity," which to this day influences the guidelines for indication for surgery [56]. In 2004, Dr. Henry Buchwald again hosted a consensus conference and published a report updating the 1991 recommendations [57].

In an effort to further promote program standardization, the ASBS developed the Center of Excellence designation in 2004 and then combined efforts with the American College of Surgeons starting in June of 2012. The first COE program was credentialed by the ASBS in 2005. Participation in such programs required surgeons to submit data on their patients to the BOLD database. The abundance of data led to subsequent publications showing the remarkable safety and efficacy of bariatric surgery when performed at accredited centers [58].

Despite the evidence supporting the benefits of bariatric surgery, the increase in demand led some insurance companies to continue to limit the coverage of such procedures due to the economic pressure resulting from their costs. On February 21, 2006, the Center for Medicare and Medicaid services (CMS) announced coverage of bariatric surgery for its beneficiaries nationwide. This gave millions of patients suffering from obesity an opportunity to seek surgical weight loss after failing medical therapy. This decision also prompted many private insurance carriers to consider the inclusion of surgery as a core benefit in their health-care plans. Initially approved procedures for Medicare and Medicaid beneficiaries included the LRYGB and the LAGB. After several years of extensive lobbying by the members of the bariatric community, the LSG was added to the list of approved procedures. The lack of universal inclusion of bariatric benefits in every health-care plan remains a disappointment for many bariatric professionals and patients.

The Scientific Advances

The development and refinement of bariatric procedures have been accompanied by the investigation of the metabolic effects of such operations. With the first reported bariatric procedure, Henrikson's patient noted a generalized improvement in her overall health despite a failure in weight loss. As early as the 1950s, surgeons observed health-related benefits associated with procedures which unintentionally induced weight loss. Patients undergoing subtotal gastrectomy with reconstruction for other indications were noted to sustain an improvement in the control of diabetes as an unexpected side effect [59].

Surgeons also witnessed a wealth of anecdotal evidence of the resolution of numerous obesity-related conditions and the metabolic syndrome. While such observations were commonplace, obesity-related research to illuminate the impact conferred by metabolic surgery upon the resolutions of such diseases was scarce. In 1980, O'Leary and colleagues published the first account of JIB positively affecting diabetes and hyperlipidemia [60]. In 1995, Pories and colleagues also published a noteworthy article underlining the effectiveness and durability of the RYGB to treat adult-onset diabetes mellitus [61]. A follow-up article from the same group showed a decrease in the progression of diabetes and decreased mortality in patients undergoing RYGB versus a nonoperative cohort [62]. The impact of the LRYGB on diabetes mellitus was further exposed in a landmark article by Schauer's group published in 2003 [63]. The provoked impact upon insulin resistance was studied and shown to be mediated by mechanisms which were independent of the actual sustained weight loss. Numerous authors also reported significant rates of resolution of hypertension, obstructive sleep apnea, hyperlipidemia, and GERD among other conditions strongly linked to obesity [64–67].

In 2004, Buchwald and colleagues published a large meta-analysis of the literature evaluating present-day bariatric surgery [68]. They reviewed 2,738 citations in the English language from 1990 to 2003. This was a landmark piece of literature which evaluated excess weight loss for the various contemporary procedures as well as the resolution rate of obesity-related comorbidities including diabetes mellitus, hyperlipidemia, hypertension, and obstructive sleep apnea. Other landmark publications included articles from the Swedish Obese Subject (SOS) study, led by Dr. Lars Sjostrom, which evaluated the impact of surgery upon the health of morbidly obese individuals when compared to standard medical therapies over several decades. This included studying the impact on diabetes, cardiovascular risk factors, lifestyle, and long-term mortality [69, 70].

The impact of consistent weight loss upon physical, social, and economic comorbidities was also studied and reported upon in publications too numerous to mention. The evidence of enhanced health and quality of life enjoyed by obese patients who underwent weight loss surgery became abundant and clear. Some of the most compelling evidence came about from well-structured randomized controlled studies, solidifying the role of surgery in the treatment of the many facets of obesity [71–75].

In 2004, Christou and colleagues published a study evaluating the impact of weight loss surgery upon the longevity of obese individuals [76]. This represented the most convincing evidence to date, that weight loss surgery dramatically impacted long-term survival. Adams and colleagues added to this in 2007, with a longitudinal study evaluating mortality of patients with morbid obesity with and without weight loss surgery over a period of 20 years [77]. This historic study added to the mounting evidence that weight loss surgery increases longevity. In March 2007, the Diabetes Surgery Summit in Rome, Italy, organized by Drs. Phil Schauer, Lee Kaplan, David Cummings, and Francesco Rubino, was the first ever global meeting of experts delineating guidelines for the utilization of surgery in the treatment of diabetes. Later in the decade, results of the mortality rates in the SOS study also showed a decrease in long-term mortality in patients with morbid obesity that underwent weight loss surgery [78].

The increased application of weight loss surgery ignited an interest in research of gastrointestinal physiologic and hormonal mechanisms. The term "metabolic surgery" has been coined to reflect the utility of surgery for the treatment of type 2 diabetes and other medical conditions strongly associated with obesity. The groundbreaking discoveries of gastrointestinal hormones mediating metabolic responses quickly confirmed that the impact of gastrointestinal surgery reached far beyond that of restriction and malabsorption. The association of decreased levels of ghrelin, a hunger hormone, with gastric bypass was one such landmark discovery by Cummings in 2002 [79]. In addition, authors such as Rubino and colleagues further elucidated the relationship between diabetes and gastrointestinal bypass [80]. To this day, these mechanisms are not fully known, and both scientists and surgeons persist in their quest to better understand the underlying physiology.

A Look to the Future

At its annual meeting in June of 2013, the American Medical Association recognized obesity as a disease. It is noteworthy that those individuals who have done so much to advance the field of bariatric and metabolic surgery are often the ones who point out that the best understanding and treatment of obesity are yet to come. There is much work left to be done in order to augment what has already been accomplished. This includes elucidating physiologic mechanisms that still remain an enigma, improving access to care for patients who would benefit from surgery, advancing surgical techniques and technology, and promoting the training of our future bariatric and metabolic surgeons.

References

1. Henrikson V. [Kan tunnfarmsresektion forsvaras som terapi mot fettsot? Nordisk Medicin. 1952;47:744]. Can small bowel resection be defended as therapy for obesity? Obes Surg. 1994;4:54–5.
2. Meyer HW. Acute superior mesenteric artery thrombosis: recovery following extensive resection of small and large intestines. Arch Surg. 1946;53(3):298–303.
3. Kremen A, Linner J, Nelson C. An experimental evaluation of the nutritional importance of proximal and distal small intestine. Ann Surg. 1954;140:439–44.
4. Payne J, DeWind L, Commons R. Metabolic observations in patients with jejunocolic shunts. Am J Surg. 1963;106:273–89.
5. Scott HW, Dean R, Shull HJ, Abram HS, Webb W, Younger RK. New considerations in use of jejunoileal bypass in patients with morbid obesity. Ann Surg. 1973;177(6):723–35.
6. Scott HW, Law DH, Sanstead HH, Lanier VC, Younger RK. Jejunoileal shunt in surgical treatment of morbid obesity. Ann Surg. 1970;171(5):770–82.
7. Buchwald H, Rucker R. The rise and fall of jejunoileal bypass. In: Nelson RL, Nyhus LM, editors. Surgery of the small intestine. Norwalk: Appleton Century Crofts; 1987. p. 529–41.
8. Griffen Jr WO, Bivins BA, Bell RM. The decline and fall of the jejunoileal bypass. Surg Gynecol Obstet. 1983;157(4):301–8.

9. Brown R, O'Leary J, Woodward E. Hepatic effects of jejunoileal bypass for morbid obesity. Am J Surg. 1974;127:53–8.

10. Deitel M, Shahi B, Anand PK, Deitel FH, Cardinell DL. Long-term outcome in a series of jejunoileal bypass patients. Obes Surg. 1993;3(3):247–52.

11. Mason E, Ito C. Gastric bypass in obesity. Surg Clin North Am. 1967;47(6):1345–51.

12. Mason E. History of obesity surgery. Surg Obes Relat Dis. 2005;1:123–5.

13. Griffen Jr W, Young V, Stevenson C. A prospective comparison of gastric and jejunoileal bypass procedures for morbid obesity. Ann Surg. 1977;186(4):500–9.

14. Sugerman HJ, Starkey JV, Birkenhauer R. A randomized prospective trial of gastric bypass versus vertical banded gastroplasty for morbid obesity and their effects on sweets versus non-sweets eaters. Ann Surg. 1987;205(6):613–24.

15. Scopinaro N, Gianetta E, Civalleri D, Bonalumi E, Bachi V. Biliopancreatic bypass for obesity: I. An experimental study in dogs. Br J Surg. 1979;66:613–7.

16. Scopinaro N, Gianetta E, Civalleri D, Bonalumi U, Bachi V. Biliopancreatic by-pass for obesity: II. Initial experience in man. Br J Surg. 1979;66:618–20.

17. Scopinaro N, Gianetta E, Adami G, Friedman D, Traverso E, Marinari G, et al. Biliopancreatic diversion for obesity at eighteen years. Surgery. 1996;119:261–8.

18. Scopinaro N, Adami G, Marinari G, Gianetta E, Traverso E, Friedman D, et al. Biliopancreatic diversion. World J Surg. 1998;22:936–46.

19. Scopinaro N. Biliopancreatic diversion: mechanisms of action and long-term results. Obes Surg. 2006;16(6):683–9.

20. Hess DS, Hess DW. Biliopancreatic diversion with a duodenal switch. Obes Surg. 1998;8:267–82.

21. Marceau P, Hould FS, Simard S, Lebel S, Bourque RA, Potvin M, et al. Biliopancreatic diversion with duodenal switch. World J Surg. 1998;22:947–54.

22. Hess DS. Biliopancreatic diversion with duodenal switch. Surg Obes Relat Dis. 2005;1:329–33.

23. Printen KJ, Mason EE. Gastric surgery for relief of morbid obesity. Arch Surg. 1973;106:428–31.

24. Gomez CA. Gastroplasty in morbid obesity. Surg Clin North Am. 1979;59:1113–20.

25. Pace WG, Martin Jr EW, Tetirick T, Fabri PJ, Carey LC. Gastric partitioning for morbid obesity. Ann Surg. 1979;190(3):392–400.

26. Long M, Collins JP. The technique and early results of high gastric reduction for obesity. Aust N Z J Surg. 1980;50(2):146–9.

27. Laws HL, Piantadosi S. Superior gastric reduction procedure for morbid obesity: a prospective, randomized trial. Ann Surg. 1981;193(3):334–40.

28. Mason EE. Vertical banded gastroplasty. Arch Surg. 1982;117:701–6.

29. Marsk R, Jonas E, Gartzios H, Stockeld D, Granstrom L, Freedman J. High revision rates after laparoscopic vertical banded gastroplasty. Surg Obes Relat Dis. 2009;5(1):94–8.

30. Tevis S, Garren MJ, Gould JC. Revisional surgery for failed vertical-banded gastroplasty. Obes Surg. 2001;21(8):1220–4.

31. Wilkinson LH, Peloso OA. Gastric (reservoir) reduction for morbid obesity. Arch Surg. 1981;116(5):602–5.

32. Steffen R. The history and role of gastric banding. Surg Obes Relat Dis. 2008;4(3):S7–13.

33. Kuzmak LI, Rickert RR. Pathologic changes in the stomach at the site of silicone gastric banding. Obes Surg. 1991;1(1):63–8.

34. Szinicz G, Muller L, Erhart W, Roth FX, Pointner R, Glaser K. "Reversible gastric banding" in surgical treatment of morbid obesity—results of animal experiments. Res Exp Med. 1989;189(1):55–60.

35. Forsell P, Hellers G. The Swedish Adjustable Gastric Banding (SAGB) for morbid obesity: 9 year experience and a 4 year follow-up of patients operated with a new adjustable band. Obes Surg. 1997;7:345–51.

36. Kuzmak LI. A review of seven years' experience with silicone gastric banding. Obes Surg. 1991;1:403–8.

37. Fox SR, Oh KH, Fox KM. Adjustable silicone gastric banding vs vertical banded gastroplasty: a comparison of early results. Obes Surg. 1993;3:181–4.

38. Broadbent R, Tracey M, Harrington P. Laparoscopic gastric banding: a preliminary report. Obes Surg. 1993;3(1):63–7.

39. Belachew M, Zimmermann JM. Evolution of a paradigm for laparoscopic adjustable gastric banding. Am J Surg. 2002;184:21S–5.

40. Fielding GA, Rhodes M, Nathanson LK. Laparoscopic gastric banding for morbid obesity: surgical outcome in 335 cases. Surg Endosc. 1999;13:550–4.

41. Ren CJ, Fielding GA. Laparoscopic adjustable gastric banding: surgical technique. J Laparoendosc Adv Surg Tech A. 2003;13(4):257–63.

42. O'Brien PE, Dixon JB, Laurie C, Anderson M. A prospective randomized trial of placement of the laparoscopic adjustable gastric band: comparison of the perigastric and pars flaccida pathways. Obes Surg. 2005;15(6):820–6.

43. Suter M, Calmes JM, Paroz A, Giusti V. A 10-year experience with laparoscopic gastric banding for morbid obesity: high complication and failure rates. Obes Surg. 2006;16:829–35.

44. Wittgrove AC, Clark GW, Tremblay LJ. Laparoscopic gastric bypass, Roux-en-Y: preliminary report of five cases. Obes Surg. 1994;4:353–7.

45. Wittgrove AC, Clark GW, Schubert KR. Laparoscopic gastric bypass, Roux-en-Y: technique and results in 75 patients with 3-30 months follow-up. Obes Surg. 1996;6:500–4.

46. Wittgrove AC, Clark GW. Laparoscopic gastric bypass, Roux-en-Y-500 patients: technique and results, with 3–60 month follow-up. Obes Surg. 2000;10(3):233–9.

47. Nguyen NT, Goldman C, Rosenquist CJ, Arango A, Cole CJ, Lee SJ, et al. Laparoscopic versus open gastric bypass: a randomized study of outcomes, quality of life, and costs. Ann Surg. 2001;234(3):279–89.

48. Higa KD, Boone KB, Ho T, Davies OG. Laparoscopic Roux-en-Y gastric bypass for morbid obesity: technique and preliminary results of our first 400 patients. Arch Surg. 2000;135(9):1029–33.

49. Schauer PR, Ikramuddin S, Gourash W, Ramanathan R, Luketich J. Outcomes after laparoscopic Roux-en-Y gastric bypass for morbid obesity. Ann Surg. 2000;232(4):515–29.

50. Ren CJ, Patterson E, Gagner M. Early results of laparoscopic biliopancreatic diversion with duodenal switch: a case series of 40 consecutive patients. Obes Surg. 2000;10:514–23.

51. Scopinaro N, Adami GF, Marnari GM. Biliopancreatic diversion: two decades of experience. In: Deitel M, editor. Update: surgery for the morbidly obese patient. Toronto: FD-Communications; 2000. p. 227–58.

52. Regan JP, Inabnet WB, Gagner M, Pomp A. Early experience with two-stage laparoscopic Roux-en-Y gastric bypass as an alternative in the super-super obese patient. Obes Surg. 2003;13:861–4.

53. Moy J, Pomp A, Dakin G, Parikh M, Gagner M. Laparoscopic sleeve gastrectomy for morbid obesity. Am J Surg. 2008;196:56–9.

54. Gagner M, Gumbs AA, Milone L, Yung E, Goldenberg L, Pomp A. Laparoscopic sleeve gastrectomy for the super-super-obese (body mass index >60kg/m²). Surg Today. 2008;38:399–403.

55. Brethauer SA, Harris JL, Kroh M, Schauer PR. Laparoscopic gastric plication for treatment of severe obesity. Surg Obes Relat Dis. 2011;7(1):15–22.

56. NIH conference. Gastrointestinal surgery for severe obesity. Consensus Development Conference Panel. Ann Intern Med. 1991; 115(12):956–61.
57. Buchwald H; Consensus Conference Panel. Bariatric surgery for morbid obesity: health implications for patients, health professionals, and third-party payers. J Am Coll Surg. 2005;200(4):593–604.
58. DeMaria EJ, Pate V, Warthen M, Winegar DA. Baseline data from American Society for Metabolic and Bariatric Surgery-designated Bariatric Surgery Centers of Excellence using the Bariatric Outcomes Longitudinal Database. Surg Obes Relat Dis. 2010;6(4): 347–55.
59. Friedman MN, Sancetta AJ, Magovern GJ. The amelioration of diabetes mellitus following subtotal gastrectomy. Surg Gynecol Obstet. 1955;100(2):201–4.
60. O'Leary JP. Overview: jejunoileal bypass in the treatment of morbid obesity. Am J Clin Nutr. 1980;33(2):389–94.
61. Pories WJ, Swanson MS, MacDonald KG, Long SB, Morris PG, Brown BM. Who would have thought it? An operation proves to be the most effective therapy for adult-onset diabetes mellitus. Ann Surg. 1995;222(3):339–50.
62. MacDonald Jr KG, Long SD, Swanson MS, Brown BM, Morris P, Dohm GL. The gastric bypass operation reduces the progression and mortality of non-insulin-dependent diabetes mellitus. J Gastrointest Surg. 1997;1(3):213–20.
63. Schauer PR, Burguera B, Ikradmuddin S, Cottam D, Gourash W, Hamad G. Effect of laparoscopic Roux-en-Y gastric bypass on type 2 diabetes mellitus. Ann Surg. 2003;238(4):467–84.
64. Gleysteen JJ. Results of surgery: long-term effects on hyperlipidemia. Am J Clin Nutr. 1992;55(2):591–3.
65. Perry Y, Courcoulas AP, Fernando HC, Buenaventura PO, McCaughan JS, Luketich JD. Laparoscopic Roux-en-Y gastric bypass for recalcitrant gastroesophageal reflux disease in morbidly obese patients. JSLS. 2004;8(1):19–23.
66. Auyang ED, Murayama KM, Nagle AP. Five-year follow-up after laparoscopic Roux-en-Y gastric and partial ileal bypass for treatment of morbid obesity and uncontrolled hyperlipidemia. Obes Surg. 2009;19(1):121–4.
67. Obeid A, Long J, Kakade M, Clements RH, Stahl R, Grams J. Laparoscopic Roux-en-Y gastric bypass: long term clinical outcomes. Surg Endosc. 2012;26(12):3515–20.
68. Buchwald H, Avidor Y, Braunwald E, Jensen MD, Pories W, Fahrbach K, et al. Bariatric surgery: a systematic review and meta-analysis. JAMA. 2004;292(14):1724–37.
69. Karlsson J, Taft C, Ryden A, Sjostrom L, Sullivan M. Ten-year trends in health-related quality of life after surgical and conventional treatment for severe obesity: the SOS intervention study. Int J Obes (Lond). 2007;31(8):1248–61.
70. Sjostrom L, Lindroos AK, Peltonen M, Torgerson J, Bouchard C, Carlsson B, et al. Lifestyle, diabetes, and cardiovascular risk factors 10 years after bariatric surgery. N Engl J Med. 2004;351(26): 2683–93.
71. Schauer PR, Kashyap SR, Wolski K, Brethauer SA, Kirwan JP, et al. Bariatric surgery versus intensive medical therapy in obese patients with diabetes. N Engl J Med. 2012;366(17):1567–76.
72. Mingrone G, Panunzi S, De Gaetano A, Guidone C, Iaconelli A, Leccesi L, et al. Bariatric surgery versus conventional medical therapy for type 2 diabetes. N Engl J Med. 2012;366(17):1577–85.
73. Ikramuddin S, Korner J, Wei-Jei L, Connett JE, Inabnet WB, Billington CJ, et al. Roux-en-Y gastric bypass vs intensive medical management for the control of type 2 diabetes, hypertension, and hyperlipidemia. JAMA. 2013;309(21):2240–9.
74. O'Brien PE, Dixon JB, Laurie C, Skinner S, Proietto J, McNeil J, et al. Treatment of mild to moderate obesity with laparoscopic adjustable gastric banding or an intensive medical program: a randomized trial. Ann Intern Med. 2006;144(9):625–33.
75. Dixon JB, O'Brien PE, Playfair J, Chapman L, Schachter LM, Skinner S, et al. Adjustable gastric banding and conventional therapy for type 2 diabetes: a randomized controlled trial. JAMA. 2008;299(3):316–23.
76. Christou NV, Sampalis JS, Liberman M, Look D, Auger S, McLean AP, et al. Surgery decreases long-term mortality, morbidity, and health care use in morbidly obese patients. Ann Surg. 2004; 240(3):416–23.
77. Adams TD, Gress RE, Smith SC, Halverson RC, Simper SC, Rosamond WD. Long-term mortality after gastric bypass surgery. N Engl J Med. 2007;357(8):753–61.
78. Sjostrom L. Bariatric surgery and reduction in morbidity and mortality: experiences from the SOS study. Int J Obes (Lond). 2008; 32(7):93–7.
79. Cummings DE, Weigle DS, Frayo RS, Breen PA, Ma MK, Dellinger EP, et al. Plasma ghrelin levels after diet-induced weight loss or gastric bypass surgery. N Engl J Med. 2002;346(21):1623–30.
80. Rubino F, Forgione A, Cummings DE, Vix M, Gnuli D, Mingrone G, et al. The mechanism of diabetes control after gastrointestinal bypass surgery reveals a role of the proximal small intestine in the pathophysiology of type 2 diabetes. Ann Surg. 2006;244(5):741–9.

5

Developing a Successful Bariatric Surgery Program

Andrew S. Wu and Daniel M. Herron

Abbreviations

ABS	American Board of Surgery
ACS	American College of Surgeons
AORN	According to the Association of Operating Room Nurses
ASMBS	American Society for Metabolic and Bariatric Surgery
BMI	Body mass index
EMR	Electronic medical record
MBSAQIP	Metabolic and Bariatric Surgery Accreditation and Quality Improvement Program
NIH	National Institutes of Health
NSQIP	National Surgical Quality Improvement Program
QI	Quality improvement
SAGES	Society of American Gastrointestinal and Endoscopic Surgeons

Introduction

Obesity, defined as a body mass index (BMI) >30 kg/m^2, is increasing in prevalence in the United States and worldwide [1]. With the desire to promote improved health amongst the obese population, bariatric surgeons are seeing a greater number of people inquiring and desiring bariatric surgery as a tool to achieve weight loss. Bariatric surgical procedures are performed in a high-risk population with many comorbid conditions and can be challenging and complex. Because the obese are at a high risk of surgical complications, the safety of bariatric surgery needs to be evaluated. One of the underlying justifications for the introduction of a designated bariatric program is that data from the National Surgical Quality Improvement Program (NSQIP) have shown that adverse outcomes and patient safety are primarily determined by the quality of the systems of care [2]. For bariatric surgery, a relationship between the surgical caseload and outcome has been suggested, and a recent article in 2011 has shown that implementation of designated bariatric surgery program leads to improved clinical outcomes [3].

We discuss a complete overview of what is necessary in developing a successful bariatric program. This begins with the requirements to get credentialed to perform bariatric surgery. Ensuring that programs develop into high-quality programs is a difficult proposition. Some evidence suggests that outcomes are better when a hospital performs over 100 cases annually, and hospitals performing less than 50 cases annually have mortality rates 4 times higher than high-volume programs [4]. We then discuss an overview of the infrastructure needed in the outpatient and inpatient setting, the personnel and surgical team who will take part in the patient care, and the resources needed for lifetime follow-up care for the patients after bariatric surgery and conclude with the costs and legal issues that a bariatric surgery program encounters.

Bariatric Surgery Credentialing and Training

A new bariatric program will generally be formed and led by a surgeon with significant experience or formal training in bariatric surgery. This is in contrast to the process in place during the 1990s, when bariatric surgery training was generally unstructured and provided informally during surgical residency. This process has become significantly more rigorous and formalized since formation of the Fellowship Council in 1997 [5]. Many fellowships with a strong or exclusive focus in minimally invasive bariatric surgery are presently available in the United States, allowing graduates of accredited 5-year surgery residencies to undergo an additional year of specialized training. Fellows completing such a fellowship who participate in 100 or more bariatric cases are eligible to apply for official recognition by the American Society for Metabolic and Bariatric Surgery (ASMBS) [6].

S.A. Brethauer et al. (eds.), *Minimally Invasive Bariatric Surgery*,
DOI 10.1007/978-1-4939-1637-5_5, © Springer Science+Business Media New York 2015

Credentialing of bariatric surgeons is the process through which individual hospitals determine that a surgeon is appropriately qualified to safely perform bariatric procedures. The credentialing process will necessarily be slightly different at every hospital. At present, there is no nationally recognized board providing certification in bariatric surgery. However, since the American Board of Surgery (ABS) does include bariatric surgery within its curriculum, most hospitals include certification by the ABS or equivalent organization as part of the bariatric surgery credentialing requirements. Detailed recommendations regarding the credentialing and recredentialing processes are provided by the American College of Surgeons (ACS) as part of the newly developed Metabolic and Bariatric Surgery Accreditation and Quality Improvement Program (MBSAQIP) jointly administered with the ASMBS. Any hospital seeking accreditation in this national quality improvement program must adhere to the program, facility, and surgeon standards outlined in the program.

A new bariatric program in the United States should develop with the goal of becoming nationally accredited by MBSAQIP. Such accreditation serves several functions. In addition to serving as a rigorous quality improvement (QI) program, the accreditation, or participation in a similar outcomes reporting program, is required by many private and public payors.

Until 2012, Bariatric Surgery Center certification included rigid volume requirements for both the hospital and the individual surgeons. In such a model, surgical volume was used as a surrogate measure of quality. The MBSAQIP program has been revised to use outcomes measures to directly assess program quality, has decrease emphasis on volume as a component of a quality composite score, and has decreased the volume requirements to be consistent with current evidence and avoid problems with access to care.

Facilities: Outpatient Office

Establishing a bariatric surgery program requires substantial infrastructure in the outpatient setting. The patient's desire for bariatric surgery begins with the initial visit in the surgery outpatient office, and thus adequate office staff training and patient education are all important for the initial encounter.

Office Staff Training

Office personnel need to be educated regarding the unique physical and psychological issues pertaining to the bariatric patient. Often times, the initial encounter is that of a phone call in which a prospective patient inquires about bariatric surgery. The office staff should engage the new patients in a professional manner and be sensitive to the use of socially unacceptable terminology. For example, the term "severely overweight" is equivalent to the expression "morbidly obese" but is viewed as being less offensive to the bariatric patient [7].

Office staff will need to understand the basics of bariatric surgery including the indications and contraindications to surgery, the various types of surgery, and the need for a truly multidisciplinary approach involving a team of physicians and consultants. Office staff are to be familiar with specific bariatric terminology such as "Roux-en-Y bypass" and "sleeve gastrectomy" and should be taught to calculate a patient's BMI. There are many resources available that the office staff has access to that are written for the layperson which provide an overview of bariatric surgery [8]. Not only will this aid in the answering of questions that patients will initially have, but this will provide an underlying framework for a screening tool to differentiate patients who indeed are candidates for surgery from those who are not. This will make the office encounter more efficient for the physician and staff when scheduling patients who are truly candidates for bariatric surgery discussion.

Patient Education Materials

With the exponential growth of informational technology via the television, public ads, and the Internet, patient access to information regarding bariatric surgery is abundant. A wide range of initial patient knowledge is seen: some patients will have already researched all there is to know about bariatric surgery and some will have none. It is important to provide all the necessary educational tools and information written and accessible to the patient for the initial visit, as a tremendous amount of preoperative education is necessary. Most bariatric centers now provide an initial informational session which is held monthly during the evening and free to the public for anyone wishing to learn about bariatric surgery. This is of significant importance as this is the most uniform and concise way for patients to start their bariatric journey and learn about the essentials of the bariatric program. Diligent work and coordination between the surgeon, bariatric team, and the marketing and public relations manager of the hospital or practice is necessary in order to provide patient awareness of an existing free informational session.

At the initial encounter in the office, packets of information should be available to give to each patient which has all of the necessary information of the bariatric experience. With the increased use of the Internet, practices should establish a website detailing everything that is in the packet for patients so that patients have permanent and public access to this on the Internet while at the same time saving distribution costs. Care should be given to making an accurate and educational website as many websites for bariatric surgery may have misleading information. If done correctly, it may be a powerful tool and invaluable educational resource for the patient [9].

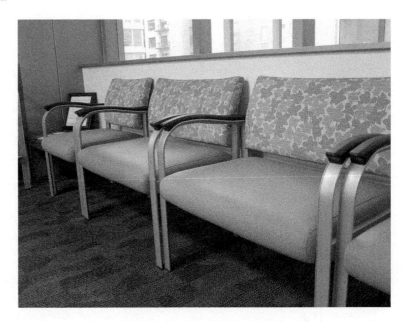

Office Furniture and Equipment

First impressions are extremely important to the patient. Thus, a clean, organized, professional, and welcoming environment for bariatric patients is absolutely essential. Deliberate thought and planning is needed to organize the waiting room and consultation room so that appropriate sized furniture for patients must be used (Figs. 1, 2 and 3) [10]. Details of specific office furniture and equipment to accommodate the bariatric surgery patient are presented in Chap. 6.

Information Systems

Because of the multidisciplinary team of physicians and providers for each individual bariatric patient, there is an extensive amount of paperwork and preoperative and postoperative visits that require documentation. Most patients will have at the minimum, four physician encounters not including the bariatric surgeon. Patients will likely have preoperative visits with their internist, cardiologist, psychologist, and nutritionist. Additional consults include gastroenterologists, endocrinologists, and pulmonologists. Each will have a documented patient encounter, and hence an organized and streamlined medical record is absolutely necessary. In addition, the postoperative visit and follow-ups for years after the surgery will accrue even more patient encounters requiring documentation. Achieving this with the traditional paper-based medical record system is feasible, but patient information will be more difficult to manage and organize. With the increased use of electronic medical records (EMRs), employing such a system significantly aids in organizing and accessing a single database which has all of the necessary patient information.

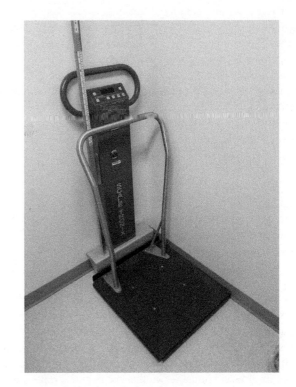

FIG. 2. An appropriate and accurate weight scale is necessary to have in the office.

Benefits of the EMR include higher-quality charting, faster charting procedures, less risk of data loss, and decreased medicolegal risk from inadequate charting [7].

For the bariatric patients, charting their weight loss or gain needs to be documented at every visit. In addition, patients who have had a gastric band placed and has routine follow-ups with band filling readjustments need to have the

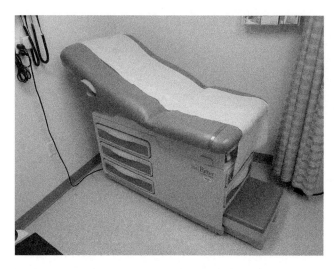

Fig. 3. Exam tables must have adequate capacity to support heavy patients.

amount of fluid placed or removed charted. Having a computerized chart and data table tracking, these changes are a much more efficient method of tracking the patient's overall course. Often times, it is beneficial to photograph patients preoperatively and again at each postoperative visit. Photos may easily be taken digitally and can be uploaded or scanned into the EMR with the consent of the patient. This may be a useful adjunct for the physician and the patient tracking the patient's weight loss progress and also may be of medicolegal value should the need arise.

Insurance Documentation

Insurance companies are mandating increasing complex prerequisites for the bariatric patient. One of the requirements that patients must undergo and prove to insurance companies is a commitment to health through personal preoperative weight loss. A bariatric candidate may not be able to have their insurance carrier cover the costs of bariatric surgery unless he or she is able to provide documentation of efforts at preoperative weight loss. An effective record keeping system such as those mentioned previously is critical to generate the paperwork necessary to facilitate the communication to the insurance companies so that there is a smooth transition without placing any additional burden on office staff.

Facilities: Hospital Infrastructure and Equipment

The growing obesity epidemic has led to an increase in patients with special obesity-related needs presenting to hospitals for care. Thus, hospitals are recognizing that facilities and structural resources appropriate for the treatment of

extremely obese patients are needed throughout their institutions [11]. Establishing a dedicated infrastructure for the bariatric patient during their inpatient stay is a critical part of their surgical experience. Evidence-based practice guidelines for specialized facilities and resources for weight loss surgery have been initially described in 2005 in a report published for the Betsy Lehman Center for Patient Safety and Medical Error Reduction and updated in 2009 [11].

Operating Room Needs

Much of the layout and organization of the operating room is standard from room to room. Specific needs for the bariatric patient include the operating bed which must be outfitted to safely hold and secure a bariatric patient. According to the Association of Operating Room Nurses (AORN) bariatric surgery guidelines, OR bariatric beds should have the capacity to hold 1,000 lb with 600 lb tilt capacity [12]. The OR tables should have side extenders, footboards, sufficient arm holders, and foam padding available for the arms, heels, and feet to prevent falls and pressure injuries. Because obese patients are not likely to be able to transfer themselves after recently having had general anesthesia, lifts or other appropriate moving devices, like an air mattress, should be utilized to facilitate easy transfer.

Since most procedures are now performed laparoscopically, special abdominal instrument sets may be needed including longer suction catheters, laparoscopic graspers, needle holders, drivers, and laparoscopes [11]. An adequately sized OR room should be used since additional space may be needed not only for patient transfer to a larger bed but also for the use of intraoperative endoscopy when performing bariatric procedures. Circulating nurses and scrub technicians should be prepared at a moments' notice should any laparoscopic case require conversion to an open procedure and have all necessary open instruments ready to use.

Inpatient Facilities

Immediately after surgery, the patient is brought to the recovery room, one that is capable of providing critical care is necessary. In addition, an available intensive care unit and a step-down area for patients are necessary should the patient require such postoperative care.

The need for specialized equipment starts in the preoperative holding area. Extra large hospital gowns, a high capacity patient scale, appropriately sized stretchers, gurneys, and wheelchairs are all needed. Appropriately sized sequential compression devices and blood pressure cuffs are required. To safely facilitate patient transfer to and from the stretcher to bed, patient rolling devices or air-assisted transfer devices such as the Hovermatt (Hovertech International, Bethlehem, PA) may be used.

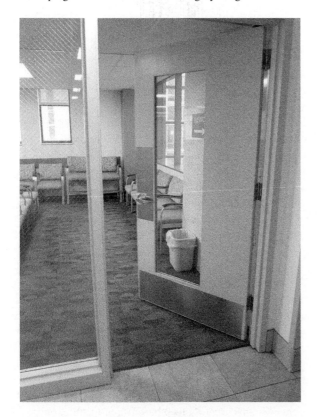

FIG. 4. Electronically powered and larger width doors as entryways either into a patient room in the hospital or in this case into the waiting area of the outpatient office are necessary.

Once out of the recovery room, patients are transferred to a regular nursing floor bed or step-down unit, if not to an intensive care unit. For obesity surgery programs, consider establishing a dedicated location, floor, or unit in the hospital to house all of the inpatient bariatric patients. This creates an environment dedicated to the care of the bariatric patient and provides a framework for specialized ancillary care having undergone special training in the nursing care of the bariatric patient. In addition, having a dedicated unit or area for these patients makes the logistics much simpler and more efficient, such as having all necessary equipment present at the particular unit.

If a dedicated floor or unit is in its construction infancy, then a blueprint for success should be carefully thought out. The actual physical requirements are more complex. Larger door widths up to 60 in. wide may be needed to accommodate larger equipment such as patient beds (Fig. 4). This includes the door to the bathroom. It is recommended that there be 5 ft of space between the foot of the bed and the walls and 5 ft between either sides of the bed and walls [13]. Space is needed for room for rolling equipment such as EKG carts, portable X-ray machines, and code carts. Bathrooms and room design will need to be constructed so that bathroom doors are at least 20 in. wide. Bathrooms should have floor mounted commodes and properly installed grab bars to prevent patient falls. Floor mounted toilets can support up to

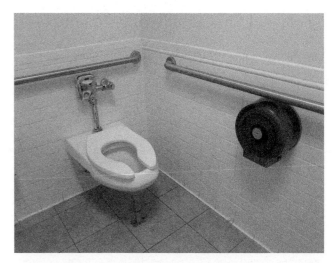

FIG. 5. Bathrooms should have floor mounted toilets with properly installed grab bars to prevent patient falls.

1,000 lb (453 kg), while most standard wall mounted commodes have a 250-lb weight limit (Fig. 5).

Most regular hospital beds can handle patients up to 440 lb; however, these beds are probably too narrow at 35 in., making it difficult for bariatric patients to reach the adjustment buttons or operate the side rails. Bariatric beds should be at least 44 in. wide and support up to 1,000 lb. The mattresses should be the low air loss type so patients will not tend to sink in their beds. The low air loss mattresses make it easier for patients to get out of bed and thus assist with preventing skin breakdown leading to sacral decubitus ulcers. It is optimal if the beds can be automatically adjusted into a chair position so patients can walk out of their beds from the seated position [11].

Many bariatric patients undergo routine postoperative upper GI contrast studies to assess their stomach pouches and proximal anastomosis [14]. Such fluoroscopy studies require a radiology table that can adequately support the heavy patient. In addition, patients may need CT scans or MRI, and similar to the fluoroscopy unit, a CT scan capable of accommodating the size of a bariatric patient may be unavailable. Backup plans for knowing which outside facilities or sites that may have the capabilities for oversized CT scanners are important.

Investment

Specialized resources for weight loss surgery require a significant investment. The average low-end per patient cost is $50,000; remodeling rooms and restocking inventory can cost up to $200,000 in 1 year. Many centers lease rather than purchase equipment, and advantages here include lower initial cost outlay and less need for storage space with the option of having more up-to-date equipment [11].

Personnel: The Bariatric Surgery Team

The bariatric surgical operation does not depend on one person, the surgeon. It involves the work of a talented team of physicians and providers working in sync to provide optimal care and long-term high-quality patient outcomes.

Surgeon

The surgeon is central to the bariatric patient's weight loss experience. The surgeon is the one whom patients want to see and talk to and the one they begin and continue their journey with. Thus it is critical that the surgeon be aware of all of the necessary planning that the bariatric patient undergoes from beginning to end. The surgeon should be in constant communication with the office staff and bariatric nurses to coordinate patient care. With many programs offering an organized patient informational session, it is recommended that a surgeon participates in these sessions in order to educate patients about bariatric surgery. During the actual patient encounter in the preoperative clinic assessment, the surgeon should personally explain to the patient a summary of the prerequisites of surgery, all of the surgical procedural options, and expectations of postoperative care and recovery. The surgeon sees the patients after surgery during their impatient stay and coordinates with consulting physicians and team members regarding their postoperative care upon discharge.

Office Personnel

The team approach begins in the office. The office may require 2 receptionists: one to check the patient in and another to confirm that their insurance covers bariatric surger. The insurance specialist is critical in assessing insurance coverage for the surgical procedure. This person should receive his or her own office as taking charge of the insurance needs and requirements is a full-time job [10].

Nurse Coordinator and Bariatric Nurse

A nurse coordinator is essential, and they may function to partake in patient care in both the clinical outpatient setting and the inpatient setting. First and foremost, they must benefit from education regarding the proper use of bariatric equipment, lifting techniques, and tailored dietary needs for these patients. The ASMBS has developed a certification program for Clinical Bariatric Nurse Specialists. In addition, the ASMBS, the AORN, and the Betsy Lehman Center for Patient Safety and Medical Error Reduction publish bariatric surgical nursing guidelines to address nursing education, practices, and certification goals, in an effort to improve patient care [15].

Dietician/Nutritionist

Registered dietitians provide patients with the information and education of the new diet that patients will be undertaking before and after bariatric surgery. They are essential for the appropriate inpatient care and long-term follow-up. They should work closely with the hospital food services to develop specialized bariatric meals that are high in protein and low in carbohydrates, fats, and sugars and are in appropriate sizes. Bariatric clear liquid diets, for example, are often different from the regular hospital clear liquid diet tray as they will have significantly less sugar. Nutritionists can also help prepare bariatric patients for the postoperative diet changes by educating patients portion control and maintenance of adequate nutrition. Without such education, patients tend to eat more fat and assume an unhealthy, unbalanced diet.

Many patients are at risk for malnutrition and should be evaluated for nutritional and vitamin deficiencies. The lifelong incidence of malnutrition after weight loss surgery can be as high as 44 % and can occur many years after the procedure [16]. This often is due to poor eating habits and poor education of what is required for the long-term process for patients attaining and maintaining a healthy well-balanced diet after bariatric surgery. In one study of 133 admissions of patients who had undergone a bariatric procedure, only 33 % of these patients were taking a multivitamin [17].

Psychologist/Psychiatrist

The mental and emotional aspects of obesity, weight loss, and weight loss surgery are an important consideration in the care of bariatric patients. Most weight loss programs in the United States require that a patient undergo a mental health evaluation prior to undergoing surgery. In fact, many insurance companies require such psychological evaluation prior to granting precertification for a bariatric procedure. Surgeons want to treat the whole person in order to increase the likelihood of a positive outcome for their patients. While 20–60 % of bariatric patients have a psychiatric disorder noted preoperatively, some psychiatric disorders are diagnosed postoperatively [18]. In addition, while some psychiatric conditions are improved with weight loss, others are made worse or become apparent with weight loss.

The psychological evaluation in the preoperative setting is the first step to ensure that the patient does not have any psychological needs that must be addressed. It is also a means for educating and introducing a patient to the expectations of their journey ahead as they proceed with surgery. Adequate time and attention should be provided for preoperative assessment of and support for psychological disorders. Patients referred for bariatric surgery are more likely than the overall population to have psychopathology such as somatization, social phobia, obsessive compulsive disorder, substance abuse/dependency, binge-eating disorder, post-traumatic stress disorder, generalized anxiety disorder, and depression [19]. In addition, a higher rate of suicide after bariatric surgery has been documented when compared to the general population [20]. While none of these is a contra-indication to surgery, these disorders should be controlled prior to undergoing surgical weight loss in an effort to reduce recidivism and produce greater sustained and successful weight loss. While many patients will only require a single preoperative visit with a mental health professional, other patients may benefit substantially from continued short-term or long-term psychotherapy. Of note, the bulk of evidence shows no relationship between preexisting axis I psychiatric diagnosis or axis II personality disorder and total weight loss. It is not certain which psychosocial factors predict success following bariatric surgery, yet many programs exclude patients who are illicit drug and/or alcohol abusers and have active uncontrolled psychosis, severe mental retardation, or lack of knowledge about the surgery [21].

Medical Consultants

Because a majority of patients getting bariatric surgery have comorbidities, it is important to have patients evaluated preoperatively regarding their medical diseases. A separate chapter in this book details the patient selection and preoperative assessment requirements.

As part of the entire bariatric surgery team, medical consultants become extremely important not only in the preoperative workup stage but in the inpatient hospital stage of their operation and most importantly adequate postoperative follow-up for the long term. Immediately after surgery, patients are most fragile to fluctuations in their hemodynamics whether it is their blood pressure or their glucose control. Many patients have hypertension and are on multiple antihypertensive medications. Many are brittle diabetics with an exact insulin regimen whom may experience drastic changes to their glucose levels in the perioperative setting. Some have sleep apnea and require careful monitoring of their pulmonary status. It is not uncommon to incorporate the medical care in the perioperative and postoperative setting with cardiologists, internists, pulmonologists, and endocrinologists to ensure that patients in the immediate postoperative setting are stable. Days after that the patient is discharged, they need to have frequent follow-up with these medical consultants to ensure continuity of care of their health.

Anesthesiologist

Most of the bariatric patients undergoing surgery have a significant number of comorbidities including complex pulmonary issues including sleep apnea, patients on CPAP or BIPAP, and patients with cardiovascular comorbidities.

The anesthesiologist must be fully cognizant of this in their preoperative anesthetic risk assessment and intraoperative management. Issues of specific concern include the airway exam and potential for difficult intravenous access. Anesthesiologists realize that a morbidly obese patient can potentially present a difficult airway and be cognizant of intubation difficulties. Insertion of a central line and/or an arterial line may be additional components necessary for safe intraoperative patient monitoring.

Many of the bariatric procedures may involve the placement of a bougie, a nasogastric tube, an anvil for a circular stapler anastomosis, or an intraoperative upper endoscopy at some point during the operation. Thus, the surgeon must always be in direct communication with the anesthesiologist to ensure that instrumentation of the oropharynx, esophagus, and down into the stomach be done smoothly and safely. Surgical staplers are often used when creating a gastric pouch in a Roux-en-Y gastric bypass or when performing a sleeve gastrectomy. It is important that any unnecessary intraluminal objects whether it is an NG tube, bougie, or temperature probe all be removed before firing the surgical stapler. The anesthesiologist must also be aware of the cardiovascular impact that persistent instrumentation of the oropharynx with these devices may cause.

House Staff/Physician Assistants

Many hospitals especially those with academic affiliations or academic centers have a team of resident physicians, fellows, and physician assistants who treat and oversee the inpatient care of the bariatric patient. In many ways, these providers are those who have constant interaction with the patient and have easy access to examine and evaluate them should these patients have any questions or should they have any medical or surgical emergency. They are the direct liaison between the patient and the surgeon who is most likely occupied elsewhere in clinic or in the operating room. The surgeon must recognize the importance of such a team because this may provide a means for a more efficient mode of patient care should an emergency necessitate a professional medical evaluation.

In-house physician assistants, nurse practitioners, or house staff should perform a postoperative checkup on the patient several hours after surgery which includes a physical exam and careful evaluation of all acute postoperative needs and orders. Although the complications of bariatric surgery are rare, when they do happen, they may be devastating with a high mortality rate especially when encountering postoperative patients with an acute anastomotic leak, bowel obstruction, or pulmonary embolus. The in-house providers must critically understand the presentations of these particular life-threatening complications so as to adequately and expediently care and treat them should they happen.

Lifetime Follow-Up, Support Groups, and Education

Weight loss surgery is a lifetime commitment to healthy eating habits and exercise. Bariatric surgery is only one of many components to achieve this. The National Institutes of Health (NIH) guidelines indicate that lifelong medical surveillance after surgical therapy is a necessity and that patients who opt for surgical intervention should be followed by a multidisciplinary team [13]. This is especially true of patients who undergo gastric banding, because they may need frequent adjustments and advice regarding choice of foods. Data has shown that inadequate adherence to follow-up care has been recognized as contributory to the development of complications after bariatric surgery. The consequences of missing appointments can lead to the late diagnosis of complications, los of a support network, and lack of reinforcement to follow the medical regimen [22].

Lifetime Follow-Up

The follow-up of patients who have had bariatric surgery includes assessments for complications, nutritional deficiencies, psychological adjustments, medical management, and weight gain. Many of the surgical and medical assessments require seeing the bariatric surgeon and the medical physicians on a timely basis.

For the first year follow-up, adherence with postoperative appointments has been shown to be associated with improved patient outcomes. One study published in 2008 identified five significant predictor variables that affect patient adherence to postoperative appointments after bariatric surgery. The predictors that indicated more likely adherence were increasing patient age, being single, and being employed. The predictors that indicated less likely adherence were self-payment for appointments and a greater BMI [23]. The long-term follow-up visits are generally scheduled for every 6 months for several years and then, by most groups, on an annual basis with the understanding that the patients can secure an immediate appointment upon request. In these visits, the following information should be recorded: weight, BMI, a review of each comorbidity that was present prior to surgery, documentation of new concerns, a list of current medications, a list of medical problems including admissions since the last visit, and laboratory studies including a hemoglobin, hematocrit, vitamin B12 level, and Hb1AC if the patient was a diabetic or demonstrated glucose impairment prior to surgery. Additional studies are ordered as indicated by additional symptoms or signs.

Seeing a nutritionist should be done more often such as every 3 months or every 6 months in order to ensure that the patient has maintained their weight and continue to eat a healthy diet. Certainly this can be tailored with every patient to their nutritional needs and weight fluctuations. This same concept applies to the psychologist/psychiatrist. Most hospitals specializing in weight loss surgery will have dedicated seminars and support groups to help further promote and continue the commitment to healthy living for bariatric patients.

Support Group Meetings

Postoperative support groups are an important aspect of a bariatric program and may improve postoperative results and limit relapse. Two nonrandomized studies have shown that patients attending support groups achieve greater weight loss than those who do not [24, 25].

Support groups can be an effective approach to the education of patients prior to surgery and to maintain strong lines of communication after the operations. In well-run groups, patients can learn from each other, not only about the surgery but also about how to adjust to changed personal relationships, how to maintain their weight, how to employ new exercise regimens into their lives, how to cook, how to apply for jobs, and how to deal with other personal concerns. Comparisons of weight loss and appearance lead to far more realistic expectations. By sharing experiences amongst people who have undergone similar journeys after bariatric surgery will shed light into living a healthier lifestyle and will mentally keep them motivated for continued success.

The models and infrastructure for support groups vary per institution. A common approach is to have the principal nurse coordinator of the practice also serve as the lead person in the support group because the patients know and trust this person. In some places, surgeons will play a role in the groups on an occasional basis so as to further promote a lifelong journey for continued healthy leaving. After introductions, a 1-h session may include a 15- to 20-min instructional talk on various pertinent subjects as plastic surgery, preparing meals, choosing clothes, and interpersonal relationships, with ample time for both questioning and shared discussions of individual experiences. In some clinics, the support groups also serve as postoperative follow-up visit opportunities. Some centers and programs employ the use of a personalized journal that each patient creates and keeps. This journal tracks the progress of each individuals' personal experience and records their weight and BMI on a quarterly basis as well as personal pictures of patients to serve as a visual reference in seeing their change over time.

Educational Seminars and Social Programs

Educational seminars are slightly different from support groups. Support groups serve as the foundation for meeting with similar patients to share and further discuss their bariatric experience. Educational seminars are those that provide additional and more in-depth knowledge about particular topics related to obesity and the bariatric experience.

The most important seminar is the preoperative informational session that patients attend which introduces them to bariatric surgery. This is a free seminar, usually one hour long, meant to educate the patient who is not familiar with bariatric surgery and who simply wants to know what it entails. It is often a seminar given by members of the bariatric team including a bariatric nurse, dietitian, and a surgeon. Topics include defining obesity, methods for weight loss without surgery, nutritional needs and changes, indications and contraindications of surgery for weight loss, expectations and inpatient experience of surgery, the various types of bariatric operations that are done with pictures and descriptions of their differences and similarities, and the postoperative experience after surgery [26]. It is at the discretion of the bariatric program to either have patients whom are interested in bariatric surgery either attend this informational seminar before seeing the surgeon in clinic or to attend it after a first encounter with the surgeon provider. Some institutions prefer having patients attend the seminar first because it will give patients the necessary information needed for the patients prior to individually coming to the first encounter with the surgeon so they have an idea of what they want or expect from surgery. In addition, this may serve to filter out patients who decide not to proceed with surgery, thus improving on the efficiency of the surgeon's outpatient practice and not losing time seeing patients who effectively are not candidates or have no desire to proceed with bariatric surgery.

There are also postoperative educational seminars and social programs that often are provided by the hospital or from community groups coordinated through the hospital which may cover other pertinent topics related to their bariatric surgery. These topics may be a more in-depth look at trends in diabetes, what is new in bariatric surgery, nutrition for the bariatric patient, or exercise techniques for the bariatric patient as an example. Social programs may interest groups from within the bariatric community that serve as a meeting place for patients with similar interests such as cooking classes for the bariatric patient or a morning walking exercise group for interested patients.

Electronic Resources

With the integration of the Internet into daily living, it is not surprising that many patients are turning to the Internet for information. Many patients use the internet to initiate their search about learning about bariatric surgery and finding a surgeon. Patients will use the Internet to first learn about weight loss techniques, healthy eating habits, and exercise regimens without having to do surgery. Bariatric practices should keep up with informational technology and dedicate time and thought into creating a personalized website which incorporates their bariatric program. A professional marketing and website designer is well worth the time and expense in creating this website because it will be a tool easily and most often accessed by the bariatric patient.

The benefits of using the Internet are that the Internet reaches many patients at one time, and travel to appointments is not an obstacle. It provides many pictures and videos to help patients understand surgery at their own individual pace. The downside to the Internet is that it does require a computer-savvy audience and it is less personal than a face-to-face discussion with a physician or nutritionist. We encourage the use of the Internet and personal website as an adjunct to the patients' bariatric experience, not a replacement.

A relatively new arena within the world of informational technology is the incorporation of the Internet as the central part of the patient's bariatric and weight loss experience after surgery. Websites may be designed to give each patient a personal login that has charting of their own progress. There may also be links for online nurses and nutritionists that may offer feedback and counseling. A study in 2003 by Tate looked at the effects of Internet behavioral counseling on weight loss in adults and showed that patients who underwent a dedicated electronic counseling treatment program requiring patients to log on weekly and submit weekly weights, food log, and exercise log had significantly increased weight loss and lower BMIs than patients without electronic counseling [27].

The web-based technology for Internet communication and education on diet and exercise has been expanding rapidly over the past 5–10 years. This has a dramatic impact on how people communicate, learn, and share information. For a bariatric practice, incorporating a personalized website should absolutely be a necessity.

Costs of Developing a Bariatric Practice

Malpractice Insurance

It is mandatory to ensure that appropriate malpractice coverage is in place prior to performing any bariatric procedures. While some insurance carriers may consider bariatric surgery to be included within general surgery coverage, many others require a separate policy or rider specifically covering metabolic and bariatric surgery. Since these policies may cost significantly more than general surgery coverage alone, this expense should be carefully evaluated early in the process of establishing a new metabolic/bariatric program.

A decade ago, it was estimated that a typical busy bariatric surgeon was sued for malpractice one to two times per year [28]. Since morbidity and mortality rates have dropped significantly since then, it is expected that malpractice expenses should decrease as well. However, while poor outcomes may be decreasing in frequency, bariatric claims are typically of high severity with potential payouts of $500,000 or more [29]. Since there is significant time lag between an occurrence and any subsequent legal action, this decrease may not be reflected in reduced premiums for a number of years, if at all.

A recent study reported the results of a survey of surgeon members of the ASMBS in which they were queried regarding their malpractice history. Although the results must be interpreted carefully, since the response rate for the survey was only 20 %, half of the surgeons reported that they had been sued at least once during their career [30]. A mean of 1.5 medical malpractice claims were filed per responding surgeon. Of these suits, 54 % were dismissed, 27 % were settled out of court, and 19 % went to trial or arbitration.

Program Expenses

There are many components to a bariatric program, including hospital and office infrastructure, hospital and office staff, as well as administrative and insurance expenses. Since these components of a bariatric program are discussed in depth elsewhere in this chapter, we will not enumerate them again here. Many of the costs, such as operating room equipment, inpatient care infrastructure, hospital nursing, etc., will necessarily be borne by the hospital. However, surgical office infrastructure and personnel costs will likely be supported by the surgical practice; these costs may become quite substantial.

At present, a nationwide trend is building in which independent surgical practices are being acquired by hospitals, hospital groups, and larger healthcare organizations. This restructuring of American surgical practice will have a strong impact on the development of a new bariatric practice. In many ways it will serve to simplify the formation of multidisciplinary programs such as a bariatric group, since many staff members in addition to the physicians and surgeons may be directly employed by the hospital. This simplification may come at the expense of decreased surgeon independence and practice control.

Conclusion

Establishing and setting up a bariatric surgery program is a major undertaking that requires a substantial amount of effort, planning, and commitment from the surgeons. It requires working with a dedicated team of providers knowledgeable in the many facets of bariatric surgery ranging from social programming, surgical education, insurance requirements, and medicolegal risks to clinical surgical care of performing the operation. Unlike acute care needs, these patients need long-term follow-up as this is critical to continued healthy living and success. Developing a program begins with coordination with a hospital to provide and establish a multidisciplinary team that includes medical providers, nutritionists, bariatric nurses, therapists, social workers, and surgeons who can provide an obese population with a specialty center, specifically a bariatric Center of Excellence dedicated to achieving weight loss through bariatric surgery.

References

1. www.cdc.gov/obesity/data/trends.html. Accessed 5 Oct 2012.
2. Khuri SF. Safety, quality, and the National Surgical Quality Improvement Program. Am Surg. 2006;72:994–8.
3. Dumon KR, Edelson PK, Raper SE, Foster-Kilgarriff K, Williams NN. Implementation of designated bariatric surgery program leads to improved clinical outcomes. Surg Obes Relat Dis. 2011;7:271–6.
4. Nguyen N, Paya M, Stevens M. The relationship between hospital volume and outcome in bariatric surgery at academic medical centers. Ann Surg. 2004;240:586–94.
5. Arregui ME. The Fellowship Council: Universal Fellowship Application and Match Service. www.fellowshipcouncil.org. 2012. https://fellowshipcouncil.org/. Accessed Nov 2012.
6. American Society for Metabolic and Bariatric Surgery. ASMBS: American Society for Metabolic and Bariatric Surgery. 2012. http://asmbs.org/. Accessed Nov 2012.
7. Herron DM. Establishing and organizing a Bariatric Surgery Program. In: Inabnet WB, DeMaria EJ, Ikramuddin S, editors. Laparoscopic bariatric surgery, vol. I. 1st ed. Philadelphia: Lippincott Williams and Wilkins; 2005. p. 23–31.
8. Thompson B. Weight loss surgery: finding the thin person hiding inside you. Tarentum: Word Association; 2003.
9. Makar B, Quilliot D, Zarnegar R, et al. What is the quality of information about bariatric surgery on the internet? Obes Surg. 2008;18(11):1455–9.
10. Frezza EE, Wachtel MS. A successful model of setting up a bariatric practice. Obes Surg. 2008;18:877–81.
11. Lautz DB, Jiser ME, Kelly JJ, et al. An update on best practice guidelines for specialized facilities and resources necessary for weight loss surgical programs. Obesity. 2009;17(5):911–7.
12. Association of periOperative Registered Nurses. AORN bariatric surgery guideline. AORN J. 2004;79:1026.
13. Jones SB, Jones DB. Obesity surgery: patient safety and best practices, vol. I. 1st ed. Woodbury: Cine-Med; 2009.
14. Toppino M, Cesarani F, Comba A. The role of early radiological studies after gastric bariatric surgery. Obes Surg. 2001;11(4):447–54.
15. Berger NK, Carr JJ, Erickson J, et al. Path to bariatric nurse certification: the practice analysis. Surg Obes Relat Dis. 2010;6:399.
16. Alvarez-Leite JI. Nutrient deficiencies secondary to bariatric surgery. Curr Opin Clin Nutr Metab Care. 2004;7:569.
17. Lizer NH, Papageorgeon H, Glembot TM. Nutritional and pharmacologic challenges in the bariatric surgery patient. Obes Surg. 2010;20:1654.
18. Greenberg I, Sogg S, Perna F. Behavioral and psychological care in weight loss surgery: best practice update. Obesity. 2009;17:880.
19. Kinzi JF, Schrattenecker M, Traweger C. Psychosocial predictors of weight loss after bariatric surgery. Obes Surg. 2006;16(12):1609–14.
20. Omalu BI, Cho P, Shakir AM. Suicides following bariatric surgery for the treatment of obesity. Surg Obes Relat Dis. 2005;1:447.
21. Bauchowitz AU, Gonder-Frederick LA, Olbrisch ME. Psychosocial evaluation of bariatric surgery candidates: a survey of present practices. Psychosom Med. 2005;67:625–832.
22. Poole NA, Al AA, Kuhanendran D. Compliance with surgical aftercare following bariatric surgery for morbid obesity: a retrospective study. Obes Surg. 2005;15:261–5.

23. Wheeler E, Prettyman A, Lenhard MJ, Tran K. Adherence to outpatient program postoperative appointments after bariatric surgery. Surg Obes Relat Dis. 2008;4:515–20.

24. Heldebrandt SE. Effects of participation in bariatric support group after Roux-en-Y gastric bypass. Obes Surg. 1998;8: 535–42.

25. Elakkary E, Elhorr A, Aziz F. Do Support groups play a role in weight loss after laparoscopic adjustable gastric banding? Obes Surg. 2006;16:331–4.

26. Angstadt J, Whipple O. Developing a New Bariatric Surgery Program. Am Surg. 2007;73:1092–7.

27. Tate DF. Effects of internet behavioral counseling on weight loss in adults at risk for type 2 diabetes. J Am Med Assoc. 2003;289(14): 1833–6.

28. Kalmbach WC. Covering your assets—estate planning. Paper presented at Master's postgraduate course, American Society for Bariatric Surgery Annual Meeting, June 18, 2003; Boston, MA.

29. Mccarthy J. Risk-management foundation. In: Jones SB, Jones DB, editors. Obesity surgery: patient safety and best practices, vol 1. 1st ed. Woodbury: Cine-Med; 2009. p. 443–62.

30. Claims common in bariatrics, but outcomes often favor surgeons. General Surgery News. 2012;39:10.

6

Essential Bariatric Equipment: Making Your Facility More Accommodating to Bariatric Surgical Patients

Hector Romero-Talamas and Stacy A. Brethauer

During the last few decades, the epidemic of obesity has been on the rise. Recent data suggests that in 2009–2010, over one-third of the adult population of the United States were obese [1]. Consequently, the number of specialized bariatric centers has also increased. Persons with morbid and super morbid obesity have special needs, which are often not met by conventional hospital equipment and furniture. Apart from the obvious size- and weight-related difficulties, the bariatric patient is often afraid of facing embarrassing situations that result from the distortion of their body contour and composition. This can be a great psychological burden, which in turn, prevents the patient from seeking medical attention when required. Moreover, there is reasonable evidence that despite the continuous implementation of antidiscrimination laws and policies, bariatric patients undergoing surgery continue to feel ignored and misinterpreted by those, who in theory, understand the genesis and mechanisms of the disease [2]. Hospitals with programs specifically addressing the surgical and medical needs of this population have an obligation to provide for their patients comfort and safety throughout their entire hospital experience. Anticipating the needs of the bariatric patient requires some experience, and meeting those needs requires some familiarity with what is available. Further, the reader is encouraged to consider this to be an ongoing endeavor of prioritizing essential and less necessary expenditures and of evaluating the results of these decisions. Guidelines and other publications are available as an aid for the new or establishing centers or practices [3–5].

This chapter is structured to answer the questions: What is bariatric equipment? Why does our facility or program need bariatric equipment? How can our program go about making our facility more accommodating to bariatric surgery patients with bariatric equipment? What are the essential equipment items that we should consider?

Definition

Broadly speaking, the term "bariatric equipment" refers to all of the "technology" utilized to administer health care to the morbidly obese population. Technology is the knowledge and application of principles involved in the production of objects for the accomplishment of specific ends [6].

In this chapter, we will further restrict our discussion to the equipment used in caring for patients undergoing bariatric surgical procedures, although much of the information is broadly applicable to caring for obese patients in any healthcare setting. Equipment can be categorized with respect to its function: diagnostic and/or therapeutic. Equipment may have a specific role in the bariatric surgical process: preoperative, operative, and postoperative. The focus of this chapter will be on the preoperative and postoperative needs. We will also discuss the needs for the bariatric patient in the emergency setting. Operative equipment and instruments are reviewed in Chap. 9.

Rationale

The concept that healing takes place in a "therapeutic patient environment" and by "putting the patient in the best condition for nature to act upon him" has been recognized for more than one century [7]. The increasing prevalence of obese and morbidly obese persons essentially mandate that healthcare facilities of all levels work toward making their facilities safe and effective for the specific needs resulting from large patient size and its accompanying comorbid conditions [8]. The combination of large size and often-limited mobility must also be taken into consideration. Moreover, there is a generalized conception that the severely obese patient has a different psychosocial profile, presumably as a result of a higher incidence of depression and isolation. This condition is frequently manifested by a high level of dependency and the presence of unrealistic expectations [9]. Safety is the most compelling reason for making your facility more accommodating to the needs of the morbidly obese patient [10, 11]. Better therapeutic and diagnostic outcomes can also be achieved with advanced planning [8, 12]. Modifications which safely enhance mobility have the additional benefit of preventing morbidity [13]. Safety for the healthcare staff is based on the need to prevent musculoskeletal injuries significantly associated with moving and physically caring for the morbidly obese patient. Many of these accidents and injuries are related to use of conventional but inadequate equipment especially for transferring and transporting patients [14–16].

Decreasing morbidity, especially that related to immobility, will enhance outcomes. Complications related to immobility include respiratory insufficiency, atelectasis, pneumonia, venous thromboembolic events, decubitus ulcers, hygiene-related skin problems, and falls [10, 11]. Other parameters that may also be affected by use of improved equipment include decreasing LOS, accidents involving obese family members, and excess nursing time used to improvise for the needs of the obese because of lack of bariatric equipment or because of inadequate space [17].

Diagnostic testing may also be hampered by inadequate equipment. Failure to perform routinely ordered tests because of patient size puts the bariatric patient at risk. Problems may be encountered in the simple measurement of blood pressure or weight without appropriate bariatric tools. Accurate results from UGI, CT scan, polysomnogram, or cardiac stress test all depend on meeting the specific needs resulting from patient size, weight, and limited mobility.

Efficiency of care is related to the availability of bariatric equipment. Prolonged waiting time for transport may be related to availability of adequate staff or equipment and wastes time, energy, and money. Enhanced satisfaction of the patient, families, and staff is clearly related to readily available and properly sized equipment. A patient who is cared for safely, efficiently, appropriately, and in a timely manner will see the facility and the caregivers as being prepared and competent. The caregivers will be better able to focus on the patient's clinical and personal needs without the distraction or even resentment generated by an increased risk of injury [13–18]. Rehabilitation may be possible only with specialized equipment including walkers or parallel bars, which accommodate the extra space and durability needed.

In 2009, an update on "Best Practice Guidelines for Specialized Facilities and Resources Necessary for Weight Loss Surgical Programs" was released. This document extends several recommendations that were written based on a thorough review of the available evidence, built in its majority by consensus and expert opinions. For the readers who are planning to or are in the process of starting a new center for the surgical management of obesity, these guidelines may prove to be an asset. They are divided into essential and optional recommendations [3] (Table 1).

TABLE 1. Bariatric facility infrastructure

Essential equipment recommendations
- Inpatient units (floor, ICU, PACU)
- Wide beds
  Standard to 440 lb
  Automated/adjustable to full sitting position
  Built-in scale
  Low air loss mattress
  Lifting/transferring equipment
  Wide commodes
  Wide wheelchairs, stretchers, walkers
  Monitoring devices
  Wide BP cuffs
  Biphasic defibrillators
  Sequential compression devices
  Emergency airway equipment
- Ambulatory facility
  Wide examination tables, bolted to floor
  Appropriately sized scales
- Radiology
  Automated wide tables with appropriate weight capacity
  CT, MRI, and interventional capability within 60 min
- Physical plant
  Dedicated floor, ICU, and PACU for bariatric patients
  Wide entrance doors to room and bathroom
  Floor-mounted toilets
  Elevators with wide doors and adequate weight capacity

Optional equipment recommendations
- Patient safety
  Inpatient units (floor, ICU, PACU)
    Wide beds
    Available to 880 lb
  Lifting/transferring equipment
    Ceiling mounted
  Monitoring equipment
    BP glove cuffs/wireless monitoring system
    Selective cardiac and apnea telemetry
  Ambulatory facility
    Wide automated examination tables
  Radiology
    In-house wide CT, MRI, and interventional facilities

Adapted from: Lautz DB, et al. (2009) Obesity (Silver Spring) 17:911-917

Investigation and Planning

The first step in initiating a bariatric clinic should be the creation of a multidisciplinary committee in which all the appropriate areas and stakeholders are represented. The committee should be in charge of evaluating the characteristics of the expected population and adapt the design of the facilities and the equipment to its specific needs. The approach that has worked the best in our experience to coordinate the implementation in bariatric equipment was the development of a bariatric task force (BTF). This can be a temporary problem-oriented group but most likely should function as a permanent committee that reviews the concerns relating to bariatric patients. Equipment and physical plant issues, in particular, will require ongoing attention (evaluation, updating, new construction, etc.). Prior to establishing the BTF, a fundamental presentation by a knowledgeable individual or group may provide an introduction to bariatric patients, equipment, surgical procedures, and surgical results for the hospital. Inclusion of department administrators goes a long way toward engendering some empathy and helps them to see why a BTF is needed. The task force should have a broad representation from all aspects of the facility—administration, parking, environmental services, transport, purchasing, nursing (intensive care units, intermediate care units, medical-surgical floors, clinics, administration, home care, bariatric coordinators, case managers, enterostomal therapy, outpatient surgery units, postanesthesia care units, operating room, and emergency room), nutrition, social work, physical therapy, radiology, cardiology, pulmonology, surgeons, and midlevel practitioners.

The first commission of the task force is to investigate the facility's assets and limitations with respect to the physical structural layout and available conventional and bariatric patient care equipment [8, 10]. Questions to ask are: How have you managed with morbidly obese patients up to this point? Which practitioners have had an interest in these patients (e.g., nurses, enterostomal therapist, physical therapist, pulmonologist)? What are the weight and width limitations of the currently available equipment starting with chairs in waiting rooms and hospital beds? Who are the vendors of bariatric equipment items already in use? What are the present policies for the utilization of bariatric equipment? What distances must the patients travel from the clinic and the acute care areas and to the diagnostic testing areas? The committee should systematically review each step of the patient's hospital experience from "home to home."

A second area of investigation should focus on what bariatric equipment is available for purchase. There are a number of reputable sources of information on products and companies. Vendors typically have websites with listings of a wide range of bariatric products with links.

A third area of investigation should focus on the characteristics of the patients expected to make up the service population in view of the hospital's prior experience with morbidly obese patients. The bariatric surgeons should be questioned with respect to their expectations for maximum and median weight and BMI. In our practice, the first 500 patients had a weight range from 190 to 473 lb (86–215 kg) with BMIs from 35 to 69. Thus contingency plans for patients greater than 500 lb (227 kg) and BMIs greater than 70 were needed, recognizing that these would represent a relatively small number.

One of the goals of these investigations will be to prioritize purchases and other adaptations in the environment. The task force should develop criteria for their utilization. For example, in our institution, we did not have a dedicated bariatric surgical floor, and there were hospital beds in the facility of a variety of vintages and models. The standard hospital beds had a variety of weight limits, 350–500 lb (159–227 kg) and widths of 34–36 in. (86–91 cm). The lowest of these weight limits had to become the maximum permitted for the use of a standard hospital bed. Similarly, the mattresses on the beds also had weight ratings, 325–400 lb

(147–182 kg). This led to the protocol that all patients with a weight over 325 lb (147 kg) and/or a BMI greater than 55 (to capture the width parameter) would require a bariatric bed [19]. Criteria-based protocols help to utilize the hospital's resources most effectively and allow for preplanning as the patient population changes [12, 13].

Essential Bariatric Equipment

Utilization of bariatric equipment does not ensure proper health care but can greatly improve the quality and safety of care [13]. Both caregivers and patients should receive specific instructions for using specialized bariatric equipment properly in order to fully benefit from the advantages, which this equipment offers.

This review of bariatric furniture and equipment which should be considered is based on available literature and the authors' experience in caring for over 4,000 bariatric surgical patients [8, 11, 12, 14, 19–24]. The following discussion will follow the surgical patient through the entire hospital course, from "home to home" which is divided clinically into the preoperative, operative, and postoperative periods. Since the operative period is discussed in detail elsewhere (see Chap. 10), this chapter reviews the equipment needs of the preoperative and postoperative morbidly obese patient.

Table 2 lists the bariatric equipment items discussed along with contact information for some of the vendors.

Preoperative

At times, patients will not be able to come to the facility by independent means and require an ambulance. The team should collect information on the ambulance services in the surrounding area and how they are equipped for the transportation of morbidly obese patients. A number of modifications can be made to ambulance equipment and to transportation protocols to assure that the service provided is a safe, efficient, comfortable, and dignified experience [18].

Transportation Equipment

When considering the transportation of obese individuals, different scenarios call for different devices. Several questions should be considered by the caregiver in charge: are there enough personnel to move the patient? Is there a weight limit to be considered for the use of the available transportation device? Will the maneuver be safe for the team and the patient? A number of devices have been designed to better address these issues.

Temporary Transfer

The first step for transporting the patient is to safely get the subject to the definitive device. In many cases, the patient is

TABLE 2. Bariatric equipment information listing

Patient transfer		
Most commonly used size: 34 in., use 39 in. for very large patients		
Hovermatt	Website: www.hovermatt.com	1-800-471-2776
AirPal	Website: www.airpal.com	1-800-633-4725
Reliant 600 Patient Lift		
Invacare Corporation	Website: www.invacare.com	1-800-333-6900
Stryker	Website: www.stryker.com	1-800-869-0770
Beds		
Bed and mattress weight capacity 1,000 lb, 39-in. mattresses		
Wheelchairs		
Size: 26-, 28-, and 30-in. widths, seat depths 22 in., 750. weight capacity		
Commode chairs		
Width 30 in., weight capacity 750 lb, seat depth 23 in.		
Invacare Corporation	Website: www.invacare.com	1-800-333-6900
KCI (BariKare)	Website: www.kci1.com	1-888-275-4524
Stryker	Website: www.stryker.com	1-800-869-0770
Shower chair		
Width 30 in., weight capacity 750 lb, seat depth 23 in.		
Hill-Rom	Website: www.hill-rom.com	1-800-445-3730
KCI	Website: www.kci1.com	1-888-275-4524
Invacare Corporation	Website: www.invacare.com	1-800-333-6900
Scales		
Weight capacity 600–880 lb		
Scale-Tronix	Website: www.scale-tronix.com	1-800-873-2001
Tanita Corp. of America	Website: www.tanita.com	(847)-640-9241
Furniture		
Nemschoff	Website: www.nemschoff.com	1-800-203-8916
Sauder Manufacturing	Website: www.saudermanufacturing.com	1-800-537-1530
Chair: Special Edition Series 30 and 40-in. widths		
Folding Chair–Lifetime Inc.	Website: www.lifetime.com	1-800-225-3865
Examination tables		
Midmark	Website: www.midmark.com	1-800-MIDMARK
United Metal Fabricators	Website: www.umf-exam.com	1-800-638-5322
Hausmann Inc.	Website: www.hausmann.com	1-888-428-7626
Stretchers		
Stryker Medical Inc.	Website: www.med.stryker.com	1-800-STRYKER
Hill-Rom Inc.	Website: www.hill-rom.com	1-800-445-3730
Gendron Inc.	Website: www.gendroninc.com	1-800-537-2521
Gowns/pants		
Size 10XL and 3XL		
Superior Pad Outfitters	Website: www.superiorpads.com	1-888-855-7970
104 in/107 in		
Calderon Textiles	Website: www.calderonhealth.com	1-888-742-1998

found to be lying on the floor or in other difficult positions as a result of a fall or an accident. In this scenario, one recommendation is the Transfer-Flat (Stryker) (Fig. 1). This vinyl device has a maximum weight capacity of 1,600 lb (727 kg) and can be operated by a maximum of 12 persons. This is a versatile aid in minimizing injuries to the transporting personnel. Another clever alternative for patient lifting is the HoverJack™ Air Patient Lift. This is a great option to lift a patient without the need of a team. This item is constructed with multiple independent air compartments that can be inflated separately until the desired height is reached (Fig. 2). Another transfer device is the HoverMatt™ Air Transfer System for lateral transfers. Since this product eliminates the necessity to lift, the caregivers' safety is ensured while maintaining patient's comfort (Fig. 3).

Wheelchairs and Stretchers

In the past, many facilities invested in oversized wheelchairs, as this was one of the first areas where it was recognized that one size does not fit all. Initially, manufacturers simply took standard wheelchair design and made them wider to accommodate the larger patients' needs. However, a good bariatric wheelchair is specifically engineered for the extra weight as well as size of the morbidly obese patient. It should come in a number of widths, 24–30 in. (60–76 cm), and have a weight capacity of at least 750 lb (340 kg) (Fig. 4).

Similarly, stretchers were not designed for the morbidly obese patient and increasing weight limit modifications have been incorporated over the years. A good stretcher for the bariatric patients will have the appropriate weight rating in

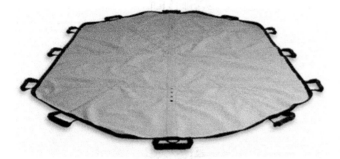

Fig. 1. The transfer-flat for bariatric patient transfer (Courtesy of Stryker, Kalamazoo, MI).

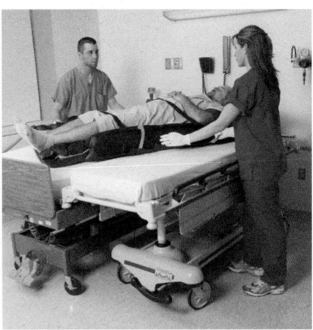

Fig. 3. HoverMatt™ Air Transfer System for lateral transfers (Courtesy of HoverTech International, Bethlehem, PA).

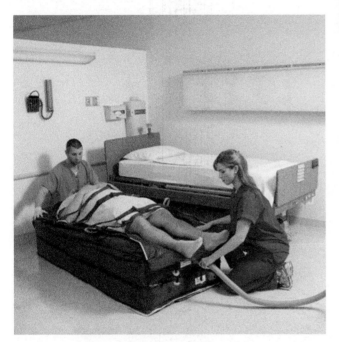

Fig. 2. HoverJack™ Air Patient Lift (Courtesy of HoverTech International, Bethlehem, PA).

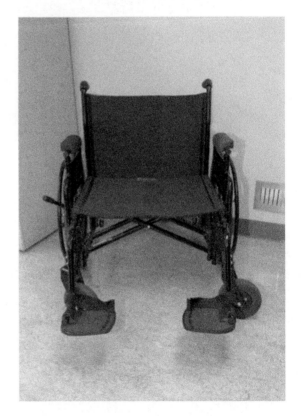

Fig. 4. Bariatric wheelchair (Invacare) (Picture Courtesy of Bariatric and Metabolic Institute, Cleveland Clinic, Cleveland, OH).

addition to adjustability of the head section and overall height. A crucial factor is the stretcher width. Space is a limiting factor in the successful passage through elevators, hallways, and doorways, but the width of the stretcher affects patient comfort and the potential for pressure morbidity. Many facilities use stretchers such as the Stryker M series with a weight limit of 500–700 lb (227–317 kg), a height range of between 20.75 and 34.5 in. (53–87 cm), and a patient surface width of 26–30 in. (66–76 cm), with side-rails-up width of 33.5–37 in. (85–94 cm). The Prime Series Stretchers by Stryker have the same weight capacity (700 lb) and include special features such as positioning controls for the patient and the caregiver. In addition, the Zoom Motorized Drive System can be incorporated to eliminate the need for manual pushing thus diminishing the risk of injuries for the transporting personnel (Fig. 5a). These are adequate for the majority of patients provided that they are not to be

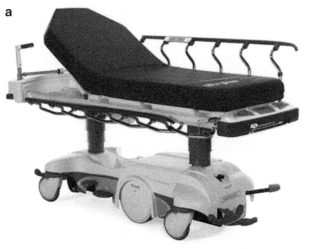

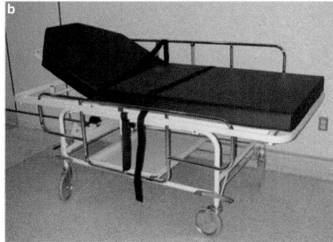

FIG. 5. (**a**) Stryker's Prime Series Stretcher plus Zoom Motorized Drive System. (Courtesy of Stryker, Kalamazoo, MI). (**b**) Bariatric gurney (Courtesy of Stryker, Kalamazoo, MI)

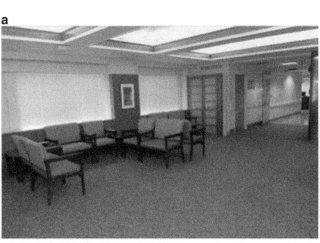

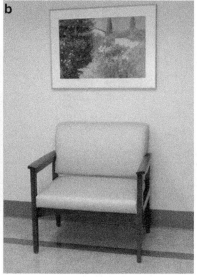

FIG. 6. (**a**) Bariatric waiting room (Courtesy of Bariatric and Metabolic Institute, Cleveland Clinic, Cleveland, OH). (**b**) Bariatric chair in vital signs area (Courtesy of Bariatric and Metabolic Institute, Cleveland Clinic, Cleveland, OH)

used for extended periods due to pressure concerns. All facilities should have the availability of a bariatric stretcher for those instances where these limitations are exceeded. A bariatric stretcher will have a weight limit of 1,000 lb (454 kg) and a patient surface width of 39 in. (99 cm) (Fig. 5b). These dimensions make it more difficult to negotiate in tight halls, elevators, and rooms, and the patient's route to critical areas should be tested in advance, including potential routes for diagnostic testing and emergencies.

Chairs

One of the common concerns of a morbidly obese patient is that they will break furniture, especially chairs or get stuck in

the chair causing them extreme embarrassment or even injury. Typically the chairs in medical office waiting rooms are not weight rated specifically or are rated up to only 300 lb (136 kg). Their widths are usually from 20 to 24 in. (50–60 cm) and often have limiting arms. A bariatric chair should have a width of between 28 and 44 in. (72 and 112 cm) and a weight rating of 600–750 lb (272–341 kg) (Fig. 6a, b). Another important factor is the height of the chair. Some morbidly obese persons are also of short stature. Adjustability of the chair height is a feature offered on some models. These chairs can be used in waiting rooms, hallways, and in the patients' rooms postoperatively.

For group information sessions or support groups, a portable and relatively inexpensive folding chair is especially helpful. There are folding chairs that have weight capacities of up to 500 lb (227 kg), are without arms, and offer flexibility in seating arrangements for discussions (Fig. 7).

Commodes

Another important facility/clinic item is the availability of an appropriate commode. The standard wall-mounted model is not safe (Fig. 8a). Additional structural support can be added under an existing wall-mounted commode to provide sufficient weight-bearing capacity. Beginning April 2000, the ANSI standard for pedestal commodes was increased to 500 lb (227 kg) (Fig. 8b). In addition, the commode will require adequate surrounding space to accommodate the morbidly obese (Fig. 8c).

Scales and Height-Measuring Devices

Easy and accurate measure of weight and height in bariatric patients is essential to calculate body mass index (BMI) and to track clinical changes associated with fluid management. A number of manufacturers have responded to this challenge with an array of products. Our team has used Scale-Tronix models. The important features of a scale are: accuracy, stability, ample standing platform, a weight limit above 750 lb (340 kg), portability, attachable height gauge, and wheelchair accessibility. These models have weight limits of 1,000 lb (445 kg). Many products come with a height measure attached. The most recent models combine all of these virtues thus offering better accessibility and portability in low-profile, heavy-duty devices (Fig. 9a, b).

Blood Pressure Monitoring (Standard Cuffs and New Technology)

It is commonly understood that an adequately large cuff size is required to get an accurate blood pressure reading. In morbidly obese patients, these measurements are difficult to obtain. The American Heart Association recommends a cuff that covers 40 % of the arm circumference and at least 80 % of the length [25]. The large adult size or the thigh size cuffs must be readily available in clinics (Fig. 10). In an effort to simplify the blood pressure measurements, alternative technologies have arisen. One example is the introduction of a wrist-mounted device that estimates blood pressure based on pulsations of the radial artery. This has proven to be a reliable tool in lean patients. Unfortunately, when compared to

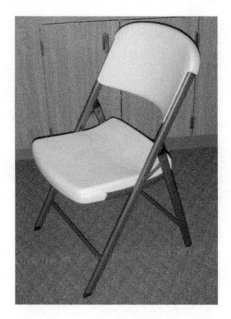

FIG. 7. Folding chair with weight limit of 500 lb

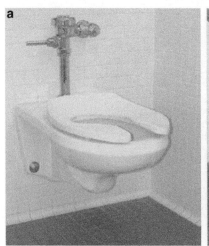 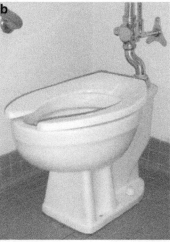 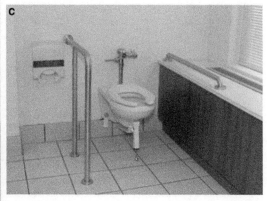

FIG. 8. (a) Wall-mounted commode. (b) Pedestal commode. (c) Handrails and adequate space around the commode (Courtesy of Bariatric and Metabolic Institute, Cleveland Clinic, Cleveland, OH)

FIG. 9. (**a**) Bariatric Portable Stand-On Scale with weight limit of 1,000 lb (Courtesy of Scale-Tronix). (**b**) Adjustable Bariatric Wheelchair Scale. (Courtesy of Scale-Tronix).

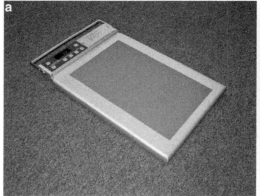
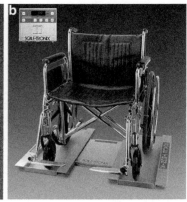

FIG. 10. Multiple sizes of blood pressure cuffs (*Source*: *Top*, Welch Allyn, Skaneateles Falls, NY, with permission; *middle* and *bottom*, American Diagnostic Corporation, Hauppauge, NY, with permission).

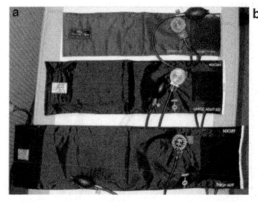
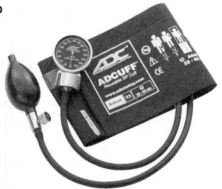

arterial catheterization, considerable differences in individual mean measurements can be observed, thus making this technology an unsuitable replacement for invasive monitoring in the intraoperative setting [26, 27].

Examination Tables

Morbidly obese persons may have difficulty ascending the examination table. Both height and stability must be taken into account. Standard examination tables are often about 33 in. (84 cm) in height with a 7 in. (18 cm) step. The obese person can destabilize the table using the step. Extra width is also required. The needs of a majority of patients are met by bariatric tables like the Midmark® Model 405 which has height adjustments from 26 to 37 in. (68–94 cm), a weight limit of 600 lb (273 kg), and a width of 26 in. (68 cm) (Fig. 11). However, the power functions of tilt and lift serve only up to 300 lb (137 kg). For those super obese patients, the availability of a bariatric examination table like the Hausmann Inc. Model 4795 is helpful. It offers a 600-lb (273 kg) weight limit, a powered height range of 20–29 in. (51–74 cm), a width of 32 in. (81 cm), and a powered back rest that rises to 75°.

X-Rays and Other Imaging Modalities

The increased prevalence of obesity and associated comorbidities mixed with the rapid spread and success of bariatric

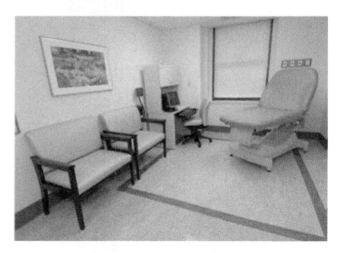

FIG. 11. Bariatric examination room and table (Courtesy of Bariatric and Metabolic Institute, Cleveland Clinic, Cleveland, OH).

surgery have elevated the need for adequate imaging equipment [28].

When obtaining standard radiographic studies in obese subjects, a number of problems, such as difficult positioning, attenuation of the X-ray beam, the presence of artifacts, and low-quality images, can arise. Certain strategies, such as increments of the radiological parameters, the use of multiple cassettes, and cassette-mapping techniques, can be useful [29]. Ultrasonography is frequently used as part of the available diagnostic tests for the management of the obese patient.

It is considered brief, inexpensive, and free of radioactivity. However, a thick abdominal wall may null all of these advantages. It is estimated that in a patient with 8 cm of subcutaneous fat, 94 % of the original sound wave is attenuated before it reaches the peritoneal cavity. A possible solution to this issue is the use of harmonic imaging. This device generates the waves within the tissue, thus increasing the penetrance of the beam. This results in better resolution and reduced artifacts [28].

Preoperative and postoperative upper GI studies and abdominal CT scans are frequently required to assess comorbid conditions, variant anatomy, and complications such as leak of the anastomosis [30]. Even in the best of circumstances, the quality of these studies may be inferior, but it is important that the patients size can be accommodated by the diagnostic facilities and equipment [31].

Fluoroscopy equipment has limitations in the image quality and weight limits regarding articulation of the table. Full articulation of most tables has a weight limit of 300 lb (137 kg). The footboards on the tables have weight limits of between 300 and 350 lb (137–159 kg) depending on the model. Larger patients' studies are often obtained in the standing position (on the floor) with a sacrifice of optimal image control. The Luminos Agile by Siemens offers a high-capacity (606 lb/275 kg) static table with a full-tilt function and high-quality imaging (Fig. 12).

The limitations with abdominal CT scanning in the bariatric patients relate to the weight limitations of the power table, the diameter of the entry port, as well as the overall imaging power. Exceeding the recommended parameters may produce considerable damage to the equipment and may be hazardous for the patient. Although CT may be considered the best imaging modality for severely obese patients, accommodating these patients may be troublesome. The body habitus of these patients makes positioning and intravenous access especially difficult. In addition, the size of the display and the quality of the image may not be appropriate [29]. Fortunately, new technologies, such as the multidetector CT with larger gantry entries (up to 90 cm) and extended field of view, are now available. Another, better example is the SOMATOM Sensation Open scan by Siemens, which combines the latest imaging technology with a large 82 cm gantry opening, ideal for CT-guided interventions in bariatric patients (Fig. 13a). The mixture of these technologies with appropriate obesity CT protocols has resulted in significant improvements in this aspect of care [32] (Fig. 13b). Even though the magnetic

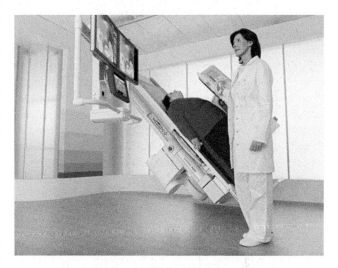

FIG. 12. The Siemens Luminos Agile Fluoroscopy System offers a high-capacity platform with full-tilt function. (Courtesy of Siemens Corporation).

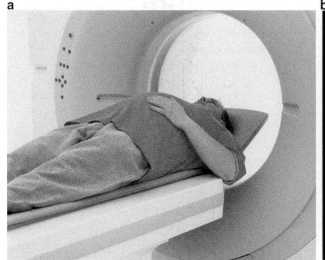

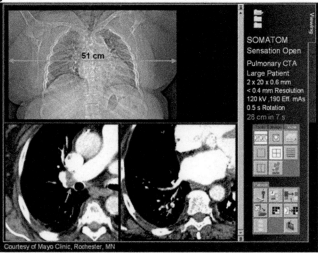

FIG. 13. (**a**) The SOMATOM Sensation Open scan by Siemens allows for simplified scanning of bariatric patients. (Courtesy of Siemens Corporation). (**b**) Clinical images from SOMATOM Sensation Open scan by Siemens. Different dosages are automatically tailored according to the patient's body shape in the topogram. (Courtesy of Siemens Corporation).

resonance imaging (MRI) could be considered a valuable diagnostic resource in the obese patients, it is seldom used in the perioperative care of bariatric patients.

Cardiac Risk Stratification Equipment

Cardiac risk stratification in high-risk morbidly obese patients in preparation for bariatric surgery has many limitations. The most frequently used SPECT myocardial perfusion study has weight limitations of about 300 lb (137 kg) due to the camera. The planar scans can be performed in patients up to 400 lb range, but the risk of false positives increases at the higher weights. Dobutamine stress echocardiogram studies can be performed on morbidly obese patients, but anatomic and operator variability decreases the accuracy and reliability. Cardiac catheterization, the gold standard in risk stratification, is difficult to perform technically due to vascular access problems and has weight limitations of 350 lb (159 kg) due to the table. A limited catheterization without table articulation or on an alternative stretcher can be performed as an alternative. These equipment weight and performance limitations leave cardiac risk stratification in obese patients in a less than optimal state especially at weights greater than 400 lb (182 kg), which can be altogether prohibitive for some studies.

Postoperative

Beds and Mattresses

Beds and mattresses are considered a cornerstone of the in-hospital experience for the bariatric patient. Their importance lies not only in the concept of comfort but also in the fact that complications such as rhabdomyolysis and skin-related problems can be prevented [33, 34]. Standard hospital beds have weight ratings between 350 and 500 lb (159–227 kg). It is important to check with the manufacturer for the weight rating according to the model(s) and vintage(s). Most recent models have weight ratings of up to 500 lb (227 kg), and this would serve the majority of patients. The standard mattress on the bed also will have a weight rating often between 300 and 500 lb (136–227 kg). They also are available in a number of different types of surfaces. It is very reasonable to routinely use a pressure reduction mattress recognizing the high risk for developing pressure ulcerations [13, 35].

The width of the patient and bed must be considered. Standard hospital beds are typically from 34 to 36 in. (86–91 cm) often with the critical care beds tending to be the narrowest. Manufactures recommend often that a patient be fitted for the need for a bariatric bed by having the patient measured lying flat. This is not often practical prior to surgery. We and others have adopted utilization of a BMI parameter to take into account the width of the patient [36]. Our criteria-based protocol calls for a bariatric bed and

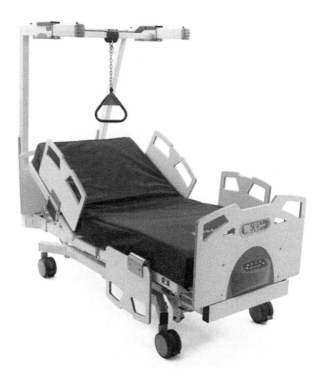

FIG. 14. Stryker's Bari 10A Bariatric Bed. Equipped with an in-bed scale, provides a 1,000 lb capacity and expandable length and width. (Courtesy of Stryker, Kalamazoo, MI).

wheelchair for those patients 325 lb (150 kg) or a BMI of 55 or greater.

Special bariatric beds offer a number of options requiring choices at the time of purchase or rental. There are two types in regard to entry—the side entry (as with standard beds) and those that allow bottom entry and some easily allow both. The side entry looks more like the standard hospital bed and may have fewer stigmas for the majority of bariatric surgical patients who are, for the most part, free to ambulate. The bottom entry beds can often be converted into a chair position to facilitate ambulation and possibly lead to fewer staff injuries related to patient ambulation. Special bariatric beds, like Stryker's Bari 10A, offer a 1,000 lb weight capacity and are expandable. This particular item is able to go from 80″ to 88″ in. length and from 36″ to 48″ in. width. It also includes an in-bed scale that can be quite useful when the patient experiences a prolonged hospital stay (Fig. 14). Other features to take into consideration are: the type of side rail adjustment, the wheels and locks, the height adjustment parameters, ability to attach over-bed trapezes, and the complexity and ease of use of the hand controls. Another important consideration is that the bed should be able to be placed in at least 45° of reverse Trendelenburg easily; this is the optimum position for pulmonary function given that many of the patients have ventilatory comorbid conditions (obstructive sleep apnea, obesity hypoventilation syndrome, and restrictive lung disease) and may in some cases require tracheotomy and ventilatory support [37].

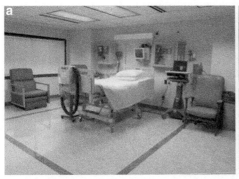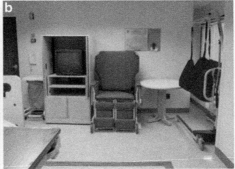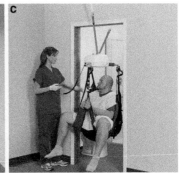

FIG. 15. (**a**) Bariatric inpatient room with adequate space around bed. (Courtesy of Bariatric and Metabolic Institute, Cleveland Clinic, Cleveland, OH). (**b**) Bariatric recliner chair in inpatient room and patient lift (*right*). (Courtesy of Bariatric and Metabolic Institute, Cleveland Clinic, Cleveland, OH). (**c**) HoverTrans® Roomer ceiling lift for horizontal room-to-room transfer. (Courtesy of HoverTech International, Bethlehem, PA).

Hospital Patient Room Layout, Equipment, and Fixtures

The design of a bariatric facility should not be solely focused on making everything "supersized." Concepts like functionality, ergonomics, dignity, and other ideas are to be considered. The layout of the hospital room is the basic building block of a bariatric nursing unit and most influential in the administering of nursing care postoperatively. A dedicated unit with a dedicated staff is most preferable but at present is not the norm. The driving force in the design and layout is the large patient size and weight requiring many pieces of oversized and extremely durable equipment (already noted) and safety in negotiating around the patient by the staff. The American Institute of Architects has recommended to plan the design, taking into consideration the following parameters: (a) average patient, 330 lb; (b) bariatric visits of 450–510 lb; (c) design target, "minimum" of 500 lb; and (d) design drop weight, 700 lb [38].

In an effort to establish industry standards, the Hill-Rom Company formed a Bariatric Room Design Advisory Board (BRDAB). They made a number of recommendations with respect to room space, target maximum weight tolerance for room equipment and fixtures, and which equipment a patient room should have [17]. They recommended 5 ft (152 cm) of space around a bed to allow for the passage of oversized equipment (Fig. 15a) that necessitates an overall room size of at least 13 ft (4 m) in width and 15 ft (4.6 m) in depth from the corridor. The opening for this space should be ideally 60 in. (152 cm) with an unequally divided leaf-swinging door, one leaf being 42 in. (107 cm). The BRDAB sets a target maximum of 1,000 lb (454 kg) as a recommendation for room equipment and fixture weight tolerance. In many cases, this would not be possible at present. They recommended that other room equipment for consideration would be a bedside chair (specification as noted in earlier section) and a lift. Lifts are essential to have available due to the high number of

staff and patient-related injuries associated with patient lifting and transfer [39]. They recommended that a mobile portable lift is most applicable due to the flexibility to accommodate the patient in any portion of the room (Fig. 15b). One example of a mobile lift is the Invacare Reliant 600 that features an electric motor and a lift of up to 660 lb (300 kg). Another option is the HoverTrans® Roomer ceiling lift. This alternative is especially valuable when it comes to room-to-room transport. It has a weight maximum capacity of 480 lb (Fig. 15c).

Hygiene Items: Toilets, Showers, and Gowns/Pants

Personal hygiene can be difficult for the bariatric surgical patient due to space issues, limited mobility, and the need for a durable environment. Toileting will require a bathroom with an opening to tolerate 60 in. (152 cm) in width, the width of the widest wheelchair. Commodes will require handrails to enable the patient to self-assist (b). For those patients with minimal mobility but able to weight bear and transfer, a bedside commode is an excellent option over use of a bedpan. These especially allow for increased safety, comfort, and dignity. These should have a width of at least 30 in. (76 cm) and a weight capacity of at least 750 lb (341 kg).

The BRDAB recommends that a shower space be at least 45 square feet (4.17 m²), large enough to accommodate the assistance of two caregivers and accommodate wheelchair access. Each patient room may not be able to have this space available, and a reasonable option for showering is a communal shower; we have utilized this concept with excellent review from the patients. The BRDAB also recommend waterproof walls and floor, with a drainage sloping floor without curbs for easy entry and exit (Fig. 16a). A portable shower chair/bench either a commode chair combination model or a stand-alone is a necessity (Fig. 16b).

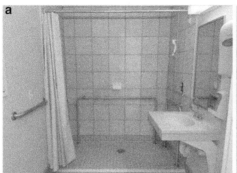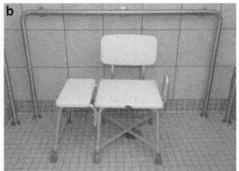

FIG. 16. (**a**) Large shower room with unobstructed access to shower. (Courtesy of Bariatric and Metabolic Institute, Cleveland Clinic, Cleveland, OH). (**b**) Shower chair (Courtesy of Bariatric and Metabolic Institute, Cleveland Clinic, Cleveland, OH).

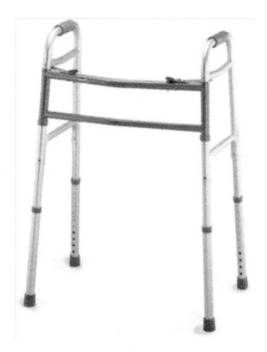

FIG. 17. A walker designed for bariatric patients has a deep and wide frame, adjustable height, and can support up to 700 lb. A wheel kit can be added on if needed. (© Invacare Corporation. Used with permission).

The availability of appropriate fitting hospital clothing is essential to safety, hygiene, and dignity. Since the morbidly obese are also not all the same size or shape, a few sizes of gowns (3X–10X) and pants (X–4X) should be readily available. The gowns should accommodate peripheral intravenous lines.

Many severely obese patients have chronic osteoarthritis affecting their back, hips, and knees. Postoperatively and upon discharge from the hospital, these patients may temporarily require a walker to avoid falls during their recovery from surgery. A walker designed specifically for the bariatric patient should be obtained. These walkers have a wide base, adjustable height, and can support up to 700 lb of weight (Fig. 17). A wheel kit can be added on to provide additional assistance with ambulation.

Periodic Reevaluation

It is important to revaluate patient anthropometric data, the equipment utilization numbers, comorbidity related to immobilization, accidents or falls involving patients, staff injuries, and overall surgical outcome data. Bariatric surgical programs including surgeons, staff, patient characteristic, and facilities will mature over time and require further evaluation of equipment needs and use criteria.

Summary

Bariatric equipment includes all of the "technology" utilized to administer health care to the morbidly obese patient. This equipment is essential in providing quality bariatric surgical care by providing for safety, reducing morbidity, and enhancing mobility thereby promoting the best possible outcomes. Further, adequately sized accommodations and equipment allow for accurate diagnostic testing and reduce stress and wasted time. These benefits promote dignity of the patients, improving satisfaction of patient, family, and staff. To achieve this, a facility must investigate their own resources and limitations, based on their current management of morbidly obese patients, survey the market in bariatric equipment, and evaluate their patient base. A BTF is a good organizational structure to coordinate this activity. Ultimately, criteria-based protocols will be developed to guide the appropriate utilization of bariatric equipment resources. These will need intermittent revision as the program matures and technology advances. The process requires and ongoing communication among clinicians and administrators and between equipment manufacturers and clinicians in the further refinement and development of additional technology to better care for the morbidly obese patient [8, 12].

References

1. Ogden CL, Carroll MD, Kit BK, Flegal KM. Prevalence of obesity in the United States, 2009-2010. NCHS Data Brief. 2012;82:1–8.

2. Kaminsky J, Gadaleta D. A study of discrimination within the medical community as viewed by obese patients. Obes Surg. 2002;12: 14–8.

3. Lautz DB, Jiser ME, Kelly JJ, Shikora SA, Partridge SK, Romanelli JR, Cella RJ, Ryan JP. An update on best practice guidelines for specialized facilities and resources necessary for weight loss surgical programs. Obesity (Silver Spring). 2009;17:911–7.

4. Whittemore AD, Kelly J, Shikora S, Cella RJ, Clark T, Selbovitz L, Flint L. Specialized staff and equipment for weight loss surgery patients: best practice guidelines. Obes Res. 2005;13:283–9.

5. Frezza EE, Wachtel MS. A successful model of setting up a bariatric practice. Obes Surg. 2008;18:877–81.

6. Gallagher S. The human element of advanced technology. Ostomy Wound Manage. 2003;49:24, 26, 28.

7. Nightingale F. Notes on nursing what it is, and what it is not. London: Harrison; 1860.

8. Foil MB, Collier MS, MacDonald Jr KG, Pories WJ. Availability and adequacy of diagnostic and therapeutic equipment for the morbidly obese patient in an acute care setting. Obes Surg. 1993;3:153–6.

9. Drake D, Dutton K, Engelke M, McAuliffe M, Rose MA. Challenges that nurses face in caring for morbidly obese patients in the acute care setting. Surg Obes Relat Dis. 2005;1:462–6.

10. Barr J, Cunneen J. Understanding the bariatric client and providing a safe hospital environment. Clin Nurse Spec. 2001;15:219–23.

11. Sarr MG, Felty CL, Hilmer DM, Urban DL, O'Connor G, Hall BA, Rooke TW, Jensen MD. Technical and practical considerations involved in operations on patients weighing more than 270 kg. Arch Surg. 1995;130:102–5.

12. Gallagher S, Arzouman J, Lacovara J, Blackett A, McDonald PK, Traver G, Bartholomeaux F. Criteria-based protocols and the obese patient: planning care for a high-risk population. Ostomy Wound Manage. 2004;50:32–34, 36, 38 passim.

13. Gallagher SM. Restructuring the therapeutic environment to promote care and safety for the obese patient. J Wound Ostomy Continence Nurs. 1999;26:292–7.

14. Nguyen NT, Moore C, Stevens CM, Chalifoux S, Mavandadi S, Wilson SE. The practice of bariatric surgery at academic medical centers. J Gastrointest Surg. 2004;8:856–60; discussion 860–851.

15. Retsas A, Pinikahana J. Manual handling activities and injuries among nurses: an Australian hospital study. J Adv Nurs. 2000;31: 875–83.

16. Gallagher S. Caring for the overweight patient in the acute care setting: addressing caregiver injury. J Healthc Saf Compl Infect. 2000;4:379–82.

17. Harrell JW, Miller B. Big challenge. Designing for the needs of bariatric patients. Health Facil Manage. 2004;17:34–8.

18. Weiss J, Perham D, Forrest J. Build your own bariatric unit: southwest ambulance creates a better way to transport obese patients. JEMS. 2003;28:36–45.

19. Gourash W. Lecture entitled bariatric equipment: making your facility more accommodating for the morbidly obese. Minimally Invasive Surgery for Morbid Obesity and GERD related topics, School of Medicine and the Minimally Invasive Surgery Center of the University of Pittsburgh Medical Center; 2001

20. Hilmer DM. Technical considerations of bariatric surgery in the super obese. Surg Technol. 1994;26:8–12. quiz 13.

21. AORN. Bariatric surgery guideline. AORN. 2004;79:1026–52.

22. Recommendations for facilities performing bariatric surgery. Bull Am Coll Surg. 2000;85:20–3.

23. Martin LF, Burney M, Faitor-Stampley V, Wheeler T, Raum WJ. Preparing a hospital for bariatric patients. New York: McGraw-Hill; 2003.

24. Martinez-Owens T. Special needs of the bariatric surgical office. New York: McGraw-Hill; 2003.

25. Veiga EV, Arcuri EA, Cloutier L, Santos JL. Blood pressure measurement: arm circumference and cuff size availability. Rev Lat Am Enfermagem. 2009;17:455–61.

26. Hager H, Mandadi G, Pulley D, Eagon JC, Mascha E, Nutter B, Kurz A. A comparison of noninvasive blood pressure measurement on the wrist with invasive arterial blood pressure monitoring in patients undergoing bariatric surgery. Obes Surg. 2009;19: 717–24.

27. Helmut H, Mandadi G, Eagon C, Pulley D, Kurz A. Intraoperative blood pressure measurement on the wrist is more accurate than on the upper arm in morbidly obese patients. Abstract presented at the American Society of Anesthesia 2004 annual meeting; 2004.

28. Modica MJ, Kanal KM, Gunn ML. The obese emergency patient: imaging challenges and solutions. Radiographics. 2011;31: 811–23.

29. Carucci LR. Imaging obese patients: problems and solutions. Abdom Imaging. 2013;38(4):630–46.

30. Blachar A, Federle MP, Pealer KM, Ikramuddin S, Schauer PR. Gastrointestinal complications of laparoscopic Roux-en-Y gastric bypass surgery: clinical and imaging findings. Radiology. 2002; 223:625–32.

31. Uppot P. How obesity hinders image quality and diagnosis in radiology. Bariatrics Today. 2005;1:31–3.

32. Uppot RN. Impact of obesity on radiology. Radiol Clin North Am. 2007;45:231–46.

33. Rush A, Muir M. Maintaining skin integrity bariatric patients. Br J Community Nurs. 2012;17(154):156–9.

34. de Menezes Ettinger JE, dos Santos Filho PV, Azaro E, Melo CA, Fahel E, Batista PB. Prevention of rhabdomyolysis in bariatric surgery. Obes Surg. 2005;15:874–9.

35. Brown S. Bed surfaces and pressure sore prevention: an abridged report. Orthop Nurs. 2001;20:30–40.

36. Fruto LV, Malancy K, Forbis J, Cochran J. Development of decision guidelines for specialty bed/mattress selection for obese patients. Ostomy Wound Manag. 1997;43:66.

37. Burns SM, Egloff MB, Ryan B, Carpenter R, Burns JE. Effect of body position on spontaneous respiratory rate and tidal volume in patients with obesity, abdominal distension and ascites. Am J Crit Care. 1994;3:102–6.

38. Andrade SD. Planning and design guidelines for bariatric healthcare. Acad J. 2006.

39. Evanoff B, Wolf L, Aton E, Canos J, Collins J. Reduction in injury rates in nursing personnel through introduction of mechanical lifts in the workplace. Am J Ind Med. 2003;44:451–7.

7

Patient Selection: Pathways to Surgery

Monica Dua, Eric P. Ahnfeldt, and Derrick Cetin

Clinical Pathways

Clinical pathways are increasingly used in various fields of surgery to create a standardized approach to maximize clinical efficiency and optimize patient outcomes [1–5]. Pathways are defined as structured multidisciplinary treatment plans which detail the routine care of the uncomplicated patient for a specific condition over a given time frame. These plans document the sequence and progression of actions needed to decrease treatment variation and provide coordination of care among different disciplines [6]. As bariatric surgery is an elective procedure, it is important that individuals considering weight-loss surgery be carefully selected and medically optimized to minimize surgical risk. Several studies have examined the impact of perioperative clinical pathways in bariatric surgery and demonstrated quality improvements and economic benefits [7]. These include reduced variability in patient care patterns [8], enhanced recovery schemes [9], decreased length of stay [5], and decreased resource utilization contributing to cost-efficient care [5, 10]. Although specific medical guidelines exist for the clinical practice of multidisciplinary care provided in support of the bariatric patient [11, 12], individual bariatric centers use different institution-specific perioperative patient evaluation protocols. We will discuss the essential components of a preoperative bariatric surgery evaluation and present a protocol for patient assessment which was developed and is currently in routine use within the Bariatric and Metabolic Institute at the Cleveland Clinic, Ohio.

Preoperative Components

Patients seeking to proceed with bariatric surgery need to be well informed and prepared for the physical and behavioral changes induced by the procedure. This educational aspect can be facilitated through group seminars or individualized counseling sessions with appropriate members of the bariatric team. Appropriate screening involves multidisciplinary care to diagnose relevant comorbidities and optimize any preexisting medical conditions. The preoperative assessment should include a thorough history and physical examination, inclusive of a focused weight history, social history, and review of systems to elicit undiagnosed conditions associated with obesity. In addition to medical consultants, patients should also be evaluated by a nutritionist to facilitate perioperative maintenance of dietary habits and a psychologist for mental health evaluation prior to surgery. Laboratory investigations and preoperative procedures should be directed at evaluating relevant risk factors or complications of obesity. Assessment by the surgical team should include a consultation with anesthesiology and the primary bariatric surgeon to discuss the recommended procedure and the potential risks and benefits of the procedure and to review the patient's knowledge and expectations about the proposed surgery.

Nutrition

Clinicians should be aware of any preexisting nutritional deficiencies in patients undergoing bariatric surgery. Consumption of high-calorie processed foods is often energy dense but nutrient poor and contributes to deficiencies in natural antioxidants, micronutrients, and vitamins [13]. Surgical weight-loss procedures are generally considered as restrictive, malabsorptive, or a combination of both; compounding these procedures with a baseline nutritional deficiency can exacerbate conditions or create new deficiencies depending on postoperative dietary intake, compliance with vitamin supplementation, and degree of malabsorption [14]. In the early postoperative period, patients are recommended to intake at minimum 60 g of protein daily; however, patients may have difficulty achieving this amount given restricted caloric intake and intolerance to protein rich

S.A. Brethauer et al. (eds.), *Minimally Invasive Bariatric Surgery*,
DOI 10.1007/978-1-4939-1637-5_7, © Springer Science+Business Media New York 2015

foods in the first 3–6 months. Regular visits with the nutritionist can provide guidance to the patient on meal plan progression, protein supplementation, and adherence to recommended nutrient supplementation.

Our standard practice after bariatric surgery is to provide supplementation with a multivitamin, vitamin B_{12}, iron, vitamin C, and calcium citrate with vitamin D. Laboratory values are drawn every 6 months for the first 2 years and continued annually unless patient presents with poor oral tolerance, evidence of dehydration, or symptoms attributable to nutrient deficiency.

Preoperative weight loss of about 10 % is frequently advocated prior to bariatric surgery [15, 16]. Whether preoperative weight loss is associated with improved postoperative weight loss has been controversial. Still and colleagues were able to demonstrate in a large cohort of 884 patients undergoing bariatric surgery that preoperative weight loss of at least 10 % was achieved in 48 % of subjects. These patients were more likely to have a decreased length of stay in the hospital postoperatively and achieve a 70 % loss of excess body weight at follow-up of 1 year [16]. Another retrospective study of 90 subjects undergoing laparoscopic gastric bypass surgery demonstrated that a preoperative weight loss of 1 % of initial weight correlated with an increase of 1.8 % of postoperative excess weight loss at 1 year [17]. In addition, preoperative weight loss of greater than 5 % also correlated significantly with shorter operative times [17]. In contrast, other studies have not demonstrated an association between pre- and postoperative weight loss with the concern that these preoperative requirements may delay surgery and contribute to patient dropout rates [18].

A separate functional aspect of preoperative weight loss relates to the technical aspect of bariatric surgery. Laparoscopic procedures in morbidly obese patients can be technically challenging given the small amount of working space in the setting of a large fatty liver and increased amount of intra-abdominal adiposity. The enlarged liver can cause difficulty with exposure at the gastroesophageal junction and is reported to be one of the more common causes for conversion to open procedure [19]. Acute preoperative weight loss has been associated with less intraoperative blood loss and a decreased frequency of deviation from the standard laparoscopic procedure [20]. Several studies have shown a reduction in liver size with different variations of low-calorie diets over a 2- to 4-week period [21–23]. Although short-term weight loss is not a prerequisite for surgery, our practice is to place patients on a 800–1,000 kcal/day liquid diet with protein shake supplementation starting 2 weeks prior to their bariatric procedure.

Mental Health Evaluation

The mental health evaluation is an essential component to the preoperative evaluation of bariatric surgery candidates due to the high prevalence of psychiatric and behavioral complications observed in this population [24]. Morbid obesity (BMI > 40) is positively associated with incidence of depression, and preoperative clinical interviews suggest that approximately 50 % of patients seeking weight-loss surgery report a lifetime history of depression [24–26]. Population studies demonstrate that up to 60 % fulfill criteria for an Axis I psychiatric disorder inclusive of mood disorders, general anxiety disorders, and substance abuse disorders [12, 27]. Contributing to this statistic is the fact that bariatric patients often report physical ailments, emotional toll, and a significant alteration in quality of life measures. Many obese individuals have suffered stereotypes throughout their life that have potential to discriminate in three important areas of living—employment, education, and health care [28]. Increased dissatisfaction with body image can also negatively impact marital relationships and sexual functioning. Eating behaviors and habits should also be reviewed with specific attention toward binge-eating disorders. Binge-eating disorder is commonly identified in bariatric surgery candidates and can contribute to postoperative weight regain if not appropriately addressed and treated [29].

Despite the necessity and frequency of preoperative psychological evaluations for bariatric surgery, consensus guidelines as to what constitutes an appropriate evaluation or psychological reasons for denial of surgery have not been established. At our institution, a multidimensional Cleveland Clinic Behavioral Rating System (CCBRS) was developed to assess patients across a variety of domains identified in published reports to be important in the preoperative psychological assessment [30]. At entry into the bariatric program, psychiatric interviews and objective psychological testing using either the Millon Behavioral Medicine Diagnostic or Minnesota Multiphasic Personality Inventory-2 Restructured Form are used to assess behavioral comorbidities [30]. The initial interview consists of a query of specific domains which are then assessed on a Likert rating scale from 5 (excellent—no concerns and no follow-up with psychology recommended unless future problems develop) to 1 (poor—inappropriate risk that very likely outweighs benefits). These ratings are given for the following nine domains of interest:

(1) *Consent*—assessment of cognitive functioning, understanding of procedure, and capacity to consent.
(2) *Expectations*—inclusive of transition of surgery, weight-loss goals, and long-term outcomes.
(3) *Social support*—assessment of patient support circle including spouse or significant other, family members, coworkers, and bariatric support group attendance.
(4) *Mental health*—assessment of psychiatric diagnosis and severity and duration of diagnosis.
(5) *Chemical/alcohol abuse/dependence*—inclusive of use, abuse, and dependency of substance, history and present use, and tobacco assessment.
(6) *Eating behaviors*—inclusive of binge eating, night eating, compensatory behaviors, problematic outcomes from previous diet attempts.

(7)*Adherence*—inclusive of adherence to previous dietary attempts, past psychological/psychiatric interventions, medical recommendations, and tobacco prohibition.

(8)*Coping/stressors*—assessment of coping resources in the context of situational stressors.

(9) *Overall impression*

The CCBRS has been demonstrated to be an internally consistent and useful tool for multidimensional psychological assessment of bariatric surgery candidates with favorable inter-rater reliability between examining psychologists. In a study of 389 bariatric surgery candidates using this rating system, most candidates (71.7 %) were deemed psychologically acceptable, a smaller subset (25.7 %) were considered guarded requiring additional treatment of requirement fulfillment prior to gaining clearance for surgery, and finally a very small percentage (2.6 %) of candidates were unable to reach candidacy [30]. Our experience using the CCBRS has improved communication between the multidisciplinary team allowing surgeons and treating physicians to review the summary of a patient's strengths and weaknesses.

Labs and Procedures

Selection of preoperative laboratory tests should be based on specific clinical indication; however, routine fasting blood glucose, lipid profile, complete blood count, and a metabolic panel are considered reasonable for the bariatric patient [12]. Baseline micronutrient and vitamin levels are useful to monitor and treat any subsequent deficiencies that may develop as a result of malabsorptive procedures. Female patients of childbearing age should have a pregnancy test.

Routine upper gastrointestinal (UGI) evaluation or abdominal ultrasound are not recommended universally and are typically at the discretion of the surgeon or treating institution. UGI contrast studies and esophagogastroduodenoscopy (EGD) are often used by surgeons in the preoperative evaluation of bariatric patients to assess for any preexisting anatomical variations or upper GI pathology. The most common findings on UGI include gastroesophageal reflux and hiatal hernia; however, typically these findings rarely lead to a change in the proposed surgical plan or cancellation [31]. Routine use of EGD for preoperative evaluation has also been controversial. The majority of findings include hiatal hernias, gastritis, esophagitis, gastric or esophageal ulceration, and Barrett's esophagus [32, 33]. Opponents of nonselective preoperative EGD suggest that in asymptomatic patients, these findings are infrequently clinically significant. However, considering that gastric bypass procedures preclude endoscopic evaluation of the gastric and duodenal mucosa postoperatively, supporters of preoperative EGD have used endoscopy to obtain baseline gastric pathology and concurrent investigation of the gastric mucosa for *H. pylori*. A small number of studies have indicated that incidence of postoperative marginal ulcer and gastrointestinal bleeding may be higher in patients infected with *H. pylori* [34, 35].

Preoperative ultrasonography of the abdomen is employed primarily to assess for gallbladder disease; obesity is a cause for the higher incidence of gallstones in bariatric patients. In addition, rapid weight loss after bariatric surgery is a well-known risk factor for gallstone formation and exacerbation; therefore, ultrasound is used to screen for patients that may benefit from concurrent cholecystectomy. Although previously, prophylactic simultaneous cholecystectomy was often performed with gastric bypass, this has largely been abandoned. The more conventional approach is to perform cholecystectomy in the presence of symptomatic gallstones, as the incidence of subsequent cholecystectomy after bariatric surgery is reported to be less than 15 % in most studies [36]. Our practice is to also use the preventative administration of ursodeoxycholic acid for 6 months postoperatively which has been shown to decrease gallstone formation during rapid weight loss [37].

Cleveland Clinic Protocol

An overview of the steps to weight-loss surgery at the Cleveland Clinic Bariatric and Metabolic Institute (BMI) are presented in Table 1. The initial patient worksheet questionnaire is a 16-page health document that requests the patient to fill out sections regarding demographics, insurance information, and weight and diet history inclusive of any previous behavioral or medical treatment for weight loss, current medications, medical and surgical history, prior bariatric surgery, psychological or emotional disorders, recent diagnostic examinations, review of systems, social history with substance abuse information, sleep apnea screen, ambulatory status, and expectations for weight loss. This questionnaire is submitted on paper or via the program's website and is then evaluated by the BMI staff for

TABLE 1. Basic steps through the program

	Description
Step 1	Complete initial patient worksheet questionnaire
Step 2	Send initial patient worksheet questionnaire to Cleveland Clinic Bariatric and Metabolic Institute Program office (paper or via website)
Step 3	Insurance coverage for weight-loss surgery
Step 4	Medical qualification for weight-loss surgery
Step 5	Appointment for the weight-loss surgery patient workshop
Step 6	Weight-loss surgery workshop or online informational seminar
Step 7	Visit with the surgeon
Step 8	Medical consultations and assessments
Step 9	Acquiring insurance pre-approval
Step 10	Scheduling the surgery date and pre-op clinic visit
Step 11	The surgery
Step 12	Follow-up visits

TABLE 2. Pathway assignment criteria

Pathway	Determination
General pathway	No life-threatening comorbidities
	Age < 60 and BMI < 60
High-risk medical	Age < 60, BMI > 60, ASA Class IV, >8 comorbid conditions (one of the 8 = diabetes or HTN), prior CV event (MI, CVA, TIA), life-threatening comorbid conditions :
	(1) Known sleep apnea, noncompliant with CPAP therapy
	(2) HgA1C > 8 %
	(3) Diabetic nephropathy, retinopathy, or neuropathy
	(4) Cirrhosis
	(5) Pulmonary HTN
	(6) Poorly managed pseudotumor cerebri
	(7) Significant coagulopathy including hx of PE, bleeding diathesis, hypercoagulable syndrome, excessive bleeding, >1 DVT, on Coumadin or Plavix
	(8) Chronic steroid therapy
	(9) O_2 dependent
	(10) Wheelchair bound
	(11) Systemic disease and poor functional capacity (MS, inflammatory bowel disease, scleroderma, SLE, cancer)
	(12) Severe venous stasis ulcers
	(13) Recent undiagnosed chest pain
High-risk psychology	Schizophrenia, bipolar disorder, suicide attempt, psych hospitalization, hx of substance abuse/dependency, eating disorder hx, binge-eating score > 26, cognitive dysfunction, mental retardation, diagnosed personality disorder, gender dysphoria, multiple psychotropics
High-risk medical/psychology	Combination of red/yellow pathway determination
Adolescent/pediatric	Age 12–18 years old
Revision	Prior bariatric surgery

determination of eligibility for weight-loss surgery according to the National Institutes of Health guidelines and current recommendations of the American Diabetes Association and International Diabetes Federation Task Force on Epidemiology and Prevention [12, 38, 39]. Once medical qualification for weight-loss surgery has been established and insurance coverage verified, patients are scheduled for a 2-h bariatric surgery workshop program. At this point, they are also triaged into one of six different clinical preoperative pathways, designated by color code and based on objective medical criteria as described in Table 2. The specific pathways of potential bariatric patients include (1) general pathway, (2) high-risk medical, (3) high-risk psychology, (4) high-risk medical/psychology, (5) adolescent/pediatric, and (6) revision pathway [40]. Common to all these pathways is a thorough history and physical examination by the bariatric surgeon and bariatric medical internist as well as the nutritional and psychology assessments.

Consultation with the bariatric surgeon includes discussion of the recommended procedure with explanation of the risks and benefits. The final decision whether treatment is offered is then based on completion of the cumulative multidisciplinary evaluation. Baseline laboratory studies include a complete blood count, comprehensive metabolic profile, type and screen, coagulation studies, liver function, lipid profile, thyroid function, glycosylated hemoglobin, ferritin levels, and vitamins. Ultrasonography of the abdomen is performed to assess for biliary tract pathology and cholelithiasis. Patients in the high-risk medical group are referred for additional investigations or consultations from other subspecialties as medically indicated, with special emphasis on cardiopulmonary assessment. Standard investigations will at minimum include a chest X-ray and electrocardiogram. Patients that demonstrate a significant cardiac history or major clinical predictors for a cardiac event (unstable coronary syndromes, decompensated CHF, significant arrhythmias, or severe valvular disease) are referred to cardiology for preoperative evaluation. Patients with poor functional capacity (<4 METS) or have at least intermediate clinical predictors for a cardiac event (mild angina pectoris, prior myocardial infarction, compensated or prior CHF, diabetes mellitus, and renal insufficiency) are often evaluated with an echocardiogram or dobutamine stress echocardiogram as indicated as well as consideration for the use of perioperative beta blockade. Patients with a BMI > 50 or an Epworth sleepiness scale > 10 are routinely referred for polysomnography and consultation with sleep medicine to evaluate need for a continuous positive airway pressure (CPAP) device [41].

The number of nutritional sessions (range 3–6 months) is typically designated by different insurance carriers. Each session should document weight, diet, exercise regimens, and overall compliance. With regard to the psychological assessment, patients under the age of 18 years are evaluated by adolescent medicine or pediatric behavioral health. Adults are seen by a team of psychologists, and recommended follow-up visits are determined depending on pathway classification after the initial interview and brief questionnaire. Patients may also be referred to behavioral health groups (Table 3) to help change behavioral, emotional, or psychological patterns that may interfere with a good surgical outcome.

Revisional bariatric surgery patients are at higher risk for operative complications; therefore, a specific pathway was created for their preoperative assessment. Available previous medical records and diagnostic studies are obtained and reviewed. In addition to the above mentioned evaluation, all patients undergo upper endoscopy and UGI barium swallow studies for complete understanding of patient anatomy and physiology prior to selecting the appropriate revision or staged procedure indicated.

Regular follow-up visits after surgery serve as a continuation of the initial assessment to help patients maintain their personal and health goals as well as evaluate compliance with lifestyle changes. The outpatient follow-up scheme is shown in Table 4. Routine follow-up appointments after bariatric surgery are scheduled at 1 week postoperatively, followed by 1 month postoperatively, and then every 3 months until 18 months at which time they return annually. Surgeons visit with the patients at the 1 week, 1 month, and annual visit. The remainders of the visits starting at the 1-month visit consist of appointments held with nutrition, psychology, and the bariatrician. Patients receive individual monitoring of diet progression, medications and nutritional supplements, exercise, blood work as needed, and disease management. The bariatrician then leads a shared appointment of patients in groups of 10–12 for 90 min to discuss relevant health-care issues in a relaxed and supportive group setting, allowing for patients to have the opportunity to talk with each other about their own experiences or concerns. Patient feedback from this type of follow-up visit has been positive as it provides companionship within the group for supportive reassurance and encouragement.

Conclusion

Candidates for bariatric surgery include patients with a $BMI \geq 40$ kg/m² or $BMI \geq 35$ kg/m² with significant obesity-related comorbidities. Recent guidelines also suggest the benefits of bariatric surgery for the treatment of diabetes refractory to medical treatment in lower BMI

TABLE 3. Specialized psychology groups

Group	Patient population	Description
BEST—start	Binge-eating behavior	Change habits associated with eating/emotional eating
		Attitudes and body image
		Eating in social situations
BEST—aftercare	Graduates of BEST—start	Prevent relapse into binge-eating behavior
GET SET—Getting Experience Today for a Successful Experience Tomorrow	Pre-bariatric surgical patients	Addresses negative thoughts associated with obesity
		Surgical options reviewed
		Expectation management
MASTERY—Managing After Surgery: Tools, Eating, Relationships and You	Post-bariatric surgical patients	Addresses post-op challenges:
		Food grievance
		New healthy coping skills
		Social eating
		Preventing relapse
Substance Risk Reduction Group	Addictive behavior	Discussion of addictive substances after surgery
		Prevent transfer of addiction
Life After Surgery	Post-bariatric surgical support group (3–6 months post-op)	Explore benefits
		Address obstacles
		Maintain long-term healthy living
		Setting motivational plans
Life After the First Year	Post-bariatric surgical support group (6–12 months post-op)	Extension of Life After Surgery for patients further out from surgery
CHANGE—Changing Habits, Attitudes, New Goals, and Exercise	Seeking nonsurgical weight management	Discuss cognitive and behavioral aspects of controlled eating
		Identify strategies for healthy lifestyle
		Coping with challenges

TABLE 4. Follow-up schedule

Time	Appointment type
1 week	Surgeon
1 month	Surgeon
	Nutrition
	Psychology
3 months	Shared medical appointment
	Bariatrician
	Nutrition
	Life-after-surgery group—psychology
6 months	Surgeon—select cases
	Shared medical appointment
	Bariatrician
	Nutrition
	Psychology as needed
	Labs required
9 months	Shared medical appointment
	Bariatrician
	Nutrition
	Psychology as needed
12 months	Surgeon
	Shared medical appointment
	Bariatrician
	Nutrition
	Psychology as needed
	Labs required

patients. Patients should be of acceptable operative risk with documented failure of nonsurgical weight-loss programs. The elective nature of bariatric surgery allows for a comprehensive preoperative evaluation to appropriately optimize medical conditions and minimize surgical risk in this patient population. It is essential that patients are well informed of nutritional goals and psychologically stable with realistic expectations. Our model screens potential bariatric candidates based on their individual risk profiles or existing comorbidities and categorizes them into specific groups to guide preoperative treatment. This has led to the development of algorithms to treat patients via a selective approach and eliminate unnecessary investigations. Institution of a preoperative clinical pathway for bariatric patients allows for a systematic, cost-effective, and customized approach to the multidisciplinary evaluation of candidates for surgery.

References

1. Lemmens L, van Zelm R, Vanhaecht K, Kerkkamp H. Systematic review: indicators to evaluate effectiveness of clinical pathways for gastrointestinal surgery. J Eval Clin Pract. 2008;14(5):880–7.
2. Schwarzbach M, Rossner E, Schattenberg T, Post S, Hohenberger P, Ronellenfitsch U. Effects of a clinical pathway of pulmonary lobectomy and bilobectomy on quality and cost of care. Langenbecks Arch Surg. 2010;395(8):1139–46.
3. Schwarzbach M, Hasenberg T, Linke M, Kienle P, Post S, Ronellenfitsch U. Perioperative quality of care is modulated by process management with clinical pathways for fast-track surgery of the colon. Int J Colorectal Dis. 2011;26(12):1567–75.
4. Yeats M, Wedergren S, Fox N, Thompson JS. The use and modification of clinical pathways to achieve specific outcomes in bariatric surgery. Am Surg. 2005;71(2):152–4.
5. Huerta S, Heber D, Sawicki MP, Liu CD, Arthur D, Alexander P, et al. Reduced length of stay by implementation of a clinical pathway for bariatric surgery in an academic health care center. Am Surg. 2001;67(12):1128–35.
6. Kinsman L, Rotter T, James E, Snow P, Willis J. What is a clinical pathway? Development of a definition to inform the debate. BMC Med. 2010;8:31.
7. Rotter T, Kinsman L, James E, Machotta A, Gothe H, Willis J, et al. Clinical pathways: effects on professional practice, patient outcomes, length of stay and hospital costs. Cochrane Database Syst Rev. 2010;3, CD006632.
8. Campillo-Soto A, Martin-Lorenzo JG, Liron-Ruiz R, Torralba-Martinez JA, Bento-Gerard M, Flores-Pastor B, et al. Evaluation of the clinical pathway for laparoscopic bariatric surgery. Obes Surg. 2008;18(4):395–400.
9. Ronellenfitsch U, Schwarzbach M, Kring A, Kienle P, Post S, Hasenberg T. The effect of clinical pathways for bariatric surgery on perioperative quality of care. Obes Surg. 2012;22(5):732–9.
10. Cooney RN, Bryant P, Haluck R, Rodgers M, Lowery M. The impact of a clinical pathway for gastric bypass surgery on resource utilization. J Surg Res. 2001;98(2):97–101.
11. SAGES Guidelines Committee. SAGES guideline for clinical application of laparoscopic bariatric surgery. Surg Obes Relat Dis. 2009;5(3):387–405.
12. Mechanick JI, Kushner RF, Sugerman HJ, Gonzalez-Campoy JM, Collazo-Clavell ML, Spitz AF, et al. American Association of Clinical Endocrinologists, The Obesity Society, and American Society for Metabolic & Bariatric Surgery medical guidelines for clinical practice for the perioperative nutritional, metabolic, and nonsurgical support of the bariatric surgery patient. Obesity (Silver Spring). 2009;17 Suppl 1:S1–70, v.
13. Kant AK. Consumption of energy-dense, nutrient-poor foods by adult Americans: nutritional and health implications. The third National Health and Nutrition Examination Survey, 1988-1994. Am J Clin Nutr. 2000;72(4):929–36.
14. Xanthakos SA. Nutritional deficiencies in obesity and after bariatric surgery. Pediatr Clin North Am. 2009;56(5):1105–21.
15. Alami RS, Morton JM, Schuster R, Lie J, Sanchez BR, Peters A, et al. Is there a benefit to preoperative weight loss in gastric bypass patients? A prospective randomized trial. Surg Obes Relat Dis. 2007;3(2):141–5; discussion 5–6.
16. Still CD, Benotti P, Wood GC, Gerhard GS, Petrick A, Reed M, et al. Outcomes of preoperative weight loss in high-risk patients undergoing gastric bypass surgery. Arch Surg. 2007;142(10):994–8; discussion 9.
17. Alvarado R, Alami RS, Hsu G, Safadi BY, Sanchez BR, Morton JM, et al. The impact of preoperative weight loss in patients undergoing laparoscopic Roux-en-Y gastric bypass. Obes Surg. 2005;15(9):1282–6.
18. Jamal MK, DeMaria EJ, Johnson JM, Carmody BJ, Wolfe LG, Kellum JM, et al. Insurance-mandated preoperative dietary counseling does not improve outcome and increases dropout rates in patients considering gastric bypass surgery for morbid obesity. Surg Obes Relat Dis. 2006;2(2):122–7.
19. Schwartz ML, Drew RL, Chazin-Caldie M. Factors determining conversion from laparoscopic to open Roux-en-Y gastric bypass. Obes Surg. 2004;14(9):1193–7.
20. Liu RC, Sabnis AA, Forsyth C, Chand B. The effects of acute preoperative weight loss on laparoscopic Roux-en-Y gastric bypass. Obes Surg. 2005;15(10):1396–402.

21. Colles SL, Dixon JB, Marks P, Strauss BJ, O'Brien PE. Preoperative weight loss with a very-low-energy diet: quantitation of changes in liver and abdominal fat by serial imaging. Am J Clin Nutr. 2006;84(2):304–11.

22. Fris RJ. Preoperative low energy diet diminishes liver size. Obes Surg. 2004;14(9):1165–70.

23. Edholm D, Kullberg J, Haenni A, Karlsson FA, Ahlstrom A, Hedberg J, et al. Preoperative 4-week low-calorie diet reduces liver volume and intrahepatic fat, and facilitates laparoscopic gastric bypass in morbidly obese. Obes Surg. 2011;21(3):345–50.

24. Wadden TA, Sarwer DB. Behavioral assessment of candidates for bariatric surgery: a patient-oriented approach. Surg Obes Relat Dis. 2006;2(2):171–9.

25. Onyike CU, Crum RM, Lee HB, Lyketsos CG, Eaton WW. Is obesity associated with major depression? Results from the Third National Health and Nutrition Examination Survey. Am J Epidemiol. 2003;158(12):1139–47.

26. Dixon JB, Dixon ME, O'Brien PE. Depression in association with severe obesity: changes with weight loss. Arch Intern Med. 2003;163(17):2058–65.

27. Sarwer DB, Cohn NI, Gibbons LM, Magee L, Crerand CE, Raper SE, et al. Psychiatric diagnoses and psychiatric treatment among bariatric surgery candidates. Obes Surg. 2004;14(9):1148–56.

28. Puhl R, Brownell KD. Bias, discrimination, and obesity. Obes Res. 2001;9(12):788–805.

29. Kalarchian MA, Marcus MD, Wilson GT, Labouvie EW, Brolin RE, LaMarca LB. Binge eating among gastric bypass patients at long-term follow-up. Obes Surg. 2002;12(2):270–5.

30. Heinberg LJ, Ashton K, Windover A. Moving beyond dichotomous psychological evaluation: the Cleveland Clinic Behavioral Rating System for weight loss surgery. Surg Obes Relat Dis. 2010; 6(2):185–90.

31. Sharaf RN, Weinshel EH, Bini EJ, Rosenberg J, Ren CJ. Radiologic assessment of the upper gastrointestinal tract: does it play an important preoperative role in bariatric surgery? Obes Surg. 2004; 14(3):313–7.

32. Sharaf RN, Weinshel EH, Bini EJ, Rosenberg J, Sherman A, Ren CJ. Endoscopy plays an important preoperative role in bariatric surgery. Obes Surg. 2004;14(10):1367–72.

33. Zeni TM, Frantzides CT, Mahr C, Denham EW, Meiselman M, Goldberg MJ, et al. Value of preoperative upper endoscopy in patients undergoing laparoscopic gastric bypass. Obes Surg. 2006;16(2):142–6.

34. Schirmer B, Erenoglu C, Miller A. Flexible endoscopy in the management of patients undergoing Roux-en-Y gastric bypass. Obes Surg. 2002;12(5):634–8.

35. Hartin Jr CW, ReMine DS, Lucktong TA. Preoperative bariatric screening and treatment of Helicobacter pylori. Surg Endosc. 2009;23(11):2531–4.

36. Swartz DE, Felix EL. Elective cholecystectomy after Roux-en-Y gastric bypass: why should asymptomatic gallstones be treated differently in morbidly obese patients? Surg Obes Relat Dis. 2005; 1(6):555–60.

37. Uy MC, Talingdan-Te MC, Espinosa WZ, Daez ML, Ong JP. Ursodeoxycholic acid in the prevention of gallstone formation after bariatric surgery: a meta-analysis. Obes Surg. 2008;18(12):1532–8.

38. Schauer PR, Rubino F. International Diabetes Federation position statement on bariatric surgery for type 2 diabetes: implications for patients, physicians, and surgeons. Surg Obes Relat Dis. 2011; 7(4):448–51.

39. Rubino F, Kaplan LM, Schauer PR, Cummings DE. The Diabetes Surgery Summit consensus conference: recommendations for the evaluation and use of gastrointestinal surgery to treat type 2 diabetes mellitus. Ann Surg. 2010;251(3):399–405.

40. Eldar S, Heneghan HM, Brethauer S, Schauer PR. A focus on surgical preoperative evaluation of the bariatric patient—the Cleveland Clinic protocol and review of the literature. Surgeon. 2011;9(5): 273–7.

41. Vana KD, Silva GE, Goldberg R. Predictive abilities of the STOP-Bang and Epworth Sleepiness Scale in identifying sleep clinic patients at high risk for obstructive sleep apnea. Res Nurs Health. 2013;36(1):84–94.

8

The Role of Behavioral Health in Bariatric Surgery

Leslie J. Heinberg and Janelle W. Coughlin

Introduction

Bariatric surgery is considered the most effective treatment for severe obesity (BMI ≥ 40 kg/m^2), resulting in an average weight loss of 35 % of initial body weight (IBW) and significant reductions in medical comorbidity [1]. This marked effectiveness has resulted in bariatric surgery becoming an increasingly common surgical procedure. However, unlike many other common surgeries, bariatric surgery is closely linked with behavior and psychosocial factors. Eating and exercise behaviors as well as psychological and social factors may have caused, exacerbated, or maintained the severe obesity necessitating surgery. Further, bariatric surgery candidates are a psychiatrically vulnerable population with a high level of psychiatric and psychosocial comorbidity [2, 3]. Additionally, bariatric surgery, and the weight loss it engenders, likely results in major changes to patients' medical status, body image, quality of life, emotional well-being, and social relationships [4]. Finally, although surgery results in significant anatomical alterations, long-term success requires significant behavioral change and necessitates individuals to adhere to permanent lifestyle alterations in diet and exercise as well as the ability to reduce reliance upon food to cope with life stressors. Although improvements are experienced by the majority of bariatric surgery patients, there is considerable variability in outcome [5]. A significant minority of individuals fail to lose the expected amount of weight. Others instead may have initial weight loss success but regain considerable weight, particularly within the first few years following surgery. Reasons for weight regain are generally not well understood. Many biological and physiological mechanisms have been posited, but the majority of putative factors relate to behavior, compliance, and psychiatric comorbidity [6–8].

Due to these challenges, mental health professionals are an essential component of the multidisciplinary assessment and treatment team at most bariatric surgery treatment centers [9]. This chapter will focus on the role of the psychologist within this multidisciplinary team. Although the focus will be on the licensed psychologist, this role can be (and often is) fulfilled by a variety of mental health professionals. The objectives of this chapter are to (1) review why behavioral health is a critical component of the bariatric team and (2) provide a review of the presurgical evaluation including psychiatric vulnerability, psychosocial comorbidity, domains that are assessed, as well as methods of assessment. Finally, the chapter will focus on areas of concern perioperatively and postoperatively.

Why Bariatric Behavioral Health?

Psychological evaluation is a widely utilized and accepted part of the multidisciplinary assessment for all weight loss surgery candidates, particularly those with a known or suspected psychiatric illness. Indeed, when bariatric programs have been surveyed, 97–98.5 % of centers endorse utilizing psychosocial interviews for their surgical candidates [9–11]. However, it may be helpful to further explore the role of mental health in weight loss surgery.

Over 20 years ago, the NIH released a consensus statement on surgery for severe obesity [4]. This statement outlined nine indications for surgery including: BMI > 40 kg/m^2 or BMI > 35 kg/m^2 with significant obesity-related comorbidities, acceptable operative risk, failure of nonsurgical weight loss programs, psychologically stable with realistic expectations, well-informed and motivated patient, supportive family/social environment, absence of active alcohol or substance abuse, and absence of uncontrolled psychotic or depressive disorder. Thus, outside of the first two indications, these criteria rely upon an understanding of the patient's psychological well-being, psychosocial functioning, behavior, and cognitions. More recently, in 2013, the American Association of Clinical Endocrinologists, the Obesity Society, and the American Society for Metabolic and Bariatric Surgery jointly published updated guidelines for the clinical practice of bariatric surgery [12]. Similar to the NIH consensus

S.A. Brethauer et al. (eds.), *Minimally Invasive Bariatric Surgery*,
DOI 10.1007/978-1-4939-1637-5_8, © Springer Science+Business Media New York 2015

statement, three of four of the listed contraindications relate to psychosocial risk. These contraindications include: reversible endocrine or other disorders that can cause obesity; current drug or alcohol use; uncontrolled, severe psychiatric illness; and lack of comprehension of risks, benefits, expected outcomes, alternatives, and lifestyle changes required with bariatric surgery.

Extreme obesity is associated with considerable psychosocial comorbidity, and patients who present for bariatric surgery are considered to be a psychiatrically vulnerable population [2, 3]. Moreover, a number of studies have demonstrated that patients burdened by depression and other psychiatric difficulties may have greater difficulty with weight loss after surgery [6, 13, 14]. As a consequence, psychological evaluation of bariatric surgery candidates has become the norm within the majority of programs. Finally, the majority of insurance companies require an assessment by a mental health professional prior to approving weight loss surgery [15].

Qualifications of the Behavioral Health Professional

The practice of behavioral health related to surgical weight loss is slowly evolving into a specific subspecialty. The 2004 *Suggestions for the Pre-Surgical Psychological Assessment of Bariatric Surgery Candidates* was published by the ASMBS and outlined minimum standards for this specialty which include: knowledge of the nature and mechanics of the various bariatric surgical procedures, the expected postoperative course, and the physiology of obesity, dieting, and weight loss [4]. In addition, they suggest that an understanding of how these factors can interact in the postoperative course is essential. Given the importance of evaluating and addressing psychiatric comorbidities, practitioners should be licensed practitioners who can assess and treat psychological conditions. Further, practitioners should have a thorough understanding of the biological, psychological, and social causes and consequences of morbid obesity and of behavioral factors that may impact weight loss and weight loss maintenance. A background in eating disorders is also preferred. Finally, we would add that professionals should be competent in weight sensitivity and present a bariatric-friendly patient environment (e.g., appropriate size furniture, scales).

Unfortunately, although most programs require one, there is significant variability in the quality of such psychosocial evaluations. Unlike specialized certifications for nursing or physicians, a standardized exam for mental health professionals has not yet been established. A recent study of ASMBS members found that the majority felt that mental health professionals working with bariatric populations should have extensive and specific knowledge of weight loss surgery, obesity, and nonsurgical management of obesity and experience

in working with these patients pre- and postoperatively [16]. The care of bariatric patients would undoubtedly be improved by better standardization across the field.

Presurgical Evaluation

As previously noted, despite the almost universality of psychological evaluation for bariatric surgery candidates, 20 years of guidelines suggesting the need for such evaluations and a substantial literature on psychosocial risk factors in this population, there is no consensus regarding how an evaluation should be conducted; the role, need, and utility of objective psychological testing [17]; or reasons for denial. Unfortunately, this has limited the ability of bariatric behavioral health to fully engage in empirical trials and has, at times, diminished the perceived value of these clinicians' roles.

In reviewing the literature, there does appear to be general agreement upon important factors to assess [18, 19]. Generally, researchers agree that a standard psychiatric interview focusing on diagnostic comorbidities is necessary but not sufficient for evaluating candidacy. In addition, a detailed assessment of eating behaviors, stress and coping, and social support are considered essential points of evaluation. Further, capacity to consent, understanding of risk and benefits of the surgery, knowledge of surgery, and expectations for weight loss, health outcomes, and psychosocial impact are largely accepted as being of additional importance.

There also appears to be consensus regarding psychosocial contraindications for weight loss surgery including: current illicit drug abuse, active/under-controlled schizophrenia or other overt psychiatric illness, severe intellectual disabilities, heavy alcohol use, severe and untreated eating disorder, lack of knowledge about surgery, severe situational stress, insufficient motivation, and lack of significant support. In studies examining rates for psychological denial of weight loss surgery, refusals for psychosocial reasons tend to range between 2 and 6 % [9, 11, 20–22]. Beyond such denials, patients may be required to complete additional treatment or delay surgery in order to stabilize a condition. Studies suggest that programs do not immediately approve patients due to psychosocial reasons up to 25 % of the time [11]. A survey of 103 psychologists who conduct presurgical psychological evaluations indicated significant variability in such decision making. Although respondents noted delaying or denying surgery for an average of 14.3 % of candidates, the range was 0–60 % [9]. Further, the benefits of delaying surgery as well as the costs due to potential loss of patients as a result of delays are largely unknown [12].

Beyond clear-cut contraindications, patients may be considered high risk psychiatrically and may be triaged into differing pathways which may require more in-depth assessment and/or treatment. Within the Cleveland Clinic's program, patients are triaged as high risk if they have a history of: schizophrenia, bipolar disorder, past suicide attempt, inpatient psychiatric hospitalization, substance abuse/dependence, history of anorexia nervosa or bulimia nervosa, cognitive dysfunction, developmental delay, personality disorder, or multiple psychiatric medications. These patients are seen initially by the psychologist rather than potentially having their visit later in the preoperative process (e.g., after initiating an insurance-mandated supervised diet). Thus, patients who may not be candidates, or who may be delayed, can be identified prior to numerous appointments with other program providers (e.g., surgical consult, sleep study, etc.).

Elements of the Psychological Evaluation

For illustrative purposes, we describe the elements that we utilize within our evaluations. Many patients are very concerned about the requirement for a psychological evaluation. Often they believe that if the professional uncovers something negative, it will adversely affect their ability to undergo surgery. Thus, the evaluation is seen as an obstacle between them and a very strongly desired outcome. As a result, it is often important to first build rapport and discuss the collaborative role of the evaluation (e.g., identifying strengths to build upon and addressing obstacles that could impact their ability to have an optimal outcome). We begin by asking what surgery they are interested in and what led to their decision to pursue weight loss surgery. Next, an assessment of their understanding of the mechanics of their surgery, expected experience, and recovery time as well as their knowledge regarding risks vs. benefits should be determined. Next, we assess their weight loss expectations; beyond weight loss, what do they expect will be different, improved, etc. following weight loss surgery? This allows the evaluator to not only assess consent and expectations but also to provide education about what to expect and what surgery can—and cannot—alter.

A comprehensive evaluation should also include a thorough eating and weight history. The patient's weight history should be determined, including lowest and highest adult weight and how these relate to current weight as well as factors that led to obesity. A thorough assessment of past weight loss strategies should be conducted focusing on what was beneficial, difficulties with adherence, and length of maintenance. During the assessment of past dietary attempts, history of purgative attempts such as vomiting and laxative and diuretic abuse should be determined. Although most patients will also see a dietitian, some assessment of the patient's typical eating pattern can be informative—particularly with focus on abnormal timing of eating, skipping of meals, etc. Such assessment segues well into an assessment of binge eating disorder. We currently follow the diagnostic criteria

from the DSM-5 [23]. Patients should be queried regarding objective binge episodes, subjective lack of control over eating during the binge episode, as well as the associated distress related to binge eating. Other disordered eating behaviors such as excessive graze eating patterns or night eating should also be assessed.

Next, we review medical comorbidities related to obesity as well as currently prescribed medications. This can lead to further discussion regarding a patient's adherence with prescribed medications or other medical recommendations (e.g., adherence with CPAP). Capacity to consent (and brief cognitive screen if needed) should also be determined with a review of memory and concentration difficulties, history of learning difficulties, special education, traumatic brain injuries, and other cognitive issues that could impact decisional capacity.

The next part of the evaluation is more consistent with a traditional psychiatric diagnostic interview. Patients are queried on their current mental state, and relevant diagnostic symptoms of psychiatric disorders are assessed. Past and current outpatient, inpatient, and psychotropic treatments are reviewed as well as past history of suicide attempts and self-injurious behavior. Family mental health history is determined and a brief trauma history is conducted. Further, a standard mental status examination is conducted.

Next, the patient's current use of nicotine, alcohol, and illicit and prescription drugs are determined. Symptoms of abuse and dependence should be determined, and any past history of alcohol and/or drug abuse/dependence or treatment should be evaluated. Other potentially problematic habits such as caffeine use, carbonation, and sugar-sweetened beverages can also be determined. All patients, including those considered low risk for alcohol abuse, should be educated about the risk for increased sensitivity and potential increased risk for abuse following surgery [24]; additional information on conducting an alcohol history in the bariatric presurgical patient can be found in a review by Heinberg et al. [25].

Support plays a crucial role in patient's adjustment and success; thus, a thorough psychosocial history is taken beginning with a review of the patient's family of origin and childhood. Next, the patient's current living situation and relationship status should be evaluated. The impact that surgery, altered eating and activity behaviors, and weight loss may have on relationships should be discussed. Patients should be queried regarding who they will share the decision with, how they will address negative commentary, and who will help care for them following surgery. A psychosocial history should also include information about patients' educational level and achievement, work history, and their plans for time off following surgery. Interpersonal, occupational, financial, legal, and other stressors should be reviewed with an assessment of coping strategies. Often, eating is listed as a primary coping method, and this can lead to early discussion about the need to identify alternative coping resources.

Physical and sedentary activity should be assessed. If patients are not currently active, it is helpful to identify any past exercise attempts, degree of adherence, and intention to exercise following surgery.

Following this interview, the evaluator should be able to at least provisionally provide a DSM-5 diagnosis and make an initial impression about the patient's relative strengths entering into weight loss surgery and make recommendations about the plan of care pre- and postoperatively. We find it most helpful to delineate between requirements—those tasks that are necessary prior to writing a clearance letter (e.g., smoking cessation, adherence with psychiatric medications, abstinence from drugs and/or alcohol) and recommendations that are not necessary but determined to be helpful (e.g., attendance at a support group, importance of bringing a support person to future appointments, wean off of carbonated beverages). Finally, as a means of summarizing the findings in a more consistent and empirical manner, the Cleveland Clinic Behavioral Rating Scale can be utilized [18]. This measure has evaluators rate patients on a 5-point scale (poor, guarded, fair, good, excellent) across 8 domains of interest (consent, expectations, social support, mental health, chemical/alcohol abuse/dependence, eating behaviors, adherence, and stress/coping) with a final overall rating ranging from excellent candidacy to poor noncandidacy.

The Perioperative Stage

Research on the perioperative phase of bariatric surgery focuses mostly on medical management issues (e.g., perioperative glycemic control, strategies for managing obstructive sleep apnea) [26, 27] and perioperative outcomes, including in-hospital mortality, complications, and length of stay [28–30]. In-hospital morbidity and mortality following bariatric surgery relate to procedure type, having open vs. laparoscopic procedures, accreditation of the bariatric surgery program, and surgical volume [28, 30].

Median inpatient length of stay following RYGB is 2–3 days, and longer procedure time, surgeon, higher BMI, being African-American, older age, and status as a Medicare/Medicaid beneficiary have all been identified as predictors of a longer inpatient length of stay [29]. Currently, we are aware of no research that has systematically assessed psychological factors associated with inpatient perioperative outcomes; however, we anticipate the Longitudinal Assessment of Bariatric Surgery-3 (LABS-3) Psychosocial study [3] will provide good insight on this issue. In the absence of strong research and guidelines on behavioral and psychological risk management during the perioperative period, the following are considerations for those providing psychological care during the inpatient phase of bariatric surgery.

Bariatric psychologists as well as inpatient mental services often need to serve as consult-liaisons (C/L) for bariatric patients. As previously noted, the bariatric surgery population is psychiatrically vulnerable with approximately one-third having a current Axis I psychiatric diagnosis. Further, the medically compromised state of surgery may exacerbate a number of symptoms and disorders. C/L behavioral health provides a comprehensive analysis of the patient's response to illness and surgical course, can help identify mental disorders or psychological response to surgery that is in need of further intervention, and can help identify effective coping mechanisms to improve outcomes and postoperative adjustment. Common reasons for consultation include: depression, agitation, hallucinations, sleep disorders, confusion, suicidal ideation, nonadherence or refusal to consent to a procedure, and a lack of organic basis for symptoms (e.g., conversion, malingering, somatization). Finally hospitalized patients are particularly vulnerable to acute confusional states. Delirium is surprisingly common and can seriously complicate the postoperative course and can lead to significant management problems.

Another concern is managing patient's psychotropic medications following surgery. In examining bariatric populations, 72.5 % of surgical candidates report a lifetime history of psychotropic medication use—almost 90 % of which were antidepressants. Further, 47.7 % were currently on at least one psychiatric medication [20]. Unfortunately, many patients are NPO for at least 24 h. If complications occur, patients may be off of important psychiatric medications for a number of days.

The Postoperative Phase

Early Behavioral Adjustments

A few studies have examined postoperative outcomes that encompass the 30 days following surgery [29, 31–33]. However, similar to the studies on perioperative outcomes outlined above, studies on short-term postsurgical outcomes have not yet focused on psychosocial factors associated with 30-day adverse events. Although serious complications in the month following bariatric surgery are rare, many patients report overlapping and often vague symptoms, like abdominal discomfort and nausea in the first year following surgery, particularly in the first 6 months. These symptoms should be followed closely and often necessitate evaluation through an upper endoscopy and upper gastrointestinal series [34]. Abdominal pain is perhaps the most commonly reported postsurgical problem, and careful evaluation for conditions such as ulcer disease, upper gastrointestinal bleed, stomal stenosis, biliary disorder, and anastomotic leak may be indicated. However, studies have shown that the majority of patients who undergo endoscopy have normal findings and symptoms such as nausea/vomiting, abdominal discomfort, and gastroesophageal reflux are more likely explained by the reduced gastric pouch not being able to accommodate larger amounts of food [34]. It is unclear what overlap these symptoms have with psychological comorbidities such as depression which may worsen pain complaints. In the first 6 months following surgery, overeating, rapid eating, brief impaction (i.e., plugging), and inadequate chewing are common. To identify behavioral explanations for pain and other gastrointestinal symptoms, a full and detailed assessment of symptoms in relation to eating behaviors is necessary. Fortunately, behaviorally induced symptoms typically resolve in the first 6 months, as patients identify the relationship between their eating behaviors and discomfort and correct the problems. During this period of adaptation and relearning, behavioral support is important and should be a standard component of postsurgical care.

Postoperative Follow-Up

It is recommended, at a minimum, that patients who undergo bariatric surgery return to the bariatric surgery program for follow-up within 1–2 weeks of surgery, 6 months postoperatively, and annually thereafter. Those who undergo AGB may return more frequently for adjustments to the band. Patients are also encouraged to participate in postoperative support groups, which are a common component of most established bariatric surgery programs. Some programs recommend more frequent follow-up with the surgical team, particularly in the first postoperative year, and offer additional services to augment postsurgical support, including support groups, nutrition groups, and shared medical and shared psychological appointments. These groups allow for support, normalizing of experiences, and sharing of knowledge and lead to greater efficiencies within a program as providers can see a number of similar patients and impart similar information in a single setting. Importantly, both follow-up with the surgical program and attendance at support groups are associated with better postoperative outcomes [35, 36]; therefore, strong recommendations should be made for ongoing follow-up, and programs should do their best to offer easily accessible postsurgical services.

Guidelines for postsurgical behavioral health services are not as well defined as presurgical guidelines; however, it is advised that patients have available to them a psychologist or other specialized mental health professional to provide support during the psychological, behavioral, and interpersonal adjustments that can occur with surgery. This is particularly true for individuals who have psychiatric conditions and could experience a worsening of psychiatric comorbidity postsurgically.

Psychosocial Adjustments

Although not well studied, it is not unusual for patients to experience some regret after surgery, particularly when experiencing pain and discomfort in the initial postoperative weeks and while reestablishing eating patterns. The process can be somewhat akin to having a baby—patients can prepare

mentally and can even be excited about the changes to come; however, the physiological and mental changes that occur after surgery can collide to produce "postsurgical blues." As with postpartum blues, it is important for this low, or blue, period to be carefully monitored and treated appropriately; however, it is our experience that patients typically move through this period within the first few postoperative weeks or months, and many do not experience it at all.

Research on the relationship between psychiatric symptoms and postsurgical outcomes, though not always easy to interpret when considered collectively, suggests that psychiatric comorbidity is associated with less favorable weight loss outcomes following bariatric surgery. This appears to be particularly true for those with more than one psychiatric diagnosis [6, 13], those with a bipolar disorder [14], and those with symptoms in the first 9 months following surgery [37]. For example, Semanscin-Doerr and colleagues found that patients who had a clinically diagnosable mood disorder at the time of their initial evaluation experienced less weight loss 1, 3, 6, and 9 months following VSG as compared to those without a psychiatric condition [14]. These findings were no longer significant at 1 year post-VSG, nor were they significant when removing those with a bipolar disorder from the analyses. Kalarchian and colleagues found that a lifetime history of a mood or anxiety disorder was associated with less weight loss 6 months following RYGB [8]. However, a current diagnosis of mood, anxiety, substance, or eating disorder at the time of presurgical psychological evaluation was not significantly associated with 6-month outcomes nor was a diagnosis of a personality disorder. In a prospective study following patients up to 3 years after RYGB, current or lifetime history of a depressive disorder did not relate to weight loss outcomes [13]. However, having more than one past or current psychiatric diagnosis (e.g., both an affective disorder and an anxiety disorder) was associated with poorer weight loss outcomes. Collectively, these studies suggest that psychiatric comorbidity, particularly multiple comorbidities or a diagnosis of bipolar disorder, may be associated with less favorable weight loss and that lifetime history, rather than diagnosis at the time of the presurgical evaluation, may be associated with poorer short-term outcomes. It is important to note, however, that this association may not exist at longer-term follow-up and that even those with less weight loss may likely be experiencing clinically significant improvements in health and will lose more weight with surgery than with more conservative interventions. Moreover, there is evidence that weight loss following surgery is associated with significant improvements in mood and quality of life [13]. Although improvements in health-related quality of life (vs. mental health-related quality of life) are more likely to occur early on (in the first 3 months following surgery) [38, 39], studies have shown improvements in a wide range of quality-of-life dimensions, including psychosocial and sexual functioning domains, 1–2 years following surgery [40, 41].

Research on interpersonal changes that occur after surgery is limited; however, clinically patients often share both positive and negative changes in their relationships. Whereas patients often find that they relate better to their family members, peers, and coworkers as they experience improvements in their sense of self and quality of life, they may also find that they struggle with their new identify and find that others treat and relate to them differently. A qualitative study by Bocchieri and colleagues nicely summarizes these issues and identifies a number of "tension-generating changes" that occur after surgery, including increased feelings of vulnerability, conflicted emotions regarding new reactions from others, and the need to develop and implement new, non-dietary means of coping with emotions [42]. Perhaps the best approach to helping patients adjust to these changes is attendance at support groups and participation in interpersonal, familial, or couples therapy. As discussed in our summary of the presurgical evaluation, assessing support is an important component of the presurgical assessment, and enlisting patients' support system can be very important postsurgically. Moreover, patients can be empowered to understand how their behaviors and success can impact significant others in their lives.

Interestingly, bariatric surgery can also have a positive impact on family members' health. One study has shown that mothers who have had surgery tend to model better eating behaviors for their children [43], and another found that family members of those undergoing surgery often experience weight loss and improved health behaviors, such as increased exercise, even though they themselves did not undergo surgery [44]. Furthermore, surgical patients who have a family member who has also undergone surgery tend to have better weight loss and follow-up than those without a family member who has also undergone surgery [45]. These studies underscore the importance and bidirectionality of family support in bariatric surgery.

Weight Loss Outcomes, Weight Regain, and Behavioral Adherence

Weight loss outcomes are often expressed as percentage of excess weight loss (% EWL = weight loss/excess weight × 100), and, on average, between the first and third postoperative years, patients lose ~70 %, 60–65 %, 55 %, and 45–50 % EWL (BPD/DS, RYGB, VSG, and AGB, respectively) [5, 46, 47]. Less data is available on shorter-term weight loss outcomes; however, a recent study conducted at Duke University examined weight loss patterns at earlier postoperative visits for those having RYGB [48]. They found that individuals who lost > 2 % EWL/week during the first 14 weeks postsurgically had the greatest chance of having better weight loss outcomes at 1 year. Moreover, they found that % EWL at month 1 significantly predicted % EWL at 12 months. Thus, identifying "underperformers" early on is important so that appropriate interventions can be identified to optimize early weight loss.

A sizeable minority (10–25 %) of bariatric surgery patients experience suboptimal weight loss, often defined as failure to lose at least 40 or 50 % EWL [49–53]. Although a number of physiological explanations can be offered, a commonly pursued explanation for less optimal weight loss following bariatric surgery is failure to adhere to and adopt the recommended lifestyle and dietary modifications required for success [54]. Weight regain following bariatric surgery is also common. The most commonly cited and longest study of bariatric surgery outcomes, the Swedish Obese Subjects Trial, has shown that, on average, RYGB and AGB patients lose ~30 % and 20 % of their IBW in the first 2 years following surgery, respectively [55]. After this period of time, weight regain is common in both procedures, with an average regain of 6–7 % of IBW at 10-year follow-up, most of which occurs between the second and sixth postsurgical years [52, 55, 56].

Only a few studies have assessed lifestyle behaviors following bariatric surgery. A recent study found that most patients adhere to the recommendation not to drink while eating, and most take their vitamins and medications as prescribed (95 %, 86 %, and 90 %, respectively) [57]. However, few (5 %) eat the recommended 5–6 meals per day, most exceed recommended portion sizes during meals and snacks (100 % and 72 %, respectively), and less than half consume the recommended servings of fruits and vegetables (≥5 per day). Furthermore, only 16 % regularly consume adequate liquids, and less than a quarter engage in ≥30 min of moderate to vigorous physical activity (MVPA) per day [57]. One study of objectively measured accelerometry data revealed that only 5 % of bariatric surgery patients are compliant with physical activity recommendations (≥150 min/week of MVPA in bouts ≥ 10 min) after surgery [58].

Recently, investigators have started to develop and assess behavioral and psychosocial interventions for patients who have undergone surgery with the goal of improving postoperative outcomes. A meta-analysis of this literature found that patients who receive postoperative interventions experience larger weight losses as compared to those who receive usual postoperative care, which does not typically include a level of ongoing behavioral support that many need to make sustained behavioral modifications necessary for success [59]. One of the most important contributions those who specialize in the behavioral health management of bariatric surgery patients can make to the field is to develop and study the efficacy of postsurgical programs designed to optimize weight and health outcomes and to ensure that patients maintain psychiatric stability.

Special Psychiatric Considerations

Psychiatric Medications

Anatomical and physiological changes that occur during and after bariatric surgery, particularly RYGB, likely affect the pharmacokinetic properties (e.g., absorption, distribution, and elimination) of medications. Alterations in these properties could affect the efficacy and tolerability of medications, which may be a point of particular concern when thinking about psychiatric medications. While a great majority of postsurgical patients are able to discontinue or decrease medications they were taking presurgically for many medical conditions (e.g., T2DM, hypertension), there is no evidence that patients should decrease or come off of psychiatric medications postsurgically. Moreover, though research in this area is limited, there is evidence of decreased absorption of a single dose of sertraline in post-RYGB patients in comparison to weight-matched nonsurgical controls [60]. Fortunately, research in this area is growing; however, to date there are no established clinical guidelines for psychiatric medication changes and/or dosage adjustments in bariatric surgery patients. In the absence of such guidelines, the following are actions that are sometimes considered by those prescribing psychiatric medications to patients who are considering or have undergone bariatric surgery: (1) switching to an immediate-release medication vs. sustained release; (2) when available, using liquid vs. tablet form; (3) when appropriate, crushing a medication vs. using in solid form; (4) when available, using an injectable medication vs. an oral medication; and (5) as possible, monitoring plasma levels of medications. While these medication adjustments could be considered, close and ongoing psychiatric management is always recommended.

Suicide Rates

The reported higher rate of suicide among bariatric patients postoperatively has been a source of significant concern within the field. These studies find a higher rate of suicide among bariatric patients postoperatively, compared to the population as a whole or to obese individuals who do not undergo weight loss surgery. Although overall mortality declines following weight loss surgery, increased deaths by accident, drug overdose, and suicide have all been documented following weight loss surgery [61–63].

One of the best controlled studies by Adams et al. compared long-term mortality rates and causes of death among over 7,000 gastric bypass patients and obese controls [61]. At a mean follow-up of 7.1 years, they found 15 suicides in surgery group vs. 5 in the control group. However the hazard ratio for suicide in the surgery group as compared to the control population was not significantly different. This suicide rate among surgical patients certainly appears to be considerably higher than the general US suicide rate of ~11/100,000. Bariatric surgery-related deaths in Pennsylvania have also been extensively studied over the last decade. Most recently, Tindle et al. reported an overall suicide rate of 6.6/10,000 in post-bariatric patients with highly differing rates for men and women (13.7 per 10,000 among men vs. 5.2 per 10,000 among women) [62]. However, in both studies the authors

were unable to determine whether participants were at higher risk of committing suicide preoperatively. Given the high prevalence of psychopathology among morbidly obese individuals and the high prevalence of past suicide attempts in bariatric candidates, it is unclear if this reflects a vulnerable population or something more specifically about the surgery [64].

Other than presurgical psychological distress, potential reasons for higher suicide rates among bariatric patients in the postoperative period include dissatisfaction with body image, alterations in metabolic biomarkers such as a decrease in serum cholesterol, and changes in the pharmacokinetics of psychotropic drugs resulting in reduced efficacy [65]. Although research should continue to identify the underlying reasons for suicide among bariatric patients, clinicians should absolutely continue to assess suicidality in this population and institute appropriate management as necessary.

Postsurgical Alcohol Abuse

Research indicates that individuals pursuing bariatric surgery have rates of lifetime alcohol use disorders (AUD) that are fairly comparable to the general population (35 % vs. 30 %, respectively) [24, 66]. However, current alcohol and substance abuse at the time of preoperative assessment is remarkably low (<1 %) compared to population norms (8.9 %), even in studies in which data collection is separate and confidential from the presurgical psychological evaluation [2]. Many patients continue to consume alcohol after surgery. A web-based questionnaire study indicated that 83 % of respondents continued to consume alcohol after RYGB, with 84 % of those drinking one or more alcoholic beverages a week and 28.4 % indicating a problem controlling alcohol use [17]. Suzuki and colleagues found that about 10 % of patients who had undergone AGB and RYGB met current diagnosis for an alcohol abuse disorder 2–5 years after surgery, rates that are similar to those in the general population [66]. The majority of these cases had a lifetime history of alcohol abuse disorders, suggesting relapses rather than new cases, and all occurred among those who had undergone RYGB, consistent with knowledge that physiological changes that occur with RYGB may change vulnerability to problematic alcohol use. More recently, longitudinal data across 10 bariatric programs and over 2,000 patients demonstrated a significant increase in AUD in the second (but not first) postoperative year and higher when compared to the year prior to surgery. A number of related risk factors were found including male gender, younger age, smoking, regular preoperative alcohol use, recreational drug use, and lower scores on social support [24]. In a study of longer-term outcomes (13–15 years) [67], an increase in alcohol abuse over time (2.6 % presurgery to 5.1 % postsurgery) but a decline in alcohol dependence was noted (10.3 % presurgery vs. 2.6 % postsurgery). In a study examining substance abuse treatment center admissions, 2–6 % of admissions were positive for a bariatric surgery history [68].

We recently described assessment techniques and strategies to provide informed consent and education on alcohol among patients preparing to having surgery [25]. Little guidance, however, has been offered regarding how to conduct postoperative screening nor how to provide specialized treatment for those who develop alcohol problems after surgery, nor has research yet addressed alcohol abuse rates following SG.

Body Image Concerns

Although overall body image is rated more positively after bariatric surgery, studies suggest that both men and women remain dissatisfied with specific body areas associated with redundant skin [69]. Rapid and substantial weight loss is often associated with hanging, redundant skin, which is aesthetically displeasing to patients and often leads to skin irritation, skin breakdown, infection, and ulcerations. Further, patients often note its effects on physical functioning, sexual functioning, posture, and difficulties with urination. Thus, patients often consider body contouring surgery to address excess skin; however, this surgery is not always covered by third-party payers and may be too expensive for patients to pursue. Setting realistic expectations about both positive and negative aesthetic changes following surgery should be part of patient's preparation. Further, helping patients adjust to significant body image disturbance (vs. dissatisfaction that does not cause interference) may be an important aspect of postsurgical psychological care.

Development of Eating Pathology and Eating Disorders

Research on the emergence of eating pathology following bariatric surgery is limited and is complicated by uncertainty over when to classify postsurgical eating behaviors as pathological, since eating behaviors in postsurgical bariatric patients will differ from the "normal" population and, thus, may appear aberrant (e.g., avoidance of certain foods to avoid dumping, markedly slowing down chewing, etc.). A recent review of pathological eating following bariatric surgery concluded that the development of full-syndrome eating disorders following surgery is rare, though serious [70]. As the rate of bariatric procedures increases nationwide, eating disorder treatment programs are increasingly faced with the challenge of developing protocols for post-bariatric patients presenting with a clinically diagnosable eating disorder and, more frequently, eating problems that do not meet classic eating disorder criteria. Although a few assessment tools exist, De Zwaan and colleagues developed a Bariatric

Surgery Version of the Eating Disorders Examination (EDE-BSV) to help differentiate between eating behaviors influenced by anatomical alterations that occur with surgery (e.g., vomiting due to food getting stuck/plugging) and those that are aberrant behaviors motivated by body image concerns (e.g., vomiting to promote weight loss or avoid weight gain) [71]. When the EDE-BSV was administered to 59 patients 18–35 months after RYGB surgery, 12 % of patients reported self-induced vomiting for weight purposes, 30 % reported chewing and spitting out food, 12 % reported nocturnal eating, and 32 % reported picking or nibbling at food. No other compensatory behaviors (e.g., laxative and diuretic use) were reported, and chewing and spitting was not reported for weight reasons but to avoid plugging. When pathological eating behaviors are suspected, referral to an eating disorder specialist is recommended, and in the case of extreme weight loss, inpatient treatment may be necessary.

Summary

Mental health professionals are considered an essential component of the multidisciplinary assessment and treatment team at most bariatric surgery treatment centers. These practitioners should have a thorough understanding of the biological, psychological, and social causes and consequences of morbid obesity and of behavioral factors that impact weight loss and weight loss maintenance following weight loss surgery. We have provided a detailed overview of components of the presurgical psychosocial evaluation of bariatric surgery patients and have summarized the literature on pre-, peri-, and postoperative management of bariatric surgery patients as related to behavioral and psychosocial risk factors. It is our strong belief that behavioral health should be an essential focus of all bariatric surgery programs and that guidelines for efficacious postoperative psychiatric behavioral support are needed to further impact bariatric surgery outcomes, including optimizing weight loss, resolving medical comorbidities, and improving quality of life and mental health status.

Review Questions

1. Which of the following is NOT a common psychological reason for denying candidates bariatric surgery?
   a. Current illicit drug abuse or dependence
   b. Binge eating disorder
   c. Active/under-controlled schizophrenia or other psychotic illness
   d. Lack of capacity to consent
   e. None of the above
   Answer: b

2. Problematic alcohol use following bariatric surgery has been linked to
   a. RYGB procedures
   b. Male gender
   c. Food addiction
   d. a and b
   e. All of the above

Answer: d

3. Poorer weight loss outcomes (as defined by % EWL) has been associated with
   a. Depression
   b. Disordered eating behaviors
   c. Bipolar disorder
   d. Total number of psychiatric diagnoses
   e. All of the above

Answer: e

References

1. Buchwald H, Oien DM. Metabolic/bariatric surgery worldwide 2008. Obes Surg. 2009;19(12):1605–11.
2. Kalarchian MA, Marcus MD, Levine MD, Courcoulas AP, Pilkonis PA, Ringham RM, et al. Psychiatric disorders among bariatric surgery candidates: relationship to obesity and functional health status. Am J Psychiatry. 2007;164(2):328–34.
3. Mitchell JE, Selzer F, Kalarchian MA, Devlin MJ, Strain GW, Elder KA, et al. Psychopathology before surgery in the longitudinal assessment of bariatric surgery-3 (LABS-3) psychosocial study. Surg Obes Relat Dis. 2012;8(5):533–41.
4. Allied Health Science Section ad hoc Behavioral Health Committee. American Society for Metabolic and Bariatric Surgery. Suggestions for the pre-surgical psychological assessment of bariatric surgery candidates; 2004.
5. Buchwald H, Avidor Y, Braunwald E, Jensen MD, Pories W, Fahrbach K, et al. Bariatric surgery: a systematic review and meta-analysis. J Am Med Assoc. 2004;292(14):1724–37.
6. Kinzl JF, Schrattenecker M, Traweger C, Mattesich M, Fiala M, Biebl W. Psychosocial predictors of weight loss after bariatric surgery. Obes Surg. 2006;16(12):1609–14.
7. Livhits M, Mercado C, Yermilov I, Parikh JA, Dutson E, Mehran A, et al. Preoperative predictors of weight loss following bariatric surgery: systematic review. Obes Surg. 2012;22(1):70–89.
8. Kalarchian MA, Marcus MD, Levine MD, Soulakova JN, Courcoulas AP, Wisinski MS. Relationship of psychiatric disorders to 6-month outcomes after gastric bypass. Surg Obes Relat Dis. 2008;4(4):544–9.
9. Walfish S, Vance D, Fabricatore AN. Psychological evaluation of bariatric surgery applicants: procedures and reasons for delay or denial of surgery. Obes Surg. 2007;17(12):1578–83.
10. Bauchowitz AU, Gonder-Frederick LA, Olbrisch ME, Azarbad L, Ryee MY, Woodson M, et al. Psychosocial evaluation of bariatric surgery candidates: a survey of present practices. Psychosom Med. 2005;67(5):825–32.
11. Fabricatore AN, Crerand CE, Wadden TA, Sarwer DB, Krasucki JL. How do mental health professionals evaluate candidates for bariatric surgery? Survey results. Obes Surg. 2006;16(5):567–73.
12. Mechanick JI, Youdim A, Jones DB, Garvey WT, Hurley DL, McMahon MM, Heinberg LJ, Kushner R, Adams TD, Shikora S, Dixon JB, Brethauer S. Clinical practice guidelines for the perioperative nutritional, metabolic, and nonsurgical support of the bariatric surgery patient—2013 update: cosponsored by American Association of Clinical Endocrinologists, the Obesity Society, and American Society for Metabolic & Bariatric Surgery. Obesity. 2013;21:S1–27.
13. de Zwaan M, Enderle J, Wagner S, Muhlhans B, Ditzen B, Gefeller O, et al. Anxiety and depression in bariatric surgery patients: a prospective, follow-up study using structured clinical interviews. J Affect Disord. 2011;133(1–2):61–8.
14. Semanscin-Doerr DA, Windover A, Ashton K, Heinberg LJ. Mood disorders in laparoscopic sleeve gastrectomy patients: does it affect early weight loss? Surg Obes Relat Dis. 2010;6(2):191–6.
15. Shikora SA, Kruger Jr RS, Blackburn GL, Fallon JA, Harvey AM, Johnson EQ, et al. Best practices in policy and access (coding and reimbursement) for weight loss surgery. Obesity (Silver Spring). 2009;17(5):918–23.
16. West-Smith L, Sogg S. Creating a credential for bariatric behavioral health professionals: potential benefits, pitfalls, and provider opinion. Surg Obes Relat Dis. 2010;6(6):695–701.
17. Buffington C. Alcohol use and health risks: survey results. Bariatric Times. 2007;4:21–3.
18. Heinberg LJ, Ashton K, Windover A. Moving beyond dichotomous psychological evaluation: the Cleveland Clinic Behavioral Rating System for weight loss surgery. Surg Obes Relat Dis. 2010;6(2):185–90.
19. Sogg S, Mori DL. The Boston interview for gastric bypass: determining the psychological suitability of surgical candidates. Obes Surg. 2004;14(3):370–80.
20. Pawlow LA, O'Neil PM, White MA, Byrne TK. Findings and outcomes of psychological evaluations of gastric bypass applicants. Surg Obes Relat Dis. 2005;1(6):523–7.
21. Tsuda S, Barrios L, Schneider B, Jones DB. Factors affecting rejection of bariatric patients from an academic weight loss program. Surg Obes Relat Dis. 2009;5(2):199–202.
22. Sadhasivam S, Larson CJ, Lambert PJ, Mathiason MA, Kothari SN. Refusals, denials, and patient choice: reasons prospective patients do not undergo bariatric surgery. Surg Obes Relat Dis. 2007;3(5):531–5.
23. American Psychiatric Association. Diagnostic and statistical manual of mental disorders. 5th ed. Arlington: American Psychiatric Association; 2013.
24. King WC, Chen JY, Mitchell JE, Kalarchian MA, Steffen KJ, Engel SG, et al. Prevalence of alcohol use disorders before and after bariatric surgery. J Am Med Assoc. 2012;307(23):2516–25.
25. Heinberg LJ, Ashton K, Coughlin J. Alcohol and bariatric surgery: review and suggested recommendations for assessment and management. Surg Obes Relat Dis. 2012;8(3):357–63.
26. Tiboni M, Zhalid Z, Powles P, Guyatt G, Anvari M. Safety of a perioperative strategy for the management of obstructive sleep apnea in bariatric surgery patients: a single Bariatric Center of Excellence experi. Pol Arch Med Wewn. 2012;122(12):641–3.
27. Bochicchio G. Perioperative glycemic control in bariatric and colorectal surgical patients. Ann Surg. 2013;257(1):15–6.
28. Nguyen NT, Nguyen B, Nguyen VQ, Ziogas A, Hohmann S, Stamos MJ. Outcomes of bariatric surgery performed at accredited vs nonaccredited centers. J Am Coll Surg. 2012;215(4):467–74.
29. Dallal RM, Trang A. Analysis of perioperative outcomes, length of hospital stay, and readmission rate after gastric bypass. Surg Endosc. 2012;26(3):754–8.
30. Gould JC, Kent KC, Wan Y, Rajamanickam V, Leverson G, Campos GM. Perioperative safety and volume: outcomes relationships in bariatric surgery: a study of 32,000 patients. J Am Coll Surg. 2011;213(6):771–7.
31. Smith MD, Patterson E, Wahed AS, Belle SH, Berk PD, Courcoulas AP, et al. Thirty-day mortality after bariatric surgery: independently adjudicated causes of death in the longitudinal assessment of bariatric surgery. Obes Surg. 2011;21(11):1687–92.
32. Dorman RB, Miller CJ, Leslie DB, Serrot FJ, Slusarek B, Buchwald H, et al. Risk for hospital readmission following bariatric surgery. PLoS One. 2012;7(3):e32506.

33. Flum DR, Belle SH, King WC, Wahed AS, Berk P, Chapman W, et al. Perioperative safety in the longitudinal assessment of bariatric surgery. N Engl J Med. 2009;361(5):445–54.

34. Subhani M, Rizvon K, Mustacchia P. Endoscopic evaluation of symptomatic patients following bariatric surgery: a literature review. Diagn Ther Endosc. 2012;2012:753472.

35. Compher CW, Hanlon A, Kang Y, Elkin L, Williams NN. Attendance at clinical visits predicts weight loss after gastric bypass surgery. Obes Surg. 2012;22(6):927–34.

36. Kaiser KA, Franks SF, Smith AB. Positive relationship between support group attendance and one-year postoperative weight loss in gastric banding patients. Surg Obes Relat Dis. 2011;7(1):89–93.

37. Ashton K, Heinberg L, Windover A, Merrell J. Positive response to binge eating intervention enhances postoperative weight loss. Surg Obes Relat Dis. 2011;7(3):315–20.

38. Vincent HK, Ben-David K, Conrad BP, Lamb KM, Seay AN, Vincent KR. Rapid changes in gait, musculoskeletal pain, and quality of life after bariatric surgery. Surg Obes Relat Dis. 2012; 8(3):346–54.

39. Pilone V, Mozzi E, Schettino AM, Furbetta F, Di MA, Giardiello C, et al. Improvement in health-related quality of life in first year after laparoscopic adjustable gastric banding. Surg Obes Relat Dis. 2012;8(3):260–8.

40. Sarwer DB, Wadden TA, Moore RH, Eisenberg MH, Raper SE, Williams NN. Changes in quality of life and body image after gastric bypass surgery. Surg Obes Relat Dis. 2010;6(6):608–14.

41. Dixon JB, Dixon ME, O'Brien PE. Quality of life after lap-band placement: influence of time, weight loss, and comorbidities. Obes Res. 2001;9(11):713–21.

42. Bocchieri LE, Meana M, Fisher BL. Perceived psychosocial outcomes of gastric bypass surgery: a qualitative study. Obes Surg. 2002;12(6):781–8.

43. Walters-Bugbee SE, McClure KS, Kral TV, Sarwer DB. Maternal child feeding practices and eating behaviors of women with extreme obesity and those who have undergone bariatric surgery. Surg Obes Relat Dis. 2012;8(6):784–91.

44. Woodard GA, Encarnacion B, Peraza J, Hernandez-Boussard T, Morton J. Halo effect for bariatric surgery: collateral weight loss in patients' family members. Arch Surg. 2011;146(10):1185–90.

45. Rebibo L, Verhaeghe P, Cosse C, Dhahri A, Marechal V, Regimbeau JM. Does longitudinal sleeve gastrectomy have a family "halo effect"? A case-matched study. Surg Endosc. 2013;27(5):1748–53.

46. Garb J, Welch G, Zagarins S, Kuhn J, Romanelli J. Bariatric surgery for the treatment of morbid obesity: a meta-analysis of weight loss outcomes for laparoscopic adjustable gastric banding and laparoscopic gastric bypass. Obes Surg. 2009;19(10):1447–55.

47. Clinical Issues Committee of the American Society for Metabolic and Bariatric Surgery. Updated position statement on sleeve gastrectomy as a bariatric procedure. Surg Obes Relat Dis. 2010;6(1):1–5.

48. Mor A, Sharp L, Portenier D, Sudan R, Torquati A. Weight loss at first postoperative visit predicts long-term outcome of Roux-en-Y gastric bypass using Duke weight loss surgery chart. Surg Obes Relat Dis. 2012;8(5):556–60.

49. Melton GB, Steele KE, Schweitzer MA, Lidor AO, Magnuson TH. Suboptimal weight loss after gastric bypass surgery: correlation of demographics, comorbidities, and insurance status with outcomes. J Gastrointest Surg. 2008;12(2):250–5.

50. DiGiorgi M, Rosen DJ, Choi JJ, Milone L, Schrope B, Olivero-Rivera L, et al. Re-emergence of diabetes after gastric bypass in patients with mid- to long-term follow-up. Surg Obes Relat Dis. 2010;6(3):249–53.

51. Barhouch AS, Zardo M, Padoin AV, Colossi FG, Casagrande DS, Chatkin R, et al. Excess weight loss variation in late postoperative period of gastric bypass. Obes Surg. 2010;20(11):1479–83.

52. Magro DO, Geloneze B, Delfini R, Pareja BC, Callejas F, Pareja JC. Long-term weight regain after gastric bypass: a 5-year prospective study. Obes Surg. 2008;18(6):648–51.

53. Snyder B, Nguyen A, Scarbourough T, Yu S, Wilson E. Comparison of those who succeed in losing significant excessive weight after bariatric surgery and those who fail. Surg Endosc. 2009;23(10): 2302–6.

54. Sarwer DB, Dilks RJ, West-Smith L. Dietary intake and eating behavior after bariatric surgery: threats to weight loss maintenance and strategies for success. Surg Obes Relat Dis. 2011;7(5): 644–51.

55. Sjostrom L. Bariatric surgery and reduction in morbidity and mortality: experiences from the SOS study. Int J Obes (Lond). 2008;32 Suppl 7:S93–7.

56. Karlsson J, Taft C, Ryden A, Sjostrom L, Sullivan M. Ten-year trends in health-related quality of life after surgical and conventional treatment for severe obesity: the SOS intervention study. Int J Obes (Lond). 2007;31(8):1248–61.

57. Thomas JG, Bond DS, Ryder BA, Leahey TM, Vithiananthan S, Roye GD, et al. Ecological momentary assessment of recommended postoperative eating and activity behaviors. Surg Obes Relat Dis. 2011;7(2):206–12.

58. Bond DS, Jakicic JM, Unick JL, Vithiananthan S, Pohl D, Roye GD, et al. Pre- to postoperative physical activity changes in bariatric surgery patients: self report vs. objective measures. Obesity (Silver Spring). 2010;18(12):2395–7.

59. Rudolph A, Hilbert A. Post-operative behavioural management in bariatric surgery: a systematic review and meta-analysis of randomized controlled trials. Obes Rev. 2013;14(4):292–302.

60. Roerig JL, Steffen K, Zimmerman C, Mitchell JE, Crosby RD, Cao L. Preliminary comparison of sertraline levels in postbariatric surgery patients versus matched nonsurgical cohort. Surg Obes Relat Dis. 2012;8(1):62–6.

61. Adams TD, Gress RE, Smith SC, Halverson RC, Simper SC, Rosamond WD, et al. Long-term mortality after gastric bypass surgery. N Engl J Med. 2007;357(8):753–61.

62. Tindle HA, Omalu B, Courcoulas A, Marcus M, Hammers J, Kuller LH. Risk of suicide after long-term follow-up from bariatric surgery. Am J Med. 2010;123(11):1036–42.

63. Omalu BI, Ives DG, Buhari AM, Lindner JL, Schauer PR, Wecht CH, et al. Death rates and causes of death after bariatric surgery for Pennsylvania residents, 1995 to 2004. Arch Surg. 2007; 142(10):923–8.

64. Windover AK, Merrell J, Ashton K, Heinberg LJ. Prevalence and psychosocial correlates of self-reported past suicide attempts among bariatric surgery candidates. Surg Obes Relat Dis. 2010;6(6): 702–6.

65. Heneghan HM, Heinberg L, Windover A, Rogula T, Schauer PR. Weighing the evidence for an association between obesity and suicide risk. Surg Obes Relat Dis. 2012;8(1):98–107.

66. Suzuki J, Haimovici F, Chang G. Alcohol use disorders after bariatric surgery. Obes Surg. 2012;22(2):201–7.

67. Mitchell JE, Lancaster KL, Burgard MA, Howell LM, Krahn DD, Crosby RD, et al. Long-term follow-up of patients' status after gastric bypass. Obes Surg. 2001;11(4):464–8.

68. Saules KK, Wiedemann A, Ivezaj V, Hopper JA, Foster-Hartsfield J, Schwarz D. Bariatric surgery history among substance abuse treatment patients: prevalence and associated features. Surg Obes Relat Dis. 2010;6(6):615–21.

69. Kitzinger HB, Abayev S, Pittermann A, Karle B, Kubiena H, Bohdjalian A, et al. The prevalence of body contouring surgery after gastric bypass surgery. Obes Surg. 2012;22(1):8–12.

70. Marino JM, Ertelt TW, Lancaster K, Steffen K, Peterson L, de Zwaan M, et al. The emergence of eating pathology after bariatric surgery: a rare outcome with important clinical implications. Int J Eat Disord. 2012;45(2):179–84.

71. de Zwaan M, Hilbert A, Swan-Kremeier L, Simonich H, Lancaster K, Howell LM, et al. Comprehensive interview assessment of eating behavior 18-35 months after gastric bypass surgery for morbid obesity. Surg Obes Relat Dis. 2010;6(1):79–85.

9

Operating Room Positioning, Equipment, and Instrumentation for Laparoscopic Bariatric Surgery

Stacy A. Brethauer and Esam S. Batayyah

Introduction

The majority of bariatric operations are now performed laparoscopically. While it may seem second nature to experienced bariatric surgeons who have established techniques, there are many different techniques and devices available to perform gastric bypass and sleeve gastrectomy safely. For the surgeon starting a bariatric program, considerable thought and planning are required to obtain the proper operating room equipment and surgical instrumentation. Frequently, the instruments used during a surgeon's fellowship are not available at their new hospital and a case must be made to obtain the equipment necessary for the surgeon to perform the operations as they did during their training. Deviations from a standardized technique and the use of unfamiliar instrumentation can be stressful and may prolong operations or affect outcomes [1, 2]. This chapter reviews specialized equipment used for patient positioning, laparoscopic access, insufflation, visualization by camera, energy sources for transection and coagulation, staplers, hand instruments, flexible endoscopy, voice activation and robotics, and a "fully integrated" operating room layout.

Morbidly obese patients present multiple obstacles and specific patient characteristics which may require modifications to the technology normally used for laparoscopic procedures. In particular excessive abdominal adiposity interferes with visualization, freedom of instrument movement and frequently requires instruments of exceptional length and strength. Laparoscopic approaches in obese surgical patients require advanced skills in intracorporeal stapling techniques, suturing techniques, hemostasis techniques, and flexible endoscopy. Comorbid medical conditions may reduce patient tolerance of intra-abdominal CO_2 and necessitate alternative means of maintaining visualization [1].

For the purposes of this chapter, it is assumed that the surgeon is familiar with the application of laparoscopic instruments and equipment as they apply to the general patient undergoing minimally invasive surgery [3, 4]. Detailed information regarding the engineering and technology behind the equipment is available from many excellent sources [5–9]. It is certainly recognized that there may be alternative equipment or approaches that are equally or more suitable and that optimal choices will change with time and the availability or newer technologies.

Patient Positioning

The main goals in the positioning of a morbidly obese patient in preparation for bariatric surgery are: safe transfer to the operating room table, neutral positioning of the major joints and extremities, avoidance of pressure injuries to skin or nerves, accessibility of the operative field by the surgical team, and security of the patient on the table [10, 11]. Due to anatomical considerations of some morbidly obese persons, standard fundamental patient positioning principles with attention to detail as well as some creativity will be needed to achieve these goals.

The patient is brought to the operating room by stretcher. We have found that lateral transfer devices which utilize hover technology (Hovermatt, HoverTech International) enable the team to move the patient to the operating table and back to the transport stretcher or bed in a secure and comfortable manner. It requires at least two staff members, one on each side of the patient with minimal lifting or pulling force. This device has decreased patient and staff injuries (Fig. 1).

During surgery, we use a supine position with legs together and arms abducted. The patient is positioned and secured at the waist with table straps. The patient is also secured at the legs with tape to keep the knees from flexing apart while in steep reverse Trendelenburg position. The patient's weight should be evenly distributed on the table without parts of the torso or limbs hanging over the side. Side rail extensions can be used to augment the width of the table.

Fɪɢ. 1. Use of lateral transfer device to move patient on and off operating table.

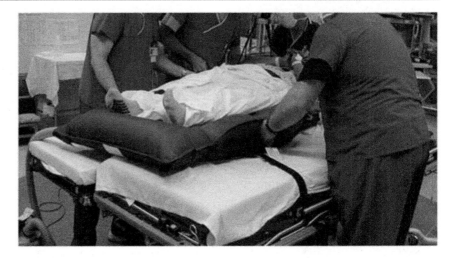

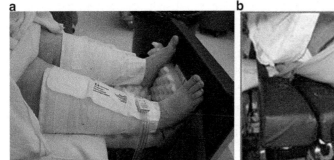
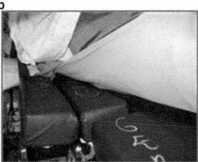
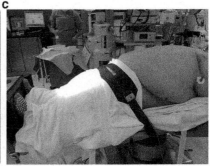

Fɪɢ. 2. Patient positioning and application of sequential compression device (**a**). Padded bed extensions should be used for larger patients (**b**). Inspect for areas of significant pressure, circulatory compromise, neutral positioning of extremities, and patient security to table prior to prepping and draping the abdomen (**c**).

Pneumatic compression devices that accommodate the super-obese patient are placed on the patient prior to induction of anesthesia [12].

After the induction of general anesthesia and endotracheal intubation, a urinary catheter is inserted (often requiring two staff members, one for retraction of skin folds and one for insertion), and a bovie grounding pad is placed usually on the anterior thigh. A foot board is placed on the table so the feet will have a secure base to rest when the patient is in extreme reverse Trendelenburg position.

The surgeon stands on the patient's right side along with the scrub nurse; the first assistant and the camera operator are on the patient's left side. The arms may be left out if adequate room is available or one or both may be tucked. Occasionally, when tucking an arm, a metal or plastic limb holder (sled) may be required to secure the arm at the side. This approach also serves to protect the arm.

The base of a stationary retractor-holding device may be attached to the table at this time. Care must be taken that it does not come in direct contact with the patient's skin to avoid pressure injury or electrocautery conduction.

Prior to prepping and draping the patient, a "final check" is important to be sure that all pressure points are avoided, especially along the side, arms, hands, head, and feet. Sequential compression devices should be placed and turned on (Fig. 2a). Table attachments must be padded appropriately to avoid pressure or nerve injuries (Fig. 2b). Security of the patient on the table and neutrality of joint positioning of the extremities are also confirmed again (Fig. 2c). Of special note is to be certain there is no undue pressure on the gluteal area. A rare complication of rhabdomyolysis has been reported, especially with patients with a BMI 60 or greater. Consequences of rhabdomyolysis include renal failure and death [13, 14]. Heating blankets are helpful in preventing hypothermia related to heat loss from evaporation and continuous insufflation, particularly during operations of long duration.

After prepping and draping the abdomen, setting up the equipment on the field, and assembling the OR team, the working field will appear as depicted in Fig. 3. Some surgeons prefer the "French" or "between the legs" positioning in which the patient's legs are abducted and the surgeon stands

FIG. 3. The operating team in their places. Primary surgeon is to the patient's right. First assistant is across from the primary surgeon. Second assistant and scrub nurse are at the foot of the bed.

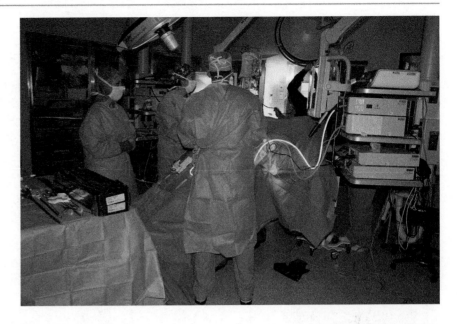

FIG. 4. Standard and long Veress needles.

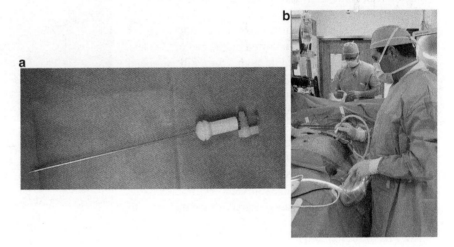

Laparoscopic Access

The Veress Needle Approach

We utilize a Veress needle to establish a pneumoperitoneum in the obese patient because it is technically very difficult to perform an open cutdown (Hasson) technique. A long-length Veress needle of 150 mm (Autosuture, Division of Tyco Healthcare) (Fig. 4a, b) is inserted using a subcostal incision in the left upper quadrant. The 2-mm needle has a spring-loaded blunt inner cannula that automatically extends beyond the needle point once the abdominal cavity has been entered. This blunt cannula has a side-hole to permit entry of CO_2 gas into the abdominal cavity. Correct position of the Veress needle after it has passed through the abdominal wall can be verified by methods such as the water drop test or by assessing CO_2 pressures and flow. In obese patients, opening intra-abdominal pressures may be high (up to 10–12 cm of H_2O).

Insertion of Trocars

In addition to being safe and reliable, trocars and cannulas for laparoscopic bariatric surgery should minimize air leaks, secure readily to the abdominal wall, allow rapid exchange of instruments of various diameters, and be of sufficient length to reach the peritoneal cavity without causing excessive disruption of the abdominal fascia. We currently use a

between them with assistants and OR technician flanking him/her. This is described in other chapters. A limitation with this approach is that there may be a little space between the legs due to the girth of the thighs or of the surgeon.

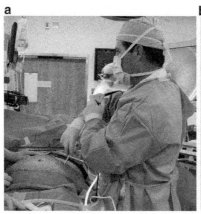
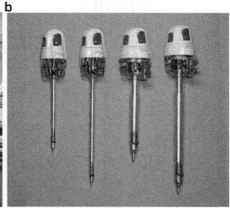

Fig. 5. (**a**) A 5-mm optical viewing trocar can be used to obtain direct access to the peritoneal cavity without pneumoperitoneum. The distinct layers of subcutaneous fat, fascia, muscle, preperitoneal fat, and the peritoneum are identified as the trocar passes through them (Endopath Xcel, Ethicon Endosurgery, Cincinnati, OH). (**b**) 5- and 12-mm trocars (100 and 150 cm lengths) (Endopath Xcel, Ethicon Endosurgery, Cincinnati, OH). These clear-tipped bladeless trocars can also be used for optical entry into the peritoneal cavity.

5-mm optical viewing trocar (Xcel, Ethicon Endosurgery, Cincinnati, OH) for initial access to the peritoneal cavity. The 5-mm scope is placed into the trocar after the camera is white balanced. The focus is adjusted on the end of the clear trocar tip. The trocar is placed through a 5-mm incision and the fatty, fascial, and muscular layers of the abdominal wall are directly visualized as the trocar passes through them (Fig. 5a). After the tip of the trocar passes through the preperitoneal fat and the peritoneum, the camera and obturator are removed, and the insufflations tubing is attached. Once adequate pneumoperitoneum is established, the remaining trocars are placed under direct laparoscopic vision. Trocars with 100-mm shafts are usually sufficient, but occasionally, extra-long trocars (150 mm) are required for the patient with an excessively thick abdominal wall (Fig. 5b).

After the insertion of the first trocar, a standard 25-gauge spinal needle can be helpful in locating the precise intra-abdominal location for the placement of additional trocars and providing preemptive analgesia with injection of local anesthetic (Fig. 6).

Insufflator

In laparoscopic surgery, exposure depends upon insufflation of the peritoneal cavity with CO_2 to create a pneumoperitoneum. The insufflator monitors the current intra-abdominal pressure and regulates the flow of CO_2 from a pressurized reservoir. A desired intra-abdominal pressure is selected and the flow of gas is automatically regulated. The front LCD screen on the insufflator displays the current intra-abdominal pressure, the preset desired pressure, the current rate of CO_2 insufflation, the volume of gas infused, and the residual volume in the CO_2 tank. Alarms signal high intra-abdominal pressures, excessive gas leak, and low gas level in the CO_2 tank. The rate of insufflation can be adjusted from 1 up to 40 L/min and higher flows are typically used. Our standard

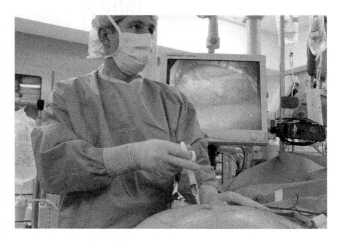

Fig. 6. Spinal needle placed through abdominal wall to help with port positioning. Local anesthetic is injected into the preperitoneal space under laparoscopic visualization prior to port placement.

preset intra-abdominal pressure is 15-mmHg, but we will intermittently use higher pressure (16–18-mmHg) when better exposure is needed or a lower pressure when instrument length is insufficient or the patient isn't physiologically tolerating higher pressures.

Gas leakage can be very troublesome during laparoscopic bariatric procedures especially if a circular stapling technique is in use. A high flow insufflator (40 L/min) is highly recommended to accommodate for gas leakage from small air leaks at port sites, instrument exchanges, and during intra-abdominal suctioning (Fig. 7).

Visualization

Technology which provides the surgeon with a clear view of the operating field has been critical to the development of advanced laparoscopic procedures. Safely and effective performance of a laparoscopic procedure is dependent upon the quality of visualization. Since the surgeon is not able to touch and palpate, a clear crisp bright image is mandatory at all times. There are no "blind" maneuvers in laparoscopy. Components that create and maintain the image have steadily improved.

There are several conditions specific to laparoscopic bariatric surgery that make obtaining an adequate image challenging. In the morbidly obese patient, the voluminous abdominal cavity expanded by the pneumoperitoneum requires more light for visualization than that required for the non-obese patient. Copious adipose tissue covering mesentery, omentum, and viscera may crowd the view and obscure the landmarks of interest. Instrumentation that will allow viewing around or over or under such objects is necessary. Additional instruments are needed to enable adequate exposure.

Laparoscope

The laparoscope uses the Hopkins rod lens system which consists of a series of quartz rod lenses and a fiber bundle surrounding the rod lens for transmission of light [5, 6]. The eyepiece of the laparoscope is connected to the camera by means of a coupler adapter.

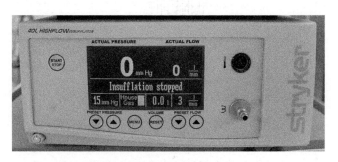

Fig. 7. High flow insufflator. Stryker.

Standard laparoscopes have a length of approximately 32 cm and have diameters that range from 2 to 10 mm. Scopes are angled to various degrees, most commonly from a 0° to 45° orientation. Angled scopes provide more flexibility in viewing internal structures and provide access to areas that would be "blind" to 0° scopes. However, they require some additional skill to operate and the angling decreases light transmission slightly.

For our bariatric procedures, we have a variety of laparoscopes available: 30° and 45° with 5 and 10 mm diameters (Fig. 8a, b) (Stryker Endoscopy). Typically we use a 5-mm 45° scope, initially at the 5-mm entrance site, to visualize the other port placements. A 10-mm diameter, 45° angled laparoscope is used for the rest of the procedure as we have found that it provides the best field of view especially in extremely obese patients. An extra-long laparoscope (45–50 cm) is sometimes necessary and very helpful in super-obese patients. Excessive abdominal wall thickness, together with a large expanded abdominal cavity, does not allow for a close-up view of distant sites (e.g., the esophagogastric junction) using the standard-size scopes. Extra-long scopes are also helpful during the use of any type of scope-holding instrument or robot which takes up functional scope length in establishing the connection.

An important scope accessory is a stainless steel scope warmer canister filled with hot sterile water for cleaning the scope and preventing lens fogging (Applied Medical) (Fig. 9).

Video Camera

Miniature lightweight cameras, weighing as little as 40 g, are now in use providing excellent resolution and color rendition which are essential for laparoscopic bariatric surgery. The miniature camera uses an LCD chip containing approximately 300,000 light-sensitive pixels on the chip surface measuring only about ½ inch on the diagonal. Three-chip cameras have become the industry standard; each chip provides one of the three primary colors: red, green, and blue.

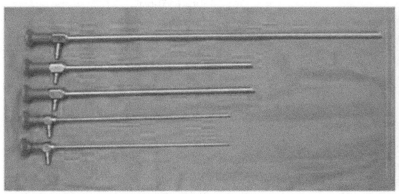
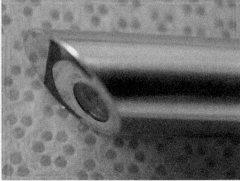

Fig. 8. Laparoscopes: angled 45° (*inset*) and 30°, 5 and 10 mm diameters and standard and long lengths.

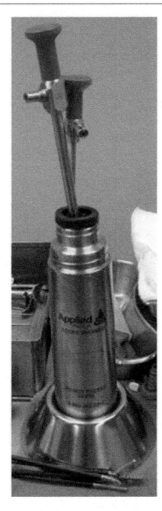

Fig. 9. Laparoscope warmer decreases fogging (Applied Medical). The laparoscope warmer should be attached to the surgical drapes for easy access.

There are a number of options for this type of equipment including the Stryker Endoscopy® 3-chip camera (Fig. 10), which has 1920 × 1080p resolution.

A C-mount endoscopic coupler permits rapid attachment of the camera to whichever scope is in use. The coupler also has a focusing knob. The camera head control buttons enable the user to adjust gain, digital zoom, and printer modalities. The camera is connected to the power supply and electronic control by cable. The system is further enhanced using voice activation technology to control adjustments of white balance, gain, shutter, and digital enhancement.

Light Source and Light Cable

Laparoscopy requires a high intensity light source for an adequate video image of the operative field. A xenon or metal halide bulb with a life span of about 250 h is typically used because these provide the desirable color temperature in the range of daylight (5,500 k). An automatic adjustment as well as a manual override is available (to over- or under-illuminate

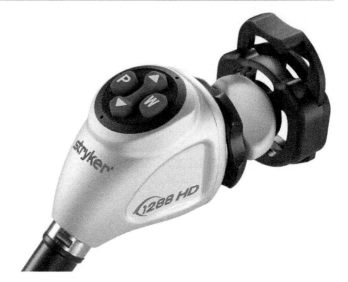

Fig. 10. Three-chip video camera (Stryker).

if needed). Interaction between the camera and the light source allows automatic adjustment of the illumination intensity with changes in light level at the camera CCD surface. This will greatly reduce annoying glare. The light is transmitted from the bulb to the scope through a fiber optic light cable which should be replaced if more than 15 % broken fibers are noted. A full benefit of the light source depends on proper connection of the cable to the light source and the telescope. The light cables should not be autoclaved and must be sterilized in either ethylene-oxide or glutaraldehyde.

Video Monitor

The video monitor providing the laparoscopic image should be of the highest quality. There are many configurations and products available. We currently utilize a flat panel digital design mounted on an overhead boom. The boom facing the operating surgeon (right side) has two screens so that endoscopic and laparoscopic images can be simultaneously displayed (Fig. 11).

Operating Tables

The operating table must provide maximum tilt and rotation and allow gravity to shift abdominal structures to allow full visualization. For bariatric procedures, the operating table must have the capacity to support super-obese patients up to the maximum weight with which the surgeon is comfortable. Many standard general purpose OR tables have weight limits of about 227 kg which are adequate for 95 % or more of the cases in most bariatric practices. It is advisable to check with the manufacturer regarding the specific weight limitations of the specific operating table model and vintage available to you. Bariatric practices which include patients with weights

Fig. 11. Dual monitors facing the operation surgeon allow for simultaneous laparoscopic and endoscopic images which is particularly useful when performing an intraoperative leak test.

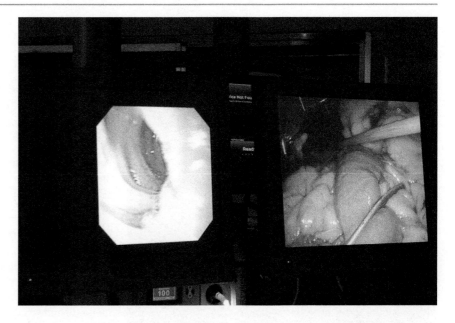

Fig. 11. Dual monitors facing the operation surgeon allow for simultaneous laparoscopic and endoscopic images which is particularly useful when performing an intraoperative leak test.

greater than 227 kg require access to an operating room table that can accommodate them safely. Many general purpose tables have been modified to accommodate the greater weight with some loss in the angle of tilt and Trendelenburg/ reverse Trendelenburg in the interest of assuring stability. This trade-off has become less necessary due to improving weight ratings and articulation in recent operating table technology. Important bed accessories include side extenders, footboards, straps, and padding to safely secure the patient to the bed and prevent injuries.

Hand Instrumentation

Grasping Instruments

Hand instruments are available with many different features and preferences. Our preference has been for "in-line" design (as opposed to a pistol grip design and for instruments where ratcheted handle control can be turned on and off along with finger-controlled rotation of the shaft. For the super-obese patient, instrument length is an important factor. Many instruments are available in standard (32 cm) and extra-long lengths (45 cm) (Fig. 12). For laparoscopic bariatric surgery, atraumatic and traumatic grasping hand instruments are needed. An atraumatic grasper is required to manipulate bowel without causing injury. We use a 5-mm atraumatic grasper "duckbill" (Snowden-Pencer) that features fine teeth and a broad tip design which provide a secure grip without traumatizing the tissue. The 5-mm "alligator" grasper (Snowden-Pencer) features tissue channels and long contoured jaws to provide secure grasping ability. It is excellent for holding the stomach and omentum.

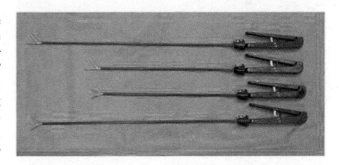

Fig. 12. Hand instrumentation: standard and long-length grasper. Traumatic graspers are shown on top and atraumatic graspers for use on the small bowel are shown at the bottom (Snowden-Pencer).

Retracting Instruments and Instrument Stabilizers

Anterior and cephalad retraction of the left lobe of the liver is required to expose the gastroesophageal junction. A number of devices work effectively for this purpose; they must be strong enough to retract large, heavy livers without trauma to the organ tissue. The 5-mm diameter Endoflex Retractor (Snowden-Pencer) is effective; it assumes a triangular configuration when tightened (Fig. 13). The retractor is usually held in a stationary position by means of an external holding device attached to the OR table such as the Fast Clamp System (Snowden-Pencer) (Fig. 14). For extremely large livers, a modification of the Endoflex liver retractor called the "Big D" type is available to help stabilize and provide exposure. Occasionally in extremely large patients, it has been necessary to use two liver retractors. In these cases, the Endoflex can be used to hold up the right and medial left lobe of the liver and a Nathanson retractor placed

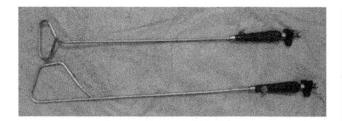

FIG. 13. 5-mm, flexible liver retractors: standard and "Big D" type.

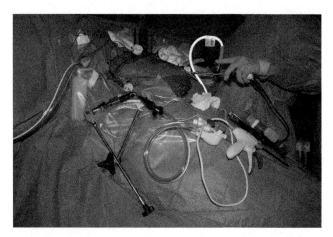

FIG. 14. Table-mounted instrument holding device used for liver retractor.

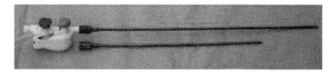

FIG. 15. Suction irrigator: standard and long-length tips (Stryker Endoscopy).

through a subxiphoid incision can be added to lift the left lateral segment upward to provide adequate working space around the upper stomach.

Suction Irrigation Devices

A suction/irrigation instrument clears the surgical field of pooling blood and keeps the abdominal cavity free from smoke and vapor. The StrykeFlow 2 (Stryker Endoscopy) is a 5-mm disposable instrument with reusable probe tips which performs the function of both suction and irrigation through a single common channel. The probe tips come in a standard (32 cm) working length as well as an extra-long (45 cm) working length which is crucial for the super-obese patient (Fig. 15). A larger diameter, 10-mm, suction tip is available and is useful when suctioning larger clots or thicker fluid from the abdominal cavity.

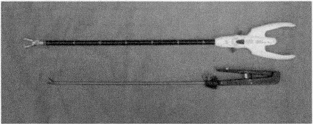

FIG. 16. Endo Stitch™ (US Surgical) and in-line laparoscopic needle driver.

Suturing Instruments

Standard laparoscopic needle drivers and sutures and suturing devices such as the Endo Stitch are suitable for laparoscopic bariatric surgery. We utilize the Endo Stitch™ (Covidien) to facilitate endoscopic suturing. The 10-mm diameter, disposable Endo Stitch™ has a double-pointed shuttle needle with the thread mounted at the center of the needle (Fig. 16). Double action jaws allow the needle to be passed back and forth by squeezing the handle and maneuvering the toggle switch eliminating regrasping and repositioning the needle. The Endo Stitch is compatible with a variety of absorbable (i.e., Polysorb™) and nonabsorbable sutures (i.e., Surgidek™). The Endo Stitch is used during the RYGBP for approximating the bowel for the enteroenterostomy and for oversewing the gastrojejunostomy (two-layer closures).

Atraumatic Bowel Clamps

The laparoscopic bowel clamp is a 10-mm diameter instrument that has long jaws with serrations that provide a secure atraumatic grip. It has a ratcheted handle for locking the jaws. It is available in a straight and curved jaw and is used to clamp the small bowel (Roux-limb) before performing endoscopy to prevent distal insufflation of the small bowel (Fig. 17).

Specialized Grasping Instruments

The fenestrated articulating grasper instrument (Snowden-Pencer) has an articulating tip which forms a gentle curve at about a 45° angle when the handles are closed (Fig. 18). The instrument can be used to help in the dissection and identification of the angle of His and the development of a passage as a guide for the stapler to use as a guide. In the retrocolic retrogastric approach, this instrument is very useful in passing the Roux-limb through the retro colic and retro gastric tunnel up to the gastric pouch before performing the anastomosis.

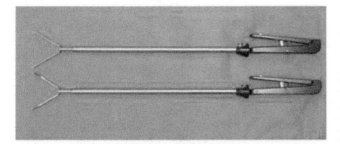

Fig. 17. Atraumatic bowel clamps: straight and curved tips.

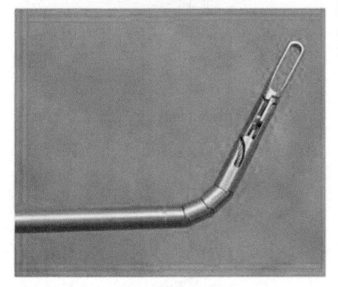

Fig. 18. Fenestrated articulating grasper helps with dissection at the angle of His.

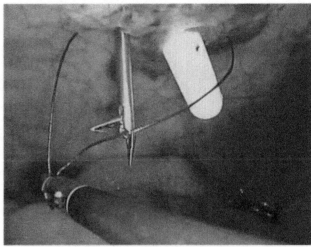

Fig. 19. Suture passer device facilitates closure of trocar sites and can be used to close small ventral hernias.

Suture Passer for Trocar Site Closure

To prevent trocar site hernias, we close all ports 10 mm or greater with a strong absorbable suture such. There are a number of devices available for passing sutures through the abdominal wall fascia. We use the Carter-Thomason CloseSure System (Inlet Medical Inc.) (Fig. 19) which facilitates full-thickness closure. It is a disposable device that comes with guides (pilots) of varying diameters and in a standard and long length to accommodate very thick abdominal walls. The angle projected by the guide allows for an adequate purchase of fascial tissue. The suture passer can also be used without the guide to ligate abdominal wall bleeders and to repair small umbilical, ventral, and incisional hernias noted at the time of laparoscopic bariatric surgery.

Other Hand Instruments

We use disposable endoscopic shears for cutting tissues when a laparoscopic scissor is needed. These shears are 5 mm with a rotating shaft and a 16-mm curved blade. A reliably sharp blade is one of its major advantages.

In the event of bleeding where a clip is needed, we use the multiload disposable clip applier with titanium clips. It is available in 5-mm and 10-mm diameter sizes. Compared to single-clip units, the multiload units considerably increase the speed and efficiency with which hemostasis can be accomplished.

Energy Sources for Transecting and Coagulation

In general laparoscopy, dividing tissues and achieving hemostasis, can be obtained with standard unipolar or bipolar electrocautery. Ultrasonic transaction and coagulation may be preferable for extremely vascular tissue such as mesentery. These devises are ultrasonically activated instruments that provide excellent tissue transection and hemostasis while eliminating the problem of electrical arc injury associated with unipolar electrocautery. The instruments have a stationary jaw and blade that vibrate at a frequency of between 55,000 and 60,000 Hz. The mechanical action of a stationary jaw and blade that vibrate at that frequency denatures collagen. This allows the formation of a coagulant which instantly seals small blood vessels. Minimal heat is generated in the tissue through friction; the lateral spread of thermal energy is 1–2 mm.

Ultrasonic instruments are available in 5 mm diameter and come in short (15.7-cm working length) and long lengths (45-cm working length) with finger-controlled rotating shaft (Fig. 20). They are activated by foot switch or by a finger-controlled button, which adjusts the blade frequency and the speed of cutting through tissue and the degree of hemostasis. These instruments produce water vapor that can obscure vision requiring intermittent evacuation of the vapor.

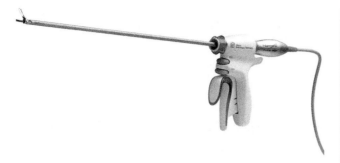

Fig. 20. Ultrasonic dissecting shears with hand controls (*inset*) (Ethicon Endosurgery, Cincinnati, OH).

During LRYGBP, we employ ultrasonic dissection liberally, especially for dissection along the lesser and greater curves of the stomach for gastric pouch creation and for making enterotomies in the stomach and small intestine, for stapler insertion, and for creating the division of the omentum in the antecolic approach.

Staplers: Linear and Circular

Linear Staplers

The laparoscopic articulating linear stapler has allowed the techniques in bariatric surgery to be performed efficiently and safely. It can be used to transect hollow viscera, to divide highly vascular tissue such as mesentery, and to create an anastomosis. We use the Endopath Echelon 60 disposable stapler (Ethicon Endosurgery, Cincinnati, OH) that applies two triple rows of staples before dividing the tissue with an advancing knife (Fig. 21). The stapler can be reloaded for use with tissues of varying thickness including a white load (2.5 mm), blue load (3.5 mm), green load (4.1 mm), and a gold cartridge that is used primarily for thicker tissue compressible to 1.8 mm. The stapler fits down a 12-mm trocar. We use the blue load to create the gastric pouch and gastrojejunostomy and the white load to divide the small bowel and mesentery and to create the jejunojejunostomy. The green load is useful for revisional bariatric surgery or in cases where the tissue is unusually thick or indurated.

Circular Staplers

A circular endoluminal stapler can be used to create the gastrojejunal anastomosis during laparoscopic RYGB. The Covidien EEA circular stapler (Covidien, Mansfield, MA) forms two rows of circular staples with an inner circular knife to create a circular anastomosis (Fig. 22). The stapler (21 or 25 mm) is typically inserted through an enlarged port

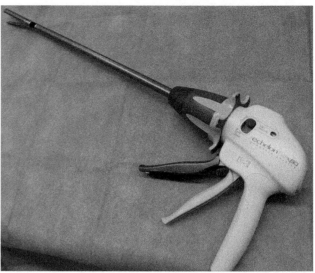

Fig. 21. Laparoscopic linear cutting stapler (Echelon 60, Ethicon Endosurgery, Cincinnati, OH).

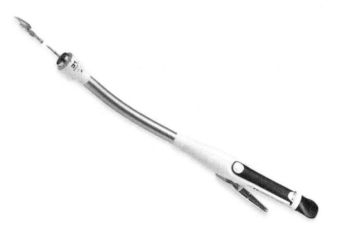

Fig. 22. An EEA stapler used to create a circular stapled gastrojejunostomy (DST Series™ EEA Stapler™. All rights reserved. Used with permission of Covidien).

site in the left upper quadrant. The anvil can be placed into the pouch using transoral or transgastric techniques. When using the transoral technique with the EEA, the anvil is attached to an orogastric tube which is used to pull the anvil into place through a gastrotomy in the pouch. The anvil rotates parallel with the shaft to facilitate transoral passage and removal.

Flexible Endoscopy

Flexible endoscopy serves several useful functions during the course of the LRYGB. A two-camera system, one each for the laparoscope and endoscope, facilitates this approach.

Both camera systems are fed through a digital mixer producing the two images on the same monitor as a "picture-in-picture" format or on adjacent screens allowing both the surgeon and the endoscopist to visualize both activities simultaneously.

At the completion of the LRYGB, a flexible endoscope is useful to examine the gastrojejunal anastomosis (Olympus GIF XQ40, Exerna CLV-160). The scope is inserted prior to completion of the closure of the gastrojejunostomy common opening when using the linear stapler anastomosis technique. This maneuver serves to stent the opening and to help gauge the diameter of the anastomosis. After the anastomosis is completed, intraluminal insufflation of the submerged anastomosis is used to inspect for air leaks. The endoscope is further useful in gauging the size and patency of the anastomosis and to examine for bleeding and viability of the gastric pouch.

Voice Activation Technology

A major new innovation in operating room procedure has been the introduction of voice control technology (Intuitive Surgical and Stryker Endoscopy). This technology provides a centralized and simplified interface for a surgeon to medical devices through voice commands. The system requires a computer control unit associated with other accessory units which are networked with multiple devices. The surgeon, who wears a wireless headphone/microphone transmitter (ATW-T75 Transmitter) (Audio-Techniques/Stryker Endoscopy) is able to control and operate the devices throughout the procedure saving time and dependency on human intermediaries. This technology allows the surgeon to voice control the camera, light source, insufflator, video/image recorder, printer, telephone, operating table, and operating room lights.

Voice-activated control is especially appropriate to bariatric laparoscopic procedures because of the multiple adjustments and readjustments of multiple complicated medical devices during the course of the operation. Safety and quality of patient care appear to be enhanced by returning focus from the technology to the patient [15].

Operating Room Layout

The organization and layout of the operating room are as crucial to efficient surgery as the equipment used. There must be an adequate space for transfer of morbidly obese patients to and from the operating table must be allowed for, including the number of personnel needed for the transfer. Vital equipment must be in easy reach without obstructing movement of the operating staff. Many teams use mobile towers to house equipment.

Over the last 5 years, operating rooms specialized for minimally invasive procedures have made significant strides.

These operating rooms employ boom technology for efficient space utilization and integrate electrical, fiber optic, computer, communication, digital, video, voice activation, and piped gas technologies. These have been called "fully integrated" or "intelligent" operating rooms. Efficient design of these operating rooms will likely improve overall operating efficiency and safety [16]. The advantages in efficiency and safety appear to justify the cost as these complex procedures become increasingly frequent in many medical centers.

Robotics

Robotic Assistance

Because of the complex scope maneuvering in the upper and mid-abdomen, surgeons must allow for a learning curve. Preliminary studies have shown that the benefit of the robotic arm is improved efficiency of motion and improved ergonomics for the surgeon at the console [17–19].

The da Vinci Surgical System is an FDA-approved laparoscopic surgical robot that is used by many surgical specialties (Fig. 23). The system is capable of performing surgical cutting, dissecting, suturing, tissue retraction as well as providing visualization. It provides improved dexterity, greater surgical precision, improved minimal access, increased range of motion due to the articulation of the arm *wrist* joints, three-dimensional image drawing, and reproducibility. A number of clinical investigators have been involved with trial of this robot in laparoscopic bariatric surgery [20, 21]. These early studies note that laparoscopic bariatric surgery using the da Vinci robot is safe and feasible but will require further investigation. Currently there is no clear outcome advantage demonstrated with the use of the robot in bariatric surgery, though many groups throughout the country use it routinely and attest to its value in performing these complex operations.

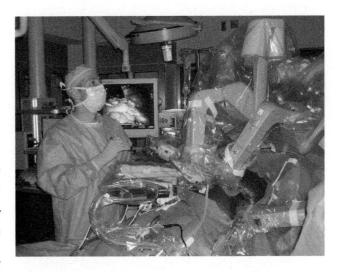

FIG. 23. Robot docked during gastric bypass procedure.

Appendix 1: Laparoscopic Roux-en-Y Gastric Bypass Reusable Instrumentation

Item name	Item #	Company	# on set
	Routine set		
Crocodile grasper (traumatic) (32 cm)	90-7064	Snowden-Pencer	2
Crocodile grasper (traumatic) (45 cm)	90-7264	Snowden-Pencer	2
Diamond jaw atraumatic dissector (32 cm)	90-7041	Snowden-Pencer	3
Diamond jaw atraumatic dissector (45 cm)	90-7271	Snowden-Pencer	3
Endo-right angle	90-7031	Snowden-Pencer	1
Right angle electrode	89-7200	Snowden-Pencer	1
Tapered curved dissector	90-7033	Snowden-Pencer	1
Hasson "S" retractor narrow	88-9113	Snowden-Pencer	1 set
Hasson "S" retractor wide	88-9114	Snowden-Pencer	1 set
Monopolar cord	88-9199	Snowden-Pencer	1
Instrument tray	88-6275	Snowden-Pencer	1
Scopes			
30° 10 mm	502-357-030	Stryker	1
45° 10 mm	502-357-045	Stryker	1
30° 5 mm	502-585-030	Stryker	1
45° 5 mm	502-585-045	Stryker	1
45° 10 mm extra long	502-657-045	Stryker	1
Scope warmer			
Scope warmer canister	C3001	Applied Medical	1
Base for scope warmer	C3002	Applied Medical	1
Seals for scope warmer	C3101	Applied Medical	1
Table-mounted instrument holding device			
Fast Clamp System	89-8950	Snowden-Pencer	1
Liver retractors			
80-mm triangular liver retractor 5 mm	89-6110	Snowden-Pencer	1
"Big D" diamond flex liver retractor	89-8216	Snowden-Pencer	1
Bowel instruments			
DeBakey clamp, straight, 10 mm	90-7052	Snowden-Pencer	1
DeBakey clamp, curved, 10 mm	90-7054	Snowden-Pencer	1
Specials			
Diamond flex articulating atraumatic grasper 40°	89-0509	Snowden-Pencer	1
Bougie 34-French or olympus endoscope bowel grasper	33331C	Storz	1
Diamond-jaw needle holder	90-7016	Snowden-Pencer	1
O'Brien LAP-BAND placer		Automated Medical Products Corp.	1
StrykeProbe and tips, 5 mm (32 and 45 cm)		Stryker Endoscopy	1

References

1. Ramanathan RC, Gourash W, Ikramuddin S, Schauer PR. Equipment and instrumentation for laparoscopic bariatric surgery. In: Deitel M, Cowan GSM, editors. Update: surgical for the morbidly obese. Toronto: FD-Communications; 2000. p. 277–90.
2. Carbonell AM, Joels CS, Sing RF, Heniford BT. Laparoscopic gastric bypass surgery: Equipment and necessary tools. J Laparoendosc Adv Surg Tech. 2003;13(4):241–5.
3. Schauer PR, Ikramuddin S, Gourash W. Laparoscopic Roux-en-Y gastric bypass: a case report at one-year follow-up. J Laparoendosc Adv Surg Tech. 1999;9:101–6.
4. Schauer PR, Ikramuddin S, Gourash W, Ramanathan R, Luketich JD. Outcomes of laparoscopic Roux-en-Y gastric bypass for morbid obesity. Ann Surg. 2000;232(4):515–29.
5. Coller JA, Murray JJ. Equipment. In: Ballantyne GH, Leahy PL, Modlin IL, editors. Laparoscopic surgery. Philadelphia: WB Saunders; 1994. p. 3–14.
6. Spencer MP, Madoff RD. Imaging. In: Ballantyne GH, Leahy PL, Modlin IL, editors. Laparoscopic surgery. Philadelphia: WB Saunders; 1994. p. 15–21.
7. Berci G, Paz-Partlow M. Videoendoscopic technology. In: Toouli J, Gossot D, Hunter JG, editors. Endosurgery. New York: Churchill Livingstone; 1996. p. 33–9.

8. Prescher T. Video imaging. In: Toouli J, Gossot D, Hunter JG, editors. Endosurgery. New York: Churchill Livingstone; 1996. p. 41–54.

9. Melzer A. Endoscopic instruments—conventional and intelligent. In: Toouli J, Gossot D, Hunter JG, editors. Endosurgery. New York: Churchill Livingstone; 1996. p. 69–95.

10. AORN Bariatric Surgery Guideline. AORN J. 2004;79(5):1026–52.

11. Schauer PR, Gourash W, Hamad G, Ikramuddin S. Operating set up and patient positioning for laparoscopic gastric bypass. SAGES Manual. Springer (in press).

12. Nguyen NT, Cronan M, Braley S, Rivers R, Wolfe BM. Duplex ultrasound assessment of femoral venous flow during laparoscopic and open gastric bypass. Surg Endosc. 2003;17:285–90.

13. Collier B, Goreja MA, Duke BE. Postoperative rhabdomyolysis with bariatric surgery. Obes Surg. 2003;13(6):941–3.

14. Mognol P, Vignes S, Chosidow D, Marmuse JP. Rhabdomyolysis after laparoscopic bariatric surgery. Obes Surg. 2004;14:91–4.

15. Luketich JD, Fernando HC, Buenaventura PO, Christie NA, Grondin SC, Schauer PR. Results of a randomized trial of HERNES-assisted versus non-HERMES-assisted laparoscopic antireflux surgery. Surg Endosc. 2002;16(9):1264–6.

16. Kenyon TAG, Urbach DR, Speer JB, Waterman-Hukari B, Foraker GF, Hansen PD, Swanstrom LL. Dedicated minimally invasive surgery suites increase operating room efficiency. Surg Endosc. 2001;15:1140–3.

17. Kavoussi LR, Moore RG, Adams JB, et al. Comparison of robotic versus human laparoscopic camera control. J Urol. 1995;154:2131–6.

18. Omote K, Feussner H, Ungeheuer A, Arbter K, Wei GQ, Siewert JR, Hirzinger G. Seof-guided robotic camera control for laparoscopic surgery compared with human camera control. Am J Surg. 1999;177:321–4.

19. Dunlap KD, Wanzer L. Is the robotic arm a cost effective tool? AORN J. 1998;68:265–72.

20. Nguyen NT, Hinojosa MW, Finley D, Stevens M, Paya M. Application of robotics in general surgery: initial experience. Am Surg. 2004;70(10):914–7.

21. Jacobsen G, Berger R, Horgan S. The role of robotic surgery in morbid obesity. J Laparoendosc Adv Surg Tech A. 2003;13(4):279–83.

10

Anesthesia for Minimally Invasive Bariatric Surgery

Cindy M. Ku and Stephanie B. Jones

Anesthetic Concerns

Airway

Difficult intubation and difficult mask ventilation are more commonly encountered in obese patients. A recent closed claims study in the United States showed that obesity was a contributing factor in more than a third of the claims related to airway management at the induction of anesthesia [1]. A national audit of airway management in the United Kingdom, published in 2011, revealed that obese patients were twice as common in reports of airway complications or difficult airway cases compared to the normal weight population, and that obesity was often not prospectively identified as a risk factor for potential difficult airway [2]. Many obese patients have an increase in neck circumference ("short thick neck"). Such body habitus along with excessive pharyngeal soft tissue may contribute to difficult mask ventilation after induction of general anesthesia. In addition, cervical fat pads often prevent the anesthesiologist from placing the patient in the hyperextended or "sniffing" position, a position that aligns the oral, pharyngeal, and laryngeal axes for optimal laryngoscopy condition. Obese patients also have a higher incidence of obstructive sleep apnea (OSA). OSA, increased neck circumference, and difficult intubation have been demonstrated to be significantly associated in the overall population [3–6]. However, a recent study of bariatric patients showed that Mallampati airway assessment score of 3 or greater and male gender were more accurate predictors of difficult intubation; on the contrary, body mass index, OSA, or neck circumference did not individually contribute to such [7]. Despite this particular finding, it remains important for the anesthesiologist to establish an airway and mechanical ventilation with the shortest period of apnea possible, due to the limited pulmonary reserve and therefore relatively high incidence of oxygen desaturation during induction of general anesthesia. Careful preoperative evaluation and planning, optimal positioning for induction, and appropriate selection of airway equipment are critical in this population.

Oxygenation and Ventilation

Not surprisingly, oxygenation and ventilation can be problematic in the bariatric population. In the normal weight patient, lung volumes are decreased in the supine position and further reduced under general anesthesia. Obese patients have impaired respiratory mechanics at baseline. Excess adipose tissue increases abdominal girth and thereby decreases the mobility of the diaphragm, while excess adipose tissue in the chest wall can further decrease respiratory system compliance and increases resistance to air flow. Restrictive pulmonary physiology results, leading to a reduction in the functional residual capacity and total lung capacity [8]. Obese patients therefore may have elevated peak airway pressures despite maximum neuromuscular blockade, and the increased intra-abdominal pressure from pneumoperitoneum during laparoscopic surgery can further exacerbate problems with ventilation, leading to hypercarbia and hypoxemia.

Obesity is a major risk factor for both OSA and obesity hypoventilation syndrome. More than 70 % of bariatric surgery patients have OSA [9, 10]. OSA is associated with multiple organ system comorbidities, including but not limited to hypertension, coronary artery disease, congestive heart failure, arrhythmias, metabolic syndrome, and impaired glucose tolerance [11, 12]. OSA is also an independent risk factor for all-cause mortality [13]. Long-term OSA with abnormal ventilatory drive leads to the obesity hypoventilation syndrome ("Pickwickian syndrome"), resulting in hypoxemia, hypercarbia, daytime somnolence, pulmonary hypertension, polycythemia, and right heart failure [8]. Such sequelae of sleep disordered breathing syndromes can be mitigated by treatment with continuous positive airway pressure (CPAP) or noninvasive positive pressure ventilation (NIPPV) prior to bariatric surgery, which will reduce the risks of perioperative complications. Effective use of CPAP

S.A. Brethauer et al. (eds.), *Minimally Invasive Bariatric Surgery*,
DOI 10.1007/978-1-4939-1637-5_10, © Springer Science+Business Media New York 2015

can reverse the abnormal ventilatory drive in patients with obese hypoventilation syndrome in 2 weeks [14], improve cardiovascular function in 3–4 weeks [15, 16], and normalize pharyngeal soft tissue anatomy in 4–6 weeks [17]. OSA patients also benefit from continuation of CPAP therapy in the immediate postoperative period, when residual anesthetic and requirement for analgesia may cause hypopnea or decrease in respiratory drive [18], without significant negative effect on surgical outcome [19].

Cardiovascular Morbidity

The obese patient is in a hypervolemic and high cardiac output state due to increased blood volume from excess adipose tissue and increased muscle mass. The increased oxygen demand is often not met by an appropriate increase in oxygen supply because of the restrictive pulmonary physiology. The resulting ventilation-perfusion mismatch can put the patient at risk of myocardial ischemia when under increased stress. In addition, metabolic syndrome is highly associated with obesity and therefore bariatric patients often have associated comorbidities, that are also risk factors for coronary artery disease such as dyslipidemia and impaired glucose tolerance. Musculoskeletal problems such as osteoarthritis are also common in the obese population due to the excessive mechanical load on the joints, leading to a vicious cycle of sedentary lifestyle and worsening obesity. Therefore the assessment of functional capacity and cardiovascular status of these patients can be challenging.

Endocrine Comorbidities

Impaired glucose tolerance and type 2 diabetes are common comorbidities in bariatric patients. Diabetes is an independent risk factor for coronary artery disease. Other consequences of diabetes, such as peripheral and autonomic neuropathy, are also of significance to the anesthesiologist. Patients with pre-existing peripheral neuropathy are at higher risk of developing perioperative neuropathy. Gastroparesis from long-term diabetes puts patients at higher risk of aspiration during induction of anesthesia.

Fluid Status and Renal Function

Renal blood flow, glomerular filtration rate, and tubular reabsorption are increased by obesity in association with the relative increase in blood volume and cardiac output. Bariatric patients may therefore be more susceptible to problems with hypovolemia, such as prerenal azotemia and acute tubular necrosis, leading to acute renal failure postoperatively. Other factors that require consideration include baseline renal function, home medications that reduce renal function such as ACE inhibitors and non-steroidal anti-inflammatory drugs

(NSAIDs), and the presence of left ventricular dysfunction [8]. The type of bariatric surgery and the expected duration are also important to take into account. In gastric banding, for example, some may consider limiting intraoperative fluids due to concerns with tissue edema. In laparoscopic gastric bypass, patients are at higher risk of developing rhabdomyolysis because of prolonged immobilization and fluid shifts; maintaining euvolemia is therefore paramount to prevent the development of acute renal failure.

Postoperative Pain Management

Appropriate postoperative analgesia can be challenging in the bariatric population because of altered pharmacodynamics of analgesics and the prevalence of OSA. The mainstay of analgesia in the immediate postoperative period is opioids. Many commonly prescribed opioids such as morphine and hydromorphone are lipophilic and therefore have a large volume of distribution. In the obese patient, the excessive adipose tissue serves as a large reservoir for lipophilic opioids. This can be particularly problematic in patients with OSA because they are more susceptible to hypoventilation from any cause or degree of respiratory depression. Many physicians are understandably wary of administering significant quantity of opioids for these patients. Appropriate postoperative monitoring, therefore, should be available to the bariatric patients. Non-opioid analgesics should be utilized when possible, as part of a multimodal analgesic plan. The patient's baseline analgesic requirement should be carefully assessed; those with chronic pain should be seen by a pain medicine specialist preoperatively to obtain recommendations for appropriate postoperative analgesic strategies.

The selection of surgical candidates for minimally invasive bariatric procedures should be meticulous because unexpected conversion from a laparoscopic to open procedure can significantly complicate postoperative pain management. Neuraxial techniques such as thoracic epidural analgesia are deemed instrumental in open upper abdominal surgeries, but can be challenging to perform in the bariatric patient even in the best of circumstances and may be nearly impossible to do in a patient with significant pain from an unanticipated open incision. The surgeon and the anesthesiologist should have a preoperative discussion of postoperative pain management when the likelihood of conversion from laparoscopic surgery to laparotomy is high, and consider placing a thoracic epidural catheter prior to induction. Ultrasound guided thoracic epidural catheter placement may be necessary in obese patients.

Preoperative Evaluation

Patients scheduled for bariatric surgery should undergo preoperative evaluation by either an anesthesiologist or a mid-level healthcare provider (nurse practitioner or physician assistant)

with extensive knowledge of the aforementioned anesthetic concerns. The timing of the preoperative evaluation should be sufficiently prior to the scheduled surgery so that additional studies or medical record review can be performed if necessary, keeping in mind that beneficial effects of certain therapies such as CPAP for OSA will take weeks to develop. The evaluation should follow pertinent existing American Society of Anesthesiologists (ASA) practice guidelines, such as Practice Guidelines for the Perioperative Management of Patients with Obstructive Sleep Apnea and the Practice Advisory for Preanesthesia Evaluation.

Medical History

A detailed history should be obtained to elicit history of prior surgery and anesthetics, history of difficult intubation, and either a personal or family history of anesthesia-specific problems such as pseudocholinesterase deficiency or malignant hyperthermia. The patient's complete medical history should be solicited, and medical records or correspondence from the bariatric surgeon, primary care physician, or bariatrician should be available for detailed review. In particular, signs and symptoms of coronary artery disease, valvular heart disease, reactive airway disease, and the patient's functional capacity should be specifically solicited. The patient's risk of having OSA should also be assessed. Several validated screening tools are available for evaluating patients for OSA. The STOP-Bang questionnaire is an eight-item validated questionnaire commonly used to screen surgical patients for OSA. The Berlin questionnaire is a widely used OSA screening tool in the primary care setting, and the ASA task force on OSA has developed a checklist by consensus. These two latter checklists have been shown to demonstrate a moderately high level of sensitivity for OSA screening when compared to the STOP-Bang questionnaire in the surgical population [20]. Symptoms of dysphagia or upper gastrointestinal bleeding should be assessed, as esophageal instrumentation using endoscopes or bougies is common in bariatric procedures and placement of orogastric or nasogastric drainage tubes for gastric decompression prior to peritoneal insufflation is commonplace. Limitations on peripheral vascular access (such as history of difficult peripheral intravenous catheter placement, amputation, lymphedema, or concern for developing such after lymph node dissection, central venous thrombus, arterial-venous fistulas) should be noted, as establishing access can be difficult and appropriate planning should be made. A list of prescription and over-the-counter medications should be reviewed. The patient should be given explicit instructions regarding his or her medications, particularly with respect to any discontinuation (such as ACE inhibitors, metformin, and anticoagulants), reduction in dosage (such as long-acting insulin analogs), or continuation with importance (such as beta-adrenergic blockers and appropriate chronic pain medications).

Physical Examination

In addition to a general physical examination with accurate height and weight, the airway examination should be thorough in order to fully prepare the patient for the operating room. The information will be helpful for the anesthesiologist to gather the appropriate airway equipment for patients with a potentially difficult airway. In addition to assessing the oropharynx using the Mallampati scale, the hyomental distance, thyromental distance, mouth opening, and mandibular prognathism should be assessed. Neck circumference or at least the habitus should be noted, as well as any limitations on the cervical range of motion and the presence of a cervical fat pad. Dentition, including any artificial implants, should be noted as well. Patients with a history of difficult intubation or those at high risk of difficult intubation should be advised of the potential need for awake fiberoptic intubation and of elevated risk of dental injury. An anesthesiologist should be available to answer specific airway management concerns and inquiries.

Laboratory Data and Studies

Preoperative laboratory testing should be guided by the type of surgery and the patient's medical history, as routine screening has not been shown to be advantageous. Preoperative tests that may need to be obtained in the bariatric patient include:

– Hemoglobin and blood type with antibody screen if significant blood loss is anticipated
– Coagulation studies if patient is anticoagulated
– Electrolytes, blood urea nitrogen, and creatinine if patient has underlying renal disease or diabetes mellitus
– Liver function tests in patients with underlying liver dysfunction such as nonalcoholic fatty liver disease or viral hepatitis
– Electrocardiogram if patient has cardiac risk factors or a history of cardiac disease. A recent ECG (within 3–6 months) in a patient with no interval symptoms should be considered to be adequate
– Chest radiograph if patient has a history of pulmonary disease
– Sleep studies (i.e., polysomnography) if the patient is at high risk of having OSA, as effective use of OSA treatment such as CPAP can help to decrease the perioperative complications from OSA by reversing some of its systemic sequelae [16–19]

Bariatric patients with underlying cardiac disease should be evaluated using the most recent American College of Cardiology/American Heart Association guidelines for preoperative evaluation for noncardiac surgery. Transthoracic echocardiogram may be of value if the patient has poor functional capacity or complains of dyspnea at baseline, although resting LV function is not a consistent predictor of perioperative ischemic events [21]. It is also important to note that transthoracic echocardiography is often limited by the body habitus of the bariatric patient and echocardiogram findings may be inaccurate. Therefore functional capacity may offer a better understanding of the patient's cardiopulmonary status. Pulmonary function tests (PFTs) may be obtained in patients with a history of poorly controlled pulmonary diseases such as asthma or chronic obstructive pulmonary disease, and are often used to monitor the medical management of such patients. It is unlikely, however, that random PFTs in bariatric patients without such history would change perioperative management of the patient.

Intraoperative Concerns and Adaptations

Vascular Access

Patients should arrive to the preoperative holding area with ample time for preparation, as obtaining peripheral vascular access can be challenging because of excessive subcutaneous adipose. A peripherally inserted central catheter (PICC line) should be considered in patients with an extensive history of extremely difficult peripheral intravenous catheter placement.

Preoperative area nursing staff can assist by applying warm compresses to the upper extremity early in the preparation process to aid the vasodilation and visualization of peripheral veins. Ultrasound-guided peripheral venous catheter placement can be valuable in these challenging patients; long peripheral venous catheters, soft-tip guidewires, transducing gels, and other equipment for ultrasound imaging should be readily available. Lastly, a central venous catheter via internal jugular or subclavian approach can be placed prior to induction if needed; ultrasound guidance can again be helpful with either approach to visualize structures given body habitus and the loss of surface landmarks.

Monitoring

All bariatric patients require standard ASA monitoring: 5-lead ECG, blood pressure, continuous pulse oximetry, end-tidal carbon dioxide, and temperature. Automated noninvasive blood pressure monitoring can be problematic because standard rectangular blood pressure cuffs may not fit the cone-shaped upper arm of the obese patient. Appropriate cuff sizing is paramount for accurate blood pressure monitoring. One can consider using commercially available conical or V-shaped blood pressure cuffs that may be compatible with preexisting anesthesia monitoring systems. Using a rectangular cuff on the forearm is a commonly accepted alternative. Invasive blood pressure monitoring via arterial cannulation may be necessary when noninvasive blood pressure measurements are not acceptable, when patient comor-

bidities (e.g., severe valvular heart disease or high suspicion of coronary artery disease) make such monitoring prudent, or when frequent blood sampling may be required. One advantage of continuous arterial blood pressure monitoring is the ability to better estimate the patient's volume status using stroke volume variation or pulse pressure variation calculations during positive pressure ventilation, assuming the presence of a sinus rhythm. Stroke volume variation can be calculated by cardiac output sensor systems; pulse pressure variation is often a built-in function in newer anesthesia monitoring systems.

Accurate monitoring of depth of neuromuscular blockade is of high importance in minimally invasive bariatric surgery and is also often difficult to achieve. Anesthesiologists understand that the body habitus of the bariatric patient requires maximum neuromuscular blockade to achieve optimal operating conditions within the abdominal cavity. The restrictive pulmonary physiology and the increased intra-abdominal pressure from the pneumoperitoneal insufflation also make a high degree of neuromuscular blockade a key factor in optimizing intraoperative ventilation. Many anesthesia providers, however, are limited to subjective measurement of the depth of neuromuscular blockade. The most common and widely available peripheral nerve stimulators require the observer to recall the magnitude of repeated nerve stimulation to determine the degree of blockade [22]. It has been shown that many patients who were deemed to be "adequately reversed" from neuromuscular blockade have residual weakness in the recovery room [23]. While some had no discernable symptoms, others required varying degree of respiratory support, ranging from placement of oral or nasal airways to CPAP or noninvasive ventilation to reintubation. In the obese patient with OSA, residual neuromuscular blockade can lead to upper airway obstruction, rapidly resulting in hypoxemia given these patients' limited pulmonary reserve. Acceleromyography is an objective method to measure neuromuscular blockade based on Newton's second law of motion (force equals mass multiplied by acceleration). Using a small piezoelectric ceramic wafer attached to the thumb, the device measures the electrical signal proportional to the acceleration of the thumb as a result of an evoked mechanical response (Fig. 1). The objective measurement allows the anesthesiologist to more accurately assess the depth of neuromuscular blockade and administer additional doses of neuromuscular blocking agents. Several models of acceleromyography devices with a simple user interface and setup are commercially available.

Urine output should be monitored and causes of oliguria should be investigated, but it should be noted that transient oliguria in the setting of peritoneal insufflation and increased abdominal pressure is common. The patient's core or near-core temperature should be monitored throughout the procedure. The most easily accessible core temperature site is the esophagus; however, esophageal temperature probes must often be removed for the surgical procedure. Alternative sites for continuous temperature monitoring include nasopharynx,

FIG. 1. Acceleromyography.
(a) Monitor indicates TOF
(train-of-four) ratio of 17 % as
the depth of neuromuscular
blockade. (b) Placement of
electrodes. Source:
AnaesthesiaUK http://www.frca.
co.uk/article.
aspx?articleid=101113. With
permission of Blue Starent.

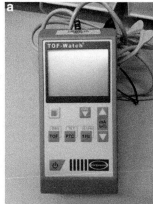
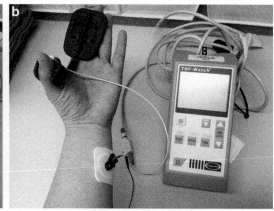

oropharynx, or rectum. Many anesthesiologists utilize bispectral index (BIS) monitoring to assess the depth of the anesthetic. While clinical trials have shown that BIS monitoring does not reduce the incidence of intraoperative awareness under anesthesia [24], it can be helpful to provide guidance if total intravenous anesthesia is utilized, especially in the United States where target-controlled infusion of intravenous anesthetic agents is not widely available.

Positioning

Prior to induction of anesthesia, the bariatric patient should be positioned on a ramp (Fig. 2) on the operating table so that the neck can be optimally extended for direct laryngoscopy. A slight head-up or reverse Trendelenburg position for preoxygenation can be helpful in recruiting additional functional residual capacity, in conjunction with CPAP [25]. The ramp for intubation can be made with multiple blankets; there are also commercially available foam and inflatable ramps. The ramp should be easily removable after the patient is anesthetized to provide good operating position; ideally the ramp should also be easily repositioned at emergence in the event of a need for reintubation. If the plan for airway management is an awake fiberoptic intubation, the patient may be placed in a sitting position for optimal oxygenation; adequate space must be available for the anesthesiologist and the necessary equipment. The patient's extremities should be properly padded and positioned to avoid positional neuropathy; patients at extremes of weight are known to be at higher risk of developing perioperative neuropathies.

Induction of Anesthesia and Airway Equipment

Induction of anesthesia should begin with ample time for preoxygenation to optimize the patient's apneic reserve and minimize hypoxemia during the apneic period. Excessive premedication should be avoided as the patient should be able to cooperate fully with preoxygenation. The operating room staff, including the surgeon, should be available to assist with securing the airway, especially in the event of unanticipated difficult airway. Bariatric operating room personnel should be educated on the basics of the difficult airway algorithm and the location of various airway devices in order to assist the anesthesiologist should such a situation arise. In addition to various direct laryngoscopy blades, an assortment of laryngeal mask airways (LMA) should be available. LMAs provide a means for manual ventilation as a rescue device and can also act as a conduit for intubation using an intubating LMA or via fiberoptic intubation using the Aintree catheter. Video laryngoscopes such as the GlideScope and the McGrath have become popular airway management alternatives to awake fiberoptic intubation. Though most commonly used after induction of anesthesia, successful awake GlideScope intubations have also been reported [26]. As a last resort in the difficult airway algorithm, cricothyrotomy kits should be available to the surgeon and the anesthesiologist. In our institution, the bariatric operating room has a dedicated difficult airway cart with some of the aforementioned devices, and cricothyrotomy kits are stocked in every anesthesia workstation.

Communication Between Operating Room Personnel

Communication between the surgeon and the anesthesiologist is of utmost importance in minimally invasive bariatric surgery, particularly at several critical points in the procedure. Peritoneal insufflation can lead to sudden dysrhythmias, with severe bradycardia being the most common [27]. Instrumentation of the esophagus—such as the removal of the nasogastric tube and esophageal temperature probe, or insertion of sizing bougies—should also be a concerted effort between the surgeon and the anesthesiologist. In addition, any concerns of bleeding on the surgical field should immediately be relayed to the anesthesiologist, as obtaining additional IV access may be difficult in the bariatric patient. An unanticipated conversion to

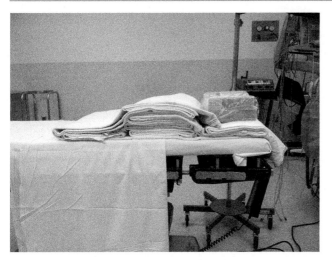

Fig. 2. Ramp with blankets for patient positioning.

open laparotomy will significantly change the postoperative course of the patient, including postoperative pain management and possibly continued mechanical ventilation in the immediate postoperative period. While many anesthesiologists in high-volume bariatric surgery centers are familiar with the steps in the surgical procedure and the usual duration, it is helpful for the surgeon to communicate with the anesthesiologist at these critical junctures. The anesthesiologist should ideally provide maximal neuromuscular blockade but still maintain the ability to adequately reverse the neuromuscular blockade at the end of the procedure. The repeat dosing of neuromuscular blockade agents at proper intervals should be guided by the use of the aforementioned peripheral nerve stimulators or acceleromyography as well as direct communication with the surgeon. A lack of peripheral nerve response to stimulation reflects greater than 90 % of neuromuscular junction acetylcholine receptor blockade, and reversal with an acetylcholinesterase inhibitor at that point is deemed to be ineffective. Such a situation at the end of the procedure may lead to inadequate neuromuscular recovery and therefore unnecessarily prolonged mechanical ventilation in the postoperative period.

Postoperative Management

Postoperative concerns after general anesthesia include pulmonary complications such as hypoxemia and hypercarbia, hemodynamic instability, hypothermia, nausea and/or vomiting, and inadequate analgesia. Of these, pulmonary complications and proper analgesia are of particular concern for bariatric patients. It has been demonstrated that obese patients, with and without OSA, experience frequent desaturations in the postoperative period after laparoscopic bariatric surgery [28]. For those with OSA, symptoms of apnea may be exacerbated by both residual anesthetic and opioid analgesics.

Bariatric patients should be extubated awake with intact airway reflexes to avoid upper airway obstruction or aspira-

tion events that can lead to hypoventilation and hypoxemia. If the patient has a diagnosis of sleep apnea and uses CPAP or NIPPV at home, the home unit should be brought to the recovery room and applied post-extubation; the device settings should be noted so that hospital devices can be used if needed. CPAP therapy should also be considered in those patients who do not have a formal diagnosis of OSA but are suspected of such during the perioperative course. Supplemental oxygen should be administered to all patients after laparoscopic bariatric surgery, and can be discontinued when patients are able to maintain their baseline oxygen saturation on room air. Some patients who fulfill all postrecovery room discharge criteria but have a mild degree of hypoxemia may be discharged to an inpatient ward with lowflow supplemental oxygen and proper monitoring, with the goal of weaning the oxygen therapy over a longer period of time. In our institution, patients with OSA who do not experience apneic episodes in the recovery room can be discharged to the inpatient ward once the standard discharge criteria are met, while those who do experience apneic episodes are kept in the recovery room until they can demonstrate at least a 30-min continuous period without apnea when left undisturbed. The ASA task force recommends continuous pulse oximetry monitoring for patients with OSA who continue to be at increased risk of respiratory compromise after discharge from the recovery room [29]; such arrangements should be readily available in facilities providing bariatric surgical services.

Because bariatric patients may be more susceptible to the respiratory depressive effects of opioid analgesics, an opioidsparing, multimodal analgesic plan is the standard model of care [30]. Surgical port sites should be infiltrated with longacting local anesthetics such as bupivacaine either prior to incision or during closure. The use of patient-controlled intravenous opioid analgesia (PCA) should be initiated in the post-anesthesia recovery unit so that hypoxemic, hypopneic, or apneic events can be quickly identified and the PCA regimen can be adjusted. Non-opioid analgesics should include acetaminophen; the intravenous formulation that has recently become available in the United States should facilitate the administration of acetaminophen as scheduled doses (usually 1 g every 6 h and not to exceed 4 g/day). Though long-term use of NSAID such as ibuprofen is discouraged due to the risk of peptic ulcer disease in the post-bariatric surgery population, short-term and limited use of intravenous NSAID such as ketorolac should be seriously considered in the immediate postoperative period. For the bariatric patients with a history of chronic pain or neuropathic pain, other non-opioid analgesics such as gabapentin can be incorporated into the analgesic plan, if not already previously prescribed by other physicians. Other agents such as intravenous ketamine infusion and transdermal clonidine can be useful adjuncts in patients experiencing difficulty with pain management; expert pain consultation should be sought in these circumstances. Lastly, regional analgesic techniques such as epidural analgesia should be considered in patients with pain that is poorly controlled by parenteral means, and in patients who have undergone open bariatric procedure, bearing in mind that the procedure may be more challenging in these patients due to body habitus and patients' difficulty with cooperation given their level of discomfort in the postoperative period.

Conclusion

The bariatric population is heterogenous; morbidly obese patients cannot be treated on a one-size-fits-all basis. However, certain key issues should be kept in mind throughout the perioperative period. These include OSA and postoperative respiratory complication risk, the presence of systemic comorbidities including cardiovascular disease and diabetes mellitus, the potential challenge of postoperative pain management, and the need for close communication between all members of the perioperative care team. It is our belief that meticulous and systematic attention to the above will lead to better outcomes for the obese patient undergoing bariatric, or other, surgical procedures.

Review Questions and Answers

1. List four reasons why airway and ventilation are significant concerns for the anesthesiologist in minimally invasive bariatric surgery.
   - Bariatric patients have limited pulmonary reserve and will desaturate very quickly following induction of anesthesia.
   - Mask ventilation and intubation can be difficult in many bariatric patients due to alterations in body habitus.
   - Obese patients have impaired respiratory mechanics which can be worsened when under general anesthesia.
   - Many obese patients have obstructive sleep apnea (OSA), which can complicate the administration of anesthetic agents and postoperative pain management.
2. Your institution has purchased disposable foam positioning ramps for the operating room, one of which has been placed on the operating table. After the anesthesiologist intubates the patient with a video laryngoscope, you ask her and other operating room personnel to remove the ramp in order to position the patient supine for the procedure. The anesthesiologist asks that the ramp be kept nearby and be inserted underneath the patient at the end of the case. Explain her rationale.
   - Video laryngoscopes and other advanced airway equipment are often used when a difficult intubation is expected or when a rapid intubation is desired so that the patient is apneic for the least amount of time, both common in bariatric patients. One of the keys to optimize intubating conditions is positioning. A ramp can

provide a head-up position that can be helpful for both preoxygenation/denitrogenation and positioning the patient's head and neck into a hyperextended "sniffing" position for laryngoscopy. It would be helpful to replace the ramp underneath the patient at the end of the case and prior to extubation in the event that the patient fails to maintain adequate spontaneous ventilation after extubation and has to be reintubated urgently.

3. You are about to place the gastric band when the pneumoperitoneum appears to be inadequate. While the circulator checks the insufflation pressure, you ask your anesthesiologist to administer additional muscle relaxant. Your anesthesiologist replies that there is no twitch on the peripheral nerve monitor, and he wants to know approximate duration of the remainder of the case. Why does the anesthesiologist want to know this information?
   - "No twitch" implies greater than 95 % neuromuscular blockade. Administering additional muscle relaxant without a detected twitch on the train-of-four monitor is unlikely to detectably increase the depth of neuromuscular blockade. Administering neuromuscular reversal agents at this point will not result in adequate muscle strength for extubation. At least one twitch (85–90 % blockade) in train-of-four monitoring is needed for successful reversal of neuromuscular blockade. Your anesthesiologist would like to provide as much muscle relaxation as possible so that pneumoperitoneum can be maintained without losing the ability to successfully reverse the blockade when needed. Therefore depending on the type of muscle relaxant used, the known pharmacodynamics of the drug, the effects demonstrated thus far in this patient, and the duration of the case, your anesthesiologist may tell you that additional relaxant is not needed and that he would like to plan ahead for relaxant reversal later in the case.

4. Your bariatric patient has a diagnosis of OSA for which he uses a CPAP (continuous positive airway pressure) device, and has undergone a laparoscopic gastric bypass procedure about 2 h ago. Your assistant had written the patient's admission orders. You are now informed by the recovery room nurse that the patient has significant pain not well controlled by the PCA (patient-controlled analgesia). His spouse had also forgotten to bring in his home CPAP device. He is on 2 L of oxygen by nasal cannula with an oxygen saturation of 95 %, and has had two episodes of apnea, both of which occurred when the he dozed off after receiving some intravenous hydromorphone bolus per the anesthesiologist's order. You have reviewed your assistant's order and note the PCA order to be intravenous hydromorphone 0.12 mg per bolus with a lockout interval of 6 min and a maximum dose of 1.2 mg/h. The nurse is wary of giving additional hydromorphone boluses because of the apneic episodes. What can be done to improve the patient's analgesia?

- The patient suffers from OSA and should resume CPAP therapy in the immediate postoperative period. You should order CPAP from the hospital's respiratory service and try to obtain home CPAP settings for quicker titration. Patients with OSA are sensitive to opioids, and therefore intravenous opioid boluses may contribute to the apneic episodes. Once the CPAP therapy is initiated, one can increase dosage of the hydromorphone PCA bolus while the patient is continuously monitored in the recovery room. Once recovery room discharge criteria are met then the patient should be discharged to the ward with continuous pulse oximetry monitoring. The need for continuous pulse oximetry monitoring can be reassessed the following day. Nonopioid analgesics such as acetaminophen should be included in the pain regimen as well.

References

1. Schumann R. Anaesthesia for bariatric surgery. Best Pract Res Clin Anesthesiol. 2011;25:83–93.
2. Woodall N, Frerk C, Cook TM. Can we make airway management (even) safer?—lessons from national audit. Anaesthesia. 2011;66 Suppl 2:27–33.
3. Brodsky JB, Lemmens HJ, Brock-Utne JG, et al. Morbid obesity and tracheal intubation. Anesth Analg. 2002;94:732–6.
4. Juvin P, Lavaut E, Dupont H, Lefevre P, Demetriou M, Dumoulin JL, Desmonts JM. Difficult tracheal intubation is more common in obese than in lean patients. Anesth Analg. 2003;97(2):595–600.
5. Benumof JL. Obstructive sleep apnea in the adult obese patient: implications for airway management. J Clin Anesth. 2001;13(2):144–56.
6. Siyam M, Benhamou D. Difficult endotracheal intubation in patients with sleep apnea syndrome. Anesth Analg. 2002;95:1098–102.
7. Neligan PJ, Porter S, Max B, et al. Obstructive sleep apnea is not a risk factor for difficult intubation in morbidly obese patients. Anesth Analg. 2009;109:1182–6.
8. Nguyen L, Jones SB. Chapter 6: obesity. In: Vacanti CA, Sikka P, Urman R, editors. Essential clinical anesthesia. Cambridge: Cambridge University; 2011.
9. Frey WC, Pilcher J. Obstructive sleep-related breathing disorders in patients evaluated for bariatric surgery. Obes Surg. 2003;13:676–83.
10. O'Keeffe T, Patterson EJ. Evidence supporting routine polysomnography before bariatric surgery. Obes Surg. 2004;14:23–6.
11. Pashayan AG, Passannante AN, Rock P. Pathophysiology of obstructive sleep apnea. Anesthesiol Clin North America. 2005;23:431–43.
12. Chung SA, Yuan H, Chung F. A systemic review of obstructive sleep apnea and its implications for anesthesiologists. Anesthesiology. 2008;107:1543–63.
13. Marshall NS, Wong KKH, Liu PY, et al. Sleep apnea as an independent risk factor for all-cause mortality: the Busselton Health Study. Sleep. 2008;31:1079–85.
14. Cartagena R. Preoperative evaluation of patients with obesity and obstructive sleep apnea. Anesthesiol Clin North America. 2005;23:463–78.
15. Tkacova R, Rankin F, Fitzgerald FS, et al. Effects of continuous positive airway pressure on obstructive sleep apnea and left ventricular afterload in patients with heart failure. Circulation. 1998;98:2269–75.
16. Golbin JM, Somers VK, Caples SM. Obstructive sleep apnea, cardiovascular disease and pulmonary hypertension. Proc Am Thorac Soc. 2008;5:200–6.
17. Ryan CF, Lowe AA, Li D, Fleetham JA. Magnetic resonance imaging of the upper airway in obstructive sleep apnea before and after chronic nasal continuous positive airway pressure therapy. Am Rev Respir Dis. 1991;144(4):939–44.
18. Neligan PJ, Malhotra G, Fraser M, Williams N, Greenblatt EP, Cereda M, Ochroch EA. Continuous positive airway pressure via the Boussignac system immediately after extubation improves lung function in morbidly obese patients with obstructive sleep apnea undergoing laparoscopic bariatric surgery. Anesthesiology. 2009;110(4):878–84.
19. Weingarten TN, Kendrick ML, Swain JM, Liedl LM, Johnson CP, Schroeder DR, Johnson BD, Sprung J. Effects of CPAP on gastric pouch pressure after bariatric surgery. Obes Surg. 2011;21(12):1900–5.
20. Chung F, Yegneswaran B, Liao P, Chung SA, Vairavanathan S, Islam S, Khajehdehi A, Shapiro CM. STOP questionnaire: a tool to screen patients for obstructive sleep apnea. Anesthesiology. 2008;108(5):812–21.
21. Fleisher LA, Beckman JA, Brown KA, Calkins H, Chaikof EL, Fleischmann KE, Freeman WK, Froehlich JB, Kasper EK, Kersten JR, Riegel B, Robb JF. 2009 ACCF/AHA focused update on perioperative beta blockade incorporated into the ACC/AHA 2007 guidelines on perioperative cardiovascular evaluation and care for noncardiac surgery: a report of the American college of cardiology foundation/American heart association task force on practice guidelines. Circulation. 2009;120(21):e169–276. Epub 2009 Nov 2.
22. Kopman A. Chapter 22: perioperative monitoring of neuromuscular function. In: Reich DL, et al., editors. Monitoring in anesthesia and perioperative care. Cambridge: Cambridge University; 2011. Cambridge Books Online. doi:10.1017/CBO9780511974083.
23. Murphy GS, Brull SJ. Residual neuromuscular block: lessons unlearned. Part I: definitions, incidence, and adverse physiologic effects of residual neuromuscular block. Anesth Analg. 2010;111(1):120–8.
24. Mashour GA, Shanks A, Tremper KK, Kheterpal S, Turner CR, Ramachandran SK, Picton P, Schueller C, Morris M, Vandervest JC, Lin N, Avidan MS. Prevention of intraoperative awareness with explicit recall in an unselected surgical population: a randomized comparative effectiveness trial. Anesthesiology. 2012;117(4):717–25.
25. Gander S, Frascarolo P, Suter M, et al. Positive end-expiratory pressure during induction of general anesthesia increases duration of nonhypoxic apnea in morbidly obese patients. Anesth Analg. 2005;100:580–4.
26. Doyle DJ. Awake intubation using the GlideScope video laryngoscope: initial experience in four cases. Can J Anaesth. 2004;51(5):520–1.
27. Valentin MD, Tulsyan N, Dolgin C. Recurrent asystolic cardiac arrest and laparoscopic cholecystectomy: a case report and review of the literature. JSLS. 2004;8(1):65–8.
28. Ahmad S, Nagle A, McCarthy RJ, Fitzgerald PC, Sullivan JT, Prystowsky J. Postoperative hypoxemia in morbidly obese patients with and without obstructive sleep apnea undergoing laparoscopic bariatric surgery. Anesth Analg. 2008;107(1):138–43.
29. Gross JB, Bachenberg KL, Benumof JL, Caplan RA, Connis RT, Coté CJ, Nickinovich DG, Prachand V, Ward DS, Weaver EM, Ydens L, Yu S, American Society of Anesthesiologists Task Force on Perioperative Management. Practice guidelines for the perioperative management of patients with obstructive sleep apnea: a report by the American society of anesthesiologists task force on perioperative management of patients with obstructive sleep apnea. Anesthesiology. 2006;104:1081–93.
30. Schug SA, Raymann A. Postoperative pain management of the obese patient. Best Pract Res Clin Anaesthesiol. 2011;25(1):73–81.

11

Postoperative Pathways in Minimally Invasive Bariatric Surgery

Rebecca Lynch, Debbie Pasini, and Adrian G. Dan

List of Abbreviations

ASMBS	American Society for Metabolic and Bariatric Surgery
BPD-DS	Bilio-pancreatic diversion with duodenal switch
COE	Center of excellence
IV	Intravenous
LAGB	Laparoscopic adjustable gastric banding
LRYGB	Laparoscopic Roux-en-Y gastric bypass
LSG	Laparoscopic sleeve gastrectomy
UGI	Upper gastrointestinal
VTE	Venous thromboembolism

Introduction

The emergence of the obesity epidemic and the advancement of minimally invasive techniques have made weight-loss operations some of the most commonly performed surgical procedures. It is estimated that over 100,000 patients undergo bariatric surgery yearly in the United States [1]. With the high prevalence of such operations, patients and third-party payers have come to expect high-quality results and value. Accreditation or participation in a national quality improvement program or center of excellence program is based upon specific criteria including standardization of a postoperative clinical care pathway. The goal is to generate high-quality outcomes by adhering to evidence-based practice recommendations. In many surgical specialties, implementation of clinical pathways affords the necessary high-quality results with reduction of cost through standardization of care [2]. Standardizing postoperative pathways in bariatric surgery has been shown to decrease length of stay and improve resource utilization without compromising patient outcome [3, 4]. This chapter focuses on the necessary components of postoperative bariatric care and the relevant scientific evidence upon which clinical pathways are structured.

Postoperative care of the bariatric patient begins following a standardized outpatient preoperative work-up and standardized procedure which are described in other sections within this text. From the operating room, the patient is immediately transported to the recovery room under the supervision of one of the operating surgeons and a member of the anesthesia team. For proper communication between clinicians, operative notes and computerized orders should be completed immediately following the procedure. Such immediate postoperative orders begin the postoperative pathway.

The majority of bariatric patients will be cared for on a surgical unit or one which also has telemetry capabilities. The necessity for telemetry is often based upon the specific patient's need for increased monitoring due to elevated risk. This includes patients with severe sleep apnea, other pulmonary conditions, cardiac dysrhythmias, and opioid sensitivity. For patients with more extensive comorbidities, or those who have undergone very lengthy or difficult operations, admission to an intensive care unit may be necessary. Upon arrival to the postanesthesia care unit and upon arrival to the designated postoperative care unit, the patient should be evaluated by the attending registered nurse. The nursing staff should be highly trained in postoperative bariatric care and recognition of the initial presenting signs for potential complications. An algorithm must be in place to facilitate communication between the nursing staff and the appropriate physician should complications and concerns arise.

Postoperative Considerations

There are several important considerations in the postoperative period. These include laboratory testing, pain management, respiratory care, venous thromboembolism (VTE) prophylaxis, radiologic evaluation, diet progression, wound care, and postoperative follow-up. Some recommendations are universal to all the common present-day bariatric procedures, while other recommendations are procedure specific. These procedures include: laparoscopic Roux-en-Y gastric bypass (LRYGB), bilio-pancreatic diversion with duodenal

S.A. Brethauer et al. (eds.), *Minimally Invasive Bariatric Surgery*,
DOI 10.1007/978-1-4939-1637-5_11, © Springer Science+Business Media New York 2015

TABLE 1. Key postoperative bariatric care components

Post-op day #0	Laboratory studies
	Resume necessary home medications in IV form
	IV pain management
	IV hydration
	Pulmonary toilet/respiratory care
	VTE prophylaxis
	Early ambulation
	Incision and drain care
	Surgeon and anesthesia postoperative evaluation
Post-op day #1	Laboratory studies
	UGI contrast study (routine or selective)
	Bariatric clear liquid diet commencement
	Resume appropriate PO home medications
	Convert to PO pain medication
	Pulmonary toilet/respiratory care
	VTE prophylaxis
	Increase ambulation
	Incision and drain care and teaching
	Postoperative patient education
	Discharge education and discharge for purely restrictive procedures (LAGB, LSG)
Post-op day #2	Laboratory studies
	Increase volume of clear bariatric liquids
	Pulmonary toilet/respiratory care
	VTE prophylaxis
	Continue ambulation
	Continue postoperative patient education
	Discharge education

switch (BPD-DS), laparoscopic sleeve gastrectomy (LSG), and laparoscopic adjustable gastric banding (LAGB) (see Table 1).

Laboratory Tests

Blood work should be obtained immediately following surgery to assess the patient's electrolyte and blood counts. In addition, patients with super morbid obesity or extended operative times should have a creatine phosphokinase level checked to rule out the possibility of gluteal compartment syndrome and rhabdomyolysis. In such patients, early intervention could be lifesaving and decrease the potential for renal damage [5].

It is critical in the immediate postoperative period to ensure that patients are adequately hydrated. Laboratory values, along with urine output and fluid balance assessment, aid the clinician in assessing adequate hydration. Routine blood work including complete blood count, basic metabolic panel, and magnesium levels should be obtained on morning rounds during the inpatient stay. The suspicion of intraluminal or intraperitoneal hemorrhage may prompt the clinician to order additional hematocrit levels and coagulation studies. Patients with known diabetes mellitus or elevated perioperative blood glucose should undergo glucose level testing while on NPO and when diet is begun. Insulin regimens frequently need to be adjusted due to altered dietary intake, highlighting the importance of close glucose monitoring [6].

Pain Management

Inadequate pain control in the postoperative period may lead to patient discomfort, dissatisfaction, and increased length of stay. It can also limit the patient's ability to take deep breaths and attain early ambulation. This can consequently contribute to other complications such as atelectasis, pneumonia, and VTE. Tachycardia may result, which can unnecessarily confound the clinical picture for the surgeon and trigger an unnecessary work-up. There must be a balance between appropriate pain management and over-sedation of the patient. Clinicians and ancillary staff must have a high index of suspicion for over-sedation and the potential cardiopulmonary consequences.

Intravenous (IV) opioids may be scheduled or delivered by patient controlled anesthesia depending on the surgeon's preference. Adjuncts to this may include IV administration of acetaminophen and ketorolac if not contraindicated. Once a clear liquid diet is started, conversion to oral pain medication is appropriate with use of IV opioids for breakthrough pain only. Strategic administration of local anesthetics using continuous delivery catheters has also been utilized by some in efforts to decrease opioid use. Abdominal binders and icing may assist in ameliorating postoperative discomfort.

Respiratory Care

The postoperative respiratory care of the bariatric patient is of paramount importance. Immediately upon arrival to the floor, patients should be provided with an incentive spirometry device and be instructed on spirometer utilization as well as coughing and deep breathing. This aggressive pulmonary toilet routine can decrease pulmonary complications such as atelectasis and pneumonia [7]. A dedicated respiratory therapist plays an important role in the pulmonary toilet regimen.

Many bariatric patients suffer from obstructive sleep apnea and proper utilization of their own CPAP or BiPAP machines is essential at all times while sleeping. Oxygen supplementation may also be necessary and O_2 saturations should be monitored in patients with known obstructive sleep apnea or other pulmonary symptoms requiring O_2. This can be done safely on a monitored floor [8].

Venous Thromboembolism Prophylaxis

Bariatric patients are predisposed to develop venous thrombosis leading to pulmonary embolism [9, 10]. Laparoscopic bariatric procedures are often associated with prolonged operative times, steep reverse Trendelenburg positioning, pneumoperitoneum pressures up to 18 mmHg, and decreased perioperative mobility. These factors further contribute to the increased risk of VTE in bariatric surgical patients. Although VTE may be infrequent, it still remains a significant postoperative cause of death in this patient population, making VTE prophylaxis crucial [11].

Preoperatively, patients may benefit from 5,000 units of subcutaneous heparin prior to inducing general anesthesia [12]. Postoperative recommendations include early ambulation, sequential venous compression devices, and aggressive hydration [13]. Additionally, chemoprophylaxis may be considered and is an acceptable practice. However, there is no level I evidence to substantiate additional benefits of chemoprophylaxis over its risks in bariatric surgery patients. Continuation of anticoagulation for approximately 1 or 2 weeks following discharge has been considered and employed in high-risk patients with super morbid obesity, known hypercoagulable state, or history of VTE [14].

Radiological Evaluation

In some practices, upper gastrointestinal (UGI) contrast study is performed routinely on postoperative day 1 to evaluate the integrity and patency of the gastrojejunostomy in LRYGB and the duodenojejunostomy in BPD-DS or the patency of a sleeve gastrectomy. A delayed film may also be performed to assess the patency of the jejunojejunostomy. However, the utility of *routine* UGI contrast studies has come into question. Several authors advocate the use of *selective* UGI contrast studies based upon each patient's clinical status, symptoms, and drain amylase level [15]. Following purely restrictive procedures, such as the LAGB and LSG, an UGI contrast study is often employed to rule out obstruction and to obtain a baseline radiograph of band position. However, some have advocated that the utility of UGI contrast studies in LAGB may be limited [16].

Dietary Progression

Patients generally remain on NPO with IV hydration on the night of surgery and are started on a bariatric clear liquid diet on postoperative day 1 [6]. For patients undergoing a routine UGI contrast study, diet is started after the study is determined to show no complication. The bariatric clear liquid diet consists of no added sugar liquids with minimal gastrointestinal residue and no carbonation or caffeine [6]. Fluid intake is usually regulated during the inpatient postoperative stay to ensure that patients are able to tolerate diet before advancement. The familiarity of the bedside nurse and patient with the dietary restrictions is essential. Patient education regarding further diet progression following discharge from the hospital should be provided. Also, patients may be encouraged to record fluid intake and keep a diet journal to improve compliance. The traditional diet advancement after discharge involves clear to full liquid, pureed, soft, and finally to a regular maintenance bariatric diet [17]. As diet is advanced, patients should continue to eat small, balanced meals with adequate protein intake in the range of 60 g/day up to 1.5 g/kg/day based on ideal body weight [6]. Commencement of vitamin and trace element education should also start before discharge.

Incision and Drain Care

As with any surgical intervention, incisional care is of high importance. All laparoscopic incisions should be carefully examined by the clinicians on a daily basis to ensure early identification of any wound infection or dehiscence. Nursing staff should be educated on early signs and symptoms of wound infection, proper drain care, and expected drain color and consistency. When a drain is present, output, color, and consistency should be accurately recorded.

TABLE 2. Potential nutritional deficiencies and postoperative monitoring after bariatric surgery [6, 17]

Nutritional deficiency	Laboratory test	Considerations
Vitamin A	Retinol	Deficiency is more likely in BPD-DS
Vitamin B1 (thiamine)	Serum thiamine	Have high index of suspicion in patients with symptoms consistent of Wernicke's encephalopathy (which may result in irreversible neurologic deficits)
Vitamin B9 (folate)	RBC folate	Must check RBC folate. A serum folate level reflects PO folate intake
Vitamin B12 (cobalamin)	Serum B12	Deficiency is common and most likely in LRYGB
Vitamin D	25 (OH) vit D	Deficiency is more likely in LRYGB and BPD-DS
Vitamin K	PT	More common in BPD-DS
Iron	Ferritin, serum iron, total iron body content	Deficiency is common
Zinc	Plasma zinc	More likely in LRYGB and BPD-DS
Protein	Serum albumin, serum total protein	

Discharge Instructions

Prior to discharge, the patient and caretakers should undergo a thorough educational session with the bariatric case manager. This gives the bariatric team a unique opportunity to reinforce the important concepts related to proper dietary compliance as well as the instructions related to home incision and drain care. Patients should be educated regarding appropriate postoperative activity and restrictions. Teaching should also include the signs and symptoms of anastomotic leak, VTE, and other potential complications. Medications and foods that need to be resumed, adjusted, or avoided can be reviewed at this time. The patient's postoperative office follow-up should be confirmed. Due to the possibility of rapid improvement in comorbidities, patients are instructed to also follow up closely with their primary care providers for medication adjustment and monitoring.

Post-hospitalization Follow-Up

The first follow-up visit, usually 1 week following the operation, serves to ensure that the patient has done well in the immediate postoperative period. It gives the clinician a chance to reevaluate the incisions, ensure the patient is adequately hydrated, and discuss the patient's current symptoms. The clinician can then determine if the patient needs further investigation for cardiac, pulmonary, hematologic, or gastrointestinal complications. Any sutures and drains are usually removed at this point. This office visit also serves as an opportunity to discuss diet progression, medication adjustment, vitamin supplementation, and activity status. A registered dietitian is involved in reinforcing the components of diet advancement and commencing nutritional supplementation.

After the first postoperative visit, bariatric patients follow up at regular intervals over the next 18 months. Visits usually occur at 1, 3, 6, 9, 12, and 18 months postoperatively with some variation amongst programs. This allows physicians to monitor weight loss, evaluate for potential complications, and provide nutritional, medical, and psychiatric support from a focused bariatric standpoint. During these visits, the patients should have appropriate laboratory studies to address potential protein, vitamin, and trace element deficiencies (see Table 2). Patients may have expected symptoms related to normal adjustment to their new anatomic and physiologic alterations. However, patients should also be monitored for early complications in this time period. These include pneumonia, anemia, VTE, anastomotic stricture, and marginal ulceration amongst others. Guidance and reassurance by the physician regarding the patient's expected weight loss may be provided. The steepness of the weight-loss curve can be discussed to help the patient understand the weight-loss expectations.

Specifically for the LAGB patient, postoperative office follow-up is more intense during the first year. Office visits may occur monthly to adjust the degree of band restriction as needed [18]. After the first year, adjustments are often spread out over longer intervals.

At 1 year to 18 months, the patient's weight loss begins to stabilize, and from this time a recommended yearly evaluation should occur. It is at this point that patients may consider body contouring, and appropriate referrals can be made. Annual follow-ups play an important role in ensuring patient compliance with diet, vitamin supplementation, and exercise regimens. A focused bariatric dietician and psychologist may be helpful and can be offered as needed. If available, a regularly scheduled bariatric support group may also serve to benefit and motivate patients. The patient should be encouraged to follow up with the bariatric office annually and indefinitely.

Conclusion

As the prevalence of obesity and its surgical treatments have increased, so have the efforts to improve postoperative outcomes. Utilization of evidence-based best practices remains of paramount importance and the implementation of standardized postoperative pathways may consistently provide a way to ensure optimal outcomes. Programs should strive to structure postoperative clinical pathways supported by the best available evidence.

References

1. Buchwald H, Oien DM. Metabolic/bariatric surgery worldwide 2011. Obes Surg. 2013;23:427–36.
2. Müller MK, Dedes KJ, Dindo D, Steiner S, Hahnloser D, Clavien PA. Impact of clinical pathways in surgery. Arch Surg. 2009; 394:31–9.
3. Huerta S, Heber D, Sawicki MP, Liu CD, Arthur D, Alexander P, et al. Reduced length of stay by implementation of a clinical pathway for bariatric surgery in an academic health care center. Am Surg. 2001;67(12):1128–35.
4. Yeats M, Wedergren S, Fox N, Thompson JS. The use and modification of clinical pathways to achieve specific outcomes in bariatric surgery. Am Surg. 2005;71(2):152–4.
5. Chakravartty S, Sarma DR, Patel AG. Rhabdomyolysis in bariatric surgery: a systematic review. Obes Surg. 2013;23(8):1333–40.
6. Mechanick JI, Youdim A, Jones DB, Garvey WT, Hurley DL, McMahon MM, et al. Clinical Practice Guidelines for the perioperative nutritional, metabolic, and nonsurgical support of the bariatric surgery patient-2013 update: cosponsored by the American Association of Clinical Endocrinologists, the Obesity Society, and American Society for Metabolic and Bariatric Surgery. Surg Obes Relat Dis. 2013;9(2):159–91.
7. Cassidy MR, Rosenkranz P, McCabe K, Rosen JE, McAneny D. I COUGH: reducing postoperative pulmonary complications with a multidisciplinary patient care program. JAMA Surg. 2013;148(8): 740–5.
8. Shearer E, Magee CJ, Lacasia C, Raw D, Kerrigan D. Obstructive sleep apnea can be safely managed in a level 2 critical care setting after laparoscopic bariatric surgery. Surg Obes Relat Dis. 2013; 9(6):845–9.
9. Stein PD, Beemath A, Olson RE. Obesity as a risk factor in venous thromboembolism. Am J Med. 2005;118:978–80.
10. Stein PD, Goldman J. Obesity and thromboembolic disease. Clin Chest Med. 2009;30:489–93.
11. Longitudinal Assessment of Bariatric Surgery (LABS) Consortium, Flum DR, Belle SH, King WC, Wahed AS, Berk P. Perioperative safety in the longitudinal assessment of bariatric surgery. N Engl J Med. 2009;361(5):445–54.
12. Agarwal R, Hecht TE, Lazo MC, Umscheid CA. Venous thromboembolism prophylaxis for patients undergoing bariatric surgery: a systematic review. Surg Obes Relat Dis. 2010;6(2):213–20.
13. The American Society for Metabolic and Bariatric Surgery Clinical Issues Committee. ASMBS updated position statement on prophylactic measures to reduce the risk of venous thromboembolism in bariatric surgery patients. Surg Obes Relat Dis. 2013;9(4):493–7.
14. Wu EC, Barba CA. Current practices in the prophylaxis of venous thromboembolism in bariatric surgery. Obes Surg. 2000;10(1):7–14.
15. Lee SD, Khouzam MN, Kellum JM, DeMaria EJ, Meador JG, Wolfe LG, et al. Selective, versus routine, upper gastrointestinal series leads to equal morbidity and reduced hospital stay in laparoscopic gastric bypass patients. Surg Obes Relat Dis. 2007;3(4): 413–6.
16. Frezza EE, Mammarappallil JG, Witt C, Wei C, Wachtel MS. Value of routine postoperative gastrographin contrast swallow studies after laparoscopic gastric banding. Arch Surg. 2009;144(8):766–9.
17. Allied Health Sciences Section Ad Hoc Nutrition Committee, Aills L, Blankenship J, Buffingtong C, Furtado M, Parrott J. ASMBS Allied health nutritional guidelines for the surgical weight loss patient. Surg Obes Relat Dis. 2008;4(5 Suppl):S73–108.
18. Favretti F, O'Brien PE, Dixon JB. Patient management after LAP-BAND placement. Am J Surg. 2002;184(6B):38–41.

12

Bariatric Surgery: Patient Safety and Quality Improvement

John M. Morton and Dan E. Azagury

Introduction

Patient safety and quality improvement are a long-standing priority for surgeons as evidenced by the tradition of participating in morbidity and mortality conference. Safety has always been the center of our attention and decision-making. So why has patient safety and quality become such an important focus in the past decade and especially in bariatric surgery? The primary answer is *information*. In this age of immediate, global, and overwhelming information, patients (and stakeholders) find themselves naturally seeking information for one of their most important decisions: their healthcare. And with the increasing availability of this information around the country and the world, your family physician's opinion is no longer a sufficient basis for referral: both patients and payers require access to objective data in order to make an informed decision.

This chapter will focus on the patient safety and quality improvement initiatives in bariatric surgery. The outline will be based on the widely accepted principles established by Avedis Donabedian whereby quality of healthcare can be assessed by measuring aspects of structure, processes, and outcomes.

Structure

Accreditation

The advent of bariatric surgery and its widespread adoption created a wide patient pool undergoing elective surgery in a high-risk population. As the number of these procedures increased, so did the direct cost to payers. Both private insurers and the Centers for Medicare and Medicaid Services initially drove the need to objectively identify high-quality providers by requiring centers performing bariatric surgery to be accredited, using their own specific criteria.

As this occurred, surgeons viewed this opportunity to support accreditation in order to build a quality system that could be used to improve patient care by providing widespread data for both scientific investigation and quality improvement projects. Even if some of the provider dynamics have recently changed, surgical quality and accreditation programs have been very successful and widely adopted. In bariatric surgery, the two main providers of accreditation—the American College of Surgeons (ACS) and the American Society for Metabolic and Bariatric Surgery (ASMBS)—have merged their accreditation system to create the Metabolic and Bariatric Surgery Accreditation and Quality Improvement Program (MBSAQIP) in 2013 [1]. MBSAQIP has recently released the inaugural standards for their joint accreditation program, and their requirement will be summarized later in this chapter.

Besides the different requirements needed for a particular accreditation, the role and benefit of accreditation itself as a quality metric have been recently debated. Indeed, after having initiated the accreditation requirement for bariatric surgery, CMS (the Centers for Medicare and Medicaid Services) has recently reversed their policy regarding bariatric centers of excellence and no longer require accreditation to perform these procedures. However, the majority of studies published since the implementation of facility certification for bariatric surgery have demonstrated improvement in outcomes.

These studies have shown:

- Up to a threefold reduction in mortality [2–5]
- Reduced inpatient, 30-day, 90-day, and 180-day complications by up to 37 %, 62 %, 24 %, and 21 % respectively [6, 7]
- Up to a 33 % reduction in reoperation rates [7]
- Lower readmission rates (10.8 % vs. 8.8 %) [5]
- Reduced cost up to 20 % [4, 7]
- Shorter length of stay of up to 1.42 days [2, 4]

Some studies do suggest that accreditation by itself does not directly improve outcomes, but other metrics like surgeon or institution volume, potentially imbedded in accreditation,

S.A. Brethauer et al. (eds.), *Minimally Invasive Bariatric Surgery*,
DOI 10.1007/978-1-4939-1637-5_12, © Springer Science+Business Media New York 2015

are actually more accurate in evaluating quality [8, 9]. They did confirm, however, a relationship with hospital volume, a metric in all accreditation programs including the Michigan Collaborative. In addition, the recent publication by Jafari et al. demonstrated a benefit for bariatric surgery outcomes rendered by accreditation that is independent of volume status [10]. Also, in a 2014 American Surgical Association presentation by Morton et al., a precise advantage of accreditation was demonstrated by accredited centers having superior rates of "failure to rescue" than nonaccredited centers [11]. This advantage makes intuitive sense in that experienced centers with appropriate personnel and resources can readily recognize and treat complications before any potentially fatal event.

Resources Needed

As mentioned previously, MBSAQIP has recently released the inaugural standards for their joint accreditation program, (http://www.mbsaqip.org/docs/Resources%20for%20 Optimal%20Care%20of%20the%20MBS%20Patient.pdf).

The requirements for accreditation fall under nine standards and essentially define two tiers in general bariatric accreditation: low-acuity centers and comprehensive centers.

Low-acuity centers perform a minimum annual volume of 25 approved metabolic and bariatric stapling operations on low-acuity patients: i.e., adults under the age 65, males with a BMI<55 and females with a BMI <60, and those who do not have either organ failure or history of organ transplant. These centers are not accredited to perform non-emergent revisional procedures but can perform all other approved bariatric procedures in this specific patient population. Comprehensive centers may perform all approved procedures including high-risk patients as well as revisional procedures.

Of the 9 described standards, 7 are core standards and 2 pertain to specific patient age (i.e., adolescents) or procedures (gastric banding). The 7 core standards are applicable to both tiers of accreditation. The differentiation in low-acuity vs. comprehensive centers is solely based on volume: low-acuity centers need to perform a minimum of 25 bariatric stapling cases per year, whereas comprehensive centers are required to perform at least 50 cases annually.

The 7 core standards are:

Standard 1: Case volume—see above

Standard 2: Commitment to quality care

- Centers must have an established bariatric committee including a director/surgeon, a coordinator, and a clinical reviewer.
- The center must maintain general facility accreditation.
- Surgeons must be credentialed in bariatric surgery according to society guidelines, must undergo annual verification, and must provide a bariatric call schedule.
- A designated clinic and inpatient area must be available and include trained nursing staff.

- A multidisciplinary specialized team must be available including nursing staff, registered dieticians, psychologists/psychiatrists, and physical therapists.

Standard 3: Appropriate equipment and instruments

- This includes every aspect of care from appropriate operating room tables and imaging equipment to blood pressure cuffs and adequate bedding, showers, toilets, etc.

Standard 4: Critical care support

- Required Advanced Cardiac Life Support (ACLS)-qualified provider, stabilization and transfer capabilities, and arrangements made if they cannot provide the level of care required by a medical event.
- This also requires established protocols and availability for bariatric patient management of nonsurgical services: anesthesia, 24/7 critical/intensive care unit, endoscopy, diagnostic and interventional radiology, and/or written transfer agreement to transfer patients to a facility providing these services.

Standard 5: Continuum of care

- Use of clinical education and perioperative protocols
- Long-term follow-up and available support groups

Standard 6: Data collection

- Data entry and reporting of all procedures

Standard 7: Continuous quality improvement process

- Maintain a collaborative between all bariatric surgeons in the institution.
- Perform at least one quality improvement initiative per year.
- Continuously monitor safety and outcomes.

Optimal Preoperative Evaluation

If national guidelines have been used to frame the indications for bariatric surgery, they remain vague as to evaluating patients in order to safely provide the best surgery to each patient. Current National Institutes of Health (NIH) guidelines for bariatric surgery date back over 20 years—1991 consensus conference on gastrointestinal surgery for severe obesity [12]—and do not provide guidance toward adequate patient evaluation. These guidelines require a BMI>40 or a BMI>35 and either high-risk comorbid conditions such as life-threatening cardiopulmonary problems, severe diabetes mellitus, or obesity-induced physical problems interfering with lifestyle. They state that patients should be able to demonstrate failed attempts at diet and exercise, be motivated and well informed, and be free of significant psychological disease.

The extent of the preoperative workup in order to assist patient/procedure selection is therefore extremely variable depending on the provider. In our view, an extensive preoperative multidisciplinary workup is necessary to assess the extent of each patient's comorbidities and guide appropriate preoperative management or procedure selection. Details of the preoperative evaluation are presented in the previous chapters.

Process

Volume Outcomes

The relationship between institution or surgeon volume and outcome has been widely held for multiple complex surgical procedures, and bariatric surgery is no exception. Multiple studies have demonstrated a relationship between outcomes and volume, with reduction in morbidity and mortality in high-volume centers. A recent systematic review covering 24 studies and over 450,000 patients confirmed this association for both institutions and surgeons. While this relationship holds true on average, it does not fully account for outcomes—this will be discussed later in this chapter (composite measures)—and some low-volume centers can have good outcomes or vice versa [2, 10, 13, 14].

An interesting aspect of volume-outcome metrics is the threshold chosen for the determination of low- vs. high-volume centers. When the first accreditation programs for bariatric surgery were established, in 2004–2005, the threshold was somewhat arbitrarily defined at 125 cases/institution/year for the centers of excellence. Today, top tier accreditation as comprehensive center requires less than half that number, and only 25 cases/year are necessary to receive low-acuity center accreditation. The current standards specify that these need to be stapling procedures. This trend is actually supported by the literature: most studies analyzing volume outcomes in bariatric surgery have either chosen 25 cases/year or 50 cases/year as their cutoff for high-volume centers and have demonstrated improved outcomes in the defined high-volume centers. It also demonstrates the enhanced safety profile of bariatric surgery over time and the impact of stapled procedures upon morbidity. Recently, Jafari et al. have studied the Nationwide Inpatient Sample reviewing laparoscopic cases between 2006 and 2010, using the new criteria (>50 stapling procedures per year): they have demonstrated a 2.5-fold increased mortality rate in low-volume centers. This new threshold could therefore improve access to care while preserving outcomes [10].

Laparoscopic Versus Open procedures

One aspect in the improvement of bariatric surgery outcomes is the widespread adoption of laparoscopy: from <2 % of procedures in 1998 to over 90 % today [15]. If the exact role of laparoscopy in the improvement of outcomes is difficult to quantify, multiple studies have demonstrated the benefits of laparoscopy, both for these procedures and for this specific patient population. By far, the most thoroughly studied procedure is the gastric bypass. From early randomized control trials to large nationwide cohort analysis with >100,000 patients, studies have demonstrated a wide range of benefits

to the laparoscopic approach [16–19]. They include reduced mortality (up to 50 % lower) and morbidity (reduced by a third) and shorter length of stay but also reduced overall cost while maintaining equivalent or better long-term weight loss. Laparoscopy also resulted in the virtual disappearance of wound-related complications such as wound infection (>10 % in open gastric bypass) or incisional hernia (>7 % in open gastric bypass).

Peri- and Postoperative Management

Ulcer Prophylaxis

Marginal ulcers after gastric bypass have a reported incidence that varies widely (0.6–16 %). If pathogenesis is still unclear, studies have demonstrated that acid exposure as well as mucosal ischemia in the pouch is likely associated with the incidence of marginal ulcers [20]. With the incidence of ulcers also decreasing with time after surgery, many centers have proceeded with proton-pump inhibitor prophylaxis [21, 22]. A recent international survey showed that nearly 90 % of bariatric surgeons prescribe prophylaxis for 30–90 days postoperatively [23]. We currently systematically prescribe 3–6 months of proton-pump inhibitors to all bariatric surgery patients. Another potential risk factor for anastomotic ulcers is the presence of *H. pylori*. Taking into account the unknown efficacy of *H. pylori* eradication after gastric bypass, *H. pylori* detection and eradication have been advocated.

Gallstone Prophylaxis

Given the increased risk of gallstone formation with rapid weight loss, multiple prevention strategies have been advocated, including prophylactic cholecystectomy at the time of surgery for either all patients or patients with asymptomatic gallstones. The discussion regarding prophylactic cholecystectomy is outside of the realm of this chapter. However, as a framework, a recent meta-analysis on >6,000 patients showed a cholecystectomy rate of 6.8 % after gastric bypass with 0 % mortality and 1.8 % morbidity [24]. Common bile duct pathologies occurred in 0.2 % of cases for common bile duct stones and 0.2 % for biliary pancreatitis. Therefore, if cholecystectomy is not performed at the time of gastric bypass surgery, ursodiol prophylaxis has been clearly demonstrated to significantly reduce the incidence of symptomatic/gallstone formation and should be advocated postoperatively. Studies have shown that ursodiol provided a reduction in gallstone formation from 32 to 2 %, and a recent meta-analysis also showed a significant reduction, with 8.8 % of patients on prophylaxis developing gallstones compared to 27.7 % for placebo [25, 26].

Outcomes

Risk Adjustment

Measures of outcomes are probably the single most useful metric for assessing quality of care in surgery. Surgery usually involves a procedure with a known or expected outcome to which results can be compared. However, heterogeneous patients with heterogeneous risk factors will provide heterogeneous results, and these data therefore need to be corrected or *adjusted* for risk factors. It is difficult, however, to establish both reliable and usable risk-adjustment models. Indeed, for example, the ACS has created the National Surgical Quality Improvement Program (NSQIP) in order to allow for the collection of data to produce risk-adjusted outcomes for quality improvement. However, in order to encompass the complexity of patients across surgical specialties, it requires a very large number of data points for risk adjustment: it notably gathers 74 preoperative and 19 intraoperative metrics. The amount and complexity of data produced is so large that NSQIP currently functions on the basis of sampling a number of procedures for each institution.

However, more recently, multiple authors have been developing procedure-specific risk-adjustment models. By reducing the heterogeneity of procedures studied, risk factors can be more specific and therefore reduced to a small number of variables without loss of predicting power. These models, called parsimonious models, make risk adjustment not only easier but also allow providers to focus their attention on the most important risk factors in order to improve outcomes. This has already been the case for colectomies, for example [27]. By nature, bariatric surgery lends itself perfectly to this type of analyses, and risk-adjusted outcomes have shown higher predictability for performance than other metrics such as hospital volume.

Composite Measures

As just mentioned, parsimonious risk-adjustment models provide a useful while still user-friendly approach without requiring unmanageable amounts of data. However, even these models do not allow to completely encompass the complexity of surgical cases, and applying these models to bariatric surgery only explained 83 % of future outcomes in institutions. Dimick et al. have recently developed composite measures for bariatric surgery. These measures combine multiple quality metrics as the ones described above in order to create a score with the highest possible predictive power of future outcomes. These composite measures include metrics such as complication rates for the given procedure but also other procedures, reoperation rates, readmissions, and hospital characteristics. Their study showed that these metrics could more accurately explain institutional variations in

complications when compared to either hospital volume or risk-adjusted complications [28–30].

Mortality

Bariatric surgery has witnessed a dramatic decrease in mortality from approximately 0.5 % before 2000 [31] to 0.06 % in the latest reports [10]. Multiple factors have probably contributed to this nearly tenfold decrease in mortality rates. As mentioned above, adoption of laparoscopy has probably played a significant role. But bariatric surgery as a specialty has witnessed an extremely rapid but heavily structured development. With the creation of the national and international society of bariatric and metabolic surgery, emphasis has been placed on allowing the rapid growth of bariatric surgery to provide for the increasing number of patients candidates for surgery in the safest possible way. A strong importance has been focused on adequate training and quality assessment and improvement.

Quality Improvement

Readmissions

As noted, over the last decade, bariatric surgery has had tremendous success in quality improvement in a highly comorbid population. Mortality rates have dropped to where bariatric surgery mortality is now equal to laparoscopic cholecystectomy [15]. A key component to this quality improvement has been the accreditation process, which is now a unified program for the American Society of Metabolic and Bariatric Surgery and the American College of Surgeons called MBSAQIP. The accreditation process has been proven to save lives, lower complications, increase access, and decrease costs [5].

The MBSAQIP accreditation program provides an ideal platform for quality improvement by maintaining a clinically derived, data registry with the ability to benchmark results and track outcomes longitudinally. As the MBSAQIP program moves forward with over 700 hospitals in place, the program will seek to find further opportunities for quality improvement. The 30-day readmission rate is an ideal outcome upon which to focus future quality improvement efforts.

Rationale

The current MBSAQIP standards require each hospital to perform at least one annual quality improvement project. In prioritizing quality improvement efforts, it is critical to find opportunities for improvement that are preventable and actionable. With mortality rates and specific complications such as anastomotic leaks becoming increasingly rare, other quality metrics must be investigated. Thirty-day readmission rates are an important quality metric. Readmission rates are a *meta*-outcome, which touch upon patient/physician satisfaction, cost, coordination of care, and complications. In addition, the Centers for Medicare and Medicaid Services, along with other payors, have made readmission rate reduction a leading initiative.

Decreasing Readmission Rates

The first aspect of process change is definition and measurement. There should be a distinction between 23 h readmissions and readmissions greater than 24 h given the difference in acuity and intervention between both types of readmissions. In addition, the readmission capture rate should include readmissions to not only the index hospital but other hospitals as well. MBSAQIP is able to accomplish both of these tasks as well as provide an opportunity to benchmark individual hospital results to national rates.

Within our program at Stanford, we determined that our 30-day readmission rates were higher than the national average at 8 %. At the inaugural Obesity Week 2013, we presented our quality improvement program for readmission reduction [32]. Preventable causes for readmission are listed here:

- Medication side effects
- Patient expectations
- Dehydration
- Nausea

Next, the following quality improvement measures were added:

- Medication reconciliation at preop visit.
- Postoperative prescriptions given at preop visit.
- Improved preop patient education/discharge planning.
- Intraoperative nausea management including IV fluids, Decadron, and propofol.
- Clinical road map/standardized order set/early ambulation.
- Provided direct phone numbers to patients.
- Clinic RN calls each patient the day after discharge.
- Same day appointments made available for any concerns.
- Discharge checklist.
- Using clinical decision unit for 23 h stays particularly for dehydration.
- 2-week post-op appointment with nutritional counseling.
- Readmission postmortem or root cause analysis for readmission.

After the implementation of these readmission measures, 30-day readmission rates dropped from 8 to 2.5 % over 18 months.

Next Steps

Quality improvement will be a critical component as MBSAQIP moves forward. Reduction in 30-day readmissions will be the first quality improvement project for MBSAQIP. With proven processes, the national goal for MBSAQIP will be to reduce readmissions within 30 days. In addition, MBSAQIP will work with establishing standardized preoperative educational modules in surgery, nursing, nutrition, psychology, and pharmacology. Other national initiative processes will include: website, toolkit, webinars/audio conferences, discharge checklist cards, and regional initiatives for large hospital chains.

Plans are for the MBSAQIP project to begin in July 2014. The name of the quality improvement project is termed *DROP* (Decreasing Readmission through Opportunities Provided). Quality improvement is a lasting legacy for bariatric surgery.

Conclusion

Deeply embedded in bariatric surgery's DNA are patient safety, quality improvement, and innovation. It is a remarkable American surgical success story that bariatric surgery has written so far. With mortality falling tenfold and 90 % of cases performed laparoscopically, it may appear that bariatric surgery has accomplished much. More remains to be done, though, and no field is better suited to the changes in healthcare than bariatric surgery. Bariatric surgery with its multidisciplinary team has its eye on the future, chin forward, and head held high with the one effective and enduring therapy for obesity.

References

1. Metabolic and bariatric surgery accreditation and quality improvement program. *mbsaqiporg*. Available at: http://www.mbsaqip.org/. Accessed March 4, 2014.
2. Hollenbeak CS, Rogers AM, Barrus B, Wadiwala I, Cooney RN. Surgical volume impacts bariatric surgery mortality: a case for centers of excellence. Surgery. 2008;144(5):736–43. doi:10.1016/j.surg.2008.05.013.
3. Nguyen NT, Hohmann S, Slone J, Varela E, Smith BR, Hoyt D. Improved bariatric surgery outcomes for Medicare beneficiaries after implementation of the medicare national coverage determination. Arch Surg. 2010;145(1):72–8. doi:10.1001/archsurg.2009.228.
4. Nguyen NT, Nguyen B, Nguyen VQ, Ziogas A, Hohmann S, Stamos MJ. Outcomes of bariatric surgery performed at accredited vs nonaccredited centers. J Am Coll Surg. 2012;215(4):467–74. doi:10.1016/j.jamcollsurg.2012.05.032.
5. Kwon S, Wang B, Wong E, Alfonso-Cristancho R, Sullivan SD, Flum DR. The impact of accreditation on safety and cost of bariatric surgery. Surg Obes Relat Dis. 2013;9(5):617–22. doi:10.1016/j.soard.2012.11.002.
6. Encinosa WE, Bernard DM, Du D, Steiner CA. Recent improvements in bariatric surgery outcomes. Med Care. 2009;47(5):531–5. doi:10.1097/MLR.0b013e31819434c6.
7. Flum DR, Kwon S, MacLeod K, et al. The use, safety and cost of bariatric surgery before and after Medicare's national coverage decision. Ann Surg. 2011;254(6):860–5. doi:10.1097/SLA.0b013e31822f2101.
8. Birkmeyer NJO, Dimick JB, Share D, et al. Hospital complication rates with bariatric surgery in Michigan. JAMA. 2010;304(4):435–42. doi:10.1001/jama.2010.1034.

9. Dimick JB, Nicholas LH, Ryan AM, Thumma JR, Birkmeyer JD. Bariatric surgery complications before vs after implementation of a national policy restricting coverage to centers of excellence. JAMA. 2013;309(8):792–9. doi:10.1001/jama.2013.755.

10. Jafari MD, Jafari F, Young MT, Smith BR, Phalen MJ, Nguyen NT. Volume and outcome relationship in bariatric surgery in the laparoscopic era. Surg Endosc. 2013;27(12):4539–46. doi:10.1007/s00464-013-3112-3.

11. Morton JM, Garg T, Nguyen NT. Does Hospital Accreditation Matter for Bariatric Surgery? Ann Surg. 2014;260(3):504–9.

12. Hubbard VS, Hall WH. Gastrointestinal surgery for severe obesity. Obes Surg. 1991;1(3):257–65.

13. Zevin B, Aggarwal R, Grantcharov TP. Volume-outcome association in bariatric surgery: a systematic review. Ann Surg. 2012;256(1):60–71. doi:10.1097/SLA.0b013e3182554c62.

14. Gould JC, Kent KC, Wan Y, Rajamanickam V, Leverson G, Campos GM. Perioperative safety and volume: outcomes relationships in bariatric surgery: a study of 32,000 patients. J Am Coll Surg. 2011;213(6):771–7. doi:10.1016/j.jamcollsurg.2011.09.006.

15. Nguyen NT, Nguyen B, Shih A, Smith B, Hohmann S. Use of laparoscopy in general surgical operations at academic centers. Surg Obes Relat Dis. 2013;9(1):15–20. doi:10.1016/j.soard.2012.07.002.

16. Nguyen NT, Goldman C, Rosenquist CJ, et al. Laparoscopic versus open gastric bypass: a randomized study of outcomes, quality of life, and costs. Ann Surg. 2001;234(3):279–89. Discussion 289–91.

17. Paxton JH, Matthews JB. The cost effectiveness of laparoscopic versus open gastric bypass surgery. Obes Surg. 2005;15(1):24–34. doi:10.1381/0960892052993477.

18. Banka G, Woodard G, Hernandez-Boussard T, Morton JM. Laparoscopic vs open gastric bypass surgery: differences in patient demographics, safety, and outcomes. Arch Surg. 2012;147(6):550–6. doi:10.1001/archsurg.2012.195.

19. Lujan JA, Frutos MD, Hernandez Q, et al. Laparoscopic versus open gastric bypass in the treatment of morbid obesity. Ann Surg. 2004;239(4):433–7. doi:10.1097/01.sla.0000120071.75691.1f.

20. Azagury DE, Abu Dayyeh BK, Greenwalt IT, Thompson CC. Marginal ulceration after Roux-en-Y gastric bypass surgery: characteristics, risk factors, treatment, and outcomes. Endoscopy. 2011;43(11):950–4. doi:10.1055/s-0030-1256951.

21. Moon RC, Teixeira AF, Goldbach M, Jawad MA. Management and treatment outcomes of marginal ulcers after Roux-en-Y gastric bypass at a single high volume bariatric center. Surg Obes Relat Dis. 2014;10:229–34. doi:10.1016/j.soard.2013.10.002.

22. Garrido Jr AB, Rossi M, Lima Jr SE, Brenner AS, Gomes Jr CAR. Early marginal ulcer following Roux-en-Y gastric bypass under proton pump inhibitor treatment: prospective multicentric study. Arq Gastroenterol. 2010;47(2):130–4.

23. Steinemann DC, Bueter M, Schiesser M, Amygdalos I, Clavien P-A, Nocito A. Management of anastomotic ulcers after roux-en-Y gastric bypass: results of an international survey. Obes Surg. 2013. doi:10.1007/s11695-013-1152-3.

24. Warschkow R, Tarantino I, Ukegjini K, et al. Concomitant cholecystectomy during laparoscopic Roux-en-Y gastric bypass in obese patients is not justified: a meta-analysis. Obes Surg. 2013;23(3):397–407. doi:10.1007/s11695-012-0852-4.

25. Sugerman HJ, Brewer WH, Shiffman ML, et al. A multicenter, placebo-controlled, randomized, double-blind, prospective trial of prophylactic ursodiol for the prevention of gallstone formation following gastric-bypass-induced rapid weight loss. Am J Surg. 1995;169(1):91–6. Discussion 96–7.

26. Stokes CS, Gluud LL, Casper M, Lammert F. Ursodeoxycholic acid and diets higher in Fat prevent gallbladder stones during weight loss: a meta-analysis of randomized controlled trials. Clin Gastroenterol Hepatol. 2013. doi:10.1016/j.cgh.2013.11.031.

27. Merkow RP, Hall BL, Cohen ME, et al. Validity and feasibility of the American college of surgeons colectomy composite outcome quality measure. Ann Surg. 2013;257(3):483–9. doi:10.1097/SLA.0b013e318273bf17.

28. Dimick JB, Osborne NH, Hall BL, Ko CY, Birkmeyer JD. Risk adjustment for comparing hospital quality with surgery: How many variables Are needed? J Am Coll Surg. 2010;210(4):503–8. doi:10.1016/j.jamcollsurg.2010.01.018.

29. Dimick JB, Staiger DO, Hall BL, Ko CY, Birkmeyer JD. Composite measures for profiling hospitals on surgical morbidity. Ann Surg. 2013;257(1):67–72. doi:10.1097/SLA.0b013e31827b6be6.

30. Dimick JB, Birkmeyer NJ, Finks JF, et al. Composite measures for profiling hospitals on bariatric surgery performance. JAMA Surg. 2014;149(1):10. doi:10.1001/jamasurg.2013.4109.

31. Balsiger BM, Kennedy FP, Abu-Lebdeh HS, et al. Prospective evaluation of Roux-en-Y gastric bypass as primary operation for medically complicated obesity. Mayo Clin Proc. 2000;75(7):673–80. doi:10.4065/75.7.673.

32. Morton JM, Sell T, Garg T, Rivas H. Utilizing national clinical data to drive quality improvement. Atlanta: Obesity Week; 2013.

13

Data Management for the Bariatric Surgery Program

M. Logan Rawlins

Abbreviations

ABS	American Board of Surgery
ASMBS	American Society for Metabolic and Bariatric Surgery
BMI	Body mass index
BOLD	Bariatric Outcome Longitudinal Database
BSCN	Bariatric Surgery Center Network
CABG	Coronary artery bypass graft
COE	Center of excellence
COPD	Chronic obstructive pulmonary disease
CPAP	Continuous positive airway pressure
CTP	Child-Turcotte-Pugh
DVT	Deep Venous Thrombosis
EEA	End to end anastomosis
GERD	Gastroesophageal reflux disease
IRB	Institutional Review Board
IVC	Inferior vena cava
MBSAQIP	Metabolic and Bariatric Surgery Accreditation and Quality Improvement Program
MBSC	Michigan Bariatric Surgery Collaborative
MI	Myocardial infarction
PCTI	Percutaneous coronary transluminal intervention
PE	Pulmonary embolus
POD	Postoperative day
PPI	Proton Pump Inhibitor
PSVT	Paroxysmal supraventricular tachycardia
SRC	Surgical Review Corporation
VTE	Venous thromboembolism

History of Database Management

As the field of bariatric surgery continues to expand and grow, the surgical treatment of morbid obesity has become more common and accepted by both medical and surgical colleagues. However, as with any emerging surgical specialty, it was subject to a barrage of criticism regarding the lack of published data to support surgical efficacy and safety. Prior to the mid-2000s, there was very little centralized data collection from surgeons regarding their results and morbidity/mortality. The drive for quality improvement, improved surgical safety, and evaluation of specific surgical procedures has pushed the field toward collection of more data for evaluation. Prior to this time, all results from bariatric surgery were limited to a few meta-analyses and published case series. Bariatric surgeons felt a great need for randomized clinical trials but more importantly centralized data collection. This data would further be utilized for certifying and accrediting surgeons and centers that perform high-volume surgery with good outcomes, which lead to the derivation of what is now known as "centers of excellence" (COEs) [1]. Data collection is also important for individual surgeons as the American Board of Surgery (ABS) now requires reporting outcomes for the maintenance of certification [2].

Many bariatric surgery programs have been recording their outcomes in private institutional databases for years; however, this data was not commonly shared outside the surgeons practice unless it was used for publications or conference presentations. Surgeons maintained these databases as it allowed them to quickly access their outcomes so they can provide patients with institution-specific rates of complications and weight loss expectations. It also allowed a system for tracking patient follow-up and reestablishing care for those with long intervals between visits. The need for these local databases will continue to exist as each institution may elect to track patient outcome variables that they deem to be important and may not be tracked nationally.

ACS-BSCN

The first national database used for center accreditation was started by the ACS in 2005 and was known as the Bariatric Surgery Center Network (BSCN) bariatric surgery database [3]. The database was a requirement to establish and maintain accreditation and 100 % capture of all data points and cases

S.A. Brethauer et al. (eds.), *Minimally Invasive Bariatric Surgery*,
DOI 10.1007/978-1-4939-1637-5_13, © Springer Science+Business Media New York 2015

was required. It was easily accessed through the internet or could be managed on a local workstation platform with electronic data transmission. All data was encrypted and de-identified to protect the confidentiality of the surgeons and patients. Programs did not incur any additional cost for the database as it was included in their credentialing fees. Post surgical guidelines were established and standardized for a minimum follow-up of 30 days, 6 months, and annually thereafter. If an institution already participated in the National Surgical Quality Improvement Project (NSQIP), this data would auto-populate into the bariatric surgery database. However, more fields were required in the bariatric database specific to these types of patients requiring more data entry than what is required into NSQIP. It was mandated that data entry be done by a trained data collector, a position ideally filled by a medically trained person or dedicated bariatric staff member. The data entry person could not be a surgeon or mid-level provider with direct patient care responsibilities in an attempt to avoid reporting bias in the data. While outcomes were monitored for the safety of the program, accreditation was closely tied to institution and surgeon volume.

ASMBS-SRC and BOLD

In 2007, the American Society for Metabolic and Bariatric Surgery (ASMBS) joined forces with the Surgical Review Corporation (SRC) to form a separate and distinct accrediting agency and bariatric database [4]. Their goals were similar to those of the ACS. The database they created was known as BOLD (Bariatric Outcomes Longitudinal Database). The guiding principles of database management and program organization were very similar to those of the ACS-BSCN. There were even features which interfaced with electronic medical records to expedite the entry of data and prevent duplication or errors in the transcription of data. One key difference in this database was the intention to use blinded data for research purposes accessed by third parties. It was thought that a large database such as this should be used to provide size and statistical power needed to study both high- and low-frequency occurrences. The database could also be easily accessed by each individual surgeon to query their own outcomes.

There were also many questions initially regarding how these databases could be used for research studies and whether they required institutional review board (IRB) approval to exist and/or be accessed. Eventually it was determined that according to 45 CFR Part 164.501, 506, these activities are implemented solely for the purpose of assessing the quality of care and do not require review by an IRB [5]. The BOLD database did undergo review through the Copernicus Group Independent Review Board prior to its inception. Nevertheless, it is still recommended that each institution wishing to review their own data via this database

and publish related results may elect or may be required to obtain approval though their own hospital IRB.

MBSAQIP

In the years that followed the initiation of two separate data collection and accrediting agencies (ACS-BSCN and SRC-ASMBS BOLD), questions were raised why there was not one centralized database and credentialing agency. There were also criticisms of a lack of evolution of the BOLD database. There were also concerns about the exclusive nature of "centers of excellence" creating a two-tiered system implying superiority and inferiority. Common goals of quality, over a simple volume-based threshold, became the new focus. This eventually led to the creation of the new ASMBS-ACS quality program known as the Metabolic and Bariatric Surgery Accreditation and Quality Improvement Program (MBSAQIP) [6, 7]. The fusion of these two programs began in April 2012. This transition was spearheaded by Robin Blackstone, MD, president of the ASMBS at that time. It was felt that the ACS database, which was a second-generation-type registry with many improvements over BOLD, would be maintained as the new centralized data collection registry. This second-generation database was considered progressive and changed over time as unnecessary data points were removed. Any data collected which did not impact quality and was not needed was no longer included. With fewer elements to report, primarily through yes and no questions, it became much easier for the program to comply. Data remains tied to NSQIP, which theoretically should strengthen it.

New requirements for data collection were also instituted under MBSAQIP with significantly important changes [8]. Data entry is required to be completed by a designated personnel who is not a patient care provider. This requirement for a single data collector at each site who was medically trained or an experienced chart abstractor became stricter with the addition of a web-based certification process. The program also created stricter definitions for adverse events so it was easier for the "Bariatric Surgery Clinical Reviewer" (BSCR) to enter this data. It was also recognized that the preferred method of data collection is by chart abstraction, not encounter forms, third-party data transmission, or real-time entry during patient visit. This does, however, create more work for the BSCR but will hopefully provide data with higher fidelity. The updated database also fixes problems such as how to correctly code comorbidity severity, complications, and revisional surgery, known to be common complaints of the BOLD database. One goal was to limit the amount of free text entries by standardizing definitions. The program also decreased the number of reportable complications and limited them to those which have an impact on risk adjustment. The comorbidity severity scale was changed to simplify the presence or absence of remission. Maintaining a patient on medications for preventative health, such as a statin or metformin, is no longer considered treating a comorbidity as these types of medications are now commonly continued on patients even when their comorbidities have significantly improved. Likewise, treatment of atrial fibrillation with a beta blocker or calcium channel blocker in a patient with previous hypertension does not preclude them from being in remission. Outcome reporting is still required at 30 days, 6 months, 12 months, and annually thereafter. New time constraints have been enforced with data entry required within 120 days of each entry data point with a system lockout after that time. Follow-up windows are also lengthened after the initial 30 days to provide some flexibility in actual visit dates. For instance, the annual follow-up data can include 6 months on either side of the surgery anniversary.

Another common problem with BOLD was data auditing [8]. BOLD data auditing used to only check the 1 year prior to recertification and only those surgeons who were COE surgeons at a facility were required to report. In the new system, facility certification takes greater precedence. In the past, BSCOE program individual surgeons were credentialed separately from the institution. Program certification could exclude particular surgeons at a facility and their data was not included. Now all surgeons' data must be included and reported at each facility. Program data audit previously only occurred every 3 years with site inspection, but programs may now also be subject to closer interval or random auditing to keep programs honest.

Tracking patient follow-up is another improvement of MBSAQIP database over BOLD. BOLD has incomplete follow-up data, as the definition of lost to follow-up only includes patients that died while all others were still considered "eligible" for follow-up years after their last data entry [8]. The new system also has an easier way to track patient follow-up with specific tracking reports. These reports show which patients are due for follow-up and when. It will also allow programs to track when patients are contacted to attempt to reestablish care and document discharge or transfer from the practice or inability to contact. Both data systems still suffer from the lack of being able to track patients as they may switch practices or have a complication treated by another provider.

The new program will also report a program's risk-adjusted outcomes compared to national risk-adjusted benchmarks, a feature not available in BOLD [8]. Comorbidity remission data is also now provided in a useful table that providers can use for quality improvement, application for hospital certifications, or insurance coverage.

Many questions have been raised regarding the fate of BOLD data [8]. While demographics were rather easy to transfer from BOLD to the new MBSAQIP database, adverse event data was too unreliable to transfer over. Data from BOLD will be returned to programs for their internal use. A public-use file will also be maintained for research purposes,

both for ongoing studies and for those wishing to access it in the future. BOLD data is also being used for state by state comparisons to evaluate access to care issues.

MBSC (Michigan Bariatric Surgery Collaborative)

There has been interest by some groups in the country to obtain a more detailed bariatric database that can be used for quality improvement and optimal outcome-based cost containment. The best example of this type of program is the MBSC, which is a clinical outcome registry formed from a regional, voluntary consortium of hospitals and surgeons that perform bariatric surgery in Michigan [9]. The project is funded by Blue Cross and Blue Shield of the Michigan/Blue Care Network and coordinated at the University of Michigan under the lead direction of Nancy Birkmeyer, PhD. Over 40 hospitals participate and data is not excluded from low-volume centers which differentiate it from the other larger national databases. Given that the guiding principle for the program is quality improvement, the group meets multiple times per year to examine their data and to design and implement changes in care that result in better outcomes for their bariatric patients. Quality improvement projects resulting from this database have led to reduction in the use of preoperative inferior vena cava (IVC) filter placement, as well as risk stratification for VTE prophylaxis [10, 11]. Their data has also contested the notion that high-volume COEs have improved outcomes compared to low-volume non-COEs [12]. This has pushed credentialing agencies to move toward outcome-based certification rather than strictly volume based.

Creating the Ideal Internal Database

It is likely that bariatric surgeons may wish to track their outcomes locally on an institutional database for easier access and customizability. This section is dedicated to how to design the ideal internal database. While listing every customizable database program is beyond the scope of this chapter, certain factors should go into the decision of which program to choose. The software should be easy to use for both input and data extraction. A modifiable entry form with user designed prompts for each different patient encounter makes data entry easier. Search functions should allow the user to identify and sort data with multiple tiers of data points and create a spreadsheet from these desired data points. The program would ideally be made by a manufacturer that is well established and will continue to be in business for some time so the product can be serviced and grow as platforms and operating systems change over time, as opposed to one

TABLE 1. Initial visit

Initial visit date

Seminar date

Patient demographics

  Name

  Date of birth

  Medical record number

  Gender

  Race

  Primary language

  Height (cm, inches)

Weight at first patient contact (kg, lb) + date

BMI at first patient contact + date

Excess body weight (calculate from ideal body weight)

Smoking (current pack per day, pack/year history, or how long ago had the patient quit smoking)

Mobility status (if not fully mobile, document immobile, or mobility aids needed)

Previous abdominal surgery history

Obesity history

  Overweight since what age

  Highest weight

  Most weight ever lost

  Attempting to lose weight for how many years

  Unsuccessful commercial diets/pills

  Current exercise regimen

  Previous weight loss operations (which one)

Obesity-related medical conditions

  Diabetes mellitus

    Type I/II

    Controlled/uncontrolled

    Controlled with diet, oral meds, or insulin

    Diabetic complications (nerve, eye, kidney, skin)

    Hemoglobin A1c and fasting blood sugar + date

  Hypertension

    Controlled/uncontrolled

    Number of and class of medications

  Hyperlipidemia

  Gastroesophageal reflux disease

    Medication treatment (PPI or H2 blocker)

    Previous surgical or endoluminal therapy

Nonalcoholic steatohepatitis or cirrhosis

Obstructive sleep apnea (sleep study, STOPBang score, CPAP)

Other non-obesity-related medical conditions

  Asthma

  COPD (home oxygen requirement)

  Coronary artery disease (h/o MI, PCTI, or CABG)

  CHF (recent EF %)

  Atrial fibrillation or PSVT

  Pacemaker

  Peripheral vascular disease

  Peptic ulcer disease (*Helicobacter pylori* status)

  Gallstones (present or history of cholecystectomy)

(continued)

TABLE 1. (continued)

Stress incontinence
Renal failure (creatinine, dialysis, transplant patient/candidate)
Cirrhosis (cause, CTP class, MELD score, transplant patient/candidate)
DVT/PE (history, previous/current treatment)
Psychological (anxiety, depression, substance abuse, suicidal, bipolar, eating disorder)
Connective tissue disorder (which one?)
Bleeding disorder (which one?)

TABLE 2. Preoperative H and P visit

Preoperative visit date
Weight + BMI
Planned procedure + date
Labs/tests
   Anemia (hemoglobin)
   Arterial blood gas
   C-reactive protein
   Creatinine
   Coagulation panel (if necessary)
   Chest X-ray
   EKG
   Vitamin/micronutrient deficiency
   H. pylori (histology, serology, stool antigen, urea breath test, CLO test)
   Upper endoscopy
   Upper gastrointestinal series

which may be obsolete in a decade or less. While each individual surgeon may wish to track uncommon data points important to them, the following tables list items every surgeon may want to include in their database. These tables are arranged according to when the data should be recorded based on patient visits in a chronological order. They include the initial visit (Table 1), the preoperative history and physical visit (Table 2), the operative encounter (Table 3), postoperative visits in the perioperative period within 30 days of surgery (Table 4), and long-term visits defined as after 30 days from the date of surgery (Table 5).

Conclusion

As the field of bariatric surgery moves forward, accurate data collection and reporting will become a critical part of any practice. Risk-adjustment models are being developed that will help surgeons, patients, and payors understand outcomes in a way that more accurately reflects the patients a specific program cares for. Whether the data is used for internal process improvement, payor reimbursement, or as part of a national accreditation program, a thoughtful and detailed approach to data collection and reporting will be necessary.

TABLE 3. Operation

Procedure performed + date
Approach (open, laparoscopic, converted to open)
Procedure changed or aborted (+reason)
OR procedure time (incision to closure) Additional OR procedures (cholecystectomy, hiatal hernia, liver biopsy, abdominal wall hernia)
Intraoperative complications
Procedure specifics
Adjustable gastric band
Band type
Allergan LAP-BAND AP standard or large
Ethicon REALIZE Band or REALIZE Band-C
Gastro-gastric sutures placed?
Gastric bypass
Roux limb length (cm)
Estimated pouch size (cc)
Banded pouch
GJ anastomosis
Linear staple (Length in cm)
Circular staple (21 vs. 25 mm EEA)
Ante-ante or retro-retro Roux limb position
Close Peterson's defect?
Intraoperative leak test (method and result)
Drain placed?
Duodenal Switch
Alimentary limb length (cm)
Common channel limb length (cm)
Sleeve bougie size (Fr)
Duodenoileostomy anastomosis
Linear staple (length in cm)
Circular staple (21 vs. 25 mm EEA)
Intraoperative leak test (method and result)
Drain placed
Sleeve gastrectomy
Initial staple fire length from the pylorus (cm)
Sleeve bougie size (Fr)
Staple line reinforcement (none vs. SEAMGUARD vs. suture imbrication)
Intraoperative leak test (method and result)
Drain placed

TABLE 4. First postoperative visit (<30 days)

Visit date + POD#
Weight
Procedure performed + date
POD#1 upper GI series result
Drain removed on POD# (if placed)
VTE prophylaxis
   Foot pumps or SCDs
   IVC filter (if yes: temporary or permanent)
   Chemical
      Type: UFH or LMWH or other
      Pre-op, intra-op, post-op, post-discharge (include dosages)
Complications
   Death (suspected cause)
   Abscess/wound infection (superficial, deep, organ space + treatment)
   Bleeding (intra-/extraluminal, reoperation, transfusion, lowest Hgb, splenectomy)
   Port-site hernia or wound dehiscence
   Respiratory (hypoxia, prolonged oxygen requirement, reintubation)
   Hospital infection (pneumonia, urinary tract, *Clostridium difficile*)
   Venous thromboembolism (DVT or PE + treatment)
   Cardiac event (MI, cardiac arrest)
   Renal failure
   Gastric bypass or duodenal switch specific complications
      Leak (site, day diagnosed, treatment)
      Bowel obstruction (location, cause, treatment)
      Stricture (location, cause, treatment)
      Anastomotic ulcer
   Sleeve gastrectomy specific complications
      Leak (site, day diagnosed, treatment)
      Stricture (location, cause, treatment)
   Adjustable gastric band specific complications
      Gastric perforation
      Band outlet obstruction
      Port-site infection
      Band slippage

TABLE 5. Follow-up visit (>30 days)

Visit date + month/years out from surgery

Procedure

Weight (include also current BMI, BMI lost, lb lost, kg lost, % EWL, % WL,
   % EBMIL)

Exercise program

Food choices

Supplementation intake

Late complications

   Gastric bypass or duodenal switch

      Bowel obstruction (location, cause, treatment)

      Stricture (location, cause, treatment)

      Anastomotic ulcer

      Nonhealing leak

      Dumping syndrome

      Vitamin/micronutrient deficiencies

   Sleeve gastrectomy specific complications

      Nonhealing leak

      Stricture (location, cause, treatment)

      Severe GERD

   Adjustable gastric band specific complications

      Band slippage

      Gastric erosion

      Port-site infection

      Band malfunction/defect (does not fill properly or leaks)

      Band intolerance/removal

Modifiable bariatric comorbidity (improved/remission—# of medications off,
   still on)

   Diabetes mellitus

      Document HbA1c levels

      Preventative metformin does not imply non-resolution

   Hypertension

      Document current blood pressure

      Preventative beta blockers does not imply non-resolution

   Hyperlipidemia

      Document lab improvement

      Preventative statin does not imply non-resolution

   Gastroesophageal reflux disease

      Symptom resolution, still on medication, reflux worse (sleeve/band)

Obstructive sleep apnea

   Off CPAP, improved symptoms

Emergency department visits (reason and number of visits)

Adjustable gastric band

   Adjustment #

   Current band volume

   Adjustment volume

   New band volume

   Hungry

   Making good food choices?

   Exercise

TABLE 5. (continued)

Yearly Labs (in order of importance depending on the type of procedure performed)
Complete blood count
Basic metabolic panel
Iron
Vitamin D
PTH
Vitamin B12
Vitamin B1
Vitamin A
Copper, selenium, zinc (for malabsorptive procedures or clinically indicated)

References

1. Surgicalreview.org [Internet]. Raleigh: Surgical Review Corporation; c2012 [cited 2012 Sept 1]. COE Program Overview. Available from: http://www.surgicalreview.org/coe-programs/overview/

2. Absurgery.org [Internet]. Philadelphia: American Board of Surgery; c2003–2012 [updated August 2012, cited 2012 Sept 1]. MOC Part 4—Practice Assessment Resources. Available from: http://www.absurgery.org/default.jsp?exam-mocpa.

3. Acsbscn.org [Internet]. Chicago: American College of Surgeons Bariatric Surgery Center Network Accreditation Network; c2010 [cited 2012 Sept 1]. Available from: http://www.acsbscn.org/Public/index.jsp.

4. Surgicalreview.org [Internet]. Raleigh: Surgical Review Corporation; c2012 [cited 2012 Sept 1]. BOLD Overview. Available from: http://www.surgicalreview.org/bold/overview/

5. Surgicalreview.org [Internet]. Raleigh: Surgical Review Corporation; c2012 [cited 2012 Sept 1]. BOLD Study Oversight. Available from: http://www.surgicalreview.org/bold/bariatric/research/study-oversight/

6. Asmbs.org [Internet]. Gainesville: American Board of Surgery; c2012 [updated 2012 August 5, cited 2012 Sept 1]. MBSAQIP Update. Available from: http://asmbs.org/2012/08/mbsaqip-update/

7. Advisory.org [Internet]. Washington: The Advisory Board Company; c2012 [updated 2012 June 29, cited 2012 Sept 1]. ASMBS 2012—COE requirements shifting to focus on quality beginning in 2013. Available from: http://www.advisory.com/Research/Technology-Insights/The-Pipeline/2012/06/ASMBS-2012-CoE-Requirements-Shifting-to-Focus-on-Quality-Beginning-in-2013.

8. Blackstone R. ASMBS Update. Bariatric Times. 2012. p. 21–24.

9. Michiganbsc.org [Internet]. Ann Arbor: Michigan Bariatric Surgery Collaborative; c2012 [cited 2012 Sept 1]. Available from: https://michiganbsc.org/Registry/

10. Birkmeyer NJ, Share D, Baser O, Carlin AM, Finks JF, Pesta CM, et al. Preoperative placement of inferior vena cava filters and outcomes after gastric bypass surgery. Ann Surg. 2010;252(2):313–8.

11. Finks JF, English WJ, Carlin AM, Krause KR, Share DA, Banerjee M, et al. Predicting risk for venous thromboembolism with bariatric surgery: results from the Michigan bariatric surgery collaborative. Ann Surg. 2012;255(6):1100–4.

12. Birkmeyer NJ, Dimick JB, Share D, Hawasli A, English WJ, Genaw J, et al. Hospital complication rates with bariatric surgery in Michigan. JAMA. 2010;304(4):435–42.

14

Sleeve Gastrectomy: Technique, Pearls, and Pitfalls

Cheguevara Afaneh and Alfons Pomp

Background

Laparoscopic sleeve gastrectomy, sometimes referred to as longitudinal gastrectomy, was initially introduced as part of the duodenal switch procedure in super obese patients in 1999 [1] and as a stand-alone procedure in 2000 [2]. It is now becoming one of the most popular bariatric procedures based on perceived simplicity of the procedure, significant improvement in comorbidity profile, and evident weight loss. Beginning in 2009 the American Society for Metabolic and Bariatric Surgery endorsed laparoscopic sleeve gastrectomy as a potential first-stage procedure for high-risk morbidly obese patients [3]. At our institution, it is now the most commonly performed bariatric procedure.

The procedure has not been universally standardized to date. At multiple points during the procedure, various technical modifications are employed by different surgeons, including using different surgical staplers, altering the diameter of the bougie, adjusting the size or volume of the sleeve and the distance from the pylorus, or by varying the type or number of stapler cartridges used, In this chapter, we describe the procedure performed at our institution.

Physiologic Changes

The efficacy of the laparoscopic sleeve gastrectomy leading to sustained weight loss and improvement in comorbidity profile is the result of various mechanisms. First, given the reduction in stomach size and volume, there is decreased alimentary intake [4]. Second, there is a significant drop in the level of the orexigenic hormone, ghrelin, which leads to anorexia. Ghrelin production is significantly reduced following laparoscopic sleeve gastrectomy as the fundus is the principal location of ghrelin function [5]. As a result, patients feel a significant reduction in hunger sensations. Nevertheless, the mechanism of sustained weight loss is most likely multifactorial and yet to be fully elucidated at this time.

Preoperative Considerations

Laparoscopic sleeve gastrectomy may be performed on those patients who qualify for bariatric surgery (i.e., meet NIH criteria and have satisfied a multi-disciplinary evaluation by a weight loss surgery team). This operation may be offered as an "initial stage" in patients who are at high risk for other more traditional bariatric operations, such as laparoscopic Roux-en-Y gastric bypass or the biliopancreatic diversion with duodenal switch procedure. Laparoscopic sleeve gastrectomy is considered for the following high-risk patients:

– Any patient with a BMI > 60 kg/m^2
– Patients with severe android ("apple-shaped") body habitus
– Significant previous intestinal surgery
– Cirrhosis (esophageal/gastric varices or severe hepatic disease may preclude all types of weight loss surgery)
– Inflammatory bowel disease
– Chronic NSAID use

After significant weight loss, these patients may undergo a "second-stage" operation with conversion to either Roux-en-Y gastric bypass or biliopancreatic diversion with duodenal switch. With excellent initial weight loss results and increasing experience with the operation, sleeve gastrectomy is now considered an appropriate stand-alone procedure in average-risk patients.

Special attention in the history and physical should elicit any signs of liver disease and cirrhosis. In diabetic patients, if there is a clinical suspicion of gastroparesis, gastric emptying studies should be considered. Patients with a history of gastroesophageal reflux require preoperative upper endoscopy to diagnose esophageal erosions or hiatal hernia and also to rule out gastric lesions, ulcers, polyps, or *Helicobacter pylori* infection. Barrett's esophagitis may be considered a contraindication to performing sleeve gastrectomy.

Electronic supplementary material: Supplementary material is available in the online version of this chapter at 10.1007/978-1-4939-1637-5_14. Videos can also be accessed at http://www.springerimages.com/videos/978-1-4939-1636-8.

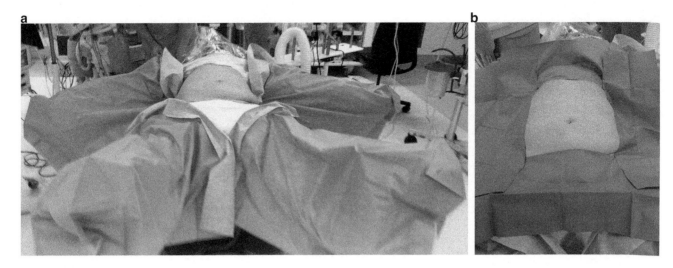

F<small>IG</small>. 1. (**a**, **b**). Patient is positioned split leg on the table as shown above with arms abducted and legs split.

Clinical Anatomy

The stomach is a well-vascularized organ that has a rich blood supply, which includes the left and right gastric arteries, the left and right gastroepiploic arteries, and the short gastric vessels. This operation involves removal of the majority of the stomach along the greater curve, leaving behind a narrow "sleeve" of stomach based along the lesser curvature with vascularization essentially derived from the left gastric artery. The vagus nerves on the lesser curve of the stomach (Latariet) remain undivided and intact.

The angle of His is given special consideration to ensure the entire left diaphragmatic crus is freed from attachments such that transection of the stomach does not leave a posterior pouch of fundus on the proximal portion of the sleeve. If a hiatal hernia is encountered, reduction (and then hiatal hernia repair) is necessary to ensure complete removal of redundant fundus.

Operative Steps

1. Anesthesia induction
   (a) The patient is positioned in reverse Trendelenburg, and a ramp is placed behind the patient's upper torso during intubation. The ramp is removed following successful intubation.
   (b) An anesthesia team experienced with the morbidly obese patient population should administer general anesthesia. These patients often have difficult airways and may require a full complement of adjunctive airway techniques, including awake fiberoptic intubation or a McGrath®- type video laryngoscope.

2. Patient positioning
   (a) The patient is positioned supine with both arms abducted and the legs split (Fig. 1). The surgeon stands between the legs with an assistant holding camera on the patient's right and an additional assistant on the patient's left.
   (b) The patient is placed in reverse Trendelenburg position throughout the entire procedure.
   (c) It is important to ensure that nothing is placed in the patient's mouth at any time, including esophageal temperature probe or nasogastric tube, unless specifically instructed by the surgeon.
   (d) A transparent part of the surgical drape over the neck and mouth is a preferred adjunct as the surgeon can then visually confirm that there is nothing in the patient's mouth.
   (e) A Foley catheter is routinely placed for this procedure.
   (f) Patients are administered perioperative antibiotics.
   (g) Surgeons also administer chemical antithrombotic prophylaxis to complement sequential pneumatic compression stockings.

3. Procedure
   (a) Pneumoperitoneum can be established via a variety of established techniques (open, visualizing trocars or Veress needle). We place trocars as shown (Fig. 1): a 15 mm trocar at the umbilicus, a 5 mm trocar in the right upper quadrant, a 5 mm trocar in the epigastrium, a 5 mm trocar in the left upper quadrant, and a 5 mm trocar in the lateral left upper quadrant. The Nathanson® liver retractor is placed via an additional 5 mm incision in the superior epigastrium. If necessary, additional 15 mm stapling trocars can be placed in the right and left upper quadrants.

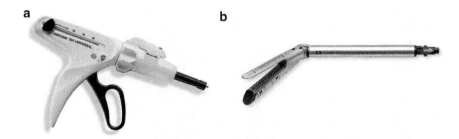

Fig. 2. (**a**, **b**). The Covidien® Endo GIA Universal Stapler is used to perform the laparoscopic sleeve gastrectomy. As shown in the lower figure, we use the Endo GIA™ Black Reload with Tri-Staple™ Technology. Used with permission of Covidien.

(b) If the stomach appears dilated (and difficult to maneuver), a nasogastric tube may be placed to evacuate the stomach. The nasogastric tube should be removed after the stomach has been emptied.

(c) The left lobe of the liver is elevated with the Nathanson® retractor, exposing pars flaccida and the vagus nerves.

(d) Using an ultrasonic scalpel, the gastrocolic omentum is divided off the greater curvature of the stomach, beginning approximately 5–6 cm proximal to the pylorus and proceeding to the angle of His at the hiatal orifice, completely mobilizing the greater curve. The entire fundus is freed posteriorly from the left crus (Fig. 2). Posterior attachments to the pancreas are also divided such that the stomach is only attached via its lesser curvature blood supply. The most efficient maneuver to achieve adequate exposure for the posterior dissection is to retract the posterior aspect of the stomach to the right with a grasper and dissect with the harmonic scalpel beneath the grasper. If present, a hiatal hernia should be reduced to ensure complete mobilization of the fundus; the hernia is then repaired (preferably by posterior apposition of the crus). A large gastric fat pad (seen especially on males) can be resected.

(e) Prior to transection of the stomach, an additional 5 mm port is placed in the midline superior to the 15 mm trocar. The camera is now placed in this position as the 15 mm port in the umbilicus will serve for introduction of the stapling device.

(f) Transection of the stomach begins on the antrum 5–6 cm proximal to the pylorus with a 60 mm long, articulating stapler using Endo GIA™ Black Reload with Tri-Staple™ Technology cartridges. The transection is oriented such that the stomach is not narrowed at the incisura (Fig. 3).

(g) After the first staple firing, a 40 F Maloney or Hurst-type bougie is placed by the anesthesia team and directed towards the pylorus along the lesser curvature. The surgeon can guide proper placement of the bougie using graspers.

(h) The remainder of the stomach transection is performed aligning the bougie against the lesser curvature to guide the resection as it proceeds towards the angle of His. Seamguard® (W.L. Gore & Associates, Inc.,

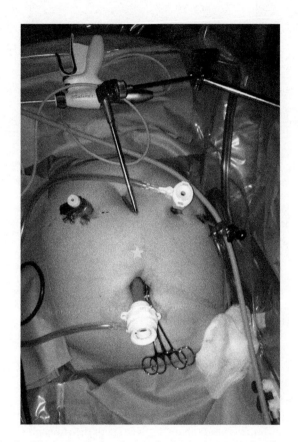

Fig. 3. The image depicts the standard port placement for a laparoscopic sleeve gastrectomy. The star demarcates where an additional 5 mm port is introduced when performing the hiatal dissection.

Flagstaff, AZ) is used for each firing after the initial of the stapling device. The Endo GIA™ Black Reload with Tri-Staple™ Technology (Covidien) cartridge can be used for the entire resection with the addition of commercially available buttress materials. Alternatively, 3.5 mm-height (blue) staples can be used in the thinner, more proximal portions of the stomach. Generally, 4–5 cartridges are necessary to complete the sleeve.

(i) The bougie is withdrawn once the sleeve is complete. A nasogastric tube is advanced into the stomach and a methylene blue leak test is performed. The pylorus is occluded using a previously fired stapling device or grasper to compress the area. If there are any areas

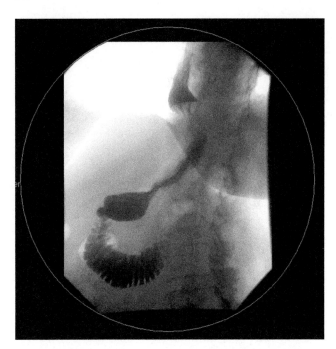

Fig. 4. The upper GI series representative image demonstrates no evidence of contrast extravasation on postoperative day 1.

of leakage, then additional absorbable sutures can be placed to reinforce the area and the leak test can be repeated.

(j) Hemostasis can be achieved along the staple line with interrupted absorbable sutures in a simple interrupted fashion or figure of eight stitches.

(k) The initial staple line without Seamguard® (W.L. Gore & Associates, Inc., Flagstaff, AZ) is oversewn with an absorbable suture to ensure adequate hemostasis.

(l) We routinely perform an omentopexy of the staple line to avoid torsion or twisting of the stomach at any point. We perform this omentopexy with 4–5 separated sutures spaced out along the entire staple line.

(m) The specimen is removed using a large Endo Catch bag via the 15 mm umbilical port and the fascia at this site is then closed. We do not routinely leave drains following a laparoscopic sleeve gastrectomy.

Postoperative Care

Patients are monitored in an appropriate setting in the post-anesthesia care unit (PACU) before transfer to the floor. All patients routinely received intravenous patient-controlled analgesia (IV PCA), and chemical antithrombotic prophylaxis is routinely administered. An upper gastrointestinal series using water-soluble contrast may be obtained on the first postoperative day to exclude leaks and evaluate gastric function and anatomy (Fig. 4). Clinical manifestations of a leak include tachycardia or dyspnea postoperatively, significant fever, oliguria, or signs of peritoneal irritation.

Patients are advanced to a bariatric clear liquid diet and progressed to pureed food on the second day. The IV PCA and Foley catheters are routinely removed on the first postoperative day. Patients are given liquid or crushed narcotic tablets dissolved in liquids. Patients are also routinely started on proton-pump inhibitors. The dietician routinely sees all patients postoperatively and reinforces dietetic modifications. Patients are usually discharged home on the second postoperative day. Solid foods are avoided for at a minimum 2 weeks postoperatively, and during that time period, patients are maintained on a pureed diet (including liquid protein supplements).

Pearls and Pitfalls

Identification of a hiatal hernia is crucial to the procedure. Complete mobilization of the fundus should be performed prior to transection to avoid missing a hiatal hernia. We always dissect the phrenoesophageal membrane and inspect the great curve of the stomach for the presence of a hiatal hernia. If identified, the dissection should proceed posteriorly to achieve appropriate approximation and closure of the crura to repair the hernia (Table 1).

Care must be taken when stapling the antrum as this tissue may be relatively thick which can cause stapler misfire or tissue fracturing. If staple line reinforcement products (buttress) are used, it may be prudent to forego them in the antral area.

When the stomach resection begins, it is extremely important to have the anesthesiologist hold the bougie in place throughout the procedure. Failure to do so may result in inadvertently pushing the bougie in a cephalic direction and unintended transection of the bougie or the stomach.

The final staple firing should veer slightly away from the gastroesophageal junction so that the esophagus is avoided. The thinner esophageal wall and absence of serosa make it vulnerable to inadequate stapler closure, which may contribute to the development of a leak.

Carefully inspect the entire gastric staple line upon completion to ensure all staples are well formed and oversew portions as necessary, especially at the junction of stapler firings.

Patients may experience significant reflux, nausea, and dysphagia, which can usually be managed with appropriate medications (ondansetron, metoclopramide, hyoscyamine sulfate) postoperatively.

Complications

The most common complications following a laparoscopic sleeve gastrectomy include leaks, strictures, bleeding, and gastroesophageal reflux disease. In most cases these complications can be successfully treated without revisional bariatric surgery, although in extreme cases additional surgical intervention is required.

TABLE 1. Advantages and disadvantages over other bariatric procedures

Advantages	Disadvantages
Maintains gastrointestinal continuity	Long staple line at risk for leak
Avoidance of implantable material	Long staple line at risk for bleeding
Avoidance of malabsorption	Typically less weight loss than bypass procedures
Convertibility to other procedures	

Based on a recent systematic review, the leak rate is anywhere between 2 and 3 % [6]. In the same review, staple line reinforcement did not affect the incidence of leaks. Leaks are usually diagnosed on upper gastrointestinal series. Postoperative patients with no abnormalities on upper gastrointestinal series, but with tachycardia and fever, require immediate operative intervention for exploration. Leaks can be classified based on timing of presentation [7]. Early leaks occur within the first 1–6 weeks. Late leaks occur after 6 weeks while chronic leaks occur after 12 weeks. Most early leaks can be adequately treated with a stent in stable patients. Leaks that fail to close following exclusion with a stent after 30 days have a very low likelihood of sealing. Unstable patients with contained or uncontained leaks require immediate operative intervention. Stenting is less likely to be successful in chronic leaks; typically these patients need operative re-intervention as often these leaks are exacerbated by a high intraluminal pressure created by a relative stenosis at the incisura. Options include bringing a Roux limb up to the leak site or conversion of the sleeve gastrectomy to a Roux-en-Y gastric bypass.

Strictures are another complication that can occur following laparoscopic sleeve gastrectomy. The incisura angularis is the site at greatest risk for stricture formation. Strictures occurring within the first 6 weeks following surgery tend to be symptomatic. The initial treatment of a stricture is simple observation if patients are minimally symptomatic. The next step can be endoscopic dilation. If that fails after 6 weeks, a seromyotomy is a surgical option [8]. The last resort is conversion of the sleeve gastrectomy to a Roux-en-Y reconstruction.

Bleeding can occur anywhere along the staple line. It is generally accepted to reinforce staple lines by oversewing the staple line or buttressing the staple line. Based on a recent review, the overall postoperative bleeding rate is between 1 and 3 % [9]. In the same review, the use of reinforcement did not significantly change the incidence of bleeding (Table 2) (Video. 1).

Acknowledgements CA: No financial disclosures and no conflicts of interest to declare.

TABLE 2. Postoperative complications

Postoperative complications
Acute leak (within 7 days)
Early leak (within 1–6 weeks)
Late leak (after 6 weeks)
Chronic leak (after 12 weeks)
Stricture
Bleeding
New-onset gastroesophageal disease

AP: Is a consultant, speaker and receives honoraria from W L Gore & Associates and also Covidien

References

1. Marceau P, Hould FS, Simard S, et al. Biliopancreatic diversion with duodenal switch. World J Surg. 1998;22:947–54.
2. Gumbs AA, Gagner M, Dakin G, Pomp A. Sleeve gastrectomy for morbid obesity. Obes Surg. 2007;17(7):962–9.
3. Clinical Issues Committee of the American Society for Metabolic and Bariatric Surgery. Updated position statement on sleeve gastrectomy as a bariatric procedure. Surg Obes Relat Dis. 2010;6(1):1–5.
4. Klok MD, Jakobsdottir S, Drent ML. The role of leptin and ghrelin in the regulation of food intake and body weight in humans: a review. Obes Rev. 2007;8:21–34.
5. Frezza EE, Chiriva-Internati M, Wachtel MS. Analysis of the results of sleeve gastrectomy for morbid obesity and the role of ghrelin. Surg Today. 2008;38:481–3.
6. Parikh M, Issa R, McCrillis A, Saunders JK, Ude-Welcome A, Gagner M. Surgical strategies that may decrease leak after laparoscopic sleeve gastrectomy: a systematic review and meta-analysis of 9991 cases. Ann Surg. 2013;257(2):231.
7. Rosenthal RJ, International Sleeve Gastrectomy Expert Panel, Diaz AA, Arvidsson D, Baker RS, Basso N, et al. International sleeve gastrectomy expert panel consensus statement: best practice guidelines based on experience of >12,000 cases. Surg Obes Relat Dis. 2012;8(1):8–19.
8. Vilallonga R, Himpens J, van de Vrande S. Laparoscopic management of persistent strictures after laparoscopic sleeve gastrectomy. Obes Surg. 2013;23(10):1655–61.
9. Knapps J, Ghanem M, Clements J, Merchant AM. A systematic review of staple-line reinforcement in laparoscopic sleeve gastrectomy. JSLS. 2013;17(3):390–9.

15

Laparoscopic Sleeve Gastrectomy: Outcomes

Stacy A. Brethauer and Esam S. Batayyah

Indications for Sleeve Gastrectomy

There are a wide variety of circumstances in which LSG (Fig. 1) has been used, and this can make outcome assessment difficult when reviewing the literature. These can be categorized according to anatomical limitations, the patient's overall risk profile, and specific medical considerations that make other bariatric procedures suboptimal. Additionally, preference for this operation among lower-risk patients and revisional patients is increasing as many surgeons and patients find this operation meeting their criteria from a risk/benefit standpoint.

Anatomical considerations include super obesity ($BMI > 60$ kg/m^2) in which there is massive hepatomegaly, a foreshortened small bowel mesentery, and bulky visceral fat and omentum. This combination of intraoperative findings results in severely limited working space or tension on the gastrojejunal anastomosis and severe torque on the laparoscopic instrumentation and may be prohibitive for proceeding with laparoscopic gastric bypass. Multiple prior abdominal surgeries, particularly prior small bowel resections, can also limit the surgeon's ability to complete a bypass procedure safely. In patients with massive abdominal wall hernias with loss of domain, it is challenging to complete a gastric bypass as they frequently have had abdominal sepsis and open abdomen in the past. The decision to proceed with LSG in these settings is often made intraoperatively based on the limitations encountered at the time of surgery.

Patients who are very high-risk surgical candidates due to advanced age, severe cardiopulmonary disease, pre- or post-organ transplant status, poor functional status, or inability to ambulate due to joint paint or a very high body mass index are potential candidates for LSG [1]. Depending on the initial BMI, some of these patients will require a second-stage operation (gastric bypass or duodenal switch) after their weight loss from the LSG plateaus.

There are also specific medical circumstances in which LSG has been used, even if the patient is not at particularly high risk for general anesthesia. These include patients with Crohn's disease, the need for chronic antiinflammatory medication use, or the need for reliable absorption of specific medication such as immunosuppressants after organ transplantation. Unlike laparoscopic Roux-en-Y gastric bypass (LRYGB), LSG allows continued endoscopic access to the common bile duct for patients with biliary disease or liver transplants.

LSG as a revisional procedure has also been reported and is discussed in Chap. 17. This is mostly described after failed laparoscopic adjustable gastric bands (LAGB), particularly if there have been a complication (e.g., esophageal dilation, chronic prolapse, or paraesophageal hernia) related to the band. Most of the reported studies include small numbers of patients with limited follow-up. Converting an uncomplicated LAGB to LSG for failed weight loss has been reported [2–4], but the best revision procedure after failed restrictive procedure is still debated. Foletto et al. [5] performed 41 band removals and simultaneous LSG, and 16 patients had interval LSG after the band was removed. The mean preoperative body mass index (BMI) was 45.7 ± 10.8 kg/m^2 and decreased to 39 ± 8.5 kg/m^2 with a mean excess BMI loss of $41.6 \% \pm 24.4 \%$ after 2 years. The postoperative complications included perigastric hematoma ($n=3$, 5.7 %), staple-line leakage ($n=3$, 5.7 %), mid-gastric stenosis ($n=1$), and death due to septic shock ($n=1$). Two patients required DS for insufficient weight loss after LSG.

The American Society for Metabolic and Bariatric Surgery's (ASMBS) 2011 updated position statement on LSG [6] recognizes this operation as a primary bariatric procedure and as a first-stage procedure in high-risk patients as part of a planned staged approach.

The ASMBS also recognizes that as with any bariatric procedure, long-term weight regain can occur and can be managed effectively with re-intervention. Reoperations for failed weight loss after LSG are necessary in 6.8 % (range, 0.7–25 %) of cases with patients receiving LSG as a stand-alone procedure and in 9.6–28.5 % of cases with

Fig. 1. (a, b). Vertical sleeve
gastrectomy. Reprinted with the
permission of the Cleveland
Clinic Center for Medical Art
and Photography.

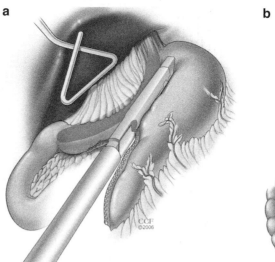
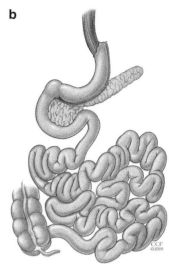

Fig. 1. (a, b). Vertical sleeve gastrectomy. Reprinted with the permission of the Cleveland Clinic Center for Medical Art and Photography.

patients undergoing LSG as a planned first-stage procedure [7], but the updated statement does not address LSG as a revisional procedure.

Outcomes Compared to Other Bariatric Procedures

Several studies have provided direct comparisons to widely accepted procedures such as LAGB and LRYGB (Table 1). Kehagias [8] randomized 60 patients with body mass index <50 (kg/m^2) to LRYGB and LSG with 3 years follow-up. The results revealed a significantly better weight loss after sleeve in the first year. At 3 years, percent excess weight loss (% EWL) was 62 % after LRYGB and 68 % after LSG ($P=0.13$), and both procedures were equally effective in the amelioration of comorbidities. Karamanakos et al. [9] performed a double-blind study comparing LSG and LRYGB that demonstrated better weight loss at 6 months (55.5 %±7.6 % vs. 50.2 %±6.5 %, $p=0.04$) and at 12 months (69.7 %±14.6 % vs. 60.5 %±10.7 %, $p=0.05$) in the LSG group. A randomized controlled trial by Himpens and colleagues [10] compared LAGB and LSG and found significantly better weight loss at 3 years after LSG (48 % vs. 66 % EWL, respectively).

Carlin et al. [11] reported data from the Michigan Bariatric Surgery Collaborative regarding the risks and benefits of LSG compared to LAGB and LRYGB. The study included 2,949 LSG patients and compared outcomes to 2,949 LAGB and 2,949 LRYGB patients who were matched for 23 baseline characteristics. Excess weight loss, complications, comorbidity remission, and QOL were assessed at 30 days, 1, 2, and 3 years postoperatively. The complication rates,

weight loss, and comorbidity improvement for LSG were intermediate between LAGB and LRYGB in this large study (Figs. 2 and 3).

Durability

A comprehensive literature review of LSG shows a mean % EWL after LSG ranging from 47 to 83 % at 2 years and 66 % at 3 years. The reported overall mean % EWL after LSG was 55 % with average follow-up less than 3 years [6] and % EWL ranging from 48 to 69 % with follow-up more than 5 years (Table 2). Most of the earlier reports using LSG included high-risk patients with a planned second-stage gastric bypass or duodenal switch. Some of these patients had sufficient weight loss and those with reduction in comorbidities with the sleeve alone did not undergo the second-stage operation for personal or insurance reasons. Eid et al. [12] reported outcomes for 74 patients who did not undergo their planned second-stage operation. Long-term follow-up data was available for 69 patients (93 % follow-up). Mean patient age at the time of surgery was 50 years and the mean preoperative BMI was 66±7 kg/m^2 (range, 43–90). Most patients had significant comorbid conditions a mean of nine (range, 2–17) per patient. The high-risk status of this patient population was demonstrated by the fact that 54 % were classified as ASA IV by the American Society of Anesthesiology, and the remaining 46 % were classified as ASA III status before surgery. The mean length of follow-up was 73 months (range, 38–95 months). Mean % EWL at 38–60 months, 61–72 months, 73–84 months, and 85–95 months was 51 %, 52 %, 43 %, and 46 %, respectively, with an overall % EWL of 48 % for the entire group. These patients provide evidence

TABLE 1. Randomized trials evaluating sleeve gastrectomy to other bariatric procedures

Author	Procedure (n)	Mean preop BMI	Follow-up	Weight loss	Conclusion
Woelnerhanssen et al. [11]	LSG (11) LRYGB (12)	LSG 45 LRYGB 47	12 months	LSG 28 % TBW LRYGB 35 % TBW	No differences in weight loss, insulin sensitivity, or effects on adipokines (adiponectin, leptin)
Kehagias et al. [8]	LSG (30) LRYGB (30)	LSG 46 LRYGB 45	36 months	LSG 68 % EWL LRYGB 62 % EWL	No differences in weight loss. LSG and LRYGB are equally safe and effective in the amelioration of comorbidities. LSG is associated with fewer postoperative metabolic deficiencies
Lee et al. [13]	LSG (30) Mini-GB (30)	LSG 30 LRYGB 30	12 months	LSG 76 % EWL Mini-GB 94 % EWL*	GB patients more likely to achieve remission of T2DM (HbA1c <6.5 %, 93 % vs. 47 %, p=0.02)
Karamanakos et al. [9]	LSG (16) LRYGB (16)	LSG 45 LRYGB 46	12 months	LSG 69 % EWL LRYGB 60 % EWL**	Greater weight loss with SG at 1 year PYY levels increased similarly after either procedure Greater ghrelin reduction and appetite suppression after SG compared with LRYGB
Himpens et al. [10]	LSG (40) LAGB (40)	LSG 39 LAGB 37	36 months	LSG 66 % EWL LAGB 48 % EWL**	Weight loss and loss of feeling of hunger after 1 year and 3 years are better after SG than LAGB. GERD is more frequent at 1 year after SG and at 3 years after GB
Peterli et al. [29]	LSG (14) LRYGB (13)	LSG 46 LRYGB 47	3 months	LSG 39 % EBMIL LRYGB 43 % EBMIL*	Both procedures markedly improved glucose homeostasis; insulin, GLP-1, and PYY levels increased similarly after either procedure

From the updated statement of the ASMBS

*P=not significant, **P<0.05

BMI body mass index, *LSG* laparoscopic sleeve gastrectomy, *LRYGB* laparoscopic Roux-en-Y gastric bypass, *LAGB* laparoscopic adjustable gastric band, *EWL* excess weight loss, *EBMIL* excess body mass index loss, *Mini-GB* Mini-gastric bypass

FIG. 2. COMORBIDITY RESOLUTION OF LSG COMPARED TO LAGB AND LRYGB (FROM CARLIN ET AL. ANN SURG MAY 2013 WITH PERMISSION).

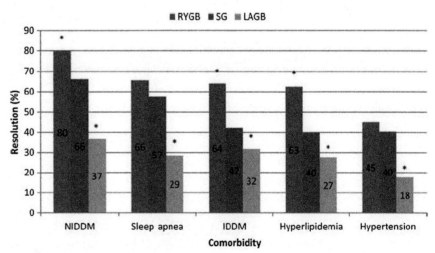

regarding the effectiveness and durability of LSG for severe obesity, even in high-risk patients.

Sarela et al. [13] reported 8–9-year follow-up data for LSG as a definitive bariatric procedure for 13 out of 20 patients. Of the remainder, 4 patients underwent revision surgery and 3 were lost to follow-up after 2 years. The small number of patients in that series did not permit statistically meaningful comparison at additional intervals. For the entire cohort, the median % EWL was 68 % (range, 18–85 %) at 8 or 9 years.

D'Hondt et al. [14] had 83 patients (81.4 %) who were eligible for long-term follow-up evaluation. Their mean

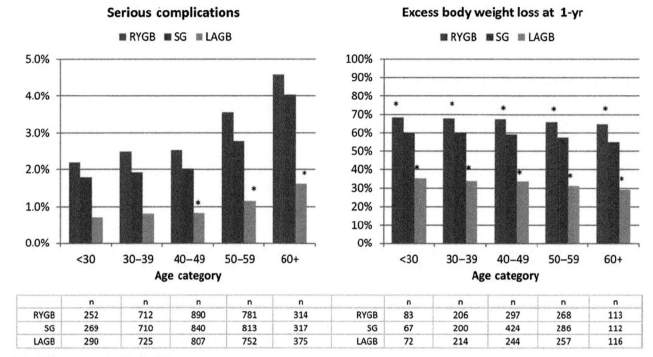

Fig. 3. Complications and weight loss of LSG compared to LAGB and LRYGB (from Carlin et al. Ann surg may 2013 with permission).

Table 2. Sleeve gastrectomy durability

Author	Patient (n)	Preoperative BMI (kg/m²)	Follow-up duration (years)	% EWL (%)
Himpens et al. [10]	41	39	6	53
Bohdjalian et al. [31]	26	48	5	55
Sarela et al. [13]	20	46	8–9	69
D'Hondt et al. [14]	23	39	6	56
Eid et al. [12]	69	66	6–8	48

Adapted from the updated ASMBS position statement on sleeve gastrectomy [3] with modification

initial body mass index (BMI) was 39.3 kg/m². No major complications occurred. At a median follow-up point of 49 months (range, 17–80 months), the mean % EWL was 72.3 %±29.3 %. For the 23 patients who reached the 6-year follow-up point, the mean % EWL was 55.9 %±25.55 %. The overall success rate (% EWL > 50 %) was 85.7 % after 4 years, 64.3 % after 5 years, and 54.5 % after 6 years. The % EWL reported by the surgeons in a survey at the Third International Summit for LSG 4 and 5 years was 57.3 % and 60.0 %, respectively [15].

Comorbidity Reduction

Diabetes is currently a major public health problem in both developed and developing countries. Like obesity, type 2 diabetes mellitus (T2DM) is a chronic disease, with increasing prevalence. T2DM is challenging to control with current therapies that include diets, drug therapy, and behavioral modification, especially in obese patients. Bariatric surgery has become a powerful tool in the management of these closely related disease processes.

Schauer et al. [16] published a randomized controlled, single-center trial, evaluating the efficacy of intensive medical therapy (IMT) alone versus medical therapy plus LRYGB versus IMT plus LSG in 150 patients with a BMI of 27–43 and an uncontrolled type 2 diabetes. Ninety-one percent of patients completed 36 months of follow-up. The proportion of patients achieving the primary end point (glycated hemoglobin level of 6.0 % or less at 36 months) was 5 % in the medical-therapy group versus 38 % in the gastric-bypass group (P < 0.001) and 24 % in the sleeve-gastrectomy group (P = 0.01). The use of glucose-lowering medications, including insulin, was lower in the surgical groups than in the medical group. Patients in the surgical groups had greater total weight loss, with reductions of 24.5 ± 9.1 % in the gastric-bypass group and 21.1 ± 8.9 % in the sleeve-gastrectomy group, as compared with a reduction of 4.2 ± 8.3 % in the medical-therapy group (P < 0.001 for both comparisons).

Lee et al. [17] evaluated in RCT the effects of mini-gastric bypass versus LSG for type 2 diabetes mellitus on lower BMI patients (mean BMI, 31.0 ± 2.9 kg/m²) with diabetes. Of the 60 patients enrolled, all completed the 12-month follow-up. Remission of T2DM was achieved by 28 (93 %) in the gastric-bypass group and 14 (47 %) in the sleeve-gastrectomy group ($P=0.02$). In this study, preoperative C-peptide levels directly correlated with remission of diabetes.

Vidal et al. [18] performed a 12-month prospective study including 39 LSG patients and 52 LRYGB patients who matched for duration and severity of T2DM. Diabetes remission was 84.6 % for both the LSG and the LRYGB patients, and there were comparable remission rates of metabolic syndrome (62 % and 67 %, respectively (NS)) 1 year after surgery. Neither weight loss nor decrease in waist circumference was associated with T2DM remission after LSG or LRYGB.

Shorter duration of T2DM and lower presurgical fasting plasma glucose or HbA1c were associated with T2DM remission. Rosenthal et al. [19] performed a retrospective review of 30 diabetic patients whom had undergone LSG. Diabetes remission at 6 months was 63 %. Patients with diabetes <5 years were found to have an 87.5 % chance of DM resolution, while those >5 years only had 35.7 % remission ($P=0.004$).

Kehagias'[9] randomized trial showed an overall prevalence of obesity-related comorbidities of 72 % (43 out of 60 patients). In the LRYGB group, 23 of the 30 patients had at least one comorbidity compared to 20 of the 30 patients who were randomized to LSG. At 3 years postoperatively, a significant improvement or resolution of comorbidities was recorded. Dyslipidemia improved at a higher rate after LRYGB and hypertension resolved at a higher rate following LSG. The rest of the studied comorbidities resolved or improved equally between groups. Sarkhosh [20] did a systematic review evaluating the impact of sleeve gastrectomy on hypertension, and LSG resulted in resolution of hypertension in 58 % of patients. On average, 75 % of patients experienced resolution or improvement of their hypertension.

A systematic review by Chiu [21] studied the effect of LSG on gastroesophageal reflux disease (GERD) and included 15 studies. Two reports analyzed GERD as a primary outcome, and 13 included GERD as a secondary study outcome. Of the 15 studies, 4 showed an increase in GERD after SG, 7 found reduced GERD prevalence after LSG, 3 included only the postoperative prevalence of GERD, and 1 did not include data on prevalence of GERD. The evidence of the effect of SG on GERD did not consolidate to a consensus.

A previous systematic review of the sleeve gastrectomy in literature revealed >60 % rates of remission or improvement in many other obesity-related comorbidities including gastroesophageal reflux, degenerative joint pain, sleep apnea, leg edema, hypertension, and hyperlipidemia [22].

Complications

One of the potential advantages of LSG is a lower complication rate compared to duodenal switch and RYGB. The effective use of LSG as a first-stage procedure in high-risk patients has provided evidence for its safety and utility in this patient population [1]. Several recent publications have evaluated the safety profile of sleeve gastrectomy in high-risk patients as well as in average-risk bariatric patients.

Although most of the data available suggest that morbidity related to LSG is lower than in LRYGB, results vary according to different studies. Results confirm that morbidity is significantly lower in patients undergoing LSG, in a nonrandomized, retrospective comparison of patients who underwent LSG ($n=216$), LAGB ($n=271$), LRYGB ($n=303$), and DS ($n=56$). Lee [23] and colleagues reported the major complication rates for these procedures as 4.6 %, 4.8 %, 10.6 %, and 39.3 % respectively ($P<0.03$). The reoperation rate for LSG was the lowest of the four procedures (2.8 %). Reoperation rates for the other procedures increased with the complexity of the operation (LAGB (4.8 %), LRYGB (8.6 %), and DS (32.1 %)). One potential weakness of this nonrandomized study is that patient selection bias may have affected the results for the different procedures.

Brethauer et al. [22] who performed a systematic review of sleeve gastrectomy outcomes reported that the complication rate among the 36 studies (2,570 patients) ranged from 0 to 23.8 %. Studies with >100 patients reported a major postoperative complication rate from 0 to 14 %. The overall 30-day mortality rate was 0.19 %. The overall rate of major complication rates were low including leaks (2.2 %), bleeding requiring reoperation or transfusion (1.2 %), and strictures requiring endoscopic or surgical intervention (0.6 %). The analysis of weight loss and complications varied depending on the patient group studied. The differences between complication rates for patient undergoing sleeve gastrectomy as a risk-reduction strategy and those undergoing LSG as a primary procedure are highlighted in Table 3.

Gastric leak and hemorrhage are the most important challenges after LSG . The long staple line of the LSG in conjunction with an increased intraluminal pressure offers a possible explanation. Shi's [24] systematic review reported the rate of major complications after LSG, such as staple-line leakage and internal bleeding (1.17 %±1.86 %, 3.57 %±5.15 %, respectively). Leaks were more common in the proximal staple line close to the gastroesophageal junction (1.6 % of cases) than at the distal staple line 0.5 % [6]. Intraluminal bleeding occurred in 2.0 % of cases and the mortality rate was 1 %.

Parikh et al. [25] analyzed the effect of various surgical techniques for LSG on the leak rate by systematically reviewing the literature and conducting a meta-analysis focusing on the relationship between leak rate and bougie size, and distance from the pylorus, and the use of buttressing material on the staple line. Hundred and ninety-eight leaks in 8,922 patients (2.2 %) were identified. The general estimating equation (GEE) model was used to calculate the odds ratio (OR) for leak and revealed that the risk of leak decreased with bougie ≥ 40 Fr (OR =0.53, 95 % CI=[0.37–0.77]; $P=0.0009$). Buttressing did not influence leak. There was no difference in % EWL between bougie <40 Fr and bougie≥ 40 Fr up to 36 months (mean % EWL 70.1; $P=0.273$), and distance from the pylorus did not affect leak or % EWL.

TABLE 3. Outcomes of sleeve gastrectomy in high-risk/staged patients versus primary procedure

	High-risk patients/staged approach	Primary procedure	All patients
Number of studies[a] (number of patients)	13 (821)	24 (1,749)	36 (2,570)
Preoperative BMI range (mean) kg/m^2	49.1–69.0 (60.0)	37.2–54.5 (46.6)	37.2–69.0 (51.2)
Postoperative BMI range (mean) kg/m^2	36.4–53.0 (44.9)	26.0–39.8 (32.2)	26.0–53.0 (37.1)
Follow-up	4 months–5 years	3 months–3 years	3 months–5 years
% Excess weight loss range (mean)	33.0–61.4 % (46.6 %)	36.0–85.0 % (60.7 %)	33.0–85.0 % (55.4 %)
Complication rate	0–23.8 % (9.4 %)	0–21.7 % (6.2 %)	0–23.8 %
All studies (mean)			
Studies with $n>100$	3.3–15.3 %	0–14.1 %	0–14.1 %
Leaks	8/686 (1.2 %)	45/1,681 (2.7 %) [+]	53/2,367 (2.2 %)
Bleeding	11/686 (1.6 %)	17/1,681 (1.0 %)	28/2,367 (1.2 %)
Strictures	6/686 (0.9 %)	9/1,681 (0.5 %)	15/2,367 (0.6 %)
Mortality	2/821 (0.24 %)	3/1,749 (0.17 %)	5/2,570 (0.19 %)

Adapted from Brethauer et al. [22]

[a]One study had clearly defined patients in both groups; $+ p=0.02$ compared to high risk group

Dapri [26] and Albanopoulos [27] compared techniques of reinforcing the staple line in LSG with suturing versus buttressing or neither. There was no significant difference in leak rates between groups. However, buttressing statistically reduced blood loss during stomach sectioning as well as overall blood loss.

Management of LSG leak patients mainly depend on their clinical condition and this is discussed in Chap. 16. Patients presenting with hemodynamic instability and uncontrolled sepsis require immediate operative management. Stable patients can be managed with percutaneous drainage, endoscopic therapy including stenting, and nutritional support. The type and duration of therapy must be individualized to allow closure of fistulas and to avoid recurrent episodes of sepsis or leak.

Mechanisms of Action

The evidence suggests that LSG effects gut hormone secretion and satiety pathways in addition to creating gastric restriction. One of the first gut hormones evaluated with LSG was ghrelin. Since ghrelin is primarily produced in the fundus of the stomach (completely resected during LSG), it is logical that ghrelin would decrease after LSG. Karamanakos et al. [9] showed that LSG suppressed fasting and postprandial ghrelin levels and attributed this decrease in ghrelin to improved postoperative satiety and greater weight loss at 1 year compared to LRYGB. The LRYGB group in this study had an initial decrease in ghrelin levels after surgery, but these levels returned to normal levels within 3 months.

Lee et al. [28] studied the treatment of patients with a low body mass index and type 2 diabetes mellitus between the two groups. LRYGB is reportedly more effective than LSG; they conclude that both procedures have strong hindgut effects after surgery, but LRYGB has a significant duodenal exclusion effect on cholecystokinin. The LSG group had lower acylated ghrelin and des-acylated ghrelin levels but greater concentrations of resistin than the LRYGB group.

In addition to evaluations of ghrelin, there are now several small studies demonstrating that gastric emptying is increased after sleeve gastrectomy. The loss of a large reservoir in the gastric fundus and body and preservation of the antral pump provide a reasonable explanation for this finding. A secondary effect of earlier distal bowel stimulation with nutrients after meals due to increased gastric emptying time may be similar to the effects seen after gastric bypass. Several mechanistic studies have demonstrated early and exaggerated postprandial peak levels of Peptide YY$_{3-36}$ and GLP-1 after LSG. GLP-1 is an incretin that stimulates insulin production and releases from pancreatic islet cells, and the increased PYY$_{3-36}$ results in satiety and reduced food intake. Karamanakos et al. [9] have independently shown that the sleeve gastrectomy does have the effect of increasing the transit time of chyme despite an intact pylorus as measured by increased postprandial PYY levels.

Peterli et al. [29] performed a randomized prospective trial with 13 LRYGB and 14 LSG patients to investigate the potential mechanism of LSG focusing on foregut and hindgut mechanisms. They found marked improvement in glucose homeostasis 1 week after surgery in both groups. This improvement was associated with early, exaggerated increases in GLP-1 secretion at 1 week, 3 months, and 1 year postoperatively in both groups. In addition to changes in GLP-1, PYY$_{3-36}$ increased significantly and ghrelin was suppressed in both groups. It is unclear whether PYY$_{3-36}$ has a direct effect on glucose homeostasis or if its effects are exhibited via appetite reduction and concomitant weight loss. Preoperatively, some patients had a blunted PYY$_{3-36}$ and GLP-1 response suggesting some "resistance" to these gut hormones in obese patients. These findings suggest that the LSG should not be viewed merely as a restrictive procedure but also as a procedure that has neurohormonal and incretin effects.

Ramon et al. [30] compared the effects of LRYGB and LSG on glucose metabolism and levels of gastrointestinal hormones such as ghrelin, leptin, GLP-1, peptide YY (PYY), and pancreatic polypeptide (PP) in morbid obese patients. This prospective, randomized study confirmed that the postprandial response of ghrelin, GLP-1, and PYY was maintained in patients undergoing LSG for 12 months after surgery and was similar to the LRYGB group results.

Adipokines are cytokines produced by adipose cell and closely linked to obesity and insulin resistance. To date, it is unclear whether the different anatomical changes of the various bariatric procedures have different effects on hormones of adipocyte origin. A prospective, randomized study by Woelnerhanssen et al. [11] compared the 1-year results of LRYGB and LSG for weight loss, metabolic control, and fasting adipokine levels. The authors confirmed a close association of specific adipokines with obesity and with the changes observed with weight loss after two different bariatric surgical procedures. The concentrations of circulating leptin levels decreased by almost 50 % as early as 1 week postoperatively and continued to decrease until 12 months postoperatively and adiponectin increased progressively. No differences were found between the LRYGB and LSG groups regarding adipokine changes.

Conclusion

The current evidence regarding sleeve gastrectomy demonstrates that it can be used safely as a primary procedure or as part of a staged approach for high-risk bariatric patients. Published early postoperative complication rates are acceptably low, and there are few long-term complications or reoperations reported after this procedure. Early and medium-term weight loss is better than laparoscopic adjustable gastric banding and is comparable to or slightly less than gastric bypass in most studies. There are growing numbers of long-term studies supporting the durability of LSG, but some patients will have weight regain that can be managed with a bypass procedure. Mechanistic studies suggest some neurohumoral effects of sleeve gastrectomy that may contribute to rapid weight loss and improved glucose metabolism.

References

1. Cottam D, Qureshi FG, Mattar SG, et al. Laparoscopic sleeve gastrectomy as an initial weight-loss procedure for high-risk patients with morbid obesity. Surg Endosc. 2006;20(6):859–63.
2. Acholonu E, McBean E, Court I, Bellorin O, Szomstein S, Rosenthal RJ. Safety and short-term outcomes of laparoscopic sleeve gastrectomy as a revisional approach for failed laparoscopic adjustable gastric banding in the treatment of morbid obesity. Obes Surg. 2009;19(12):1612–6. doi:10.1007/s11695-009-9941-4. PMID: 19711138.
3. Dapri G, Cadière GB, Himpens J. Feasibility and technique of laparoscopic conversion of adjustable gastric banding to sleeve gastrectomy. Surg Obes Relat Dis. 2009;5(1):72–6. doi:10.1016/j.soard.2008.11.008. Epub 2008 Nov 27. PMID: 19161936.
4. Iannelli A, Schneck AS, Ragot E, Liagre A, Anduze Y, Msika S, Gugenheim J. Laparoscopic sleeve gastrectomy as revisional procedure for failed gastric banding and vertical banded gastroplasty. Obes Surg. 2009;19(9):1216–20. doi:10.1007/s11695-009-9903-x. Epub 2009 Jun 27. PMID: 19562420.
5. Foletto M, Prevedello L, Bernante P, Luca B, Vettor R, Francini-Pesenti F, Scarda A, Brocadello F, Motter M, Famengo S, Nitti D. Sleeve gastrectomy as revisional procedure for failed gastric banding or gastroplasty. Surg Obes Relat Dis. 2010;6(2):146–51. doi:10.1016/j.soard.2009.09.003. Epub 2009 Sep 15.
6. ASMBS. Updated Position Statement on Sleeve Gastrectomy as a Bariatric Procedure. Revised 10/28/2011. http://asmbs.org/2011/12/sleeve-gastrectomy-as-a-bariatric-procedur/
7. Fischer L, Hildebrandt C, Bruckner T, Kenngott H, Linke GR, Gehrig T, Büchler MW, Müller-Stich BP. Excessive weight loss after sleeve gastrectomy: a systematic review. Obes Surg. 2012;22(5):721–31. doi:10.1007/s11695-012-0616-1.
8. Kehagias I, Karamanakos SN, Argentou M, Kalfarentzos F. Randomized clinical trial of laparoscopic Roux-en-Y gastric bypass versus laparoscopic sleeve gastrectomy for the management of patients with BMI < 50 kg/m2. Obes Surg. 2011;21(11):1650–6.
9. Karamanakos SN, Vagenas K, Kalfarentzos F, Alexandrides TK. Weight loss, appetite suppression, and changes in fasting and postprandial ghrelin and peptide-YY levels after Roux-en-Y gastric bypass and sleeve gastrectomy: a prospective, double blind study. Ann Surg. 2008;247(3):401–7.
10. Himpens J, Dapri G, Cadière GB. A prospective randomized study between laparoscopic gastric banding and laparoscopic isolated sleeve gastrectomy: results after 1 and 3 years. Obes Surg. 2006;16(11):1450–6.
11. Carlin AM, Zeni TM, English WJ. The comparative effectiveness of sleeve gastrectomy, gastric bypass, and adjustable gastric banding procedures for the treatment of morbid obesity. Ann Surg. 2013;257(5):791–7.
12. Eid GM, Brethauer S, Mattar SG, Titchner RL, Gourash W, Schauer PR. Laparoscopic sleeve gastrectomy for super obese patients: forty-eight percent excess weight loss after 6 to 8 years with 93 % follow-up. Ann Surg. 2012;256(2):262–5.
13. Sarela AI, Dexter SP, O'Kane M, Menon A, McMahon MJ. Long-term follow-up after laparoscopic sleeve gastrectomy: 8–9-year results. Surg Obes Relat Dis. 2012;8(6):679–84. doi:10.1016/j.soard.2011.06.020.
14. D'Hondt M, Vanneste S, Pottel H, Devriendt D, Van Rooy F, Vansteenkiste F. Laparoscopic sleeve gastrectomy as a single-stage procedure for the treatment of morbid obesity and the resulting quality of life, resolution of comorbidities, food tolerance, and 6-year weight loss. Surg Endosc. 2011;25(8):2498–504.
15. Deitel M, Gagner M, Erickson AL, Crosby RD. Third International Summit: Current status of sleeve gastrectomy. Surg Obes Relat Dis. 2011;7(6):749–59. doi:10.1016/j.soard.2011.07.017. Epub 2011 Aug 10.
16. Schauer PR, Bhatt DL, Kirwan JP, et al. Bariatric surgery versus intensive medical therapy for diabetes-3-year outcomes. N Engl J Med. 2014;370(21):2002–13.
17. Lee WJ, Chong K, Ser KH, Lee YC, Chen SC, Chen JC, Tsai MH. Chuang LM Gastric bypass vs sleeve gastrectomy for type 2 diabetes mellitus: a randomized controlled trial. Arch Surg. 2011;146(2):143–8. doi:10.1001/archsurg.2010.326.
18. Vidal J, Ibarzabal A, Romero F, et al. Type 2 diabetes mellitus and the metabolic syndrome following sleeve gastrectomy in severely obese subjects. Obes Surg. 2008;18(9):1077–82.

19. Rosenthal R, Li X, Samuel S, et al. Effect of sleeve gastrectomy on patients with diabetes mellitus. Surg Obes Relat Dis. 2009;5(4):429–34.

20. Sarkhosh K, Birch DW, Shi X, Gill RS, Karmali S. The impact of sleeve gastrectomy on hypertension: a systematic review. Obes Surg. 2012;22(5):832–7. doi:10.1007/s11695-012-0615-2.

21. Chiu S, Birch DW, Shi X, Sharma AM, Karmali S. Effect of sleeve gastrectomy on gastroesophageal reflux disease: a systematic review. Surg Obes Relat Dis. 2011;7(4):510–5.

22. Brethauer SA, Hammel JP, Schauer PR. Systematic review of sleeve gastrectomy as staging and primary bariatric procedure. Surg Obes Relat Dis. 2009;5(4):469–75.

23. Lee CM, Cirangle PT, Jossart GH. Vertical gastrectomy for morbid obesity in 216 patients: report of two-year results. Surg Endosc. 2007;21(10):1810–6.

24. Shi X, Karmali S, Sharma AM, Birch DW. A review of laparoscopic sleeve gastrectomy for morbid obesity. Obes Surg. 2010;20(8):1171–7. doi:10.1007/s11695-010-0145-8. PMID: 20379795.

25. Parikh M, Issa R, McCrillis A, Saunders JK, Ude-Welcome A, Gagner M. Surgical strategies that may decrease leak after laparoscopic sleeve gastrectomy: a systematic review and meta-analysis of 9991 cases. Ann Surg. 2013;257(2):231–7. doi:10.1097/SLA.0b013e31826cc714. PMID: 23023201.

26. Dapri G, Cadière GB, Himpens J. Reinforcing the staple line during laparoscopic sleeve gastrectomy: prospective randomized clinical study comparing three different techniques. Obes Surg. 2010;20(4):462–7. doi:10.1007/s11695-009-0047-9. Epub 2009 Dec 11.

27. Albanopoulos K, Alevizos L, Flessas J, Menenakos E, Stamou KM, Papailiou J, Natoudi M, Zografos G, Leandros E. Reinforcing the staple line during laparoscopic sleeve gastrectomy: prospective randomized clinical study comparing two different techniques. Preliminary results. Obes Surg. 2012;22(1):42–6.

28. Lee WJ, Chen CY, Chong K, Lee YC, Chen SC, Lee SD. Changes in postprandial gut hormones after metabolic surgery: a comparison of gastric bypass and sleeve gastrectomy. Surg Obes Relat Dis. 2011;7(6):683–90. doi:10.1016/j.soard.2011.07.009. Epub 2011 Jul 31.

29. Peterli R, Steinert RE, Woelnerhanssen B, Peters T, Christoffel-Courtin C, Gass M, Kern B, von Fluee M, Beglinger C. Metabolic and hormonal changes after laparoscopic Roux-en-Y gastric bypass and sleeve gastrectomy: a randomized, prospective trial. Obes Surg. 2012;22(5):740–8.

30. Ramón JM, Salvans S, Crous X, Puig S, Goday A, Benaiges D, Trillo L, Pera M, Grande L. Effect of Roux-en-Y gastric bypass vs sleeve gastrectomy on glucose and gut hormones: a prospective randomised trial. J Gastrointest Surg. 2012;16(6):1116–22.

31. Bohdjalian A, Langer FB, Shakeri-Leidenmühler S, Gfrerer L, Ludvik B, Zacherl J, Prager G. Sleeve gastrectomy as sole and definitive bariatric procedure: 5-year results for weight loss and ghrelin. Obes Surg. 2010;20(5):535–40. doi:10.1007/s11695-009-0066-6. Epub 2010 Jan 22. PMID: 20094819.

16

Laparoscopic Sleeve Gastrectomy: Management of Complications

Pornthep Prathanvanich and Bipan Chand

Abbreviations

BMI	Body mass index
CT	Computerized tomography
EWL	Excess weight loss
GEJ	Gastroesophageal junction
GERD	Gastroesophageal reflux disease
LSG	Laparoscopic sleeve gastrectomy
Post-LSG GL	Postoperative laparoscopic sleeve gastrectomy gastric leak
RYGB	Roux-en-Y gastric bypass
SEMS	Self-expandable metallic stent
SG	Sleeve gastrectomy
SIRS	Systemic inflammatory response syndrome

Introduction

Laparoscopic sleeve gastrectomy (LSG) has become an important modality in the treatment of morbid obesity. The mechanisms of weight loss include caloric restriction and hormonal alterations. Reduction of ghrelin level occurs secondary to resection of the gastric fundus. LSG was originally performed as the restrictive component of the duodenal switch procedure and also as a bridge procedure to laparoscopic Roux-en-Y gastric bypass. In 1993, Almogy et al. [1, 2] performed open sleeve gastrectomy (SG) in super-obese male patients (BMI>55) who were older than 55 years. In 1999, Gagner and Patterson performed the first LSG as part of a duodenal switch procedure at Mount Sinai Hospital in New York [3]. Recently, LSG has gained more popularity as an independent bariatric procedure after reports showing

effective, safe, and timesaving procedure. It currently accounts for more than 5 % of all bariatric operations performed worldwide [4]. A recent report from the bariatric outcomes longitudinal database (BOLD) demonstrated that between June 2007 and May 2009, LSG was the third most common bariatric procedure performed in the United States [5] (Video 1).

Several important studies have been published showing the mean excess weight loss that ranges between 52 and 61 % with follow-up of at least 5 years [6]. Brethauer et al. [7] reported a systematic review of 36 studies of sleeve gastrectomy (SG) as both a staging and primary bariatric procedure. The mean preoperative BMI from the 1,749 patients undergoing SG as a primary procedure was 46.6 kg/m^2 (range, 37.2–54.5). The mean percent excess weight loss (EWL) was 60.4 % (range, 36.0–85.0 %), and the overall complication rate of all reports ranged from 0 to 21.7 % (mean, 6.2 %). Although the LSG has been shown to effect significant weight loss with a low complication rate, LSG has a specific significant morbidity pattern including gastric staple-line leak, gastric fistula, bleeding, and obstruction or stricture. The lesser common surgical adverse effects of the procedure are rise in the incidence of gastroesophageal reflux and nutrient deficiencies (Table 1).

Gastric Leak (GL)

Leaks are the most concerning and potentially life-threatening complication after LSG.

Definition of Terms and Classification of Gastric Leak

A leak is the egress of gastrointestinal contents through a suture or staple line into a cavity. Thus, luminal content can exit through the gastrointestinal wall freely into the peritoneal cavity or can collect next to an anastomosis or

Electronic supplementary material: Supplementary material is available in the online version of this chapter at 10.1007/978-1-4939-1637-5_16. Videos can also be accessed at http://www.springerimages.com/videos/978-1-4939-1636-8.

TABLE 1. Complications of laparoscopic sleeve gastrectomy

Early complications
- Gastric leak
- Gastric fistula
- Bleeding
- Obstruction/stricture

Late complications
- GERD
- Nutrient deficiencies

TABLE 2. Incidence of gastric leak after LSG

Authors	Year	Patients (n)	Proportion of gastric leaks (%)
Johnston et al.	2003	100	1
Hann et al.	2005	130	0.7
Hamoui et al.	2006	118	0.8
Cottam et al.	2006	126	2
Roa et al.	2006	62	2
Lalor et al.	2007	148	1
Nocca et al.	2007	163	6
Weiner et al.	2007	120	3
Lee et al.	2007	216	1
Serra et al.	2007	993	0.6
Mui et al.	2008	70	1
Rubin et al.	2008	120	0
Skrekas et al.	2008	93	4.3
Lalor PF et al.	2008	148	0.7
Moy et al.	2008	135	1.4
Kasalicky et al.	2008	61	0
Arias et al.	2009	130	0.7
Burgos et al.	2009	214	3.2
Casella et al.	2009	200	3
Stroh C et al.	2009	144	7
Sanchez et al.	2009	540	2
Frezza et al.	2009	53	3.7
Menenakos et al.	2009	261	4
Armstrong et al.	2010	185	0
Ser et al.	2010	118	3.39
Csendes et al.	2010	343	4.66
Dapri et al.	2010	75	5
Lacy et al.	2010	294	4
Ser et al.	2010	118	3
Srinivasa et al.	2010	253	2
Bellanger et al.	2011	529	0

suture or staple line [8]. Gastric leak has also been described in terms of:

1. Time to diagnosis

Poujoulet et al. classified these leaks based on the period in which they appear:

Early: leaks that appear between the first and third day after surgery

Intermediate: leaks that appear between the fourth and seventh day after surgery

Late: those that appear more than eight days after surgery [8]

Regimbeau et al. [9] also classified gastric leak, post-LSG as either *early onset* (postoperative day 1–7) or *delayed onset* (after postoperative day 8)

2. Site of leakage

Identification of the gastric leak site is based on anatomic thirds (upper, middle, or distal third of the remaining stomach)

3. Clinical aspect

The clinical presentation has been described in terms of systemic signs of inflammation and sepsis (tachycardia >100/min, hyperthermia >38 °C), peritonitis (diffuse abdominal tenderness), pulmonary symptoms (cough and expectoration), and intra-abdominal abscess (localized abdominal tenderness). A clear treatment algorithm should be established based on the patient's status: stable or unstable and controlled or uncontrolled leak. Patients who are manifesting signs of sepsis or instability should be managed operatively. Laparoscopy or laparotomy should include drainage and washout of the infected collection

Incidence of Postoperative Laparoscopic Sleeve Gastrectomy Gastric Leak (Post-LSG GL)

Gastric leaks represent one of the most dangerous complications of bariatric surgery. In the literature, the incidence of GL after LSG ranges from 0 to 7 % [9–11] (Table 2). Most leaks appear in the proximal third of the stomach, close to the gastroesophageal junction or near the angle of His. Burgos et al. [12] reported 85.7 % of leaks in the proximal third and only 14.3 % in the distal third. A.A. Saber et al. [11] analyzed 29 publications using a MEDLINE search and

reported on 4,888 patient records. The mean BMI ranged from 34 to 65.4 kg/m², and all 29 studies documented a leak rate, which ranged from 0 to 7 %. The mean leak rate for all 29 studies was 2.4 %, which accounted for 115 leaks in 4,888 cases of sleeve gastrectomy. There did appear to be a higher leak rate in patients with a BMI > 50 kg/m².

Six studies specifically addressed super-obese patients with a mean BMI > 50 kg/m². In the super obese, the mean leak rate was 2.9 % or 23 leaks of 771 patients compared with the leak rate of only 2.2 % (92/4,117) for those with mean BMI < 50 kg/m² (not significant $P > 0.05$).

Causes of Post-LSG GL

It is possible that these types of proximal leaks (i.e., those at the gastroesophageal junction or near the angle of His) have multiple different etiologies. One plausible theory is that the final staple line is placed across the gastroesophageal junction or distal esophagus causing poor staple-line configuration. Another more likely is the vascular theory. As Basso et al. explains [13], the cardias (distal esophagus and esophagogastric junction) are supplied in the right and anterior side by branches of the left gastric artery and left inferior phrenic artery. The posterior left side is vascularized mainly by fundic

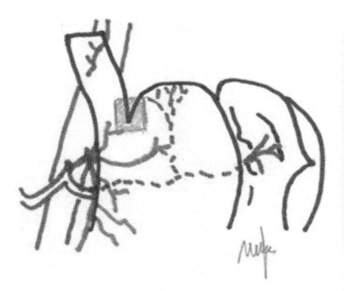

FIG. 1. Critical area of vascularization (LGA: Lt gastric artery). Reproduced with permission from *OBES SURG 2012*;22:182-187. Technical controversies in laparoscopic sleeve gastrectomy.

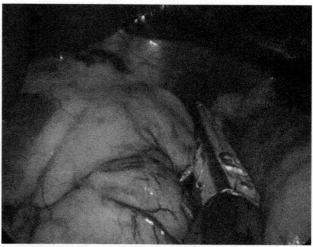

FIG. 2. Proximal staple line away from the gastroesophageal junction. Reproduced with permission from *OBES SURG 2012*;22:182-187. Technical Controversies in Laparoscopic Sleeve Gastrectomy.

branches of the splenic artery and, if present, by the posterior gastric artery. The arterial supply of the esophagus is segmental. Complete dissection of the fundus requires division of the short gastric vessels, of the posterior gastric artery, and of the phrenic branches when present. A "critical area" of vascularization may occur laterally, just at the esophagogastric junction at the angle of His (Fig. 1) (Video 2).

They describe a resection line avoiding the critical area by leaving 1–2 cm of gastric remnant just at the gastroesophageal junction to avoid the area described (Fig. 2).

Nocca et al. described particular caution at this same region in those patients who had previously undergone adjustable gastric band and were undergoing conversion to sleeve gastrectomy. The concern was due to the increased fragility of gastric tissue from the fibrosis after contact with the silicone band [14]. Bellanger et al. [15] describes two basic principles for minimizing leaks. The first and most important is to avoid creating a stenosis at the level of the angular incisures, and the second (as previously described) is to avoid resection too close to the esophagus in the area of the cardia. The mid-sleeve stenosis (at the incisura) can be from a truly stenotic lumen (Fig. 3) or, more commonly, twisting or kinking of the sleeve at the incisura that causes a functional obstruction (Figs. 4 and 5). This relative downstream obstruction in the setting of a proximal leak can lead to a persistent fistula that does not resolve with conservative management. Yehoshua et al. [16] showed that high intraluminal pressure and low compliance of the gastric tube may be the main cause of leak and fistulas in this area.

Patient factors described in the literature, with a greater incidence of leak, include older age, BMI > 60 kg/m², malnutrition, and a history of laparoscopic gastric banding. Some authors distinguish between mechanical and ischemic causes

of post-LSG GL. Baker et al. [17] suggest that fistulas on the staple line may have multiple causes, but these can be divided into two categories: mechanical-tissular causes and ischemic causes. In both situations, intraluminal pressure exceeds tissular and suture line resistance, thus causing the fistula. Classic ischemic fistulas tend to appear between 5 and 6 days after surgery, when the wall healing process is between the inflammation phase and fibrotic phase. When the cause is mechanical tissular, fistulas are usually discovered before this period, that is, within the first 2 days after surgery.

Incomplete Staple-Line Formation [17, 18]

Staple size must be selected appropriately for the tissue on which it is to be used. This is necessary to allow for proper staple formation while in turn achieving optimal staple-line strength and tissue compression. Undersizing staple cartridge increases the risk for inadequate staple formation or can lead to excessive tissue compression. This can exceed the tissue's tensile strength, leading to tearing and perforation. Incomplete staple-line formation occurs when a blue cartridge is used on thick gastric tissue. Greater staple height loads, such as green load cartridges (Ethicon), should be used on thick stomach as they are designed to be stronger (wider diameter) and form longer leg lengths (open, 5.5 mm; closed, 2.0 mm) when compared with blue load cartridges (open, 3.85 mm; closed, 1.5 mm)

Full thickness over sewing past affixed staple line may increase the risk of tearing at the point of suture penetration in the distended gastric pouch (Fig. 6). This effect is not likely to be significant in low pressure areas.

Finally, care must be taken while firing the stapler near the angle of His. Migration of the stapler with incorporation

FIG. 3. Upper GI contrast study
showing extravasation of contrast
from the upper stomach into the
left subphrenic space (**a**).
Stenosis of the midportion of the
sleeve is present where the
barium tablet is lodged (**b**)
(*arrow*). Reprinted with
permission from Obes Surg
2012; vol 20, issue 9. Gastric
Leak After Laparoscopic Sleeve
Gastrectomy.

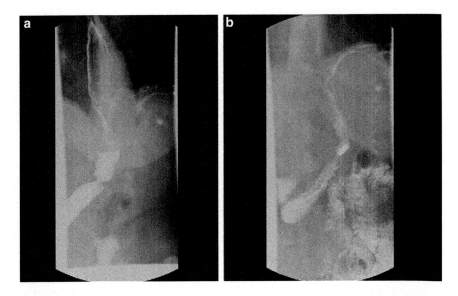

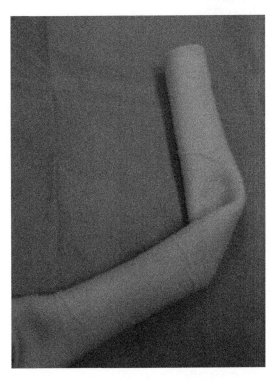

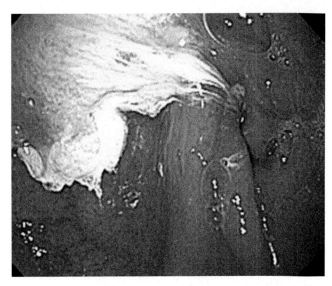

FIG. 5. Endoscopic view demonstrating the functional stenosis.
Reproduced with permission from *SURG ENDOSCOPY 2012*;
26:738-746. Management options for symptomatic stenosis after
laparoscopic vertical sleeve gastrectomy in the morbidly obese.

FIG. 4. Representation of the spiral sleeve. The functional stenosis
is caused by twisting of the sleeve. Reproduced with permission
from *SURG ENDOSCOPY 2012*;26:738–746. Management options
for symptomatic stenosis after laparoscopic vertical sleeve gastrectomy in the morbidly obese.

This formation must achieve adequate staple formation
and yet avoid tearing the tissue.

Diagnosis for Post-LSG GL

A high index of suspicion and early identification of leaks
after LSG are critical to achieving an acceptable outcome
after this complication. Unexplained tachycardia, fevers,
abdominal pain, or persistent hiccups after the procedure
should alert surgeons to investigate for a leak (Table 3).

The signs and symptoms of the patients who develop a
leak are similar to patients with other types of abdominal
infections. However the clinical presentation of gastric leak
ranges from the patient being completely asymptomatic

of the esophagus can weaken the staple line because of the
weaker nature of esophageal tissue. Bunching of fundus or a
thick fundus can also lead to leaks if inadequate staple formation or tissue shearing occurs. The ultimate goal in staple
formation is to produce mechanically sound staple lines,
which can withstand pertinent pressure forces until the tissue
response endows significant strength overtime.

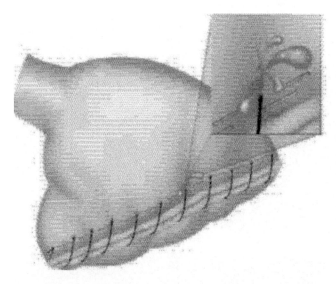

FIG. 6. Oversewing causing leaks when the pouch is distended and suture bowstrings and tissue tear.

TABLE 3. Potential signs of post-LSG GL

A high index of suspicion
1. SIRS
– Unexplained tachycardia (>100/min)
– Fever (>38 °C)
2. Abdominal pain
– Diffuse abdominal tenderness (diffuse peritonitis)
– Intra-abdominal abscess (localized peritonitis)
3. Pulmonary symptoms (subphrenic abscess or complex bronchogastric fistula)
– Cough
– Expectoration
– Persistent hiccups

(identified by fluoroscopic study) to the presentation of peritonitis, septic shock, multiorgan failure, and death. Burgos et al. report a series of 7 leaks in 214 patients (3.3 %), of which 5 patients presented abdominal pain, fever, tachycardia, tachypnea, and increased laboratory signs of infection. They observed that tachycardia is an initial sign of early leak [12]. Casella et al. reported leaks in 3 % of 200 patients. In general, the symptomatology was abdominal pain, vomiting, and fever; only one patient was asymptomatic [19]. According to Tan et al. [20] and de Aretxabala et al. [21], early-onset GL presents with severe, sudden abdominal pain (together with fever, nausea, and vomiting), whereas delayed-onset GL is usually of a more insidious nature (with gradually increasing abdominal discomfort and fever). Patients with early-onset GL show signs of sepsis caused by gastrointestinal contents in the peritoneal cavity, and they require at least a surgical lavage and the placement of drains. For patients with delayed-onset GL, fluid frequently collects near to the stomach and does not spread to the rest of the cavity. Four clinical presentations have approximately the same frequency: systemic signs of inflammation, peritonitis,

abscess, and pulmonary symptoms. Pulmonary symptoms can be caused by a subphrenic abscess (in both early- and delayed-onset GL) or complex bronchogastric fistula (delayed-onset GL). Medical and surgical teams must be aware of initial, atypical presentations or those occurring during follow-up: [1] bronchogastric fistulas (revealed by chronic cough and managed with a pulmonary lobectomy [2], acute hematemesis revealing a left gastric artery aneurysm associated with fistula and self-expandable metallic stent (SEMS), and [3] a typical Wernicke–Korsakoff syndrome linked to vitamin deficiency in patients who are, in fact, subjected to long-term fasting.

Investigation

If the surgeon becomes concerned about a leak and a drain was left in place at the time of surgery, the drain fluid can be sent for an amylase level. If the fluid amylase level is much higher than normal serum levels (in the 1,000s), this suggests that saliva is entering the drain. Regardless of the drain amylase level, early imaging is warranted if clinical suspicion of a leak exists. An upper gastrointestinal contrast study is frequently used postoperatively to assess the presence of a gastric leak as well as demonstrate patency of the sleeve gastrectomy. In general, a water-soluble contrast material is used (Gastrografin). While standing, the patient swallows 20 mL of Gastrografin and radiographs are taken. The characteristics of a tubularized stomach (i.e., dimensions, emptying, and the presence or absence of leak or stricture) are then evaluated (Figs. 7 and 8). In case of doubt, or in order to increase sensitivity, abdominal computerized tomography (CT) scan can be performed. CT scan can provide additional information in regard to fluid collections or abscess in the left upper quadrant (Figs. 9 and 10) or the presence of subdiaphragmatic air (Fig. 11).

Abdominal CT scan should be performed with intravenous and oral contrast material. It is useful to identify the postoperative normal anatomy and the presence of complications after sleeve gastrectomy. Findings suggestive of GL are extravasation of contrast agent through the wall of the gastric sleeve, accumulation adjacent to the sleeve, free intra-abdominal liquid, free intra-abdominal gas, and residual contrast agent in the drainage tube.

Management of Post-LSG GL (Fig. 12)

Interventional options include surgery (laparoscopy or laparotomy with abdominal washout, abdominal drainage close to the staple line, and feeding jejunostomy), endoscopic procedures (self-expandable metallic stents (SEMS), clips, biological glue, pigtail drains, and T-tube gastrostomy drain), and radiological procedures (percutaneous drainage).

The management of the leak depends on the patient's clinical condition. The surgeon managing this complication

FIG. 7. Normal images after
LSG. (**a**) Contrast study:
S gastric sleeve; (**b**) CT image:
S gastric sleeve; *arrow* shows
gastric staple line.

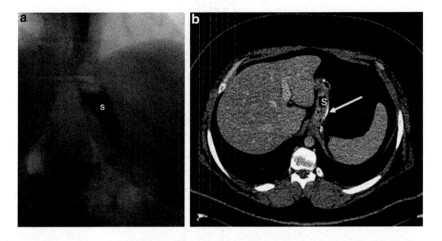

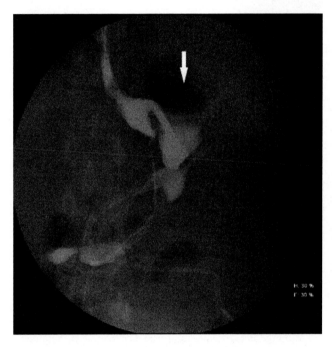

FIG. 8. An upper gastrointestinal contrast radiograph showing
proximal gastric leak. A cavity is observed adjacent to the stomach
(*white arrow*). Reproduced with permission from *OBES SURG
2011*; 21:1232-1250. Gastric Leak After Sleeve Gastrectomy:
Analysis of Its Management.

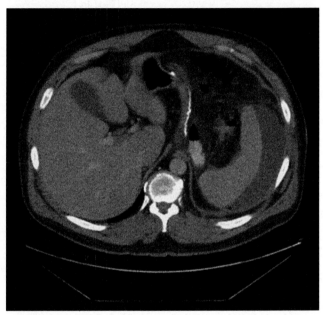

FIG. 9. Abdominal CT scan showing the staple line of the sleeve
gastrectomy with contrast extravasation proximally into an extraluminal collection immediately adjacent to the gastric sleeve staple
line. Reproduced with permission from *OBES SURG 2010*;20:1289-
1292. The Use of Endoscopic Stent in Management of Leaks After
Sleeve Gastrectomy.

must have a clear treatment strategy or algorithm based on
the patient's status, the duration of the leak, and the resources
available.

If the leak presents as a well-defined abscess several days
or weeks after surgery and the patient is clinically stable, percutaneous image-guided drainage (Fig. 13) or pigtail drainage
(Fig. 14), antibiotics, and nutritional support with parenteral
nutrition or a nasojejunal tube is appropriate. If drainage is
adequate, endoluminal therapies can be used to facilitate closure of the leak. This process often includes placement of
endoscopic clips, fibrin glue (Fig. 15), or bioabsorbable fistula
plugs and endoluminal stenting across the leak. Stenting has
been shown to be effective in small series of selected cases, but

results can be variable depending on the size and duration of
the leak. Although placement of self-expanding, covered, or
partially covered stents (Polyflex or WallFlex stents, Boston
Scientific, Natick, MA) may be beneficial, the current stent
technology is not ideal for this anatomy. The difficulty is in the
two different lumen diameters and the curvature of the gastric
lumen (Fig. 16). Before attempts at stenting, the extraluminal
collection must be adequately addressed in all cases, and surgical placement of drains with washout of the infected field is
often warranted to promote closure of the leak. Because successful outcomes after stenting often occur in carefully
selected patients, evidence is currently insufficient to make
any broad claims that stenting accelerates or promotes closure

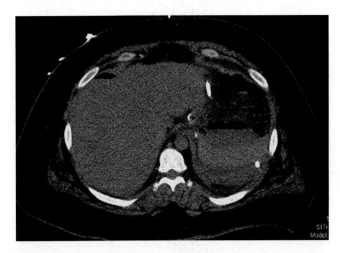

FIG. 10. CT scan showing a left upper quadrant abscess after post-LSG GL.

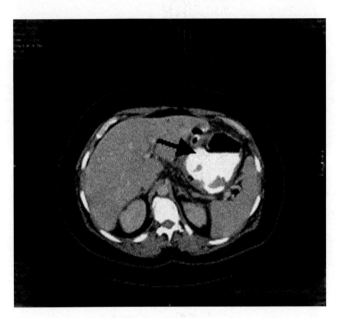

FIG. 11. CT scan showing a contained leak after laparoscopic sleeve gastrectomy. Arrow is abscess with free air, blood, and debris.

of leaks for all patients. Nevertheless, stenting may be a useful therapeutic adjunct in some patients and is associated with acceptable risk.

One advantage of stent placement in these patients is that it may allow patients to resume oral intake while the leak heals.

Patients who are manifesting signs of sepsis or are unstable should be managed operatively with laparoscopy or laparotomy (Fig. 17). Drainage and washout of the infected collection and wide drainage of the area is the primary goal of the operation. Primary closure of the defect can be performed if discovered early. Direct primary closure of the defect with or without sealants should be reserved for cases that were diagnosed early (within 24–48 h) and have good

tissue viability. Closed suction or sump drains should be placed and the omentum can be sewn over the defect to help contain the contamination. If the patient is stable during the case, a feeding jejunostomy should be placed for long-term enteral access.

In contrast to a Roux-en-Y gastric bypass (RYGB), LSG leaks are more difficult to manage and tend to be more chronic in nature. Proximal leaks (Fig. 18) may be differentiated from distal ones due to the quality of material that may be seen in the drain. Proximal leaks often have saliva and gastric acid, while distal leaks may additionally drain bile. In proximal leaks the use of drains (surgical or percutaneous) plus alimentary support should be initiated. Complementary to the adequate drainage, the use of endoscopic procedures like fibrin sealant in combination with somatostatin and placement of endoluminal stents have promising results. There are less reports on the management of distal leaks; however, the same principles as previously described should be applied (Fig. 19). Rosenthal et al. [22] presented a case report with a distal and proximal disruption of the staple line. A T-tube gastrostomy with a large proximal and distal limb was placed into the most distal area of disruption. After thorough oversewing and drainage of the proximal site and T tube (distal), a feeding jejunostomy was placed. Four weeks postoperatively, the T tube was removed after the patient had a negative Gastrografin study and tolerated oral fluids with a clamped T tube. Persistent leaks (both proximal and distal) may require conversion to a low pressure system such as RYGB.

Another important factor when treating proximal or distal leaks is to rule out distal obstruction, in particular at the incisura. If present, an EGD and endoscopic deployment of a covered stent across the leak site and obstruction will both cover the leak and more importantly decrease the pressure in the gastric lumen (Figs. 20 and 21).

"Treatment success" was defined as absence of contrast agent leakage in CT and endoscopic evaluations after permanent, covered SEMS, T-tube, or pigtail drains had been removed.

In contrast, "treatment failure" was defined as the need for radical surgery for persistent GL (total gastrectomy or Roux-en-Y gastroenterostomy at the site of GL).

Several principles should be followed when an esophageal stent is considered for management of a gastric leak after sleeve gastrectomy. First, an endoscopy must be performed to evaluate the site of the leak, the size of the leak, and the viability of the conduit. Gastric leaks at the proximal and mid-aspect of the gastric sleeve are the only leaks that are amenable to endoscopic treatment with stent. A leak at the distal staple line of the gastric sleeve, near the gastric antrum, will not be amenable to endoscopic stenting as the stent may be too small in diameter and would not provide appropriate sealing of the defect and potentially lead to a higher degree of migration. The selection of the size of the stent is based on evaluation of the gastric sleeve diameter at the time of endoscopy. Another strategy to minimize stent

Postoperative Sleeve Gastrectomy

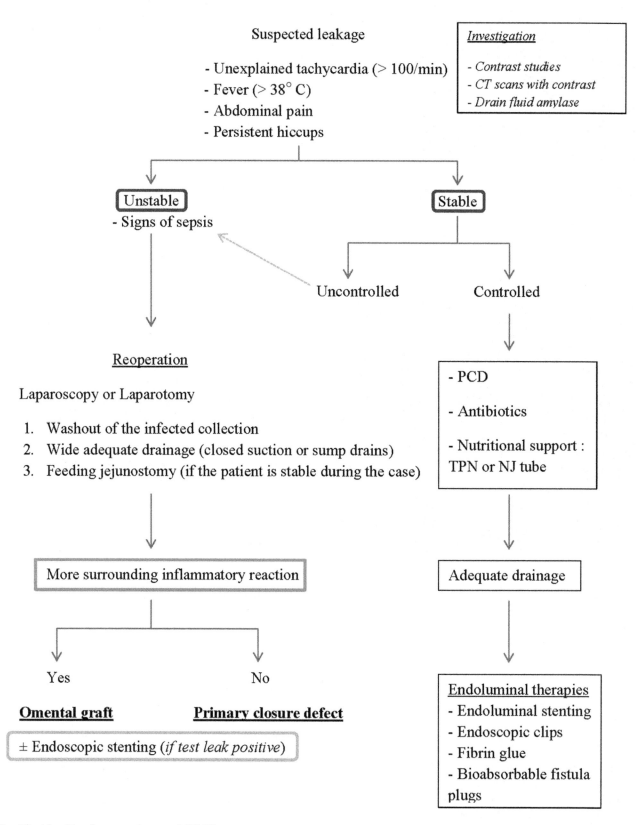

Fig. 12. Algorithm for managing post-LSG GL.

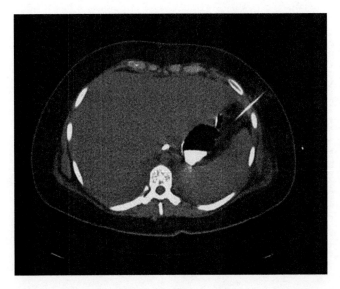

FIG. 13. Percutaneous drainage to drain a collection adjacent to the remnant stomach. Reproduced with permission from *OBES SURG 2011*;21:1232-1250. Gastric Leak After Sleeve Gastrectomy: Analysis of Its Management.

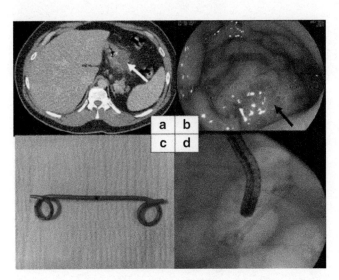

FIG. 14. Delayed-onset gastric leak. (**a**) A fluid collection bulging in the stomach (*white arrow*). (**b**) Fluid collection bulging in the stomach (*black arrow*). (**c**) A pigtail drain. (**d**) Abdominal X-ray showing two pigtail drains after the endoscopic procedure. Reproduced with permission from *OBES SURG 2012*:22;712-720. Is There a Place for Pigtail Drains in the Management of Gastric Leaks After Laparoscopic Sleeve Gastrectomy?.

migration is to use a longer stent whereby the distal aspect of the stent is rested along the wall of the gastric antrum which preclude the stent from luminal migration (Table 4).

Serra and colleagues [23] reported on the use of coated self-expanding stents for management of leaks after sleeve gastrectomy in three patients with control of leaks in 66 % of cases.

Casella et al. [25] reported the use of endoscopic stent for leak at the gastroesophageal junction after sleeve gastrectomy in five patients with complete healing occurring in all patients, suggesting that the staple-line leak can be safely and successfully managed without reoperation in patients with hemodynamic stability (rate of success of 100 %). Eubanks et al. [24] reported a success rate of 84 %. Tan et al. reported a success rate for closure of only 50 % due to stent-related complications. Other studies have suggested routine stent removal no later than 6 weeks in order to avoid tissue hyperplasia and difficult extraction. Tolerance to stents is variable (nausea, vomiting, drooling, and retrosternal discomfort) but tends to disappear after the first few days. Covered SEMS also present significant morbidity–mortality, with migration being one of the main concerns (Fig. 22). The high migration rate has been explained by the "abnormal" placement of the stent along the last portion of the esophagus and the gastric pouch. The type of stent used may also lead to higher rates of migration. Fully covered stents will have the greatest degree of migration while less covered stents will have a greater degree of tissue ingrowth.

Gastric Fistula

A chronic fistula (Fig. 23) after LSG is a challenging problem. If a leak or gastrocutaneous fistula persists for months despite adequate surgical drainage, endoluminal therapy, and nutritional support, the patient's gastrointestinal anatomy should be evaluated for a distal obstruction or stricture. Reoperation may be the only solution. Several surgical options have been reported. Therapy may include resection of fistula and proximal stomach with the creation of a Roux-en-Y esophagojejunostomy, bringing a Roux limb up and creating a gastrojejunal anastomosis directly on the leak site, placing a jejunal patch over the leak site, or placing a T tube into the leak site. Evidence is insufficient to support one approach over another, and the type of salvage procedure should be determined by the patient's anatomy and the surgeon's judgment and experience.

Bleeding Complications

The incidence of staple-line hemorrhage has been reported to be 0–8.7 % [27]. Common sites of bleeding include the sleeve staple line, the short gastric vessels, the spleen, and the omental vessels that have been divided during the dissection of the greater curvature. When bleeding is identified, conservative management including stopping anticoagulation and appropriate fluid or blood resuscitation is usually sufficient in most of cases [28, 29]. Bleeding complications requiring reoperation occur less than 2 % of the time after LSG [30]. Laparoscopic stapling devices have become pivotal tools in the field of laparoscopic

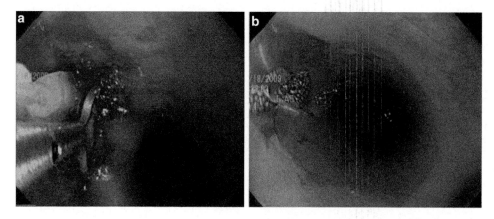

FIG. 15. Endoscopic placement of (**a**) fibrin glue and (**b**) clips across a small leak at the gastroesophageal junction after sleeve gastrectomy followed by placement of a stent across the leak.

FIG. 16. (**a, b**). Schematic illustration of gastric anatomy after sleeve gastrectomy with stent in situ and shows a small persistent leak of contrast refluxing up around the stent (*arrow*).

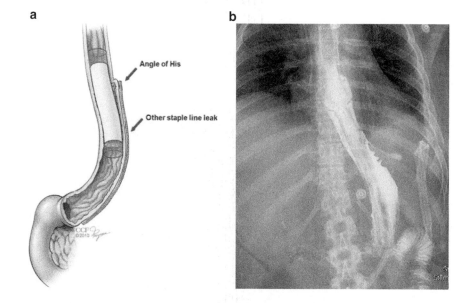

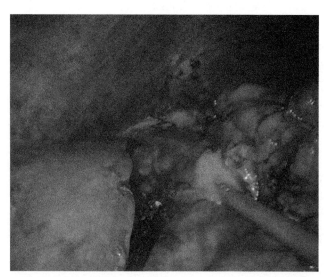

FIG. 17. Reintervention. Abscess drainage. Reproduced with permission from *OBES SURG 2010*;20:1306-1311. Gastric Leak After Laparoscopic Sleeve Gastrectomy.

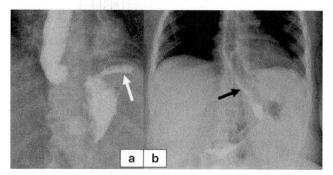

FIG. 18. (**a**) Gastrografin esophagography with gastric leak on the upper third of the staple line (*white arrow*). (**b**) Abdominal X-ray showing two covered SEMS inserted in order to bypass the gastric leak (*black arrow*). Reproduced with permission from *OBES SURG 2012*:22;712-720. Is There a Place for Pigtail Drains in the Management of Gastric Leaks After Laparoscopic Sleeve Gastrectomy?.

FIG. 19. (**a**) First postoperative day. Gastrografin swallow showing drains (A), proximal leak (B), and T-tube gastrostomy drain distal leak (C). (**b**) Gastrografin swallow 6 months after surgery.

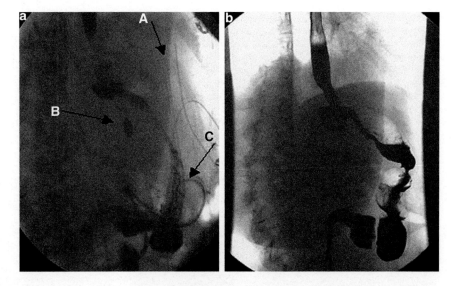

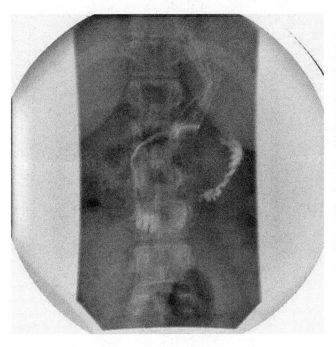

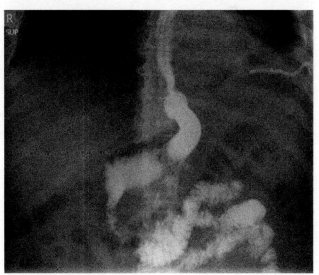

FIG. 20. Upper gastrointestinal contrast study showing a stent deployed for treatment of a proximal staple-line leak and a partial obstruction at the mid-aspect of the gastric sleeve. Note that there is a bending of the stent at its midpoint due to the stricture in the gastric sleeve. The stent protects the leak and allows contrast to pass through the stricture into the duodenum. Reproduced with permission from *OBES SURG 2010*;20:1289-1292. The Use of Endoscopic Stent in Management of Leaks After Sleeve Gastrectomy.

FIG. 21. Upper gastrointestinal contrast study on day 7 after stent deployment showing good contrast flow from esophagus through the stent into the gastric antrum. No evidence of proximal leak was observed. A percutaneous drain was placed to drain a subphrenic collection. Reproduced with permission from *OBES SURG 2010*;20:1289-1292. The Use of Endoscopic Stent in Management of Leaks After Sleeve Gastrectomy.

bariatric surgery. However, they are also associated with complications such as leak, bleeding, fistula, and technical failure, even though these complications are uncommon. In theory, reinforcing the staple line should increase its strength and help decrease the incidence of complications associated with staple lines. Furthermore, there

seems to be no reason to believe that reinforcement would lead to harmful effects. Although the importance of staple-line reinforcement in bariatric operations has been described in the literature, it remains controversial in LSG. The majority of papers that report on staple-line reinforcement in bariatric procedures are related to its use in laparoscopic gastric bypass.

The options for reinforcement include oversewing the staple line, application of fibrin glue sealants, and incorporation of buttressing materials. Staple-line buttressing has been

TABLE 4 Endoscopic stent for gastric leak after laparoscopic sleeve gastrectomy

Author	Year	Number of patients	Number of covered SEMS	Success rate (%)	Migration rate (%)
Serra et al.[23]	2007	3	7	66	14
Eubanks et al. [24]	2008	19	34	84	58
Casella et al. [19]	2009	5	11	100	9
Tan et al. [20]	2010	14	8	50	25
Pequignot et al. [10]	2011	25	50	84	8
Chand et al. [26]	2010	6	6	66	17

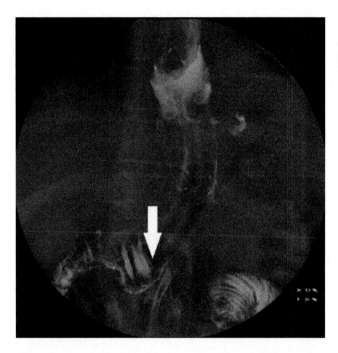

FIG. 22. Migration to the antrum of endoluminal stent (*white arrow*). Reproduced with permission from *OBES SURG 2011*;21:1232-1250. Gastric Leak After Sleeve Gastrectomy: Analysis of Its Management.

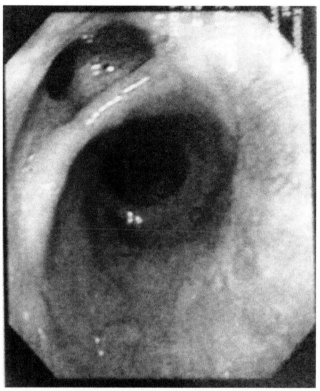

FIG. 23. Endoscopic image of gastrocutaneous fistula.

developed to improve staple-line strength by increasing the tissue thickness, resulting in decreased bleeding and risk of leak. In the bariatric literature their use remains controversial. Few published papers exist that compare the incidence of staple-line leakage or hemorrhage to that of nonreinforced staple lines in LSG procedures.

Choi et al. [31] performed a meta-analysis of eight articles (two RCTs and six cohort studies; Table 5). There were 1,335 patients in the eight studies (507 patients in the control groups and 828 patients in the intervention groups). Although there was no significant effect of overall reinforcement of the staple line in this meta-analysis, reinforcement with a buttress seemed to decrease staple-line hemorrhage (Fig. 24). On the other hand, reinforcing the staple line with oversewing may increase the risk of staple-line hemorrhage, although this result had no statistical significance.

In a subgroup analysis of this meta-analysis, reinforcing the staple line with a buttress may decrease the risk of staple-line hemorrhage and overall complications, but it is not clear whether it decreases the risk of staple-line leak after LSG. It was also unclear if the effect of reinforcing the staple line with oversewing showed any advantage when compared to the control group in regard to leak, hemorrhage, and overall complications. In addition, it could lead to strictures of the gastric sleeve and cause tears of the suture line (Fig. 7). In practice, according to Gagner's report [27], 65.1 % of 106 surgeons who participated in the Second International Consensus Summit for Sleeve Gastrectomy in 2009 answered that they reinforced the staple line of the gastric tube. Of these, 50.9 % reinforced the staple line with oversewing, 42.1 % used a buttress, and 7 % did both.

TABLE 5 Characteristics and outcomes of the included trials

Trials	Country and year	Type of study	Reinforcement			Type of reinforcement	Control		
			Leak	Hemorrhage	Overall		Leak	Hemorrhage	Overall
Consten et al.	USA, 2004	Cohort	0/10	0/10	0/10	Buttressing	0/10	2/10	3/10
Silecchia et al.	Italy, 2009	Cohort	–	–	4/29	Oversewing	–	10/56	
Sanchez-Santos et al.	Spain, 2009	Cohort	10/381	2/381	14/381	Combined	8/159	2/159	14/159
Ser et al.	Taiwan, 2010	Cohort	0/78	2/78	8/78	Oversewing	4/40	0/40	6/40
Dapri et al.	Belgium, 2010	RCT	1/25	–	3/25	Oversewing	1/25	–5/25	
			2/25		6/25	Buttressing	1/25	–	5/25
Daskalakis et al.	Germany, 2011	Cohort	3/144	4/144	9/144	Buttressing	7/86	6/86	14/86
Stamou et al.	Greece, 2011	Cohort	2/96	0/96	2/96	Buttressing	4/91	3/91	12/91
Musella et al.	Italy, 20111	RCT	1/40	4/40	9/40	Oversewing	2/40	2/40	4/40

OBES SURG 2012;22:1206-1213. Reinforcing the Staple Line During Laparoscopic Sleeve Gastrectomy: Does It Have Advantages? A Meta-analysis. Reprinted with permission

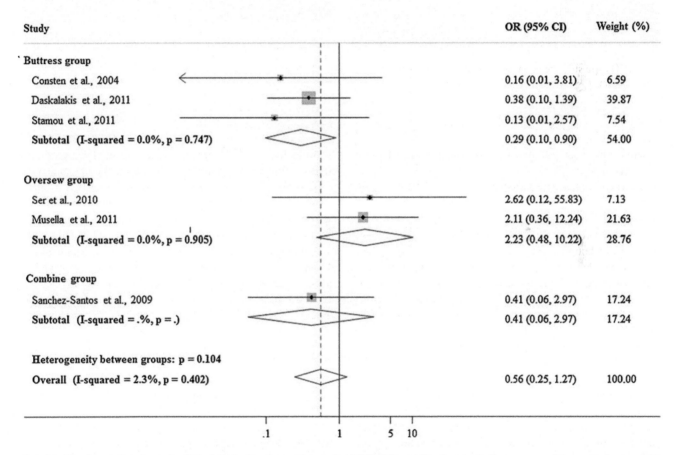

FIG. 24. The forest plot shows the OR of staple-line hemorrhage after LSG of the reinforcing staple-line group and the control group with fixed-effect-model meta-analysis (OR, odds ratio). Reproduced with permission from *OBES SURG 2012*;22:1206-1213. Reinforcing the Staple Line During Laparoscopic Sleeve Gastrectomy: Does It Have Advantages? A Meta-analysis.

Obstruction and Strictures

Sleeve stenosis can occur due to unintentional narrow tubularization of the stomach. It currently is reported to occur in 0.26–4 % of LSG operations [7, 32, 33]. This may underestimate the true incidence of stenosis in current practice because early published series of LSG tended to use larger bougies with the intention of two-stage weight loss. In a recent review of 36 studies evaluating LSG as a primary and staged procedure, Brethauer et al. [7] demonstrated that the rate of postoperative strictures requiring endoscopic or operative intervention was 0.6 % in studies with more than 100

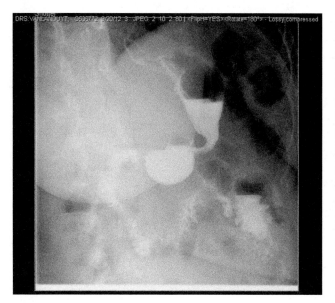

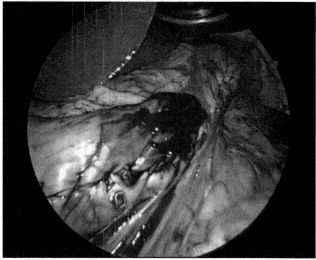

FIG. 26. Hematoma after sleeve gastrectomy.

FIG. 25. Gastric stricture at incisura angularis after sleeve gastrectomy (*arrow*).

patients. The most common site of luminal narrowing is at the incisura (Fig. 25).

Some authors have reported that the stenosis rate does not correlate with bougie size used. For example, Cottom et al. [34] reported using 46- to 50-Fr bougies with a stenosis rate of 3.9 %, whereas Lalor et al. [35] reported using either a 44- or 52-Fr bougie with a stenosis rate of only 0.7 %. This suggests another technical cause independent of bougie size contributing to the stenosis rate. Notably, Cottom et al. [34] stated that by changing their overall technique from imbricating the staple line to covering it with fibrin glue caused their stenosis rate to disappear.

This type of stenosis most likely occurred due to overnarrowing of the sleeve at the incisura. Care must be taken to leave plenty of tissue anteriorly in this area, especially when the sleeve starts closer to the pylorus. Narrowing here can occur as the clinician begins to "cut the corner" even with a larger bougie in place due to over-retraction of the greater curvature during stapling. The process of retracting the greater curvature where tension is progressively applied can cause stretch on the stomach during division. Once the bougie is removed, the stomach will recoil, resulting in a narrowing. Although true strictures can occur, this problem after LSG is typically not a true mucosal or luminal stricture as much as it is an angulation or kinking of the stomach in this area. This functional obstruction presents as persistent dysphagia to solids and liquids, with nausea and vomiting. When creating the SG initially, this complication can be prevented through avoiding sharp angulation of the staple line and allowing for adequate lumen size as the stapler approaches the incisura.

A twisted or spiral sleeve is another cause of symptomatic stenosis. Progressive rotation of the staple line in an anterior to posterior plane can lead to a narrowing despite a fairly normal luminal diameter. This curve can make passage of enteric contents difficult, resulting in a functional stenosis. This often is demonstrated by easy passage of the endoscope or balloon dilator through the narrowed area. Much like a clown twisting a straight balloon, an anterior twist at the incisura can result in a functional stenosis (Fig. 4). An endoscope can pass through by pushing and twisting in the same direction, and a balloon dilator can be used to open the stenosis. However, the stenosis returns at withdrawal of the endoscope or deflation of the balloon dilator. A functional sleeve stenosis also can result from external sources such as a hematoma (Fig. 26) that causes the sleeve to scar in a kinked manner. Such complications should be promptly treated (Video 3).

The management algorithm (Fig. 27) of patients who have undergone LSG with persistent nausea, vomiting, or dysphagia. First, an UGI contrast study should be obtained. If this study demonstrates an abnormal finding or if the symptoms persist over time, an esophagogastroduodenoscopy should be performed with anticipation of performing a dilation. Repeat dilation can be performed as long as the patient demonstrates improvement in oral tolerance. Placement of a stent also can be considered, although a stent often is poorly tolerated by the patient due to pain and discomfort. Failure of progression to a normal diet warrants consideration of operative revision to an RYGB. Clinical significant short-segment stenoses may be treated successfully with endoscopic balloon dilation and stent. Long-segment stenoses are less likely to respond to

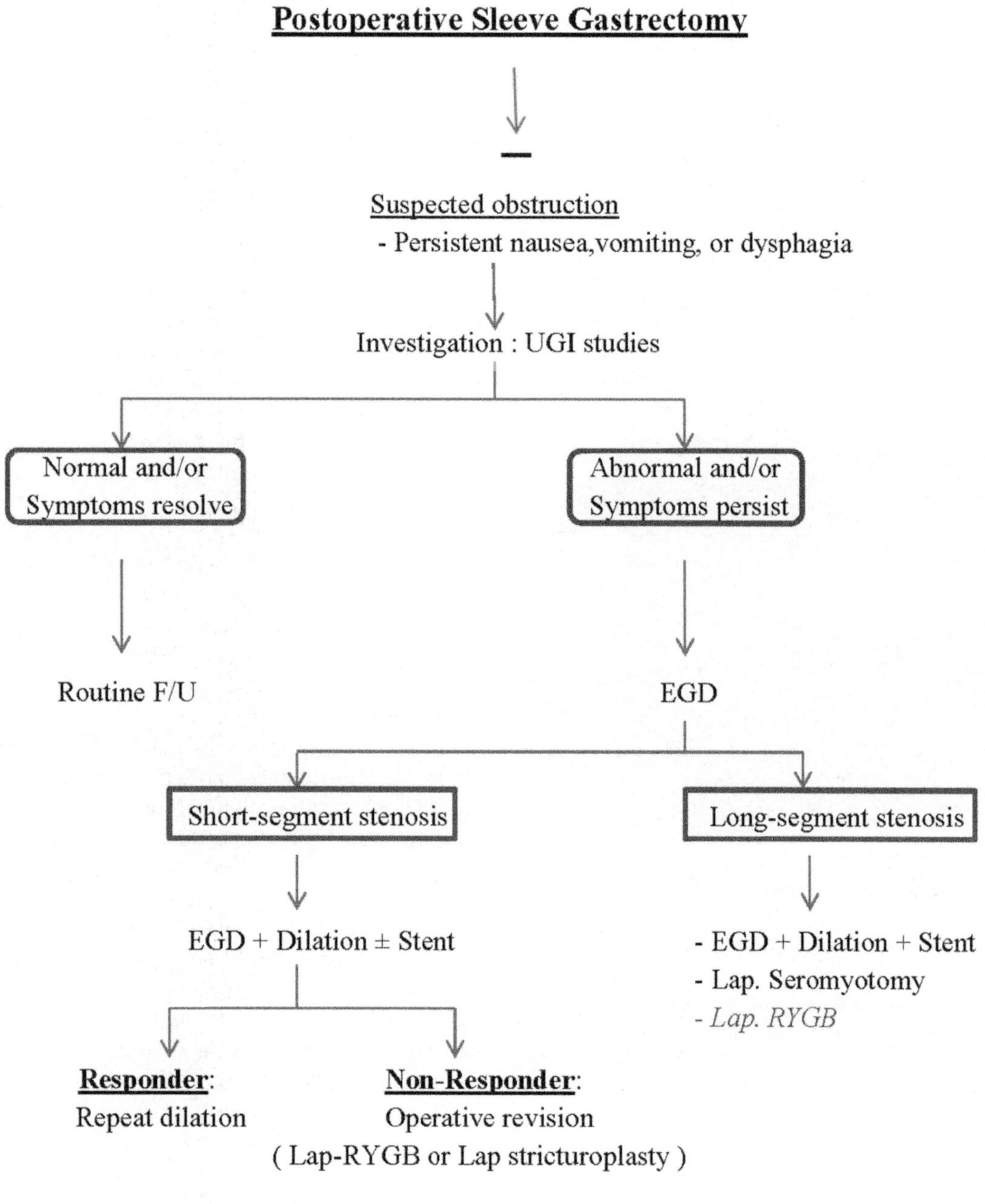

Postoperative Sleeve Gastrectomy

Suspected obstruction
- Persistent nausea, vomiting, or dysphagia

Investigation : UGI studies

| Normal and/or Symptoms resolve | | Abnormal and/or Symptoms persist |

Routine F/U   EGD

| Short-segment stenosis | | Long-segment stenosis |

EGD + Dilation ± Stent

- EGD + Dilation + Stent
- Lap. Seromyotomy
- *Lap. RYGB*

Responder: Repeat dilation

Non-Responder: Operative revision
(Lap-RYGB or Lap stricturoplasty)

FIG. 27. Algorithm for managing post-LSG obstruction.

endoscopic techniques and may ultimately require conversion to Roux-en-Y gastric bypass.

Post-LSG GERD

GERD remains a concern after LSG and has a very wide clinical spectrum of manifestation. There is probably a continuum from mild reflux that may respond well to PPIs, through severe symptomatic reflux that may need a deployment of full treatment options (high-dose PPIs, propulsive medications, and behavioral and lifestyle changes) (Fig. 28). Severe symptoms may also include an inability to ingest oral food requiring hospitalization for assisted feeding and possible reoperation. Therefore, the true incidence of this complication after sleeve gastrectomy is unknown. The works that do report the incidence cite numbers from as low as 0.1 % for prolonged vomiting and 0.2 % for delayed gastric emptying [36] to as high as 13–30 % [37]. Symptomatic GERD has been reported to occur in 7.8–20 % of patients at 12–24 months after LSG in a selected series of more than 100 patients. At the Second and the Third International

Consensus Summits for Sleeve Gastrectomy, reflux disease was reported to occur in 6.5 % and 17 % of patients, respectively, after sleeve gastrectomy. Most studies reported an increase in reflux symptoms during the first year following sleeve gastrectomy, followed by a gradual decrease in symptoms up the third postoperative year.

Even Wernicke–Korsakoff syndrome has been reported after sleeve gastrectomy (SG) due to prolonged vomiting [38]. This wide variation in incidence may also lead to variations in diagnosing criteria. Most authors report prescribing PPIs for different periods of time to SG patients. Often

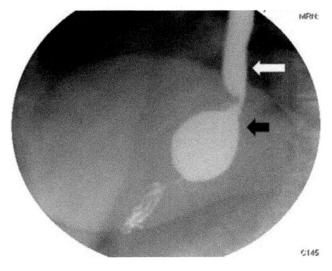

FIG. 28. UGI study revealing a dilated upper part of the sleeve (*black arrow*), with an immediate passage to the lower part. The contrast has retained in the fundus area and reflux up to the mid esophagus was observed (*white arrow*). Reproduced with permission from *OBES SURG 2010*;20:140-147. Dilated Upper Sleeve Can be Associated with Severe Postoperative Gastroesophageal Dysmotility and Reflux.

early improvement of GERD symptoms occurs after LSG, but late onset of GERD symptoms has also been reported. In a report by Himpens and colleagues [38] with 6-year follow-up, the overall incidence of new-onset GERD (defined as symptoms requiring proton pump inhibitor use) was 26 %. The investigators attribute some of the new-onset GERD symptoms to the appearance of a neofundus (dilated pouch of fundus at the proximal sleeve) (Fig. 29) that occasionally requires reoperation. In patients in whom this dilated fundus was resected, GERD symptoms improved. Anatomical changes in the angle of His and GEJ area and retention of the fundus may play an important role in postoperative sleeve emptying. The more fundus left behind, the higher the propensity of the stomach to distend, especially in view of a functional obstruction. Larger retained fundus will produce more gastric acid, and this in turn may result in larger amount of acid available for refluxing into the esophagus (Fig. 30). It is clear that in cases where the fundus has been left behind, the anatomy of the gastroesophageal junction was disturbed to a lesser degree. The fundal dilatation probably represents the retention of the fundus at the operation while trying to avoid injury to the area of the esophagogastric junction or incomplete release of the posterior fundus.

Since sleeve gastrectomy is still a relatively recent technique, the knowledge regarding the true incidence of new-onset GERD is still evolving. More investigations regarding the physiology of the procedure in terms of emptying, acid production, and reflux mechanisms are needed to draw more conclusions. Until that knowledge is available, a cautious approach to patients with preoperatively suspected motility disorders should be exercised. Patients suspected to have this kind of dysfunction should be studied by esophageal manometry or nuclear emptying studies and may be better candidates for alternative operations, such as the gastric bypass. Patients should be advised preoperatively about the possibility of this complication. If this

FIG. 29. Retained fundus functioning as diverticula. Reproduced with permission from *OBES SURG 2010*;20:140-147. Dilated Upper Sleeve Can be Associated with Severe Postoperative Gastroesophageal Dysmotility and Reflux.

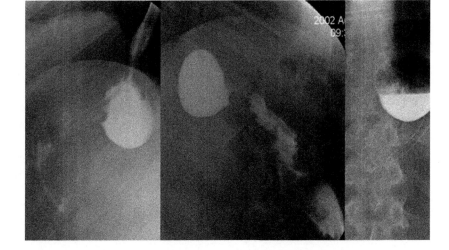

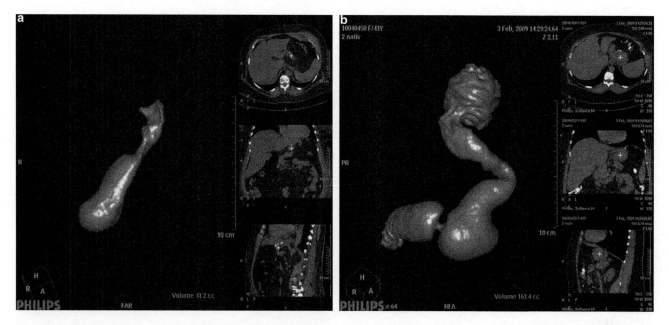

Fɪɢ. 30. (**a**) Virtual CT after sleeve gastrectomy third postoperative day: normal finding after calibration with 42-Fr tube. (**b**) Virtual CT after sleeve gastrectomy: surgical mistake with fundus in place (uncompleted resection).

complication has occurred, conservative approach is usually successful, but sometimes, a conversion to other procedure (RYGB) can be curative.

Treatment Post-LSG GERD

Treatment options are divided into conservative therapy, endoluminal modalities, and surgical options. Obviously, the simple fibrotic stricture or complete obstruction should be excluded by swallow study or endoscopy. But even in the absence of complete anatomical occlusion, there may be a functional obstruction, where the propulsive force of the stomach and esophagus is not enough to clear the content downstream. In those cases, endoscopic dilatation may be beneficial. Conservative measures are directed at reducing acid production and improvement of gastric and esophageal motility and acid clearance. Psychological and diet counseling are of utmost importance on the way to success.

Surgical options can be directed at improvement of gastric emptying and decrease of acid production. Since there is no fundic tissue available, the possibility of fundoplication is nonexistent. Ligamentum teres cardiopexy has been described. Re-sleeve will decrease the acid production, but there are no studies reporting objective data of the gastric acidity before and after the sleeve gastrectomy. The best possible operation is probably a conversion to Roux-en-Y gastric bypass. This will improve emptying and divert the acid gastric content to the small bowel. A seromyotomy is an

alternative for the mechanical and anatomical stenosis of the sleeve (Fig. 31).

Seromyotomy [38] is a difficult procedure but may resolve the problem of symptomatic dysphagia and appearance of de novo GERD symptoms. During this procedure, dissection is performed by hook electrocautery.

This tool and technique allows for a meticulous dissection of the successive muscular layers of the stomach, with very short electrical bursts near the submucosa area. Usually, bleeding encountered during dissection can be controlled by applying pressure with a closed blunt grasper. The goal is to achieve a myotomy 1 cm beyond the stenosis both proximally and distally. If gastric perforation occurs, it can be treated by interrupted intracorporeal absorbable sutures and omentoplasty. The efficacy of the treatment should be assessed by insufflation of air in the stomach. The edges of the myotomized region should easily open up with air insufflation at the end of the procedure. Symmetry of the SG, by observation of a cylindrical gastric tube, should be achieved (Figs. 32 and 33). If after the seromyotomy, an hourglass deformation still remains, and conversion to another bariatric procedure should be considered.

Jorge et al. [37] identified three technical errors that explain most cases of GERD after sleeve gastrectomy: relative narrowing at the junction of the vertical and horizontal parts of the sleeve, dilation of the fundus, and persistence of a hiatal hernia. When they routinely removed the fundus (leaving only enough to allow oversewing), they corrected hiatal hernias when found and avoided relative narrowing or

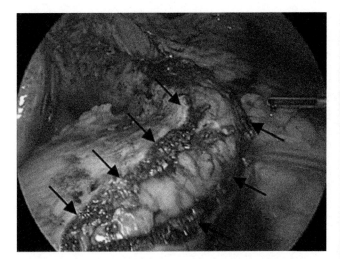

FIG. 31. Final view of laparoscopic seromyotomy. Reproduced with permission from *OBES SURG 2009*;19:495-499. Laparoscopic Seromyotomy for Long Stenosis After Sleeve Gastrectomy with or Without Duodenal Switch.

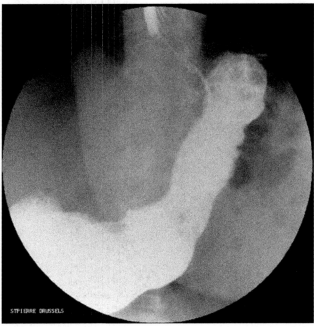

FIG. 33. Postoperative laparoscopic seromyotomy barium swallow: resolution of the stricture. Reproduced with permission from *OBES SURG 2009*;19:495-499. Laparoscopic seromyotomy for long stenosis after sleeve gastrectomy with or without duodenal switch.

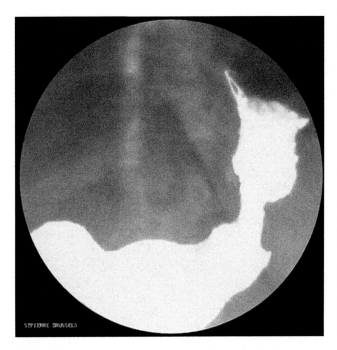

FIG. 32. Preoperative barium swallow: stricture of the SG at the incisura angularis with GERD symptoms. Reproduced with permission from *OBES SURG 2009*;19:495-499. Laparoscopic Seromyotomy for Long Stenosis After Sleeve Gastrectomy with or Without Duodenal Switch.

torsion of the sleeve; they observed a sharp decrease in the need for postoperative endoscopy to investigate food intolerance or symptoms of GERD. The results of their study show a very low incidence of GERD (1.5 %) at 6–12 months after LSG.

Nutrient Deficiencies After LSG

It has been suggested that LSG has a minimal impact on macronutrients as it does not alter the site of their absorption in the small intestine [39]. Gehrer et al. compared the nutritional deficiencies occurring after LSG and laparoscopic RYGB and observed nutritional deficiencies in 57 % of patients. In particular, after LSG the following deficiencies were observed: folate in 22 %, iron in 18 %, and vitamin B12 in 18 % [40]. Laboratory parameters should be monitored regularly to detect early nutritional deficiencies and to initiate appropriate therapies.

A significant number of patients may develop vitamin B12 deficiency after LSG. Therefore, it is likely that, without supplementation, vitamin B12 deficiencies can occur, especially more than 2 years after operation due to empting of vitamin B12 storage. Therefore, a general vitamin B12 supplementation is advisable to avoid pernicious anemia and to prevent neuropathic pain [41]. This complication could be attributed to fundus resection, which is the most abundant part of the stomach with parietal cells that release intrinsic factor essential for vitamin B12 absorption. Also, PPI (proton pump inhibitor) use might have played an additive role in the development of vitamin B12 deficiency by reducing acidity.

Folate can be absorbed throughout the intestine, especially in the jejunum, and therefore folate deficiency is less common after LSG [42]. A very small amount of folate is stored by the body, and a constant supply of a diet containing foods that are sources of folic acid is necessary to maintain serum concentrations. The best sources of folate are viscera, beans, and green leafy vegetables. Some investigators have reported that low folate levels reflect nonadherence to multivitamin supplementation because the amount of supplemented folic acid properly corrects low serum folate levels. Hakeam et al. reported folate deficiency after surgery, and though patients in this study received a daily supplement containing 0.2-mg folic acid following LSG, folate levels deteriorated throughout the study period. Therefore, patients undergoing LSG might require more than the RDA of folic acid to maintain normal folate levels. This could be attributed to the diet changes after surgery [43]. Also, more attention has to be directed to folic acid and vitamin B12 in females planning to get pregnant after LSG, as folic acid and vitamin B12 deficiency during pregnancy in general population has been linked to the increased risk of neonatal neural tube defects. Close monitoring of vitamin B12 and folate levels is important, and an adequate supplementation is necessary to maintain these parameters in the normal range for all the follow-up period.

Hakeam et al. found a low incidence of iron deficiency (4.9 %) and of anemia (1.6 %) 12 months after surgery [43]. After 1 year, the impact of this bariatric surgery on iron indices was negligible. Therefore, iron supplementation appears unnecessary in nonanemic patients undergoing LSG at least in the interval of 6–12 months after surgery.

Bone metabolism can change during the first year after LSG. Part of this change is explained by the weight loss itself due to the loss of pressure on the weight-bearing bones, thus losing a potent stimulant for bone preservation. Furthermore, normal levels of vitamin D are essential for an adequate intestinal calcium uptake. A shortage in vitamin D eventually leads to a negative calcium balance and causes a compensatory rise in PTH to promote bone resorption. Aarts et al. reported normal calcium levels 1 year after LSG but suboptimal levels of vitamin D, although on daily multivitamin supplementation [44]. Calcium supplementation is important in the first 6 months in the multivitamin formula and it is sufficient to maintain normal plasma values during the follow-up period. Patients with deficiencies in albumin, vitamin D, or calcium have a higher risk of developing osteoporosis; therefore, it is recommended that appropriate supplementations be initiated, even if the concentrations of these parameters are only slightly decreased.

PTH levels should be determined to diagnose secondary hyperparathyroidism.

Moreover, supplementation of zinc should be based on symptoms (hair loss, immune deficiency, dry skin). High zinc intake reduces absorption of copper and iron. Zinc and calcium should be taken at different times because zinc reduces calcium absorption. Supplementation of selenium is not generally necessary because postoperative deficiencies normalize on their own without supplementation, and an adequate, varied food intake seems to be sufficient.

Regular determination of laboratory parameters should be performed 3 and 6 months after the operation and semiannually thereafter; if the patient's weight stabilizes, laboratory parameters should be determined once a year.

Conclusion

LSG is an accepted bariatric procedure that can be used for many different patient populations. It has been effectively used as part of a staged risk-management strategy for high-risk patients and has gained popularity as a primary bariatric procedure. The evidence supporting the safety and efficacy of SG continues to increase and long-term data are emerging that report excess weight loss greater than 50 %. There is not yet a standard technique for this procedure. Heterogeneity includes the size of the bougie, beginning site of resection, and reinforcement of the staple line. The solution may lie in finding a suitable size at which the pressure of the tube is not excessive and the restriction is sufficient for obtaining good weight loss results without increasing the risk of complications.

Attractive features of LSG are rapid weight loss, comorbidity reduction, and avoidance of long-term complications of bypass procedures or implantable devices. Concerns remain regarding the risks of leaks, the long-term incidence of GERD symptoms, and the weight loss durability beyond 5 years. Management of leaks after LSG is a formidable challenge for the bariatric surgeon, and early diagnosis followed by a multidisciplinary treatment strategy is key.

Review Questions and Answers

Questions

1. What are the potential causes of post-LSG gastric leak?
   (a) Large hiatal hernia
   (b) Use of a large-size bougie
   (c) Mid-sleeve stenosis
   (d) Staple line near GE junction
   (e) Staple on the migratory crotch staple

2. What are the signs and symptoms of post-LSG GL?
   (a) Persistent hiccups and chronic cough
   (b) Persistent dysphagia with nausea and vomiting
   (c) Diffuse abdominal tenderness
   (d) Unexplained tachycardia (>100/min)
   (e) Localized abdominal tenderness

3. What are the common sites of post-LSG bleeding?
   (a) Mesocolon
   (b) Sleeve staple line
   (c) Short gastric vessels
   (d) Spleen
   (e) Liver

4. What are the treatment options of post-LSG obstruction?
   (a) EGD + dilatation ± stent
   (b) Laparoscopic stricturoplasty
   (c) Laparoscopic RYGB
   (d) Laparoscopic feeding jejunostomy
   (e) Laparoscopic seromyotomy

Correct Answers

1. c, d, e
2. a, c, d, e
3. b, c, d
4. a, b, c, e

References

1. Almogy G, Crookes PF, Anthone GJ. Longitudinal gastrectomy as a treatment for the high-risk super-obese patient. Obes Surg. 2004;14(4):492–7.
2. Marquez MF, Ayza MF, Lozano RB, et al. Gastric leak after laparoscopic sleeve gastrectomy. Obes Surg. 2010;20:1306–11.
3. Gagner M, Patterson E. Laparoscopic biliopancreatic diversion with duodenal switch. Dig Surg. 2000;17:547–66.
4. Buchwald H, Oien DM. Metabolic/bariatric surgery worldwide 2008. Obes Surg. 2009;19:1605–11.
5. Demaria EJ, Pate V, Warthen M, Winegar DA. Baseline data from American Society for Metabolic and Bariatric Surgery: designated bariatric surgery centers of excellence using the bariatric outcomes longitudinal database. Surg Obes Relat Dis. 2010;6:347–55.
6. Brethauer SA. Sleeve gastrectomy. Surg Clin North Am. 2011;91:1265–79.
7. Brethauer SA, Hammel JP, Schauer PR. Systematic review of sleeve gastrectomy as staging and primary bariatric procedure. Surg Obes Relat Dis. 2009;5:469–75.
8. Bruce J, Krukowski ZH, Al-Khairy G, et al. Systematic review of the definition and measurement of anastomotic leak after gastrointestinal surgery. Br J Surg. 2001;88(9):1157–68.
9. Lalor PF, Tucker ON, Szomstein S, et al. Complications after laparoscopic sleeve gastrectomy. Surg Obes Relat Dis. 2008;1:33–8.
10. Pequignot A, Fuks D, Verhaeghe P, et al. Is there a place for pigtail drains in the management of gastric leaks after laparoscopic sleeve gastrectomy? Obes Surg. 2012;22:712–20.
11. Aurora AR, Khaitan L, Saber AA. Sleeve gastrectomy and the risk of leak: a systematic analysis of 4,888 patients. Surg Endosc. 2012;26:1509–15.
12. Burgos AM, Braghetto I, Csendes A, et al. Gastric leak after laparoscopic-sleeve gastrectomy for obesity. Obes Surg. 2009;19:1672–7.
13. Basso N, Casella G, Rizzello M, et al. Laparoscopic sleeve gastrectomy as first stage or definitive intent in 300 consecutive cases. Surg Endosc. 2011;25(2):444–9.
14. Nocca D, Krawczykowsky D, Bomans B, et al. A prospective multicenter study of 163 sleeve gastrectomies: results at 1 and 2 years. Obes Surg. 2008;18(5):560–5.
15. Bellanger DE, Greenway FL. Laparoscopic sleeve gastrectomy, 529 cases without a leak: short-term results and technical considerations. Obes Surg. 2011;21(2):146–50.
16. Yehoshua RT, Eidelman LA, Stein M, et al. Laparoscopic sleeve gastrectomy—volume and pressure assessment. Obes Surg. 2008;18(9):1083–8.
17. Baker RS, Foote J, Kemmeter P, et al. The science of stapling and leaks. Obes Surg. 2004;14(10):1290–8.
18. Heniford BT, Matthews BD, Sing RF, et al. Initial results with a stapled gastrojejunostomy for the laparoscopic isolated Roux-en-Y gastric bypass. Am J Surg. 2000;179:476–81.
19. Casella G, Soricelli E, Rizello M, et al. Nonsurgical treatment of staple line leaks after laparoscopic sleeve gastrectomy. Obes Surg. 2009;19:821–6.
20. Tan JT, Kariyawasam S, Wijeratne T, et al. Diagnosis and management of gastric leaks after laparoscopic sleeve gastrectomy for morbid obesity. Obes Surg. 2010;20:403–9.
21. de Aretxabala X, Leon J, Wiedmaier G, et al. Gastric leak after sleeve gastrectomy: analysis of its management. Obes Surg. 2011;21:1232–7.
22. Court I, Wilson A, Benotti P, et al. T-tube gastrostomy as a novel approach for distal staple line disruption after sleeve gastrectomy for morbid obesity: Case report and review of the literature. Obes Surg. 2010;20:519–22.
23. Serra C, Baltasar A, Andreo L, et al. Treatment of gastric leaks with coated self-expanding stents after sleeve gastrectomy. Obes Surg. 2007;17:866–72.
24. Eubanks S, Edwards CA, Fearing NM, et al. Use of endoscopic stents to treat anastomotic complications after bariatric surgery. J Am Coll Surg. 2008;206:935–8.
25. Stroh BC, Birk D, Flade KR, et al. Results of sleeve gastrectomy-data from a nationwide survey on bariatric surgery in Germany. Obes Surg. 2009;19:632–40.
26. Yimcharoen P, Heneghan HM, Tariq N, et al. Endoscopic stent management of leaks and anastomotic strictures after foregut surgery. Surg Obes Relat Dis. 2011;7:628–36.
27. Gagner M, Deitel M, Kalberer BA, et al. The second international consensus summit for sleeve gastrectomy. Surg Obes Relat Dis. 2009;5:476–85.
28. Albanopoulos K, Alevizos L, Flessas J, et al. Reinforcing the staple line during laparoscopic sleeve gastrectomy: prospective randomized clinical study comparing two different techniques. Preliminary results. Obes Surg. 2012;22:42–6.
29. Gill RS, Switzer N, Driedger M, et al. Laparoscopic sleeve gastrectomy with staple line buttress reinforcement in 116 consecutive morbidly obese patients. Obes Surg. 2012;22:560–4.
30. Simon TE, Scott JA, Brockmeyer JR, et al. Comparison of staple-line leakage and hemorrhage in patients undergoing laparoscopic sleeve gastrectomy with or without seamguard. Am Surg. 2011;77:1665–8.
31. Choi YY, Bae J, Hur KY, et al. Reinforcing the staple line during laparoscopic sleeve gastrectomy: does it have advantages? A meta-analysis. Obes Surg. 2012;22:1206–13.
32. Parikh A, Alley JB, Peterson RM, et al. Management options for symptomatic stenosis after laparoscopic vertical sleeve gastrectomy in the morbidly obese. Surg Endosc. 2012;26:738–46.

33. Zundel N, Hernandez JD, Galvao Neto M, Campos J. Strictures after laparoscopic sleeve gastrectomy. Surg Laparosc Endosc Percutan Tech. 2010;20:154–8.

34. Cottam D, Qureshi FG, Mattar SG, et al. Laparoscopic sleeve gastrectomy as an initial weight-loss procedure for high-risk patients with morbid obesity. Surg Endosc. 2006;20:859–63.

35. Lalor PF, Tucker ON, Szomstein S, et al. Complications after laparoscopic sleeve gastrectomy. Surgery Obes Rel Dis. 2008;4: 33–8.

36. Keidar A, Appelbaum L, Schweiger C, et al. Dilated upper sleeve can be associated with severe postoperative gastroesophageal dysmotility and reflux. Obes Surg. 2010;20:140–7.

37. Daes J, Jimenez ME, Said N. Laparoscopic sleeve gastrectomy: symptoms of gastroesophageal reflux can be reduced by changes in surgical technique. Obes Surg. 2012;22(12):1874–9.

38. Dapri G, Cadiere GB, Himpens J. Laparoscopic seromyotomy for long stenosis after sleeve gastrectomy with or without duodenal switch. Obes Surg. 2009;19:495–9.

39. Capoccia D, Coccia F, Paradiso F, et al. Laparoscopic gastric sleeve and micronutrients supplementation: Our experience. Journal of Obesity. 2012;1–5.

40. Gehrer S, Kern B, Peters T, et al. Fewer nutrient deficiencies after laparoscopic sleeve gastrectomy (LSG) than after Laparoscopic Roux-Y-gastric bypass (LRYGB)-a prospective study. Obes Surg. 2010;20(4):447–53.

41. Pech N, Meyer F, Lippert H, et al. Complications, reoperations, and nutrient deficiencies two years after sleeve gastrectomy. Journal of Obesity. 2012;1–9.

42. Bloomberg RD, Fleishman A, Nalle JE, et al. Nutritional deficiencies following bariatric surgery: what have we learned? Obes Surg. 2005;15(2):145–54.

43. Hakeam HA, O'Regan PJ, Salem AM, et al. Impact of laparoscopic sleeve gastrectomy on iron indices: 1 year follow-up. Obes Surg. 2009;19(11):1491–6.

44. Aarts EO, Janssen IMC, Berends FJ. The gastric sleeve: losing weight as fast as micronutrients? Obes Surg. 2011;21:207–11.

17
Sleeve Gastrectomy as a Revisional Procedure

Raul J. Rosenthal

Introduction

Recently, laparoscopic sleeve gastrectomy (LSG) has been used as a revisional option for previously failed bariatric surgeries, including gastric banding (GB), vertical banded gastroplasty (VBG), and biliopancreatic diversion with duodenal switch (BPD-DS). Among these, LSG for failed GB has received the most attention because of the increasing number of GB being performed and high rates of failure after the procedure. There are several revisional options for failed GB, such as revision of the original surgery or converting to another operation, either restrictive or malabsorptive [1]. Although many experts currently agree that Roux-en-Y gastric bypass (RYGB) is the best option to convert a failed GB, LSG is also regarded as an acceptable alternative [2]. In this chapter, we review general aspects of LSG as a revisional treatment modality, particularly after failed GB.

Rationale

The definition of *failure* in bariatric surgery is still controversial, but it is usually constituted by the following: (1) weight gain or weight loss failure defined as <25 % excess weight loss (EWL) within 2 years of follow-up [3] and (2) development of complications after the surgery.

The adequacy of replacing a failed restrictive procedure with another restrictive procedure is open to debate [4]. The rationale for the above-mentioned is that sufficient weight loss should not be expected when replacing a failed procedure with a comparable one that has a similar mechanism of action. Therefore, conversion of the failed restrictive procedure to a malabsorptive or combined procedure has been the preferred strategy by most surgeons [2, 3]. Since some

Electronic supplementary material: Supplementary material is available in the online version of this chapter at 10.1007/978-1-4939-1637-5_17. Videos can also be accessed at http://www.springerimages.com/videos/978-1-4939-1636-8.

consider LSG a restrictive procedure [5, 6], the feasibility of performing LSG as a revisional procedure for failed GB, a purely restrictive procedure, has been controversial.

Despite being considered a restrictive procedure, LSG has been demonstrated to have other mechanisms of action such as anorexia and dumping syndrome [7, 8]. According to recent studies [9–11], weight loss and improvement in comorbidities in patients who underwent LSG seem to result not only from reduction of the gastric volume but also from neurohormonal changes. Plasma levels of ghrelin, a peptide hormone that stimulates appetite, decrease significantly after LSG as it removes the gastric fundus where most of the ghrelin-producing cells are located [9]. An increase in other gut hormones, such as GLP-1 and peptide-YY, has also been reported to play a key role in the effects after LSG [10, 11]. In addition, rapid gastric emptying is seen after LSG due to alterations in the contractility of the proximal stomach and the absence of receptive relaxation [7]. These nonrestrictive benefits, including changes in hormone levels and gastric emptying time, differentiate LSG from a purely restrictive procedure. Therefore, LSG seems to be a reasonable revisional option for a failed restrictive procedure, although the exact hormonal mechanism and true nature of LSG are still being studied.

Indications

When we consider a bariatric surgery that has failed, revisional options should be considered but only after a thorough nutritional and psychological evaluation has been performed,

LSG has been used as a revisional procedure after the failure of GB, VBG [12, 13], and BPD-DS [14]. Common reasons for performing LSG after those procedures include inadequate weight loss, band slippage, band erosion, and esophageal dilatation. The short-term safety and efficacy of LSG as a revisional treatment modality for the above indications has been reported (Table 1) [1, 3, 4, 12–25]. Nevertheless, it is hard to define indications for which revisional LSG should be

TABLE 1. Indications of revisional laparoscopic sleeve gastrectomy

Reasons of performing revisional LSG
Weight loss failure
Intolerable symptoms
Band slippage
Band erosion
Band infection
Esophageal dilatation
Esophageal motility disorder
Good candidates for revisional LSG
Patients who prefer the procedure
Patients considered high risk
Patients contraindicated for malabsorptive procedure (inflammatory bowel disease, severe small bowel adhesions)
Patients on anticoagulants
Heavy smokers
Patients with a BMI of 35–40 without comorbidities
Patients with a BMI of 30–35 with associated comorbidities
Morbidly obese adolescent or elderly
Patients requiring a second surgical procedure (e.g., kidney or liver transplantation, joint replacement)
Relative contraindications for revisional LSG
Severe GERD with aspiration pneumonia, Barrett's dysplasia, chronic cough
Eroded band

performed as the first choice, because of the presence of various feasible options and the lack of comparative studies or long-term results after LSG. When it comes to failed GB, re-banding or band removal in the case of band-related problems and conversion to RYGB are the most frequent revisional strategies currently used [26]. Although consensus on the use of LSG for weight loss failure after GB was not reached at the recent expert panel meeting [2], many surgeons still consider LSG as a valid option for failed GB due to its level of technical ease, safety, and effectiveness. Furthermore, there is a group of patients that would be good candidates for conversion to LSG as listed in Table 1 [2, 4, 16]. As a result, revisional LSG can be performed for various reasons of failure and helpful for some patients in particular, although more studies are needed.

Surgical Procedure

The aim of this operation is to create a restriction and reduce the size of the stomach to about a 150 cm³ tube by resecting the greater curvature [27]. Surgical technique of revisional sleeve gastrectomy is basically similar to that of the primary sleeve gastrectomy except for a few points, and it is performed laparoscopically unless severe intraoperative complications occur. Patients need perioperative antibiotics and thromboprophylaxis with preoperative subcutaneous heparin injection and pneumatic anti-embolic stockings. In the operating room, patients are placed in the supine position and receive general anesthesia via endotracheal intubation. The abdominal cavity is accessed through a 1 cm supraumbilical incision using an optical trocar. Pneumoperitoneum is created using carbon dioxide insufflation to a pressure of 15 mmHg. Accessory trocars are placed in the subxiphoid

area and right and left upper quadrants. The access port of the band is removed during placement of the left upper quadrant trocar. Adhesiolysis is performed particularly between the left liver lobe and the anterior wall of the stomach until the liver is retracted cranially. It is our recommendation to keep the band in place until the band capsule has been divided, the fundoplicature has been taken down, and both right and left crus of the diaphragms have been clearly dissected. Then, the posterior band capsule that is on the gastric wall is dissected and excised in order to facilitate staple closure and transection of the stomach.

The greater curvature of the stomach is dissected with a harmonic scalpel dividing the short gastric vessels from 2 to 6 cm proximal to the pylorus up to the gastroesophageal junction. A bougie is inserted transorally to the level of the distal stomach to size the sleeve, and 32–36 F is generally thought to be an optimal bougie size [2]. Linear cutting staplers are used to vertically transect the stomach, creating a gastric sleeve with an estimated capacity of 100–150 mL. When transecting the stomach, it is important to start 2–6 cm proximal to the pylorus and to maintain a reasonable distance from the gastrointestinal junction on the last firing [2]. Many surgeons usually prefer to start 6 cm proximal to the pylorus to leave most of the gastric antrum for its pumping and emptying action [12]. Although the stapler heights can vary according to tissue thickness, nothing less than green load (2.0 mm) should be used when performing revisional LSG [2]. The staple line is oversewn by absorbable suture or buttressed with a collagen-like material to prevent bleeding and leaks. After thorough hemostasis, a drain is placed in the subhepatic space. The stomach specimen and band are removed through the supraumbilical trocar site. Then the trocar sites are closed.

In patients with previous LAGB, special attention should be given to the upper third of the sleeve [4], where the tissue is thickened due to the fibrous capsule around the band. Transecting the stomach at this point can result in either poor union with leakage or poor healing [15]. If a surgeon shifts the transection plane laterally to avoid stapling the thickened scar tissue, LSG may not guarantee the complete removal of the gastric fundus. However, it is important to remove the whole gastric fundus to expect nonrestrictive benefits of LSG. Therefore, stapling the thickened scar tissue when making the upper part of the sleeve is unavoidable, and using the tallest staples is strongly recommended to make it a safe procedure [4]. There is a hypothesis that removal of the band with an interval of 3–6 months prior to LSG could reduce the complications, because this interval can help to reduce the chronic inflammatory response around the previously banded area and prevent incomplete stapling or complications. Nevertheless, consensus is not yet reached because there has been no strong data so far to support it [4]. It is our opinion that an absolute contraindication to a one-step conversion of GB to LSG is when bands are eroded or patients developed severe GERD with episodes of aspiration pneumonias.

Outcomes

Feasibility

Our experience at the Cleveland Clinic Florida included 13 cases of revisional LSG from 2005 to 2009 [4]. The mean operative time was 120 min (range 85–180 min) and mean hospital stay was 5.5 days (range 2–20 days). According to other series with over 400 cases, the mean operative time was 90–140 min and the mean hospital stay was 1–6 days, which were comparable to those of the primary LSG and shorter than those of the RYGB after failed GB [1, 3, 4, 12, 13, 15, 17–25]. Almost all cases were completed laparoscopically, with only 6 out of over 400 cases converted to open surgery mainly due to large incisional hernia or extensive adhesion.

Safety and Complications

Of the 13 cases performed at CCF, we had no mortality, and two major complications—a staple line leak requiring repair and drainage on postoperative day (POD) 3, and a postoperative acute gastric outlet obstruction in a patient 2 years after removal of an eroded gastric band that had to be converted to an RYGBP on POD 4. According to other studies, there was only one mortality reported out of over 400 cases due to multi-organ failure from septic shock, and overall complication rate was approximately 0–32 % [1, 3, 4, 12, 13, 15, 17–25]. A recent systematic review of the relevant articles reported that the weighted mean of complication rates of revisional LSG after failed GB was 4.1 % [28]. Commonly reported complications are listed in Table 2. Among those, the most prevalent complications were leaks, strictures, bleeding, and gastroesophageal reflux disease (GERD) [2]. Leak is one of the major complications of both primary and revisional LSG with long staple lines. The thick area around the pylorus is predisposed to leak. Esophagogastric junction is also vulnerable to leak, because an excessive traction applied during stapling the stomach leaves the tissue under tension [13]. For a revisional LSG, leak becomes a bigger problem in the upper part of the stomach due to the high probability of incomplete stapling of the thickened scar tissue around the previously banded area and compromised blood supply at

Table 2. Short- and long-term complications

Leakage/gastric fistula
Bleeding
GERD
Stricture
Hiatal hernia of sleeve
Incisional hernia
Intra-abdominal collection
Acute gastric outlet obstruction

the esophagogastric junction after dissecting the left crus. The ischemia or trauma during the initial procedure also contributes to a leak after the revision. Stricture is usually developed at the incisura angularis of the stomach, which would be prevented by using a bougie. Although the complication rate of LSG is lower than that of RYGB, GERD is more frequently seen after LSG than RYGB. Medical therapy with proton pump inhibitors is a treatment of choice in patients with new-onset GERD. In addition, bleeding along the staple line would be prevented by the use of staple line reinforcement with either oversewing or buttressing.

Many studies reported that the overall complication rate of revisional LSG was slightly higher compared to the primary LSG [4, 13, 17, 21, 24], although others showed no significant difference [20, 22, 25]. The possible discrepancy of complication rates between primary and revisional LSG reported by the former studies can be explained by the following technical problems of the revisional LSG: (1) difficulty of stapling the thickened scar tissue, (2) possible damage of compromised tissue when dissecting the adhesions around the previous band, and (3) compromised vascular supply to the superior part of the stomach due to dissection of the left crus. In contrast, complications occurred less frequently after LSG compared to revisional RYGB or BPD-DS. One systematic review estimated the complication rates of revisional LSG, RYGB, and BPD-DS after failed GB were 4.1 %, 10.7 %, and 24.4 %, respectively [28]. The absence of any anastomosis in case of LSG may be the reason for its being safer than malabsorptive surgeries [12, 23]. To summarize, these results support an acceptable level of safety of revisional LSG.

Effectiveness

In our study, mean excess BMI loss at 2, 6, 12, and 18 months were 28.9, 64.2, 65.3, and 65.7 %, respectively. The results of other selected studies are summarized in Table 3. Excess weight loss and expected excess BMI loss were 42.7–53 % and 46.8–65 % at 12–14 months of follow-up, respectively. These results were maintained at 24–36 months after the procedure, although not all of the patients completed the follow-up. Obesity-related comorbidities were improved or even resolved after revisional LSG in a majority of the treated patients. According to the studies that compared the results of primary and revisional LSG, the extent of weight loss after the two procedures was not significantly different [20, 22, 25]. Furthermore, considering that sufficient weight loss was achieved after revisional LSG in the patients who had failed to lose weight after the previous restrictive procedure, LSG seems not to be a mere restrictive procedure and can be used as a valid revisional option for the failed restrictive surgery.

However, it is hard to conclude whether weight loss can be sustained for a long time after performing revisional LSG, since long-term results have not yet been reported. Moreover,

R.J. Rosenthal

TABLE 3. Outcomes of revisional sleeve gastrectomy

	n	Previous surgery	Mean weight loss			Obesity-related comorbidities (%)	Complication rate (%)
			Follow-up	% EWL	% EBMIL		
Dapri	27	GB	18.6 mo[a] (1–59)	34·8		Resolution: 45	3·7
Iannelli	41	GB VBG	13.4 mo[a] (1–36)	42·7	47·4	Resolution: 38 Improvement: 23	12·2
Uglioni	29	GB	12 mo 24 mo 36 mo		65 63 60	–	24·1
Foletto	57	GB VBG	24 mo		41·6		12·2
Jacobs	32	GB VBG	26 mo[a] (5–40)	60	53·1	–	3·1
Goitein	46	GB	2 mo 6 mo 12 mo 24 mo 36 mo	24 37 53 51 48		–	6
Berende	51	GB VBG	13.8 mo[a] (2–46)		49·3	Resolution: 32 Improvement: 28	25
Rebibo	46	GB	6 mo 12 mo 24 mo	28·8 47·4 53·1	26·3 46·8 53·4		8·7

[a]Mean value

GB gastric banding, *VBG* vertical banded gastroplasty, *mo* month, *yr* year, *EWL* excess weight loss, *EBMIL* excess BMI loss

LYGB and BPD-DS are currently thought to be more effective in achieving adequate weight loss after failed GB than LSG. These are the reasons why many surgeons use RYGB as a primary revisional option for failed GB, even with the several advantages of LSG. Upcoming studies with longer follow-up results will help us to arrive at a more definitive conclusion on the effectiveness of revisional LSG.

Pros and Cons

The following are advantages of LSG. It might be safer than gastric bypass since the procedure is less technically demanding, does not require several anastomoses, and does not alter the bowel continuity. The operative time and hospital stay are shorter, and the rates of mortality and morbidity are lower than those of malabsorptive surgeries [1, 3, 4, 12, 13, 15, 17–25]. Problems related to small bowel tension do not occur after LSG. LSG can be generally done laparoscopically, even in the case of an extremely obese patient. It can preferably be used for the patients with conditions that preclude gastric bypass. Furthermore, as the procedure preserves the pylorus of the stomach, patients are less likely to have dumping syndrome and it maintains access to the biliary tract. There are so far no reports that have documented malabsorptive problems or deficiencies of minerals and vitamins other than vitamin B12.

However, there are also disadvantages. Because the staple line is long and involves thickened scar tissue where the band was previously placed, serious complications can occur, such as leak and bleeding. Another problem is that complete resection of the fundus during LSG can be challenging in the patients with failed GB, because gastro-gastric sutures sometimes can create strong adhesions between the inferior aspect of the liver and the anterior gastric wall in the fundal region [15]. Furthermore, GERD is more common in LSG than the bypass surgery. Therefore, careful attention to these issues is necessary when performing this procedure and managing the patients postoperatively. Last but not least, long-term effectiveness of revisional LSG has not yet been reported.

Conclusion

Recently, LSG has been performed as a revisional option for failed GB, VBG, and BPD-DS. LSG as a revisional treatment modality has been performed most often after failed gastric banding, as a result of the fact that gastric banding has been the most popular bariatric procedure performed worldwide. Performing revisional LSG for patients who failed to lose weight after receiving restrictive procedures is reasonable because LSG facilitates weight loss through a nonrestrictive as well as a restrictive mechanism. Although GB is currently regarded as the best option for failed GB, advantages of LSG, such as level of technical ease and relative safety, make it a promising alternative. Furthermore, LSG can preferably be performed on patients with conditions that preclude gastric bypass. Short-term results support that LSG is a feasible revisional procedure for failed GB. More studies are required to evaluate its safety and effectiveness in the long term (Video 1).

References

1. Jacobs M, Gomez E, Romero R, Jorge I, Fogel R, Celaya C. Failed restrictive surgery: is sleeve gastrectomy a good revisional procedure? Obes Surg. 2011;21(2):157–60. PMID: 21113685, Epub 2010/11/30. eng.

2. Rosenthal RJ, Diaz AA, Arvidsson D, Baker RS, Basso N, Bellanger D, et al. International Sleeve Gastrectomy Expert Panel Consensus Statement: best practice guidelines based on experience of >12,000 cases. Surg Obes Relat Dis. 2012;8(1):8–19. PMID: 22248433, Epub 2012/01/18. eng.

3. Patel S, Eckstein J, Acholonu E, Abu-Jaish W, Szomstein S, Rosenthal RJ. Reasons and outcomes of laparoscopic revisional surgery after laparoscopic adjustable gastric banding for morbid obesity. Surg obes Relat Dis. 2010;6(4):391–8. PMID: 20655021.

4. Acholonu E, McBean E, Court I, Bellorin O, Szomstein S, Rosenthal RJ. Safety and short-term outcomes of laparoscopic sleeve gastrectomy as a revisional approach for failed laparoscopic adjustable gastric banding in the treatment of morbid obesity. Obes Surg. 2009;19(12):1612–6. PMID: 19711138, Epub 2009/08/28. eng.

5. Updated position statement on sleeve gastrectomy as a bariatric procedure. Surg Obes Relat Dis. 2012;8(3):e21–6. PMID: 22417852.

6. Baltasar A, Serra C, Perez N, Bou R, Bengochea M, Ferri L. Laparoscopic sleeve gastrectomy: a multi-purpose bariatric operation. Obes Surg. 2005;15(8):1124–8. PMID: 16197783, Epub 2005/10/04. eng.

7. Melissas J, Daskalakis M, Koukouraki S, Askoxylakis I, Metaxari M, Dimitriadis E, et al. Sleeve gastrectomy-a "food limiting" operation. Obes Surg. 2008;18(10):1251–6. PMID: 18663545, Epub 2008/07/30. eng.

8. Tzovaras G, Papamargaritis D, Sioka E, Zachari E, Baloyiannis I, Zacharoulis D, et al. Symptoms suggestive of dumping syndrome after provocation in patients after laparoscopic sleeve gastrectomy. Obes Surg. 2012;22(1):23–8. PMID: 21647622, Epub 2011/06/08. eng.

9. Langer FB, Reza Hoda MA, Bohdjalian A, Felberbauer FX, Zacherl J, Wenzl E, et al. Sleeve gastrectomy and gastric banding: effects on plasma ghrelin levels. Obes Surg. 2005;15(7):1024–9. PMID: 16105401, Epub 2005/08/18. eng.

10. Basso N, Capoccia D, Rizzello M, Abbatini F, Mariani P, Maglio C, et al. First-phase insulin secretion, insulin sensitivity, ghrelin, GLP-1, and PYY changes 72 h after sleeve gastrectomy in obese diabetic patients: the gastric hypothesis. Surg Endosc. 2011;25(11):3540–50. PMID: 21638183, Epub 2011/06/04. eng.

11. Dimitriadis E, Daskalakis M, Kampa M, Peppe A, Papadakis JA, Melissas J. Alterations in gut hormones after laparoscopic sleeve gastrectomy: prospective clinical and laboratory investigational study. Ann Surg. 2012;26. PMID: 23108120, Epub 2012/10/31. Eng.

12. Iannelli A, Schneck AS, Ragot E, Liagre A, Anduze Y, Msika S, et al. Laparoscopic sleeve gastrectomy as revisional procedure for failed gastric banding and vertical banded gastroplasty. Obes Surg. 2009;19(9):1216–20. PMID: 19562420, Epub 2009/06/30. eng.

13. Berende CA, de Zoete JP, Smulders JF, Nienhuijs SW. Laparoscopic sleeve gastrectomy feasible for bariatric revision surgery. Obes

14. Gagner M, Rogula T. Laparoscopic reoperative sleeve gastrectomy for poor weight loss after biliopancreatic diversion with duodenal switch. Obes Surg. 2003;13(4):649–54. PMID: 12935370, Epub 2003/08/26. eng.

15. Bernante P, Foletto M, Busetto L, Pomerri F, Pesenti FF, Pelizzo MR, et al. Feasibility of laparoscopic sleeve gastrectomy as a revision procedure for prior laparoscopic gastric banding. Obes Surg. 2006;16(10):1327–30. PMID: 17059742, Epub 2006/10/25. eng.

16. Roa PE, Kaidar-Person O, Pinto D, Cho M, Szomstein S, Rosenthal RJ. Laparoscopic sleeve gastrectomy as treatment for morbid obesity: technique and short-term outcome. Obes Surg. 2006;16(10):1323–6. PMID: 17059741, Epub 2006/10/25. eng.

17. Nocca D, Krawczykowsky D, Bomans B, Noel P, Picot MC, Blanc PM, et al. A prospective multicenter study of 163 sleeve gastrectomies: results at 1 and 2 years. Obes Surg. 2008;18(5):560–5. PMID: 18317859, Epub 2008/03/05. eng.

18. Dapri G, Cadiere GB, Himpens J. Feasibility and technique of laparoscopic conversion of adjustable gastric banding to sleeve gastrectomy. Surg Obes Relat Dis. 2009;5(1):72–6. PMID: 19161936, Epub 2009/01/24. eng.

19. Frezza EE, Jaramillo-de la Torre EJ, Calleja Enriquez C, Gee L, Wachtel MS, Lopez Corvala JA. Laparoscopic sleeve gastrectomy after gastric banding removal: a feasibility study. Surg Innov. 2009;16(1):68–72. PMID: 19074467, Epub 2008/12/17. eng.

20. Uglioni B, Wolnerhanssen B, Peters T, Christoffel-Courtin C, Kern B, Peterli R. Midterm results of primary vs. secondary laparoscopic sleeve gastrectomy (LSG) as an isolated operation. Obes Surg. 2009;19(4):401–6.

21. Foletto M, Prevedello L, Bernante P, Luca B, Vettor R, Francini-Pesenti F, et al. Sleeve gastrectomy as revisional procedure for failed gastric banding or gastroplasty. Surg Obes Relat Dis. 2010;6(2):146–51. PMID: 19889585, Epub 2009/11/06. eng.

22. Sabbagh C, Verhaeghe P, Dhahri A, Brehant O, Fuks D, Badaoui R, et al. Two-year results on morbidity, weight loss and quality of life of sleeve gastrectomy as first procedure, sleeve gastrectomy after failure of gastric banding and gastric banding. Obes Surg. 2010;20(6):679–84. PMID: 19902316, Epub 2009/11/11. eng.

23. Goitein D, Feigin A, Segal-Lieberman G, Goitein O, Papa MZ, Zippel D. Laparoscopic sleeve gastrectomy as a revisional option after gastric band failure. Surg Endosc. 2011;25(8):2626–30. PMID: 21416182, Epub 2011/03/19. eng.

24. Gagniere J, Slim K, Launay-Savary MV, Raspado O, Flamein R, Chipponi J. Previous gastric banding increases morbidity and gastric leaks after laparoscopic sleeve gastrectomy for obesity. J Visc Surg. 2011;148(3):e205–9. PMID: 21700522, Epub 2011/06/28. eng.

25. Rebibo L, Mensah E, Verhaeghe P, Dhahri A, Cosse C, Diouf M, et al. Simultaneous gastric band removal and sleeve gastrectomy: a comparison with front-line sleeve gastrectomy. Obes Surg. 2012;12. PMID: 22790710, Epub 2012/07/14. eng.

26. Gagner M, Gumbs AA. Gastric banding: conversion to sleeve, bypass, or DS. Surg Endosc. 2007;21(11):1931–5. PMID: 17705071, Epub 2007/08/21. eng.

27. Gianos M, Abdemur A, Rosenthal RJ. Understanding the mechanisms of action of sleeve gastrectomy on obesity. Bariatric Times. 2011;8(5 suppl):4–6.

28. Elnahas A, Graybiel K, Farrokhyar F, Gmora S, Anvari M, Hong D. Revisional surgery after failed laparoscopic adjustable gastric banding: a systematic review. Surg Endosc. 2012;31. PMID: 22936440, Epub 2012/09/01. Eng.

18

Laparoscopic Gastric Plication

Almino Cardoso Ramos, Lyz Bezerra Silva, Manoel Galvao Neto,
and Josemberg Marins Campos

Introduction

There is clear evidence in the literature on the long-term positive impact of bariatric surgery as primary therapy for obesity and its comorbidities. The main mechanisms through which bariatric surgery achieves its outcomes are traditionally related to the restriction of food intake, reduction in the absorption of ingested foods, or a combination of both [1].

The gastric volume reduction has been used for the last 50 years as a bariatric surgical procedure, initially with Mason gastroplasty, the vertical banded gastroplasty, gastric segmentation, gastric banding, Magenstrasse and Mill, and more recently the sleeve gastrectomy. Nowadays adjustable gastric banding (AGB) and laparoscopic sleeve gastrectomy (LSG) are the restrictive approaches commonly used in obese patients. Although these procedures have proven to be good options for selected patients, they are not without significant complications, such as erosion or slippage of the gastric band or leaks, reflux, and stricture in LSG.

The placement of an implantable device or the irreversible resection of gastric tissue, however, has limited the acceptance of AGB and LSG. LSG also has high costs because of the use of staplers, motivating the search for a cheaper and effective technique. Laparoscopic greater curvature gastric plication (LGCP) is gaining ground in the treatment of morbid obesity, looking to replicate the results of LSG with fewer complications.

In 1969 Kirk et al. described safe weight loss in rats by invagination of greater curvature of the stomach [2], followed by Tretbar et al. in 1976, describing gastric plication as a weight reduction procedure, done in an open approach [3]. In 1981, it was described by Wilkinson and Peloso, adding gastric wrapping with a mesh [4].

Current technique of LGCP consists of infolding the greater curvature to reduce stomach volume by placement of rows of nonabsorbable sutures. After evaluation of Nissen fundoplication, a procedure done to treat gastroesophageal reflux disease, an association with significant postoperative weight loss was showed [5]. This paper motivated a study done by Fusco et al., using gastric plication in Wistar rats, observing a significant weight loss when compared with control and sham groups [6]. Fusco et al. also compared anterior gastric wall plication with greater curvature gastric plication in rats, obtaining better results with the procedure done in the greater curvature [7]. These results are in agreement with initial clinical reports by Brethauer et al., who demonstrated an increased weight loss in patients receiving LGCP when compared to plication of the anterior surface [8]. In 2007, Talebpour et al. presented his technique, initially named total vertical gastric plication, better known today as laparoscopic greater curvature plication [9].

The primary advantages motivating the proposition of the use of LGCP as a current bariatric procedure were:

- Consistent weight loss based in animal and clinical studies
- No foreign body (band, ring)
- No gastric or intestinal resection
- No intestinal bypass
- Potential reversibility
- Can be augmented with more extensive procedures
- Decreased risk of leaks
- Lower cost

The neuroendocrine mechanisms that affect weight loss and resolution of comorbidities in LGCP have been explored by a few authors. Fried et al. report a 54.5 % diabetes resolution, and a 42.5 % improvement, with reduction in the number of medications and better metabolic markers, mirroring findings of adjustable gastric banding. Mean HbA_{1c} was 5.1 ± 1.3 (initial 6.4 ± 1.4), and mean glycemic level was reduced to 112 ± 38.8 mg/dL (initial 162 ± 62.7) [10]. Talebpour et al. report 70 % and 95 % diabetes resolution after 6 months and 1 year, respectively [11].

Electronic supplementary material: Supplementary material is available in the online version of this chapter at 10.1007/978-1-4939-1637-5_18. Videos can also be accessed at http://www.springerimages.com/videos/978-1-4939-1636-8.

Technique

There is no standardized technique for LGCP. Patient positioning on the operating table is standard in the literature, in an anti-Trendelenburg position at 30°, with the operator between legs and two assistants on each side of the patient [12]. Four to five trocars placed in the upper abdomen have been described among all authors [13]. As there is no intention to use stapler, there is no necessity for the 12 mm trocar.

The calibration of the gastric tube, as in sleeve gastrectomy, is probably the most controversial technical issue in LGCP. Surgeons have been using different ways to calibrate the stomach plication: with bougies, scopes, the EndoFLIP® (Crospon Inc., Galway, Ireland) that is an especial calibration device, and even the feeling of the surgeon as to look for the best calibration. Bougies are the most common calibration method and the size ranges from 32 to 48 Fr, with intraoperative EGD being used by Brethauer et al., having the additional benefit of visualizing the imbrications intraluminally [8]. Different energy sources are described for greater curvature mobilization, including the Ultracision Harmonic Scalpel (Ethicon Endo-Surgery, Cincinnati, OH), Ligasure Vessel Ligation System (Covidien, Boulder, CO), or even diathermy [13]. It is important to consider that in comparison with sleeve gastrectomy, where the greater curvature will be resected, in LGCP it will be maintained and plicated so it is advised to work with the energy ligation source far from the gastric wall, avoiding necrosis, ulcer, or perforation after the procedure due to ischemic lesions.

Menchaca et al. demonstrated durability of serosa-to-serosa plication in dogs, with a variety of fastening devices, obtaining good results, except for the staple-suture combination. The authors concluded that the durability of the plication is dependent on continuous fixed serosal apposition by the fastening modality at multiple points along the fold, with multiple rows of fasteners, and fastener spacing of less than 2.5 cm within a row producing more durable outcomes [14].

Ramos et al. preferred dissection of the angle of His exposing the crura as the first step of the operation, whereas in the larger studies of Skrekas et al. and Andraos et al. it was the final step of the dissection of the greater curvature of the stomach [15–17]. Mobilization of the greater curvature is performed using either a LigaSure Vessel Ligation System™ (Covidien, Boulder, CO) or an Ultracision Harmonic™ scalpel (Ethicon Endo-Surgery, Inc., Cincinnati, OH) initially by opening the greater omentum at the transition between the gastric antrum and gastric body. A bougie is used for calibration; Skrekas et al. used a diameter of 36 Fr, while Andraos et al. and Ramos et al. used 32 Fr bougies [15–17].

The gastric plication is initiated by imbricating the greater curvature applying a first row of extramucosal stitches which guide subsequent rows created with extramucosal running suture lines. The first row stops 3 cm from the pylorus.

Imbrication of the fundus is a challenging part of the procedure, mainly in patients with redundant fundus. The suture starts close to the His angle and it is important to take care not to overplicate, avoiding a big fold that can migrate to the esophagus causing obstruction. This reduction results in a stomach shaped like a large sleeve gastrectomy. Choice of suture material (absorbable versus nonabsorbable and monofilament versus multifilament) and interrupted or running suture varies among surgeons, but the use of multifilament sutures for the first row of interrupted sutures, and nonabsorbable monofilament for the subsequent lines of running sutures appears to be more common [12]. Following the recommendations done by Menchaca et al. [14], a 2 cm maximum distance between sutures is used by most authors. An intraoperative methylene blue leak test was performed in most studies, without drain placement [12]. Brethauer et al. prefer to use scope to check the patency and integrity of the tube in the end of the procedure [8].

The technique used by Ramos et al. was [15]:

- Patient under general anesthesia, in supine position, legs open.
- Closed pneumoperitoneum achieved with a five-trocar technique similar to that employed in laparoscopic Nissen fundoplication.
- Trocar placement: one 10 mm trocar above and slightly to the right of the umbilicus for the 30° laparoscope; one 10 mm trocar in the upper right quadrant (URQ) for passing the needle, suturing, and for the surgeon's right hand; one 5 mm trocar also in the URQ below the 10 mm trocar at the axillary line for the surgeon's assistant; one 5 mm trocar below the xyphoid appendices for liver retraction; and one 5 mm trocar in the upper left quadrant (ULQ) for the surgeon's left hand.
- Procedure begins with dissection of the angle of His and removal of the pad in this location.
- Careful dissection of the gastric greater curvature using the Ultracision Harmonic ™ scalpel (Ethicon Endo-Surgery, Inc., Cincinnati, OH) and opening of the greater omentum at the transition between the gastric antrum and gastric body.
- Greater curvature vessels dissected distally up to the pylorus and proximally up to the angle of His.
- Gastric plication initiated by imbricating the greater curvature over a 32 Fr bougie and applying a first row of extramucosal interrupted stitches of 2-0 Ethibond™ (Ethicon Inc., Somerville, NJ, USA) sutures.
- Two subsequent rows created with extra-mucosal running suture lines of 2-0 Prolene™ (Ethicon Inc., Somerville, NJ, USA). More recently they changed this to running suture with Ethibond™ (Ethicon Inc., Somerville, NJ, USA), due to patients presenting rupture of the prolene suture (Figs. 1 and 2).
- Leak test performed with methylene blue.
- No drains are placed.

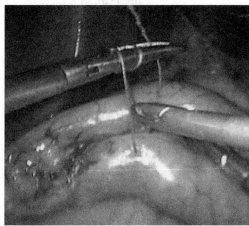 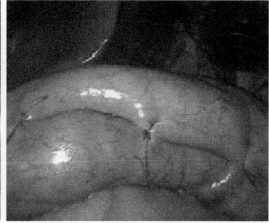

Fig. 1. Sequence of intraoperative pictures of initial suture line with interrupted nonabsorbable suture (modified from 15).

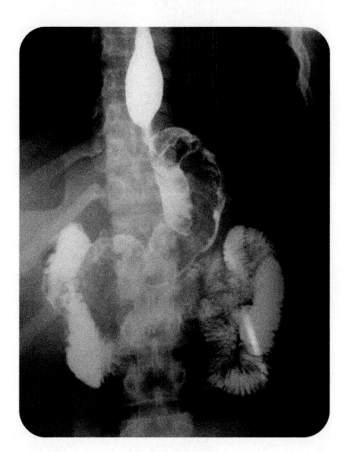

Fig. 2. Upper GI series of LGCP procedure.

Results

In a systematic review involving seven published articles, encompassing 307 patients who underwent LGCP, the mean operative time ranged from 40 to 150 min. Hospital stay length ranged between 1.3 and 1.9 days. Excess weight loss (EWL) at 6 months ranged from 54 to 51 %, while at 12

months it ranged from 67 to 53.4 %. The longest follow-up was 3 years [8, 9, 13, 15, 16, 18–20].

Universal exclusion criteria varied including pregnancy, previous bariatric or gastric surgery, hiatal hernia, uncontrolled diabetes, cardiovascular risks, history of eating disorders, medical therapy for weight loss within the previous 2 months, or any other condition that constitutes a significant risk of undergoing the procedure [12]. A BMI > 50 kg/m^2 was defined as an exclusion criterion for the Brethauer et al. and Skrekas et al. series [8, 16].

In the study by Ramos et al., 42 patients were operated, with a mean operative time of 50 min and a mean hospital stay of 36 h. No intraoperative complications were documented. The procedure was recommended to patients with morbid obesity, with mean BMI of 41 kg/m^2. Mean percentage EWL was 20 % EWL at 1 month (42 patients), 32 % EWL at 3 months (33 patients), 48 % EWL at 6 months (20 patients), 60 % EWL at 12 months (15 patients), and 62 % EWL at 18 months (9 patients) (Fig. 3). In the first postoperative week, however, nausea, vomiting, and sialorrhea occurred in 20 %, 16 %, and 35 % of patients, respectively. In all cases, these symptoms were resolved in no more than 2 weeks. No weight regain was recorded during the follow-up period [15]. In the follow-up of this group of patients, the stabilization of the weight loss in between 18 and 24 months is common, and they start to gain some weight in the third year post-surgery. By the end of the third year after the procedure, the mean EWL was 48 %, much similar with our results with adjustable gastric banding [21].

Talebpour et al. in 2012 published the longest gastric plication follow-up in medical literature, with a case series involving 800 patients, with an average time of follow-up of 5 years (range 1 month–12 years). Different techniques of plication were used. One-row plication was performed during the first 6 years of experience, followed by 6 years of two-row plication. The mean excess weight loss was 70 %

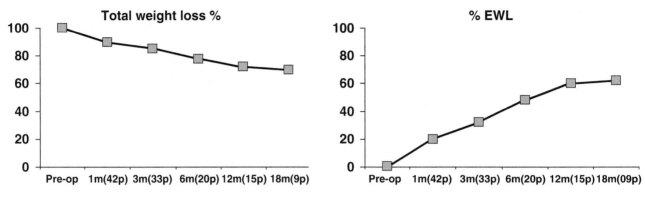

Fig. 3. Mean percentage of total weight loss and excess weight loss with LGCP procedure, in 1, 3, 6, 12, and 18 months (modified from 15).

(40–100 %) after 24 months (n=356) and 55 % (24–100 %) after 5 years (n=134). Weight regain was a complaint in 31 % of cases after the 12-year follow-up. Outside displacement of plicated fold was seen in 25 out of 38 cases of regain or failure that were reoperated. They concluded that the main reason for weight regain and failure group consisted of cases with wrong selection of technique, mainly males without good motivation. Reoperation was required in 8 patients (1 %), due to complications like microperforation, obstruction, and vomiting following adhesion of His angle. Complications were more common with the one-row plication technique. The authors concluded that the percentage of EWL in LGCP is comparable to other restrictive methods, with 1.6 % of complications, 31 % weight regain, and a lower financial cost [11].

It is important to note that Talebpour et al. used strict inclusion criteria. Gastric plication was selected for cases with potential for continuous diet and exercise after operation. In cases with less motivation, gastric bypass or a malabsorptive technique was chosen [11].

In a study focused on weight loss and type 2 diabetes outcomes, LGCP was performed in 55 morbidly obese diabetic patients, with a 1-year follow-up. BMI ranged from 35 to 52 kg/m^2 (mean 43.5 kg/m^2). Mean EWL was 35 % (30–65 %) after 12 months, with a mean BMI of 38 kg/m^2. A total of 23 % of patients stopped losing weight 6 months after the procedure, and 11 % began regaining about 14 % (12–20 %) of their EWL 9 months after the procedure. Mean HbA1c was 7.5 % (5.5–8 %) after 12 months. All patients were on oral diabetes medications preoperatively, and none had more than 5 years of disease. No patients stopped their diabetes medications after surgery. These results may indicate that LGCP has a weaker metabolic effect compared with other restrictive procedures [22]. Skrekas et al., on the other hand, showed inadequate weight loss (EWL<50 %) in 21.48 % and failure (EWL<30 %) in 5.9 % [16].

Complications

It is likely that LGCP reduces the possibility of gastric leaks. Talebpour and Amoli report one case of a gastric leak associated with a more aggressive version of LGCP, which the authors attributed to excessive vomiting in the early postoperative period [9]. In the study by Ramos et al. the adverse events described by patients were minor, such as nausea, vomiting, and hypersalivation, which were resolved quickly [15]. These events may be related to the severity of the restriction induced by the invagination of the greater curvature and/or edema caused by venous stasis. A key difference between LGCP and LSG is the presence of the endoluminal fold. Qualitative endoscopic findings suggesting that the greater curvature fold gets smaller may be related with the resolution of the initial edema, although the radiological findings did not reveal significant dilation of the LGCP at 6 months [15].

In the systematic review done by Abdelbaki et al., 8 % developed complications, with individual author complication ranging from 7 to 15.3 %. Nausea and vomiting occurred in all studies, ranging from mild to moderate, usually resolving within 1–2 weeks. Twenty patients (6.5 %) were readmitted, of whom 14 (4.6 %) required reoperation, mostly due to gastric obstruction [13].

Skrekas et al. had three cases of acute gastric obstruction, in a series of 135 patients [16]. In one of them, the fundus prolapsed in between the sutures, which was reduced and reinforced with sutures. The other two had serous fluid collection within the cavity formed by the gastric plication, both of which treated with reversal of plication. The overall complication rate in the case series was 8.8 % (12/135), including vomiting (n=4), GI bleeding (n=2), and abdominal pain attributed to a micro-leak from the suture line (n=2), one patient had a portomesenteric thrombosis leading to partial jejunal necrosis, and the three cases of gastric obstruction already described. Brethauer et al. had to reoperate on the first patient in their series due to a gastric obstruction 2 days after surgery [8].

Tsang et al. report a case of complete gastric obstruction after LGCP. At laparoscopy, no evidence of gastric necrosis or suture line leak/perforation was found. The plication sutures were removed and the stomach unfolded [20].

In one analysis of early complications in 120 patients submitted to LGCP, the major intraoperative complication was bleeding, with hemostasis achieved in all cases without the need for blood transfusion ($n=13$). During postoperative week 1, nausea, vomiting, sialorrhea, and minor hematemesis occurred in 40 %, 25 %, 22 %, and 15 % of patients, respectively. Symptoms disappeared spontaneously within 4–5 days and patients returned to normal activities 5–7 days postoperatively. In the first postoperative month, complications were mainly due to the complete obstruction of the residual gastric pouch by fold edema (5 %), extrinsic compression by intramural gastric hematoma (2 %), or elastic gastric effect of suturing and gastric tube distortion (0.8 %). Peritonitis, which occurred in one patient on POD 3 from gastric leak, was managed laparoscopically by suturing the leak hole and cleaning the whole peritoneal cavity [17].

Watkins published a case report of a 29-year-old patient who underwent LGCP, with intraoperative EGD showing a symmetric plication with an appropriately sized lumen. Postoperatively, the patient experienced liquid dysphagia, consistent with gastric edema. She was discharged home on the second POD after slight improvement. On POD 3, she returned to the emergency room with severe abdominal pain and dyspnea. An abdominal CT showed free intraperitoneal air, and the patient suffered respiratory failure. Surgical exploration revealed significant gastric necrosis in the fundus of the stomach, extending from high on the cardia down along the greater curvature to the midbody of the stomach, with a large perforation. The plication was converted to a stapled sleeve gastrectomy. Patient was discharged in good conditions. The likely cause of this complication was a lack of blood flow to the gastric wall due to edematous compression, similar to the high pressures of abdominal compartment syndrome. Although the endoscopic appearance of the initial operation was good, it likely became too tight with the edema that ensued [19].

Hii et al. report an unusual complication after LGCP: gastrogastric herniation. The patient had an AGB, with unsatisfactory weight loss, and after analysis, it was decided to do a plication below the band. At operation, the peri-band gastroplasty was undone and the greater curvature mobilized before being plicated, from below the existing band to 6 cm from the pylorus with a single row of interrupted nonabsorbable monofilament sutures, without the use of a bougie. Postoperatively the patient experienced severe nausea and vomiting, treated with antiemetics and dexamethasone to minimize edema in the intraluminal fold of stomach. The symptoms persisted, and an EGD showed a tight plication,

that still allowed passage of the endoscope. Despite a feeding tube being placed, symptoms persisted and the patient was reoperated. Laparoscopy revealed two gastrogastric hernias protruding through the imbrication stitch. The stitch was removed, showing viable tissue, allowing for a reimbrication, done with an 11 mm gastroscope in place, acting as a bougie. Patient was discharged tolerating diet. The probable causes of this complication were plication done too tight, with vomiting creating a high intraluminal pressure, and placement of too widely separated plication sutures. The authors recommend that gastric plication should be performed over a bougie, with sutures placed 1–2 cm apart [23].

A gastric perforation was described in a patient with a prior Nissen fundoplication (not taken down during LGCP procedure), happening immediately after discharge due to noncompliance with suggested food restrictions. The patient was not able to vomit, likely due to the intact Nissen fundoplication and the substantial increase in intragastric pressure. On emergency reoperation, the stitches were found to be broken, with gastric leak and peritonitis. In the same study, another major complication happened in a patient who had a gastric band and underwent LGCP to correct weight regain. An abundance of fibrous tissue adherent to the band and scarring surrounding the band area were observed. The band was removed and plication performed below the affected region. Three days following discharge patient returned with symptoms of peritonitis. On reoperation an area of partial stomach wall necrosis below the original band site was found. The authors suggest that previous surgery may limit a patient's ability to vomit and should be considered a relative contraindication to subsequent LGCP [10].

LGCP as an Adjuvant of AGB

The possibility of postoperative weight regain after LGCP still remains debatable, with most studies only showing short-term follow-up. A novel technique developed aiming to increase weight loss and prevent weight regain is the laparoscopic adjustable gastric banded plication (LAGBP) [24].

Twenty-six morbidly obese patients underwent LAGBP, preoperative mean BMI of 39.4 kg/m² (35–50.7). Swedish band placement was performed using the standard *pars flaccida* technique. The band was wrapped around the proximal gastric pouch, and two anterior gastrogastric sutures were placed to prevent slippage. A gastric plication was done using a 36 Fr bougie as calibration, with continuous seromuscular nonabsorbable sutures creating a single-layer plication along the greater curvature. Mean total operative time was 87.3 ± 22.6 min. There were no intraoperative complications. One patient presented prolonged vomiting, treated conservatively. Two patients required reoperation, due to gastrogastric intussusception and tube kinking at the subcutaneous layer. Mean EWL at 6 months was 41.3 % ($n=18$) and 59.5 % at 12 months ($n=5$) [24].

Plication as Revisional Surgery

Although some authors have been proposing and discussing the possibility of using the gastric plication concepts in revisional surgery to decrease dilated pouches, revise the size of gastric sleeves, and plicate stomachs after removing bands, there are no consistent data in the literature supporting this recommendation and there is necessity of more data and follow-up.

Conclusion

The advantages for the proposition of the gastric greater curvature plication are the decreased invasiveness with no resection, no cutting, no stapling, reversibility, and decreased risk of leaks, looking for the same results of sleeve gastrectomy, based in a low cost technique. Although these benefits were initially attractive, the excess body weight loss has been much more comparable to that achieved with adjustable gastric banding. Though rare, the risk of gastric leaks after LGCP exists, attributable to excessive intragastric pressure in the early postoperative period, due to various causes.

The mechanisms of LGCP have not yet been studied. Since gastric resection is not performed, it is unlikely that the ghrelin levels will decrease in the same way they do after LSG. Brethauer et al. suggest that LGCP leads to good hunger control, but in a lesser degree than what is observed after LSG [8].

In 2011 the American Society for Metabolic and Bariatric Surgery issued a statement regarding LGCP, with the following recommendations [25]:

- Gastric plication procedures should be considered investigational at present. This procedure should be performed under a study protocol with third-party oversight (local or regional ethics committee, institutional review board, data monitoring and safety board, or equivalent authority) to ensure continuous evaluation of patient safety and to review adverse events and outcomes.
- Reporting of short- and long-term safety and efficacy in the medical literature is strongly encouraged. Data from these procedures should also be reported to a program's center of excellence database.
- Any marketing or advertisement for this procedure should include a statement to the effect that this is an investigational procedure.

Current evidence regarding LGCP is scant and mostly described in a few studies with small series of patients and a short follow-up. Additional studies are needed to determine its effectiveness and safety as a primary operation for obesity (Video 1).

References

1. DeMaria EJ. Bariatric surgery for morbid obesity. N Engl J Med. 2007;356(21):2176–83.
2. Kirk RM. An experimental trial of gastric plication as a means of weight reduction in the rat. Br J Surg. 1969;56(12):930–3.
3. Tretbar LL, Taylor TL, Sifers EC. Weight reduction. Gastric plication for morbid obesity. J Kans Med Soc. 1976;77(11):488–90.
4. Wilkinson LH, Peloso OA. Gastric (reservoir) reduction for morbid obesity. Arch Surg. 1981;116(5):602–5.
5. Neumayer C, Ciovica R, Gadenstatter M, Erd G, Leidl S, Lehr S, et al. Significant weight loss after laparoscopic Nissen fundoplication. Surg Endosc. 2005;19(1):15–20.
6. Fusco PE, Poggetti RS, Younes RN, Fontes B, Birolini D. Evaluation of gastric greater curvature invagination for weight loss in rats. Obes Surg. 2006;16(2):172–7.
7. Fusco PE, Poggetti RS, Younes RN, Fontes B, Birolini D. Comparison of anterior gastric wall and greater gastric curvature invaginations for weight loss in rats. Obes Surg. 2007;17(10):1340–5.
8. Brethauer SA, Harris JL, Kroh M, Schauer PR. Laparoscopic gastric plication for treatment of severe obesity. Surg Obes Relat Dis. 2011;7(1):15–22.
9. Talebpour M, Amoli BS. Laparoscopic total gastric vertical plication in morbid obesity. J Laparoendosc Adv Surg Tech A. 2007;17(6):793–8.
10. Fried M, Dolezalova K, Buchwald JN, McGlennon TW, Sramkova P, Ribaric G. Laparoscopic greater curvature plication (LGCP) for treatment of morbid obesity in a series of 244 patients. Obes Surg. 2012;22(8):1298–307.
11. Talebpour M, Motamedi SM, Talebpour A, Vahidi H. Twelve year experience of laparoscopic gastric plication in morbid obesity: development of the technique and patient outcomes. Ann Surg Innov Res. 2012;6(1):7.
12. Kourkoulos M, Giorgakis E, Kokkinos C, Mavromatis T, Griniatsos J, Nikiteas N, et al. Laparoscopic gastric plication for the treatment of morbid obesity: a review. Minim Invasive Surg. 2012;2012:696348.
13. Abdelbaki TN, Huang CK, Ramos A, Neto MG, Talebpour M, Saber AA. Gastric plication for morbid obesity: a systematic review. Obes Surg. 2012;22(10):1633–9.
14. Menchaca HJ, Harris JL, Thompson SE, Mootoo M, Michalek VN, Buchwald H. Gastric plication: preclinical study of durability of serosa-to-serosa apposition. Surg Obes Relat Dis. 2011;7(1):8–14.
15. Ramos A, Galvao Neto M, Galvao M, Evangelista LF, Campos JM, Ferraz A. Laparoscopic greater curvature plication: initial results of an alternative restrictive bariatric procedure. Obes Surg. 2010;20(7):913–8.
16. Skrekas G, Antiochos K, Stafyla VK. Laparoscopic gastric greater curvature plication: results and complications in a series of 135 patients. Obes Surg. 2011;21(11):1657–63.
17. Andraos D, Ziade D, Achcouty R, Awad M. Early complications of 120 laparoscopic greater curvature plication procedures. Bariatric Times. 2011;8(9):10–5.
18. Pujol Gebelli J, Garcia Ruiz de Gordejuela A, Casajoana Badia A, Secanella Medayo L, Vicens Morton A, Masdevall Noguera C. Laparoscopic Gastric Plication: a new surgery for the treatment of morbid obesity. Cir Esp. 2011;89(6):356–61.
19. Watkins BM. Gastric compartment syndrome: an unusual complication of gastric plication surgery. Surg Obes Relat Dis. 2011;10.
20. Tsang A, Jain V. Pitfalls of bariatric tourism: a complication of gastric plication. Surg Obes Relat Dis. 2011;28.
21. Toouli J, Kow L, Ramos AC, Aigner F, Pattyn P, Galvao-Neto MP, et al. International multicenter study of safety and effectiveness of

Swedish Adjustable Gastric Band in 1-, 3-, and 5-year follow-up cohorts. Surg Obes Relat Dis. 2009;5(5):598–609.

22. Taha O. Efficacy of laparoscopic greater curvature plication for weight loss and type 2 diabetes: 1-year follow-up. Obes Surg. 2012;22(10):1629–32.

23. Hii MW, Clarke NE, Hopkins GH. Gastrogastric herniation: an unusual complication following greater curve plication for the treatment of morbid obesity. Ann R Coll Surg Engl. 2012; 94(2):e76–8.

24. Huang CK, Lo CH, Shabbir A, Tai CM. Novel bariatric technology: laparoscopic adjustable gastric banded plication: technique and preliminary results. Surg Obes Relat Dis. 2012;8(1):41–5.

25. Clinical Issues Committee. ASMBS policy statement on gastric plication. Surg Obes Relat Dis. 2011;7(3):262.

19

Laparoscopic Adjustable Gastric Banding: Technique

George Fielding

Standard Technique

After induction of general anesthesia and placement of inflatable pressure garments on the legs to minimize the risk of deep vein thrombosis, the abdomen is prepped and draped in the usual way. The patient is given subcutaneous heparin and a prophylactic antibiotic after induction.

I perform the surgery with the patient flat, in moderate reverse Trendelenburg position. I stand on the patient's right side, with my assistant and the scrub nurse opposite me.

Access to the abdomen is gained with an optical viewing port and a zero-degree laparoscope via an incision 1 cm below the end of the left costal margin. Once the abdomen is insufflated, a 30° scope is used for the rest of the procedure. A Nathanson liver retractor is placed via an incision over the xiphisternum. Three ports are placed in a line across the abdomen from the Optiview port—a 5 mm, a 15 mm, and another 5 mm—which is at the end of the right costal margin.

I use an Allergan AP Standard band for all women, irrespective of size, and for smaller men who are not diabetic. I use an Allergan AP Large for most men, due to their increased intra-abdominal fat. I make that determination before we start the case, and insert the band through the 15 mm port as soon as it's in place.

All the instruments should be extra long, at least 45 cm. A soft grasper is inserted through the right 5 mm port, to be used by the surgeon. Another is placed through the left 5 mm port. This grasper is passed to the top of the stomach, over the omentum. The handle is pushed towards the head, causing the tip of the grasper to sweep towards the feet, taking the omentum with it, thus putting the fundus on stretch, and exposing the hiatus and gastroesophageal junction. The assistant holds that grasper steady with their left hand during

Electronic supplementary material: Supplementary material is available in the online version of this chapter at 10.1007/978-1-4939-1637-5_19. Videos can also be accessed at http://www.springerimages.com/videos/978-1-4939-1636-8.

the entire procedure, maintaining an excellent exposure. A hook dissector is placed through the 15 mm port.

The first step is to assess the hiatus. It is essential to repair any hiatal hernia, or crural defect, no matter how small. We at NYU have shown that it significantly reduces the need for reoperation to treat reflux. Some surgeons do a crural repair in every case.

Using the hook, the peritoneum over the left crus of the diaphragm is divided, and the fundus completely mobilized off the diaphragm (Fig. 1). This is done by a combination of hook and blunt dissection, always pushing the tissue towards the feet. Once the left crus is exposed, the dissection continues across the front of the esophagus to the right crus. There will often be a thickened peritoneal reflection over the front of the esophagus, which is pushed superiorly along the esophagus. The right crus is then exposed in a similar fashion (Fig. 2). In many cases, all that is required is to close the crura anteriorly, using a 0 Prolene figure-of-8 suture. If there is a true, large hiatal hernia, it is better to repair it posteriorly, behind the esophagus. I use mesh reinforcement for large or paraesophageal hernias. I prefer the shaped Cook mesh, which I hold in place posteriorly with ProTacks, and anteriorly with sutures. It is important not to use tacks anteriorly, due to the risk of injuring the pericardium. It's worth stating that even a very large paraesophageal hernia is not a contraindication to a band.

Attention is then turned to placing the band. The lesser omentum is incised over the caudate lobe of the liver. The right crus always disappears into a small fat pad, where it meets the left crus. The point of dissection is right at that fat pad. A small incision is made there with the hook. There is a beautiful plane behind the esophagus starting at that point. It is essential for the assistant to maintain the sweeping retraction of the fundus. The surgeon's left hand grasper is then gently inserted into the small incision and passed behind the esophagus, to emerge in front of the left crus (Fig. 3), often going behind the spleen. There should be no resistance at all when the grasper is passed. If there is, it's usually that the fundus is being inadequately retracted, or that it has not

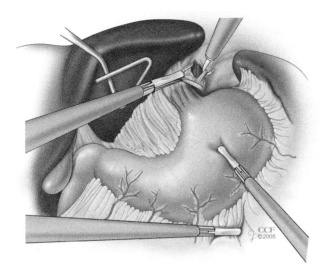

FIG. 1. Exposure of the angle of His. The lateral segment of the left lobe of liver is retracted upwards. The omental fat has been retracted downwards and the fundus is drawn downward by the assistant. The diathermy hook is opening the peritoneum over the left crus. Copyright CCF, with permission.

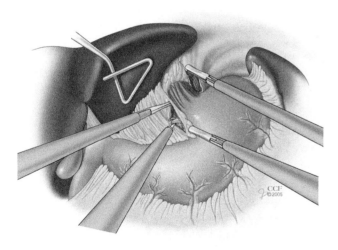

FIG. 2. Exposure of the right crus. Hiatal hernia, if identified, should be reduced and repaired. Copyright CCF, with permission.

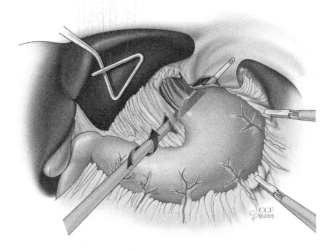

FIG. 3. The peritoneum has been opened and a tunnel developed using the grasper. The instrument should be passed easily without resistance. Copyright CCF, with permission.

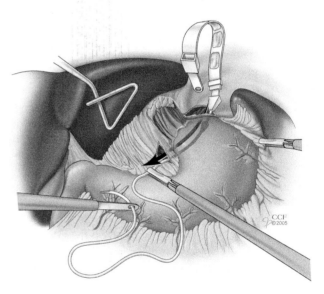

FIG. 4. The tubing is pulled through the tunnel to position the band in place. Copyright CCF, with permission.

been adequately mobilized off the left crus. The key maneuver is for the surgeon to keep their left hand grasper completely horizontal. There is a natural tendency for the tip of the grasper to slide anteriorly, a tendency that should be avoided.

The tubing of the band is brought up and grasped, then drawn behind the esophagus (Fig. 4). The band is locked (Fig. 5). The end of the tubing should come across in front of the liver like a spear, going easily into its socket. The key to locking the band is to do it gently, keeping the parts in the same plane. Any rotation will cause the silicon to lock.

There are two schools of thought about band fixation, either none at all or to use gastrogastric sutures.

Martin Fried, from Prague, has advocated using no sutures. From January to September 2006, he randomized 100 patients undergoing banding to group 1 ($n=50$, ≥ 2 imbrication sutures) or group 2 ($n=50$, no imbrication sutures).

The 3-year EWL was 55.7 % ± 3.4 % and 58.1 % ± 4.1 % for groups 1 and 2, respectively. The body mass index at 3 years was 34.0 ± 5.8 kg/m^2 and 30.3 ± 6.4 kg/m^2 (range 1.2–6.2) for groups 1 and 2, respectively ($P<0.01$). He found that slippage occurred in 1 patient (2.2 %) and 1 patient (2.0 %) and migration in 1 patient (2.2 %) and 1 patient (2.0 %) in

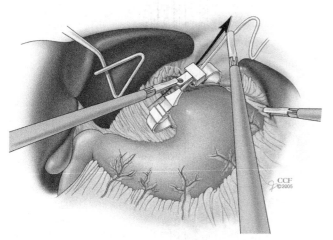

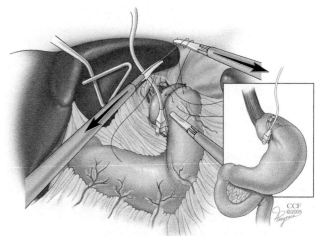

Fig. 5. The band is locked in place. Copyright CCF, with permission.

Fig. 6. Completion of anterior fixation with avoidance of bringing the gastric wall against the buckle of the band. Copyright CCF, with permission.

groups 1 and 2, respectively (P=NS). Martin concluded that the band is effective and safe with and without imbrication sutures.

Paul Super, from Birmingham, England, has taken the opposite view. Between April 2003 and June 2007, he performed banding in 1,140 consecutive patients. He used a gastropexy suture in addition to the two routine gastro-gastro tunnel sutures in all cases. The gastropexy picks up four bites of fundus and brings it to the diaphragm near the left crus. Excess percent BMI loss in these patients at 36 months was 58.9 %. Slippage with urgent readmission occurred in one patient (0.08 %) at 5 months. Two partial slippages were noticed at 12 and 18 months, respectively.

Both these approaches have delivered great results. Our choice has been to incorporate what Paul Super does by using a 2-0 Prolene to do a gastropexy, then another to do a running gastrogastric suture over the band, stopping 1 cm from the buckle (Fig. 6). I then add another gastropexy below the band, the Patterson stitch, devised by Emma Patterson, of Portland, Oregon. It's definitely belt and braces, but if it helps reduce slip, it's worth it.

The tubing is then brought out through the 15 mm port and attached to the port. A small disk of mesh is sutured to the back of the port. The port is then placed on the deep fascia, where the mesh sticks and fixes the port in position.

The wounds are closed with Monocryl and the patient sent to the recovery room, ready to start their weight loss journey.

Single Incision Band Surgery

Surgeons have recently been performing many surgical procedures, including appendectomy, cholecystectomy, fundoplication, Heller myotomy, distal gastrectomy, segmental colon resection, laparoscopic adjustable gastric band

(LAGB), sleeve gastrectomy, and Roux-en-Y gastric bypass (RYGB) through single incision laparoscopic surgery (SILS) or, in the case of gastric procedures, a single working incision, and another for liver retraction. The obvious benefit is cosmesis, especially if the incision is placed inside the umbilicus.

At NYU, we performed a retrospective review of 1,644 LAGBs performed at our institution between November 1, 2008 and November 30, 2010. Of these, 756 were performed as SILS bands (46 %) and 888 as non-SILS (54 %) with the standard 4–5 trocar incisions.

In our initial experience, we limited SILS to women with lower BMIs. As our experience grew, we included men and women with higher BMIs. We excluded patients with any incision at the umbilicus. A relative exclusion was a long torso, where the distance from xiphoid process to umbilicus was greater than 26 cm, as it would impact on the ease of instruments reaching the diaphragm with any mobility. We still prefer standard technique in men with BMI over 50 due to the difficulty retracting omentum and peri-gastric fat.

When starting to use SILS, we did it in a stepwise fashion, gradually removing ports and moving to the umbilical approach over at least 20 cases. This allowed us to develop some facility with the crossed-hands and limited angulation technique required for SILS.

Our SILS technique uses a single periumbilical 3–4 cm incision with placement of a 12 mm trocar via the Hassan technique under direct vision. The band is placed through a 1 cm incision at the base of the umbilical stalk. This is exactly the same incision we have used for thousands of laparoscopic general surgery operations. The band is inserted into the abdomen prior to placement of the 12 mm trocar through the 1 cm umbilical defect. Then, two 5 mm ports are placed to the right and left of the 12 mm trocar to minimize clashing. These trocars are staggered in length: on the right side a long trocar and the left side a short one, flush with the skin. Liver retraction is obtained either via the same infraumbilical incision (Genzyme liver retractor) or via a subxiphoid percutaneous method (Nathanson liver retractor).

The band is placed via the standard pars flaccida technique. Once all ports are inserted, a left-handed grasper is used to retract the greater curvature, exposing the angle of His. Electrocautery, held in the right hand, is used to divide the phrenoesophageal ligament and mobilize the angle of His, exposing the left crus. If a hiatal hernia or dimple in the crura is appreciated, the hiatus is fully dissected and the hernia is repaired. The gastrohepatic ligament is then divided, and the right crus exposed. A flexible grasper held in the right hand is then curved and inserted at the base of the right crus into a retrogastric tunnel, exiting at the angle of His. The band is pulled through, locked, and fixed using a 2-0 nonabsorbable gastrogastric running plication suture. Finally, the tubing is pulled out through the left-sided 5 mm trocar. The fascial defect is closed using a 0 Vicryl suture in a figure-of-eight manner and the port is attached and fixed to the anterior fascia, to the right of the umbilicus.

The mean operating time of an SILS band was 44.7 ± 20 min (12–179 min), compared to 51.1 ± 19.6 min for non-SILS bands (15–147 min). This difference was found to be statistically significant ($P < 0.001$). Over the 2-year follow-up, 37 patients (5 %) in the SILS group and 22 patients (3.7 %) in the non-SILS patients had reoperations for port complications and band slip. One SILS patient developed an umbilical hernia.

Can SILS LAGB be done? Certainly. The data in our study confirm that the two techniques are equitable in terms of operating time, complications, and outcomes.

Should it be done? Yes, but only if the surgeon finds the technique interesting, is prepared to carefully accumulate the necessary skill set, and feels that the cosmetic benefit is worth the extra trouble and difficulty. Triangulation of instruments is the key to an easy day in the operating room doing laparoscopic surgery. It becomes second nature and governs all port positions. SILS does away with triangulation. The jump from 5-port LAGB placement to one or two ports is challenging. To this end, we recommend a staged approach to starting SILS LAGB surgery. This explains why we have so many non-SILS cases over the time period, most from the first year. Our practice now is to perform SILS in the majority of our cases.

In an attempt to maximize triangulation, our preference is to use individual ports in the same incision. We have tried all available SILS port systems and found that they all restrict movement much more than do individual ports. It is also nice to use one's normal ports and instruments. This technique also reduces fascial incision size. The incision we use is 1 cm at the base of the umbilical stalk. We don't incise fascia at all. We have used the same incision for thousands of general

laparoscopic operations for over 20 years, and there is minimal risk of umbilical hernia. It needs to be 1 cm to allow nontraumatic insertion of the lap band. This is in contrast to the incision size needed for all available SILS ports.

The key with SILS is to become comfortable with crossed-hands operating and operating with hands almost in parallel. SILS is definitely more difficult than standard laparoscopy, and many surgeons will think it's not worth the extra time and trouble. That being said, when you have developed those skills, it's very satisfying to be able to offer a patient an operation with scars that are almost invisible at 3 months. Given that the only benefit of this technique seems to be cosmetic, we prefer to hide the incision in the umbilical crease, rather than place it in a more visible superior position. The addition of a tiny xiphoid incision for the Nathanson liver retractor barely diminishes this benefit, especially in men with body hair.

It must seem strange that a SILS operation can be quicker than a 4- or 5-port technique. We gradually accumulated our skill set, such that by the second year, we were able to perform these surgeries in a very timely manner. The lower time probably reflects having to place fewer ports and close fewer wounds. We have no explanation as to why the SILS group did better with weight loss. One possible, though very nebulous, idea is that they were more motivated and enthusiastic in their follow-up after they saw their good cosmetic outcome.

SILS is a step forward for patients if they are worried about their scars. The main benefit is that the total experience for the patient is better. This is especially so for women who don't have body hair to hide incisions. This is important after bariatric surgery and it removes the need to explain incisions until patients are comfortable discussing their surgery, enhancing their privacy and comfort zone. This cosmetic benefit is also very valuable for African-Americans who are more prone to keloid scarring.

Many patients comment favorably on the incision at follow-up, feeling that it has enhanced their overall experience. The joy of laparoscopic surgery is that we help people without hurting them too much. Now we can do it without leaving them easily visible incisions. Using what we have learned from SILS bands, we have extended our experience to include Roux-en-Y gastric bypass, sleeve gastrectomy, Heller myotomy, and Nissen fundoplication.

We have found the SILS band placement is a valid technique, with outcomes at least as good as those with standard LAGB. If time is taken to gradually accumulate the different skill sets required to operate this way, by starting in a staged fashion, and excluding patients with a very long torso, or males with a high BMI, there would seem to be a benefit to the patients, in an improved overall experience. Its difficulty, though, should not be underestimated.

Conclusion

Band surgery is gentle. The risks are very low and if the band is placed properly, and if hiatal hernias are fixed, the need for reoperation is small (Video 1).

Bibliography

1. Fielding GA, Allen JW. A step-by-step guide to placement of the LAP BAND adjustable gastric banding system. Am J Surg. 2002;184(6B):26S–30.
2. Hernia Gulkarov I, Wetterau M, Ren CJ, Fielding GA. Hiatal hernia repair at the initial laparoscopic adjustable gastric band operation reduces the need for reoperation. Surg Endosc. 2008;22(4):1035–41.
3. Dixon AF, Dixon JB, O'Brien PE. Laparoscopic adjustable gastric banding induces prolonged satiety: a randomized blind crossover study. J Clin Endocrinol Metab. 2005;90(2):813–9.
4. O'Brien PE, Macdonald L, Anderson M, Brennan L, Brown WA. Long-term outcomes after bariatric surgery: fifteen-year follow-up of adjustable gastric banding and a systematic review of the bariatric surgical literature. Ann Surg. 2013;257(1):87–94.
5. Weichman Weichman K, Ren C, Kurian M, Heekoung A, Casciano R, Stern L, et al. The effectiveness of adjustable gastric banding: a retrospective 6-year U.S. follow-up study. Surg Endosc. 2011; 25(2):397–403.
6. Fried M, Dolezalova K, Sramkova P. Adjustable gastric banding outcomes with and without gastrogastric imbrication sutures: a randomized controlled trial. Surg Obes Relat Dis. 2011;7(1): 23–31.
7. Singhal R, Kitchen M, Ndirika S, Hunt K, Bridgwater S, Super P. The "Birmingham stitch"—avoiding slippage in laparoscopic gastric banding. Obes Surg. 2008;18(4):359–63.

20

Laparoscopic Adjustable Gastric Banding: Outcomes

Jaime Ponce and Wendy A. Brown

Introduction

The laparoscopic adjustable gastric banding (LAGB) procedure involves the placement of an adjustable silicone band around the very upper part of the stomach immediately below the gastroesophageal junction. The level of restriction can be adjusted by adding or removing saline from the band via a subcutaneous port fixed to the anterior rectus sheath.

LAGB is the safest of the bariatric procedures [1, 2] with minimal mortality and morbidity. It can be performed as an overnight stay or same-day procedure in even the largest of patients.

The mechanism of action of the LAGB is the induction of early satiation (food satisfaction) with a small meal followed by a longer period of satiety (between-meal lack of hunger). Studies have shown that delay in gastric emptying is not the main mechanism of action and there is a lack of correlation between over-restriction and satiety [3]. Similarly, the band should not physically limit significantly food transit and there should be negligible food found above the band after a meal if the band is correctly adjusted [4]. A range of hormones including insulin, leptin, ghrelin, pancreatic polypeptide, and peptide YY do not play a significant role in LAGB function [5, 6]. It is hypothesized that the mechanical effects of the band and the passage of food bolus through this area of band resistance can generate myoenteric pressure signals [7]. Signals from these receptors may be important in both meal termination and satisfaction, and provide an important sense of well-being, although the functional roles of these receptors remain poorly understood [8].

Ongoing improvements in band placement and postoperative management have reduced morbidity as well as short-term and long-term complications. There have been a number of changes to the procedure of LAGB placement and aftercare since the original description. The surgical technique has been modified, and the majority of LAGB are now placed by the pars flaccida approach rather than the perigastric approach [9]. A randomized controlled trial comparing these techniques demonstrated fewer long-term complications with the pars flaccida approach than the perigastric approach along with a shorter operating time [10].

As the understanding of the mechanism of action of the LAGB has improved, so have aftercare programs. An optimal program will provide regular follow-up focusing on educating patients about correct food choices, small serving sizes, and emphasizing the importance of eating slowly and chewing the food well. Band adjustments should focus on the induction of early and prolonged satiety and when this is achieved, weight loss is optimal. Hunger and food seeking behavior suggests that the band is under-filled. Symptoms of reflux and an inability to eat solid food suggest the band is over-adjusted and that fluid should be removed [3].

Outcomes of LAGB surgery can be measured by change in weight, comorbidity, quality of life, long-term survival, and cost-effectiveness. The need for revisional surgery is another important outcome, and this must be considered in the context of the safety of the revision as well as the effect of the revision on weight, health, and well-being.

Weight Loss Outcomes

Weight loss after gastric banding is typically very steady at 0.5–1 kg/week. This means that weight loss progresses over a 2- to 3-year period and then stabilizes, usually in the range of 40–55 % EWL. Medium- and long-term (4- to 15-year follow-up) outcomes have been reported by individual series showing a great variation in weight loss results from 33 to 70 % EWL [11, 12] (Tables 1 and 2).

The weight loss following LAGB is gradual, 0.5–1 kg per week, and optimal outcomes require lifelong follow-up [13]. Follow-up is more intensive in the first year, with most patients requiring 6–8 visits [14, 15]. After the first year, most patients only require six monthly or annual visits. This model of care fits with the management of obesity as a chronic disease, and has been shown to be cost-effective [16–18].

S.A. Brethauer et al. (eds.), *Minimally Invasive Bariatric Surgery*,
DOI 10.1007/978-1-4939-1637-5_20, © Springer Science+Business Media New York 2015

There have been two prospective multicenter Food and Drug Administration-monitored clinical trials in the United States. The Lap-Band trial A [19] recruited patients from 1995 to 1998 in eight centers; 259 out of 292 patients had the band implanted laparoscopically by perigastric dissection. The average EWL was 26.5 % at 6 months, 34.5 % at 12 months, 37.8 % at 24 months, and 36.2 % at 36 months. The very high incidence of gastric prolapse and slippages was attributed to the learning curve, as most of the surgeons involved were inexperienced laparoscopic surgeons, as well as the use of the perigastric dissection rather than pars flaccida. There was also a lack of effective follow-up, with an average of only 1.2 adjustments in the first year. The majority of patients were adjusted by radiologist based on a contrast swallow evaluation rather than tailoring the adjustment to the patient's sensation of satiety. There was no good band-specific patient education program.

The Swedish Band clinical study [20] recruited 276 patients in 12 centers in 2003. All patients were implanted laparoscopically by pars flaccida technique. This trial included centers with both large and no experience with gastric banding management. The mean % EWL at 3 years was 41.1 %.

TABLE 1. Gastric banding short- and medium-term weight loss (1–8 years)

Study	% Excess weight loss					
	1 year	2 years	3 years	4 years	5 years	8 years
FDA trials						
Lap-Band A[a] [19] (1995–2001)			36			
Swedish Band [20] (2003–2006)			41			
Randomized studies						
Angrisani et al. [21]					47	
Nguyen et al. [22]				45		
O'Brien et al.[b] [23]		87				
Dixon et al.[b] [25]		62				
O'Brien et al. [24]		73				
Dixon et al. [26]		40				
Systematic reviews						
Buchwald et al. [27]		47				
O'Brien et al. [13]	43		57		54	59
Cunneen et al. [28]			50–56			

FDA Food and Drug Administration

[a]Perigastric technique

[b]Body mass index between 30 and 40 kg/m^2

There have been two prospective randomized clinical studies comparing gastric banding with the gastric bypass. Angrisani [21] randomized 51 patients and allocated them to undergo either banding ($n=27$) or gastric bypass ($n=24$). At 5 years after the procedure, the band patients had an average % EWL of 47.5 % vs. 66.6 % for the gastric bypass group. In a similar study, Nguyen [22] randomized and followed 86 patients with gastric banding and 111 with gastric bypass. The % EWL at 4 years was 45 % vs. 68 %, respectively.

There have been four randomized controlled trials assessing the effectiveness of LAGB with conservative weight loss programs, with all showing substantially better weight loss and comorbidity resolution in the surgical arm [23–26]. In the initial trial, patients with a body mass index between 30 and 40 kg/m^2 the gastric banding group showed 87 % EWL compared with the conservative arm 22 % EWL at 2 years of follow-up [23].

There have been several meta-analyses and systematic reviews of the literature that included a significant number of gastric band patients. Buchwald et al. [27] published a large bariatric surgery meta-analysis and systematic review that included 136 studies with 3,873 LAGB patients with the majority of the studies having 2 years or less follow-up reported. The mean EWL was 47.5 %. O'Brien et al. [13] extracted reports out of the English literature with more than 100 patients and at least 3-year follow-up. 4,456 band patients were analyzed, and EWL at 1, 3, 5, and 8 years was 42.6 %, 57.5 %, 54 %, and 59.3 %, respectively. Finally, Cunneen et al. [28] published a systematic review comparing data available on the two bands: a total of 129 studies (33 with Swedish band data and 104 with Lap-Band data). The 3-year mean Swedish and Lap-Band EWL was 56.4 % and 50.2 %, respectively, without statistically significant difference.

There have been seven case series reporting long-term (≥10 year) outcomes [29–34]. The weighted mean at maximum follow-up was 51.7 % EWL (Table 2) [12].

Comorbidity and Quality of Life Outcomes

Weight loss following LAGB surgery is accompanied by improvements in, or normalization of, insulin sensitivity and glycemia, obesity-related dyslipidemia, type 2 diabetes, non-

TABLE 2. Gastric banding long-term outcomes (≥10 years) [12]

Author	Number of patients	Follow-up %	Revisions or reversals (%)	Follow-up (years)	Number of patients at maximum years	Excess weight loss at maximum years (%)
Miller et al. [32]	554	92	8	10	154	59
Favretti et al. [29]	1,791	91	19	11	28	38
Lanthaler et al. [31]	276	80	53	10	Not reported	60
Naef et al. [33]	167	94	20	10	28	49
Himpens et al. [30]	154	54	60	12	36	48
Stroh et al. [34]	200	84	26	12	15	33
O'Brien et al. [12]	3,227	81	43	15	54	47

alcoholic fatty liver disease, sleep disturbance including obstructive sleep apnea and daytime sleepiness, ovulatory function and fertility in women with polycystic ovary syndrome, reflux disease, joint disease, hypertension, and depression among others. The degree of resolution or improvement is variable depending on several factors including percentage of weight loss, severity, and duration of the disease [35, 36].

The improvement in diabetes following weight loss after LAGB is related to the combined effects of improvement in insulin sensitivity and pancreatic beta-cell function associated to weight loss and decreased caloric intake [37]. As beta-cell function deteriorates progressively over time in those with type 2 diabetes, early weight loss intervention should therefore be a central part of initial therapy in severely obese subjects who develop type 2 diabetes [38].

In a randomized controlled trial of LAGB versus optimal conventional therapy in recently diagnosed (<2 years) type 2 diabetes, a clear benefit was shown for the surgical approach [25]. There was remission of diabetes (normal serum glucose, HbA1c<6.2 % while taking no hypoglycemic therapy) in 73 % of the surgical group and 13 % of the conventional group. There were no serious adverse events in either group.

A large series of 102 type 2 diabetic patients with an average BMI 46.3 kg/m^2 documented 40 % resolution (no medication requirement, with HbA1c <6 and/or glucose <100 mg/dL) at 5 years follow-up after LAGB. The mean duration of the diabetes before surgery was 6.5 years [39].

There is evidence of a reduction in both systolic and diastolic blood pressure (BP) following weight loss in association with LAGB [40]. The outcomes of 147 consecutive hypertensive patients at 12 months after LAGB demonstrated that 80 patients (55 %) had resolution of the problem (i.e., normal BP and taking no antihypertensive therapy), 45 patients (31 %) were improved (less therapy and easier control), and 22 patients (15 %) were unchanged [35]. In a study of 189 hypertensive patients treated by LAGB [41], there was resolution of hypertension (normal pressures, off therapy) in 60 % at 12 months and 74 % at 2 years. The fall in blood pressure is sustained to at least 4 years after surgery [42].

There are major improvements in sleep quality, excessive daytime sleepiness, snoring, nocturnal choking, and observed obstructive sleep apnea with weight loss following LAGB surgery. Obstructive sleep apnea and other sleep disturbances have been studied in 313 patients prior to LAGB and repeated at one year after operation in 123 of the patients [43]. There was a high prevalence of significantly disturbed sleep in both men (59 %) and women (45 %). Observed sleep apnea was decreased from 33 to 2 %, habitual snoring from 82 to 14 %, abnormal daytime sleepiness from 39 to 4 %, and poor sleep quality from 39 to 2 %. However, in a recent randomized controlled trial comparing LAGB to conservative weight loss, despite a marked difference in weight loss, the change in the apnea-hypoxia index (AHI) was not statistically significantly different between groups, reducing by 14 events

per hour in the conservative group and 25.5 events per hour in the surgical group [26].

Quality of Life

One large prospective study evaluated QOL after LAGB surgery using the Medical Outcome Study Short Form-36 (SF-36) health survey, which includes both physical and psychosocial dynamics [40]. Among the 459 patients, all of these areas significantly improved after surgery. The patients' QOL within 1 year of LAGB was closer to that of normal community values, and this finding was sustained throughout the 4 years of the study. Similarly in QOL measured as part of an RCT comparing LAGB to conservative weight loss, major benefits were seen across all domains [23].

Long-Term Mortality Outcomes

There are several studies that have examined long-term mortality in patients undergoing bariatric surgery, including LAGB, and comparing this to matched community controls. The range of reduction of medium-term mortality is 64–72 % giving a combined reduction in medium-term mortality of approximately 50 % [44].

An Australian group of 966 patients achieved a mean weight loss of 22.8 % 2 years after LAGB and, when compared with a matched community cohort at a mean of 5 years follow-up, had an adjusted 72 % lower risk of death [45]. Similarly, an evaluation of 821 LAGB patients in Italy documented a 64 % lower risk of death 5 years post-LAGB [46].

Cost-Effectiveness Outcomes

There are a number of studies that have demonstrated that over time LAGB surgery is not only cost-effective, but is delivering direct health cost savings [16, 17, 47]. In a recent study using US health care claims data from over 7,000 LAGB patients compared with a propensity score matched control group with a BMI greater than 35 kg/m^2, there were modest sustained savings in the LAGB group, but continuing cost increases in the control group. The net costs of banding had been reduced to zero in 4 years after band placement. In a subgroup with type 2 diabetes having LAGB surgery, net costs reduced to zero in just over 2 years [48]. Similar analyses in Europe have also demonstrated cost savings following band placement [49].

Revisional Surgery

The long-term need for revisional procedures following LAGB is 8–60 % [12]. In a published series of 3,227 patients who had undergone LAGB from 1994 to 2011 [12], there was 47.1 % EWL at 15 years ($N=54$; 95 % CI=8.3) and 62 % EWL at 16 years ($N=14$; 95 % CI=13.6). Revisional procedures were performed for proximal enlargement (26 %), erosion (3.4 %), and port and tubing problems (21 %). The band was explanted in 5.6 %. The need for revision decreased as the technique evolved, with 40 % revision rate for proximal gastric enlargements in the first 10 years, reducing to 6.4 % in the past 5 years. The revision group showed a similar weight loss to the overall group beyond 10 years. There was no perioperative mortality for the primary placement or for any revisional procedures.

Impact of Different Methods of Band Placement

Perigastric Dissection

The perigastric pathway was the traditional dissection for placement of the band. One significant problem with this dissection was the band placement through the lesser sac cavity just at the apex. The smooth peritonealized surface of the posterior wall of the stomach could be drawn across the band in response to force (i.e., vomiting) creating a posterior gastric prolapse. The perigastric technique was used in early experience and, along with steep learning curves on the part of the surgeons and early deficiencies in postoperative management protocols, probably contributed to poor results in some centers. In a prospective randomized comparison study [10] between both techniques, the perigastric technique patients had significantly higher incidence of prolapse (mainly posterior) compared with the pars flaccida group (16 % vs. 4 % at 2-year follow-up). Longer follow-up of the perigastric technique, up to 12 years, has demonstrated a high incidence of posterior pouch enlargements and band erosions were encountered [12, 30]. The perigastric approach should be considered a historical technique that has almost disappeared in published clinical practices.

Band Placement Without Gastro-Gastric Plication

Few authors have suggested the placement of a gastric band without gastro-gastric plication. In this technique the band is being placed in a similar fashion as described in the pars flaccida dissection. Care is taken to make very minimal dissection at the angle of His creating a small opening just big enough for the dissector. Also during the retrogastric dissection, meticulous attention is given to the creation of a very narrow retrogastric tunnel before the introduction of the laparoscopic adjustable gastric band. It has been suggested that the narrow and tight posterior tunnel will hold the band in the appropriate position avoiding

slippage. No gastro-gastric imbrication sutures are placed. Slow and very gradual adjustments with careful monitoring to avoid vomiting may help to prevent band displacement.

Two randomized control studies comparing this technique with the traditional placement with imbrication plication sutures have been published with opposite results. In the first one, Fried et al. [50] compared 50 patients in each group showing no difference in band slippages or erosions at 3-year follow-up. In the second one, Lazzati et al. [51] studies 81 patients divided into two groups and early termination of the study was documented secondary to three early slippages in the non-plication group. This technique needs to be studied further and it is not well accepted within the bariatric surgery community.

Summary

The LAGB helps to develop early satiation following a small meal followed by a prolonged period of satiety. Weight loss is variable ranging from 36 to 56 % of the excess body weight at 3–5 years and an average of 48 % at long-term follow-up ($\geq$10 years) with a need for both of revision and removals.

Type 2 diabetes resolution can be achieved in 40–56 % at 2–5 years follow-up and it is dependent on weight loss, and severity and duration of diabetes before surgery. Other comorbidities and quality of life also improve.

There is a 64–72 % lower risk of death at 5 years after the LAGB and the cost-effectiveness is significant, with net costs of banding reduced to zero in 4 years after band placement.

Review Questions and Answers

1. The LAGB helps to develop early satiation by:
   a. Limiting significantly the food transit
   b. Decreasing the ghrelin levels
   c. Altering the levels of several gastrointestinal hormones
   d. Generating myoenteric pressure signals

ANSWER: d

Studies have shown that delay in gastric emptying is not the main mechanism of action and there is a lack of correlation between over-restriction and satiety. The band should not physically limit significantly food transit. There is negligible food found above the band after a meal with the band correctly adjusted to induce satiety. A range of hormones including insulin, leptin, ghrelin, pancreatic polypeptide, and peptide YY do not play a significant role in LAGB function. It is hypothesized that the mechanical effects of the band and the passage of food bolus through this area of band resistance can generate myoenteric pressure signals. Signals from these receptors may be important in both meal termination and satisfaction, although the functional roles of these receptors remain poorly understood.

2. Weight loss after LAGB:

   a. Is achieved completely during the first year after surgery
   b. Has not been documented beyond 5 years
   c. Dependent in great part to an effective follow-up program
   d. Is similar to nonsurgical medical weight loss therapy

ANSWER: c

Weight loss after gastric banding progresses over a 2- or even 3-year period and then stabilizes, usually in the range of between 40 and 55 % of excess weight. Several studies have documented outcomes beyond 5 years. Weight loss outcomes are correlated with a need for lifelong follow-up with regular band adjustments. There have been randomized controlled trials assessing the superior effectiveness of LAGB vs. conservative weight loss programs.

3. The comorbidities of obesity following LAGB:

   a. Do not change
   b. Improve substantially
   c. Do not translate to an improved mortality risk
   d. Are not associated with a cost-benefit

ANSWER: b

There is an improvement in all comorbidities of obesity following LAGB and this translates to an improved risk ratio for mortality as well as a cost-benefit to the community.

4. Revisional surgery after LAGB:

   a. Is required by an average of 28 % of patients 10 years after the primary procedure
   b. Has a higher mortality than the primary procedure
   c. Leads to poor weight loss compared with prior to the procedure
   d. Conversion to an alternative bariatric procedure should be preferred

ANSWER: a

While there is an 8–60 % need for revision at 10 years post LAGB, this is consistent with the reoperation rate for any bariatric procedure as well as the revision rate for other procedures performed for benign disease (reflux, joint prosthesis). Revisions can be performed safely, and the weight loss following a revision usually resumes the pre-revision trajectory. Conversion to an alternative procedure should be considered if the lower esophageal sphincter complex is ineffective [52].

References

1. Flum D, Belle S, King W, et al. Perioperative safety in the longitudinal assessment of bariatric surgery. N Engl J Med. 2009;361: 445–54.
2. Chapman AE, Kiroff G, Game P, et al. Laparoscopic adjustable gastric banding in the treatment of obesity: a systematic literature review. Surgery. 2004;135:326–51.
3. Burton PR, Yap K, Brown WA, et al. Changes in satiety, supra- and infraband transit, and gastric emptying following laparoscopic adjustable gastric banding: a prospective follow-up study. Obes Surg. 2011;21(2):217–23.
4. Burton PR, Yap K, Brown WA, et al. Effects of adjustable gastric bands on gastric emptying, supra- and infraband transit and satiety: a randomized double-blind crossover trial using a new technique of band visualization. Obes Surg. 2010;20:1690–7.
5. Dixon AF, Dixon JB, O'Brien PE. Laparoscopic adjustable gastric banding induces prolonged satiety: a randomized blind crossover study. J Clin Endocrinol Metab. 2005;90:813–9.
6. Dixon AF, le Roux CW, Ghatei MA, Bloom SR, McGee TL, Dixon JB. Pancreatic polypeptide meal response may predict gastric band-induced weight loss. Obes Surg. 2011;21:1906–13.
7. Kampe J, Stefanidis A, Lockie SH, et al. Neural and humoral changes associated with the adjustable gastric band: insights from a rodent model. Int J Obes (Lond). 2012;27:25.
8. Berthoud HR. Vagal and hormonal gut-brain communication: from satiation to satisfaction. Neurogastroenterol Motil. 2008;1:64–72.
9. Fielding GA, Allen JW. A step-by-step guide to placement of the LAP-BAND adjustable gastric banding system. Am J Surg. 2002; 184:26S–30.
10. O'Brien PE, Dixon JB, Laurie C, Anderson M. A prospective randomized trial of placement of the laparoscopic adjustable gastric band: comparison of the perigastric and pars flaccida pathways. Obes Surg. 2005;15:820–6.
11. Ponce J, Dixon JB. Laparoscopic adjustable gastric banding. Surg Obes Relat Dis. 2005;1:310–6.
12. O'Brien PE, McDonald L, Anderson M, Brown WA. Long term outcomes after bariatric surgery: fifteen year follow up of adjustable gastric banding and a systematic review of the bariatric surgical literature. Ann Surg. 2013;257(1):87–94.
13. O'Brien P, McPhail T, Chaston T, Dixon J. Systematic review of medium-term weight loss after bariatric operations. Obes Surg. 2006;16:1032–40.
14. Shen R, Dugay G, Rajaram K, Cabrera I, Siegel N, Ren CJ. Impact of patient follow-up on weight loss after bariatric surgery. Obes Surg. 2004;14:514–9.
15. Weichman K, Ren C, Kurian M, et al. The effectiveness of adjustable gastric banding: a retrospective 6-year U.S. follow-up study. Surg Endosc. 2011;25:397–403.
16. Keating CL, Dixon JB, Moodie ML, et al. Cost-effectiveness of surgically induced weight loss for the management of type 2 diabetes: modeled lifetime analysis. Diabetes Care. 2009;32: 567–74.
17. Keating CL, Dixon JB, Moodie ML, Peeters A, Playfair J, O'Brien PE. Cost-efficacy of surgically induced weight loss for the management of type 2 diabetes: a randomized controlled trial. Diabetes Care. 2009;32:580–4.
18. Vos T, Carter R, Barendregt J, et al. Assessing cost-effectiveness in prevention (ACE–prevention): final report. University of Queensland and Deakin University; 2010.
19. Ren CJ, Horgan S, Ponce J. US experience with the LAP-BAND system. Am J Surg. 2002;184:46S–50.
20. Phillips E, Ponce J, Cunneen SA, et al. Safety and effectiveness of realize adjustable gastric band: 3-year prospective study in the United States. Surg Obes Relat Dis. 2009;5:588–97.

21. Angrisani L, Lorenzo M, Borrelli V. Laparoscopic adjustable gastric banding versus Roux-en-Y gastric bypass: 5-year results of a prospective randomized trial. Surg Obes Relat Dis. 2007;3:127–32; discussion 32–3.

22. Nguyen NT, Slone JA, Nguyen XM, Hartman JS, Hoyt DB. A prospective randomized trial of laparoscopic gastric bypass versus laparoscopic adjustable gastric banding for the treatment of morbid obesity: outcomes, quality of life, and costs. Ann Surg. 2009;250:631–41.

23. O'Brien P, Dixon J, Laurie C, et al. Treatment of mild to moderate obesity with laparoscopic adjustable gastric banding or an intensive medical program: a randomized trial. Ann Intern Med. 2006; 144:625–33.

24. O'Brien PE, Sawyer SM, Laurie C, et al. Laparoscopic adjustable gastric banding in severely obese adolescents: a randomized trial. JAMA. 2010;303:519–26.

25. Dixon JB, O'Brien PE, Playfair J, et al. Adjustable gastric banding and conventional therapy for type 2 diabetes: a randomized controlled trial. JAMA. 2008;299:316–23.

26. Dixon JB, Schachter LM, O'Brien PE, et al. Surgical vs conventional therapy for weight loss treatment of obstructive sleep apnea: a randomized controlled trial. JAMA. 2012;308:1142–9.

27. Buchwald H, Avidor Y, Braunwald E, et al. Bariatric surgery: a systematic review and meta-analysis. JAMA. 2004;292:1724–37.

28. Cunneen SA, Phillips E, Fielding G, et al. Studies of Swedish adjustable gastric band and Lap-Band: systematic review and meta-analysis. Surg Obes Relat Dis. 2008;4:174–85.

29. Favretti F, Segato G, Ashton D, et al. Laparoscopic adjustable gastric banding in 1,791 consecutive obese patients: 12-year results. Obes Surg. 2007;17:168–75.

30. Himpens J, Cadiere GB, Bazi M, Vouche M, Cadiere B, Dapri G. Long-term outcomes of laparoscopic adjustable gastric banding. Arch Surg. 2011;146:802–7.

31. Lanthaler M, Aigner F, Kinzl J, Sieb M, Cakar-Beck F, Nehoda H. Long-term results and complications following adjustable gastric banding. Obes Surg. 2010;20:1078–85.

32. Miller K, Pump A, Hell E. Vertical banded gastroplasty versus adjustable gastric banding: prospective long-term follow-up study. Surg Obes Relat Dis. 2007;3:84–90.

33. Naef M, Mouton WG, Naef U, Kummer O, Muggli B, Wagner HE. Graft survival and complications after laparoscopic gastric banding for morbid obesity—lessons learned from a 12-year experience. Obes Surg. 2010;20:1206–14.

34. Stroh C, Hohmann U, Schramm H, Meyer F, Manger T. Fourteen-year long-term results after gastric banding. J Obes. 2011;128451:22.

35. Dixon JB, O'Brien PE. Changes in comorbidities and improvements in quality of life after LAP-BAND placement. Am J Surg. 2002;184:S51–4.

36. Chen SB, Lee YC, Ser KH, et al. Serum C-reactive protein and white blood cell count in morbidly obese surgical patients. Obes Surg. 2009;19:461–6.

37. Dixon JB, Dixon AF, O'Brien PE. Improvements in insulin sensitivity and beta-cell function (HOMA) with weight loss in the severely obese. Diabet Med. 2003;20:127–34.

38. Buchwald H, Estok R, Fahrbach K, et al. Weight and type 2 diabetes after bariatric surgery: systematic review and meta-analysis. Am J Med. 2009;122:248–56.

39. Sultan S, Gupta D, Parikh M, et al. Five-year outcomes of patients with type 2 diabetes who underwent laparoscopic adjustable gastric banding. Surg Obes Relat Dis. 2010;6:373–6.

40. Dixon JB, Dixon ME, O'Brien PE. Quality of life after lap-band placement: influence of time, weight loss, and comorbidities. Obes Res. 2001;9:713–21.

41. Ponce J, Haynes B, Paynter S, et al. Effect of Lap-Band-induced weight loss on type 2 diabetes mellitus and hypertension. Obes Surg. 2004;14:1335–42.

42. O'Brien PE, Brown WA, Dixon JB. Obesity, weight loss and bariatric surgery. Med J Aust. 2005;183:310–4.

43. Dixon JB, Schachter LM, O'Brien PE. Sleep disturbance and obesity: changes following surgically induced weight loss. Arch Intern Med. 2001;161:102–6.

44. Dixon J. Survival advantage with bariatric surgery: report from the 10th international congress on obesity. Surg Obes Relat Dis. 2006; 2(6):585–6.

45. Peeters A, O'Brien PE, Laurie C, et al. Substantial intentional weight loss and mortality in the severely obese. Ann Surg. 2007; 246:1028–33.

46. Busetto L, Mirabelli D, Petroni ML, et al. Comparative long-term mortality after laparoscopic adjustable gastric banding versus nonsurgical controls. Surg Obes Relat Dis. 2007;3:496–502.

47. Cremieux PY, Buchwald H, Shikora SA, Ghosh A, Yang HE, Buessing M. A study on the economic impact of bariatric surgery. Am J Manag Care. 2008;14:589–96.

48. Finkelstein EA, Allaire BT, Burgess SM, Hale BC. Financial implications of coverage for laparoscopic adjustable gastric banding. Surg Obes Relat Dis. 2011;7:295–303.

49. Anselmino M, Bammer T, Fernandez Cebrian JM, Daoud F, Romagnoli G, Torres A. Cost-effectiveness and budget impact of obesity surgery in patients with type 2 diabetes in three European countries(II). Obes Surg. 2009;19:1542–9.

50. Fried M, Dolezalova K, Sramkova P. Adjustable gastric banding outcomes with and without gastrogastric imbrication sutures: a randomized controlled trial. Surg Obes Relat Dis. 2011;7:23–31.

51. Lazzati A, Polliand C, Porta M, et al. Is fixation during gastric banding necessary? A randomised clinical study. Obes Surg. 2011; 21:1859–63.

52. Burton PR, Brown WA, Laurie C, Hebbard G, O'Brien PE. Predicting outcomes of intermediate term complications and revisional surgery following laparoscopic adjustable gastric banding: utility of the CORE classification and Melbourne motility criteria. Obes Surg. 2010;20:1516–23.

21
Laparoscopic Adjustable Gastric Banding: Long-Term Management

Christine Ren Fielding

Immediate Postoperative Management

Postoperative care after LAGB is usually straightforward. Most patients are observed in a regular ward room. Patients with documented or suspected obstructive sleep apnea may require additional monitoring or a continuous positive airway pressure (CPAP) device. Prophylaxis for thromboembolism may include sequential compression devices, compression stockings, and/or anticoagulation therapy. Early ambulation is always encouraged.

Early postoperative retching and vomiting by the patient should be avoided. Just as in Nissen fundoplication, acute vomiting after surgery can result in an acute gastric prolapse with band slip. Anterior gastrogastric suture disruption may be a potential sequela. Aggressive antiemetic therapy should be instituted in the operating room. An intraoperative intravenous cocktail of ondansetron (Zofran)/metoclopramide (Reglan)/ketorolac (Toradol)/acetaminophen is administered prior to extubation. An additional intravenous antiemetic is given liberally during the first 24 h. Both the patient and the nursing staff are instructed on the importance of emesis prevention after surgery. Pain management involves subcutaneous injection of skin incisions with 0.25 % Marcaine. Intravenous ketorolac and acetaminophen are administered as a standing order every 6 h, with subcutaneous or oral narcotic for breakthrough pain.

Patients may be kept in the hospital overnight or discharged the same day, depending on their medical status, pain control, and presence or absence of nausea. A postoperative esophagram documents normal, rapid esophageal emptying, no extravasation of contrast, and adequate band placement, lying in an 8 o'clock to 2 o'clock position (Fig. 1). In addition, it provides the surgeon with a baseline esophagram to document band positioning for comparison with future studies. Gastrografin is used in case a perforation is found. A gastric pouch should not be seen since the band is not filled.

If the esophagram shows delayed emptying, the normal clinical progression is for increased swelling to occur over 48 h. These patients can usually swallow their saliva. It is advised to keep the patient NPO with intravenous hydration and anti-inflammatory medication (i.e., ketorolac, steroids). In contrast, complete obstruction on the film is always associated with inability to swallow saliva, and these patients do not recover with conservative measures. They must return to the operating room for laparoscopic revision. Most commonly, cutting the gastrogastric sutures, manipulating the band, and removing more perigastric fat give a good result. Placement of a larger band (LAPBAND™ APL) may also be helpful in these circumstances. In addition, an unrecognized hiatal hernia may result in a greater amount of gastric tissue incorporated into the band, leading to obstruction. In this case, the hernia must be mobilized and reduced, the crura repaired, and the band placed in the proper position; otherwise the patient will be unable to tolerate adjustments in the future.

Patients are seen in the office 10–14 days after surgery for their first follow-up, to check their wounds and reiterate dietary guidelines.

Postoperative Dietary Guidelines

Due to the possible correlation between early vomiting and gastric prolapse [1, 2], patients are placed on a diet that progresses from liquids to solids over the first 6 weeks after surgery. For weeks 1 and 2 the diet is thin liquids—any fluid that is thin enough to go through a straw. For weeks 3 and 4 the diet is pureed foods—foods that do not need to be chewed, as if the patient did not have teeth. For weeks 5 and 6 the diet is soft and flaky solid foods and crunchy foods, specifically excluding dry/tough chicken, overcooked steak, and doughy bread, which tend to form a large bolus that cannot traverse through the narrow band stoma. Patients are counseled to eat very slowly, chew their food thoroughly, and to avoid eating and drinking simultaneously, as to not outpace the emptying of the food through their band, which if occurs will result in regurgitation or vomiting.

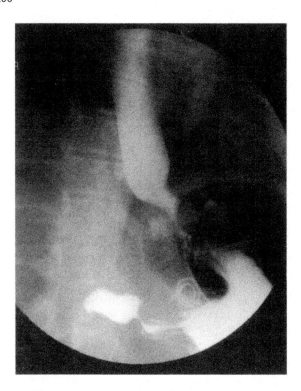

Fig. 1. Normal postoperative esophagram.

Nutritional deficiencies have not been reported after LAGB, perhaps because the operation is purely restrictive. However, patients are encouraged to take a fortified daily chewable or liquid multivitamin. More importantly, patients should already have the nutritional knowledge and skills to make healthy food choices before any bariatric surgery, including LAGB. Patients are told that high-calorie liquids and soft foods, such as chocolate and ice cream, are physically easy to eat but will lead to weight regain or weight loss failure.

The most important dietary counseling that LAGB patients need is *how* to eat—slowly and chewing thoroughly. They must learn how to put the fork down between bites. Most importantly, they must recognize when they are full, and then stop eating. This is a new skill for morbidly obese patients. Even an extra bite will make them regurgitate. Counseling on social eating and food choices is greatly appreciated by patients, since this is usually their greatest source of anxiety, particularly in young adults and teenagers as they start dating. Diurnal variation in esophageal motility may play an important role in dysphagia and appears to vary according to time of day and amount of emotional stress. Dysphagia is common when patients are eating in a stressful situation, mostly because they are typically distracted and have eaten quickly without chewing. They are counseled to have a yogurt, soup, or a protein drink during stressful times. Breakfast is sometimes difficult; therefore a liquid meal is encouraged.

Band Adjustments

The mechanisms by which LAGB works include decreasing appetite, creating satiety with a smaller amount of food, and behavior modification [3]. This is a direct function of a small gastric pouch (10–15 mL) and a narrow stomal opening that slows gastric emptying (12 mm). The LAGB acts in this capacity through external constriction of the stomach, which is gradually tightened in accordance with each individual's needs. If no constriction is created, no satiety is reached, and no weight is lost. Therefore, weight loss after LAGB is contingent on band adjustment. The band is useless if adjustments are not performed. Both patient and surgeon must understand this; otherwise weight loss will be suboptimal, the operation ineffective, and the surgery a wasted effort.

The band is left empty when initially placed. The first adjustment is performed 6 weeks postoperatively. This allows time for a capsule to form around the band and makes its position around the stomach more secure. Adjustments should be made while patients are eating solid food. The band is meant to work with solid food, specifically to maintain stretching of the gastric pouch to create an early sense of satiety. An appropriately adjusted band also acts as an appetite suppressant. A sense of hunger, increased appetite, and increased snacking are signs that the band is not appropriately tightened. Soft and liquid foods empty faster than solids, and thus more can be ingested before the feeling of satiety is reached. Thus, a band that is too tight will make solid food ingestion difficult, but easy for creamy sugary liquids. This is an example of maladaptive behavior and may necessitate band loosening.

There are two general strategies to band adjustment: in-office adjustment using a clinical algorithm and radiographic adjustment under fluoroscopic guidance. Each has its advantages and disadvantages. In-office adjustments are quick and inexpensive, but require frequent visits due to inaccuracy of the adjustment. Radiographic adjustments are more cumbersome and expensive, but require fewer visits due to the more accurate adjustment visualized under fluoroscopy.

The maximum recommended amount of saline that a gastric band accommodates depends on the band type. The Lap-Band System™ (Allergan, Irvine, CA) comes in five different types of bands which hold various maximum recommended volumes as shown in Table 1. Similarly, the Realize™ Band System (Ethicon Endosurgery, Cincinnati, OH) comes in two types and sizes. In addition to maximum recommended volume capacity, Table 1 shows the typical average volume range where a patient would eventually be when optimally adjusted.

TABLE 1 Types of adjustable gastric bands available in the USA

Band type	Maximum recommended volume (mL)	Average volume range (mL)
Allergan (Irvine, CA)		
LAPBAND 9.75	4	2.5–3
LAPBAND 10	4	2.5–3
LAPBAND VG	11	9–10.5
LAPBAND APS	10	5.5–7.0
LAPBAND APL	14	8–10.5
Ethicon Endosurgery (Cincinnati, OH)		
REALIZE	9	7.5–8.5
REALIZE-C	11	8.5–10.5

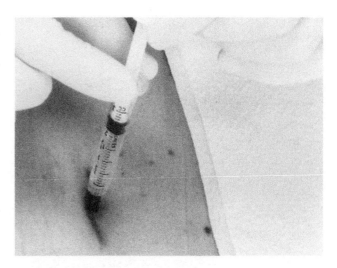

FIG. 2. IN-OFFICE PERCUTANEOUS ACCESS OF PORT (SALINE-FILLED SYRINGE ATTACHED TO NON-CORING NEEDLE).

Office-Based Adjustment

There are two aspects to band adjustments: locating the access port and determining the volume of saline to be used. When the procedure is performed in the office, the port is located by palpation. The band is adjusted by percutaneously accessing the port with a non-coring needle and subsequently injecting sterile saline, which tightens the band. Withdrawal of saline results in band loosening with subsequent decreased restriction. The skin is cleansed with alcohol, and a non-coring needle on a pre-filled syringe filled with the desired amount of saline is introduced through the skin into the access port (Fig. 2). Successful port access is confirmed by feeling the needle hit the metal base of the access port and having free reflux of saline back into the syringe. Use of any needle other than a non-coring needle may result in damage to the access port septum and subsequent leak of saline. Local anesthetic is unnecessary, as it is more painful than the needle itself. Having the patient lie on the examination table and lift his or her head up off the examination table while tensing the abdominal muscles can assist in feeling the port. Sometimes having the patient stand up will use gravity to drop the pannus and make the port more apparent.

Locating the port can be challenging in patients who have a large amount of subcutaneous fat, particularly women and individuals with a body mass index (BMI) greater than 60. An extra-long needle may be necessary to reach the port. An X-ray can be obtained to localize and mark the port (Fig. 3). The learning curve for port localization using palpation is surprisingly long and may take up to 100 cases. Our experience has shown that on review of our first 200 consecutive gastric band patients (69 % female, mean BMI 48.7), 660 adjustments were performed in the office (74 % by a nurse practitioner and 26 % by a physician) [4]. Twenty-eight (4.2 %) adjustments were unsuccessfully performed by a nurse practitioner and required physician assistance. Twelve of those attempts (1.8 %) on nine patients required radiographic guidance to localize the access port. All nine patients were women who were in the first 75 patients adjusted.

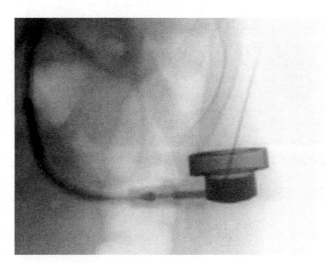

FIG. 3. X-RAY USED TO FIND ACCESS PORT.

The decision to tighten, loosen, or leave the band alone is based on three variables: hunger, weight loss, and restriction. A properly adjusted band induces the lack of hunger and appetite suppression. It should also induce a prolonged sense of satiety that lasts longer than 2 h after a meal. Weight loss should be constant and gradual over the course of 18–36 months.

The goal rate of weight loss is 6–10 lb/month. Lack of weight loss reflects too large a portion intake, and suboptimal satiety and hunger control, indicating the band needs tightening. The Green Zone chart (Fig. 4) [5] is an invaluable visual chart which educates the patient on the role of the band as a tool towards weight loss, and involves the patient in the decision-making process towards band adjustment. As shown, the Yellow Zone describes the patient as hungry between meals, eating large portions and not losing weight. The patient in the Yellow Zone requires an adjustment to move him/her towards the Green Zone which represents the

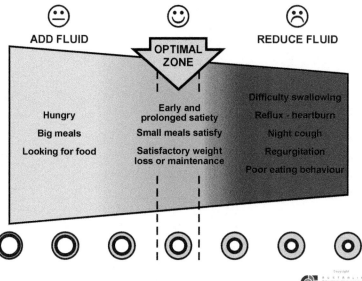

optimal situation: good appetite control, satiety with small portions, and weight loss. A patient in the Green Zone requires no band tightening or loosening. However if a patient experiences night cough, frequent regurgitation despite eating very slowly, and subsequent maladaptive eating of high-calorie soft foods, then he/she is in the Red Zone and needs to have the band loosened. Having a large framed poster of the Green Zone in the exam room is very helpful and an excellent investment towards patient education and care. It is also important for both clinician and patient to understand that the band can be adjusted at any time throughout the lifetime of the banded patient, and is not limited to a certain amount of time since surgery. For example, if a patient has been in the Green Zone for 5 years, but progressively develops increased hunger, he/she can have an adjustment in order to return to the Green Zone.

The amount of saline to inject when the patient is in the Yellow Zone is based on experience based on trial and error. In order to provide a template for new clinicians, a clinical algorithm was designed at NYU and is used as a basic general guide to use for the 9.75 cm LAPBAND SYSTEM (Allergan, Irvine, CA) (Table 1) [6] which holds a maximum recommended capacity of 4 mL. With experience, the clinician can modify this algorithm in regard to volume of saline added, particularly depending on the type of band the patient has. For example, in a band with 10 mL maximum recommended capacity, the first adjustment may be 3 mL, with subsequent increments of 1 mL.

If saline is already present, it can be aspirated into the syringe to document any loss of volume that may have occurred. However, routine aspiration of all saline from band is not recommended due to the increased restriction patients can feel soon after. Instead, the pre-planned volume of saline

should be present in the syringe, and only a small amount of saline should be allowed to reflux into the syringe in order to confirm access into the port. Therefore, complete aspiration of all saline in the band system should be reserved for times when a device leak is suspected.

After each adjustment, patients drink a cup of water to ensure that they do not have outlet obstruction. Any gurgling noises will likely lead to obstruction in the next 1–3 days. Interestingly, we have found that the band gets slightly tighter 1–2 days after an adjustment. Therefore, we have our patients stay on liquids for 2 days, pureed foods for 2 days, and then solid foods by the fifth day after adjustment.

At NYU, we perform our adjustments in the office and see our patients every 4–6 weeks for weight and appetite evaluation. The program is structured for patients to return for regular weigh-ins, progress evaluation, adjustments, nutritional reinforcement, and most importantly, behavioral counseling. We have found that frequent patient follow-up has a significant impact on percent excess weight loss (% EWL) achieved in just 1 year. Patients who return more than six times in the first year after LAGB lose an average of 50 % EWL, as compared with those who return six times or less, who lose 42 % EWL [6]. The average number of adjustments in the first year was 4.5 and in the second year was 2 (Fig. 5).

High patient volume resulting from this postoperative follow-up regimen is accommodated with the use of a dedicated nurse practitioner. This may reflect not only utilization of the restrictive properties of the band to its full potential but also the added behavioral counseling and emotional support that patients receive with each visit. The typical patient requires an average of 4–10 adjustments in the first year, and then 1–3 adjustments each year thereafter.

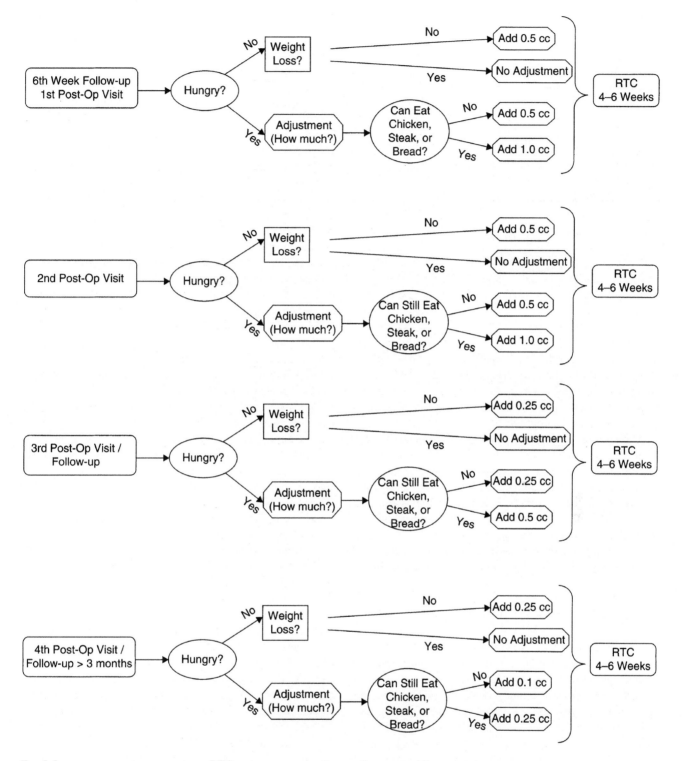

FIG. 5. IN-OFFICE ADJUSTMENT ALGORITHM. RTC, RETURN TO CLINIC. *SOURCE*: SHEN ET AL. [6] WITH PERMISSION.

Radiographically Guided Adjustment

Real-time fluoroscopy allows for rapid localization of the port to assist in percutaneous access. The needle can be observed simultaneously as the skin is punctured and the port accessed. Again, free reflux of saline into the syringe confirms successful access. Fluoroscopy also allows for visualization of the esophagus, gastric pouch, band, diameter of outlet, and integrity of tubing/port system. There is no standardized rate of esophageal emptying or outlet diameter that correlates with the perfect adjustment. There is also no evidence to suggest that a given outlet diameter correlates

TABLE 2. Radiographic criteria for adjustment

Consider fluid removal	Consider fluid addition
Stenosis of the outlet (with maladaptive eating behavior[a])	Wide outlet (>8 mm)
Esophageal dilatation (>2×)	Immediate passage of the barium swallow (one peristaltic wave)
Esophageal atony	
Esophageal emptying of the barium swallow in >4–5 peristaltic waves	
Reflux	
Pouch dilatation with insufficient emptying	

[a]Consumption of high-calorie liquid or soft foods, often induced by an overly tight band
Source: Favretti et al. [7], with permission

with dysphagia or clinical symptoms. Table 2 shows suggested radiographic criteria for adjustments as published by Favretti et al. [7].

However, what fluoroscopy does show is outlet obstruction, esophageal dilatation, gastric pouch dilatation, band slippage/prolapse, reflux, and malfunctioning band or malpositioned band. These are situations that would require immediate intervention such as loosening the band. This may be helpful since not all of these abnormalities are necessarily reflected in clinical symptoms.

Although the number of follow-up visits and adjustments are much fewer, the cost and effort required are greater. The surgeon must coordinate with a radiology facility for use of the fluoroscopy; this can be time-consuming and costly. Unless the surgeon's office has a mobile fluoroscopy unit such as a C-arm, the average time to perform an adjustment is 15–20 min. High-volume centers can decrease this time to 10 min. In addition, the patient does not receive the repetitive emotional and behavioral counseling from the caregiver.

Complaints and Symptoms

Dysphagia to solid food is the most common postoperative complaint. It usually relates to the patient's (1) eating too quickly; (2) swallowing too large a bolus of food; (3) swallowing poorly chewed food; (4) eating food that does not break down with chewing, especially steak; (5) eating food that congeals together, such as white bread; and (6) eating while anxious or angry. Most patients inadvertently forget that they have a band, eat too quickly but subsequently pay more attention to the behavioral modification of eating more mindfully. Reinforcement of behavioral modification can be accomplished with techniques such as using a 30-s timer to prolong the time between swallowed bolus and taking the next mouthful. Educating the patient to avoid performing other tasks such as talking on the phone or driving while eating can help with mindful eating. However, some patients simply fail to learn from these experiences and persist with

noncompliant behaviors. Chest pain from acute esophageal dilation will occur every time. This becomes very unpleasant for the patient and can be difficult for the surgeon to manage. Figure 6 reviews recommended management of some common complaints.

Stomal obstruction from food causes pain. Initially, this severe central chest pain and salivation can be frightening. Once patients recognize it, though, they are much less concerned. The simplest course of action is to induce vomiting, which will liberate the obstructing plug. It is actually regurgitation that occurs, rather than vomiting. Immediate resolution of pain is experienced. Patients should then stay on liquids for the rest of the meal, as mucosal swelling within the band can occur. Use of carbonated drinks to free the obstructing plug is to be avoided, as the pain becomes severe when the gas expands within the obstructed esophagus.

Recurrent regurgitation or vomiting can result in local mucosal edema within the outlet; patients are advised to stay on clear liquids for the following 24 h after any such event. If the food remains stuck and they are unable to tolerate any liquids, even their own saliva, they must call their surgeon. The band requires immediate deflation, with removal of saline to allow passage of the obstructing bolus. The band can be readjusted after 2 days.

Dysphagia and regurgitation is often worst early in the morning, improves during the day, and is rarely present in the evening. This relates to the diurnal function of esophageal motility. Many patients are best served by having a liquid breakfast, such as a cup of coffee followed by a protein shake, that they can sip slowly on the way to work. This eliminates much of the early morning stress. Explanations of these mechanisms greatly assist band patients to understand some of the difficulties they may experience and reduce the ever-present fear of failure.

Dysphagia is certainly affected by emotional issues. Anger, anxiety, or state of upset can cause esophageal spasm. Often patients who experience a death in the family, an ill loved one or loss of a job, will notice increased food intolerance. Temporary loosening of the band will relieve the dysphagia, and the band can be re-tightened once the stress passes. Sex hormones can also affect esophageal motility and lower esophageal sphincter pressure whereby female patients may notice a correlation between dysphagia and a certain time in their menses. Again, making the patient aware of these variations in perceived band "tightness" can reduce frustration and help develop strategies to avoid vomiting. One very important subgroup is young people who are dating; their newfound confidence after weight loss will evaporate if they are seen to be having difficulty eating or actually vomiting. These young people need special advice: start with a beverage to help relax; choose foods they know they can eat, such as soup, risotto, or flaky fish; and resist pressure to eat more. Eat slowly. They may have a sip of wine as they eat, just as they would do normally. This allows them to fit in with their friends and to be more comfortable dating.

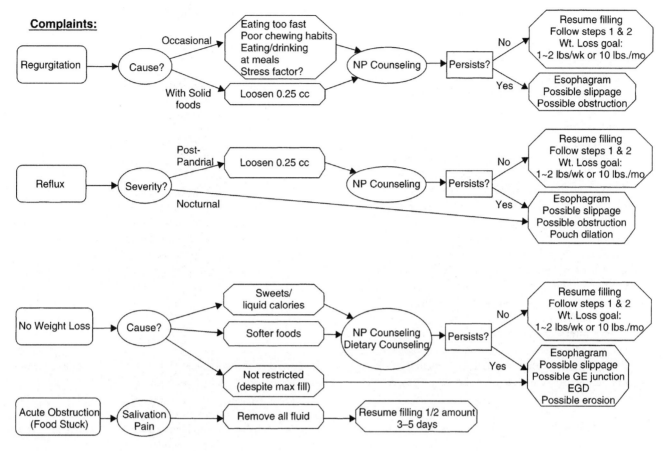

FIG. 6. COMMON COMPLAINTS ALGORITHM. *GE* GASTROESOPHAGEAL, *EGD* ESOPHAGOGASTRODUODENOSCOPY.

Reflux is not uncommon and occurs when (1) the band is too tight, (2) there is gastric prolapse with band slip, (3) there is an undiagnosed hiatal hernia, or (4) there is abnormal esophageal motility. These are indistinguishable clinically but can be diagnosed by esophagraphy. The severe end of the spectrum is nocturnal regurgitation, reflux, and night cough, often presenting as sleeplessness combined with recent-onset asthma, or even aspiration pneumonia. This is more commonly seen with gastric prolapse/band slip. Initial appropriate treatment entails removing fluid from the band, and then diagnosing the etiology of reflux. Upper endoscopy is often necessary to diagnose a hiatal hernia, and if present requires surgical reduction and repair with or without mesh. Occasionally, a band slip or a hiatal hernia cannot be diagnosed by either esophagram or upper endoscopy and require exploratory laparoscopy. Band slippage and pouch dilation require surgical reduction of the gastric prolapse and repositioning of the band if the patient has had a satisfactory weight loss. However, if the patient has experienced suboptimal weight loss at the time of band slippage, pouch dilation, or hiatal hernia diagnosis, consideration should be made to convert the patient to Roux-en-Y gastric bypass.

Reflux or heartburn not associated with a band slippage or hiatal hernia is suspected to be caused by esophagitis due to: (1) pills or (2) chronic regurgitation. Due to the narrowed stoma outlet into the stomach created by compression of the band, pills larger than 1 cm will have delayed transit through the band and increased contact with the esophageal mucosa. Large pills (>2 cm), pills with an acidic pH foundation (i.e., doxycycline, ferrous sulfate, ascorbic acid, NSAIDs, antidepressants), sustained-released pills, and gelatin-coated pills are all common causes of pill esophagitis [8]. Behavioral contributors include taking several pills in a handful, drinking minimal or no fluid when taking pills, and taking pills prior to lying down for sleep. In the case of pill esophagitis in the LAGB patient, the band should be loosened for 1–3 weeks, and the patient treated with sucralfate elixir. Offending pills should be changed to smaller size, non-sustained release, or liquid formulation, to be taken one at a time with plenty of liquid at least 2 h prior to bedtime, preferable before a meal. The band can be re-tightened with resolution.

Chronic regurgitation from an overtightened band or from behavioral non-modification (i.e., eating too fast) can similarly result in esophagitis. With esophagitis contributing to esophageal dysmotility, esophageal dilation may be seen on esophagram and requires band loosening. Proton-pump inhibitors or histamine blockers can be helpful. Patients who cannot tolerate the restriction of the band and adopt a maladaptive eating behavior may benefit from band removal and possible revision to a bypass procedure.

Weight loss outcomes after LAGB are subject to greater variation due to the many factors which contribute to weight loss. The most common reason for poor weight loss is a suboptimally adjusted band as mentioned earlier, followed by device leak either from the port, the tubing, or the band itself. Presuming that the device system is intact and the patient is in the "Green Zone," other factors may come into play. Eating due to emotional reasons, most commonly depression, rather than physical hunger is a common culprit. Colles et al. found that LAGB patients who have less physical hunger have a reduced total energy intake and greater weight loss, as compared to those who reported minimal hunger control [9]. However, "emotional" hunger, eating in response to negative emotional states, and continuing to eat despite feeling full were forms of "non-hungry eating" related to higher reports of hunger and poorer weight outcomes. Eating may become "self-medication" to avoid confronting difficult feelings, which can subsequently have negative effects on weight loss after any type of bariatric surgery [10]. These patients would benefit from psychological counseling to identify and manage this disorder as a means to optimize weight loss outcomes and emotional health.

Nutritional Evaluation

Nutritional deficiencies have not been identified to be a problem after LAGB due to the purely restrictive nature of the operation. However, it is good practice to check a full battery of laboratory tests including iron, folate, thiamine, vitamin B12, vitamin D, and calcium on an annual basis. Menstruating females are at highest risk of anemia due to decreased food and nutrient intake. Pregnancy or illness may change the nutritional requirements and can be addressed with band loosening.

Counseling

Patients should understand that achieving weight loss requires commitment to follow-up and behavioral modification. They need to make changes to their nutrition, their manner of eating and levels of activity. While LAGB is not as "foolproof" as Roux-en-Y gastric bypass (RYGBP) or sleeve gastrectomy, it can be just as effective in the long term. Patients must understand that they cannot have it both ways: They will not be able to eat the same way or the same things after surgery and still lose weight. The weight loss is gradual, due to the gradual nature of the restriction. A program approach is the most successful way of achieving significant maintained weight loss.

TABLE 3. Postoperative eating tips

1	Eat when hungry
2	If not hungry, do not eat
3	Eat slowly
4	Chew thoroughly
5	Learn to put your fork down between bites
6	Size of the meal should be the same as the palm of your hand
7	Do not try to finish everything on the plate
8	Do not eat and drink at the same time
9	All beverages should have 0 calories
10	Order an appetizer instead of an entree at a restaurant

Support groups and ongoing psychotherapy can be helpful after any bariatric surgery for the patient to adjust to the loss of food, new self-image, and change in eating behavior. However, the greatest help can come from the surgeon listening to the patient and applying some of these basic principles (Table 3).

Conclusion

The LAGB is the safest surgical tool available to assist morbidly obese patients in losing weight. The keys to its success are appropriate surgical technique, prolonged follow-up, regular adjustments, and, perhaps most importantly, an understanding of the changes that go with having a band. Its adjustability is its greatest strength. When the patient attends regularly for follow-up, and the surgeon uses adjustments wisely based on satiety, weight loss, and any other symptoms, the LAGB will deliver very satisfactory weight loss results.

Review Questions and Answers

1. The best place to adjust a gastric band is:

    a. In the operating room
    b. In the office
    c. In the radiology suite
    d. b and c

    The answer is (d). Band adjustments can be performed either in the office or in the radiology suite under fluoroscopy. Both are valid ways to perform adjustments as long as they are done on a regular basis until the patient reaches the Green Zone.

2. A patient who is 3 years after LAGB comes in complaining of coughing in her sleep for the past 3 weeks. Her last band adjustment was over a year ago. What is the first test you order?

    a. Chest CT
    b. CBC

c. Esophagram

d. Upper endoscopy

The answer is (c). Night cough means that the band is too tight and the patient is suffering from reflux. Since she did not have her band recently tightened, the cause of band obstruction is from either a band slippage, a hiatal hernia, or from decreased esophageal motility secondary to esophagitis. An esophagram is a simple test which will show the band position, pouch size, pouch emptying, esophageal diameter, and emptying.

3. The most common cause of vomiting after gastric banding is:

a. Eating too fast

b. Not chewing thoroughly

c. Having the band too tight

d. Eating tough meat

e. All of the above

The answer is (e). Vomiting in an LAGB patient is more regurgitation of undigested food rather than vomitus, and is most often due to behavioral causes such as eating too fast and not chewing properly. Reinforcement of behavioral modification is helpful. Sometimes the band is over-tightened, and this creates a very small stoma which may even be too tight for liquids to pass. In this case the band needs to be loosened.

References

1. Fielding GA. Reduction in incidence of gastric herniation with LAP-BAND: experience in 620 cases. Obes Surg. 2000; 10:136.
2. Dargent J. Pouch dilatation and slippage after adjustable gastric banding: is it still an issue? Obes Surg. 2003;13:111–5.
3. Dixon AF, Dixon JB, O'Brien PE. Laparoscopic adjustable gastric banding induces prolonged satiety: a randomized blind crossover study. J Clin Endocrinol Metab. 2005;90(2):813–9.
4. Dugay G, Ren CJ. Laparoscopic adjustable gastric band (Lap-Band) adjustments in the office is feasible-the first 200 cases. Obes Surg. 2003;13:192 [abstr].
5. Dixon JB, Straznicky NE, Lambert EA, Schlaich MP, Lambert GW. Laparoscopic adjustable gastric banding and other devices for the management of obesity. Circulation. 2012;126(6):774–85.
6. Shen R, Dugay G, Rajaram K, Cabrera I, Siegel N, Ren CJ. Impact of patient follow-up on weight loss after bariatric surgery. Obes Surg. 2004;14:514–9.
7. Favretti F, O'Brien PE, Dixon JB. Patient management after LAP-BAND placement. Am J Surg. 2002;184:38S–41S.
8. Winstead NS, Bulat R. Pill esophagitis. Curr Treat Opt Gastroenterol. 2004;7:71–6.
9. Colles SL, Dixon JB, O'Brien PE. Hunger control and regular physical activity facilitate weight loss after laparoscopic adjustable gastric banding. Obes Surg. 2008;18:833–40.
10. Beck NN, Mehlsen M, Stoving RK. Psychological characteristics and associations with weight outcomes two years after gastric bypass surgery: postoperative eating disorder symptoms are associated with weight loss outcomes. Eat Behav. 2012;13(4): 394–7.

22

Laparoscopic Adjustable Gastric Banding: Management of Complications

Paul O'Brien

Abbreviations

% EWL	% Excess weight lost
AP	Advanced platform (Lap-Band AP)
CT	Computerized tomography
DVT	Deep vein thrombosis
IGLEs	Intraganglionic laminar endings
LAGB	Laparoscopic adjustable gastric band
LECS	Lower esophageal contractile segment
LES	Lower esophageal sphincter
NERD	New, explore, repair, dissect
NIH	National Institutes of Health
RCT	Randomized controlled trial
RYGB	Roux-en-Y gastric bypass

Introduction

The laparoscopic adjustable gastric band (LAGB) has proved to be a remarkably safe procedure in the perioperative period. Considering that the patient is severely obese and usually suffering multiple medical comorbidities of obesity, the LAGB procedure can be done with minimal risk of mortality and very few early adverse events. This is a testament to the simplicity and gentleness of the procedure and the superior physiological competence of the severely obese who, until the later stages of their disease, manage to function adequately while carrying 100 lb or more of excess baggage through each day, a feat most of us would be quite unable to do.

However late adverse events are relatively common and these could be seen to represent a central weakness of the LAGB. We argue that some level of maintenance will always be required when seeking to provide a permanent control of a chronic disease. The procedure needs to remain effective over decades rather than years. It is unrealistic to expect that a treatment applied today will remain perfect without some repairs and maintenance for the remainder of the patient's life. There are revisional needs for all bariatric surgical

procedures and indeed for all procedures treating chronic problems, including cardiac surgery for ischemic heart disease and joint replacement surgery for degenerative joint diseases. . While reversal of a bariatric procedure should be counted as failure, revision to correct or repair should not. It is a part of the process of care.

The challenge is to minimize the need for revisional procedures and to ensure that, when a late adverse event occurs, it is quickly and accurately evaluated and treated optimally. This chapter provides a heavy focus on prevention and on managing the adverse events that have not been prevented.

Perioperative Mortality

There is a mortality risk with any surgery and this risk was strongly evident for bariatric surgery prior to the general use of the laparoscopic approach. Pories et al. [1] reported a perioperative mortality of 1.9 % of the 605 patients treated by open gastric bypass. The mortality occurring at the level of community surgery is probably higher than at the major academic centres. Flum and Dellinger used the Washington State Comprehensive Hospital Abstract Reporting System database and the Vital Statistics database to evaluate 30-day mortality of all people having an RYGB procedure in that state during the period 1987–2001 [2]. Of 3,328 procedures there were 64 deaths, a mortality rate of 1.9 %. This period included both laparoscopic and open surgery and could be seen to reflect community practice.

The overall mortality has decreased in more recent years, particularly with the widespread use of a laparoscopic surgical approach. Death after LAGB is rare and the two major systematic reviews of the literature that examined mortality rates show that death after LAGB is in the order of 0.05–0.02 %, an incidence that is 10–15 times less likely than after RYGB [3, 4]. At our Centre for Bariatric Surgery in Melbourne, we have performed more than 7,000 primary LAGB procedures and have performed more than 1,000

S.A. Brethauer et al. (eds.), *Minimally Invasive Bariatric Surgery*,
DOI 10.1007/978-1-4939-1637-5_22, © Springer Science+Business Media New York 2015

revisional LAGB procedures without any 30-day mortality or any later death related to the LAGB procedure.

The most definitive evaluation of mortality currently available is derived from the Longitudinal Assessment of Bariatric Surgery (LABS) study report in 2009 [5]. This NIH-sponsored study of bariatric surgery involved 10 sites, carefully selected for their expertise and experience. The 30-day rate of death was monitored closely. There were 4,776 patients who had RYGB ($N = 3412$), LAGB ($N = 1198$) or other procedures unspecified in the report ($N = 166$). There were 15 deaths in the RYGB group, 6 after a laparoscopic approach and 9 after an open approach. There were no deaths in the LAGB group of patients. The difference was highly significant.

Early Complications

The Longitudinal Assessment of Bariatric Surgery study serves also to inform on early adverse events for the two major bariatric procedures of RYGB and LAGB. Not surprisingly, the incidence of adverse events mirrored the perioperative mortality rates. Using a composite end point of death, DVT or pulmonary embolism, re-intervention or failure to be discharged by 30 days, they identified 189 who were positive to that end point, 177 in the RYGB group (5.2 %) and 12 in the LAGB group (1.0 %), a difference that was highly significant [5].

The adverse events after LAGB include infection at the access port site, infection in the region of the band, intraabdominal haemorrhage and perforation of the upper stomach. With good knowledge of the anatomy, careful dissection and appropriate prophylaxis against infection and deep venous thrombosis, perioperative adverse events should remain very uncommon.

Management

Adverse events that are specific to the band include perforation of the upper gut and infection at the access port site. Other complications are part of the general range of events that can occur with abdominal surgery and are covered adequately elsewhere.

Perforation of the upper stomach or distal esophagus is a rare but potentially lethal event. Suspicion of such an event should be raised whenever a patient is unwell after the procedure. Clinical features could include tachycardia, elevated temperature, abnormal level of pain and signs of marked upper abdominal tenderness or even of peritonitis. There is usually an elevated white cell count and C-reactive protein level. Do not hesitate to investigate such a patient. CT scan with a Gastrografin meal is the initial test of choice.

Laparoscopy should follow if the imaging does not reveal a problem but the suspicion remains. Remove the band whenever an abnormal fluid collection is present. Unless there is an obvious defect visible, do not explore further trying to find and repair a defect as you are more likely to make matters worse. Better to irrigate, place a closed drainage system and get out. The band can be replaced at 3 months after the problem has settled.

Infection around the access port should be separated from a superficial cellulitis of the access port incision. The latter will settle with antimicrobial therapy. The infection around the access port will not settle until the port is removed. Clinically it is not usually a florid infection with elevated temperature and marked swelling and redness. More likely, it presents as an initial mild local inflammatory picture, followed by a discharge from the wound that will persist until the port is removed. It carries the risk of an ascending contamination along the tubing, leading to low grade inflammation around the band itself and eventual erosion of the band.

Early but not urgent removal of the access port is indicated. At operation wash the area copiously with an appropriate antiseptic, plug the tubing with the plug available in the tubing repair kit, push the tubing well back into the peritoneal cavity and leave the wound open to heal by secondary intention. Replace the port after all healing has occurred, usually at 2–3 months.

Late Adverse Events

All bariatric procedures have a maintenance requirement. In a systematic review of all bariatric surgical reports with 10 or more years of follow-up [6], the revisional surgery rate was a median of 24 % and it was not different between procedures. Eight LAGB reports provided data on revisional surgery. The median value was 26 % with a range of 8–60 %. The median rate for the six RYGB reports that provided data was 22 % with a range of 8–38 %.

Late adverse events after LAGB can be divided into three groups of problems: proximal gastric enlargements which include anterior and posterior prolapse and symmetrical enlargement, erosion of the band into the stomach, and tubing and port problems.

Late adverse events have been relatively common after LAGB but are decreasing. Table 1 shows the total revisional procedure in 3,227 patients treated by myself and my colleague, Dr. Wendy Brown, over a 15-year period [6]. The total period has been subdivided into three, a perigastric era, a pars flaccida era and a Lap-Band AP era. For proximal enlargements, there was no difference between the first and second era and a dramatic reduction with the introduction of the Lap-Band AP system. The incidence of erosion decreased progressively through the three eras.

TABLE 1. Total revisional procedures during the follow-up period (adapted from O'Brien et al., Ann Surg 2013 [6])

	Total period	Perigastric era	Pars flaccida era	Lap-Band AP era
Dates and numbers	1994–2011 (N=3227)	1994–2000 (N=931)	2001–2005 (N=926)	2006–2011 (N=1370)
Enlargements	840 (26 %)	375 (40 %)	377 (41 %)	88 (6.4 %)
Erosions	110 (3.4 %)	79 (8.5 %)	20 (2.2 %)	11 (0.8 %)
Port/tubing	666 (21 %)	281 (30 %)	304 (33 %)	81 (5.9 %)
Explanations	181 (5.6 %)	92 (9.9 %)	59 (6.4 %)	30 (2.2 %)

Proximal Gastric Enlargements

Etiology

Proximal gastric enlargements occur because the band has been placed incorrectly, a part of the gastric wall slips through the band or there is stretching of the stomach or esophagus above the band. The central driver for all enlargements, whether they are posterior prolapse, anterior prolapse, and symmetrical enlargement, is the pressure generated by eating too quickly or taking too big a bite. It is essential that each bite must transit the area of the band before another bite is taken. With correct placement of the band, there is only a virtual stomach present. A typical barium study after placement shows no actual volume reservoir. With eating, space needs to be created for the food before it transits the band into the stomach below. This will generate a force. The two key variables that determine that force are the volume of food present and the rapidity of eating. As the force seeks to create space, any weakness in fixation will be displayed.

Posterior prolapse was seen with the perigastric pathway of placing the band, which often passed across the upper reaches of the lesser sac. The smooth and extensive peritonealized posterior gastric surface was the most likely to slip under the stress of eating, creating a posterior slip. This greater level of posterior weakness protected any deficiency in the anterior fixation and so anterior slips were relatively rare at that time. A randomized controlled trial involving 200 LAGB patients in which the perigastric pathway was compared with the pars flaccida pathway, which always places the band above the lesser sac, showed complete prevention of posterior prolapse by the pars flaccida approach [7].

Physiology and Pathophysiology of the LAGB

An understanding of the anatomy and physiology of the upper stomach when a band is present is needed to understand the mechanisms for proximal gastric enlargements and thereby to prevent them.

The LAGB should be placed at the very top of the stomach, around the cardia and within 1 cm of the esophagogastric junction. The primary mechanism of action of the LAGB

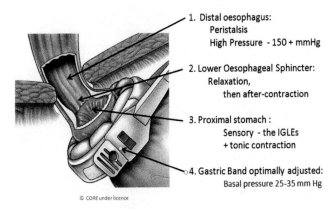

1. Distal oesophagus:
   Peristalsis
   High Pressure - 150 + mmHg

2. Lower Oesophageal Sphincter:
   Relaxation,
   then after-contraction

3. Proximal stomach :
   Sensory - the IGLEs
   + tonic contraction

4. Gastric Band optimally adjusted:
   Basal pressure 25-35 mm Hg

© CORE under licence

FIG. 1. The four components of the lower esophageal contractile segment (LECS) (© CORE under licence, with permission).

is by the induction of a sense of satiety, a lack of appetite or hunger [8]. There are two components to this—satiety and satiation.

Satiety is the state of not being hungry. It is achieved for the LAGB patient by adding or removing of fluid from the system to change the degree of compression of the band on the gastric wall. When this compression is optimal, it induces a sense of satiety which is present throughout the day. Although some hunger may develop at times during the day, there is a general reduction of appetite, less interest in food and less concern about not eating.

Satiation is the resolution of hunger with eating. For the LAGB patient, it is induced by each bite of food as it passes across the band. When the band is optimally adjusted, each bite is squeezed across by esophageal peristalsis, generating increased pressure on that segment of the gastric wall. This reduces any appetite that may have been present and induces a feeling of not being hungry after eating a small amount. The combination of these effects allows the person to eat three or less small meals per day.

Figure 1 shows the components of the lower esophageal contractile segment (LECS), an entity first described by Dr. Paul Burton from extensive study of the physiology of the gastric band [9]. It brings together the key elements that together generate early onset of satiation after eating. The distal esophagus squeezes each bite of food to the stomach proximal to the band. The lower esophageal sphincter relaxes to allow passage and then contracts to maintain the forward pressure. The proximal segment of stomach maintains tonic

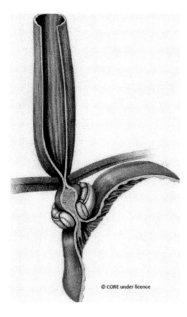

Fig. 2. A small bite of food is being squeezed across the band, thereby compressing the vagal afferents and generating a feeling of satiety (© CORE under licence, with permission).

contraction and detects the pressure increase. The band maintains an optimal compression to provide sufficient resistance to stimulate afferent signals but not sufficient to stop transit. There should be no restrictive component for normal functioning of the LAGB.

The optimally adjusted LAGB modifies the normal transit of a food bolus into the stomach. With normal swallowing, a food bolus is carried by esophageal peristalsis down the esophagus. The lower esophageal sphincter (LES) relaxes and the bolus passes intact smoothly into the stomach. The LES facilitates the final transfer with an aftercontraction. With the band in its correct place with only 1 cm of cardia above the upper edge of the band and with the band optimally adjusted (exerting a pressure of between 25 and 35 mmHg on the gastric lumen [10]), the esophagus must generate stronger peristalsis, and the after contraction of the LES becomes more important. The bolus is squeezed through by these forces. It takes between two and six squeezes to achieve complete transit of a single small bite. This may take up to 1 min [11].

Figure 2 shows a small bite of food in transit. The aftercontraction of the LES is evident. Just part of each bite will transit on each peristaltic sequence. The remainder will reflux into the body of the distal esophagus, generate a secondary peristalsis wave, and a further squeeze will occur. After several squeezes the bite will have passed. Importantly, each squeeze generates signals to the satiety centre of the hypothalamus. The signalling of both satiety and satiation to the arcuate nucleus of the hypothalamus does not appear to be mediated by any of the hormones known to arise from the cardia as none has been shown to be increased in a basal state after band placement and none increases postprandially [12].

Vagal afferents are the more probable mediators and, among these, the intraganglionic laminar endings (IGLEs) demonstrate the characteristics needed to subserve this role [13, 14].

A second swallow should not commence until all of the previous bite has passed totally into the stomach below the band or stretching of the upper stomach and distal esophagus will occur. If such stretching occurs repeatedly, disruption of the lower esophageal contractile segment and eventually persisting enlargement will occur.

Classification of Proximal Enlargements

Posterior Slip

When pressure from eating too quickly or taking too big a bite occurs, the weakest link in the chain will show up first. When the LAGB was initially placed along the perigastric pathway, the weakest link was the posterior wall of the stomach and a posterior slip or prolapse occurred. The large smooth posterior surface of the stomach could easily slide through the band to create a pouch above. On a barium meal the band was seen to have moved from a diagonal to a vertical position and the gastric pouch was lying to the patient's right side of the band. This problem was detected very soon after the introduction of the Lap-Band [15]. A range of technical changes were introduced without important effect until there was a change from the perigastric pathway to the pars flaccida pathway. By this change, the band no longer was passing across the upper reaches of the lesser sac but rather through the tissues posterior to the esophagus and the weakness was removed. A randomized trial comparing to two pathways showed elimination of the posterior slip [7].

Anterior Slip

With change to the pars flaccida approach, the next weakest link was shown to be the lateral, or less often the medial, aspect of the anterior fixation. Anterior prolapse became the common form of proximal enlargement. In this case the band was seen on plain X-ray to lie transversely and the enlargement was seen on barium meal to lie above and to the patient's left of the band.

Symmetrical Gastric Enlargement

More recently, with the exercise of greater care in completing the anterior fixation, there is generally no weak area posteriorly or anteriorly. If the patient eats too big a volume or too rapidly or the adjustment is excessive, the force simply stretches what is there and, in time, a symmetrical enlargement develops (Fig. 3). If there is too much stomach above the band from the time of the initial placement, as occurs with an unrecognized hiatal hernia, this enlargement occurs more readily.

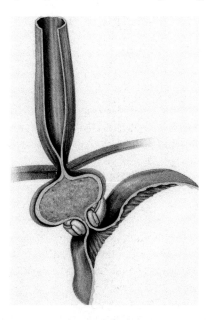

FIG. 3. The bite is too large or a second bite has been taken before the first bite has completed transit. There is a proximal enlargement disrupting the action of the lower esophageal contractile segment (© CORE under licence, with permission).

Focal Esophageal Enlargement

A variant of the symmetrical enlargement that is important to recognize is the focal enlargement of the distal esophagus. This will occur in the same setting as symmetrical gastric enlargement when there is too little stomach proximal to the band to expand. The importance of its recognition lies in its management. Revision with replacement of the band above the enlargement is not appropriate and removal of the blocking effect of the band by removal of fluid or possibly removal of the band is required.

Diagnosis of Proximal Enlargements

Each of the forms of proximal gastric enlargement presents clinically as a problem of stasis at the distal esophagus, the principal symptoms being reflux, especially at night, heartburn, vomiting, and food intolerance. There are no "normal" symptoms after LAGB. If your patient has the symptoms mentioned above, there are only three possibilities. The band is too tight, they are eating too quickly or too big a bite and they have a proximal enlargement. All three may be present.

Diagnosis of proximal enlargements is generally achieved by barium meal. A small volume of dilute barium will demonstrate the anatomy as present. However, the abnormal anatomy may be intermittent, occurring only with eating. A stress barium meal is needed to define this problem [16]. For symmetrical enlargements, upper gastrointestinal endoscopy is required to separate the esophageal and gastric enlargements.

If the symptoms persist in spite of removal of fluid from the band, the problem is treated by laparoscopic removal and replacement of the band along a new path above the previous one. It has proven to be a safe procedure, requiring no more than an overnight hospital stay, and has rarely been associated with a second enlargement, and the patients' weight loss pattern remains on the track they were initially following [6].

Treatment: Nonsurgical

The first two steps in all patients having symptoms are the reduction of fluid in the band and reinforcement of the need to eat small bites slowly. If the clinical suspicion is that the last adjustment was too much, reduction of a small volume, perhaps 0.3 mL or less is sufficient to give relief, and the patient can proceed with their weight loss process. For the more severe symptoms of an acute block, such as a bolus of food sticking and copious vomiting being present, it is preferable to remove a greater volume of fluid, 2–3 mL, check that normal swallowing now occurs and then begin to replace the fluid after a period of rest for several days. If symptoms are not relieved or recur, proceed to barium meal.

If the barium meal shows a proximal enlargement, remove all fluid from the band, wait 1 month and repeat the barium study. Generally there will be a return to normal anatomy. Reinforce the eating rules with the patient, advise of the tendency to recurrence if they are not very careful and then begin the stepwise replacement of the fluid to a level to achieve satiety. Approximately 50 % of our patients need no further action and continue on their weight loss program. If recurrence of symptoms occurs in the months or years after the conservative approach, we will generally discuss revision of the band with repositioning along a new pathway above the enlargement.

Anterior gastric slips are more likely to cause acute problems and are less likely to resolve with a conservative approach. Although we will seek to relieve the problem in some by removal of all fluid and review with barium meal at one month, we are more likely to proceed directly to surgical revision. If there is a marked enlargement and upper abdominal tenderness, this should be done urgently as perforation of the acute anterior slip has occurred. If the symptoms are more modest, early elective revision is planned.

Treatment: Surgical

The primary approach to revisional surgery is for removal of the band and replacement of the band along a new pathway just below the esophagogastric junction. If the primary band was a Lap-Band AP, the same band is generally used. All other bands are converted to a Lap-Band AP.

There are several key technical points in the revisional procedure to which we attach the acronym NERD:

- **New**: Always remove the band and create a new pathway. Do not seek to undo the previous anterior fixation. It is not necessary as the new pathway will be well above that area. Sometimes, especially with anterior slips, you will be tempted to simply reduce the slip. It can often be reduced quite easily and everything looks fine. But a recurrence is likely [17]. Don't even consider it.
- **Explore** the hiatus. Always dissect the crura. Approximate the crura if laxity is present.
- **Reduce** any hiatal hernia fully. Be sure you can see intra-abdominal esophagus.
- **Dissect** the soft tissue membrane in front of the upper stomach down to visible gastric wall sufficient to provide a path for the band. As you have already dissected the esophagus, you can now see the transition from esophagus to stomach and therefore are able to correctly position the band, the upper margin of which should be at 1 cm below that point. You need to be sure to maximize the compressive effect of the band on the vagal afferents in the underlying gastric wall by removing the buffering effect of that soft tissue layer.

Prevention of Proximal Enlargements

There will always be a need for some revisional surgery and all who care for bariatric surgical patients should be able to diagnose and manage adverse events as they arise. Yet the need for revision can be reduced and this is particularly so for the proximal enlargements. Although there are technical factors that have an influence, proximal enlargements primarily arise when the patient eats too big a bite or eats too quickly. Every bite must pass the band before the next bite is swallowed.

The optimal result from LAGB will come from an effective partnership between you and your patient. You both have three responsibilities. You must place the band safely and securely in the correct position. You must make sure your patients have access to a competent aftercare program and you must be sure your patients are appropriately instructed in what they must do. Your patients must follow the rules regarding eating, they must follow the rules regarding exercise and activity and they must come back to the aftercare program permanently.

We have brought together all the information that the patient needs into a book, "The Lap-Band Solution: A Partnership for Weight Loss" [18]. The book details the "Eight Golden Rules" and includes a DVD of these rules showing, through animations, how the band works and why the rules are what they are. This book/DVD has proved to be very valuable in developing the partnership we seek and in reducing the problems of proximal enlargements.

Some key points in minimizing the problem of proximal enlargements:

- Use a proven LAGB. There are many on the market (outside the USA). Only use a device that has been proven to be effective and safe.
- Do anterior fixation. There is a conflicting literature. It is simple and almost certainly harmless. Why save a few minutes in the operating room and risk having to reoperate later.
- Adjust the band to a level of satiety sufficient to achieve your weight loss targets over a 2- to 3-year period. Do not tighten excessively or push for rapid weight loss.
- The patient must eat small amounts—three or less meals a day, half a cup volume of food (125 mL; 125 mg) at each meal, use a small plate, fork, and spoon. Enjoy the flavours, the tastes and the textures of the food during that time.
- The patient should eat good food that is protein containing, nutritious, tasty and attractive. They should enjoy eating more after the band than before—by focussing on the quality of the food, not the quantity.
- The patient should eat slowly. Each bite should be chewed until it is mush, usually 15–20 s of chewing. Swallow it and then wait 1 min for that bite to completely cross the band before another bite is taken. Use a timer if necessary to reinforce the slowness that is essential.

Erosions

Erosion of the LAGB into the lumen of the stomach is an uncommon and surprisingly mild and manageable in most cases. As the cause is still unclear, erosion can be expected to continue albeit at a low rate. Nevertheless, the bariatric surgeon performing LAGB will see the patient with an eroded band occasionally and needs to know how to make the diagnosis, how to determine an appropriate management pathway and what outcomes can be expected.

Incidence

Erosion of the gastric band into the lumen of the stomach was initially described as a complication of LAGB in 1998 [19]. Subsequent reports have varied widely in their descriptions of possible etiology, incidence, clinical presentation, and management options.

In 2011, we reported a systematic literature review of erosions after LAGB [20]. We focussed on incidence, etiology, clinical presentation, treatment, complications, and weight loss. Twenty-five studies of LAGB reported 231 erosions in 15,775 patients (overall incidence of 1.46 %). The mean number of patients per study was 631 (±486) and the mean follow-up was 3.73 (±2.4) years. There was a wide variation in incidence ranging from 0.2 % in a study by Ren and Weiner of 444 patients followed for 2 years [21] to a prevalence of 11.1 % in a report of 90 patients treated by Westling et al. and also followed for 2 years [22]. The incidence of erosions was found to be related to surgeon experience. In four reports involving less than 100 patients, there were 27 erosions in a total of 270 patients (10 %) compared to 180 erosions in 12,978 patients (1.386 %) in the remaining 21 reports [20]. Multiple regression analysis showed that erosion rate was inversely related to the number of patients treated and number of years of surgeon experience ($r^2 = 0.186$).

In a study of our own experience, Dr. Wendy Brown reviewed 2,986 patients who had LAGB during a 15-year period [23]. A total of 100 erosions were experienced by 85 patients (2.85 %) at a median time of 33 months from initial surgery to the erosion (range 11–170 months). The rate of erosion was highest when the band was placed by the perigastric approach at 6.7 %. Since the adoption of the pars flaccida approach, the rate of erosion has decreased to 1.1 % and has been less than 1 % during the last seven years.

Etiology

The causes of erosion remain uncertain. Certainly, for erosion presenting soon after placement of the LAGB, it could be considered likely to be a result of gastric wall trauma at the time of placement. Most erosions present after this time. In our series of 100 erosions [23], the earliest presentation was at 11 months.

Putative causes for erosion include tearing of the gastro-gastric sutures, excessive tightness of the anterior wrap, overfilling of the band and infection secondary to access port infection. The pars flaccida pathway for band placement appears to be less likely to be associated with erosion than the perigastric pathway [23]. There have been no data to suggest that taking gastric irritants such as nonsteroidal anti-inflammatory drugs, smoking or alcohol is relevant.

Clinical Presentation and Diagnosis

The clinical presentation of LAGB erosion is almost always relatively mild [23]. Loss of the sense of satiety with increased hunger, stronger appetite and weight regain is the commonest mode of presentation. Mild epigastric pain is common whereas severe pain and/or evidence of peritonitis are rare. Additional presentations include port site infection and missing fluid from the band due to balloon disruption The essential diagnostic modality is upper gastrointestinal endoscopy which should be sought whenever unexplained weight regain and loss of satiety or late port infection are noted.

Management

The current recommended approach is for band removal after erosion is laparoscopic, with repair of the gastric wall and subsequent replacement of the band at least 3 months later.

Treatment is most commonly by removal of the band, repair of the stomach and later band replacement. Other options include removal alone or conversion to another procedure. In our series, weight loss was retained after treatment of the erosion with a mean weight loss at final follow-up of 50.3 % EWL [23].

For an endoscopic approach it has been advised to wait until at least the buckle of the band is in the stomach [24]. This may require a long delay and multiple endoscopies, and the scarring may prevent endoscopic removal. Because of the lengthy endoscopic procedural times, the significant failure rate and the further need for hospital admission and anesthesia for port removal, we do not generally use endoscopic removal [23, 25].

Access Port/Tubing Problems

A range of problems can arise from the tubing connecting the band to the access port. It has been rare to have a leak from the band itself or from the port. The incidence of these problems during a 15-year period for over 3,000 patients is shown for our patients in Table 1. Most commonly, there have been breaks in the tubing at its junction with the metal connection to the port. Needlestick injury to the tubing, perforation of the tubing due to rubbing on a firm structure such as the anterior rectus sheath and rotation of the port occur less frequently. Technical improvements in the design of the attachment of the tubing to the port and better training to avoid needlestick injury have been associated with a lower incidence in recent times.

Diagnosis is confirmed by noting loss of fluid on more than one occasion. If there has been only a small loss of fluid or possible confusion about the volume that should be present, a volume check on two or more occasions, ideally by the same person, is important to avoid unnecessary exploration. We have found that imaging of the system with injected contrast has been unhelpful. It has failed to detect slow leaks and it has been misleading in identifying the site of leakage. It is not recommended. If there is complete loss of fluid with a test injection, it is possible that the tubing has separated completely at the break with return of the proximal end to the abdominal cavity. A plain abdominal X-ray is then performed on the morning of the planned port replacement to determine if an initial laparoscopy and retrieval of the tubing need be undertaken.

As the problem is almost always in the vicinity of the access port, the surgical plan is to mobilize the port, identify the cause and replace the port and adjacent tubing. We proceed to band replacement only if there is a leak demonstrated to be present but is occurring proximal to the exposed port and tubing after full mobilization.

Review Questions and Answers

1. An optimal tightness of the adjustable band occurs when:

    (a) Solid food sits above the band to give a sense of fullness
    (b) Liquids can pass with some resistance across the band
    (c) There is little appetite for food throughout the day
    (d) Barium imaging shows slow transit
    (e) A small amount of food satisfies any hunger
        (c) and (e) are correct

2. The following are true regarding proximal gastric enlargements above the band:

    (a) All enlargements are associated with slippage of the stomach from below
    (b) Anterior prolapse can develop into an acute surgical emergency
    (c) Posterior prolapse is largely prevented by use of the pars flaccida pathway
    (d) Symmetrical enlargement of the stomach can be distinguished from a symmetrical enlargement of the esophagus by barium swallow
    e. Most symmetrical enlargements will resolve by removing fluid from the band
        (b), (c) and (e) are correct

3. Erosion of the gastric band into the lumen of the stomach:

    (a) Is likely to occur in about 1 % of patients
    (b) Is due to adjusting the band too tightly
    (c) Is the commonest cause of an acute abdomen in someone with a gastric band
    (d) Can be effectively treated by removal of the band and later replacement
    (e) Removal of the band by endoscopic technique is simpler and safer than laparoscopic approach
        (a) and (d) are correct

References

1. Pories WJ, Swanson MS, MacDonald KG, Long SB, Morris PG, Brown BM, Barakat HA, deRamon RA, Israel G, Dolezal JM, et al. Who would have thought it? An operation proves to be the most effective therapy for adult-onset diabetes mellitus. Ann Surg. 1995;222:339–50.

2. Flum DR, Dellinger EP. Impact of gastric bypass operation on survival: a population-based analysis. J Am Coll Surg. 2004;199:543–51.

3. Chapman A, Kiroff G, Game P, Foster B, O'Brien P, Ham J, Maddern G. Laparoscopic adjustable gastric banding in the treatment of obesity: a systematic review. Surgery. 2004;135:326–51.

4. Maggard MA, Shugarman LR, Suttorp M, Maglione M, Sugerman HJ, Livingston EH, Nguyen NT, Li Z, Mojica WA, Hilton L, Rhodes S, Morton SC, Shekelle PG. Meta-analysis: surgical treatment of obesity. Ann Intern Med. 2005;142:547–59.

5. Flum DR, Belle SH, King WC, Wahed AS, Berk P, Chapman W, Pories W, Courcoulas A, McCloskey C, Mitchell J, Patterson E, Pomp A, Staten MA, Yanovski SZ, Thirlby R, Wolfe B. Perioperative safety in the longitudinal assessment of bariatric surgery. N Engl J Med. 2009;361:445–54.

6. O'Brien P, McDonald L, Anderson M, Brennan L, Brown WA. Long term outcomes after bariatric surgery: fifteen year follow up after gastric banding and a systematic review of the literature. Ann Surg. 2013;257(1):87–94.

7. O'Brien PE, Dixon JB, Laurie C, Anderson M. A prospective randomized trial of placement of the laparoscopic adjustable gastric band: comparison of the perigastric and pars flaccida pathways. Obes Surg. 2005;15:820–6.

8. Dixon AF, Dixon JB, O'Brien PE. Laparoscopic adjustable gastric banding induces prolonged satiety: a randomized blind crossover study. J Clin Endocrinol Metab. 2005;90:813–9.

9. Burton PR, Brown WA, Laurie C, Hebbard G, O'Brien PE. Mechanisms of bolus clearance in patients with laparoscopic adjustable gastric bands. Obes Surg. 2010;20:1265–72.

10. Burton PR, Brown WA, Laurie C, Richards M, Hebbard G, O'Brien PE. Effects of gastric band adjustments on intraluminal pressure. Obes Surg. 2009;19:1508–14.

11. Burton PR, Yap K, Brown WA, Laurie C, O'Donnell M, Hebbard G, Kalff V, O'Brien PE. Changes in satiety, supra- and infraband transit, and gastric emptying following laparoscopic adjustable gastric banding: a prospective follow-up study. Obes Surg. 2011;21:217–23.

12. Pournaras DJ, Le Roux CW. The effect of bariatric surgery on gut hormones that alter appetite. Diabetes Metab. 2009;35:508–12.

13. Berthoud HR. Vagal and hormonal gut-brain communication: from satiation to satisfaction. Neurogastroenterol Motil. 2008;20 Suppl 1:64–72.

14. Zagorodnyuk VP, Chen BN, Brookes SJ. Intraganglionic laminar endings are mechano-transduction sites of vagal tension receptors in the guinea-pig stomach. J Physiol. 2001;534:255–68.

15. O'Brien PE, McMurrick P. Posterior gastric wall prolapse after lap-band placement. Obes Surg. 1995;5:247 [Abstract].

16. Burton PR, Brown WA, Laurie C, Korin A, Yap K, Richards M, Owens J, Crosthwaite G, Hebbard G, O'Brien PE. Pathophysiology of laparoscopic adjustable gastric bands: analysis and classification using high-resolution video manometry and a stress barium protocol. Obes Surg. 2010;20:19–29.

17. Manganiello M, Sarker S, Tempel M, Shayani V. Management of slipped adjustable gastric bands. Surg Obes Relat Dis. 2008;4:534–8; discussion 538.

18. O'Brien P. The lap-band solution: a partnership for weight loss. Melbourne: Melbourne University Publishing; 2011.

19. Weiner R, Emmerlich V, Wagner D, Bockhorn H. Management and therapy of postoperative complications after "gastric banding" for morbid obesity. Chirurg. 1998;69:1082–8.

20. Egberts K, Brown WA, O'Brien PE. Systematic review of erosion after laparoscopic adjustable gastric banding. Obes Surg. 2011;21:1272–9.

21. Ren CWM. Favorable early results of gastric banding for morbid obesity: the American experience. Surg Endosc. 2004;18:543–6.

22. Westling A, Bjurling K, Ohrvall M, Gustavsson S. Silicone-adjustable gastric banding: disappointing results. Obes Surg. 1998;8:467–74.

23. Brown W, Egberts KJ, Franke-Richard D, Thodiyil P, Anderson MA, O'Brien PE. Erosions following laparoscopic adjustable gastric banding: diagnosis and management. Ann Surg. 2013;257(6):1047–52.

24. Neto M, Ramos AC, Campos JM, Murakami AH, Falcao M, Moura EH, Evangelista LF, Escalona A, Zundel N. Endoscopic removal of eroded adjustable gastric band: lessons learned after 5 years and 78 cases. Surg Obes Relat Dis. 2010;6:423–7.

25. O'Brien P. Comment on: Endoscopic removal of eroded adjustable gastric band: lessons learned after 5 years and 78 cases. Surg Obes Relat Dis. 2010;6:427–8.

23

Laparoscopic Adjustable Gastric Banding: Controversies

George Fielding

Bariatric surgery is a blessing for morbidly obese people. Nothing else really works. All the currently available bariatric procedures work to varying degrees and all have their problems. I currently perform all these procedures, and my patients have reaped the rewards of surgery and suffered the tribulations that can go with them—leaks after bypass and sleeve, band slips and erosions, malnutrition after BPD, weight regain, and failure after all of them. In the main though, most patients do well and are happy. Patients play an important role in the selection of their operation and the risks and benefits of all procedures should be explained to help them make this sometimes difficult decision.

Laparoscopic adjustable gastric banding (LAGB) has been a successful choice for the treatment of morbid obesity by many bariatric surgeons around the world, since its introduction in 1994. After its approval in 2001 in the USA by the Food and Drug Administration (FDA), the use of the lap band increased and has given patients an alternative treatment to the Roux-en-Y gastric bypass (RYGBP) and more recently the sleeve gastrectomy. The LAGB does not involve any bowel anastomosis, staple line complications, or risk of leaks. It is also adjustable and easily removable, both characteristics that are appealing to patients considering bariatric surgery. After its introduction to the USA in 2001, LAGB had similar popularity to that achieved in Australia and Europe, rivaling gastric bypass as the most common bariatric operation. In recent years though, that popularity has somewhat declined, particularly with the increasing interest in sleeve gastrectomy. Several factors have influenced that change, some real, some due to different perceptions of the value of gastric banding.

The Main Controversy: Should We Still Do the Band?

Obesity is currently the second largest cause of preventable death in the USA and a devastating disease, with its incidence and associated complications rising exponentially every year. There are more morbidly obese people in the USA than the total population of Australia. There are more in India than the total population of the USA. It's overwhelming. Surgery is currently the most effective proven treatment to control this epidemic, yet so few people who need it come for it.

LAGB surgery, and its postoperative management, as it is done today, bears very little resemblance to how it was done 10 years ago. Successful modification in the technique of band implantation, especially use of the pars flaccida technique, and hiatal hernia repair/cruroplasty at the initial operation, has substantially reduced the need for reoperation after band placement [1, 2]. Changes in band technology, especially use of wider, lower pressure bands result in further reductions. We understand that the band works primarily by controlling hunger and increasing feelings of satiety, rather than as a punitive, restrictive procedure [3, 4]. We have modified our adjustment strategies accordingly, aiming to keep patients in the "Green Zone," as described by Dixon and O'Brien. We teach patients to eat slowly, telling them that they can't live with a band as if they don't have one. With all this, long-term patient satisfaction has matched the reduction in need for band revision and removal, compared to patients who had their bands inserted in the late 1990s and early 2000s.

The LAGB delivers satisfactory weight loss, provided the band is adjusted properly. The percentage excess weight loss (%EWL) after LAGB has been reported at 55 % after 5 years [5]. Lanthaler et al. report %EWL of 64 % out to 10 years [6]. O'Brien reviewed 3,227 patients treated by laparoscopic adjustable gastric band placement between September 1994 and December 2011 [7]. Seven hundred fourteen patients had completed at least 10 years of follow-up. Follow-up was intact in 78 % of those beyond 10 years. There was no perioperative mortality for the primary placement or for any revisional procedures. There was a mean of 47.0 % EWL ($n=714$; 95 % CI=1.3) for all patients who were at or beyond 10-year follow-up. The band was explanted in 5.6 %. In Weichman et al.'s recent study of

S.A. Brethauer et al. (eds.), *Minimally Invasive Bariatric Surgery*,
DOI 10.1007/978-1-4939-1637-5_23, © Springer Science+Business Media New York 2015

2,909 patients from New York, %EWL after 6 years was 47 % [8]. The %EWL 3 years after surgery was 52.9 %, which was sustained thereafter to 47 % at 6 years. In multivariate models, increased number of office visits, younger age, female gender, and Caucasian race were significantly associated with a higher maximum %EWL. Of these patients, 363 (12.2 %) experienced one or more complications. The most common complications were band slip (4.5 %) and port-related problems (3.3 %). Other complications were rare. Only 7 patients (0.2 %) had band erosion. Eleven patients (0.4 %) underwent reoperation for weight gain. A total of 10 deaths (0.34 %) occurred during the study period. Three patients died within 30 days of surgery. Two of these deaths (0.06 %) were related to surgery, and 1 resulted from a motor vehicle accident. Seven patients died of causes unrelated to surgery during the course of the study. LAGB is a safe procedure with few early or late complications. Mortality is very rare.

In 2003, Weiner published data on 984 LAGB patients, including 100 patients with over 8-year follow-up, for whom he had 90 % follow-up [9]. They had 59 % EWL, and their body mass index (BMI) fell from 47 to 32 kg/m^2. He showed that it is an effective treatment.

If one reviews the literature concerning longer follow-up of LAGB, it seems that one can expect about 50 % EWL out to 10 years, with 50 % of patients achieving 50 % EWL, with very low risk to the patient.

We often hear that the gastric bypass (RYGB) is the "gold standard" for bariatric surgery. There is actually very little long-term data for gastric bypass. The best 10-year follow-up is from Kelvin Higa [10]. A total of 242 patients underwent RYGB surgery from February 1998 to April 1999. The office follow-up rate was 33 % at 2 years and only 7 % at 10 years. An additional 19 % had telephone follow-up at 10 years. The mean excess weight loss was 57 % at 10 years. Only 67 % of patients had 50 % EWL. Furthermore, 86 (35 %) had ≥1 complication during follow-up. The internal hernia rate was 16 %, and the gastrojejunal stenosis rate was 4.9 %. Of the 242 patients, 136 (51 %) had nutritional testing at least once after postoperative year 1. Of these 136 patients, only 24 (18 %) had remained nutritionally intact during follow-up. The weight loss is not that dissimilar to LAGB patients, there is a high long-term complication rate, and most patients had nutritional deficiencies. What's more, this is in the 26 % with documented follow-up.

Himpens et al. reviewed 126 consecutive patients treated with RYGB between January 1, 2001, and December 31, 2002 [11]. Seventy-seven patients (61.1 %) were available for evaluation after 9.4±0.6 years. Initial BMI was 40.3±7.5 kg/m^2. There was no postoperative mortality. Some 9 % of the patients suffered from internal herniation, despite the closure of potential hernia sites. With time, the patients regained weight; percentage of excess BMI lost was 56.2±29.3 %, down from a maximum of 88.0±29.6 % at 2.0 years. RYGB was effective for diabetes control in 85.7 % of the affected patients, but, surprisingly, 27.9 % developed new-onset diabetes.

Long-term data for the sleeve tells a similar story. Himpens has published his data on 53 patients who had laparoscopic sleeve gastrectomy between November 2001 and October 2002 [12]. There were 41 patients in follow-up, and 11 received an additional malabsorptive procedure at a later stage because of weight regain. In the 30 patients receiving only sleeve gastrectomy, there was a 3-year %EWL of 77.5 % and 6+ year %EWL of 53.3 %. The differences between the third and sixth postoperative year were statistically significant in both groups. New gastroesophageal reflux complaints appeared in 21 % of patients.

In another study, Sarela found, in 20 patients out to 9 years, that 3 were lost and 4 converted to another procedure [13]. Of the remaining 13 patients, 55 % had 50 % EWL.

Surgery for massive super obesity is a formidable challenge. No existing open or laparoscopic procedure reduces mean BMI below 30 from a starting point above 55. Eid and Schauer recently presented a group of 74 super obese patients, with a mean BMI of 66 (43–90) having sleeve gastrectomy between January 2002 and February 2004, with a mean 6-year follow-up [14]. Mean EWL at 72, 84, and 96 months after LSG was 52 %, 43 %, and 46 %, respectively, with an overall EWL of 48 %. The mean BMI decreased from 66 (43–90) to 46 kg/m^2 (22–73).

Years ago, I presented a group of 76 super obese patients, with a mean BMI of 69 (60–104) having had LAGB [15]. Five patients had a BMI > 100 kg/m^2. BMI fell from 69±6.2 to 49±7.73 at 1 year to 37±4.45 at 3 years and this was maintained at 4 and 5 years. BMI in 13 patients with >5-year follow-up was 35.09±5.3 kg/m^2 (27–44).

Weight loss with LAGB in this group of massive super obese patients was similar to all other surgical techniques. In total contrast, Marmuses's group from France has just published very disappointing results in a group of 35 men (18.8 %) and 151 women (81.2 %), with a mean BMI of 55.06 kg/m^2 (range: 50–74.4) who had LAGB between September 1995 and December 2007 [16]. The mean follow-up was 112.5 months with a minimum of 28 months and a maximum of 172 months. The follow-up rate was maintained at 89 % at 10 years. At 10 years there was a band removal rate of 52.2 % (47 of 90 patients), a failure rate of 22 % (7 of 33 patients) of those who still had their band in place, and a median BMI of 43.43 kg/m^2. No one really knows why there is such disparity in reported outcomes with the band. It may be due to a preference to remove bands rather than revise them when there is reflux or variations in follow-up.

Weiner performed 937 sleeves between October 2001 and December 2010, with 0.4 % mortality [17]. Of the 937 patients, 17 (1.8 %) experienced staple line leakage. From 2005 to 2010, 106 secondary procedures were performed. Insufficient weight loss or weight regain was the indication in 88 cases. Sixteen (15 %) patients had severe gastroesophageal reflux which was resolved by RYGB.

In conclusion, long-term data for LAGB, sleeve, and RYGB demonstrates a remarkable similarity—about 50 % EWL—and a substantial need for reoperation.

This then leaves patients with a choice. Many patients base that choice on safety, if there is a similar benefit. In 2004, Ren et al. asked 469 consecutive patients what was the reason for their choice of operation [18]. Safety of the operation (43 %) was the highest rated factor in choosing LAGB. RYGB was preferred due to "lack of a foreign body," "inability to cheat," and "dumping." Duodenal switch (BPD/DS) was selected in 11 % of patients, primarily because of "durability of the weight loss" (51 %).

Patients care about safety. The one indisputable feature that separates the LAGB from other procedures is its safety with operative mortality in the order of 1/2,000. Nguyen et al. recently reviewed 10,151 bands admitted in University Healthcare Consortium (UHC) hospitals between January 2007 and December 2009 [19]. There was a mean length of stay of 1.2 days and 3 deaths (0.03 %).

Chakraverty et al. performed a search of all comparative studies of LAGB and other procedures and found five level one randomized controlled trials [20]. Their conclusion was that LAGB delivered satisfactory weight loss and was much safer, with fewer complications and shorter stay, and thus may be preferable to patients. Gould reviewed 32,509 bariatric procedures, of which 58 % were laparoscopic RYGB and 21 % LAGB. Mortality was 0.09 % vs. 0.02 % ($P<0.05$) and inpatient complications 4 % vs. 1.6 % ($P<0.1$) [21]. Finks, reviewing the Michigan Bariatric Collaboration data of 25,469 patients found that 644 patients had a serious complication and that sleeve was 2.46 times and RYGB 3.58 times as likely as LAGB to have a complication [22]. In a review of 322 super obese patients, Parikh found that 27 patients had a major complication. LAGB had 4.7 % and RYGB 11.3 % [23].

If one was to apply mortality rates of 0.02 % and 0.3 % to the 23 million people in the USA with a BMI over 35, the difference is 4,500 dead people after surgery with a band, compared to 70,000 after a bypass. It is the fear of death after bypass or sleeve that prevents so many people from coming for bariatric surgery.

Saunders et al. reviewed 2,823 consecutive bariatric patients. Of these 165 (5.8 %) patients required 184 (6.5 %) readmissions within 30 days of their operation [24]. LAGB had the lowest patient readmission rate of 3.1 % compared to RYGB 7.3 %. LAGB decreased the odds for readmission. The same authors then assessed 1-year readmission rates for 1,939 patients and found that LAGB was 12.7 % and RYGB 24 % [25].

The issue with band vs. sleeve is slightly different. There is a similar safety differential as with a bypass. The real problem is leak after the sleeve, a complication that typically has a very protracted recovery, unlike anything seen after LAGB and only rarely after bypass. In published literature up to 2012, leak rates range from 0 to 2.5 %. Aurora reviewed 4,888 sleeve patients, with a leak rate of 2.4 %, most of which happened after discharge [26]. Weiner showed a leak rate of 1.8 % in 937 patients [15]. Sakran showed 44 (1.5 leaks in 2,834 patients, all but 1 after discharge [27]. The leaks had a median closure of 40 days (1–270 days).

What a patient has to be told, quite simply, is that if you have a sleeve, based on current data, the chance of dying after a sleeve is five times that of a band. The patient will have a 1/40 chance of a leak, which takes an average of 40 days to close. You also have a 1/5 chance of needing a conversion to another procedure by 5 years. After all that, the weight loss at 5 years is the same as with a well-adjusted band.

Follow-Up

Given that it's much safer and delivers similar weight loss long term as a bypass or a sleeve, why is there controversy about using the band? The answer lies in the need for a high level of long-term maintenance and the need for band revision. Long-term follow-up is the weak point of all bariatric operations. With the band, far more than the other procedures, it determines success or failure. In 2004, Shen et al. reviewed 216 LAGB and 139 RYGB operations performed between October 2000 and September 2002 [28]. Of these patients, 186 LAGB patients and 115 RYGBP patients were available for 1-year follow-up. Of the LAGB patients, 130 (70 %) returned 6 or less times in the first year and achieved 42 % EWL, and 56 patients (30 %) returned more than 6 times and had 50 % EWL ($P=0.005$). Overall %EWL after RYGBP was 66.1 %. Some 53 patients (46 %) returned 3 or less times in the first year, achieving 66.1 % EWL. A further 62 patients (54 %) returned more than 3 times after surgery and achieved 67.6 % EWL ($P=NS$). They showed that patient follow-up plays a significant role in the amount of weight lost after LAGB, but not after RYGBP. It still holds true today. Patient motivation and surgeon commitment for long-term follow-up is critical for successful weight loss after LAGB surgery.

This is the key to the whole issue of band vs. other procedures. A successful outcome after LAGB requires a substantial input from patient and surgeon. An unadjusted band won't work. There needs to be relatively open access to the surgeon and their team. Patients need to be able to come in if they are hungry or have a problem. This open-door policy is somewhat at odds with the traditional surgical model, as is the long-term follow-up. At NYU, we see patients once a month for the first 18 months, and then in reducing intervals after that. We see them yearly after 5 years. We have peripheral clinics to make access easier. Adjustments are done by the surgeons and by practice extenders such as RNs, PAs, and NPs. It's a lot of work. It's probably the main issue facing bariatric surgeons who wish to do LAGB surgery. With the newer bands, modern surgical techniques, and understanding of the Green Zone, more and more patients are doing well, with fewer problems. Eventually there is a very large patient load. One simply needs to decide if one wants it. The payoff is the low morbidity, low risk, effective surgery one can offer our patients. But if you want successful outcomes, you have to do the work. If this is daunting or cannot be accommodated into practice, then it's probably best not to do LAGB surgery.

Revisions

The major long-term concern with the LAGB is the need for reoperation, usually due to severe reflux following band slip or pouch dilatation. Several European papers have shown high band removal/revision rates at 10 years. This has led these authors to suggest that surgeons should abandon the LAGB. The two strongest publications suggesting the band is less satisfactory are from Himpens and Romy.

Himpens et al. reviewed 151 consecutive patients who had LAGB between January 1, 1994, and December 31, 1997, with follow-up of 54.3 % (82 of 151 patients) at 12 years [29]. The biggest surprise was that 28 % experienced band erosion, which is markedly outside all other reported ranges. Seventeen percent of patients had their procedure switched to laparoscopic RYGBP. Thirty-six patients (51.4 %) still had their band, and their mean excess weight loss was 48 % (range: 38–58 %). Overall, the satisfaction index was good for 60.3 % of patients. It is crucial when contemplating this paper to realize that this was at the very start of the band experience, with small high pressure bands, placed low on the stomach, without hiatal hernia repairs, and before any real understanding of Green Zone adjustment theory. That being said, many patients in this group continue to do well with their band.

In a very well-structured paper, Romy et al. reviewed 422 matched patients after LAGB and RYGB [30]. Follow-up was 92.3 % at the end of 6 years, which is extraordinary. Early morbidity was higher after RYGB than after LAGB (17.2 % vs. 5.4 %; $P<0.001$). Weight loss was quicker, maximal weight loss was greater, and weight loss remained significantly better after RYGB until the sixth postoperative year. However, both groups did very well. RYGB patients had 78.5 % EWL and LAGB patients 64.8 %. Maximal weight loss was achieved 18 months after a gastric bypass procedure, while maximum weight loss was achieved on average 36 months after gastric banding. At 6 years, there were more failures (BMI>35 or reversal of the procedure/conversion) after LAGB (48.3 % vs. 12.3 %; $P<0.001$). There were more long-term complications (41.6 % vs. 19 %; P 0.001) and more reoperations (26.7 % vs. 12.7 %; $P<0.001$) after LAGB. There was very little description of what the complications were.

At first blush, there seems to be a major difference between the two groups in Romy's paper—78.5 % vs. 65 % EWL. However, in a 5′5″, 270 lb woman (BMI 45), it is a difference of 17 lb. Is 17 lb, at 6 years, worth the risk?

Achieving 65 % EWL with the LAGB is excellent—it represents 100 lb weight loss for the 5′5″, 270 lb woman, with a BMI of 45.

The other issue arising from these two excellent papers is the need for revision, and whether to revise the slipped band or remove it. It's important to distinguish band removal due to weight loss failure from band removal due to symptoms of reflux, or, more rarely, erosion. Many centers have taken the position of removing the band to treat reflux and a slip, as well as failure and performing bypass or sleeve. Our position at NYU has been to revise bands for reflux and remove them, if the patient wants, for weight loss failure. Beitner has recently reviewed 3,876 patients treated by LAGB at NYU from January 1, 2001, to June 30, 2009 [31]. There were 411 patients that had the band revised for pouch-related problems (10.6 %). Of these, 9 subsequently had the band removed and 12 were converted to another bariatric procedure. An additional 31 patients were converted to another bariatric procedure without a revisional procedure beforehand. Thus 390 patients were included in the analysis of weight outcomes after revision. There were no procedure-related deaths. The 30-day patient complication rate for all reoperations was 0.5 %. Late complications (erosion) occurred in 0.5 % and 29 patients (7.4 %) required a second revision. The initial weight and BMI were 124.06±21.28 kg and 44.80±6.12 kg/m^2. At reoperation, weight, BMI, and %EWL were 89.18±20.51 kg, 32.25±6.50 kg/m^2, and 54.13±21.80 %. Reoperation occurred at a mean of 33.67±33.27 months after the primary procedure. Mean operating time was 67.02±30.50 min and length of hospital stay was 1.11±0.92 days. The band was repositioned in 252 patients (64.6 %) and replaced in 109 patients (27.9 %). Twenty-nine patients (7.4 %) had hiatal hernia repair alone. Weight, BMI, and %EWL were 92.24±20.22 kg, 33.32±6.41 kg/m^2, and 48.81 % 12 months post revision and 92.42±19.91 kg, 33.53±6.25 kg/m^2, and 47.50±22.91 % 24 months post revision. Weight loss was sustained both at 12 months and 24 months after reoperation and did not differ from those without reoperation at the same length of time after primary banding. Importantly, we found that if a patient has lost weight with a band, they will maintain that weight loss after revision. If they have done less well, revising the band will not change that. The choice to remove the band and convert to another procedure is then the patient's. Patient satisfaction with the band was not affected by reoperation. Reoperation for pouch-related problems after LAGB can be achieved with minimal morbidity. Reoperation neither affects weight loss nor patient satisfaction after LAGB.

We also found that incidence of band revision has fallen significantly over the last 5 years, with the newer bands, and improved understanding of band physiology. O'Brien has found the same thing in his series of 3,227 patients, of whom 714 were at more than 10 years [7]. Revisional procedures were performed for proximal enlargement (26 %), erosion (3.4 %), and port and tubing problems (21 %). The need for revision decreased as the technique evolved, with 40 % revision rate for proximal gastric enlargements in the first 10 years, reducing to 6.4 % in the past 5 years. The revision group showed a similar weight loss to the overall group beyond 10 years.

Revising a band is a safe procedure. It is certainly much safer than converting to bypass or sleeve. Worni et al. reviewed 66,303 patients after RYGB—63,171 (95.3 %) having a primary bypass and 3,132 patients (4.7 %) RYGB after removal of LAGB [32]. Patients having bypass after a band had more intraoperative complications (OR: 2.3, $P=0.002$) and postoperative complications (OR: 8.0, $P<0.001$), were at higher risk of reoperations/reinterventions (OR: 6.0, $P<0.001$), and had increased length of hospital stay.

Rebibo et al. compared primary sleeve gastrectomy (259) with sleeve and band removal (46) [33]. The indication for surgery was renewed weight gain or insufficient weight loss in 68 % of these cases. The complication rate was 8.6 % in the band out group and 8 % in the primary sleeves. The fistula rates in the two groups were 4.3 and 3.4 %, respectively ($P=0.56$). Foletto et al. reviewed 41 patients who had concurrent band removal and sleeve, and 16 who had band removal followed by an interval sleeve. One patient died of multiple organ failure from septic shock [34]. Three patients (5.7 %) developed a perigastric hematoma, 3 (5.7 %) had leaks, and 1 had mid-gastric short stenosis. The median hospital stay was 5 days. The mean BMI at revisional sleeve was 45.7 and had decreased to 39 after 2 years. Two patients required a duodenal switch for insufficient weight loss. Iannelli et al. reviewed 41 patients who had conversion of LAGB to sleeve [35]. Indication for revisional surgery was insufficient weight loss in all the cases. There was no mortality, but 5 patients (12.2 %) developed complications (high leak, 1 patient; intra-abdominal abscess, 3 patients; and complicated incisional hernia, 1 patient). At 13 months, %EWL was 42.7 %, and 6 patients needed a further procedure due to failed weight loss.

What should a surgeon offer their patient who has problems after a band? If the issue is failed weight loss and the patient wants further help, the band should be removed and another procedure offered, with the understanding that there is a real risk of substantial complications. However, if reflux secondary to slip or pouch dilatation or hiatal hernia is the issue, the band can be safely revised, and the patient can continue to have a successful outcome.

Does the Band Work in Diabetics?

There is little doubt that BPD/BPDDS is the most effective procedure for diabetics, but it is only rarely performed, due to its complexity and long-term malnutrition issues. The RYGB is also very effective. Schauer has recently described this very clearly [36]. Medical therapy alone was compared to RYGB or sleeve gastrectomy in 150 obese patients with uncontrolled type 2 diabetes and an average HBA1C 1 of 9.2 ± 1.5 %. The primary end point was the proportion of patients with an HBA1C level of 6.0 % or less 12 months after treatment. The proportion of patients with the primary end point was 12 % (5 of 41 patients) in the medical therapy group vs. 42 % (21 of 50 patients) in the RYGB group ($P=0.002$) and 37 % (18 of 49 patients) in the sleeve group ($P=0.008$). The use of drugs to lower glucose, lipid, and blood pressure levels decreased significantly after both surgical procedures but increased in patients receiving medical therapy only.

Can LAGB offer anything similar? Parikh et al. analyzed 282 bariatric patients with diabetes mellitus (218 LAGB, 53 RYGB, and 11 BPD/DS) [37]. Preoperative age (46–50 years), BMI (46–50; calculated as kg/m^2), race and gender breakdown, and baseline oral hypoglycemic (82–87 %) and insulin requirements (18–28 %) were comparable among the three groups ($P=NS$). Percentage excess weight loss at 1, 2, and 3 years was 43, 50, and 45 % for LAGB and 66, 68, and 66 % for RYGB. At 1 and 2 years, the proportion of patients requiring oral hypoglycemics postoperatively was 39 and 34 % for LAGB and 22 and 13 % for RYGB ($P=NS$). At 1 and 2 years, the proportion of patients requiring insulin postoperatively was 14 and 18 % for LAGB and 7 and 13 % for RYGB ($P=NS$). Despite the disparity in %EWL between LAGB and RYGB, the authors found that the rate of resolution of diabetes mellitus is equivalent.

Dixon et al. performed a randomized controlled trial in 60 obese patients (BMI >30 and <40) with recently diagnosed (<2 years) type 2 diabetes, between conventional diabetes therapy with a focus on weight loss by lifestyle change and LAGB [38]. Remission of type 2 diabetes was achieved by 22 (73 %) in the surgical group and 4 (13 %) in the conventional therapy group. Surgical and conventional therapy groups lost a mean of 20.7 % and 1.7 % of weight, respectively, at 2 years ($P<0.001$). Remission of type 2 diabetes was related to weight loss ($R^2=0.46$, $P<0.001$) and lower baseline HbA1c levels (combined $R^2=0.52$, $P<0.001$). Participants randomized to surgical therapy were more likely to achieve remission of type 2 diabetes through greater weight loss.

Dixon then sourced 35 studies from Scopus, MEDLINE, and EMBASE published from 2000 through May 2011 that provided some details of diabetes status before and after LAGB [39]. Weight loss was progressive over the first 2 years with a weighted average of 47 % excess weight loss at 2 years. Remission or improvement in diabetes varied from 53 to 70 % over different time periods. Results were broadly consistent, demonstrating clinically relevant improvements in diabetes outcomes with sustained weight loss in obese people with type 2 diabetes following LAGB surgery.

Sultan et al. assessed 102 patients with type 2 diabetes mellitus who had LAGB between January 2002 and June 2004 [40]. During that time, 631 patients had a band surgery, giving an incidence of diabetes of 16.2 %. Of the 102 patients,

7 were excluded because 2 had had the band removed early, and 5 patients had died; 2 of cancer and 3 of unknown causes. The mean duration of the diabetes diagnosis before surgery was 6.5 years. The mean preoperative BMI was 46.3 and had decreased to 35.0 by 5 years, an EWL of 48.3 %. Of 94 patients, 83 (88.3 %) were taking medications preoperatively, with 14.9 % taking insulin. At 5 years postoperatively, 33 (46.5 %) of 71 patients were taking medications, with 8.5 % taking insulin. The mean fasting preoperative glucose level was 146.0 mg/dL, and it decreased to 118.5 mg/dL at 5 years ($P=0.004$). The mean HbA1c level was 7.53 preoperatively and was 6.58 at 5 years ($P<0.001$). Overall, diabetes had resolved (no medication requirement, with HbA1c <6 and/or glucose <100 mg/dL) in 40 % and had improved (use of fewer medications and/or fasting glucose levels of 100–125 mg/dL) in 43 %. The combined improvement/remission rate was 83 %.

Even though it may not be quite as effective as RYGB, LAGB is an excellent tool for the treatment of morbidly obese patients with diabetes.

Conclusion

It's now 18 years since the LAGB was first used to help morbidly obese patients. Much has changed in that time. Larger, softer, lower pressure bands are placed higher on the stomach, often with a concomitant crural or hiatal hernia repair. Bands are adjusted slowly, aiming to control hunger, and increase satiety, rather than act purely as a restrictive tool. All bariatric operations have their strengths and weaknesses. The band's strength is it's safety, adjustability, and ease of removal. Its weakness is the need for reoperation. However, that problem is decreasing in frequency with the changes mentioned above. Band revision is safer than alternate procedures. A band can be safely revised, and patients then continue their journey to control their weight. All the various procedures can and do fail. If a band fails, alternate procedures can be offered. LAGB is still a very effective weight loss tool. Given the enormous surge in obesity, it will remain attractive to many patients who are nervous of more aggressive procedures and their complications. Adequate band adjustment in long-term follow-up is the cornerstone of success with a lap band.

References

1. Fielding GA, Allen JW. A step-by-step guide to placement of the LAP-BAND adjustable gastric banding system. Am J Surg. 2002;184(6B):26S–30S.
2. Hernia Gulkarov I, Wetterau M, Ren CJ, Fielding GA. Hiatal hernia repair at the initial laparoscopic adjustable gastric band operation reduces the need for reoperation. Surg Endosc. 2008;22(4):1035–41.
3. Dixon AF, Dixon JB, O'Brien PE. Laparoscopic adjustable gastric banding induces prolonged satiety: a randomized blind crossover study. J Clin Endocrinol Metab. 2005;90(2):813–9.
4. Colles SL, Dixon JB, O'Brien PE. Hunger control and regular physical activity facilitate weight loss after laparoscopic adjustable gastric banding. Obes Surg. 2008;18(7):833–40. doi:10.1007/s11695-007-9409-3.
5. Biagini J, Karam L. Ten years experience with laparoscopic adjustable gastric banding. Obes Surg. 2008;18(5):573–7.
6. Lanthaler M, Aigner F, Kinzl J, Sieb M, Cakar-Beck F, Nehoda H. Long-term results and complications following adjustable gastric banding. Obes Surg. 2010;20(8):1078–85.
7. O'Brien PE, Macdonald L, Anderson M, Brennan L, Brown WA. Long-term outcomes after bariatric surgery: fifteen-year follow-up of adjustable gastric banding and a systematic review of the bariatric surgical literature. Ann Surg. 2013;257(1):87–94.
8. Weichman K, Ren C, Kurian M, Heekoung A, Casciano R, Stern L, et al. The effectiveness of adjustable gastric banding: a retrospective 6-year U.S. follow-up study. Surg Endosc. 2011;25(2):397–403.
9. Weiner R. Outcome after laparoscopic adjustable gastric banding—8 years experience. Obes Surg. 2003;13(3):427–34.
10. Higa K, Ho T, Tercero F, Yunus T, Boone KB. Laparoscopic roux-Y gastric bypass: 10 year follow up. Surg Obes Relat Dis. 2011;7(4):516–25.
11. Himpens J, Verbrugghe A, Cadière GB, Everaerts W, Greve JW. Long-term results of laparoscopic Roux-en-Y gastric bypass: evaluation after 9 years. Obes Surg. 2012;22(10):1586–93.
12. Himpens J, Dobbeleir J, Peeters G. Long-term results of laparoscopic sleeve gastrectomy for obesity. Ann Surg. 2010;252(2):319–24.
13. Sarela AI, Dexter SP, O'Kane M, Menon A, McMahon MJ. Long-term follow-up after laparoscopic sleeve gastrectomy: 8-9-year results. Surg Obes Relat Dis. 2012;8(6):679–84.
14. Eid GM, Brethauer S, Mattar SG, Titchner RL, Gourash W, Schauer PR. Laparoscopic sleeve gastrectomy for super obese patients: forty-eight percent excess weight loss after 6 to 8 years with 93% follow-up. Ann Surg. 2012;256(2):262–5.
15. Fielding GA. Laparoscopic adjustable gastric banding for massive superobesity (>60 body mass index kg/m²). Surg Endosc. 2003;17(10):1541–5.
16. Arapis K, Chosidow D, Lehmann M, Bado A, Polanco M, Kamoun-Zana S, Pelletier AL, Kousouri M, Marmuse JP. Long-term results of adjustable gastric banding in a cohort of 186 super-obese patients with a BMI≥ 50kg/m². J Visc Surg. 2012;149(2):e143–52.
17. Weiner RA, Theodoridou S, Weiner S. Failure of laparoscopic sleeve gastrectomy-further procedure? Obes Facts. 2011;4 Suppl 1:42–6.
18. Ren CJ, Cabrera I, Rajaram K, Fielding GA. Factors influencing patient choice for bariatric operation. Obes Surg. 2005;15(2):202–6.
19. Nguyen N, Hohmann S, Nguyen XM, et al. Outcome of laparoscopic adjustable gastric banding and prevalence of band revision and explantation at academic centers, 2007–2009. Surg Obes Relat Dis. 2012;8(6):724–8.
20. Chakravarty PD, McLaughlin E, Whittaker D, Byrne E, Cowan E, Xu K, Bruce DM, Ford JA. Comparison of laparoscopic adjustable gastric banding (LAGB) with other bariatric procedures; a systematic review of the randomised controlled trials. Surgeon. 2012;10(3):172–82.
21. Gould JC, Kent KC, Wan Y, Rajamanickam V, Leverson G, Campos GM. Perioperative safety and volume: outcomes relationships in bariatric surgery: a study of 32,000 patients. J Am Coll Surg. 2011;213(6):771–7.
22. Finks JF, Kole KL, Yenumula PR, English WJ, Krause KR, Carlin AM, Genaw JA, Banerjee M, Birkmeyer JD, Birkmeyer NJ, Michigan Bariatric Surgery Collaborative, from the Center for Healthcare Outcomes and Policy. Predicting risk for serious complications with bariatric surgery: results from the Michigan Bariatric Surgery Collaborative. Ann Surg. 2011;254(4):633–40.
23. Parikh MS, Laker S, Weiner M, Hajiseyedjavadi O, Ren CJ. Objective comparison of complications resulting from laparoscopic bariatric procedures. J Am Coll Surg. 2006;202(2):252–61.

24. Saunders JK, Ballantyne GH, Belsley S, Stephens D, Trivedi A, Ewing DR, Iannace V, Capella RF, Wasielewski A, Moran S. Schmidt HJ.30-day readmission rates at a high volume bariatric surgery center: laparoscopic adjustable gastric banding, laparoscopic gastric bypass and vertical banded gastroplasty-Roux y gastric bypass. Obes Surg. 2007;17(9):1171–7.

25. Saunders J, Ballantyne GH, Belsley S, Stephens DJ, Trivedi A, Ewing DR, Iannace VA, Capella RF, Wasileweski A, Moran S, Schmidt SJ. One year readmission rates at a high volume bariatric center: laparoscopic adjustable gastric banding, laparoscopic gastric bypass and vertical banded gastroplasty-roux y gastric bypass. Obes Surg. 2008;18(10):1233–40.

26. Aurora AR, Khaitan L, Saber AA. Sleeve gastrectomy and the risk of leak: a systematic analysis of 4,888 patients. Surg Endosc. 2012;26(6):1509–15.

27. Sakran N, Goitein D, Raziel A, Keidar A, Beglaibter N, Grinbaum R, Matter I, Alfici R, Mahajna A, Waksman I, Shimonov M, Assalia A. Gastric leaks after sleeve gastrectomy: a multicenter experience with 2,834 patients. Surg Endosc. 2012;27(1):240–5.

28. Shen R, Dugay G, Rajaram K, Cabrera I, Siegel N, Ren CJ. Impact of patient follow-up on weight loss after bariatric surgery. Obes Surg. 2004;14(4):514–9.

29. Himpens J, Cadiere GB, Bazi M, Vouche M, Cadiere B, Dapri G. Long-term outcomes of laparoscopic adjustable gastric banding. Arch Surg. 2011;146(7):802–7.

30. Romy S, Donadini A, Giusti V, Suter M. Roux-en-Y gastric bypass vs gastric banding for morbid obesity: a case-matched study of 442 patients. Arch Surg. 2012;147(5):460–6.

31. Beitner M, Ren-Fielding C, Kurian M, Schwack B, Skandarajah A, Thomson B, Baxter A, Fielding G. Sustained weight loss after gastric banding revision for pouch-related problems. Ann Surg. 2014;260(1):81–6.

32. Worni M, Ostbye T, Shah A, Carvalho E, Schudel IM, Shin JH, Pietrobon R, Guller U. High risks for adverse outcomes after gastric bypass surgery following failed gastric banding: a population-based trend analysis of the United States. Ann Surg. 2013;257(2):279–86.

33. Rebibo L, Mensah E, Verhaeghe P, Dhahri A, Cosse C, Diouf M, Regimbeau JM. Simultaneous gastric band removal and sleeve gastrectomy: a comparison with front-line sleeve gastrectomy. Obes Surg. 2012;22(9):1420–6.

34. Foletto Foletto M, Prevedello L, Bernante P, Luca B, Vettor R, Francini-Pesenti F, et al. Sleeve gastrectomy as revisional procedure for failed gastric banding or gastroplasty. Surg Obes Relat Dis. 2010;6(2):146–51.

35. Iannelli A, Schneck AS, Ragot E, Liagre A, Anduze Y, Msika S, Gugenheim J. Laparoscopic sleeve gastrectomy as revisional procedure for failed gastric banding and vertical banded gastroplasty. Obes Surg. 2009;19(9):1216–20.

36. Schauer PR, Kashyap SR, Wolski K, Brethauer SA, Kirwan JP, Pothier CE, Thomas S, Abood B, Nissen SE, Bhatt DL. Bariatric surgery versus intensive medical therapy in obese patients with diabetes. N Engl J Med. 2012;366(17):1567–76.

37. Parikh M, Ayoung-Chee P, Romanos E, Lewis N, Pachter HL, Fielding G, Ren C. Comparison of rates of resolution of diabetes mellitus after gastric banding, gastric bypass, and biliopancreatic diversion. J Am Coll Surg. 2007;205(5):631–5.

38. Dixon JB, O'Brien PE, Playfair J, Chapman L, Schachter LM, Skinner S, Proietto J, Bailey M, Anderson M. Adjustable gastric banding and conventional therapy for type 2 diabetes: a randomized controlled trial. JAMA. 2008;299(3):316–23.

39. Dixon JB, Murphy DK, Segel JE, Finkelstein EA. Impact of laparoscopic adjustable gastric banding on type 2 diabetes. Obes Rev. 2012;13(1):57–67.

40. Sultan S, Gupta D, Parikh M, Youn H, Kurian M, Fielding G, Ren-Fielding C. Five-year outcomes of patients with type 2 diabetes who underwent laparoscopic adjustable gastric banding. Surg Obes Relat Dis. 2010;6(4):373–6.

24

Gastric Bypass: Transoral Circular-Stapled Gastrojejunostomy Technique

Abdulrahim AlAwashez and Matthew Kroh

Introduction

Denans invented the first mechanical device designed for bowel anastomosis. It consisted of an inner cylinder and two shorter outer rings that when placed together resulted in necrosis of the compressed tissue and bonding of the adjacent healthy tissue. Much has changed since this initial description of stapling devices and currently there are many types of surgical staplers [1].

In 1969 Mason reported the first application of gastric stapling as a surgical procedure-induced weight loss [2]. The maturation of stapling devices and bariatric surgery as a field has been facilitated by the minimally invasive era. In 1993 Wittgrove et al. reported the first laparoscopic gastric bypass. For the most critical step of their procedure, creation of the gastrojejunal anastomosis (GJ), they used the smallest (21-mm) circular stapling device on the market with a transorally placed anvil. This technique was partly derived from placement of the percutaneous endoscopic gastrostomy (PEG) tube [3].

Laparoscopic Roux-en-Y gastric bypass (LRYGB) is the most commonly performed operation for morbid obesity in the United States. Three main different techniques are widely used with good results for performing the gastrojejunal anastomosis, including the linear-stapled anastomosis, hand-sewn anastomosis, and circular-stapled anastomosis [3–5].

Though practice patterns are always in flux, most surgeons use the circular stapler technique (66 %) to create the gastrojejunal anastomosis, followed by the hand sewn (18 %) and linear stapler (16 %) [6].

The selection of a particular anastomotic technique is usually based on the surgeon's preference and none of these approaches are considered as a standard. The circular-stapled anastomosis has been our preference. Our technique as well as outcomes of this technique is discussed in this chapter.

Technique

After standard preoperative preparation, access to the abdominal cavity is accomplished using an optical 10-mm trocar under vision with a zero-degree laparoscope in the left upper periumbilical area. Once the peritoneal cavity is entered, carbon dioxide is insufflated, and the optic is changed to a 45° camera. A brief diagnostic laparoscopy examination is performed and additional four trocars are placed as well as a Nathanson liver retractor. The left upper quadrant trocar is 15 mm in size and this is the site that the circular stapler is eventually inserted through (Figs. 1 and 2).

Pouch Reconstruction

The patient is placed in extreme reverse Trendelenburg position and attention is turned to the hiatus. We start the procedure by dissecting off the phrenoesophageal fat to expose the left pillar of the diaphragm using hook electrocautery. With the help of the pneumoperitoneum, dissection continues laterally closer to the greater curvature until the first branch of short gastric vessel is reached. This limited dissection facilitates pouch construction by mobilizing the most cephaled part of the lateral pouch. We then open the pars flaccida and perform a blunt dissection to expose the posterior gastric wall. A 3.5-mm cartridge load of 60-mm linear stapling device with staple-line buttress material is used to take the descending branch of the left gastric vessels. The buttress allows for easy maneuverability of the pouch without actually grasping tissue. A single load of 60-mm (3.5-mm cartridge) stapler in a horizontal orientation, and 2–3 vertical applications typically complete the pouch. It is important when firing the vertical loads to avoid crossing the previous staple line and to ensure that the stapler is lateral to the angle

S.A. Brethauer et al. (eds.), *Minimally Invasive Bariatric Surgery*, DOI 10.1007/978-1-4939-1637-5_24, © Springer Science+Business Media New York 2015

FIG. 1. Operating room setup for gastric bypass. Copyright CCF.

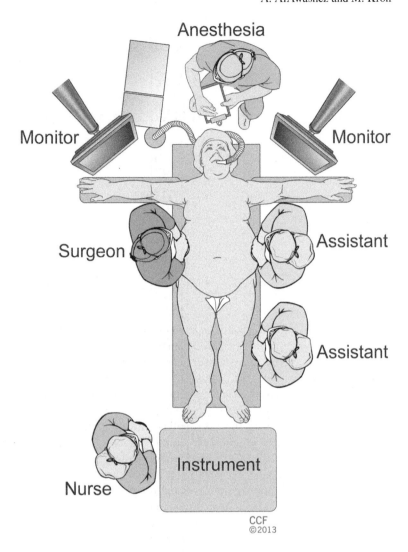

of His when firing the final load. This approximately 30 cm^3 vertically oriented pouch will be sufficient in size to admit the anvil of the 21-mm circular stapler. The staple line is inspected for quality of staple application and for any bleeding. Hemostasis is important as hematoma formation on the staple line could cause staple-line dehiscence and gastric pouch leak.

The Roux and Biliopancreatic Limb Constructions

Once the pouch is completed, we construct the Roux and biliopancreatic limbs. The patient is placed in a supine position. The omentum and transverse colon are gently swept cephalad to identify the ligament of Treitz. The duodenum is identified and confirmed by the adjacent IMV. We then measure 40–50 cm from the ligament of Treitz and divide the small bowel using a linear cutter stapler with 2.5-mm cartridge load. To achieve more mobility of the Roux limb, the small-bowel mesentery is further divided with ultrasonic shears with care taken to avoid devascularizing the biliopancreatic limb or to approach too close to the root of the mesentery. A 150-cm Roux limb is then measured out and a side-to-side jejunojejunostomy is fashioned between the biliopancreatic limb and the common channel. After stay sutures are placed, a single firing of a white 60-mm linear stapler makes the anastomosis and the common enterostomy is closed with hand-sewn running absorbable suture. The mesenteric defect is closed with a hand-sewn running, locking permanent suture. The omentum is then split with ultrasonic shears in preparation for transmission of the Roux limb in an antecolic position.

Gastrojejunostomy Anastomosis

For transoral placement of the anvil, we use the Orvil package (Covidien, Mansfield, MA), which consists of a 21-mm anvil with the head pre-tilted and the tip attached to an oral

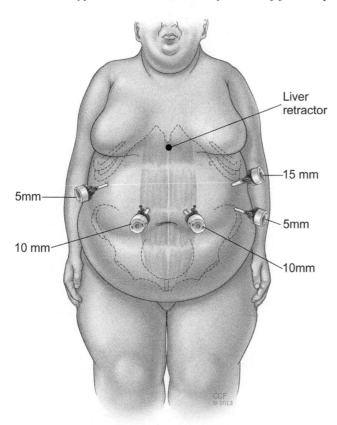

FIG. 2. Port placement for circular-stapled gastrojejunostomy technique. Copyright CCF.

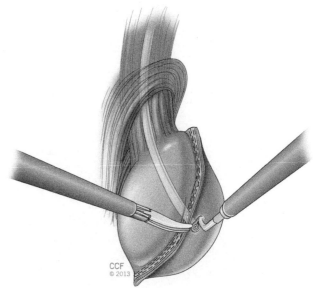

FIG. 3. Hook cautery is used to make a small gastrotomy posterior to the horizontal staple line on the pouch. The tube can be gently advanced against the gastric wall to position the opening correctly. Copyright CCF.

gastric tube. The tube is passed similar to an orogastric tube downward until it protrudes against the pouch. Gentle manipulation is used to direct the tip of the tube to the chosen place for the gastrotomy. During the oral passage, it is important to ensure that the anvil does not get caught on the teeth or the endotracheal tube at the narrowest area of the anvil's transit, which is at the level of the balloon. Application of a jaw thrust and control of the endotracheal tube are important when introducing the anvil.

Once advanced, hook electrocautery is used to make a small gastrotomy against the tip of the tube that is pushed gently downward (Fig. 3). The oral gastric tube is advanced through the gastrotomy and it is pulled out through the trocar while applying a gentle counter-traction on the pouch (Fig. 4). We prefer to make our gastrotomy immediately posterior to the horizontal staple line. The stitch that has kept the anvil head in a tilted position is cut, and the tube is detached from the anvil and passed off the surgical field.

In preparation for the placement of the 21-mm circular stapler, a retractable sterile sleeve is fashioned around the tip of the circular stapler to minimize the skin wound contamination upon removal. The 15-mm port site at the left upper quadrant is dilated then the circular stapler is inserted directly through the skin. The Roux limb is then brought up to gastric pouch without any undue tension and traced back to the jejunojejunostomy to check for any twist. The Roux limb staple line is excised and the circular stapler is introduced into the lumen of the Roux limb through the enterotomy and advanced several centimeters inside the lumen. The spike of the stapler is then advanced to penetrate the Roux limb wall on the antimesenteric side. The stem of the anvil is then grasped by the surgeon and united to the spike. The circular stapler is closed slowly while the assistant maintains the orientation of the Roux limb during stapler closure. Once it is fired, the stapler is opened and rotated as it is withdrawn from the formed anastomosis. The previously placed sterile sleeve is then retracted over the tip, covering the contaminated end. The stapler is withdrawn from the abdomen and the 15-mm port is reinserted. The enterotomy is closed with an application of the linear stapling device leaving a very short candy cane. A medial and a lateral absorbable suture are placed at each side of the anastomosis and the tails are left intentionally long. In addition to help to minimize any tension on the anastomosis, these sutures can be used to rotate and bring the posterior staple line anteriorly for inspection in case of a bleeding or a leak. The anterior anastomosis line is hand oversewn with additional interrupted sutures.

Endoscopy and Leak Test

The Roux limb is then occluded, the abdomen is filled with saline, and diagnostic upper endoscopy is performed. Pouch configuration and size are examined. The gastrojejunostomy is evaluated for patency, bleeding, and disruption.

FIG. 4. The orogastric tube is pulled through a laparoscopic port to deliver the anvil into the pouch. Copyright CCF.

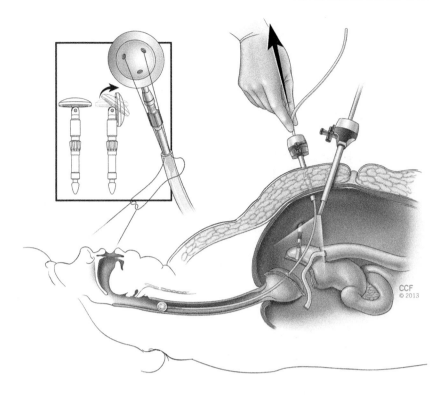

Gentle insufflation also allows for laparoscopic detection of leak by examining for any bubbles. We routinely leave a channel drain at the gastrojejunostomy.

Outcomes

The overall 30-day mortality for bariatric surgical procedures is less than 1 % [7].

Among both early and late complications, anastomotic leaks remain one of the most challenging complications. The rate of anastomotic leak in RYBG is 1.5–6 % and can be as high as 35 % in revisional surgery [8].

Carrasquilla et al. have reported a low incidence of leaks at 0.1 %. Their technique involves the antecolic and antegastric approach and the use of a circular stapler for the gastroenterostomy [9].

Most leaks occur early in the first week after surgery but can occur up to a few weeks later. If not diagnosed in a timely fashion, the mortality rate increases dramatically. Early clinical symptoms of a leak are subtle and require clinical vigilance for signs such as low-grade fevers, sustained tachycardia, or respiratory distress. If a leak is suspected clinically, emergent surgical exploration should be performed even if imaging is negative, given the rapid progression to sepsis in the severely obese patient.

The surgical principles in treating a leak include providing broad-spectrum antibiotic coverage, identification and repair of the defect, irrigation and control of contamination, wide drainage of the contaminated area and providing enteral access for feeding. Percutaneous drainage of a contained fluid collection may be an option in patients who are stable [10].

Giordano et al. performed a meta-analysis comparing linear versus circular stapler technique with a primary outcome of gastrojejunal anastomosis leak. Eight studies involving 1,321 patients were retrieved and included in this study. All eight studies reported results on gastrojejunostomy leakage, and pooled analysis did not show significant difference between the two groups (RR, 1.03; 95 % CI, 0.36–2.93; p 0.95) [11].

Bleeding

Significant bleeding after gastric bypass was observed more following laparoscopic versus open GBP. The overall rate is 0.6–4 % [12].

Early bleeding typically occurs from one of the anastomotic or staple lines. It is most commonly intraluminal. Tachycardia, a decreased hematocrit, and melena are the most common presentations. Intraluminal bleeding typically resolves without surgical intervention, but may require transfusion of blood products. For ongoing bleeding with high transfusion requirements, endoscopic intervention is appropriate. Laparoscopic exploration and oversewing of the staple line, occasionally with concomitant endoscopy, is the definitive treatment in patients who fail endoscopic management or for intraluminal bleeding not amenable to endoscopic therapy.

Nguyen et al. reported that 3.2 % of patients who underwent a LRYGB with creation of the gastrojejunostomy anastomosis with a circular stapler developed postoperative hemorrhage in 24 h after surgery. Recent meta-analysis comparing linear versus circular stapler technique to evaluate this issue showed no significant differences between the groups in the incidence of stomal ulcer or postoperative bleeding [11].

Wound Infection

Some authors have reported an increased frequency of wound infection with circular stapler, related to the extraction of the contaminated handpiece through a port [13].

The rate of infection at the abdominal wall site could be reduced down to 1 % by protecting the wound with a plastic sheet and this is our preferred technique [14].

Gastrojejunal Strictures

Among the most significant postoperative complications are gastrojejunal (GJ) anastomotic strictures. There is considerable variability in stricture rates between different surgical techniques with an incidence of 1–31 % in some series [13, 15].

Overall, the gastrojejunal stenosis rate is higher in laparoscopic gastric bypass compared with open technique [12].

Creation of the GJ anastomosis can be accomplished via a hand-sewn technique or utilization of a linear or circular stapler (either 21 or 25 mm in diameter).

A 2008 online survey of American Society for Metabolic and Bariatric Surgery revealed that the circular stapler technique is the most commonly used technique by bariatric surgeons to construct the gastrojejunostomy. Furthermore, an increasing number of surgeons use this technique compared with a prior survey [16].

In an Internet-based survey, Madan et al. reported on the preferred surgical technique for GJ: 43 % of the surgeons performed a circular-stapled technique, while 41 % prefer linear stapling, and 21 % prefer the totally hand sewn.

Selection of a particular technique to create the gastrojejunal anastomosis is based on a range of factors. The 21-mm circular-stapled anastomosis has been our preference. It gives a uniformly reproducible 12-mm diameter stoma that delays gastric pouch emptying. The success of the gastric bypass as a weight loss procedure depends somewhat on its restrictive component that results from creation of a small pouch to restrict food intake combined with a narrow outlet to limit pouch emptying and hence, inducing the feeling of the satiety. This involves the appearance of stenosis with an incidence ranging from 3 to 27 % [17].

Even within anastomotic technique categories, there is significant variability in stricture rates. This variation in rates may be partly explained by how the stricture is defined or diagnosed among the surgeons and the endoscopists [14, 18].

The etiology of stricture formation is uncertain, although tissue ischemia, excessive scarring from undetected leakage, gastric acid hypersecretion, and increased tension on the gastrojejunal anastomosis are believed to have major roles. Gastroesophageal reflux disease and age have been shown to be statistically significant independent predictors of stricture [19].

With circular staplers, several studies have published higher rates of GJ strictures, with the highest rates specifically with the 21-mm circular staplers. However, we believe that the most important factor that influences potential stricture development is surgeon experience and technique.

Carter et al. describe a series of 654 consecutive RYGB performed open or laparoscopically. Univariate analysis revealed that surgeon experience was a risk factor for stricture formation for the first 50 gastric bypasses [20].

Perugini et al. reported a decrease in the rate of anastomotic stricture from 17 to 4 % from their first 100 patients compared with their second 100 patients with the same anastomotic technique [21].

Suter and his group were able to reduce their stricture rates to 0.8 % after introducing a slight modification of their surgical technique by encompassing the pouch horizontal staple line in the circular staple line [18].

Whether the higher stricture rate with circular staplers reflects procedures performed on the steep portion of the laparoscopic gastric bypass learning curves is another consideration. Investigators from McGill looked at a series of 201 consecutive LRYGB performed by a single surgeon. They noticed that the anastomotic stricture rates decreased from 11.9 % in the first 67 patients to 3.0 % in the remaining patients (p 0.01) [21].

Since 1993 and throughout their program's history, Wittgrove and his group have maintained a rate around 3.8 % utilizing the 21-mm circular stapler [23].

This rate of stricture is among the lowest seen with the 21-mm circular stapler and is comparable to the lowest rates of all techniques reported in the recent literature. With early dilation of 12–15 mm proving to be an effective and safe treatment for strictures, most patients have resolution of symptoms after only one therapeutic endoscopy [24–26].

Nontechnical factors have also been implicated in postoperative stricture formation. Takata et al. propose that ischemia, excessive scar formation, and gastric hypersecretion can all promote stricture formation. Importantly, smoking and NSAID use are considered modifiable risk factors for gastrointestinal strictures.

Several other factors may lead to a higher stricture rate, including demographic attributes, comorbid disease, and the use of nonabsorbable Lembert sutures to reinforce the gastrojejunostomy [27].

Patients typically present several weeks after surgery with nausea, vomiting, dysphagia, gastroesophageal reflux, and eventually an inability to tolerate oral intake.

The majority of strictures occur within the first 4–6 weeks after surgery, and some strictures occur later and are generally related to smoking or medication usage [28].

The diagnosis is usually established by endoscopy or with an upper gastrointestinal series. The definition of a stricture varies between clinicians, which could explain the variability in the reported stricture rates.

Endoscopic balloon dilation is usually successful, with dilation at 15 mm proving to be an effective and safe treatment for strictures; most patients have resolution of symptoms after only one therapeutic endoscopy [29].

Peifer et al. reported their experience with endoscopic management of anastomotic strictures in 43 of 801 patients receiving open or laparoscopic RYGB [30]. Strictures were dilated to 15 mm with no perforations or clinically significant bleeding. Ninety-three percent of the strictures were managed with 1 or 2 endoscopic sessions. Dilation to at least 15 mm did not affect weight loss at 1 year compared with weight loss in the group without a stricture.

Nguyen and his group noticed no difference in the percentage of excessive body weight loss 1 year postoperatively when comparing stricture versus non-stricture groups and between 21-mm and 25-mm groups [28].

Modification and Alternative Techniques

Most of the technical modifications of circular-stapled gastroenterostomy involve anvil placement. The major difficulty in the transoral technique is passage of the anvil through the upper esophageal sphincter. Multiple maneuvers have been used to facilitate the transoral passage of the anvil including neck extension, jaw thrust, and deflation of the endotracheal tube balloon. It is very rare that maneuvers fail or anvil passage results in injury. Wittgrove et al. reported no esophageal injury in the first 1,400 patients using this technique. However, complications including hypopharyngeal perforation have been reported [31].

With this concern and in an attempt to improve the transoral technique for placement of the anvil, Gagner and colleagues manually tilted the head of the anvil to facilitate its passage through the hypopharynx and upper esophageal sphincter. The tilted configuration of the anvil improved the ease of transoral passage. In 2006, a pre-tilted anvil (Orvil, Autosuture, Norwalk, CT, USA) was developed specifically for the purpose of transoral delivery.

Several studies have looked at anastomotic complications between 21-mm and 25-mm circular staplers and their successful endoscopic management. Analysis of individual small trials comparing 21-mm and 25-mm circular-stapled laparoscopic gastrojejunal (GJ) anastomosis demonstrates that 21-mm technique was associated with increased symptomatic stenosis. However, most of these studies have limited demographic data and methodology concerns that make it difficult to assess the effect of confounding variables. These series began with the use of a 21-mm circular stapler

and then later the groups switched to a 25-mm stapler. This introduces potential bias of a learning curve [32].

For patients who developed a stricture, no significant difference was found in the requirement for postoperative endoscopic balloon dilation in both groups [28].

The internal anastomotic diameter of a 21-mm versus 25-mm circular stapler is approximately 12 and 16 mm, respectively. The 4-mm difference in diameter changes the cross-sectional area from 113 to 201 mm [33].

Also, differences in circular staplers should be considered. Depending on the manufacturer, there may be a difference in internal diameter of 1 mm between similarly sized staplers. For example, the Ethicon Endosurgery Inc. (Cincinnati, OH) 25-mm circular stapler has an internal diameter of 16.4 mm compared with the 15.3-mm diameter of a Covidien (Norwalk, CT) circular stapler. The difference of 1.1-mm diameter between the two 25-mm staplers correlates to a 14.7 % larger cross-sectional area (211 mm^2 versus 184 mm^2). Whether this difference is important enough clinically to affect the stricture rate or restrictive component of weight loss is unclear.

The Orvil (Covidien, Mansfield, MA) EEA stapler, which has been available since 2006, also has an outer diameter of 25 mm but an internal diameter of 16.9 mm [34].

Despite the possible advantage of a lower stricture rate using 25-mm circular staplers, there are some drawbacks with its use. It requires a larger skin and fascial incision that may result in more postoperative pain. Also placing the 25-mm circular stapler into the end of the small intestine can be challenging because of the larger diameter. Additionally, the larger anvil may carry a higher risk of pharyngeal or esophageal injury from the transoral placement of the anvil.

Another modification that was suggested to reduce the anastomotic complication was the reinforcement of the gastrojejunal anastomosis staple line utilizing buttressing material. Jones and associates found a significant reduction in anastomotic strictures using a 25-mm circular-stapled gastrojejunal anastomosis with a bioabsorbable material. They suggest that the staple-line reinforcement reduces anastomotic complications by reducing tension on the staple line by the even distribution of force and by buttressing against small defects that may have been present within the staple line [35].

When Hope and his group analyzed circular-stapled anastomoses with and without Seamguard (Gore, Flagstaff, AZ) in a porcine model, they found a decrease in collagen content with Seamguard-stapled anastomosis and no difference in vascularity, adhesions, or inflammation at 1 week. It is unknown whether the decrease in collagen at 1 week has an impact on a future anastomotic stricture formation [36, 37].

Another technique that some bariatric surgeons used to avoid the transoral route is the transabdominal technique for placement of the anvil [38, 39].

However, this technique has some drawbacks including the need to enlarge the trocar site to accommodate the anvil and construction of the gastrotomy for anvil insertion and subsequently its closure. Due to limitations of transoral and transgastric anvil passage, some surgeons use linear and hand-sewn gastrojejunostomy techniques [40].

First described by Higa in 2000, the hand-sewn gastrojejunostomy anastomosis is becoming more common as surgeons improve their laparoscopic technical skills [41].

In addition to being less expensive and less prone to stenosis, the advantage of lower bleeding rate compared with the mechanically performed anastomosis makes it preferable in spite of its technical high demands [41].

The evidence comparing linear-stapled versus circular-stapled laparoscopic gastrojejunostomy anastomosis in morbid obesity surgery is only documented in a few small trials. Recently Penna et al. performed a pooled analysis of these individual small trials. They included 9 trials comprising 9,374 patients (2,946 linear versus 6,428 circular). They noticed an increase in the rate of GJ stricture associated with circular-stapled anastomosis and a reduced rate of wound infection, bleeding, and operative time associated with linear stapling. No significant differences appeared for the other outcomes. The author suggests these results need to be interpreted cautiously with a number of potential biases influencing these findings [42].

Several retrospective studies comparatively analyzed the three anastomotic techniques. The advantage of one technique over another is determined mainly by the surgeon's skill and experience. When such an anastomosis is performed, the classic general surgical principles are probably still the most important ones [13].

Regardless of the technique used to construct the anastomosis, unnecessary manipulation of the small bowel and gastric pouch, improper positioning of the gastrojejunal anastomosis, added tissue dissection, poor stapler manipulation, and improperly placed Lembert sutures may all lead to early technical errors causing anastomotic complications.

Conclusion

The creation of the gastrojejunal anastomosis is a challenging step during LRYGB. There are several effective techniques for performing the gastrojejunostomy in bariatric surgery. None of these techniques are considered as a standard. However, the transoral circular-stapled gastrojejunostomy is an efficient and reproducible construct for use in LRYGB.

References

1. McGuire J, Wright IC. Surgical staplers a review. J R Coll Surg Edinb. 1997;42(1):1–9.
2. Mason EE, Ito C. Gastric bypass. Ann Surg. 1969;170(3):329–39.
3. Wittgrove AC, Clark GW, Tremblay LJ. Laparoscopic gastric bypass, roux-en-Y. Preliminary report of five cases. Obes Surg. 1994;4(4):353–7.
4. Schauer PR, Sayeed I. Laparoscopic surgery for morbid obesity. Surg Clin North Am. 2001;81(5):1143–79.
5. Higa KD, Bone KB, Ho T. Complications of the laparoscopic Roux-en-Y gastric bypass1,040 patients—what have we learned? Obes Surg. 2000;10(6):509–613.
6. Finks JF, Carlin A, Share D, O'Reilly A, Fan Z, Birkmeyer J, et al. Effect of surgical techniques on clinical outcomes after laparoscopic gastric bypass—results from the Michigan Bariatric Surgery Collaborative. Surg Obes Relat Dis. 2011;7(3):284–9.
7. DeMaria EJ, Pate V, Warthen M, Winegar DA. Baseline data from American Society for Metabolic and Bariatric Surgery-designated Bariatric Surgery Centers of Excellence using the Bariatric Outcomes Longitudinal Database. Surg Obes Relat Dis. 2010;6(4):347–55.
8. Gonzalez R, Murr MM. Anastomotic leaks following gastric bypass surgery. In: Jones DB, Rosenthal R, editors. Weight loss surgery: a multidisciplinary approach. Edgemont: Matrix Medical Communications; 2008. p. 369.
9. Carrasquilla C, English WJ, Esposito P, Gianos J. Total stapled, total intra-abdominal (TSTI) laparoscopic Roux-en-Y gastric bypass: one leak in 1000 cases. Obes Surg. 2004;14(5):613–7.
10. Gonzalez R, Sarr MG, Smith CD, Baghai M, Kendrick M, Szomstein S, et al. Diagnosis and contemporary management of anastomotic leaks after gastric bypass for obesity. J Am Coll Surg. 2007;204(1):47–55.
11. Giordano S, Salminen P, Biancari F, Victorzon M. Linear stapler technique may be safer than circular in gastrojejunal anastomosis for laparoscopic Roux-en-Y gastric bypass: a meta-analysis of comparative studies. Obes Surg. 2011;21(12):1958–64.
12. Nguyen NT, Goldman C, Rosenquist CJ, Arango A, Cole CJ, Lee SJ, Wolfe BM. Laparoscopic versus open gastric bypass: a randomized study of outcomes, quality of life, and costs. Ann Surg. 2001;234(3):279–89.
13. Gonzalez R, Lin E, Venkatesh KR, Bowers SP, Smith D. Gastrojejunostomy during laparoscopic gastric bypass. Analysis of 3 techniques. Arch Surg. 2003;138(2):181–4.
14. Alasfar F, Sabnis AA, Liu RC, Chand B. Stricture rate after laparoscopic Roux-en-Y gastric bypass with a 21-mm circular stapler: the Cleveland Clinic experience. Med Princ Pract. 2009;18(5):364–7.
15. Lujan JA, Frutos MD, Hernandez Q, Cuenca JR, Valero G, Parrilla P. Experience with the circular stapler for the gastrojejunostomy in laparoscopic gastric bypass (350 cases). Obes Surg. 2005;15(8):1096–102.
16. Madan AK, Harper JL, Tichansky DS. Techniques of laparoscopic gastric bypass: on-line survey of American Society for Bariatric Surgery practicing surgeons. Surg Obes Relat Dis. 2008;4(2):166–73.
17. Frutos MD, Luján J, García A, Hernández Q, Valero G, Gil J, Parrilla P. Gastrojejunal anastomotic stenosis in laparoscopic gastric bypass with a circular stapler (21 mm): incidence, treatment and long-term follow-up. Obes Surg. 2009;19(12):1631–5.
18. Suter M, Donadini A, Calmes JM, Romy S. Improved surgical techniques for laparoscopic Roux-en-Y gastric bypass reduces complications at the gastrojejunostomy. Obes Surg. 2010;20(7):841–5.
19. Blackstone RP, Rivera LA. Predicting stricture in morbidly obese patients undergoing laparoscopic Roux-en-Y gastric bypass: a logistic regression analysis. J Gastrointest Surg. 2007;11(4):403–9.
20. Carter JT, Tafreshian S, Campos GM, Tiwari U, Herbella F, Cello JP, Patti MG, Rogers SJ, Posselt AM. Routine upper GI series after gastric bypass does not reliably identify anastomotic leaks or predict stricture formation. Surg Endosc. 2007;21(12):2172–7.
21. Perugini RA, Mason R, Czerniach DR, Novitsky YW, Baker S, Litwin DE, Kelly JJ. Predictors of complication and suboptimal weight loss after laparoscopic Roux-en-Y gastric bypass. Arch Surg. 2003;138(5):541–6.

22. Andrew CG, Hanna W, Look D, McLean AP, Christou NV. Early results after laparoscopic Roux-en-Y gastric bypass: effect of the learning curve. Can J Surg. 2006;49(6):417–21.

23. Rondan A, Nijhawan S, Majid S, Martinez T, Wittgrove AC. Low anastomotic stricture rate after Roux-en-Y gastric bypass using a 21-mm circular stapling device. Obes Surg. 2012;22(9):1491–5.

24. Dresel A, Kuhn JA, Westmoreland MV, Talaasen LJ, McCarty TM. Establishing a laparoscopic gastric bypass program. Am J Surg. 2002;184(6):617–20.

25. Wittgrove AC, Clark GW. Laparoscopic gastric bypass, Roux en-Y-500 patients: technique and results, with 3–60 month follow-up. Obes Surg. 2000;10(3):233–9.

26. Mathew A, Veliuona MA, DePalma FJ, Cooney RN. Gastrojejunal stricture after gastric bypass and efficacy of endoscopic intervention. Dig Dis Sci. 2009;54(9):1971–8.

27. Takata MC, Ciovica R, Cello JP, Posselt AM, Rogers SJ, Campos GM. Predictors, treatment, and outcomes of gastrojejunostomy stricture after gastric bypass for morbid obesity. Obes Surg. 2007;17(7):878–84.

28. NguyenNT SCM, Wolfe BM. Incidence and outcome of anastomotic stricture after laparoscopic gastric bypass. J Gastrointest Surg. 2003;7(8):997–1003.

29. Go MR, Muscarella P, Needleman BJ, Cook CH, Melvin WS. Endoscopic management of stomal stenosis after Roux-en-Y gastric bypass. Surg Endosc. 2004;18(1):56–9.

30. Peifer KJ, Shiels AJ, Azar R, Rivera RE, Eagon JC, Jonnalagadda S. Successful endoscopic management of gastrojejunal anastomotic strictures after Roux-en-Y gastric bypass. Gastrointest Endosc. 2007;66(2):248–52.

31. Nguyen NT, Wolfe BM. Hypopharyngeal perforation during laparoscopic Roux-en-Y gastric bypass. Obes Surg. 2000;10(1):64–7.

32. Markar SR, Penna M, Venkat-Ramen V, Karthikesalingam A, Hashemi M. Influence of circular stapler diameter on postoperative stenosis after laparoscopic gastrojejunal anastomosis in morbid obesity. Surg Obes Relat Dis. 2012;8(2):230–5.

33. Carrodeguas L, Szomstein S, Zundel N, Lo Menzo E, Rosenthal R. Gastrojejunal anastomotic strictures following laparoscopic Roux-en-Y gastric bypass surgery: analysis of 1291 patients. Surg Obes Relat Dis. 2006;2(2):92–7.

34. Gould JC, Garren M, Boll V, Starling J. The impact of circular stapler diameter on the incidence of gastrojejunostomy stenosis and weight loss following laparoscopic Roux-en-Y gastric bypass. Surg Endosc. 2006;20(7):1017–20.

35. Jones WB, Myers KM, Traxler LB, Bour ES. Clinical results using bioabsorbable staple line reinforcement for circular staplers. Am Surg. 2008;74(6):462–7.

36. Hope WW, Zerey M, Schmelzer TM, Newcomb WL, Paton BL, Heath JJ, et al. A comparison of gastrojejunal anastomoses with or without buttressing in a porcine model. Surg Endosc. 2009;23(4): 800–7.

37. Dolce CJ, Dunnican WJ, Kushnir L, Bendana E, Ata A, Singh TP. Gastrojejunal strictures after Roux-en-Y gastric bypass with a 21-mm circular stapler. JSLS. 2009;13(3):306–11.

38. de la Torre RA, Scott JS. Laparoscopic Roux-en-Y gastric bypass: a totally intraabdominal approach—technique and preliminary report. Obes Surg. 1999;9(5):492–8.

39. Murr MM, Gallagher SF. Technical considerations for transabdominal loading of the circular stapler in laparoscopic Roux-en-Y gastric bypass. Am J Surg. 2003;185(6):585–8.

40. DeMaria EJ, Sugerman HJ, Kellum JM, Meador JG, Wolfe LG. Results of 281 consecutive total laparoscopic Roux-en-Y gastric bypasses to treat morbid obesity. Ann Surg. 2002;235(5): 640–7.

41. Higa KD, Boone KB, Ho T, Davies OG. Laparoscopic Roux-en-Y gastric bypass for morbid obesity: technique and preliminary results of our first 400 patients. Arch Surg. 2000;135(9):1029–33.

42. Penna M, Markar SR, Venkat-Raman V, Karthikesalingam A, Hashemi M. Linear-stapled versus circular-stapled laparoscopic gastrojejunal anastomosis in morbid obesity: meta-analysis. Surg Laparosc Endosc Percutan Tech. 2012;22(2):95–101.

25

Gastric Bypass: Transgastric Circular Stapler Technique

Jaisa Olasky and Daniel B. Jones

Since the first description of laparoscopic Roux-en-Y gastric bypass in 1994, surgeons have performed the gastrojejunal anastomosis using a circular end-to-end anastomosis (EEA) stapled technique. The circular stapled method may be favored as it allows for construction of a very small gastric pouch and represents a safe, consistent, and relatively simple method of anastomosis. In a study published in 2007, authors surveyed bariatric surgeons on their usual practice for creating the gastrojejunal anastomosis. The percentage of surgeons using the circular stapler, linear stapler, and hand-sewn technique was 43 %, 41 %, and 21 %, respectively. Surgeons using the circular stapler used either a 21- or 25-mm size anvil. This particular report, however, did not investigate whether the anvil was placed transabdominally or transorally [1].

Initially, the gastrojejunostomy was created by a transoral technique in which the circular stapler anvil was introduced orally using endoscopic guidance [2, 3]. This technique required an experienced endoscopist to advance the endoscope into the gastric pouch. Next, a venous catheter was used to pass a guidewire into the gastric pouch for endoscopic retrieval. The pull wire was then attached to the EEA anvil and advanced in an antegrade fashion from the mouth through the esophagus and into the gastric pouch in a technique similar to that used to perform a percutaneous endoscopic gastrostomy (PEG) tube. This required temporary deflation of the balloon of the endotracheal tube and lifting the patient's head and jaw anteriorly to allow the anvil to pass into the distal esophagus. Although large series have reported no anvil-related complications, other surgeons have noted significant injuries associated with the transoral technique [4, 5]. Proprietary differences among EEA manufacturers may prevent universal application of the transoral approach.

It has been suggested that various anvil stem lengths and the use of a spiked anvil may contribute to difficulty passing the EEA anvil and to esophageal injury [4]. Trouble navigating the anvil at the level of the cricopharyngeus muscle as well as complications including esophageal perforation and gastric wall injuries have led surgeons to develop a transgastric technique for anvil placement [6–9]. In addition to safety, other potential advantages of the transgastric technique include obviating the need for the surgeon to perform endoscopy, avoidance of wound contamination with oral flora, and reduced risk of inadvertent endotracheal tube migration or dislodgment during manipulation of the anvil through the esophagus.

A number of transgastric techniques have evolved. Among the alternatives, transgastric anvil placement may be performed either by using a balloon cholangiogram catheter to position the anvil as described by De la Torre [7] and Scott et al. [6], or by first creating the gastric pouch and opening the end [7, 9]. We prefer the latter technique, in which the anvil, attached to a suture is inserted directly into the pouch. The needle of the attached suture is passed from within the stomach to a selected site on the gastric pouch. The suture is then used to pull the anvil through the pouch wall and the pouch gastrotomy is closed.

In a simplified technique, the intended gastric pouch may be first sized by inflating a 15-mL gastric balloon at the level of the gastroesophageal junction (Fig. 1). A gastrotomy is performed on the anterior wall of the stomach. A 25-mm EEA anvil with an attached looped suture is placed within the abdominal cavity through one of the port sites. The suture is then held with a 45-cm, modified Maryland grasper (Jones Perforator, Stryker Endoscopy, San Jose, CA) and advanced through the gastrotomy (Fig. 2) [10]. Using the tip of the grasper to penetrate the gastric wall, the suture is advanced at the selected anastomotic site within the area of the proposed gastric pouch. The suture is pulled anteriorly to allow the anvil spike to advance through the gastric wall.

Next, the pouch is fashioned using several firings of a laparoscopic gastrointestinal anastomosis (GIA) stapler.

Electronic supplementary material: Supplementary material is available in the online version of this chapter at 10.1007/978-1-4939-1637-5_25. Videos can also be accessed at http://www.springerimages.com/videos/978-1-4939-1636-8.

S.A. Brethauer et al. (eds.), *Minimally Invasive Bariatric Surgery*,
DOI 10.1007/978-1-4939-1637-5_25, © Springer Science+Business Media New York 2015

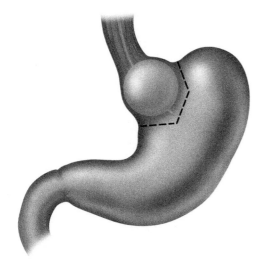

FIG. 1. Sizing the pouch and the intragastric balloon. Reprinted with permission, Ciné-Med Publishing, Inc. Adapted from Atlas of Metabolic and Weight Loss Surgery, Copyright © 2010.

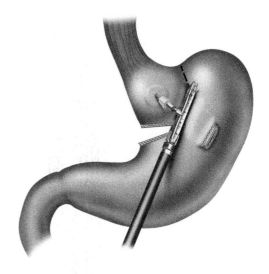

FIG. 3. Gastric division. Reprinted with permission, Ciné-Med Publishing, Inc. Adapted from Atlas of Metabolic and Weight Loss Surgery, Copyright © 2010.

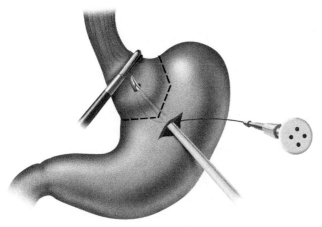

FIG. 2. Transgastric end-to-end anastomosis (EEA) anvil placement. Reprinted with permission, Ciné-Med Publishing, Inc. Adapted from Atlas of Metabolic and Weight Loss Surgery, Copyright © 2010.

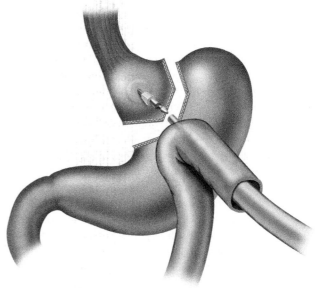

FIG. 4. EEA placement. Reprinted with permission, Ciné-Med Publishing, Inc. Adapted from Atlas of Metabolic and Weight Loss Surgery, Copyright © 2010.

We currently use the articulating Endo GIA Ultra Universal Stapler with the 3.5-mm purple tri-staples (Covidien, Mansfield, MA) (Fig. 3). As with any stapled gastrojejunostomy, care must be taken to ensure that no tubes, such as nasogastric tubes or temperature probes, remain within the stomach before creating the pouch, as they are at risk for division by the GIA stapler. Such an oversight may result in staple-line disruption, leak, and retained tube fragment.

The gastrotomy is approximated with three tacking sutures and closed with an application of the Endo GIA Universal Straight Stapler with the blue 3.5-mm load (Covidien, Mansfield, MA). Finally, the EEA is placed through a port site and once within the Roux limb it is mated with the anvil (Fig. 4). We use a 25-mm anvil with the Tilt-Top feature that increases the ease of removal (Premium Plus

CEEA Stapler, Covidien, Mansfield, MA). Before deploying the EEA, the mesentery of the Roux limb should be inspected to ensure that it is oriented properly. The EEA is fired and removed.

The open end of the Roux limb is then excised again using the Endo GIA Universal Stapler but with the shorter, 2.5-mm white staples (Fig. 5). The anastomosis is reinforced with several absorbable horizontal mattress sutures in order to decrease tension. The gastrojejunostomy is then tested for leaks by injecting methylene blue via a nasogastric tube. Alternatively, endoscopic insufflation may be performed,

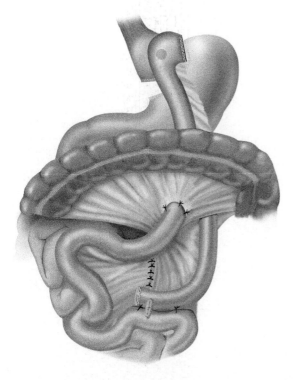

FIG. 5. Completed gastric bypass. Reprinted with permission, Ciné-Med Publishing, Inc. Adapted from Atlas of Metabolic and Weight Loss Surgery, Copyright © 2010.

evaluating the anastomosis by air leak test. On postoperative day 1, we routinely order an upper gastrointestinal (UGI) contrast study to evaluate for leaks, although recent data suggests that this practice may not be cost effective [11, 12].

Success with either the transgastric or transoral technique should be expected to be comparable as they result in a technically similar gastroenteric anastomosis. Series data suggest that outcomes following circular stapled gastroenteric anastomosis are similar to those after hand-sewn or linear stapled anastomosis. Using the EEA, anastomotic leak rates following gastric bypass have ranged from 1.3 to 2.2 % [3, 13]. The leak rates among studies employing hand-sewn and linear stapled gastroenteric anastomoses have been similar (2–5.1 %) [14–16].

Anastomotic strictures may result from local ischemia, undue tension, or a technically narrow anastomosis. Such strictures may be managed safely with either pneumatic balloon or bougie dilation, thus averting the need for further surgical intervention [17]. Although some reports suggest a higher incidence of gastrojejunal stricture following circular stapled anastomosis, larger series have demonstrated acceptable rates of stenosis overall (1.6–6.9 %) [3, 18]. The data also shows that the increased risk is largely due to the use of smaller diameter anvils, which have no weight loss advantage over a larger anvil [19]. In patients where a 21-mm anvil was used, the stricture rate ranged from 9 to 26 %, while the 25-mm anvil stricture rate was 2.9–10 % [20–22]. In one study of 200 patients where 21-mm anvils were compared to

25-mm anvils, patients with smaller anvil diameters had an increased rate of symptoms leading to endoscopy and presented with these symptoms significantly earlier [23]. Based on the above data, the 25-mm anvil is recommended. In our experience, the stricture rate from June 2011 through June 2012 was 8.57 % [24]. All of the patients presented within the first 60 postoperative days and responded well to endoscopic dilation. To date, we have never revised the anastomosis as the result of a stricture.

Some surgeons who use the circular stapler have reported success with biological staple reinforcements. The data is limited; however, in a study of 596 patients whose anastomosis was created with a reinforced 25-mm anvil EEA, the strictures requiring intervention were 0.67 % in the reinforced group as compared to 9.41 % in the non-reinforced group [25]. Long-term data is needed before this can be routinely recommended.

All surgeons that use the various industry EEA devices may not universally apply transoral anvil placement. The transgastric approach allows for direct placement of a large diameter anvil at the intended anastomotic site without endangering the esophagus or requiring endoscopy [26] (Video Error! Reference source not found.).

References

1. Madan AK, Harper JL, Tichansky DS. Techniques of laparoscopic gastric bypass: online survey of American Society for Bariatric Surgery practicing surgeons. Surg Obes Relat Dis. 2008;4(2): 166–72.
2. Wittgrove AC, Clark GW, Tremblay LJ. Laparoscopic gastric bypass, Roux-en-Y: preliminary report of five cases. Obes Surg. 1994;4:353–7.
3. Wittgrove AC, Clark GW. Laparoscopic gastric bypass, Roux-en-Y 500 patients: technique and results, with 3–60 month follow-up. Obes Surg. 2000;10:233–9.
4. Wittgrove AC, Clark GW. Laparoscopic gastric bypass: endostapler transoral or transabdominal anvil placement. Obes Surg. 2000;10:376.
5. Wittgrove AC, Clark GW. Combined laparoscopic/endoscopic anvil placement for the performance of the gastroenterostomy. Obes Surg. 2001;11:565–9.
6. Scott DJ, Provost PD, Jones DB. Laparoscopic Roux-en-Y gastric bypass: transoral or transgastric anvil placement? Obes Surg. 2000; 10:361–5.
7. De la Torre RA, Scott JS. Laparoscopic Roux-en-Y gastric bypass: a totally intra-abdominal approach—technique and preliminary report. Obes Surg. 1999;9:492–8.
8. Nguyen NT, Wolfe BM. Hypopharyngeal perforation during laparoscopic Roux-en-Y gastric bypass. Obes Surg. 2000;10:64–7.
9. Teixeira JA, Borao FJ, Thomas TA, Cerabona T, Artuso D. An alternative technique for creating the gastrojejunostomy in laparoscopic Roux-en-Y gastric bypass: experience with 28 consecutive patients. Obes Surg. 2000;10:240–4.
10. Schneider BE, Provost PD, Jones DJ. Obesity surgery—laparoscopic Roux-en-Y and gastric banding procedures. In: Jones D, Wu JS, Soper NJ, editors. Laparoscopic surgery: principles and procedures. St. Louis: Quality Medical Publishing; 2004.
11. Sims TL, Mullican MA, Hamilton EC, Provost DA, Jones DB. Routine upper gastrointestinal gastrografin swallow after laparoscopic Roux-en-Y gastric bypass. Obes Surg. 2003;13:66–72.

12. Hamilton EC, Sims TL, Hamilton TT, Mullican MA, Jones DB, Provost DA. Clinical predictors of leak after Roux-en-Y gastric bypass. Surg Endosc. 2003;17:679–84.

13. Nguyen NT, Goldman C, Rosenquist CJ, et al. Laparoscopic versus open gastric bypass: a randomized study of outcomes, quality of life, and costs. Ann Surg. 2001;234:279–91.

14. Higa KD, Boone K, Ho T. Complications of the laparoscopic Roux-en-Y gastric bypass: 1,040 patients: what have we learned? Obes Surg. 2000;10:509–13.

15. De Maria EJ, Sugerman HJ, Kellum JM, Meador JG, Wolfe LG. Results of 281 consecutive total laparoscopic Roux-en-Y gastric bypass to treat morbid obesity. Ann Surg. 2002;235:640–7.

16. Schauer PR, Ikramuddin S, Gourash W, Ramanathan R, Luketich J. Outcomes after laparoscopic Roux-en-Y gastric bypass for morbid obesity. Ann Surg. 2000;232:515–29.

17. Barba CA, Butensky M, Lorenzo M, Newman R. Endoscopic dilation of gastroesophageal anastomosis stricture after gastric bypass. Surg Endosc. 2003;17:416–20.

18. Gonzalez R, Lin E, Venkatesh KR, Bowers SP, Smith CD. Gastrojejunostomy during laparoscopic gastric bypass: analysis of 3 techniques. Arch Surg. 2003;138:181–4.

19. Markar SR, Penna M, Venkat-Ramen V, Karthikesalingam A, Hashemi M. Influence of circular stapler diameter on postoperative stenosis after laparoscopic gastrojejunal anastomosis in morbid obesity. Surg Obes Relat Dis. 2012;8(2):230–5.

20. Alasfar F, Sabnis AA, Liu RC, Chand B. Stricture rate after laparoscopic Roux-en-Y gastric bypass with a 21-mm circular stapler: the Cleveland Clinic experience. Med Princ Pract. 2009;18(5):364–7.

21. Nguyen NT, Stevens CM, Wolfe BM. Incidence and outcome of anastomotic stricture after laparoscopic gastric bypass. J Gastrointest Surg. 2003;7(8):997–1003.

22. Suggs WJ, Kouli W, Lupovici M, Chau WY, Brolin RE. Complications at gastrojejunostomy after laparoscopic Roux-en-Y gastric bypass: comparison between 21- and 25-mm circular staplers. Surg Obes Relat Dis. 2007;3(5):508–14.

23. Fisher BL, Atkinson JD, Cottam D. Incidence of gastroenterostomy stenosis in laparoscopic Roux-en-Y gastric bypass using 21- or 25-mm circular stapler: a randomized prospective blinded study. Surg Obes Relat Dis. 2007;3(2):176–9.

24. ACS BSCN Bariatric Surgery Database.

25. Scott JD, Cobb WS, Carbonell AM, Traxler B, Bour ES. Reduction in anastomotic strictures using bioabsorbable circular staple line reinforcement in laparoscopic gastric bypass. Surg Obes Relat Dis. 2011;7:637–43.

26. Jones DB, Maithel SK, Schneider BE. Atlas of minimally invasive surgery. Woodbury: Cine-Med; 2006. p. 298–332.

26

Laparoscopic Gastric Bypass: Hand-Sewn Gastrojejunostomy Technique

Kelvin D. Higa and Cyrus Moon

The minimally invasive revolution began in 1993 when Wittgrove, Clark, and Tremblay first performed a proximal gastric bypass laparoscopically [1]. Later, they were able to show that this technique was viable and produced weight loss and reduction in comorbidities equal to or better than many *open* series [2]. Discussed elsewhere in this text, the laparoscopic/endoscopic anvil placement technique for creation of the gastrojejunal anastomosis was the foundation for most other procedures that followed. Initial anastomotic leakage rates of up to 5 % were observed [3]; however, the rates decreased with experience [4].

In 1999, de la Torre and Scott [5] published a series of laparoscopic Roux-en-Y gastric bypass procedures using a totally intra-abdominal approach for the formation of the gastrojejunal anastomosis with a circular stapler [5]. Champion, and later Schauer et al. [6], developed the linear cutter technique that obviates the need for transoral passage of instrumentation, thus avoiding the potential for esophageal injury while creating a stable, calibrated anastomosis.

In 1996, my group began the development of the hand-sutured technique because of our concerns regarding failure rates of stapled anastomoses; we performed our first procedure in 1998 [7]. The design of the procedure paralleled the open Roux-en-Y procedures that we were performing. Based on this experience and extrapolation of theories of gastric pouch formation [8], we adopted the basic configuration described by MacLean et al. [9]. Knowing that small changes in anatomy or technique might have pronounced effects in short- and long-term results and complications, it was important for us to emulate the open configuration as closely as possible, given the limitations of available laparoscopic instrumentation at that time.

The basis for this technique is the formation of a linear, vertically oriented pouch excluding the distensible fundus of the stomach. This provides a serviceable platform for which a hand-sewn anastomosis to the Roux limb can be performed. This technique has been reproduced and adopted by many centers, but is not as popular as the stapled techniques. The long learning curve and inexperience with advanced laparoscopic suturing are the major drawbacks. However, once mastered, these techniques enable the surgeon to resolve almost all complications related to bariatric surgery, or other complex foregut surgery for that matter, laparoscopically, and with a greater degree of precision. This technique also allows the surgeon to achieve an operative efficiency that surpasses the open equivalent.

With the discovery and delineation of enteric hormones, such as gastrin, GLP-1, and PYY, the hypothesized mechanisms of action of the gastric bypass fit better with our long-standing clinical observations [10]. The effect on the individual patient, by whatever means, is reproducible—but these proposed mechanisms also explain the variability of the response of each individual as well as the consistent response of the group given the wide range of anatomic variabilities in the anatomic construct.

Gastric reservoir volumes can vary widely among different surgeons, as much as 500 %; yet, this variance does not appear to affect weight loss outcomes. Likewise, creating a 150-cm Roux limb does not impart greater effect than that one of 75 cm. Although there are studies that have shown the short-term benefit of pouch and/or stoma reduction and lengthening of the Roux limb to enhance weight loss, results have been inconsistent, without long-term benefit.

The best predictor of success seems to be the genetic similarity among related individuals, rather than environmental factors [11]. The performance of the gastric bypass may not be influenced as strongly by the compliance of the patient as it seems to be with the adjustable gastric band and may be predetermined by the genetic and biological nature of each individual patient.

S.A. Brethauer et al. (eds.), *Minimally Invasive Bariatric Surgery*,
DOI 10.1007/978-1-4939-1637-5_26, © Springer Science+Business Media New York 2015

Operative strategy, therefore, is the same as it was described by Mason in 1966 [12]—to achieve the anatomic effect of proximal alimentary diversion, with the least side effects and complications with long-term control of weight and medical comorbidities safely and cost-effectively.

This chapter will describe our technique of laparoscopic gastric bypass; although the adoption of a hand-sewn gastro-jejunal anastomosis is somewhat unique, the reader should pay attention to the operative strategy and port placement that makes this approach reproducible and adaptable to nearly all patient situations.

Preparation for Surgery

The treatment of morbid obesity requires a dedicated multi-disciplinary team consisting of a surgeon, psychologist, nutritionist, physical therapist, anesthesiologist, and others. More importantly, the patient must be an active participant in the bariatric surgical program if optimal outcomes are to be achieved. Optimization of preoperative nutrition and cardio-pulmonary performance is advisable and can help to limit one of the major causes of laparoscopic conversions—hepatic enlargement limiting visualization of the proximal stomach. Preoperative weight reduction, although limited in long-term management alone, may be quite helpful in decreasing the size of the liver and the amount of intraperito-neal fat preoperatively, thus enabling the surgeon to safely perform the procedure laparoscopically while establishing sound nutritional and exercise habits beneficial after surgery. Universal mandatory medical weight management imposed by some insurance carriers in order to qualify for surgery has no scientific basis.

Bowel preparation is unnecessary. A liquid diet 24 h before surgery will prevent the possibility of retained food in the stomach from obstructing the jejunojejunal anastomosis immediately after surgery, a potential cause of acute gastric distention [13].

Bariatric patients are at moderate risk for perioperative venous thromboembolism [14]. Prophylaxis in the form of mechanical (sequential compression boots and early ambula-tion) and pharmacologic (subcutaneous fractionated or unfractionated heparin) is advised. Traditional parenteral antibiotic prophylaxis is standard.

Positioning of the patient in the operating room must include attention to the prevention of pressure sores and neuropathy. Dedicated operative tables must be weight rated appropriately with lateral extensions available to accommodate larger patients. Protocols for patient transfer and other safety issues should be included as part of a hospital-wide awareness program.

Surgical Procedure

Optimal port placement allows for dissection of the small bowel without compromising the exposure of the proximal stomach. Extremes of size can be challenging: adequate space to allow the formation of the Roux limb in smaller patients can be as problematic as the inadequate length of instrumentation and difficulties associated with visualization of the proximal stomach in larger patients. Interestingly, authors describe various approaches and port locations to solve these issues while maintaining the critical nature of their particular port placement. We use five ports (Fig. 1). This arrangement also allows for concomitant cholecystec-tomy if indicated.

Trocar placement is a critical step toward a safe and suc-cessful operation. Most authors describe external landmarks such as the umbilicus or xiphoid to determine placement. However, obese patients have a high degree of abdominal wall thickness with corresponding varying degrees of rigid-ity. Also, the size of the liver and presence of previous opera-tions and their associated internal adhesions will determine the initial and subsequent trocar placements. Therefore, we feel it better to place the trocars based on internal anatomy, rather than external landmarks. In this way, triangulation and visualization will be preserved, accommodating for varia-tions in the size of the liver or length of the patient's torso.

Attention must not only be given to individual trocar placement but also the angle in which the trocar enters the skin. Some individuals' thick, muscular abdominal walls do not allow for the range of motion necessary to achieve the objective, forcing re-direction of the trocar internally, through the same skin incision but different fascial opening, or by placement of another trocar. In general, the optimal placement is to orient all trocars toward the midline, pointing to the base of the mesocolon.

Extra-long trocars may be necessary and although some surgeons prefer to limit the number of 12-mm trocars (neces-sary to accommodate stapling devices), this may limit proper stapler orientation and compromise the anatomic construct. The hernia risk is minimized by either closing the trocar defects or, preferably, using non-bladed trocars without fas-cial closure to minimize postoperative pain.

Our trocar placement scheme is as follows; it illustrates the rationale necessary for consistency of this technique and represents an evolutionary process that has taken over 12 years to develop:

1. Initial trocar (12 mm)—Left, upper quadrant, subcostal, mid-clavicular line. This is often an optical entry without prior insufflation. The rationale is that many patients have

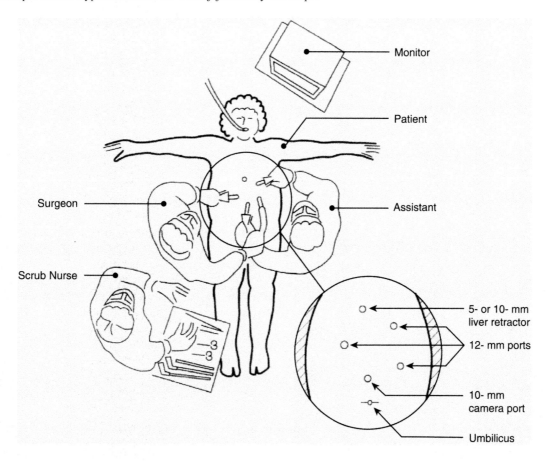

Fɪɢ. 1. Position and port placement.

had previous procedures, pelvic or otherwise—this area is rarely affected with intra-abdominal adhesions from common open procedures. This allows dissection of midline adhesions, inspection of the size of the liver, and determination of the best level for the primary optical port. This will also be the primary port for vertical stapling of the gastric pouch. Once adhesions are mobilized, then the optical port can be thoughtfully placed as to see the ligament of Treitz as well as the hiatus without having to "turn around." Also, by keeping the initial entry away from the midline, the vena cava and aorta are not as vulnerable to injury.

2. Primary optical trocar (12 mm)—Its placement has been described above. Optimal placement allows for forward visualization of the proximal small bowel and the hiatus. Once this trocar is placed, the camera is moved to this port for subsequent trocar placement. I have not found the current 5-mm scopes to provide enough light delivery and therefore resolution for optimal visualization in most patients.

3. Right-sided trocar (12 mm)—This trocar must be placed thoughtfully just as all others. Exterior landmarks are irrelevant. It must come in below the liver edge, just to the right of the midline so as to be able to triangulate on the hiatus as well as the ligament of Treitz; therefore, it should be angled toward the root of the mesocolon, rather

than perpendicular to the abdominal wall. It must be 12 mm to accommodate the stapler that will define the inferior gastric pouch.

4. Left-inferior trocar (12 mm)—This is often at the same level as the primary optical trocar and in the same line as the initial trocar. This will be the primary stapler entry site for the jejunojejunostomy and, along with the right upper quadrant trocar, will triangulate very well for a comfortable manual gastrojejunostomy.

5. Liver retractor—The most consistent placement appears to be the subxiphoid. A 5-mm trocar can be used here, depending on the liver retractor of choice. We have found that a simple 5-mm instrument or similar device will provide excellent exposure and therefore is often placed without a trocar, through direct puncture, as it will not be removed until the end of the case.

The Bypass

The omentum is displaced cephalad to expose the ligament of Treitz. In patients whose omentum is adherent to pelvic structures or involved in an incarcerated ventral hernia, we

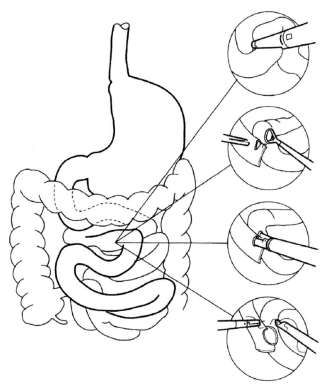

Fig. 2. Formation of the Roux limb and jejunojejunostomy.

prefer to incise the gastrocolic omentum and open the transverse mesocolon from above, thus exposing the ligament of Treitz directly. Ventral hernias are repaired at a later date when optimal weight loss and nutrition ensure a greater degree of primary success, and the use of prosthetic mesh is not compromised by contamination of enteric contents.

The proximal jejunum is transected with a 2.5–3.8-mm linear stapler, depending on the thickness of the bowel.

The mesentery is divided with the harmonic scalpel. The Roux limb is measured and a side-to-side linear anastomosis is performed (Fig. 2). Typically, the length of the Roux limb can be up to 150 cm without an associated increased incidence of malabsorptive complications [15]; however, our data showed no difference in the outcomes of using a 150-cm Roux limb in the super obese (BMI > 50 kg/m²) as opposed to a 100-cm Roux limb in patients with BMI < 50 kg/m² [16]. We therefore use a 100-cm Roux limb for all patients. The enterotomy is closed with a single layer of absorbable suture. The mesenteric defect must be closed with a continuous, nonabsorbable suture to limit the possibility of internal herniation.

The Roux limb is passed through a retrocolic tunnel and fixed to the transverse mesocolon with nonabsorbable sutures, which also includes closing the Petersen's space, again, to help prevent possible internal herniation. Alternatively, we also utilize an antecolic route for the Roux limb, depending on individual patient anatomy.

There are times when the mesocolon is uncomfortably short and will not allow for the safe passage of a retrocolic Roux limb. In these rare instances, the decision to route the Roux limb antecolic must be made before the transection of the jejunum. This site must be more distal from the ligament of Treitz, typically 50–100 cm, to limit the tension on the gastrojejunal anastomosis. By lengthening the biliopancreatic limb, iron and calcium absorption may be less efficient, and the incidence of these deficiencies may be theoretically increased or more difficult to manage with oral supplementation alone.

When routing the Roux limb antecolic, the omentum can be left intact, displaced to the right of the patient, or divided. When dividing the omentum, it is best to begin at the colon and work distally, to avoid devascularization of the omentum—and a potential reoperation.

Controversy exists as to whether the large resultant Petersen's space associated with an antecolic Roux limb requires closure. Clearly, these patients are still at risk for intestinal volvulus [17]. Therefore, our philosophy is to eliminate the risk of postoperative bowel obstruction rather than simply settling for a reduction in the incidence; leaving these spaces open makes little sense [18].

The liver retractor is now placed to allow dissection of the proximal stomach. Occasionally, a very large liver will not allow for sufficient visualization—an indication for open conversion. However, displacement of the liver to the right, rather than anterior, will allow sufficient exposure in the largest of patients. Alternatively, the surgeon may decide to abort the procedure, evaluate the cause of hepatic enlargement (usually steatosis), and institute therapy (medical weight reduction) in anticipation of performing the procedure at a later time under more ideal circumstances. In this way, surgical restraint and proper judgment may reduce the morbidity associated with these operations.

The Pouch

The pouch is formed by sequential firing of a laparoscopic linear cutter, a stapling device around a 34-Fr. orogastrically placed bougie (Fig. 3). The first firing is horizontal, introducing the stapler from the RUQ port. Beginning no more than 5 cm distal to the esophagogastric junction, using 3.8- to 4.1-mm cartridges, depending on stomach thickness, it is important to orient the stapler slightly cephalad to angulate the stapler line. Subsequent firings are vertically oriented to the angle of His, introducing the stapler from the LUQ port. By using this port configuration, extra-long staplers are unnecessary for the majority of patients.

One of the critical steps in the creation of the gastric pouch is posterior visualization at the level of the hiatus. Many surgeons will "bluntly" dissect behind the stomach, but given the variable level of adhesions to the pancreas and the splenic vessels, this is unwise. Optimally, it is better to

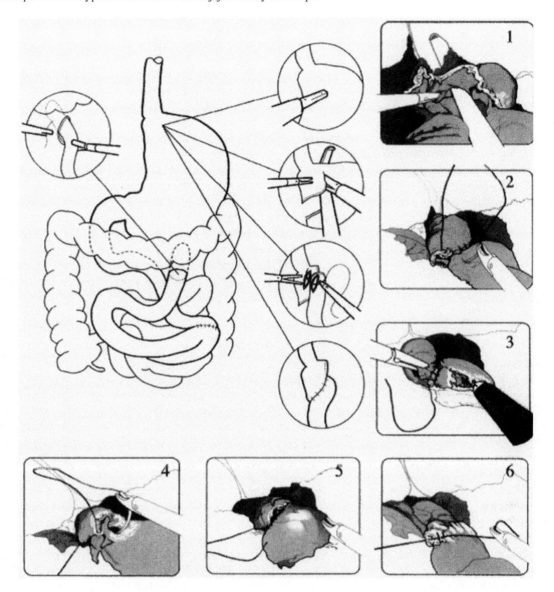

Fig. 3. Formation of the gastric pouch and gastrojejunostomy.

enter the lesser sac through the gastrocolic omentum and free the posterior gastric adhesions up to the esophageal hiatus. This protects the pancreas and the occasional tortuous splenic artery from inadvertent injury. After this, the lesser curve, perigastric dissection can be performed with more confidence and placement of the stapler more precisely as not to "twist" the stomach pouch. This occurs when posterior gastric adhesions prevent the initial horizontal stapler from capturing equal amounts of anterior and posterior gastric wall. The resultant twist is not as critical as in the gastric sleeve but is not aesthetically pleasing.

Controversy exists as to whether or not to dissect the hiatus and repair a hiatal hernia when present. Autopsy studies show that a hiatal hernia is present in up to 70 % of individuals, similar to our observations. However, dissection of the hiatus can add additional time and potential complications to an already complicated procedure. Our studies have not shown that preoperative endoscopy accurately predicts the absence of a hiatal hernia; the only way to determine its presence is through circumferential dissection of the esophagus. The absence of the "anterior" dimple is not reliable as the hernia space is often taken up by a large paraesophageal lipoma that can be easily reduced into the abdomen once identified. Once identified, the hiatal hernia is best repaired posteriorly.

The question remains: "Is it important to repair every hiatal hernia at the time of gastric bypass?" The answer is not clear. If one assumes that precise dissection and formation of the gastric pouch is important to limit postoperative complications, then it would be appropriate to absolutely identify the location of the gastroesophageal junction, often hidden in a "sea of fat," to better perform more consistent reconstruction.

It has been our observation that almost 100 % of patients we have reoperated after gastric bypass have a significant hiatal hernia at the time of reoperation—something not appreciated at the time of the first intervention.

Dissection of the hiatus and repair of the hiatal hernia along with removing the fat pad overlying the angle of His may allow for more precise and consistent pouch formation and subsequent better long-term performance and lower complications, but this has not been proven. Although this may add up to 5–10 min of operative time, which is significant, the added exposure may make for a safer operation. Each surgeon will need to evaluate this perception in the context of his or her individual experience and skill level. Suffice it to say, to perform a good laparoscopic gastric bypass, the surgeon must be expert at hiatal dissection.

The Anastomosis

The formation of the gastrojejunostomy begins with a running posterior, exterior layer of 3-0 polyglactin (Vicryl) sutures. Beginning distally and sewing proximally, the antimesenteric side of the Roux limb is approximated to the inferior staple line of the gastric pouch, incorporating the staples in the suture line. Enterotomies are performed on the gastric pouch and Roux limb adjacent to the suture line. A second posterior, full-thickness, running suture line is performed and continued anteriorly beyond the termination of the first posterior suture.

Two anterior suture lines are run from the distal anterior aspect of the enterotomy, the first being full thickness and the second seromuscular. Before the completion of the anastomosis, the 34-F tube is carefully inserted across the anastomosis to help calibrate the opening as well as provide assurance of a patent anastomosis. The anterior sutures are tied with their respective posterior counterparts.

The anastomosis and proximal staple lines can be tested with blue dye, air insufflation via the orogastric tube, or operative endoscopy. The port sites are inspected for bleeding on withdrawal of the trocars, and the skin is closed with simple absorbable monofilament sutures.

Postoperative Management

Perioperative antibiotics are continued for 24 h, while thromboembolism prophylaxis continues until the patient is discharged. Analgesia is in the form of patient-controlled narcotic delivery systems and intravenous ketorolac or acetaminophen. Oral narcotics are offered when clear liquids are tolerated. Metoclopramide is administered routinely and a variety of antiemetic pharmacologic agents are available for nurses to use at their discretion.

Routine postoperative contrast studies add little to the management of these patients and serve only to delay discharge

secondary to nausea [19]. A normal postoperative upper gastrointestinal (UGI) study should not preclude the surgeon's intervening based on clinical suspicion of a leak [20].

Patients are started on clear liquids on the day of surgery and are required to ambulate with assistance. Preoperative oral medications can be resumed as soon as the patient can tolerate clear liquids. Almost all patients are discharged by the second postoperative day; the majority leave on the first postoperative day.

Patients are continued on a clear liquid diet for 1 week and slowly advanced to solids over a 3- to 4-week period. Patients are instructed to take either an H2 blocker or proton pump inhibitor for 30 days. Routine follow-up visits are at 1, 3 weeks, and quarterly for the first year and then on a yearly basis. Ongoing nutritional, emotional, and exercise counseling and support groups are provided. Complete nutritional assessment occurs on a yearly basis or when symptoms or clinical suspicion dictates.

Results

Long-term data regarding gastric bypass have been lacking due to the complexity of issues regarding follow-up. Himpens [21] reported a 9-year data consistent with the long-term open gastric bypass data that was comparable to our 10-year data (Table 1) [22]. Although we experienced poor follow-up, there was no difference in outcomes between patients who consistently followed up in our office and those who did not; so it is not unreasonable to extrapolate our results.

Early complication rates and operative times suffer from a very steep learning curve. This is dependent not only on the initial experience of the surgeon but also on the surgeon's ability to organize a systematic method of approaching this complex operation. Efficiency as a result of preparedness of the operative team is critical. Our data suggest that performing more than 100 procedures as the primary surgeon may be necessary for this learning process.

Management of Early Complications

The most common complication in our series is stenosis of the gastrojejunal anastomosis. This has remained constant at 4.9–5.21 % (Table 2) and responds well to endoscopic balloon dilation. Patients complain of regression or intolerance of diet advancement at about the third postoperative week. The etiology of this phenomenon is unclear and appears unrelated to the method of gastrojejunostomy (Table 3). Rarely does it occur at the level of the mesocolon or jejunojejunostomy. These locations do not respond to endoscopic dilation and must be repaired operatively. At times, a recurrent gastrojejunal stenosis also requires operative attention.

The second most common complication in our series is that of internal hernias and bowel obstructions (Table 4).

TABLE 1. Comparison of published data

Investigator	Patients (n)	Follow-up (years)	Patients eligible for follow-up (n)	Patients at follow-up, n (%)	%EWL	Postoperative BMI (kg/m²)
Jones [23]	352	10	71	36 (51)	62	30
Pories et al. [24]	608	10	NR	158 (NR)	55	35
Sugerman et al. [25]	1,025	10–12	361	135 (37)	52	36
Christou et al. [26]	272	12	272	161 (59)	68	38
Higa et al. [22]	242	10	242	65 (27)	57	33
Himpens et al. [21]	126	9	126	77 (61)	63	30

TABLE 2. Complications of 242 study patients and 65 patients evaluated during POY 10

Morbidity	242 study patients, n (%)	65 patients evaluated during POY 10, n (%)
Early		
Incomplete division of the stomach	4 (1.7)	
Staple-line failure	2 (0.8)	
Thermal injury with perforation	1 (0.4)	
Marginal ulcer perforation	1 (0.4)	
Bleeding, observation	1 (0.4)	1 (1.5)
Deep venous thrombosis	1 (0.4)	
Stenosis, gastrojejunostomy	12 (5.0)	4 (6.2)
Stenosis, mesocolon	1 (0.4)	
Fever	1 (0.4)	
Readmission	5 (2.1)	1 (1.5)
Hypoglycemia	1 (0.4)	1 (1.5)
Central pontine myelinolysis	1 (0.4)	
Subtotal	31 (12.8)	7 (10.8)
Late		
Internal hernia	39 (16.1)	
Marginal hernia	11 (4.5)	5 (7.7)
Gastrogastric fistula	1 (0.4)	1 (1.5)
Biliary requiring cholecystectomy	17 (7.0)	12 (18.5)
Alcohol dependency	6 (2.5)	5 (7.7)
Other substance abuse	1 (0.4)	
Hernia, trocar	3 (1.2)	1 (1.5)
Subtotal	78 (32.2)	24 (36.9)
Total	109 (45.0)	31 (47.7)

Data in parentheses are percentages
POY postoperative year

TABLE 3. Incidence of gastrojejunal stenosis

Author	n	Stenosis: n (%)
Wittgrove et al. [4]	1,000	40 (4.0)
Schauer et al. [6]	275	13 (4.7)
Higa et al. [33]	1,500	73 (4.9)
Champion et al. [34]	63	4 (6.3)
De Maria et al. [35]	281	18 (6.6)

TABLE 4. Internal hernia data (2,805 patients)

Location	n	Percent
Mesocolon	61	2.2
Jejunojejunostomy	41	1.5
Petersen's	13	0.5
Multiple sites	13	0.5
Total	128	4.6

These may occur immediately postoperatively or many years after the procedure. Primarily due to migration of bowel through an open mesenteric defect, this phenomenon can be difficult to detect in the absence of overt bowel obstruction. Often, patients complain of intermittent, severe, postprandial abdominal pain, but noninvasive radiographic studies are completely normal in at least 50 % of cases. Diagnostic laparoscopy must be performed based on clinical suspicion, and reduction and repair of the defects are straightforward [28].

The prevention of internal hernias requires meticulous closure of all potential defects with a nonabsorbable suture material. Some surgeons have brought the Roux limb antecolic in hopes that the most common cause of small bowel obstruction, that of transmesocolic herniation, is eliminated. However, the large resulting Petersen's space and the jejunal mesentery defects are still potential sites that need to be addressed [29]. Our current internal hernia rate has stabilized at 1 %, utilizing nonabsorbable continuous closure of all potential hernia spaces.

Proximal anastomotic leaks or staple-line disruptions are tolerated poorly by the bariatric patient. Leaks are often subtle in their initial presentation; the only indication may be sustained tachycardia (>120/min). Typical symptoms of abdominal pain, fever, or leukocytosis can be indistinguishable from cardiac events, pulmonary embolism, acute gastric distention, or hemorrhagic shock. Morbidly obese patients have little cardiopulmonary reserve; therefore, time to treatment is critical. Workup and evaluation must be expeditious and directed by clinical suspicion. If a leak is suspected, reexploration, usually laparoscopically, is the only definitive method to rule it out.

At surgery, there should be an attempt to identify and repair the defect, knowing that it will sometimes fail. Operative endoscopy is often helpful in identifying the leak and evaluating the repair. Drainage is essential, and enteric access via a gastrostomy tube in the gastric remnant can be established at this time. This prevents gastric distention and can later be used as a conduit for nutritional support.

Venous thromboembolism is the primary cause of death in most series. Surprisingly, given the physical attributes of the patient population, comorbid conditions, and nature of the operation (position, prolonged operative times, and so forth), this is a rare occurrence. The use of both mechanical and pharmacologic prophylaxis along with early mobilization made possible by the elimination of incisional

pain likely contributes to these outcomes. The use of prophylactic vena cava filters should be limited to patients
with previous pulmonary embolism or significant pulmonary hypertension.

Management of Late Complications

The use of tobacco or nonsteroidal analgesic agents contributes to marginal ulceration. Patients present with abdominal
pain, dyspepsia, and occasionally bleeding. The diagnosis
can be made radiographically, but endoscopy is often
required for evaluation and treatment of an associated gastrojejunal stenosis or for control of bleeding.

Perforated marginal ulcers are amenable to laparoscopic intervention. The absence of significant intra-abdominal adhesions
and the anterior location of the anastomosis allow for a relatively simple closure and omental patch. Operative endoscopy
is helpful in these cases to rule out gastrogastric fistulas and to
evaluate the gastrojejunal anastomosis and repair.

Protein, vitamin, and mineral deficiencies are relatively
common [30]. Although most nutritional issues can be prevented by simple vitamin and calcium supplementation, few
patients are compliant. This continues to be a challenge as
well as long-term follow-up for most programs.

Inadequate initial weight loss and weight recidivism are
often attributable to the lack of patient compliance and/or
participation in postoperative programs. However, as the
pathophysiology of the disease of obesity is as poorly understood as our surgical interventions, to assign blame to the
individual is irrational. The durability of our interventions,
alone, indicates a biological rather than mechanical mechanism—we should expect a response curve similar to all interventions. This is exactly what we observe—up to 20 % of
patients fail to obtain their target weight or resolve their
comorbidities; the majority do well, as some have extraordinary results. This is unpredictable and adds to the frustration
shared by the patient and surgeon.

Clearly, the concept of obesity as a chronic disease should
mandate a multidisciplinary and lifelong approach to therapy. This includes the possibility of secondary surgical procedures for selected patients who do not achieve correction
or stabilization of medical comorbid conditions. Attempts at
the enhancement of the existing anatomy through additional
"restriction," such as downsizing the pouch and/or anastomosis, have been disappointing. This observation underscores the biological rather than mechanical mechanism of
the proximal gastric bypass.

References

1. Wittgrove AC, Clark GW, Tremblay LJ. Laparoscopic gastric
   bypass, Roux-en-Y: preliminary report of five cases. Obes Surg.
   1994;4:353–7.
2. Wittgrove AC, Clark GW. Laparoscopic gastric bypass: a five-year
   prospective study of 500 patients followed from 3–60 months. Obes
   Surg. 1999;9:123–43.
3. Wittgrove AC, Clark GW, Schubert KR. Laparoscopic gastric
   bypass, Roux-en-Y: technique and results in 75 patients with 3–30
   month follow-up. Obes Surg. 1996;6:500–4.
4. Wittgrove AC, Endres JE, Davis M, et al. Perioperative complications in a single surgeon's experience with 1,000 consecutive laparoscopic Roux-en-Y gastric bypass operations for morbid obesity.
   Obes Surg. 2002;12:457–8 (abstr L4).
5. de la Torre RA, Scott JS. Laparoscopic Roux-en-Y gastric bypass:
   a totally intra-abdominal approach: technique and preliminary
   report. Obes Surg. 1999;9:492–8.
6. Schauer PR, Ikramuddin S, Gourash W, et al. Outcomes after laparoscopic Roux-en-Y gastric bypass for morbid obesity. Ann Surg.
   2000;232:515–29.
7. Higa KD, Boone KB, Ho T, et al. Laparoscopic Roux-en-Y gastric
   bypass for morbid obesity: technique and preliminary results of our
   first 400 patients. Arch Surg. 2000;9:1029–33.
8. Mason EE, Maher JW, Scott DH, et al. Ten years of vertical banded
   gastroplasty for severe obesity. In: Mason EE, guest editor; Nyhus
   LM, editor-in-chief. Surgical treatment of morbid obesity. Problems
   in general surgery series, Vol. 9. Philadelphia: Lippincott, 1992.
   p. 280–9.
9. MacLean LD, Rhode BM, Forse RA. Surgery for obesity: an update
   of a randomized trial. Obes Surg. 1995;5:145–50.
10. Evans S, Pamuklar Z, Rosko J, Mahaney P, Jiang N, Park C,
    Torquati A. Gastric bypass surgery restores meal stimulation of the
    anorexigenic gut hormones glucagon-like peptide-1 and peptide
    YY independently of caloric restriction. Surg Endosc. 2012;26(4):
    1086–94.
11. Hatoum IJ, Greenawalt DM, Cotsapas C, Reitman ML, Daly MJ,
    Kaplan LM. Heritability of the weight loss response to gastric
    bypass surgery. J Clin Endocrinol Metab. 2011;96(10):1630–3.
12. Mason EE, Ito C. Gastric bypass in obesity. Surg Clin North Am.
    1967;47:1345–51.
13. Higa KD, Boone KB, Ho T. Complications of the laparoscopic
    Roux-en-Y gastric bypass: 1,040 patients—what have we learned?
    Obes Surg. 2000;10:509–13.
14. Westling A, Bergvist D, Bostrom A, et al. Incidence of deep venous
    thrombosis in patients undergoing obesity surgery. World J Surg.
    2000;26:470–3.
15. Brolin RE, Kenler HA, Gorman JH, Cody RP. Long-limb gastric
    bypass in the super obese: a prospective randomized trial. Ann
    Surg. 1991;215:387–95.
16. Champion JK. Small bowel obstruction after laparoscopic Roux-
    en-Y gastric bypass. Obes Surg. 2002;12:197–8 (abstr 17).
17. Khanna A, Newman B, Reyes J, Fung JJ, Todo S, Starzl TL. Internal
    hernia and volvulus of the small bowel following liver transplanta-
    tion. Transpl Int. 1997;10(2):133.
18. Iannelli A, Facchiano E, Gugenheim J. Internal hernia after laparo-
    scopic Roux-en-Y gastric bypass for morbid obesity. Obes Surg.
    2006;16:1265–71.
19. Singh R, Fisher B. Sensitivity and specificity of postoperative upper
    GI series following gastric bypass. Obes Surg. 2003;13:73–5.
20. Sims TL, Mullican MA, Hamilton EC, et al. Routine upper gastro-
    intestinal Gastrografin swallow after laparoscopic Roux-en-Y gas-
    tric bypass. Obes Surg. 2003;13:66–72.
21. Himpens J, Verbrugghe A, Cadiére G, Everaerts W, Greve J. Long-
    term results of laparoscopic Roux-en-Y gastric bypass: evaluation
    after 9 years. Obes Surg. 2012;22:1586–93.
22. Higa KD, Ho T, Tercero F, Yunus T, Boone KB. Laparoscopic
    Roux-en-Y gastric bypass: 10-year follow-up. Surg Obes Relat Dis.
    2011;7:516–25.
23. Jones K. Experience with the Roux-en-Y gastric bypass, and com-
    mentary on current trends. Obes Surg. 2000;10:183–5.

24. Pories W, Swanson M, MacDonald K. Who would have thought it? An operation proves to be the most effective therapy for adult-onset diabetes mellitus. Ann Surg. 1995;222:339–50.

25. Sugerman HJ, Wolfe LG, Sica DA, Clore JN. Diabetes and hypertension in severe obesity and effects of gastric bypass-induced weight loss. Ann Surg. 2003;237:751–8.

26. Christou NV, Look D, Maclean LD. Weight gain after short- and long-limb gastric bypass in patients followed for longer than 10 years. Ann Surg. 2006;244:734–40.

27. Schauer PR, Ikramuddin S, Hammad G, et al. The learning curve for laparoscopic Roux-en-Y gastric bypass in 100 cases. Surg Endosc. 2003;17:212–5.

28. Higa K, Ho T, Boone K. Internal hernias after laparoscopic Roux-en-Y gastric bypass: incidence, treatment and prevention. Obes Surg. 2003;13:350–4.

29. Schweitzer MA, DeMaria EJ, Broderick TJ, Sugerman HJ. Laparoscopic closure of mesenteric defects after Roux-en-Y gastric bypass. J Laparoendosc Adv Surg Tech A. 2000;10(3):173–5.

30. Rhode BM, MacLean LD. Vitamin and mineral supplementation after gastric bypass. In: Deitel M, Cowan G, editors. Update: surgery for the morbidly obese patient. Toronto: FD-Communications; 2000.

31. Schauer PR. Physiologic consequences of laparoscopic surgery. In: Eubanks WS, Soper NJ, Swanstrom LL, editors. Mastery of endoscopic surgery and laparoscopic surgery. Philadelphia: Lippincott Williams & Wilkins; 2000. p. 22–38.

32. Nguyen NT, Lee SL, Goldman C, et al. Comparison of pulmonary function and postoperative pain after laparoscopic vs open gastric bypass: a randomized trial. J Am Coll Surg. 2001;192:469–76.

33. Higa K, Ho T, Boone K. Laparoscopic Roux-en-Y gastric bypass; technique and 3-year follow-up. J Laparoendosc Adv Surg Tech A. 2001;11:377–82.

34. Champion JK, Hunt T, DeLisle N. Laparoscopic vertical banded gastroplasty and Roux-en-Y gastric bypass in morbid obesity. Obes Surg. 1999;9:123–44.

35. DeMaria EJ, Sugerman HJ, Kellum JM, et al. Results of 281 consecutive total laparoscopic Roux-en-Y gastric bypasses to treat morbid obesity. Ann Surg. 2002;235:640–7.

27

Laparoscopic Gastric Bypass Using Linear Stapling Technique

Bruce D. Schirmer

Roux-en-Y gastric bypass (RYGB), originally described by Mason [1] as a loop technique, was later modified by him to a Roux limb, the technique of which was further popularized by Griffin [2]. MacLean [3] and others confirmed that dividing the stomach was superior to simply stapling it, eliminating the potential for staple line breakdown causing loss of restrictive capacity of the operation. Gastric bypass then underwent few major revisions until Wittgrove and Clark [4] first described the operation being performed laparoscopically. That is the approach now used in the vast majority of procedures.

The operation has been the gold standard procedure for bariatric surgery since the 1970s in the United States. It has proven to provide durable weight loss through largely a restrictive mechanism. The small proximal gastric pouch restricts food intake dramatically initially. Adaptation allows the pouch to empty more quickly, and later patients may and do eat more. Long-term success is maintained only with a change in patient diet and exercise habits. These are often easily adapted during the first year after surgery when weight loss is dramatic, appetite is suppressed, food intake is limited, and patients experience a major change in overall well-being, body habitus improvement, improvement of major associated medical problems, and improvement in activities of daily living. Most patients are motivated enough by these improvements to maintain these gains through revised eating and exercise habits. A minority, however, may regain weight as time passes.

While simple restriction certainly explains the major reason for weight loss and thereby improvement of weight-associated medical problems, the anatomy of RYGB also produces profound improvement in some medical problems, especially type II diabetes, that weight loss alone cannot

account for the changes (Pories article [5]). RYGB causes loss of the pyloric restriction of slow release of food into the duodenum. Rapid passage of food into the Roux limb will produce dumping syndrome if the food is highly osmotic (sweets especially). It has also been shown that the rapid passage of food into the more distal gut will cause the release of GLP-1 with consequent improvement of insulin sensitivity and thereby type II diabetes (Mason or some other articles about GLP-1 release and action [6, 7]). The complete picture of the metabolic effects of RYGB on carbohydrate metabolism, fat metabolism, and gut adjustments to digestion is still being studied, and certainly will be more complex than just the changes in GLP-1 release. Effects on satiety, gut flora alteration, and changes in the inflammatory response contributing to metabolic syndrome are all areas that will contribute to understanding the effectiveness and changes that occur after performance of RYGB.

While it would be optimal for comparing outcomes to have all RYGB operations performed in a standard fashion, unfortunately that has not been the evolution of the operation. Surgeons all have some variability in how they perform the procedure. Some have placed a restrictive band [8] or an adjustable band [9] around the proximal gastric pouch. Other variables include the length of the Roux limb, anatomic positioning of the Roux limb relative to the stomach and transverse colon, size of the proximal gastric pouch, size of the gastrojejunal anastomosis between that pouch and the Roux limb, and the way in which this anastomosis is created.

Despite these variations in the actual performance of RYGB, the main principles that are important to the successful performance of the operation have emerged as being food restriction and bypassing the proximal gut with rapid pouch emptying. Anatomically, then, the operation should be constructed so as to maximize these principles. The performance of the operation as I perform it at the University of Virginia will now be briefly described, emphasizing the use of the linear stapling technique for performance of the proximal anastomosis (the gastrojejunostomy) of the operation. This technique is now my standard method of performing the

Electronic supplementary material: Supplementary material is available in the online version of this chapter at 10.1007/978-1-4939-1637-5_27. Videos can also be accessed at http://www.springerimages.com/videos/978-1-4939-1636-8.

operation to date, but I evolved to it over many years, having done a circular anastomotic technique in the past. The linear stapling technique will be described, after which the reasons for favoring it will be given.

While the complete description of performing RYGB is given in other chapters, this chapter will briefly describe the procedure aside from the emphasis on the creation of the gastrojejunostomy so that the reader may reproduce it if desired. Port placement, Roux limb position, and creation of the gastric pouch all are done in a manner so as to be compatible with and optimize the creation of the linear-stapled gastrojejunostomy using this approach.

Port Placement

The advent of articulating linear staplers has caused us to modify our port placement slightly. The surgeon now may more easily use a right-hand-dominant stapling technique, and the left-hand port does not need to be a 12-mm size. The adjustability of the stapler now allows the surgeon to more easily work with both ports located in the right upper quadrant. The assistant still benefits from having one 12-mm port in the left upper quadrant, as we do a double-stapling technique for the distal anastomosis (jejunojejunostomy). A second 5-mm port for the assistant is located lower in the left upper quadrant. The 12 mm camera port is located in the umbilical region, with some variability based on body habitus. For a longer torso individual, for example, a supraumbilical location is needed. A liver retractor is placed in the epigastric region. Port placement is shown in Fig. 1.

Distal Anastomosis

This is performed first, as the patient is already supine. A variable-length Roux limb is created, based on patient BMI and visceral adiposity. Greater levels of one or both parameters are an indication for a longer Roux limb (150 cm or longer range). The linear stapler (white load) is used to divide the bowel and the harmonic scalpel is used to divide the mesentery down to near its base, mobilizing the Roux limb as much as possible yet avoiding too deep a division of the mesentery to cause hemorrhage from major and larger proximal mesenteric vessels. Once the length of Roux limb is determined, a linear double-stapling technique (two white loads) with suturing of the stapler defect is used for the distal anastomosis. The mesenteric defect is then closed using a running permanent suture.

Passing the Roux Limb

In order to create a retrocolic and retrogastric anastomosis, a defect is created in the transverse colon mesentery as it is displayed on a stretch. The area just to the left and above the

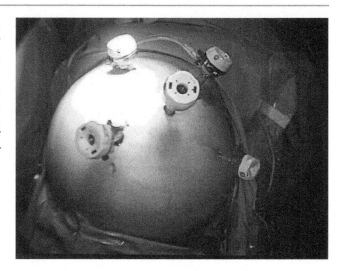

FIG. 1 Placement of ports for laparoscopic Roux-en-Y gastric bypass with linear stapling technique

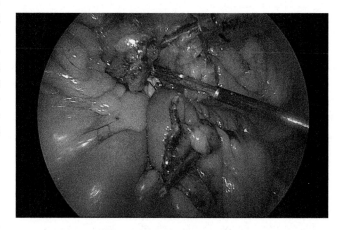

FIG. 2 Passing the Roux limb through the transverse colon mesentery for a retrocolic-retrogastric placement of the Roux limb

ligament of Treitz is often relatively avascular, being to the patient's left of the middle colic vessels. Variability in the mesenteric arcade exists, and this step is performed with a harmonic scalpel. Once the mesenteric opening has been created, the stomach is grasped and pulled down to the level of the defect, and the retrogastric space is cleared of adhesions if present. Then the Roux limb is passed into the retrogastric space (Fig. 2). It is critical to keep the mesentery of the Roux limb correctly oriented and prevent the limb from twisting, which would result in ischemia and breakdown of the anastomosis. We usually attach a Penrose drain to the most proximal end of the Roux limb to help with this passing of the Roux limb into the retrogastric space as well as later retrieval from that space.

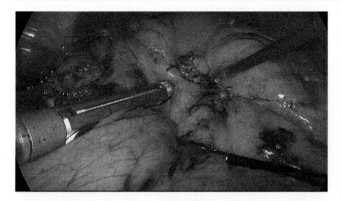

FIG. 3 Creation of the proximal gastric pouch starts 1–3 cm above the *incisura* on the lesser curvature side of the stomach. (**a**) First staple firing; (**b**) subsequent staple firing

Creation of the Proximal Gastric Pouch

This step is performed using the linear stapler, beginning by first stapling at right angles to the lesser curvature above the *incisura*, with the length of the pouch determined by each patient's anatomy. Excellent mobilization of the Roux limb and a smaller patient allow the pouch to be created beginning more proximal on the lesser curvature, perhaps 5–6 cm below the gastroesophageal junction (Fig. 3). However, we have found with larger patients or patients with less mobile Roux limbs that creation of a longer proximal gastric pouch, even down to the *incisura* if necessary, is safer and allows a tension-free anastomosis while still preserving excellent weight loss. Indeed, the proximal gastric pouch in these patients begins to resemble the proximal portion of a sleeve gastrectomy. The surgeon and anesthesiologist must remember that removal of all tubes within the gastric lumen is mandatory before the initiation of gastric stapling and division.

Details of the Linear-Stapled Gastrojejunostomy

Once the gastric pouch has been created, the distal stomach is elevated along its newly created staple line to look into the retrogastric region. This allows identification of the Penrose drain and the Roux limb. The drain is used to draw the limb up adjacent to the proximal gastric pouch, with the staple line facing inferiorly toward the patient's feet (Fig. 4). The very end of the Roux limb is usually less mobile than the several inches beyond it, and thus this slightly more distal part of the Roux limb is more easily brought up adjacent to the proximal portion of the gastric pouch. Beginning 6–7 cm from the end of the Roux limb, the side of the Roux limb adjacent to the gastric pouch is sewn to the gastric pouch staple line, with the suture ending at the proximal end of the Roux limb and the inferior end of the gastric pouch, which are now adjacent to each other (Fig. 5). The Penrose drain is removed as this suturing occurs. The end of the suture line is left long temporarily.

Once the Roux limb is thus secured to the proximal pouch, then the anesthesiologist passes an Ewald tube, which is a gastric lavage tube that is 36 Fr in size. This tube is advanced carefully under monitored observation by both the surgeon and the anesthesiologist, so it can be positioned with the tip at the distal end of the proximal gastric pouch and no further (to avoid injury to the pouch). Then the harmonic scalpel is used to create a gastrotomy, using the Ewald tube as a backstop (Fig. 6). We have found that creation of a full-thickness gastrotomy of adequate size is essential to facilitating the insertion of the jaw of the stapler for the anastomosis. One must avoid creation of a false passage within the wall of the stomach which may occur if an inadequate opening not completely through the mucosa is created. An opening is made in the Roux limb directly opposite the gastrotomy. Then a blue load of the 45-mm linear stapler is inserted full length into the two openings (Fig. 7), creating an anastomosis with one

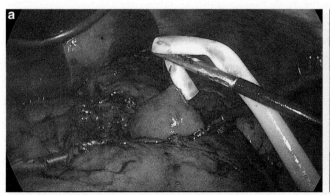

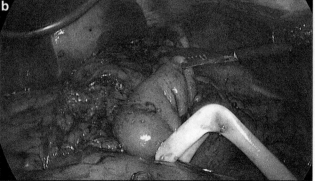

FIG. 4 Passing the Roux limb using the Penrose drain to bring the proximal end of the Roux limb down and adjacent to the distal end of the proximal gastric pouch

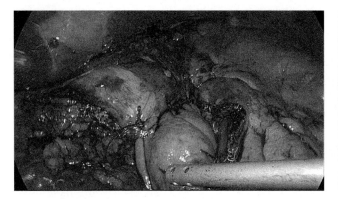

Fɪɢ. 5 The Roux limb has now been sewn to the side of the proximal gastric pouch to align them appropriately for the anastomosis

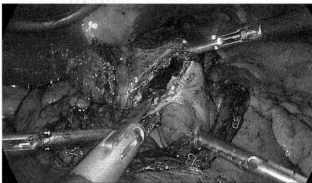

Fɪɢ. 8 The stapler defect is now closed beginning at the end where the stapler was inserted, as this area of the defect is most difficult to expose and best closed first. A running suture is used to close the defect

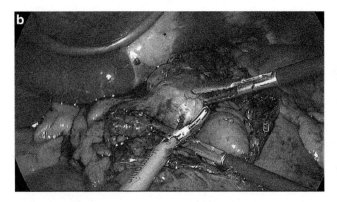

Fɪɢ. 6 Creating the gastrotomy in the proximal gastric pouch using the harmonic scalpel

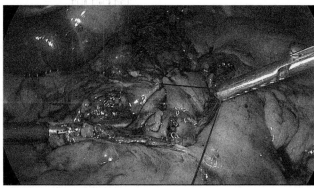

Fɪɢ. 9 The first suture line is reinforced with a second suture line, beginning distally beyond the staple line and sewing toward the camera

suturing this opening beginning inferiorly at the inferior intersection of the stomach and jejunum is best, since this area is best accessed and the sutures are most accurately placed here if it is done first, whereas visualization is limited if it is the final area of closure (Fig. 8). Thus our suture line for closure runs superiorly starting at the inferior edge of the anastomosis.

Once the stapler defect has been closed, we have our anesthesiologist again advance the Ewald tube, this time stopping the tip just 1 cm beyond the anastomosis into the Roux limb lumen. Then the sutured closure of the staple defect is oversewn with a running suture beginning at the portion of the anastomosis furthest away, running the oversewing suture toward the surgeon and in turn imbricating the first suture line (Fig. 9). The end of the initial suturing of the stomach to jejunum which was left long is used to tie to and anchor this imbrication suture once it has reached that suture, marking the proximal end of the anastomosis. Finally, once the oversewing is completed, we use the Ewald tube to perform an on-table methylene blue dye test (120 mL via the

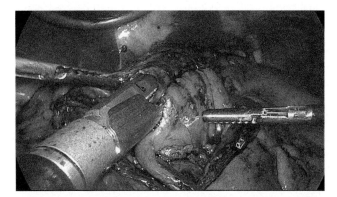

Fɪɢ. 7 The jaws of the stapler have been inserted into the stomach and Roux limb to create the linear-stapled gastrojejunostomy

firing of the stapler. We strive to achieve inserting the stapler to its full length as this creates an adequate-sized anastomosis which is large enough to prevent structuring postoperatively. The Ewald tube is of course pulled back several inches prior to inserting the stapler. Once the stapler has been fired, the stapler defect is then sewn closed. We have found that

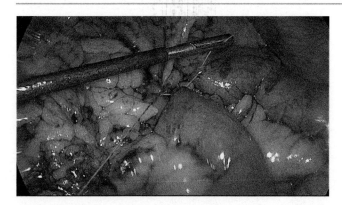

FIG. 10 The mesenteric defect in the retrocolic and retrogastric approach is best closed using a purse-string type suture of permanent suture material to include Roux limb, jejunum next to the ligament of Treitz, and both sides of the transverse colon mesentery

TABLE 1. Incidence of stenosis and other complications using circular (cs) versus linear (ls) technique for gastrojejunostomy in performing laparoscopic gastric bypass

	cs	ls
# patients	247	630
# stenoses	43	6
% stenosis	17.4	1.0*
Post-op month	3.1±1.1	7.2±5.9
Leak	3 (1.2 %)	2 (0.3 %)
Marginal ulcer	8 (3.2 %)	5 (0.8 %)#

University of Virginia data 1996–2004. *$p < 0.001$, #$p < 0.05$

TABLE 2. Weight loss (% excess weight loss for patients undergoing laparoscopic gastric bypass using circular stapling (cs) versus linear stapling (ls) technique for gastrojejunostomy)

	cs	ls
% EWL 1 year post-op	64.9±1.6	64.4±0.8
% EWL 2 years post-op	69.4±1.8	67.2±1.6
% EWL 3 years post-op	65.3±2.0	63.8±3.1

University of Virginia data 1996–2004. p = ns all categories

tube under forced pressure) to confirm the lack of any leaks of the pouch or staple line closure. The Ewald tube is then removed.

Closure of Mesenteric and Port Defects

The location of the Roux limb using this technique places it directly to the patient's left of the ligament of Treitz as it enters the transverse colon mesentery. This facilitates using a permanent suture to tack the Roux limb to the proximal jejunum at the ligament of Treitz using several nonabsorbable sutures. We have termed the initial such suture the "triple stitch" since it includes both pieces of bowel and the transverse colon mesentery in the 2 o'clock and 10 o'clock areas of the opening. It is thus a small purse-string type suture (Fig. 10). A second suture 1–2 cm (no further) inferiorly on the bowel is used to again suture bowel to bowel. A third (or more if preferred but we find one usually suffices) is used to tack the 4 o'clock position of the mesenteric opening to the adjacent surface of the Roux limb.

We routinely close all 12-mm port sites with a single absorbable 0 weight suture using a simple suture passer technique. We have had no incisional hernias using this approach.

Rationale for the Linear Stapling Technique

In our experience, the reduction of postoperative anastomotic stenosis from the circular stapling technique to the linear stapling technique was absolutely astounding. Table 1 summarizes the changes in the incidence of complications observed in the first 630 patients undergoing linear stapling versus our initial experience of 247 patients undergoing circular stapling. Whereas we experienced a 17 % incidence of proximal anastomotic stricture requiring endoscopic or fluoroscopic balloon dilation postoperatively after using a circular stapling technique, we, and more importantly our patients, have enjoyed less than a 1 % incidence of stenosis since using the linear stapling technique. The difference in these incidences was markedly statistically significant. The incidence of marginal ulcers was also observed to be significantly lower. The incidence of leaks, though, was not significantly lower for the linear stapling technique, although the absolute percentage was lower. Post-op stenosis after the circular stapling technique tended to occur slightly earlier after lap RYGB, but this difference was also not statistically significant.

Our long-term weight loss data (Table 2) show that the use of the linear stapler to perform what is likely a technically larger anastomosis did not detract from postoperative weight loss. Both groups lost a comparable amount of weight. These data also speak volumes to deflate the persistent myth in the bariatric literature that maintaining the size of the proximal anastomosis as small as possible both initially and long term is optimal for good weight loss. In fact, since we endoscope our own patients most commonly for postoperative symptoms and problems, it has become quite evident over the years that the size of the anastomosis does not directly correspond to the success of the patient in terms of weight loss. Restricting gastric pouch size does seem to be important. Anastomotic size does not. In fact, the rapid emptying of food contents into the jejunum, which produces some of the beneficial effects on carbohydrate metabolism from release of GLP-1 and other hormones, is further facilitated by a larger anastomosis.

What does seem to make the ultimate difference in long-term outcomes after lap RYGB is not anastomotic size itself, but rather the patient's adoption of new eating and exercise habits based on the initial results the operation was able to deliver to them.

Summary

The use of a linear stapling technique to perform the gastrojejunostomy of the laparoscopic RYGB has, in our experience, been associated with a significantly lower incidence of postoperative anastomotic stenosis. Weight loss using this technique is equally as good as a circular stapling technique, to which it was compared in our experience. We therefore advocate the use of the linear stapling technique as being technically easier and producing better outcomes for patients undergoing laparoscopic RYGB (Video 1).

References

1. Mason EE, Ito C. Gastric bypass in obesity. Surg Clin North Am. 1969;47:1345–51.
2. Griffin WO, Young VL, Stevenson CC. A prospective comparison of gastric and jejunoileal bypass procedures for morbid obesity. Ann Surg. 1977;186:500–9.
3. MacLean LD, Rhode BM, Nohr CW. Late outcome of isolated gastric bypass. Ann Surg. 2000;231:524–8.
4. Wittgrove AC, Clark WG, Tremblay LJ. Laparoscopic gastric bypass, Roux-en-Y: preliminary report of five cases. Obes Surg. 1994;4:353–7.
5. Pories WJ, Swanson MS, MacDonald KG, et al. Who would have thought it? An operation proves to be the most effective therapy for adult-onset diabetes mellitus. Ann Surg. 1995;222:339–52.
6. Falken Y, Hellstrom PM, Holst JJ, et al. Changes in glucose homeo-stasis after Roux-en-Y gastric bypass surgery at day three, two months, and one year after surgery: role of gut peptides. J Clin Endocrinol Metab. 2011;96:2227–35.
7. Brubaker PL. Minireview: update on incretin biology: focus on glucagon-like peptide-1. Endocrinology. 2010;151:1984–9.
8. Fobi MA, Lee H, Felahy B, et al. Choosing an operation for weight control, and the transected banded gastric bypass. Obes Surg. 2005; 15:114–21.
9. Bessler M, Dauid A, Kim T, DiGiorgi M. Prospective randomized trial of banded versus nonbanded gastric bypass for the super obese: early results. Surg Obes Relat Dis. 2007;3:480–5.

28

Outcomes After Laparoscopic Gastric Bypass

Bruce D. Schirmer

Open RYGB

RYGB has been shown to improve survival in patients who undergo it versus those who do not [3–6]. The estimated increase in longevity for a man having the operation is 12 years and for a woman is 9 years.

Improvement in many comorbid medical problems occurs in over 70 % of patients for most problems and reaches or approaches 90 % for many. Venous stasis ulcers disappear at a 90 % rate, and hyperlipidemia is resolved at a rate of 70 %. Hypertension is resolved in 50–65 % of cases. Obstructive sleep apnea (OSA) is improved in at least that high a percentage, although the definition of remission in that disease is still controversial. Data from a major review of the published experience of open RYGB by Buchwald [7] are shown in Table 1.

Among the especially powerful accomplishments of RYGB has been its ability to produce rapid remission of type 2 diabetes in severely obese patients with that disease [8]. The remission rate is as high as 80 % or more for patients with disease of 5 years' duration or less. This is a huge consideration for the patient who has begun insulin therapy. The remission of type 2 diabetes after gastric bypass has become the focus of much of the shift from considering RYGB more as a metabolic than a bariatric operation [9]. There is an entire chapter devoted to this topic in this text, and the reader is referred to it for the details of this particular metabolic action of RYGB. It should also be noted that there are also now good data to support extending the indications for performing RYGB for patients with type 2 diabetes who have a BMI between 30 and 35 [10].

Improvement in vital organ function and improvement in obesity-related organ dysfunction is also well documented after RYGB. Patients with nonalcoholic fatty liver disease (NAFLD) have been shown to benefit from RYGB. Postoperatively, based on biopsy analysis, RYGB produced a 93 % incidence of improvement in liver score and at times reversed fibrosis (20 %) and inflammation (37 %) [11].

Cardiovascular disease has also been shown to be improved after gastric bypass. Observations of the improvement in hypertension have been made since the operation has been monitored, and improvement in measured cardiac function has been more recently emphasized in the literature [12]. Cardiac function has been shown to be reversibly improved in adolescents with left ventricular hypertrophy and dilatation after undergoing LRYGB [13].

Pulmonary function has been documented to improve as well after RYGB. Hewitt et al. [14] showed long-term improvement in pulmonary function as measured by spirometry in 101 patients who had undergone RYGB. Nguyen et al. [15] showed similar findings in a similar sized group of patients as well, documenting the changes were evident as quickly as 3 months after surgery.

OSA is almost certainly underdiagnosed in the morbidly obese patient population. Hallowell et al. [16] showed that when routine testing was done for OSA preoperatively, a significant percentage of patients had undiagnosed disease. The incidence of patients felt to have OSA by clinical criteria versus routine testing rose from 56 to 91 %. This high percentage of undiagnosed patients may thus mitigate the already impressive incidence of improvement or resolution of OSA in the many studies after RYGB. Marti-Valeri et al. [17] reported that 86 % of patients no longer needed CPAP 1 year after RYGB. Patients with severe OSA may not be able to wean completely off their CPAP but often have their disease state ameliorated to moderate disease. They also may appear clinically less symptomatic than they prove to be with strict testing [18]. In large database reviews, OSA was seen to be improved in 66 % of patients after RYGB in the BSCN database [19]. The NSQIP data show a 70 % improvement nationally in OSA for patients undergoing LRYGB [20].

Degenerative joint disease is perhaps the most frequent comorbid medical problem found in patients who are candidates for bariatric surgery. However, its resolution or improvement is much more difficult to quantify as it is very

S.A. Brethauer et al. (eds.), *Minimally Invasive Bariatric Surgery*,
DOI 10.1007/978-1-4939-1637-5_28, © Springer Science+Business Media New York 2015

TABLE 1. Outcomes for bariatric operations

	LAGB	RYGB	BPD/DS
% EWL	47.5	61.6	70.1
% mortality	0.1	0.5	1.1
% morbidity	10–25	13–38	27–33
% nutritional morbidity	0–10	15–25	40–77

LAGB laparoscopic adjustable gastric banding, *BPD/DS* biliopancreatic diversion/duodenal switch. Adapted from Buchwald et al. [7]

much symptom based without objective parameters of measurement. Certainly, however, all bariatric surgeons are witnesses to frequent testimonies by patients of marked improvement in their joint and back pain. Improved mobility is enjoyed by many of the patients and often conversions from wheelchair-bound to ambulatory status are not infrequently seen in this patient population after RYGB.

Gastroesophageal reflux disease (GERD) is symptomatically present in mild degrees in approximately one half of patients with severe obesity and has been objectively proven to be present in 55 % in one study [21]. In another study in which anatomic and physiologic assessments were done of patients planning RYGB, the incidence of GERD was 64 % [22]. In that study, the incidence of postoperative GERD decreased to 33 % and median acid exposure of the esophagus from 5.1 to 1.1 %. The improvement postoperatively was somewhat decreased by a persistent and new onset of regurgitation in some patients. RYGB offers an anatomic advantage to treating this disease, in that the large-volume stomach is no longer connected to the esophagus. Instead, the very-small-volume proximal gastric pouch can be the only source of acid reflux. As a result, the incidence of resolution or improvement of GERD after RYGB is quite high. This has actually made RYGB the treatment of choice for patients with severe GERD and a BMI over 40. Resolution of symptoms in that patient population postoperatively is high and moreover is higher in the long term than patients treated with antireflux surgery, who due to their obesity and its associated increase in intra-abdominal pressure develop recurrence of symptoms and hiatal hernia more frequently than normal-weight individuals.

Venous stasis ulcers were shown by Sugerman et al. [23] to be effectively treated with RYGB in over 90 % of cases. These patients, however, were noted to have higher risk factors, more severe comorbidities, and higher death and complication rates than the general population of patients undergoing RYGB.

Pseudotumor cerebri is present in perhaps 1 % of patients with morbid obesity. However, when present, it is especially well treated with bariatric surgery. Reports of its almost 100 % resolution of RYGB have been documented in the literature [24]. The key to its treatment is appreciation by a neurologist or neurosurgeon of the value of weight loss in eliminating the condition.

Pseudotumor cerebri as well as stress urinary incontinence, another condition which responds well to weight loss therapy,

represent diseases among the spectrum of comorbid medical problems which have been hypothesized by Sugerman to arise from increased abdominal pressure [25]. The fact that there is an inflammatory component to many of these comorbid problems, as a result of the pressure, further supports this hypothesis. Metabolic studies have now shown inflammatory components to the cardiovascular, glucose intolerance, renal dysfunction, and hyperlipidemia dysfunction present in the severely obese patient population. The metabolic syndrome is characterized by a constellation of medical conditions, all of which are felt to include an inflammatory component in their etiology. The metabolic syndrome is well treated by RYGB, with resolution in 45 % of patients reported in one large series of diverse backgrounds [26].

In one recent study, LRYGB was shown to decrease the measured amount of urinary and serum inflammatory markers, as well as mean arterial pressure. It is hypothesized by the authors that the improvements seen in renal function, proteinuria, and hypertension after RYGB are related to weight loss-induced decrease in these inflammatory factors [27].

Overall quality of life has been measured in numerous reports of patients undergoing open and LRYGB. Schauer et al. [28] showed an improved quality of life for patients undergoing LRYGB, and Nguyen et al. [29] showed that SF-36 and BAROS score improvement was even greater than the improvement seen after open RYGB.

Open gastric bypass has traditionally provided patients with weight loss in the range of 60–70 % of excess weight at 1 year after surgery. Studies looking at outcomes from the era of open surgery reported this figure to be in the 60–65 % range [7]. Longer-term follow-up data show that some patients regain weight. However, the recidivism of weight regain tends to decrease after 10 years, and studies have shown that RYGB and other procedures produce long-term durable weight loss [5, 8].

Mortality after open RYGB was traditionally reported as between 1 and 2 % in the literature [30, 31]. A combination of many factors has now caused that number to have dropped to one-tenth its value in current practice.

Complications after open RYGB were also reported as being higher than they are today. The differences, however, could be variable depending on whether a study included long-term complications such as incisional hernia, bowel obstruction, and marginal ulcer, to name a few common ones. The transition from open surgery to laparoscopic surgery drastically reduced the serious wound complications and virtually eliminated the problem of incisional hernia after RYGB. The latter, in our institutional experience, was approximately 33 % if patients were followed carefully for a decade. Table 2 shows data from the University of Virginia comparing the first 5 years of our laparoscopic experience with performing gastric bypass versus the previous 15 years' experience with open surgery. Notable is the decrease in postoperative wound and incisional hernia complications, which consequently results in a huge difference in the overall complication rates of RYGB versus LRYGB. The second

TABLE 2. Outcomes for laparoscopic versus open RYGB (University of Virginia 1994–2004)

Characteristics	LRYGB	ORYGB	p value
Number of patients	765	363	
Preoperative BMI (kg/m^2)	50.9±0.3	57.5±0.5	<0.001
Number of comorbidities	2.7±0.1	3.6±0.1	<0.001
30-day mortality	2 (0.3 %)	6 (1.7 %)	<0.02
Overall complications	111 (14.5 %)	208 (57.3 %)	<0.001
Reoperation	67 (8.8 %)	150 (41.3 %)	<0.001
Incisional hernia	13 (1.7 %)	123 (33.9 %)	<0.001
Wound infection	14 (1.8 %)	27 (7.4 %)	<0.001

LRYGB laparoscopic Roux-en-Y gastric bypass, ORYGB open Roux-en-Y gastric bypass. Adapted from Schirmer B, Schauer P. The Surgical Management of Obesity. In: Schwartz's Principles of Surgery. 9th edition. McGraw Hill Medical, New York, 2010, pp. 949–978

TABLE 3. Factors which are likely responsible for the improvement in outcomes of gastric bypass over the past decade

1. Use of a laparoscopic approach to perform the operation
2. Change in patient population to include patients with lower BMI and less comorbidities
3. Increased volume of the procedure resulting in increased surgeon experience
4. Increased institutional experience
5. Centers of excellence programs monitoring outcomes
6. Centers of excellence programs improving facilities and practicing quality improvement
7. Perioperative protocols and best practices to limit complications

important observation is that patients who underwent open RYGB were generally heavier and had more comorbid medical problems than those undergoing LRYGB. This phenomenon likely has, to some extent, contributed to the decrease in incidence of morbidity and mortality after gastric bypass as well as other bariatric and metabolic operations.

Institutions besides our own reported an open RYGB complication rate in the 15–25 % range, depending on how such complications were defined and classified. Recent databases on LRYGB give the complication rates as being between 11.79 % for the BOLD database [32] and 15 % for the NSQIP database for cases done from 2007 to 2010 [19]. Current NSQIP 30-day complication rates for gastric bypass are as low as 4.7 % for 21,557 entered cases [20].

Laparoscopic RYGB

Outcomes after LRYGB are remarkably improved over those of open RYGB of a decade ago by a decrease in the complication rates associated with performance of the procedure. The effectiveness of LRYGB in resolving comorbid medical problems has also been more carefully documented in larger patient populations. Metabolic syndrome resolved in 48.7 % of cases in one large database of over 4,000 patients from the Kaiser Permanente system [26]. A large meta-analysis of the bariatric literature that included open gastric bypass (57 % of cases) showed resolution of type 2 diabetes in 80.3 % of patients who had that condition preoperatively [33]. The ACS BSCN database for cases performed from 2007 to 2010 showed a resolution or improvement of diabetes in 83 % of patients, hypertension in 79 %, OSA in 66 %, and GERD in 70 % of patients undergoing LRYGB at 1-year follow-up for 14,491 cases [19]. Current MBSAQIP database reduction in morbidities over time for the year 2012 demonstrated comparable reductions, within 10 % for all the above parameters. The reduction in hyperlipidemia was 61 % and for musculoskeletal disease 61.5 % [34].

Surgical therapy has been measured against best medical therapy in treating type 2 diabetes in the STAMPEDE trial [35]. In that trial, best medical therapy resulted in only 5 %

of patients receiving medical therapy achieving a glycated hemoglobin level of 6.0 % or less, while 38 % of patients undergoing LRYGB achieved it, a highly significant difference. In the Diabetes Surgery Study randomized trial, patients who had LRYGB added to maximal medical therapy for diabetes, hypertension, and hyperlipidemia achieved a 49 % rate of achieving goal objectives of treatment for those diseases, whereas the medically treated patients achieved only a 19 % rate of success [36].

LRYGB has produced equal or in some reports even superior weight loss to open RYGB. In the first large series reported on the use of laparoscopy to perform gastric bypass, Schauer et al. [28] reported an 83 % excess weight loss (EWL) at 2 years after surgery. Since the operation is virtually the same as the open procedure, it is likely that any improvements in this parameter are due in part to patient population changes, as well as improvements in surgeon experience and the technology to be able to perform the procedure efficiently. Studies that have looked at weight loss relative to BMI have usually shown patients in the higher BMI categories will not lose as high a percentage of their excess weight as those in lower BMI categories [24]. This observation persists today with the most recent such reports [26]. This likely relates to decreased mobility, increased medical problems, and other issues relative to the larger patients. LRYGB produces an average BMI loss of 11.87 for the first year after surgery based on the ACS BSCN data [19]. Our institutional 5-year follow-up data have shown an EWL of 64 % at 5 years after surgery for LRYGB. Studies in the literature are generally in this range.

The marked decrease in operative mortality and morbidity for LRYGB over the past decade is likely multifactorial. Potential contributing factors are listed in Table 3. Mortality after LRYGB has decreased significantly from 1 to 2 % reported a decade ago for open surgery to the most recent reports of databases from centers of excellence programs. The most recent report from the BOLD database showed a mortality of 0.15 % for gastric bypass, both open and laparoscopic, from a database of 81,751 reported RYGB patients with 30-day follow-up [37]. The LABS database showed it to be 0.2 % [38]. Nguyen et al. [39] reported the rate of in-hospital mortality for 23,812 patients undergoing LRYGB at accredited centers of excellence to be 0.06 %.

TABLE 4. Incidence of complications specific to gastric bypass

Anastomotic leak [19]	0.8 %
Hemorrhage [42]	1 %
Marginal ulcer [40]	1–3 %
Internal hernia obstruction [41]	3.8–8.5 %
Stenosis of gastrojejunostomy [43]	1–17 %
Iron deficiency [44, 45]	15–50 %
Vitamin B12 deficiency [44]	11 %

The BSCN database report showed the 30-day complication rate for nearly 15,000 LRYGB cases to be 5.91 % [19]. Bariatric-specific complications listed in that report were all low, generally lower than those reported in single-center reports from the previous decade. This may be largely a factor of the 30-day limit in collecting data on complications. The only complications noted to be above 1 % within the first month were fluid and electrolyte disturbances and stenosis causing obstruction. The most concerning complications which do occur after LRYGB include a 1 % incidence of anastomotic leak (0.78 % in the BSCN database) [19], a 1–2 % incidence of venous thromboembolism, and a less than 1 % incidence of pulmonary embolism. Pulmonary embolism and sepsis are the leading causes of postoperative death after LRYGB. Table 4 gives a summary of major complications seen after LRYGB based on data from the literature. Given the lower overall complication rates that are now being reported in the past 5 years, these numbers may be an overestimation of the incidences of the various complications. Some of them are also derived from reports where open and laparoscopic RYGB were performed.

Although large databases such as the BSCN and the BOLD databases are not as accurate in capturing adverse events and complications after 30 days, the new MBSAQIP database does report the incidence of reoperations for LRYGB for successfully followed patients. For the year 2012, that number was 5.9 % [34].

A few of the complications specific to and common after LRYGB warrant slight further discussion. Anastomotic leaks are the most feared complication after LRYGB, because they can at times present initially with a single unalarming symptom such as tachycardia. A high index of suspicion is always appropriate when a leak is being considered, and operative therapy is the safest option if in doubt in terms of treatment. Operative drainage, repair if possible, and provision of an enteral feeding access are the hallmarks of the operative treatment of an anastomotic leak.

Marginal ulcers have been reported at an incidence between 3 and 15 %, with this wide variability likely based on the degree to which the problem is investigated. Treatment is usually medical, but smoking inhibits ulcer healing rates dramatically [40]. Preoperative smoking is a contraindication for performing LRYGB in some surgeons' practices.

The long-term risk of bowel obstruction appears to be approximately in the 5–7 % range, with at least half of cases being internal hernias. Failure to close mesenteric defects increases the chance of such hernias, but unfortunately doing so does not preclude their occurrence either [41]. It must be emphasized that, due to the risk of internal hernias, a patient who has had a LRYGB and who presents with abdominal pain and signs of a mechanical bowel obstruction *must be emergently evaluated for likely bowel obstruction, and urgent surgery is indicated. Conservative therapy is inappropriate and risks the potential for severe bowel ischemia.* When surgery is performed, the approach is to define the intestinal anatomy retrograde, beginning at the terminal ileum, to allow positive identification of loops of bowel and their relationship. Bowel obstruction is the single most concerning long-term complication after LRYGB.

Postoperative hemorrhage after LRYGB is usually intra-abdominal and of small enough quantity that it is self-limited, with a transfusion incidence of approximately 3–4 %. Hemodynamic instability obviously warrants reoperation, and hematemesis is also an indication for return to the operating room for endoscopic injection of bleeding from the Gastrojejunostomy. Revising the anastomosis is not usually necessary or desirable as a treatment for this complication. Hemorrhage was observed in approximately 1 % of patients in review of a large series of over 4,000 patients undergoing LRYGB [42].

The incidence of anastomotic stenosis is variable and is related to the type of anastomotic stapler used. Circular staplers have a significantly higher risk of postoperative stenosis than do linear staples. Our institutional experience to this effect is given in detail in the chapter on Linear Stapling Technique for Gastrojejunostomy in this book. We observed a decrease in the incidence of stenosis from 17.4 to 1 % with a linear stapling technique. Stenosis at the gastrojejunostomy is amenable to endoscopic balloon dilatation as an effective therapy in most cases [43].

Postoperative nutritional complications after LRYGB are largely based on patient compliance with taking recommended vitamins and vitamin supplements postoperatively. Patients are at risk for iron deficiency after LRYGB. Traditionally there has been a reported incidence of iron deficiency of 20–40 % after gastric bypass. Recent studies have shown between a 15 % [44] and a 50 % [45] incidence of postoperative iron deficiency after RYGB. Vitamin B12 has been noted to be deficient after LRYGB as well, at 11 % in one study [44]. Actual neurologic deficit from B12 deficiency is extremely rare after LRYGB. Vitamin D is low in a high percentage of the population in general—it was deficient in 57 % of patients at baseline in a review by Toh et al. [44]. The incidence is felt to be even higher in the morbidly obese. Thus its routine measurement and supplementation when levels are low is an appropriate guideline. There is no clear evidence that LRYGB worsens the incidence of vitamin D deficiency.

Summary

Outcomes after LRYFB have improved dramatically in the last decade since it became common to perform Roux-en-Y gastric bypass using a laparoscopic approach. Mortality rates have decreased tenfold. Morbidity rates have decreased and are more than halved if one considers the high incidence of incisional hernias and wound problems that are nearly completely eliminated using a laparoscopic approach. LRYGB has shown at least as if not more effectiveness against treating obesity-related medical diseases, with high efficacy for most of those conditions. A number of factors have helped accomplish these achievements, and consistent measurement of outcomes, quality improvement and best practice programs, and centers of excellence systems which now exist are likely to result in potentially even further improvements in the overall delivery of care to patients with severe obesity and related comorbid medical problems.

References

1. NIH conference. Gastrointestinal surgery for severe obesity. Consensus Development Conference Panel. Ann Int Med. 1991; 115:956–61.
2. Ecinosa WE, Bernard DM, Du D, Steiner CA. Recent improvements in bariatric surgery outcomes. Med Care. 2009;47(5): 531–5.
3. Christou NV, Sampalis JS, Liberman M, et al. Surgery decreases long-term mortality, morbidity, and health care use in morbidly obese patients. Ann Surg. 2004;240:416–24.
4. Adams TD, Gress RE, Smith SC, et al. Long-term mortality after gastric bypass surgery. N Engl J Med. 2007;357(8):753–61.
5. Sjostrom L, Narbro K, Sjostrom CD, et al. Effects of bariatric surgery on mortality in Swedish obese subjects. N Engl J Med. 2007;357:741–52.
6. MacDonald Jr KG, Long SD, Swanson MS, et al. The gastric bypass operation reduces the progression and mortality of non-insulin dependent diabetes mellitus. J Gastrointest Surg. 1997;1:213–20.
7. Buchwald H, Avidor Y, Braunwald E, et al. Bariatric surgery. A systematic review and meta-analysis. JAMA. 2004;292:1724–37.
8. Pories WJ, Swanson MS, MacDonald KG, et al. Who would have thought it? An operation proves to be the most effective therapy for adult-onset diabetes. Ann Surg. 1995;222:339–50.
9. Rubino F, Kaplan LM, Schauer PR, Cummings DE. Diabetes Surgery Summit Delegates. The Diabetes Surgery Summit consensus conference: recommendations for the evaluation and use of gastrointestinal surgery to treat type 2 diabetes mellitus. Ann Surg. 2010;25:399–405.
10. DeMaria EJ, Winegar DA, Pate VW, et al. Early postoperative outcomes of metabolic surgery to treat diabetes from sites participating in the ASMBS bariatric surgery center of excellence program as reported in the Bariatric Outcomes Longitudinal Database. Ann Surg. 2010;252:559–66.
11. Mattar SG, Velcu LM, Rabinovitz M, et al. Surgically-induced weight loss significantly improves nonalcoholic fatty liver disease and the metabolic syndrome. Ann Surg. 2005;242:610–20.
12. Kokkinos A, Alexiandou K, Liaskos C, et al. Improvement in cardiovascular indices after Roux-en-Y gastric bypass or sleeve gastrectomy for morbid obesity. Obes Surg. 2013;23:31–8.
13. Michalsky MP, Raman SV, Teich S, et al. Cardiovascular recovery following bariatric surgery in extremely obese adolescents: preliminary results using Cardiac Magnetic Resonance (CMR) imaging. J Pediatr Surg. 2013;48:170–7.
14. Hewitt S, Humerfelt S, Sovik TT, et al. Long-term improvements in pulmonary function 5 years after bariatric surgery. Obes Surg. 2014;24:705–11.
15. Nguyen NT, Hinojosa MW, Smith BR, et al. Improvements of restrictive and obstructive pulmonary mechanics following laparoscopic bariatric surgery. Surg Endosc. 2009;23:808–12.
16. Hallowell PT, Stellato TA, Schuster M, et al. Potentially life-threatening sleep apnea is unrecognized without aggressive evaluation. Am J Surg. 2007;193:364–7.
17. Marti-Valeri C, Sabate A, Masdevall C, Dalmau A. Improvement of associated respiratory problems in morbidly obese patients after open Roux-en-Y gastric bypass. Obes Surg. 2007;17:1102–10.
18. Lettieri CJ, Eliasson AH, Greenburg DL. Persistence of obstructive sleep apnea after surgical weight loss. J Clin Sleep Med. 2008;15:33–40.
19. Hutter MM. First report from the American College of Surgeons Bariatric Surgery Center Network: laparoscopic sleeve gastrectomy has morbidity and effectiveness positioned between the band and the bypass. Ann Surg. 2011;254:410–20.
20. American College of Surgeons. National Surgery Quality Improvement Program. Accessed April 2014
21. Frezza EE, et al. Symptomatic improvement in gastroesophageal reflux disease (GERD) following laparoscopic Roux-en-Y gastric bypass. Surg Endosc. 2002;16:1027–31.
22. Madolosso CAS, Gurski RR, Callegari-Jacques SM, et al. The impact of gastric bypass on gastroesophageal reflux disease in patients with morbid obesity. Ann Surg. 2010;251:244–8.
23. Sugerman HJ, Sugerman EL, Wolfe L, et al. Risks and benefits of gastric bypass in morbidly obese patients with severe venous stasis disease. Ann Surg. 2001;234:41–6.
24. Jamal MK, DeMaria EJ, Johnson JM, et al. Impact of major comorbidities on mortality and complications after gastric bypass. Surg Obes Relat Dis. 2005;1:511–6.
25. Sugerman HJ. Comment on: correlations between intra-abdominal pressure and obesity-related co-morbidities. Surg Obes Relat Dis. 2009;5:528–9.
26. Coleman KJ, Huang YC, Koebnick C, et al. Metabolic syndrome is less likely to resolve in Hispanics and non-Hispanic blacks after bariatric surgery. Ann Surg. 2014;259:279–85.
27. Fenske WK, Dubb S, Bueter M, et al. Effect of bariatric surgery-induced weight loss on renal and systemic inflammation and blood pressure: a 12-month prospective study. Surg Obes Relat Dis. 2013;9:559–68.
28. Schauer PR, Ikrammudin S, Gourash W, et al. Outcomes after laparoscopic Roux-en-Y gastric bypass for morbid obesity. Ann Surg. 2000;232:515–29.
29. Nguyen NT, Goldman C, Rosanquist CJ, et al. Laparoscopic versus open gastric bypass: a randomized study of outcomes, quality of life, and costs. Ann Surg. 2001;234:279–91.
30. Flum DR, Salem L, Elrod JA, et al. Early mortality among medicare beneficiaries undergoing bariatric surgical procedures. JAMA. 2005;294:1903–8.
31. DeMaria EJ, Portenier D, Wolfe L. Obesity surgery mortality risk score: proposal for a clinically useful score to predict mortality risk in patients undergoing gastric bypass. Surg Obes Relat Dis. 2007;3:134–40.
32. Pratt GM, Learn CA, Hughes GD, et al. Demographics and outcomes at American Society for Metabolic and Bariatric Surgery Centers of Excellence. Surg Endosc. 2009;23:795–9.
33. Buchwald H, Estok R, Fahrbach K, et al. Weight and type 2 diabetes after bariatric surgery: systematic review and meta-analysis. Am J Med. 2009;122:248–56.

34. Metabolic and Bariatric Surgery. Accreditation and Quality Assurance Program Database. Accessed April 2014

35. Schauer PR, Batt DL, Kirwan JP, et al. Bariatric surgery versus intensive medical therapy for diabetes—3 year outcomes. N Engl J Med. 2014;370:2002–13.

36. Ikramuddin S, Korner J, Lee WJ, et al. Roux-en-Y gastric bypass versus intensive medical management for the control of type 2 diabetes, hypertension, and hyperlipidemia: the Diabetes Surgery Study randomized clinical trial. JAMA. 2013;309:2240–9.

37. Benotti P, Wood CG, Winegar D, et al. Risk factors associated with mortality after Roux-en-Y gastric bypass surgery. Ann Surg. 2014;259:123–30.

38. Flum DR, Belle SH, King WC, Longitudinal Assessment of Bariatric Surgery (LABS) Consortium, et al. Perioperative safety in the longitudinal assessment of bariatric surgery. N Engl J Med. 2009;361:445–54.

39. Nguyen NT, Masoomi H, Laugenour K, et al. Predictive factors of mortality in bariatric surgery: data from the nationwide inpatient sample. Surgery. 2011;150:347–51.

40. Moon RC, Texeira AF, Goldbach M, Jawad MA. Management and treatment outcomes of marginal ulcers after Roux-en-Y gastric bypass at a single high volume bariatric center. Surg Obes Relat Dis. 2014;10:229–34.

41. Obeid A, McNeal S, Breland M, et al. Internal hernia after laparoscopic Roux-en-Y gastric bypass. J Gastrointest Surg. 2014;18:250–5.

42. Heneghan HM, Meron-Edlar S, Yenumula P, et al. Incidence and management of bleeding complications after gastric bypass surgery in morbidly obese. Surg Obes Relat Dis. 2012;8:729–35.

43. Schirmer B, Erenoglu C, Miller A. Flexible endoscopy in the management of patients undergoing Roux-en-Y gastric bypass. Obes Surg. 2002;12:634–8.

44. Toh SY, Zarshenas N, Jorgensen J. Prevalence of nutrient deficiencies in bariatric patients. Nutrition. 2009;25:1150–6.

45. Obinwanne KM, Frederickson KA, Mathiason MA, et al. Incidence, treatment, and outcomes of iron deficiency after laparoscopic Roux-en-Y gastric bypass: a 10-year analysis. J Am Coll Surg. 2014;246–52.

29

Laparoscopic Gastric Bypass: Management of Complications

Emanuele Lo Menzo, Samuel Szomstein, and Raul J. Rosenthal

Introduction

Roux-en-Y gastric bypass (RYGB) remains the gold standard for surgical weight loss, constituting over half of the procedure performed. In fact, the number of RYGBs increased by 125 % from 2004 to 2007 in US academic centers [1]. Also, the approach to gastric bypass changed overtime with currently an excess of 85 % of gastric bypasses performed laparoscopically. The extensive number of procedures performed via the laparoscopic approach as well as the implementation quality improvement initiatives has contributed to increase the safety and has improved outcomes. Nevertheless, several complications are still commonly encountered after RYGB, not only by the bariatric surgeon, but also by the general surgeon, gastroenterologist, and primary care provider.

This chapter will review some of the most common complications encountered after gastric bypass surgery, with complications divided into intraoperative and postoperative.

Intraoperative

The intraoperative complications include technical problems such as bleeding, staple misfiring, positive air leak test, and nontechnical and anesthesia complications such as myocardial infarction, deep vein thrombosis, arrhythmias, allergic reactions, peripheral neuropathies, and rhabdomyolysis (Table 1).

Electronic supplementary material: Supplementary material is available in the online version of this chapter at 10.1007/978-1-4939-1637-5_29. Videos can also be accessed at http://www.springerimages.com/videos/978-1-4939-1636-8.

Technical

Staple Misfiring

Not accounting for the manufacturing defects of the actual stapling device, the rest of the staple line misfiring is due to incorrect choices or inappropriate use of the device itself. The key elements in avoiding these problems are adequate choice of cartridge staple heights (especially if buttressing material is used), avoidance of bunched up tissue within the jaws of the stapler, careful evaluation of the crossing of staple lines, and appropriate tissue compression time. In general, all the staple lines should be carefully evaluated, and when in doubt, redo stapling or oversewing should be implemented.

Positive Air Leak Test

Intraoperative air leak test of the Gastrojejunal anastomosis is currently considered the standard of care during gastric bypass surgery. The different types of leak test include pneumatic (either by gastric tube or endoscope) or blue dye (usually methylene blue).

As previously described by others, the reproducible air leak is the one that requires intervention [2]. If the actual location of the air leak is clearly recognized, suture closure with adjuncts of omental patch or fibrin glues or sealants is acceptable. However, if the site is not clearly identifiable, or the former intervention is ineffective, redoing the anastomosis is mandatory. Furthermore, drainage of the area should be considered even by surgeons who do not routinely drain anastomosis. Under these circumstances the need for remnant gastrostomy tube should be individualized, and it should be

Table 1. Intraoperative complications of RYGB

Technical
Bleeding
Staple misfire
Positive air leak test
Anesthesia/medically related complications
Peripheral neuropathy
Rhabdomyolysis
Venous thromboembolism
Cardiac arrhythmias, CAD
Hypertensive crisis
Hypoxia, hypercarbia
Malignant hyperthermia
Allergic reaction

considered in the reoperative cases. Also, it is the authors' strong belief that a postoperative upper gastrointestinal (GI) study is beneficial in this scenario both from a clinical and medical legal standpoint.

Anesthesia/Medically Related Complications

Peripheral Neuropathies

Most of these perioperative peripheral neuropathies are due to traction or compression injuries at the time of patient positioning in the operative table. The most common locations are the brachial plexus (overextension of the arms on the arm boards), ulnar neuropathy (from compression at the elbow), and lower extremities neuropathy. The main symptom is usually paresthesia. The mechanism of nerve injury is usually neuropraxia, due to the injury to the endoneurial capillaries with resulting edema and conduction block. Since there is no degeneration of the axon, the return of sensation is rapid and usually complete within 1 week or less. When the trauma is more significant and causes segmental demyelinization, the functional recovery occurs within few months.

A rare but typical peripheral neuropathy is meralgia paresthetica [3]. This is caused by the compression of the lateral cutaneous nerve against the inguinal ligament. Symptoms vary from hypersensitivity and paresthesia to pain in the lateral anterior aspect of the thigh. This typically occurs after laparoscopic procedures and tends to resolve spontaneously with conservative treatment. Occasionally a local nerve block may be helpful in reducing symptoms.

Rhabdomyolysis (RML)

Rhabdomyolysis is a syndrome caused by injury to the skeletal muscle. In most cases the pathogenesis is due to ischemia-reperfusion syndrome causing sarcolemmal damage of the skeletal muscle and resulting in the release of proteins and renal tubules damage. Besides the well-known acute renal insufficiency, RML can cause severe hyperkalemia, hypocalcemia, compartment syndrome, disseminated intravascular coagulation, cardiac arrhythmias, and even death. Its incidence has been reported between 12.9 and 37.8 % [4]. Contributing risk factors for the development of RML are male gender, higher BMI (>50 kg/m^2), current therapy with statins, operative time >4 h, and the use of propofol injection. Propofol infusion syndrome is very rare, but it is more frequent in obese patients due to the lipophilic characteristics of the drug. Careful padding of all pressure points, early patient mobilization, and reduction of operating room time can contribute to the prevention of this syndrome. The diagnosis is both clinical and biochemical (increased CPK levels five times higher than the normal and the presence of myoglobin in the urine). The treatment is mostly supportive with aggressive fluid resuscitation, correction of electrolytes abnormalities, and, in some cases, alkalinization of the urine.

Other common early complications related to anesthesia and the medical aspects of obesity, such as cardiac complications, venous thromboembolic events, hypoxia/hypercarbia, hyperglycemia, and hypertensive crisis, are outside the scope of this chapter and will be addressed elsewhere.

Postoperative

The postoperative complications of gastric bypass surgery can be divided into acute (7 days), early (7 days–6 weeks), late (6–12 weeks), and chronic (>12 weeks).

Acute (7 Days) and Early (7 Days–6 Weeks)

Leaks

Leaks remain the second leading cause of death after RYGB surgery. Potential sites of leaks include the Gastrojejunal anastomosis, gastric pouch, gastric remnant, the jejunal blind end, and the Jejunojejunal anastomosis. Approximately 70–80 % of the leaks occur at the Gastrojejunal anastomosis, 10–15 % at the gastric pouch, 5 % at the Jejunojejunal anastomosis, and 3–5 % at the excluded stomach. Factors involved in the development of these leaks include tension, ischemia, and staple misfiring. Different techniques have been described for the Gastrojejunal anastomosis using a circular stapler, linear stapler (with stapled or hand-sewn closure of the anterior wall), and completely hand sewn. The available data comparing the techniques has never been able to convincingly show the difference in leak rates of the three techniques. A recent collaborative study showed an increased incidence of hemorrhage and wound infection with the circular stapled technique [5]. The other variable potentially involved in the degree of tension on the anastomosis is the route of the Roux limb. Although it is true that the retrocolic-retrogastric route is the shortest one, leak rates between this technique and the antecolic-antegastric one have not been definitively proven to be different. Only one study was able to demonstrate a significant difference with higher leak rates of the antecolic (3 %) versus the retrocolic (0.5 %) [6]. Some of the risk factors associated with higher incidence of leaks include male gender, super morbid obesity, age >55 years, and revisional procedures [6].

Unquestionably, an early diagnosis and treatment significantly affects the patient outcome, not only in terms of hospital, and in particular ICU stay, but also in terms of survival. It is then important to have a degree of suspicion, even when the workup remains negative. Common, but not uniformly present, signs and symptoms of leak include sustained tachycardia, abdominal pain, fever, nausea and vomiting, oliguria, hemodynamic instability, and sense of impending doom. The diagnosis can be obtained or confirmed by radiographic modalities such as contrast upper gastrointestinal fluoroscopic evaluation (UGI) or CT scan. Although the specificity of the UGI is very high for GJ leaks, its sensitivity is only in the 20 % range [7]. CT scan adds sensitivity to the diagnosis of GJ leaks because of the ability to show not only contrast extravasation and extraluminal collections but also indirect signs of leak, such as surrounding inflammatory changes, intra-abdominal free air, and left pleural effusion. Also, the CT scan is able to show additional sites of potential leaks, such as the gastric remnant, JJ anastomosis, gastric remnant distention, etc. Occasionally, the diagnosis of leak is made by the character of the fluid obtained from the intraoperative drain. In these circumstances a specific, but not sensitive, adjunct diagnostic modality is the use of oral dye, such as methylene blue.

The goals of treatment are antibiotic treatment, bowel rest, control of secretions, wide drainage, and early nutrition. Although the standard means of obtaining these goals is by operative intervention, the hemodynamic status of the patient and the time of occurrence of the leak might dictate a nonoperative approach. During the operative approach, the key steps include extensive irrigation; repair of the leak, if feasible and safe; placement of enteral access distal to the leak site; and extensive closed suction drain placement. Based on the surgeon's individual skills and experience, these steps can be either accomplished laparoscopically or via an open approach. Whenever the patient's hemodynamic status allows, the local sepsis control can be accomplished via percutaneous drainage or with the drains previously placed at the time of surgery. It is important in these cases to continue to monitor symptom progression, as failure of nonoperative treatment has been reported in 12 % of the cases [7]. Regardless of the approach utilized, the mortality of a leak remains high (10 %) [8].

TABLE 2. Etiology of gastrogastric fistulae. Modified frovm R. Rosenthal et al. [10]

Iatrogenic
Previous anastomotic leaks
Type of operation
Gastric tissue migration
Marginal ulcer and perforation
Foreign body erosion

Gastrogastric (GG) Fistula

Gastrogastric fistula (GGF) refers to an abnormal communication between the excluded gastric pouch and the gastric remnant. The incidence of GGF varies between 0 and 46 % in the literature [9]. In our own experience, the incidence has been 1.2 % [10]. Overall the incidence of GGF, similar to other complications after gastric bypass, has been steadily decreasing. Reasons for the dramatic reduction include better instrumentation, improved techniques, and increased experience among surgeons performing these procedures.

Common presenting symptoms include nausea, vomiting, and epigastric pain, which are present in approximately 80 % of patients. Up to 53 % of patients will have a marginal ulcer or a complication of it (bleeding, perforation) as presenting symptoms. Another subset of patients will present with failure of weight loss or weight regain. The latter category of patients, upon further questioning, always report some element of nausea or vomiting, epigastric pain, or a history of marginal ulcers.

The time of onset and location of GGF vary significantly depending on etiology (Table 2). In fact, GGF can be classified into 6 categories based on their etiology [11], including the following:

1. *Iatrogenic*. This is the result of a technical error and omission of completely dividing the gastric pouch from the gastric remnant. They typically occur near the gastroesophageal junction, where the angle of His could be difficult to visualize, especially in larger male patients.
2. *Previous leaks at the Gastrojejunal anastomosis*. This is the result of a contained or subclinical leak treated nonoperatively. Consequently, the inflammatory cavity can eventually erode into the gastric remnant. Due to the etiology of this particular complication, the fistulae are located at the level of the Gastrojejunal anastomosis.
3. *Type of operation*. This type of fistula is now rarely seen since the accepted method of gastric pouch creation is complete division of the gastric pouch from the remnant.
4. *Gastric tissue migration*. In this case gastric tissue will migrate and reattach to the remnant, even in the absence of an inflammatory process. This is shown to be the case even when interposed omentum or jejunum is being utilized as a barrier.
5. *Marginal ulceration and perforation*. The presence of a deep ulcer will result in tissue injury and ischemia.

This, in addition to potential migration of foreign bodies such as staples, might create a path for passage of cells in both directions, which eventually will lead to a communication between the pouch and the excluded stomach.

6. *Foreign body erosion*. This type of GGF might occur in patients who had, at the time of their primary bypass, placement of a ring to prevent anastomotic dilatation. Over time the ring can erode in the pouch and/or in the adjacent gastric remnant.

The diagnosis of GGF is usually based on symptoms and confirmed either by endoscopy or upper GI study. The upper endoscopy is unfortunately positive in approximately half of the patients. The most sensitive test, however, remains the upper GI study. This is commonly performed in different patient's positions, including decubitus. Additional information can also be obtained by an abdominal CT scan, such as gastric remnant distention with gas and contrast.

The initial treatment is medical and consists of protein pump inhibitors, with the addition of sucralfate in case of a documented concomitant ulcer. The aim of the treatment is to reduce the acid production in the gastric remnant, which is now enhanced by the presence of food. In the presence of a marginal ulcer responding to medical therapy and in the absence of additional symptoms, observation and reevaluation in 6 weeks is acceptable. The minority of patients that do not respond adequately to medical treatment and present with weight regain or failure of weight loss will require additional interventions. Some authors advocate endoscopy as a first-line therapeutic intervention, claiming no increased complication if a future revisional surgery is necessary [12]. Unfortunately, although often technically feasible, endoscopic closure has a very high recurrence rate. The success rate is inversely proportional to the diameter of the fistula itself. Fistulae larger than 1 cm have a much less chance of remaining closed after endoscopic treatment. Endoscopic techniques include injection or fibrin glue, plasma coagulation, clipping, stenting, and various endoscopic suturing techniques.

A much more effective treatment, although more invasive, is surgical intervention. The type of approach is dictated by the type of fistula. It is important to not only address the anatomic abnormality but also to understand the physiologic derangement, if any, that led to the fistula in the first place. In the case of acid hypersecretion and chronic marginal ulcer, pouch trimming and redo Gastrojejunostomy are fundamental. In the case of refractory marginal ulcer with proven acid hypersecretion in the pouch, a truncal vagotomy might be added. Remnant gastrectomy has also been advocated by our group as a treatment option for GGF [12]. In the cases of fistulae related to the failure of separation of the remnant from the gastric pouch, simple stapling across the previously undivided gastric bridge will be appropriate. This is especially true when the fistula is not in proximity of the Gastrojejunal anastomosis. A thorough knowledge of the anatomy of the previous gastric bypass, as well as a review of the previous operative reports, helps in strategizing the surgical approach. Whenever Gastrojejunal anastomosis resection has to be carried out, it is important to have information about the length of the Roux limb and its location in relationship to the stomach and colon. In fact, resecting the pouch and the anastomosis without having enough Roux limb length to achieve a tension-free new anastomosis will require revision of the Jejunojejunostomy to a more distal position as well. It is then important to have a thorough preoperative evaluation both by EGD and upper GI study to acquire as much information as possible concerning the gastric pouch size, the anastomotic status, and the Roux limb length.

Postoperative Hemorrhage

Postoperative hemorrhage has been reported in 1.9–4.4 % of gastric bypass procedures [13]. The bleeding could be either intraluminal or extraluminal, and it usually originates from the staple lines of the GJ or JJ anastomosis, gastric remnant, or gastric pouch. Although some mostly retrospective studies showed decreased incidence of postoperative bleeding with staple line reinforcement, a recent meta-analysis of three randomized trials reports no difference in bleeding episodes [14]. It is important to use standardized postoperative protocols to avoid system errors and automatic DVT prophylaxis anticoagulation administration before a full patient assessment. The signs and symptoms vary based on the entity of the bleeding from mild tachycardia to signs of hypovolemic shock with hypotension and oliguria. It is important to remember that intraluminal bleeding can also determine intestinal obstruction and devastating complications (anastomotic leak, gastric remnant perforation) even if the bleeding is self-limiting. Whenever intestinal obstruction is suspected, imaging studies with upper GI contrast study and CT scan are warranted. Although most of the immediate postoperative hemorrhages are self-limiting and can be managed with blood product transfusion, stopping anticoagulation, and aggressively correcting coagulation derangements, the presence of hemodynamic instability or the continuous requirement of blood transfusion is an indication for immediate intervention. In the early postoperative period, the role of endoscopy for the evaluation of intraluminal bleeding is limited to the evaluation and potential treatment of the Gastrojejunal anastomosis. More aggressive endoscopic procedures (enteroscopy and double-balloon enteroscopy) to evaluate Jejunojejunostomy and gastric remnant should be reserved for late postoperative bleeding. Whenever endoscopic intervention is not feasible or appropriate, operative intervention should not be delayed. The hemodynamic status of the patient along with the surgeon's comfort level will determine if a laparoscopic or laparotomic approach is chosen. Often the intra-abdominal source of bleeding is not found, but hematoma evacuation and washout expedites the patient's recovery. In the presence of an intraluminal bleeding source, the affected anastomosis can be approached directly or intraluminally via an adjacent enterotomy.

Small Bowel Obstruction

Although small bowel obstruction can occur at anytime after gastric bypass, up to 48 % occur within the first month [15]. Based on the location the obstruction can be classified into the following: type A, when the alimentary limb is affected; type B, when the biliopancreatic limb is obstructed; and type C, common channel obstruction [13].

Early postoperative obstruction can further be divided into mechanical or functional.

Mechanical

Common sites of mechanical obstruction are the Gastrojejunostomy, the Jejunojejunostomy, the mesenteric defects, and the port sites.

Stenosis at the anastomotic site is usually due to postoperative edema and tends to resolve in 24–48 h. It is important to avoid vomiting and retching during this phase in order to prevent aspiration and anastomotic disruption. Antiemetics, inhibitors of acid secretions, and possible tube decompression, with nasogastric tubes carefully placed under fluoroscopic guidance, are helpful in the expectant management of these patients. This is especially true if a non-complete obstruction is present. In cases of complete obstruction or whenever the clinical picture does not improve, technical issues are involved and anastomotic revision is necessary. Intraluminal clots from recent staple line bleeding have also been described as a cause of early mechanical obstruction.

Radiographic evaluation is essential in the diagnosis. It is important to evaluate not only the site of obstruction but also the status of the proximal bowel or stomach. In fact, certain obstructions can determine a closed loop obstruction picture and cause gastric remnant perforation. The presence of gastric remnant distention has to be carefully evaluated, and it can be the only apparent sign of a distal obstruction. The intervention varies based on the type and degree of distention. Purely air-filled remnant without any bowel dilatation can be observed with sequential X-rays, as long as the patient is asymptomatic. Most of the time this finding is related to a transient "vagal stunning" and it is self-limited. Metoclopramide can be utilized with variable results in this case, as long as distal obstruction has been ruled out. If the patient is symptomatic, left shoulder pain, hiccups, retching, or percutaneous or operative decompression is in order. Whenever the gastric remnant is fluid filled, the most likely cause is the presence of a distal obstruction. Early intervention is usually recommended in this case. Percutaneous decompression is not advised because it will not resolve the distal obstruction, and the intraluminal fluid will likely leak around the insertion site, as this is typically not buttressed against the abdominal wall. Acute Gastrojejunostomy strictures are rare and they are mostly related to technical errors. The initial treatment is observation to allow edema resolution. If after a reasonable waiting period (4–5 days) there is no improvement, endoscopic dilatation or redo anastomosis is indicated. Early endoscopic dilatation might be necessary but has to be conservative in the immediate postoperative period. There is no data to establish when it is too early to perform endoscopic dilatation. Our group has safely performed endoscopic dilatation as early as 7 days postoperatively [16]. Usually the patient can then be kept on a mostly liquid diet until 4–6 weeks after surgery and be submitted to a more aggressive and safer endoscopic dilatation. Early strictures (7 days–6 weeks) are usually ischemic in origin or due to foreign bodies (suture or staples extrusion) or marginal ulcers.

Internal hernias can cause mechanical obstruction in the early/acute phase, or more likely, late/chronic after the visceral fat diminishes as a result of effective weight loss. They are the most common cause of bowel obstruction after laparoscopic RYGB. Their incidence has been reported in up to 9 % of the cases. The potential mesenteric spaces through which internal hernias occur vary based on the configuration of the bypass reconstruction. Typically after retrocolic-retrogastric bypass, three defects are present, including transverse mesocolon, Petersen's (between the Roux limb and the transverse mesocolon), and mesenteric defect at the Jejunojejunostomy. One of the advantages claimed by the proponents of the antecolic-antegastric reconstruction technique is the decreased incidence of internal hernias, as a mesocolic defect is not created. Although it is widely accepted to close some or all of the defects with nonabsorbable sutures, other authors report similar incidence of hernias without any closure. Other important factors that likely affect the incidence of internal hernias are the division of the mesentery, the length of the limbs, and the orientation of the Jejunojejunostomy. In fact, some authors have suggested that the counterclockwise rotation of the Roux limb reconstruction causes fewer internal hernias (in particular at the Petersen's space) than the clockwise rotation [17].

If the ability to perform gastric bypass laparoscopically has significantly decreased the incidence of wound infection and hernias, it has opened the possibility for potential acute postoperative port site hernias with obstruction. The reported incidence of port site hernias is 0.74 % for all laparoscopic procedures and 0.57 % after bariatric surgery [18]. Current recommendations call for closure of trocars >10 mm in diameter. However, in obese patients, 12 mm ports from radially dilating non-bladed trocars, especially if off the midline, are not routinely closed, based on level II data. Port site hernias are often difficult to diagnose simply by physical exam because of the patient body habitus and the common presence of port site tenderness and occasional seromas.

A liberal use of CT scan can reliably identify the condition, which requires prompt re-exploration.

Also, reconstruction configuration errors (Roux-en-O) determine mechanical obstruction. This type of configuration error occurs when the biliopancreatic limb is mistakenly anastomosed to the gastric pouch. The typical presentation includes abdominal pain, nausea, bilious vomiting, and rapid weight loss. Although sometimes the clinical presentation is quite dramatic with a picture of proximal small bowel obstruction, at times all the diagnostic modalities (contrast upper GI and CT scan) can be normal. Additional radiographic studies that can assist in the diagnosis are fluoroscopic examination with contrast directly injected in the gastric remnant (when access via a gastrostomy tube if preset) and hepatobiliary iminodiacetic acid scan (HIDA). The latter test can unequivocally show the radionuclide excreted in the duodenum reflux back into the gastric pouch and esophagus.

Functional

Besides the mild generalized ileus that can be encountered after laparoscopy, the majority of functional obstructions occur at the level of the gastric remnant. The severity varies from just mild dilatation of the remnant in an asymptomatic patient to impending remnant perforation with nausea, hiccups, shoulder pain, and secondary vomiting. Most of the cases are self-limiting and are due to the previously mentioned "vagal stunning." In these cases, medical treatment with metoclopramide and close observation with follow-up imaging are sufficient. In the cases of symptomatic remnant distention, percutaneous or operative drainage is mandatory. As previously mentioned, the drainage method has to be dictated by the clinical scenario and the imaging findings.

Late (6–12 Weeks) and Chronic (>12 Weeks)

Late complications after gastric bypass could be secondary to surgical or anatomical abnormalities or secondary to nutritional or metabolic derangements.

Surgical or Anatomical

Internal Hernias (IH)

As previously reviewed, internal hernia can occur at any stage postoperatively. Although the etiology of the late types remains unclear, speculations exist on the role of loss of intra-abdominal fat after weight loss surgery. Interestingly, IH are reported by both authors who close mesenteric defects, as well as those who do not [19]. The incidence of IH is clearly greater after laparoscopic gastric bypass than open, likely secondary to the paucity of intra-abdominal adhesions after the former approach. The symptoms can be those of a typical bowel obstruction or more subtle of intermittent crampy abdominal pain episodes. The imaging study of choice is the CT scan, which often reveals evidence of partial bowel obstruction and more direct signs of IH (swirl sign of the mesentery, malposition of the Jejunojejunostomy either supramesocolic or to the right of the midline). Imaging studies could be normal in up to 30 % of cases, which is probably due to the intermittent nature of the herniation. Whenever enough clinical suspicion exists, diagnostic exploration should not be delayed even in the presence of negative preoperative imaging evaluation. In fact, the potential consequences of a missed internal hernia with volvulus around the SMA and potential central mesenteric ischemia are catastrophic. During the exploration, especially if done laparoscopically, even if the site of IH herniation is apparent, the direction of the volvulus might not be. The safest approach is to run the small bowel retrograde from the terminal ileum, in order to sort out the orientation of the mesentery and derotating the volvulus. In the presence of permanent vascular impairment of the small bowel, prompt conversion to open and appropriate resection is indicated. After reduction of the hernia is reduced, the mesenteric defects should be closed with permanent sutures.

Marginal Ulcers (MU), Stricture

Marginal ulcers and stricture are analyzed together due to the frequent coexistence and similar etiology. The incidence of marginal ulceration has been reported between 1 and 16 %, whereas the incidence of strictures has been estimated in up to 27 % [20]. Several factors have been associated with their pathogenesis, including ischemia, acid exposure, foreign body at the anastomotic site, medications, and tobacco. Acid hypersecretion could either be primary or secondary to a GGF, as previously mentioned. The technique utilized to construct the anastomosis might play a role in the incidence of stricture. Some evidence exists that an anastomosis done with a circular stapler has a higher incidence of stricture. The antecolic-antegastric route of the Roux limb has been suggested to create more tension and tissue ischemia, but has never definitely been proven to affect the incidence of MU or stricture. The use of absorbable sutures at the anastomosis decreases the incidence of both MU and strictures compared to permanent ones.

In general, conflicting evidence exists on the role of drugs—such as nonsteroidal anti-inflammatory agents, steroids, and tobacco—on the pathogenesis of MU. Even though the direct association between *Helicobacter pylori* and MU is controversial, the number and severity of complications of MU in patients *Helicobacter pylori* negative or with eradicated infection is significantly inferior.

The treatment of MU is primarily medical with acid suppression with protein pump inhibitors combined with cytoprotective agents (sucralfate). Approximately one third of the patients will require surgical intervention either because of intractability or complications (i.e., bleeding, perforation, or stricture) of MU. The type of procedure is dictated by the indication. In general, the bleeding should be treated endoscopically, and in case of failure or recurrence, oversewing the ulcer bed is the treatment of choice. In cases of hemodynamic stability, Gastrojejunal resection with reanastomosis ± vagotomy might play a role. Perforations are usually treated with Graham patch alone, or primary closure with omental patch, and only rarely anastomotic resection with new anastomosis is feasible or indicated. Anastomotic strictures are largely managed by endoscopic dilatation (either using through-the-scope balloon dilators or bougie dilators) with a high success rate. The need for surgical revision has been reported in less than 1 % of cases [20].

Intussusception

Intussusception is a much more rare cause of mechanical obstruction after gastric bypass. Its reported incidence is between 0.07 and 0.15 %, and it seems to occur with equal frequency after open and laparoscopic approach. Intussusception more frequently occurs in women after significant weight loss. Almost invariably the site of intussusception is around the Jejunojejunal anastomosis, and no lead points are usually identified. Its pathogenesis remains unclear, and both functional and mechanical causes have been advocated. Among the functional ones, Ver Steeg et al. speculated that the presence of a new ectopic pacemaker focus in the Roux limb combined with the natural duodenal pacer determines a very high-amplitude wave that predisposes to intussusception [4]. Mechanical factors that have been proposed in the etiopathogenesis of intussusception are adhesions, focal inflammation, suture line of the Jejunostomy, long mesentery, and sudden increase of intra-abdominal pressure. The clinical presentation can be acute with intermittent abdominal pain, vomiting, occasional bloody bowel movements, or chronic with spontaneous reduction and relapsing crampy abdominal pain.

Physical examination is often normal, and the diagnosis is mostly based on the patients' history and symptoms. Imaging studies can confirm the clinical suspicion, but can be unrevealing. The most reliable imaging study is the CT scan with oral contrast with the typical "target" sign, but its accuracy is only 80 % [6].

As is the case for other causes of bowel obstruction after gastric bypass, the intervention is almost invariably surgical and it should be expeditious in order to avoid disastrous consequences. Nasogastric decompression has to be used cautiously as it can lead to perforation at the Gastrojejunostomy as well as a false sense of decompression. In fact, even if the Roux limb can be temporarily decompressed, the biliopancreatic limb and gastric remnant do not improve with such intervention.

As far as the preferred surgical approach, the surgeon's experience and comfort level should dictate if the surgery is laparoscopic or open. If the laparoscopic approach is chosen, prompt conversion to open laparotomy is necessary in the presence of vascular compromised bowel, or in case of massive bowel dilatation that prevents adequate visualization. The goals of surgery include reduction of the intussusception and inspection of the viability of the intussusceptum and prevention of recurrence. No consensus exists on how to decrease recurrences. If no additional procedures are done, the chance of recurrence is nearly 100 %, whereas plication of the common channel to the biliopancreatic limb and resection and reconstruction of the Jejunostomy decrease the recurrence rates to 40 % and 12 %, respectively.

Associated Pathologies (Nephrolithiasis, Cholelithiasis, Adhesions)

Abdominal pain after gastric bypass could be attributed to many different factors. Besides the aforementioned causes, nephrolithiasis, cholelithiasis, and adhesions can cause varied degree of abdominal pain.

Several studies have reported an increased incidence of nephrolithiasis after RYGB (7 %). Although the pathogenesis is not entirely understood, it has been demonstrated that post-gastric bypass patients present with hyperoxaluria from increased intestinal absorption. This phenomenon seems to be related to the preferred binding of intestinal calcium to higher-level fatty acid than to oxalate, which will leave free oxalate available for reabsorption.

It is well known that rapid weight loss from malabsorptive procedures facilitates formation of gallstones. The mechanism of increased risk of cholelithiasis remains unclear. Several potential reasons have been postulated. Rapid weight loss can determine an increased cholesterol excretion in the bile, resulting in an imbalance among its components determining lithogenic bile. There is also evidence that the increased gallbladder secretion of mucin, prostaglandins, and arachidonic acid seen in these patients could contribute to gallstone formation. Of the patients who develop gallstones after gastric bypass, only 7–16 % became symptomatic enough to require surgical intervention. It is important, however, to promptly recognize and treat this small percentage of patients in order to avoid the complications of gallstone disease. This is particularly true because of the more difficult endoscopic access to the biliary tree after gastric bypass. Although the use of ursodeoxycholic acid has shown reduction of gallstone formation after gastric bypass, this is not accepted as a standard practice, and prophylactic cholecystectomy at the time of gastric bypass in asymptomatic patients with gallstones is no longer advocated.

Nutritional or Metabolic

Nutritional and metabolic consequences after gastric bypass, such as anemia, vitamin deficiencies, and macronutrients and micronutrients malnutrition, are outside the scope of this chapter and will be discussed in Chap. 31. Nevertheless, the hypoglycemic syndrome is an increasingly reported nutritional complication after gastric bypass, and it is worth discussing in this chapter.

Hypoglycemic Syndrome

The presence of postprandial hypoglycemic episodes after gastric bypass has been described with an increased frequency. Based on its distinction from insulinomas and its hyperinsulinemic pathogenesis, the suggested name for this condition is noninsulinoma pancreatogenous hypoglycemic syndrome (NIPHS). Histologically, patients exhibit diffuse β-cell hyperplasia along with diffuse hypertrophy of islet cells. In addition to the classic Whipple's triad of insulinomas, NIPHS classically presents with postprandial neuroglycopenic episodes, negative 72-h fasting test, lack of imaging evidence of pancreatic lesions, and positive arterial calcium stimulation test. These patients should be distinguished from the reactive hypoglycemia secondary to dumping syndrome, as the former group presents neuroglycopenic episodes and lacks additional gastrointestinal symptoms.

Among the etiologic factors, a rapid progression of carbohydrates into the small intestine might play a role, and in fact, this condition has been described in post-vagotomy patients who did not have RYGB. Also, a postoperative increase in GLP-1 has been advocated as a pathogenetic factor. Dietary modifications (carbohydrate restriction) are usually ineffective, contrary to cases of late dumping syndrome. Medical suppression of insulin secretion (diazoxide, octreotide), α-glucosidase inhibitors (acarbose), and calcium channel blocker (verapamil) have limited efficacy. Currently the most effective treatment is partial pancreatectomy. The extent of the pancreatectomy, however, is controversial. It seems that more conservative resections carry a higher chance of persistent hypoglycemia, whereas the more extensive the resection, the higher the likelihood of diabetes. Regardless of the extent of the resection, a significant percentage of patients will have recurrent symptoms, but can be managed medically.

Conclusion

The increased experience with gastric bypass and the more widely accepted implementation of the laparoscopic technique have determined a significant reduction of complications. However, gastric bypass remains a complex procedure not only from a technical standpoint but also from its lifelong postoperative management prospective. The close follow-up of the increasing number of patients is essential to prevent and treat the complications early, some of which can have devastating consequences. The widespread awareness and knowledge of these complications and their identification and treatment is important, as many patients will present at a center other than where they had their bariatric operation (Video **Error! Reference source not found.**).

Electronic Supplementary Material

Below is the link to the electronic supplementary material. Video 1 Laproscopic transection of gastro-gastric fistula with oversewing of the gastric remnant and pouch (MOV 1301462 kb)

Review Questions and Answers

Questions

1. Which one of the following is not commonly found in rhabdomyolysis (RML) post gastric bypass?

   A. Elevated serum creatine phosphokinase (CPK)
   B. Myoglobinuria
   C. Anesthesia with propofol
   D. Female gender

2. Regarding gastroesophageal leak the following is true:

   A. Tachycardia is invariably present
   B. Upper GI study is as sensitive as CT scan
   C. Upper GI study is more specific than CT scan
   D. Every Gastrojejunal anastomotic leak requires surgical re-intervention

3. A 47-year old woman with a history of laparoscopic gastric bypass 2 years ago presents with intermittent periumbilical pain and vomiting. The CT scan and physical exam are unremarkable. Which is the best next step?

   A. EGD
   B. Upper GI
   C. Diagnostic laparoscopy
   D. Nutritional consult

Answers

1. D. Male gender, higher BMI (>50 kg/m^2), current therapy with statins, operative time >4 h, and the use of propofol injection have been associated with increased incidence of rhabdomyolysis. The diagnosis is both clinical and biochemical (increased CPK levels five times higher than the normal, and the presence of myoglobin in the urine). The treatment is mostly supportive with aggressive fluid resuscitation, correction of electrolytes abnormalities and, sometimes, alkalinization of the urine.

2. C. Although the specificity of the UGI is very high for GJ leaks, its sensitivity is only 20 %. CT scan adds sensitivity to the diagnosis of GJ leaks because of the ability to show not only contrast extravasation and extraluminal collections, but also indirect signs of leak, such as surrounding inflammatory changes, intraabdominal free air, and left pleural effusion.

3. C. Intermittent abdominal pain and vomiting after laparoscopic gastric bypass can be due to either an internal hernia or intussusception. The CT scan can be negative in up to 30 % of cases. The best diagnostic and therapeutic intervention is a diagnostic laparoscopy.

References

1. Hinojosa MW, Varela JE, Parikh D, Smith BR, Nguyen XM, Nguyen NT. National trends in use and outcome of laparoscopic adjustable gastric banding. Surg Obes Relat Dis. 2009;5(2):150–5.

2. Kligman MD. Intraoperative endoscopic pneumatic testing for gastrojejunal anastomotic integrity during laparoscopic Roux-en-Y gastric bypass. Surg Endosc. 2007;21(8):1403–5.

3. Frantz DJ. Neurologic complications of bariatric surgery: involvement of central, peripheral, and enteric nervous systems. Curr Gastroenterol Rep. 2012;14(4):367–72.

4. Ettinger JE, MarcíliodeSouza CA, Azaro E, Mello CA, Santos-Filho PV, Orrico J, et al. Clinical features of rhabdomyolysis after open and laparoscopic Roux-en-Y gastric bypass. Obes Surg. 2008;18(6):635–43.

5. Edwards MA, Jones DB, Ellsmere J, Grinbaum R, Schneider BE. Anastomotic leak following antecolic versus retrocolic laparoscopic Roux-en-Y gastric bypass for morbid obesity. Obes Surg. 2007;17(3):292–7.

6. Ballesta C, Berindoague R, Cabrera M, Palau M, Gonzales M. Management of anastomotic leaks after laparoscopic Roux-en-Y gastric bypass. Obes Surg. 2008;18(6):623–30.

7. Gonzalez R, Sarr MG, Smith CD, Baghai M, Kendrick M, Szomstein S, et al. Diagnosis and contemporary management of anastomotic leaks after gastric bypass for obesity. J Am Coll Surg. 2007;204(1):47–55.

8. Cucchi SG, Pories WJ, MacDonald KG, Morgan EJ. Gastrogastric fistulas. A complication of divided gastric bypass surgery. Ann Surg. 1995;221(4):387–91.

9. Flicker MS, Lautz DB, Thompson CC. Endoscopic management of gastrogastric fistulae does not increase complications at bariatric revision surgery. J Gastrointest Surg. 2011;15(10):1736–42.

10. Cho M, Kaidar-Person O, Szomstein S, Rosenthal RJ. Laparoscopic remnant gastrectomy: a novel approach to gastrogastric fistula after Roux-en-Y gastric bypass for morbid obesity. J Am Coll Surg. 2007;204(4):617–24.

11. Griffith PS, Birch DW, Sharma AM, Karmali S. Managing complications associated with laparoscopic Roux-en-Y gastric bypass for morbid obesity. Can J Surg. 2012;55(5):329–36.

12. Tucker ON, Escalante-Tattersfield T, Szomstein S, Rosenthal RJ. The ABC System: a simplified classification system for small bowel obstruction after laparoscopic Roux-en-Y gastric bypass. Obes Surg. 2007;17(12):1549–54.

13. Rosenthal RJ. Dilating the stenotic gastrojejunostomy after laparoscopic Roux-en-Y gastric bypass for morbid obesity: when things go wrong. J Gastrointest Surg. 2009;13(9):1561–3.

14. Nandipati KC, Lin E, Husain F, Srinivasan J, Sweeney JF, Davis SS. Counterclockwise rotation of Roux-en-Y limb significantly reduces internal herniation in laparoscopic Roux-en-Y gastric bypass (LRYGB). J Gastrointest Surg. 2012;16(4):675–81.

15. Owens M, Barry M, Janjua AZ, Winter DC. A systematic review of laparoscopic port site hernias in gastrointestinal surgery. Surgeon. 2011;9(4):218–24.

16. Ver SK. Retrograde intussusception following Roux-en-Y gastric bypass. Obes Surg. 2006;16(8):1101–3.

17. Edwards MA, Grinbaum R, Ellsmere J, Jones DB, Schneider BE. Intussusception after Roux-en-Y gastric bypass for morbid obesity: case report and literature review of rare complication. Surg Obes Relat Dis. 2006;2(4):483–9.

18. Simper SC, Erzinger JM, McKinlay RD, Smith SC. Retrograde (reverse) jejunal intussusception might not be such a rare problem: a single group's experience of 23 cases. Surg Obes Relat Dis. 2008;4(2):77–83.

19. Matlaga BR, Shore AD, Magnuson T, Clark JM, Johns R, Makary MA. Effect of gastric bypass surgery on kidney stone disease. J Urol. 2009;181(6):2573–7.

20. Mathavan VK, Arregui M, Davis C, Singh K, Patel A, Meacham J. Management of postgastric bypass noninsulinoma pancreatogenous hypoglycemia. Surg Endosc. 2010;24(10):2547–55.

30
Gastric Bypass as a Revisional Procedure

Luigi Angrisani and Michele Lorenzo

Obesity is a multifactorial disease expanding worldwide. Obesity is frequently associated with several comorbidities or life-threatening diseases. Three hundred million obese were predicted in 2025 by the World Health Organization (WHO) [1]. Conservative treatment seems to be ineffective in most of these patients with disappointing results, and diet and lifestyle changes are effective only for a short period but are unable to sustain the long-term weight loss [2].

Over the last decades, bariatric surgery has been shown to be effective in the long-term treatment in this kind of patients [3, 4]. The rationale of bariatric surgery is based on a gastric volume restriction (restrictive surgery) or absorption intestinal capacity reduction (malabsorptive surgery) or a combination of both. Restrictive procedures particularly the laparoscopic adjustable gastric banding gained popularity because of its relatively low complexity and adjustability in combination with low morbidity and mortality rates [4–6]. Moreover LAGB is totally reversible after band removal. And the stomach regains its normal anatomy. At the moment, the vertical banded gastroplasty is no longer utilized (Figs. 1, 2, and 3).

Despite good results in the first postoperative period, the restrictive procedures have several limitations such as gastric pouch dilation, intragastric migration, band slippage, and gastrogastric fistulas [7–10]. Furthermore, over time a number of patients have inadequate weight loss or weight regain [7–9].

These problems of restrictive procedures run parallel with a similar increase in revisional procedures. The revisional bariatric surgical procedures are mainly indicated for the development of an acute or chronic complication or a side effect of the primary bariatric procedure, metabolic and nutritional sequelae, or the absence of postoperative weight loss or weight regain after a successful period, untreatable with conservative approach [11–17].

The laparoscopic Roux-en-Y gastric bypass (LRYGB) during the last years gained wide consensus as one of the procedure of choice as revisional bariatric procedure after restrictive primary operations [8, 12, 16, 18, 19].

Preoperative Workup

The preoperative workup is the same with the multidisciplinary evaluation done for all the bariatric surgical procedure. During the workup the patient compliance to adhere to follow-up was also stated. Particular attention is due to recognize any band-related or previous gastric complication that can delay the time of the surgical approach for several days or more.

Surgical Procedure

Revisional Surgery After Vertical Banded Gastroplasty [18, 20–26]

After clearing all adhesions, the gastric band is identified. In some cases with dense anterior adhesions, this may be facilitated by getting into the lesser sac and behind the stomach from the greater curve to first find the band in an area with less fibrosis and scarring. When possible, the gastroplasty vertical staple line is identified as well. A window must then be created into the lesser sac, on the lesser curve side of the stomach and proximal to the gastric band. The lesser curve neurovascular bundle should be preserved, and this window should be created as close to the gastric wall as possible. Once this dissection is complete, a linear stapler with a thick tissue cartridge is fired transversely on the gastric pouch and fundus proximal to the band. An esophageal bougie (38–42 French) is passed until it abuts the newly created proximal transverse staple line. The bougie is maneuvered as close as possible to the lesser curve of the pouch, and a linear stapler is fired multiple times until the new gastric pouch is completely isolated and divided from the remnant stomach. It is important to avoid crossing the original gastroplasty staple line when creating the pouch. By crossing staple lines and incorporating tissue of vastly different thicknesses in the same staple line, the potential for staple line failure increases.

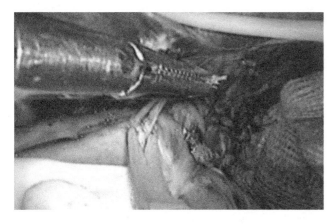

FIG. 1. Laparoscopic gastric band removal: gastrogastric stitches were cut.

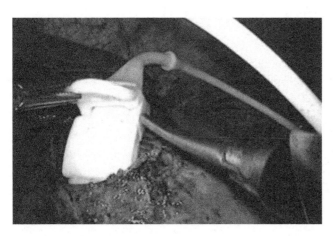

FIG. 2. Laparoscopic gastric band removal: the band was gently freed by the adhesion.

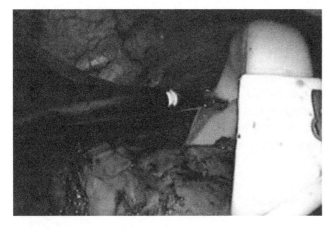

FIG. 3. Laparoscopic gastric band removal: the band was cut and removed.

There is an additional possibility of leaving a small cuff of stomach on either the remnant stomach or the gastric pouch that does not communicate with either lumen. For this reason, it is mandatory to stay very close to lesser curve bougie and typically resect the fundus of the remnant stomach along with

the band and the original staple lines. For open cases, a hand-sewn gastrojejunostomy, using absorbable sutures, was performed. In laparoscopic cases, the gastrojejunostomy is created by passing the anvil to a 25-mm circular stapler (DST Series™ EEA™ OrVil 25-mm device, Covidien, Norwalk, CT) transorally. Several experiences reported the same limb length as in primary LRYGB: a 50-cm biliopancreatic limb and a 100- or 150-cm Roux limb, depending on the patient's BMI.

Revisional Surgery After LAGB [8, 16, 19, 26–29]

After band deflation the first step is to identify the gastric band and its orientation. The fibrous tissue that covers the band is removed, and the port-connection tube is cut and pulled out of the abdomen. Then the band is sectioned, freed by the remaining adhesions, and gently extracted into a port. The gastric bypass can be performed during the same laparoscopic session or after several weeks according to both the surgeons' experience and patients' conditions.

The patient is positioned in the reverse Trendelenburg lithotomy position. A closed carbon dioxide pneumoperitoneum is created, and 6 trocars (5 of 12 mm and 1 of 5 mm) are inserted. The balloon gastric bougie (Inamed-Allergan) is placed transorally in the stomach and inflated with 30 mL of a saline solution, and the stomach is retracted backward by the anesthesiologist to reach the cardioesophageal junction. Dissection is started at its equator in the perigastric space between the neurovascular bundle of Latarjet and the lesser curvature of the stomach using the harmonic scalpel (Ultracision, Ethicon Endo-Surgery, Cincinnati, OH). The retrogastric space is entered, and gastric transection performed by multiple linear staples fired in sequence up to the angle of His. The 30–45 Endocutter (Ethicon Endo-Surgery, Cincinnati, OH) and 35-, 45-, and 60-mm Endo GIA (US Surgical, Tyco Healthcare) were used interchangeably when available and as required. The flip-top anvil of a 25-mm circular stapler (CEEA, US Surgical, Tyco Healthcare) is advanced transorally into and through the proximal gastric pouch using a modified nasogastric tube anvil apparatus. The Roux limb is constructed by transecting the small bowel 40–60 cm from the ligament of Treitz. A jejunotomy on the alimentary limb is created, and the circular stapler is introduced transabdominally and advanced into the lumen of the jejunum to create an antecolic, antegastric end-to-side gastrojejunostomy. The jejunotomy is closed with a 60-mm linear stapler. The presence of a gastrojejunostomy leak is tested by injecting 40–60 mL of methylene blue through the nasogastric tube previously positioned into the temporarily clamped alimentary limb. A side-to-side jejunojejunostomy is performed with a 45-mm linear stapler through a jejunotomy 100–150 cm distal to the gastrojejunostomy. The anastomosis is completed using 2-0 polydioxanone continuous suture (LAPRA-TY, Johnson & Johnson, Cincinnati, OH).

The closure of the Peterson space with nonabsorbable stitches is routine. Also, drainage of the gastroenteroanastomosis and enteroenteroanastomosis is done in all cases.

Some authors have described a new technique with band left in situ and the small bowel anastomosed with the stomach above the band.

Redo Timing

The question of performing a revisional procedure from gastric banding to gastric bypass in one or two steps is controversial. The authors supporting the two-step approach indicate mainly technical reasons due to tissue quality and adhesions [12]. A two-step approach is also indicated in case of LapBand complications as intragastric migration or gastric pouch dilation because of the difficulty in finding adequate and healthy gastric tissue for the gastrojejunostomy. There are some reports suggesting that stricture rates are higher when the anastomosis is created to thick, scarred gastric tissue [19, 30].

The authors who support the single-step approach suggest that it is preferable because it avoids weight regain during the time between the band removal and the revisional bypass and avoids a second general anesthesia [11, 19, 30]. Moreover the fibrosis resulting from gastric band seems not to influence the technical results if the band is totally deflated 1 month before the conversion and if the fibrous band on the stomach is totally excised.

Results of Revisional LRYGB After VBG and LAGB

Vertical Banded Gastroplasty

Vertical banded gastroplasty was the most popular bariatric procedure in the 1980s and early 1990s. It was largely abandoned owing to the poor long-term weight loss results and the high rate of complications requiring revisional bariatric surgery. The most common causes of failure of vertical banded gastroplasty requiring a redo surgery were the dehiscence of the staple line, a switch to a wrong eating pattern with concomitant weight regain, pouch dilation, and intractable gastroesophageal reflux [11]. In two studies with patients followed for 10 years or more, a high rate of revisional procedure was reported. Marsk and colleagues observed that after a mean follow-up of 3 years almost 21 % of VBG-operated patients had required a revisional surgery either for insufficient weight loss or complications [22]. For the same reasons, Belsiger and colleagues in 10 years reported the rate of 17 % of revisional procedure [21]. The conversion in LRYGB was considered by most authors to be the most suitable procedure. Shouten and colleagues found that weight loss following

VBG conversion to LRYGB was highly dependent on the indications for revision with better results in patients with insufficient weight loss [23]. Several other experiences confirm this observation. Gagné and colleagues reported that laparoscopic conversion of VBG in LRYGBP was feasible with acceptable weight loss, but the rate of surgical complication was high (38 %) [16–18, 20].

Laparoscopic Adjustable Gastric Banding

The results of redo LRYGB are largely studied in LAGB. Ardestani and colleagues compared band revision versus Roux-en-Y gastric bypass conversion [27]. After laparoscopic adjustable gastric banding, they observed that patients who have experienced successful weight loss with LAGB with band complications will have satisfactory outcomes with band revisions (i.e., band repositioning) maintaining the excess weight loss. Patients with inadequate weight loss with LAGB after conversion to LRYGB can experience better weight loss. Other authors have suggested that revisional procedure is less effective than primary LRYGBP [31, 32].

In a recent systematic review by Coblijn and colleagues, the perioperative mortality of LRYGBP after LAGB in 478 patients was zero [12]. The overall complication rate was 8.5 % and ranged from minor complications as wound infection to major complication as perforation and bleeding. The most common short-term complication was wound infection (3.5 %); less frequent were bleeding (1.8 %) and anastomotic leakage (0.9 %). Long-term complications were considered by Coblijn and colleagues, those which occur later than 30 days postoperatively [12]. Overall rate of patients with one or more complications was 8.9 %. The most common complication was the gastrojejunostomy stenosis (6.5 %), followed by marginal ulceration (1 %). The rate of laparotomic conversion was 2.4 % mainly due to adhesions. The mean incidence in this review was 6.5 % and mainly due to bleeding, staple line leakage, intestinal obstruction, stenosis, and internal hernia.

Another advantage of the revisional bypass is the disappearance of esophageal motility disorders and gastroesophageal reflux symptoms related to restriction and diaphragmatic crus enlargement [19, 33, 34]. Moreover, after revision with LRYGB, a radical improvement of several comorbidities as type II diabetes is observed [19, 35].

These data indicates that LRYGBP as a revisional procedure after restrictive bariatric surgery is safe with low complication rate and mortality not different from LRYGBP as a primary procedure. Potentially the revisional procedure can be more difficult than primary procedure, above all for the adhesions. This is probably true for vertical banded gastroplasty, not for LAGB, because the area around the stomach can be damaged and scarred. The conversion rate varied (0–23 %) according to several experiences [12, 19].

Additionally, the rate of leakage of LRYGBP after LAGB was 0.9 %, and after primary bypass the rate is reported between 0.4 and 5 % [12, 36]. The reoperation rate in revisional LRYGBP was 6.5 %, higher than the reoperation rate in primary procedures (3.2 %) [12, 36].

Conclusion

Several options are available after failed and/or complicated bariatric restrictive procedures as vertical banded gastroplasty and laparoscopic adjustable gastric banding. LRYGB seems at the moment to be the best surgical procedure in terms of safety and weight loss results. However, it must be underlined that redo bariatric surgery results in higher morbidity and reoperation rates than primary procedure. The timing and the technical options of LRYGB are still a matter of concern, and long-term data in this field are poor or lacking. Based on the current evidence, these revisional procedures should be performed by experienced bariatric surgeons.

References

1. WHO: Director General. Life in the 1st century: a vision for all. Geneva: World Health Organization; 1998.
2. Colquitt JL, Picot J, Loveman E, et al. Surgery for obesity. Cochrane Database Syst Rev. 2009;(2):CD003641.
3. Chapman AE, Kiroff G, Game P, et al. Laparoscopic adjustable gastric banding in the treatment of obesity: a systematic literature review. Surgery. 2004;135:326–51.
4. Buchwald H, Oien DM. Metabolic/bariatric surgery worldwide 2011. Obes Surg. 2013;23:427–36.
5. Angrisani L, Furbetta F, Doldi SB, et al. Lap Band®—Adjustable Gastric Banding System. The Italian experience with 1863 patients operated on 6 years. Surg Endosc. 2003;17:409–12.
6. O'Brien PE, MacDonald L, Anderson M, Brennan L, Brown WA. Long-term outcomes after bariatric surgery: fifteen-year follow-up of adjustable gastric banding and a systematic review of the bariatric surgical literature. Ann Surg. 2013;257:87–94.
7. Di Lorenzo M, Furbetta F, Favretti F, et al. Laparoscopic adjustable gastric banding via pars flaccida vs perigastric positioning. Technique, complications and results in 2529 patients. Surg Endosc. 2010;24:1519–23.
8. Angrisani L, Borrelli V, Lorenzo M, et al. Conversion of LapBand to Gastric bypass for dilated gastric pouch. Obes Surg. 2001;11:232–4.
9. Elnahas A, Graybiel K, Farrokhyar F, et al. Revisional surgery after failed laparoscopic adjustable gastric banding: a systematic review. Surg Endosc. 2012;27:740–5.
10. Di Lorenzo N, Lorenzo M, Furbetta F, et al. Intragastric gastric band migration-erosion: an analysis of multicenter experience on 177 patients. Surg Endosc. 2013;27:1151–7.
11. Himpens J, Dapri G. Redo bariatric procedure. In: Frezza E, Gagner M, Li MKW, editors. International principles of laparoscopic surgery. Woodbury: Cine-Med, Inc.; 2010. p. 393–404.
12. Coblijn UK, Verveld CJ, van Wagensveld BA, Lagarde SM. Laparoscopic Roux-en-Y gastric bypass or laparoscopic sleeve gastrectomy as revisional procedure after adjustable gastric band. A systematic review. Obes Surg. 2013;23:1899–914.
13. Gumbs AA, Pomp A, Gagner M. Revisional bariatric surgery for inadequate weight loss. Obes Surg. 2007;17:1137–45.
14. Angrisani L, Lorenzo M, Santoro T, et al. Videolaparoscopic treatment of gastric banding complications. Obes Surg. 1999;9:58–62.
15. Angrisani L, Lorenzo M, Santoro T, et al. Follow up of lap-band complications. Obes Surg. 1999;9:276–8.
16. Gonzales R, Gallagher SF, Sarr MG, Murr MM. Gastric bypass as a revisional procedure. In: Schauer PS, Schirmer BD, Brethauer SA, editors. Minimally invasive bariatric surgery. New York: Springer; 2007. p. 301–10.
17. Suter M. Revisional surgery for failed restrictive procedures in morbidly obese patients. In: Parini U, Nebiolo PE, editors. Bariatric surgery. Multidisciplinary approach and surgical techniques. Aosta: Musumeci Ed; 2007. p. 376–405.
18. Gagné DJ, Dovec E, Urbandt JE. Laparoscopic revision of vertical banded gastroplasty to Roux-en-Y gastric bypass: outcomes of 105 patients. Surg Obes Relat Dis. 2011;7:495–9.
19. Maud R, Poncet G, Boulez J, Mion F, Espalieu P. Laparoscopic gastric bypass for failure of adjustable gastric banding: a review of 85 cases. Obes Surg. 2011;21:1513–9.
20. Tevis S, Garren MJ, Gould JC. Revisional surgery for failed vertical banded gastroplasty. Obes Surg. 2011;21:1220–4.
21. Balisinger B, Poggio JL, Mai J, et al. Ten and more years after vertical banded gastroplasty as primary operation for morbid obesity. J Gastrointest Surg. 2000;4:598–605.
22. Marsk R, Jonas E, Gartzios H, et al. High revision rates after laparoscopic vertical banded gastroplasty. Surg Obes Relat Dis. 2009;5:84–98.
23. Schouten R, van Dielen FMH, van Gemert WG, et al. Conversion of vertical banded gastroplasty to Roux-en-Y gastric bypass results in restoration of the positive effect on weight loss and co-morbidities. Evaluation of 101 patients. Obes Surg. 2007;17:622–30.
24. Mognol P, Chosidow D, Marmuse JP. Roux-en-Y gastric bypass after failed vertical banded gastroplasty. Obes Surg. 2007;17:1431–4.
25. Boomberg RD, Urbach DR. Laparoscopic Roux-en-Y gastric bypass for severe gastroesophageal reflux after vertical banded gastroplasty. Obes Surg. 2002;12:408–11.
26. Angrisani L, Lorenzo M, Borrelli V. Laparoscopic adjustable gastric banding versus Roux-en-Y gastric bypass. 5-Years results of a prospective randomized trial. Surg Obes Relat Dis. 2007;3:127–32.
27. Ardestani A, Lautz DB, Tavakkolizadeh A. Band revision versus Roux-en-Y gastric bypass conversion as salvage operation after laparoscopic adjustable gastric banding. Surg Obes Relat Dis. 2011;7:33–7.
28. Meesters B, Latten G, Timmermans L, Schouten R, Greve JW. Roux-en-Y gastric bypass as revisional procedure after gastric banding: leaving the band in place. Surg Obes Relat Dis. 2012;8:717–22.
29. Victorzon M. Revisional bariatric surgery by conversion to gastric bypass or sleeve. Good short-term outcomes at higher risks. Obes Surg. 2012;22:29–33.
30. Radtka III JF, Puleo IA, Wang L, Cooney RN. Revisional bariatric surgery: who, what, where, and when? Surg Obes Relat Dis. 2010;6:635–42.
31. Zingg U, McQuinn A, DiValentino D, et al. Revisional vs primary Roux-en-Y gastric bypass. A case matched analysis: less weight loss in revision. Obes Surg. 2010;20:1627–32.
32. Deylgat B, D'Hondt M, Pottel H, et al. Indications, safety and feasibility of conversion of failed bariatric surgery to Roux-en-Y gastric bypass: a retrospective comparative study with primary laparoscopic Roux-en-Y gastric bypass. Surg Endosc. 2012;26:1997–2002.

33. Angrisani L, Iovino P, Lorenzo M, et al. Treatment of morbid obesity and gastroesophageal reflux with hiatal hernia by Lap-Band. Obes Surg. 1999;9:396–8.

34. Weber M, Muller MK, Michel JM, et al. Laparoscopic Roux-en-Y, but not rebanding, should be proposed as rescue procedure for patients with failed laparoscopic gastric banding. Ann Surg. 2003;238:827–33.

35. Rubino F, Gagner M, Gentileschi P, et al. The early effect of the Roux-en-Y gastric bypass on hormones involved in body weight regulation and glucose metabolism. Ann Surg. 2004;240:236–42.

36. Flum DR, Belle SH, King WC, et al. Perioperative safety in the longitudinal assessment of bariatric surgery. N Engl J Med. 2009; 361:445–54.

31

Laparoscopic Gastric Bypass: Nutritional Management After Surgery

Kelli C. Hughes, Rebecca N. Puffer, and Mary B. Simmons

Introduction

Gastric bypass surgery is a well-documented and widely accepted medical treatment for obesity. The importance of complete preoperative nutrition evaluation and postoperative nutrition education and management is critical to patient health and success. Clearly defined protocols should be established within a bariatric program to provide patients with comprehensive education and follow-up.

The Roux-en-Y gastric bypass (RYGB) limits food intake and induces malabsorption to produce weight loss by creating a small stomach pouch and bypassing the duodenum along with a portion of the proximal jejunum. Patients who chose to have weight loss surgery need to be ready and able to make long-term lifestyle changes and commit to lifelong vitamin and mineral supplementation. Because the amount of food that can be eaten is limited and nutrients are not fully absorbed, patients are at risk for developing a variety of macro- and micronutrient deficiencies. Nutrition guidelines should be explained at the onset of surgery consideration and reiterated at every phase of the process. This chapter will outline postoperative nutrition and supplementation requirements as well as review possible nutrient deficiencies, symptoms, and treatment for deficiencies should they occur. In addition, this chapter will address postoperative nutrition evaluation and follow-up protocols for nutrition care. It is important to provide continuous monitoring and adequate support to patients after surgery to ensure that they understand and are following program guidelines.

After any weight loss surgery, an ongoing commitment to appropriate food choices, portions, eating habits, and physical activity is essential to maximize weight loss and to maintain a healthy weight. Patients often have numerous habits that need to be permanently changed in order for this to happen. While this should be addressed extensively in the preoperative education and screening process, patients generally require a structured weight loss and maintenance program that includes continuous contact, accountability, and support in order to transition from a dieting mindset to an understanding and acquisition of permanent lifestyle change.

The Role of Nutrition Education

In 1991, the National Institutes of Health issued a consensus statement on Gastrointestinal Surgery for Severe Obesity in which patient selection criteria for gastric bypass were set [1]. This statement specifies that patients should be well informed, motivated, and able to participate in long-term follow-up. A multidisciplinary team approach including medical, surgical, psychiatric, and nutrition experts was recommended to educate, counsel, and monitor these patients. Many professional organizations and others have since issued statements on the care and management of surgical weight loss patients that highlight the importance of patient education and the role of a nutrition expert [2–8].

Because the RYGB procedure results in a restricted diet and nutrient malabsorption, patients must follow specific nutrition guidelines to be successful and prevent complications. These guidelines are not simply for the postsurgical recovery period but rather are permanent lifestyle and behavior changes that will require lifelong assessment, counseling, and support [2, 5, 9]. Registered dietitians (RDs) have assessment and counseling skills as well as nutrition expertise that lend themselves to this patient population and their long-term need for education and support [6].

The American Society for Metabolic and Bariatric Surgery (ASMBS) and the Academy of Nutrition and Dietetics professional practice guidelines highlight that nutrition management begins well before surgery with preoperative assessment and comprehensive education [3, 5]. Early education can ensure that patients are appropriate candidates for surgery and will be successful after surgery [3]. Pre- and postoperative therapy to modify eating behaviors, promote lifelong behavior change, and adjust to postsurgery diet and supplement requirements should be well planned and led by the RD [2, 5, 10]. Comprehensive education enables patients to acquire greater knowledge and understanding of obesity, energy balance, and self-management skills [7].

The goals of nutrition education should be to help patients ingest adequate energy and nutrients for healing, to preserve

S.A. Brethauer et al. (eds.), *Minimally Invasive Bariatric Surgery*,
DOI 10.1007/978-1-4939-1637-5_31, © Springer Science+Business Media New York 2015

lean body mass while experiencing rapid weight loss, and to minimize complications or undesirable symptoms while maximizing weight loss [3, 4, 11]. Achieving these goals requires consistent, long-term follow-up with the bariatric dietitian to provide individualized education and support. Current practice for postsurgical follow-up with the bariatric team is a postoperative check at 2–4 weeks and then routine follow-up at 3 months, 6 months, 12 months, and annually thereafter [3, 6, 7, 11, 12]. In addition, nutrition-focused individual or group meetings at more frequent intervals, especially within the first 2 years after surgery, are essential for optimal health and weight loss [6, 12]. Table 1 outlines the suggested components of nutrition follow-up.

Nutrition Management Guidelines

Diet Texture Progression

The postoperative diet is a staged progression to ensure adequate nutrient intake and tolerance after RYGB. While no standardized recommendations exist across bariatric surgery programs, the need for standardization has been recognized [12]. Typically, patients are given a sugar-free, clear liquid diet after surgery and advanced to full liquid/pureed food, then mechanical soft foods followed by solid food/regular diet over a period of time, taking into consideration individual tolerance and needs [3, 6, 10–14].

Clear liquids are recommended for 1–2 days after RYGB, as is common with many types of surgery, and should be sugar-free, low calorie, and non-carbonated. The clear liquid diet is not intended to meet nutrition needs as patients are typically still in the hospital and getting intravenous fluids.

After clear liquids, a combination of full liquids and pureed foods are recommended for 3–4 weeks (see Table 2).

TABLE 1. Suggested nutrition follow-up assessment

Anthropometric	Current height, weight, body mass index
	Total weight loss since surgery
	Total percent of excess weight loss since surgery
Supplements	Compliance with vitamin and mineral recommendations
Diet	Usual diet recall
	Diet progression and consistency of foods
	Protein intake
	Fruit and vegetable intake
	Fluid intake
	Meal schedule
	Portion size
	Food tolerance
Behavior	Separate eating and drinking
	Eating habits (speed, size of bites, chewing)
	Physical hunger vs. psychological hunger
	Coping mechanisms and stress management
	Weight maintenance strategies
Physical activity	Type, amount, and frequency
Goal setting	Patient-directed goals

Liquids should be sugar-free, non-carbonated, and low fat. Foods in this stage of the diet have a thin, smooth consistency to minimize pressure on the staple lines and sutures. Solid foods can be blended with liquids to attain the pureed consistency, or patients may choose to use baby foods. At this stage, and for those that follow, high-quality protein intake is of utmost importance and should comprise the majority of each meal.

The soft diet is introduced approximately 1 month after surgery and prescribed for 1–4 weeks (see Table 3). Patients should be able to tolerate all full liquids and pureed foods without pain or regurgitation before advancing to soft foods. Soft foods must be well cooked, moist, ground, shredded, or otherwise able to be chewed into mush when eaten. Protein foods are the priority at meals and can be supplemented with small amounts of fruit, vegetable, or starch.

The regular bariatric diet incorporates all consistencies of foods and is begun 4–8 weeks after surgery (see Table 4). Tolerance of the regular diet will vary widely among patients. Introduction of solid foods should be monitored carefully by both the patient and the bariatric team and done over a period of weeks and months. It is helpful to try one new solid food at a time when the regular diet is first introduced. Once a wide variety of foods are well tolerated, choosing solid, dense foods will result in greater satiety from small portions, thus maximizing weight loss. Meals continue to be predominantly protein based.

Calorie Balance and Macronutrients

In all stages of the post-RYGB diet, the goal is to produce a substantial caloric deficit while maintaining an adequate intake of essential macro- and micronutrients [6]. Because the patient's intake is significantly restricted and the absorption of the nutrients they ingest is hindered by RYGB, the diet must be well designed to meet nutrient needs and prevent deficiencies. As mentioned above, it is essential that patients are thoroughly educated about the ways in which their diet can both keep them healthy and optimize weight loss before they proceed with surgery.

Protein

Protein intake after surgery should be the primary nutrition goal for a number of reasons. During periods of rapid weight loss, the body will lose not only fat but also lean body mass. In order to preserve as much lean body mass as possible, patients must ingest a much higher percentage of their diet as protein than either fat or carbohydrate. The benefits of preserving muscle mass are increased metabolism and ability to burn calories. Additionally, high-quality protein sources in the diet provide the components for protein synthesis in the body, prevent protein deficiency, slow digestion, and therefore increase satiety [15].

TABLE 2. Blended/pureed

	Foods allowed	Foods to avoid
Protein	Lean fish, tuna, poultry, beef or pork; tofu; eggs or egg substitute; cooked beans; reduced-fat, smooth peanut butter; liquid protein supplements	Fried or breaded meat; meat with visible fat; processed meat
Dairy	Fat-free (skim) or 1 % milk; light yogurt; nonfat powdered milk; low-fat cottage cheese; low-fat or nonfat cheese; low-fat soymilk	Flavored milk; 2 % or whole milk; ice cream; regular yogurt with sugar; regular cheese
Fruit and vegetables	Applesauce; mashed potatoes; other cooked fruit and vegetables without seeds or skins	Raw fruit and vegetables
Starches	Oatmeal; grits; cream of wheat	Bread and rolls; cold cereals; pasta and rice
Other	Sugar-free gelatin; sugar-free fat-free pudding; sugar-free popsicles	Chewing gum; sweets and desserts

TABLE 3. Soft foods

	Foods allowed	Foods to avoid
Protein	Lean, soft, and moist meats (fish, tuna, poultry, or pork); soft tofu; eggs or egg substitute; soft, low-fat casseroles with soft vegetables; reduced-fat, smooth peanut butter; liquid protein supplements	Crunchy peanut butter; meat that is dry, tough, or chewy; processed meat
Dairy	Fat-free (skim) or 1 % milk; light yogurt; nonfat powdered milk; low-fat cottage cheese; low-fat or nonfat cheese; low-fat soymilk	Flavored milk; 2 % or whole milk; ice cream; regular yogurt with sugar; regular cheese
Fruit and vegetables	Fruit and vegetables without seeds or hulls that have been cooked soft; soft unsweetened canned fruits or vegetables; fresh soft fruit	Raw vegetables; fresh, crunchy fruits; fruit and vegetables with tough skins or seeds
Starches	Oatmeal, grits, and cream of wheat	Bread and rolls; cold cereals
Other	Sugar-free gelatin; sugar-free fat-free pudding; sugar-free popsicles; light mayonnaise; light or fat-free salad dressing; cooking spray	Chewing gum; sweets and desserts; butter; oils; regular mayonnaise; regular salad dressing

TABLE 4. Solids

	Foods allowed	Foods difficult to tolerate	Foods to avoid
Protein	Lean, moist meats; beans; nuts; eggs or egg substitutes; tofu; vegetarian meat substitutes	Tough or dry meat	Fried or breaded meat; fast-food meat; meat with skin or visible fat; processed meat
Dairy	Fat-free (skim) or 1 % milk; light yogurt; low-fat cottage cheese; low-fat or nonfat cheese; low-fat soymilk		Flavored milk; 2 % or whole milk; ice cream; regular yogurt with sugar; regular cheese
Fruit	Fresh; canned in juice; frozen; cooked without sugar	Fruits with skin or tough peels; dried fruit	Fruit with added sugar; canned in syrup
Vegetables	Fresh; no salt added canned; frozen; cooked without added fat	Raw vegetables with tough skins or seeds	Fried or breaded vegetables; vegetables with sauces or added fat
Starches	Dry or toasted whole grain bread; whole grain crackers; baked tortillas; oatmeal; grits; cream of wheat; cold cereal without added sugar; soft cooked potatoes, whole wheat pasta; brown rice	Soft breads and rolls; breads with nuts, seeds, or dried fruit; cold cereal with dried fruit or nuts; rice; pasta	Doughnuts; pastries; white bread; sugary cold cereal; instant noodle or potato dishes; French fries
Other	Sugar-free gelatin; sugar-free fat-free pudding; sugar-free popsicles; light mayonnaise; light or fat-free salad dressing; cooking spr	Chewing gum; popcorn; spicy foods	Fried or greasy foods; cream-based soups; fast food; sweets and desserts; butter; oils; regular mayonnaise; regular salad dressing

It is generally recommended that patients consume 60–80 g of protein per day as soon as their diet has been advanced from clear liquids [3, 8, 9, 11, 12, 14]. Some programs use 1.0–1.5 g/kg ideal body weight to calculate protein needs which generally results in a similar total protein intake [3, 13]. This is slightly higher than the current Dietary Reference Intake of 46–56 g per day for normal adults. In order to meet this protein goal, a patient would need to eat approximately 8–10 oz of lean meat per day or the equivalent of other high-protein foods. While this may be possible in later stages of the diet, for several weeks or months immediately after surgery, liquid protein supplements will likely be necessary to meet this goal. The 60–80 g daily protein intake is ideally distributed evenly throughout the day at 3–5 h intervals and at least three meals [16].

An important consideration to promote optimal health after RYGB is the type and quality of protein. Not all sources or types of protein will be digested or absorbed equally after surgery, and patients will benefit greatly from choosing the highest quality proteins, especially with regard to protein supplements. Two factors that influence protein quality are their indispensable (essential) amino acids (IAA) content and their branched-chain amino acids (BCAA) content. The nine IAAs are those which the body cannot synthesize and therefore must be supplied from the diet. Three of these IAAs are called BCAAs due to their structure and uniquely contribute to both protein synthesis and metabolic function, as compared to the other IAAs that are involved in only one of those functions [16]. This distinction makes the BCAAs protein powerhouses for bariatric patients.

Given these factors, the highest quality whole food protein sources are low-fat milk products (whey and casein proteins), soy, and eggs (egg-white protein). Meat, fish, poultry, beans, and legumes have slightly lower IAA and BCAA contents but are still high-quality protein sources. Grains and nuts also contribute protein to the diet, but are not the best sources of high-quality proteins [16]. With respect to protein supplements, those made from whey, casein, or soy proteins, either as the whole protein or protein isolates, are the gold standard for bariatric patients. Whey protein supplements especially contain all the IAAs and therefore BCAAs are soluble in the stomach and rapidly digested [3]. These types of protein supplements are widely available and affordable for patients and should be used to help patients meet protein goals immediately after surgery. Collagen-based protein supplements do not contain the necessary IAAs and may not be easily digested and absorbed in RYGB patients and so should not be recommended [3].

Fat

For optimal food tolerance and weight loss, dietary fat should be limited in the post-RYGB diet. The fat in foods contributes more than twice as many calories as the equivalent amount of either protein or carbohydrate, thus hindering weight loss. High-fat foods, especially those that are greasy or fried, are often poorly tolerated after RYGB and can cause a number of unpleasant gastrointestinal symptoms. Patients should be advised to limit added fats such as butter, margarine, regular mayonnaise and salad dressing, gravy, cream sauce, oils, cream cheese, and sour cream and choose low-fat, light, or fat-free versions when possible [14]. A helpful guideline is to read food labels and avoid all foods with >5 g total fat per serving.

Carbohydrates

Like protein, the type and quality of carbohydrate in the bariatric diet is important. While a patient's meals will be predominantly protein, the goal is not a carbohydrate-free diet as is popular in many weight loss programs. Complex, high-fiber carbohydrate foods such as fruit, vegetables, and whole grains are recommended as a small part of every meal for the RYGB patient. These foods will slow digestion and increase satiety as well as provide essential vitamins and minerals.

By contrast, simple, rapidly digested carbohydrate foods such as sweets, processed or refined grains, added sugars, and sugar-sweetened beverages should be avoided. Not only do these foods contribute significant calories with no real nutrient benefits but the digestion of these after RYGB can result in dumping syndrome. Dumping syndrome occurs when a meal containing large amounts of sugar empties quickly into the small bowel which causes a fluid shift into the bowel. This results in symptoms such as nausea, bloating, abdominal cramps, and explosive diarrhea [6]. In order to avoid dumping syndrome and excess calories, all food should have <10 g of sugar per serving. Patients can obtain this information by reading food labels. Artificial sweeteners such as NutraSweet®, Splenda®, Sweet'N Low®, and stevia-based sweeteners are acceptable substitutes for real sugar. They will not cause dumping syndrome and will help with weight loss and maintenance since they contain very few calories.

Behavior Modification

RYGB surgery necessitates a whole lifestyle transformation. The gastrointestinal system must be retrained with the diet progression as the body adjusts to altered digestion and metabolism. Perhaps more challenging though is the psychological retraining involved in learning new eating habits and patterns, recognizing hunger signals, and establishing a new relationship with food. Bariatric patients will benefit greatly from understanding what specific habits and guidelines to follow as well as the rationale behind those guidelines in language and concepts they can understand. This education will improve compliance with the complex guidelines and provide motivation to make the best possible nutrition choices after surgery [3].

The goal of behavior guidelines is to promote optimal nutrient intake while minimizing adverse side effects from food intolerance and maximizing weight loss. Some details of nutrition guidelines will vary between bariatric programs; however, general recommendations are well established and widely used [6, 7, 9, 11–14]. The key nutrition guidelines are summarized in Table 5.

Overall, the RYGB diet requires planning and scheduling. Meal times and content should be planned in order to meet nutrient goals, avoid grazing or mindless eating, regulate metabolism, and ensure that the meal plan is realistic and feasible for an individual patient's lifestyle. It is very difficult, for example, to guarantee an intake of 60 g of protein with a restricted meal size without planning which foods and what amounts will be eaten throughout a given day. The diet

TABLE 5. Nutrition behavior guidelines for RYGB

Meal planning	Eat every 3–5 h
	Eat 4–6 times a day
	Schedule meal times
	Plan meal content ahead of time
	Keep a food journal
Diet content	60–80 g protein per day, distributed evenly throughout the day
	Limit added fats and sugars
	Choose foods with < 5 g total fat and < 10 g sugars per serving
	When diet has progressed to solid foods, choose moist, solid foods and limit soft, mushy foods
Portion size	1/4–1/2 cup meals during pureed and soft food stages
	1/2–1 cup meals during solid food stage
	Measure foods before eating
Eating habits	Eat protein foods first
	Include 1/8–1/4 cup fruit and/or vegetables at all meals
	Meals should last 20–30 min; eat slowly
	Cut food into small bites
	Chew food very well
Fluids	Drink 48–64 oz sugar-free, non-carbonated fluids per day
	Do not drink from 30 min before until 30–60 min after eating

TABLE 6. Guidelines for supplementation after RYGB

Supplement	Dose
Multivitamin complete	Twice daily
Calcium citrate with vitamin D	1,500 mg daily
Iron (ferrous gluconate)[a]	325 mg daily (36 g elemental iron)
Vitamin B12	500 mcg daily

[a]Only if menstruating or advised by bariatric team

signs and symptoms of nutrient deficiencies, laboratory assessment, and causes and prevalence of deficiency as well as treatment. Table 6 outlines recommended supplementation after RYGB.

Patient Instructions

- Avoid men's formula vitamins and "silver" vitamins.
- Calcium should be taken in 500 mg doses.
- Avoid taking iron and calcium together because they compete for absorption.
- Avoid taking calcium and multivitamin together because the multivitamin contains iron.

Vitamin B12

Vitamin B12 is absorbed mainly in the terminal ileum. It has a key role in nervous system function, DNA synthesis, and red blood cell formation. Signs and symptoms of a vitamin B12 deficiency include paresthesias, ataxia, glossitis, fatigue, and coordination disorders. Serum vitamin B12 is the most commonly used indicator of a deficiency. However, elevated methylmalonic acid and homocysteine levels may be more sensitive indicators of a vitamin B12 deficiency [17].

The cause of vitamin B12 deficiency following RYGB is multifactorial. Initially, the release of vitamin B12 from protein-containing foods is incomplete due to a decrease in hydrochloric acid from decreased stomach size. This decrease in stomach size also decreases the amount of intrinsic factor available to bind with vitamin B12 for absorption in the terminal ileum. Food intolerances or avoidance of vitamin B12-rich foods such as meat and fortified cereals is another cause of possible vitamin B12 deficiency following RYGB. Lastly, small bowel bacterial overgrowth (SBBO) following RYGB may cause a low vitamin B12 level due to the utilization of the vitamin by the bacteria [18].

Vitamin B12 deficiency has been noted as early as 6 months following RYGB [19]. The incidence of deficiency has been reported between 7 and 37 % [19–23]. Treatment of a vitamin B12 deficiency has been suggested at 350–550 mcg per day by mouth (PO) or 1,000 mcg/week for 8 weeks PO and then 1,000 mcg/month intramuscularly (IM) [3, 20, 24].

progression is intentionally slow, and each meal should be a slow, thoughtful process of taking small bites, chewing well, paying attention to hunger and satiety cues, and limiting portions to 1/4 to one cup depending on diet stage. The slowed pace greatly improves tolerance, especially of solid foods, and prevents overeating. For adequate hydration, 48–64 oz of sugar-free, non-carbonated fluids are required per day. Fluids should not be consumed within 30 min of meals, again to improve food tolerance and also to promote satiety. Drinking with a meal can enable foods to be moved from the stomach into the bowel more quickly. This results in larger meals and decreased satiety which hinders weight loss.

Micronutrient Deficiencies Following Gastric Bypass

Due to the restrictive and malabsorptive nature of the RYGB, vitamin and mineral deficiencies can occur. Some of the more common deficiencies include those of calcium, vitamin D, iron, and vitamin B12. More case reports are being published of some less well-known deficiencies including thiamine and copper deficiencies, so clinicians should be aware of signs and symptoms of nutrient deficiencies and screen when appropriate. It should be noted that rates of deficiency in the literature may be skewed due to an inconsistency in testing methods and normal lab ranges. In addition, since certain vitamin levels are not routinely monitored, rates of deficiency of these nutrients may be underreported. The following section provides guidelines for supplementation,

Iron

Iron absorption is most efficient in the duodenum and proximal jejunum. Iron plays a role in oxygen transportation, DNA synthesis, and immunity. The most common signs of iron deficiency include microcytic anemia, fatigue, headache, exercise intolerance, pica, and also oral manifestations including stomatitis and glossitis. Laboratory assessment of iron deficiency should include percent saturation, ferritin, serum iron, and total iron-binding capacity. It should be noted that ferritin is an acute-phase reactant and may be elevated with infection, inflammation, and chronic disease [3].

In addition to bypassing the main site of absorption, iron deficiency can be caused by a decrease in hydrochloric acid which is needed to convert ferric iron into the ferrous state. Iron-rich foods such as meat may be avoided following RYGB which can exacerbate iron deficiency. It has been noted that menstruating women are at increased risk of iron deficiency and may require additional supplementation [21, 24, 25].

The prevalence of iron deficiency has been documented at 20–52 % [19, 20, 23, 25]. Treatment with 50–65 mg of elemental iron 2–4 times a day has been suggested [3, 25]. The absorption of iron is improved with vitamin C, so a 250 mg vitamin C supplement should be considered [26, 27]. Iron supplementation can cause gastrointestinal symptoms that may deter patients from continuing supplementation. Starting with half of a dose and increasing or taking with food may improve tolerance and compliance.

Calcium and Vitamin D

The ileum and jejunum are the main sites of vitamin D absorption, and calcium is preferentially absorbed in the duodenum and proximal jejunum. The most well-known function of calcium and vitamin D is maintenance of proper bone mineralization. Calcium also has a role in blood coagulation, muscle contraction, nerve functioning, and blood clotting. Unlike other vitamin deficiencies that show clear outward signs and symptoms, deficiencies of calcium and vitamin D are less easy to detect without testing. Muscle spasms, joint pain, malformed teeth, and frequent bone breaks may indicate a deficiency. The most accurate blood test to diagnose a vitamin D deficiency is 25-hydroxy vitamin D. Serum calcium should not be used as a marker of bone health. A decrease in serum calcium would not be expected until severe osteoporosis has set in [3]. An elevated parathyroid hormone (PTH) can be indicative of increased bone turnover and should be used in place of serum calcium. A DEXA scan would be ideal in determining actual bone density. However, this test is more expensive and not as easily accessible for the majority of patients.

In addition to bypassing the main site of absorption, deficiencies of calcium and vitamin D can be caused by decreased availability of vitamin D due to sequestering in fat mass and decreased exposure to sunlight. A negative body image may prevent morbidly obese individuals from exposing skin to sunlight which facilitates the conversion of cholesterol to vitamin D. Inadequate bile salt mixing would also cause decreased absorption of vitamin D, and use of proton pump inhibitors can decrease the absorption of calcium [28]. Lastly, since being overweight is protective of bone status, simply losing weight can increase risk of bone demineralization [29].

It should be noted that vitamin D deficiency is prevalent even before weight loss surgery with reports of 16–57 % deficiency before surgery [23, 30–32]. The rate of vitamin D deficiency following RYGB has been reported at 30–73 % [20, 22, 23, 33, 34]. An increase in PTH has been seen in 30–69 % [33, 35, 36].

Supplementing calcium with vitamin D in 500–600 mg doses totaling 1,500–2,000 mg calcium daily has been suggested [3]. Vitamin D supplementation may consist of 50,000 IU weekly for up to 8 weeks [3].

Copper

Absorption of copper occurs in the stomach and proximal duodenum. A copper deficiency can be exhibited by neurologic symptoms such as polyneuropathy, myelopathy, and ataxia as well as neutropenia and anemia. Some neurologic damage may be irreversible. One of the main signs of a copper deficiency in several case reports following RYGB is a progressive decrease in ambulation [37–40]. Given the similarity in signs and symptoms of copper and vitamin B12 deficiencies, checking vitamin B12 and copper when these symptoms occur may be warranted. A copper deficiency can be confirmed with a serum copper lab test. Some are suggesting using ceruloplasmin as a marker of copper deficiency [41].

The decrease in stomach size as well as bypassing the duodenum in the RYGB is the main cause of copper deficiency. High doses of zinc supplementation can cause a copper deficiency due to competition for absorption [3, 39]. In addition, not all multivitamin/multimineral supplements contain copper or adequate amounts of copper, which can further increase the potential for a deficiency in the RYGB population.

Copper is not a standard lab test performed, so accurate rates of deficiency are difficult to obtain and the incidence is likely underreported. Gletsu-Miller found a 9.6 % deficiency rate out of 136 patients [41]. Most of the reports in the literature are case reports following RYGB. There is no globally accepted repletion rate for copper deficiency. One recommendation for repletion includes 1.0–2.5 mg IV copper for 3–6 days followed by 6–8 mg PO [37, 38, 42]. Rudnicki suggests 6 mg elemental copper daily for 1 week then 4 mg per day for the second week then 2 mg per day thereafter [43].

Thiamine

Thiamine is absorbed in the jejunum and proximal ileum. One may suspect thiamine deficiency with memory changes, paresthesia, muscle cramps, irritability, neuropathy, and gait ataxia. The most severe form of a thiamine deficiency is Wernicke's encephalopathy which includes ataxia, ophthalmoplegia, nystagmus, and confusion. The effects of a thiamine deficiency may be irreversible, so early detection is key. Serum thiamine is most often used for diagnostic purposes. Erythrocyte transketolase has been recommended as a more accurate marker of thiamine levels; however, access to this test may be limited [3, 27].

Thiamine deficiency is most commonly seen in the setting of protracted vomiting following RYGB [44]. Multiple vitamin noncompliance and malabsorption are other causes of deficiency. A diagnosis of SBBO is another potential cause of thiamine deficiency [27].

Clements reported the incidence of thiamine deficiency as 11–18 % [22]. Two reviews have been published reporting 32 and 84 cases of Wernicke's encephalopathy respectively [45, 46]. There are a few points to note with diagnosis and treatment of a thiamine deficiency. First, results of a serum thiamine may take up to a week to obtain. Additional damage may be done between the time blood is drawn and until the results are received. Given that thiamine is a water-soluble vitamin, one may consider treating a deficiency if it is suspected before receiving confirmation via blood work. Secondly, thiamine plays an important role in energy metabolism and has a short half-life of 9–18 days [3]. Thiamine deficiency is often seen with intractable vomiting. Patients presenting with this symptom will frequently be given IV fluid, often dextrose. The infusion of dextrose will further deplete thiamine stores, so thiamine repletion should be started before infusing carbohydrate-containing fluids. Treatment includes 50–200 mg per day IV or IM for 5–7 days or until symptoms resolve [3, 43, 47, 48]. Koch has suggested repletion with doses as high as 250 mg IM [27].

Zinc

Zinc absorption occurs mainly in the duodenum and proximal jejunum. Zinc has a major role in metabolism, wound healing, cell division, enzyme function, and immunity [3]. A zinc deficiency may be suspected with hypogeusia, poor wound healing, diarrhea, hair loss, glossitis, dermatitis, and cheilitis [3]. There is some question on the most accurate marker of zinc deficiency [49, 50]. Serum zinc levels have been used to report deficiency rates in the RYGB population [31, 51]. A zinc deficiency may result from intolerance of zinc-rich foods such as meat. Fat malabsorption may also cause a zinc deficiency following RYGB [3].

Zinc levels are not assessed on a regular basis among the RYGB population. Studies have reported a rate of zinc deficiency of 6–36 % following RYGB [31, 51]. There is limited data on appropriate treatment levels for a zinc deficiency. Supplementing elemental zinc with 30–50 mg daily or every other day has been suggested [36, 52, 53]. Sixty milligrams of elemental zinc twice per day has also been suggested [3]. More research is needed to determine an appropriate supplementation level for zinc.

Folate

Folate is absorbed mainly in the duodenum; however, adaptation after RYGB can allow absorption throughout the small bowel [3]. Folate functions in the body in red blood cell maturation, DNA synthesis, and prevention of neural tube defects. Folate deficiency may be suspected with megaloblastic anemia, diarrhea, cheilosis, glossitis, and thrombocytopenia. Red blood cell folate is preferred as a marker of deficiency compared with serum folate [3]. In addition, it has been proposed that homocysteine will be elevated with a folate deficiency which can aid in diagnosis [3].

A folate deficiency following RYGB may be caused by multiple vitamin noncompliance and avoidance or intolerance of enriched starches. Stores of folate can be depleted in as short as a few months without supplementation [3].

A wide range of folate deficiency has been reported in the RYGB population with rates of 0–35 % [19, 23, 25]. Of note, folate levels can be elevated with SBBO [18, 52]. Treatment of a deficiency has been proposed at 400 mcg to as high as 5 mg daily [3, 25, 27, 52].

Additional Nutrients

Much less common micronutrient deficiencies have also been reported in the RYGB population to include selenium, vitamin C, and vitamin A [22, 53–56] There is limited data on these deficiencies, but since they have been reported following RYGB, one should be aware and monitor for signs of deficiency.

Weight Maintenance

It is well documented that the majority of patients who undergo RYGB experience some weight regain. According to the literature, in 30–50 % of patients, the amount of weight gained 2–5 years after surgery ranges between 8 and 15 % as compared to the patients' lowest weight [57–60]. Data and follow-up beyond 5 years is minimal. This typical weight regain does not negate the clinical improvements seen between 24 and 60 months after surgery.

The ASMBS defines a successful surgery as weight loss of at least 50 % of excess weight 18–24 months after surgery [4]. Surgical failure rates range from 5 to 7 % and increase with super-obese patients to 20–33 %. Follow-up studies also indicate that weight regain increases with additional years out from surgery [60]. Surgical failure and excessive weight regain are associated with the return of comorbidities, decreased physical activity, and decreased quality of life. With data beyond 5 years lacking, it is difficult to assess the long-term ability of patients to maintain their weight loss. However, current data indicate a need for bariatric surgery programs to develop and implement maintenance protocols in order to support patients' long-term efforts to keep excess weight off.

Maintenance programs directed at helping patients stay at a healthy weight after their postsurgical weight loss has ceased should include a plan for long-term nutrition counseling, continued contact with the healthcare team, and accountability [61]. This type of follow-up should continue to include the basic nutrition tenants that have been taught and reinforced prior to surgery and during the weight loss phase. Below is an example of a maintenance program implemented at a large university hospital (see Table 7).

The predictors below should be assessed and addressed prior to surgery, during the weight loss phase, and in the long-term maintenance phase. The remainder of this section will be dedicated to looking at each ongoing predictor of successful weight maintenance and how it might be addressed as part of the patients' maintenance efforts.

TABLE 7. Outline of maintenance program

Time out from surgery	Healthcare team follow-up action
12 months	Standard follow-up visit Referral to outpatient nutritionist for maintenance meal planning Maintenance packet given to patient Schedule 6-month follow-up phone call
18 months	RD follow-up call to patient—check weight, protein intake, supplements, maintenance plan, exercise, 24-h food recall. Assess and make recommendations for improvements and set goals
24 months	Standard follow-up visit Check on progress with goals set on the phone Problem solve and set new goals as needed Schedule six-month follow-up phone call
30 months	RD follow-up call to patient—check weight, protein intake, supplements, maintenance plan, exercise, 24-h food recall. Assess and make recommendations for improvements and set goals with patient. Determine need for additional support and follow-up
3–5 years and beyond	Standard follow-up visit

Baseline predictors of postoperative weight regain [58, 59]:

- Increased food urges and binging
- Decreased sense of well-being/depression
- Addictive behaviors
- Presence of binge-eating disorders
- Higher BMI

Ongoing predictors of successful weight maintenance [58, 59, 61–63]:

- Involvement with support groups
- Self-monitoring
- Regular follow-up
- Diet quality
- Physical activity
- Nutrition counseling and RD contact

Involvement with Support Group

Regular attendance at support group meetings results in greater weight loss and increased chances of long-term maintenance according to several studies [65–69]. Research shows that continued contact and accountability with other patients and healthcare providers as well as additional behavioral and emotional support help patients stay on track with following program guidelines and sustaining behavior change after surgery. Bariatric centers of excellence are required to provide a support group for their patients; however, all programs, no matter the size, would benefit from providing ongoing programming outside of medical visits. Ideally, a support group would involve all professionals that are part of the healthcare team including doctors, nurses, RDs, behavioral health, and exercise physiology. With new technologies and increasing availability of Internet access, online support groups provide a meaningful way to connect for patients who live too far to engage in physical meetings.

Self-Monitoring

Self-monitoring of weight, food intake, and physical activity are key mechanisms for weight maintenance according to patients who have lost large amounts of weight, surgically and through diet and exercise. The necessity of all forms of self-monitoring has been consistently demonstrated in the literature, as an invaluable part of any weight loss and maintenance effort [60, 70–77]. Weight loss surgery alone, without personal responsibility for monitoring and behavior change, results in weight regain in many patients. Regular self-weighing helps patients stay in touch with the reality of what they are eating and what is happening with their weight.

Keeping food records and measuring portions assists with tracking calorie, fat, and protein intake, which is important for good nutrition but also for staying within an appropriate calorie level to maintain a stable weight. Activity records help with planning exercise and making it a regular habit. During pre- and postoperative education, weight graphs and food and activity records should be provided for patient reference and use. The role of self-monitoring should be presented as an essential part of the patients' responsibility from the first education session and regularly thereafter. There are also many electronic tools and web sites for self-monitoring that have helped patients be more successful in this area.

Regular Follow-Up

Adherence to regular follow-up protocol is directly linked to long-term success with bariatric patients [58, 59, 78]. Most programs schedule regular follow-up with patients after their surgery, but the length between visits varies and patient adherence decreases over time.

Continued contact, accountability, repetition of guidelines, and reinforcement of patient success all play a vital role in continued motivation and success. Presenting follow-up requirements prior to surgery so patients understand the commitment involved helps create "buy-in" for multiple appointments and increases commitment to following the program. At each visit, the patient should see the doctor and RD. If other healthcare professionals such as behavioral health or exercise physiologist are a part of the bariatric team, patients should see them regularly as well. If not, appropriate referrals should be made as needed.

Diet Quality

Diet quality should be examined at each visit and assessed for adherence to program guidelines. The National Weight Loss Registry (NWLR) compared the eating habits of patients who lost weight with diet and exercise vs. patients who had bariatric surgery. Surgical patients reported more fast food, increased fat intake, and less dietary restraint. They were also more likely to skip breakfast [64]. Other studies have shown post-bariatric patients to have increased consumption of sweets as well as excessive intake of calories. These patients also report insufficient intake of high-quality foods such as lean meats, eggs, fruits, and vegetables [58, 59]. Nonsurgical weight loss patients must practice and maintain dietary restraint and consistently eat a high-quality diet while restricting calories in order to produce weight loss, while patients who undergo weight loss surgery may not need to follow diet guidelines as strictly in order to lose weight. However, when weight loss ceases, if these patients have not implemented a permanent lifestyle change, they may be more likely to eat larger portions and return to poor eating habits, resulting in weight regain. The idea of permanent behavior change should be introduced and supported during all stages of the program in order to facilitate the maintenance effort.

Physical Activity

Regular physical activity is another component of a successful maintenance effort. The importance of regular, sustained physical activity is widely supported in the literature, as well as in practical evidence, as an essential part of weight loss and maintenance. In studies of those maintaining a large weight loss, exercise and self-monitoring are consistently reported as behaviors of successful maintainers [59, 64, 70–73, 76, 77, 79]. The NWLR data show that 90 % of participants who have kept off large amounts of weight exercise approximately one hour daily and engage in higher intensity activities [64, 80]. This increases the expenditure of overall calories, which can offset the increase in calorie intake and supports the overall commitment to healthy lifestyle choices. According to the American College of Sports Medicine (ACSM) expending >2,000 kcal per week is recommended for prevention of weight regain [81].

A large portion of the bariatric population is unable to exercise safely or comfortably. Many are awaiting other surgeries that will allow them to exercise more regularly, such as joint replacement or back surgery. For some, body habitus is all together preventative of activity outside of daily living (ADLs), and others cannot even perform ADLs without assistance. For the population who legitimately cannot exercise, seated exercise and physical therapy are viable options. It is important to have these patients engage in some sort of presurgery mobility to assist with conditioning as well as establish a routine and habits that can be built upon and continued after surgery. For other patients, embarrassment or dislike of exercise can inform a host of excuses for not being physically active. Problem solving and setting realistic goals to begin and continue with regular physical activity is important. Many programs utilize an exercise physiologist to work with their patients in overcoming barriers to exercise.

It is important to emphasize regular exercise and provide guidelines as a nonnegotiable part of a bariatric program. Continued support and accountability in this area is directly related to successful maintenance [59, 64, 70–74, 76, 77, 79]. The ACSM recommends moderate intensity cardiovascular exercise for ≥30 min ≥5 times a week for a total of ≥150 min per week. Resistance training of major muscle groups and stretching is recommended at least twice a week [81]. Setting smaller goals for patients to work up to this level of exercise is helpful. The ACSM position on exercise states, "Behaviorally based exercise interventions, the use of behavior change strategies, supervision by an experienced fitness instructor, and exercise that is pleasant and enjoyable can improve adoption and adherence to prescribed exercise programs" [81]. Bariatric program exercise guidelines should be clearly stated during preoperative education as well as monitored at all follow-up visits.

Nutrition Counseling and RD Contact

The degree of nutrition counseling and RD contact has also been cited as a postsurgical determinant of weight loss maintenance. Most patients report adequate nutrition counseling and follow-up immediately after surgery. However, as time passes, attendance for nutrition follow-up decreases dramatically. In several studies, lack of nutrition counseling after surgery is significantly associated with weight regain [57, 59, 82]. A clear plan for nutrition follow-up should be established preoperatively, and follow-up should be encouraged as an essential part of weight maintenance. Freire et al. reported that 47 % of patients studied reported never receiving nutrition follow-up in spite of being given specific instructions for when they should see the RD [59]. Magro and Ward-Kamar found 60 and 90 % of patients, respectively, in their studies never had nutritional follow-up after surgery [57, 82]. Papalazarou et al. demonstrated that providing nutrition and physical activity guidance as part of a lifestyle intervention after surgery results in increased weight loss and maintenance at 3 years [62].

Nutrition counseling immediately postsurgery and in the long term (2–5+ years) is an important mechanism to ensure a successful weight loss outcome of RYGB and other bariatric surgeries. Scheduling nutrition assessment and education by an RD at each follow-up visit ensures consistent and comprehensive reinforcement of and accountability for adherence to nutrition guidelines. Nutrition management after gastric bypass requires long-term follow-up that includes nutrition education, physical activity, and behavioral modification. Multidisciplinary bariatric aftercare is more likely to result in greater initial weight loss, better overall nutritional health, and increased rates of weight maintenance.

Review Questions and Answers

1. Which of the following are common nutrient deficiencies after RYGB?

   A. Calcium
   B. Vitamin D
   C. Iron
   D. Vitamin B12
   E. All of the above

Answer: E

2. Findings associated with zinc deficiency include all of the following except:

   A. Poor wound healing
   B. Hair loss
   C. Glossitis
   D. Ataxia
   E. Dermatitis

Answer: D

3. Which of the following is not a predictor of successful weight maintenance after RYGB?
   A. Involvement with support groups
   B. Time spent online
   C. Regular follow-up visits
   D. Physical activity

Answer: B

References

1. NIH conference. Gastrointestinal Surgery for Severe Obesity. Consensus Development Conference Panel. Ann Intern Med. 1991;115:956–61.
2. Seagle HM, Strain GW, Makris A, Reeves RS. Position of the American Dietetic Association: weight management. J Am Diet Assoc. 2009;109(2):330–46.
3. Aills L, Blankenship J, Buffington C, Furtado M, Parrot J. ASMBS allied health nutritional guidelines for the surgical weight loss patient. Surg Obes Relat Dis. 2008;4:S73–108.
4. Mechanick JI, Kushner RF, Sugerman HJ, Gonzalez-Campoy JM, Collazo-Clavell ML, Guven S, et al. American Association of Clinical Endocrinologists, The Obesity Society, and American Society for Metabolic and Bariatric Surgery Medical Guidelines for Clinical Practice for the perioperative nutritional, metabolic, and nonsurgical support of the bariatric surgery patient. Surg Obes Relat Dis. 2008;4(Suppl):S109–84.
5. Sheipe M. Breaking through obesity with gastric bypass surgery. Nurse Pract. 2006;31(10):12–4. 17, 18, 21.
6. Kulick D, Hark L, Deen D. The bariatric surgery patient: a growing role for registered dietitians. J Am Diet Assoc. 2010;110:600–7.
7. Ziegler O, Sirveaux MA, Brunaud L, Reibel N, Quilliot D. Medical follow-up after bariatric surgery: nutritional and drug issues. General recommendations for the prevention and treatment of nutritional deficiencies. Diabetes Metab. 2009;35(62):544–57.
8. Heber D, Greenway FL, Kaplan LM, Livingston E, Salvador J, Still C. Endocrine and nutritional management of the post-bariatric surgery patient: an Endocrine Society Clinical Practice Guideline. J Clin Endocrinol Metab. 2010;95(11):4823–43.
9. Rickers L, McSherry C. Bariatric surgery: nutritional considerations for patients. Nurs Stand. 2012;26(49):41–8.
10. McGlinch BP, Que FG, Nelson JL, Wrobleski DM, Grant JE, Collazo-Clavell ML. Perioperative care of patients undergoing bariatric surgery. Mayo Clin Proc. 2006;81(10 Suppl):S25–33.
11. McMahon MM, Sarr MG, Clark MM, Gall MM, Knoetgen 3rd J, Service FJ, et al. Clinical management after bariatric surgery: value of a multidisciplinary approach. Mayo Clin Proc. 2006;81(10 Suppl):S34–45.

12. Cummings S, Isom K. Bariatric surgery: time to standardize nutritional care. Presented at: The American Dietetic Association's Food & Nutrition Conference & Expo, San Diego (2011 Sep 26)

13. Elliot K. Nutritional considerations after bariatric surgery. Crit Care Nurs Q. 2003;26(2):133–8.

14. Parkes E. Nutritional management of patients after bariatric surgery. Am J Med Sci. 2006;331(4):207–13.

15. Flatt JP. The biochemistry of energy expenditure. In: Bray GA, editor. Recent advances in obesity research. London: Newman; 1978. p. 211–28.

16. Frank L. Why we promote protein intake and exercise in our bariatric patients: biological drivers behind the scene. Presented at: ASMBS 29th Annual Meeting, San Diego (2012 Jun 18)

17. Sumner AE. Elevated methylmalonic acid and total homocysteine levels show high prevalence of Vitamin B-12 deficiency after gastric surgery. Ann Intern Med. 1996;124:469–76.

18. Zaidel O, Lin HC. Uninvited guests: the impact of small intestinal bacterial overgrowth on nutritional status. Pract Gastroenterol. 2003;27:27–34.

19. Vargas-Ruiz AG, Hernandez- Rivera G, Herrera MF. Prevalence of iron, folate and vitamin B12 deficiency after laparoscopic Roux-en-Y gastric bypass. Obes Surg. 2008;18:288–93.

20. Brolin RE, LaMarca LB, Kenler HA, Cody RP. Malabsorptive gastric bypass in patients with superobesity. J Gastrointest Surg. 2002;6:195–205.

21. Brolin RE, Gorman JH, Gorman RC, Petschenik AJ, Bradley LJ, Kenler HA, Cody RP. Are vitamin B12 and folate deficiency clinically important after Roux-en-Y Gastric bypass? J Gastrointest Surg. 1998;2:436–42.

22. Clements RH, Katasani VG, Palepu R, Leeth RR, Leath TD, Roy BP, et al. Incidence of vitamin deficiency after laparoscopic Roux-en-Y gastric bypass in a university hospital setting. Am Surg. 2006;72:1196–204.

23. Toh SY, Zarshenas N, Jorgenson J. Prevalence of nutrient deficiencies in bariatric patients. Nutrition. 2009;25:1150–6.

24. Rhose BM, Arseneau P, Cooper BA, Katz M, Gilfix BM, MacLean LD. Vitamin B-12 deficiency after gastric surgery for obesity. Am J Clin Nutr. 1996;63:103–9.

25. Brolin RE, Gorman JH, Gorman RC, Petschenik AJ, Bradley LB, Kenler HA, Cody RP. Prophylactic iron supplementation after Roux-en-Y gastric bypass. Arch Surg. 1998;133:740–4.

26. Marion M, Russell MK, Shikora SA. Clinical nutrition for the surgical patient. Sudbury: Jones and Bartlett; 2008.

27. Koch T, Finelli F. Postoperative metabolic and nutritional complications of bariatric surgery. Gastroenterol Clin N Am. 2010;39:109–24.

28. Ming S, Gornichec RS. Therapeutic treatment options for osteoporosis in the surgical weight loss population. Bariatric Times. 2011;8(4):8–10.

29. Valtueña Martínez S. Obesity and osteoporosis: effect of weight variation on bone mass. Nutr Hosp. 2002;17 Suppl 1:49–54.

30. Gemmell K, Santry HP, Prachand VN, Alverdy JC. Vitamin D deficiency in pre-operative bariatric surgery patients. Surg Obes Relat Dis. 2009;5:54–9.

31. Madan AK, Orth WS, Tichansky DS, Ternovits CA. Vitamin and trace mineral levels after laparoscopic gastric bypass. Obes Surg. 2006;16:603–6.

32. Coupaye M, Puchaux K, Bogard C, Msika S, Jouet P, Clerici C, Larger E, Ledoux S. Nutritional consequences of adjustable gastric banding and gastric bypass: a 1-year prospective study. Obes Surg. 2009;19:56–65.

33. Flores L, Martinez Osaba MJ, Andreu A, Moize V, Rodriguex L, Vidal J. Calcium and vitamin D supplementation after gastric bypass should be individualized to improve or avoid hyperparathyroidism. Obes Surg. 2010;20:738–43.

34. Fish E, Beverstein G, Olson D, Reinhardt S, Garren M, Gould J. Vitamin D status of morbidly obese bariatric surgery patients. J Surg Res. 2010;164:198–202.

35. Slater GH, Ren CJ, Seigel N, Williams T, Barr D, Wolfe B, et al. Serum fat-soluble vitamin deficiency and abnormal calcium metabolism after malabsorptive bariatric surgery. J Gastrointest Surg. 2004;8:48–55.

36. Gehrer S, Kern B, Peters T, Christoffel-Courtin C, Peterli R. Fewer nutrient deficiencies after laparoscopic sleeve gastrectomy (LSG) than after laparoscopic Roux-Y-Gastric bypass (LRYGB)—a prospective study. Obes Surg. 2010;20:447–53.

37. Kumar N, McEvoy KM, Ahlskog E. Myelopathy due to copper deficiency following gastrointestinal surgery. Arch Neurol. 2003;60:1783–5.

38. Griffith DP, Liff DA, Zeigler TR, Esper GJ, Winton EF. Acquired copper deficiency: a potentially serious and preventable complication following gastric bypass surgery. Obesity. 2009;17:827–31.

39. O'Donnell KB, Simmons M. Early-onset copper deficiency following Roux-en-Y gastric bypass. Nutr Clin Pract. 2011;26:66–9.

40. Naismith R, Shepard J, Weihl C, Tutlam N, Cross A. Acute and bilateral blindness due to optic neuropathy associated with copper deficiency. Arch Neurol. 2009;66:1025–7.

41. Gletsu-Miller N, Broderius M, Frediani JK, Zhao VM, Griffith DP, Davis Jr SS, et al. Incidence and prevalence of copper deficiency following roux-en-y gastric bypass surgery. Int J Obes. 2011;36:328–35.

42. Shahidzadeh R, Sridhar S. Profound copper deficiency in a patient with gastric bypass. Am J Gastroenterol. 2008;103:2660–2.

43. Rudnicki SA. Prevention and treatment of peripheral neuropathy after bariatric surgery. Curr Treat Options Neurol. 2010;12:29–36.

44. Frank L. Bariatric Beriberi: Thiamin deficiency in Bariatric patients. Bariatric Times. 2011;8:14.

45. Singh S, Kumar A. Wernicke's encephalopathy after obesity surgery: a systemic review. Neurology. 2007;68:807–11.

46. Aasheim E. Wernicke's encephalopathy after Bariatric surgery: a systemic review. Ann Surg. 2008;238:714–20.

47. Ambrose ML, Bowden SC, Whelan G. Thiamin treatment and working memory function of alcohol-dependant people: preliminary finding. Alcohol Clin Exp Res. 2001;25:112–6.

48. Bloomberg RD, Fleishman A, Nalle JE, Herron DM, Kini S. Nutritional deficiencies following Bariatric surgery: what have we learned? Obes Surg. 2005;15:145–54.

49. King JC. Zinc: an essential but elusive nutrient. Am J Clin Nutr. 2011;94(Suppl):679s–84s.

50. Cominetti C, Garrido Jr AB, Cozzolino SM. Zinc nutritional status of morbidly obese patients before and after Roux-en-Y gastric bypass: a preliminary report. Obes Surg. 2006;16:448–53.

51. Gong K, Gagner M, Pomp A, Almahmeed T, Bardaro SJ. Micronutrient deficiencies after laparoscopic gastric bypass: recommendations. Obes Surg. 2008;18:1062–6.

52. Bal BS, Finelli FC, Shope TR, Koch TR. Nutritional deficiencies after bariatric surgery. Nat Rev Endocrinol. 2012;8(9):544–56.

53. Davies D, Baxter JM, Baxter JN. Nutritional deficiencies after Bariatric surgery. Obes Surg. 2007;17:1150–8.

54. Eckert MJ, Perry JT, Sohn VY, Boden J, Martin MJ, Rush RM, Steele SR. Incidence of low vitamin A levels and ocular symptoms after Roux-en-Y gastric bypass. Surg Obes Relat Dis. 2010;6:653–7.

55. Simmons M. Modern-Day Scurvy: a case following gastric bypass. Bariatric Nursing Surg Patient Care. 2009;4:139–44.

56. Strohmayer E, Via M, Yanagisawa R. Metabolic management following Bariatric surgery. Mt Sinai J Med. 2010;77:431–5.

57. Magro D, Geloneze B, Delfini R, Pareja B, Callejas F, Pareja J. Long-term weight re-gain after gastric bypass: a 5-year prospective study. Obes Surg. 2008;18:648–51.

58. Odom J, Zalesin K, Washington T, Miller W, Hakmeh B, Zaremba D, et al. Behavioral predictors of weight re-gain after bariatric surgery. Obes Surg. 2010;20:349–56.

59. Freire R, Borges M, Alvarez-Leite J, Correia M. Food quality, physical activity and nutritional follow-up as determinant of weight re-gain after roux-en-y gastric bypass. Nutrition. 2012; 28:53–8.

60. Buchwald H, Avidor Y, Braunwald E, Jensen M, Pories W, Fahrback K. Bariatric surgery: a systematic review and meta-analysis. JAMA. 2008;292:1724–37.

61. Peacock J, Zizzi S. An assesment of patient behavioral requirements pre- and post-surgery at accredited weight loss surgical centers. Obes Surg. 2011;21:1950–7.

62. Papalazarou A, Yannakoulia M, Davouras S, Komesidou V, Dimitriadis G, Papakonstantinou A, et al. Lifestyle intervention favorably affects weight loss and maintenance following obesity surgery. Obesity. 2010;18:1348–53.

63. Forbush S, Nof L, Echternach J, Hill C, Rainey J. Influence of activity levels and energy intake on percent excess weight loss after roux-en-y gastric bypass. Obes Surg. 2011;21:1731–8.

64. Bond D, Phelan S, Leahey T, Hill J, Wing R. Weight-loss maintenance in successful weight losers: surgical vs non-surgical methods. Int J Obes. 2009;33:173–80.

65. Song Z, Reinhardt K, Buzdon M, Liao P. Association between support group attendance and weight loss after roux-en-y gastric bypass. Surg Obes Relat Dis. 2008;4(2):100–3.

66. Orth W, Madan A, Taddeucci R, Coday M, Tichansky D. Support group meeting attendance is associated with better weight loss. Obes Surg. 2008;18(4):391–4.

67. Saunders R. Post-surgery group therapy for gastric bypass patients. Obes Surg. 2004;14(8):1128–31.

68. Marcus J, Elkins G. Development of a model for a structured support group for patients following bariatric surgery. Obes Surg. 2004;14(1):103–6.

69. Hildebrandt S. Effects of participation in bariatric support group after roux-en-y gastric bypass. Obes Surg. 1998;8(5):535–42.

70. Neve M, Morgan P, Collins C. Behavioural factors related with successful weight loss 15 months post-enrollment in a commercial web-based weight-loss programme. Public Health Nutr. 2012;15(7): 1299–309.

71. Wang J, Sereika S, Chasens E, Ewing L, Matthews J, Burke L. Effect of adherence to self-monitoring of diet and physical activity on weight loss in a technology-supported behavioral intervention. Patient Prefer Adherence. 2012;6:221–6.

72. Akers JD, Cornett RA, Savla JS, Davy KP, Davy BM. Daily self-monitoring of body weight, step count, fruit/vegetable intake, and water consumption: a feasible and effective long-term weight loss maintenance approach. J Acad Nutr Diet. 2012;112(5):685–92.

73. Reyes N, Oliver T, Klotz A, Lagrotte C, Vander Veur S, Virus A, Bailer B, et al. Similarities and differences between weight loss maintainers and re-gainers: a qualitative analysis. J Acad Nutr Diet. 2012;112(4):499–505.

74. Conroy M, Yang K, Elci O, Gabriel K, Styn MA, Wang J, et al. Physical activity self-monitoring and weight loss: 6-month results of the SMART trial. Med Sci Sports Exerc. 2011;43(8):1568–74.

75. Butryn M, Phelan S, Hill J, Wing R. Consistent self-monitoring of weight: a key component of successful weight loss maintenance. Obesity. 2007;12:3091–6.

76. McGuire M, Wing R, Klem M, Hill J. Behavioral strategies of individuals who have maintained long-term weight losses. Obes Res. 1999;7(4):334–41.

77. Wing R, Hill J. Successful weight loss maintenance. Annu Rev Nutr. 2001;21:323–41.

78. Mathus-Vliegen E. Long-term health and psychosocial outcomes from surgically induced weight loss: results obtained in patients not attending protocolled follow-up visits. Int J Obes. 2009;31:299–307.

79. Welch G, Wesolowski C, Piepul B, Kuhn J, Romanelli J, Garb J. Physical activity predicts weight loss following gastric bypass surgery: findings from a support group survey. Obes Surg. 2008;18(5):517–24.

80. Klem M, Wing R, McGuire M, Seagle H, Hill J. A descriptive study of individuals successful at long-term maintenance of substantial weight loss. Am J Clin Nutr. 1997;66:239–46.

81. Jakicic J, Clark K, Coleman E, Donnelly J, Foreyt J, Melanson E, et al. Appropriate Intervention strategies for weight loss and prevention of weight re-gain for adults. Med Sci Sports Exer. 2001; 33:2145–56.

82. Warde-Kamar J, Rogers M, Fancbaum L, Laferrere B. Calorie intake and meal patterns up to 4 years after Roux-n-Y gastric bypass surgery. Obes Surg. 2004;14:1070–9.

32

Laparoscopic Malabsorptive Procedures: Technique of Duodenal Switch

Giovanni Dapri, Guy-Bernard Cadière, and Jacques Himpens

Patient and Team's Positioning

General anesthesia is realized and patient is positioned in the supine position with legs apart. The patient is carefully strapped to the operative table and both arms are placed in abduction. Shoulder supports are used and extreme care is taken to pad the pressure points and joints with foam cushions. The surgeon stands between the patient's legs, with the camera person to the patient's right and the assistant to the patient's left (Fig. 1).

Trocars' Positioning

The following six abdominal trocars are placed: a 10 mm trocar (T1) 20 cm distal to the xiphoid process for the 30° optical system, a 5 mm trocar (T2) on the left anterior axillary line about 5 cm distal to the costal margin, a 12 mm trocar (T3) on the midclavicular line in the left upper quadrant between the first and second trocars, a 12 mm trocar (T4) on the right midclavicular line in the right upper quadrant, a 5 mm trocar (T5) distal and to the left of the xiphoid process, and a 5 mm trocar (T6) to the left of the midline in the lower abdomen (Fig. 2).

Sleeve Gastrectomy

This procedure can be performed using two methods: lateral-to-medial and medial-to-lateral approaches [3]. The patient is placed in the reversed Trendelenburg position.

Electronic supplementary material: Supplementary material is available in the online version of this chapter at 10.1007/978-1-4939-1637-5_32. Videos can also be accessed at http://www.springerimages.com/videos/978-1-4939-1636-8.

Lateral-to-Medial Approach

After identification of the crow's foot, an oblique line is marked on the anterior gastric surface with the coagulating hook, between the end of the gastric vessels both on the lesser and greater curvatures, at the level of the most distal vessels in the direction of the pylorus. The lesser sac is opened through a window made in the greater omentum within the epiploic vessels, 3 cm lateral to the marked line and close to the greater curvature of the stomach. This window is extended in a caudal direction until the marked line first and then cranially to the direction of the left diaphragmatic pillar, to completely dissect the greater omentum off the greater curvature. Coagulating hook, bipolar shears, or harmonic shears can be used. The dissection ends after the left diaphragmatic pillar is reached. All retrogastric adhesions are divided. Two first firings of the linear stapler (green/black load) are introduced through the T4 and divide the greater curvature in the direction of the crow's foot. The linear stapler is placed with its extremity close to the terminations of the gastric vessels on the lesser curvature. A third firing of the linear stapler (green/black load) is introduced through the T3 and transect the stomach parallel to the lesser curvature. After this last firing of the stapler, the anesthesiologist pushes down an orogastric tube of 36 Fr, in order to guide the gastric transection. The stomach is sectioned from the antrum up to the fundus at the level of the angle of His using other firings of the linear stapler (T3) (gold/purple load) (Fig. 3a). The resected stomach is left in the left upper quadrant and it is extracted in the plastic bag at the end of the procedure through the enlargement of the T3. Different options are available to manage the staple line. The staple line can be left without sutures or without the use of buttressing material; the staple line can be oversewn by two converting running sutures using absorbable material; only some stitches are placed between the terminations of the staple lines; buttressing material is used for firings of the stapler [4].

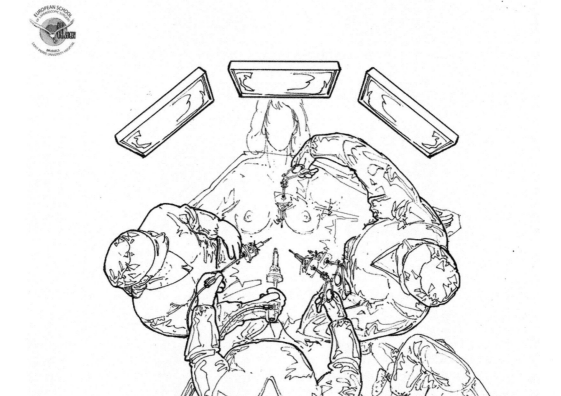

FIG. 1. Sleeve gastrectomy and beginning of duodenal switch: patient and team's positioning.

Medial-to-Lateral Approach

After the stomach is marked between the crow's foot and the pylorus, the lesser sac is opened just enough to allow the introduction of linear stapler through the T4. Two firings of the linear stapler (green/black load) are fired taking the extremity of the stapler close to the terminations of the gastric vessels on the lesser curvature. After sectioning the stomach at the level of the incisura angularis, the anesthesiologist pushes down the 36 Fr orogastric tube to guide the gastric transection in the direction of the angle of His. Further firings of the linear stapler (T3) (gold/purple load) are kept parallel to the lesser curve (Fig. 3b), and all the posterior gastric adhesions are divided. Before the last firing of the stapler, the angle of His is freed from bottom to top and vice versa; the stomach is sectioned placing the stapler lateral to the left pillar and without tension. The greater omentum is dissected from the transected greater curvature of the stomach, using the coagulating hook, bipolar shears, or harmonic shears. The resected stomach and the staple line are managed as described above.

Duodenal Switch

Laparoscopic duodenal switch is a technically difficult procedure, demanding considerable laparoscopic skill, accompanied by the possibility of intraoperative complications and characterized by postoperative morbidity. Superobese ($50 < BMI < 60$ kg/m^2) and super-superobese ($BMI > 60$ kg/m^2)

patients are often affected by arterial hypertension, diabetes type II, sleep apnea, degenerative joint, cardiovascular, pulmonary, and metabolic diseases that put them at adversely increased surgical risks. In order to decrease the morbidity and mortality, and the overall risk of perioperative complications, it has been reported [5] to separate this procedure into two steps: sleeve gastrectomy first and biliopancreatic diversion later. In this way, patients submitted to sleeve gastrectomy can achieve a sustained weight loss

and reduce the severity of obesity-related comorbidities, and after an interval time between 6 months and 2 years, the procedure of duodenal switch can be performed under safer conditions [6].

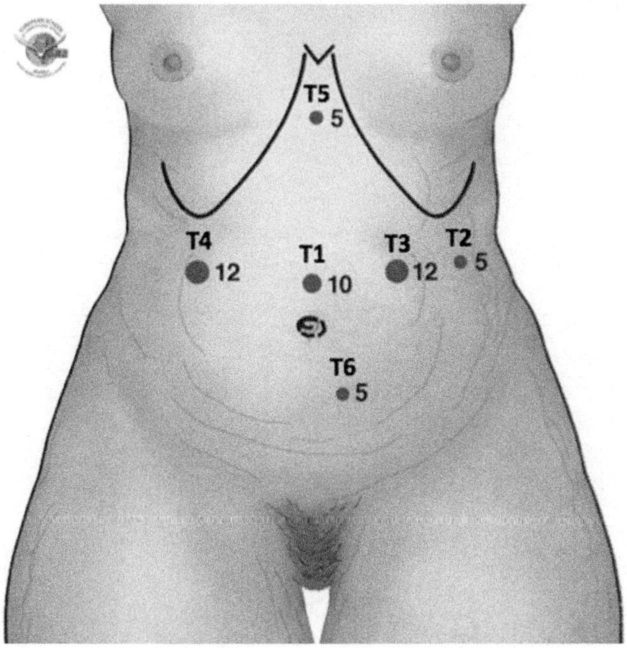

Cholecystectomy and Duodenal Section

Cholecystectomy is performed and the specimen is extracted in a plastic bag through the T3 at the end of the procedure. The duodenum can be sectioned using two methods:

- *Posterior approach*: the antrum is held up and all the retrogastric adhesions from the antrum to the pylorus are divided by the coagulating hook. A passage just anteriorly to the pancreatic head and gastroduodenal artery is created with gentle dissection in the direction of the common bile duct. The superior and inferior edges of the duodenum are freed and a piece of cotton tissue tape is used to encircle the duodenum. The tape facilitates in holding the first duodenum upwards for insertion and firing of the linear stapler (blue/purple load) through the T3 (Fig. 4a). The duodenum is divided.
- *Anterior approach*: after identification of the pylorus, the anterior peritoneal sheet at the superior border of the first duodenum, across from the common bile duct, is dissected by the coagulating hook. A passage between the above first duodenum and the pancreatic head is created under vision. The first duodenum is encircled by a piece of cotton tissue tape. The tape is taken up in order to permit the introduction of the linear stapler (blue/purple load) through the T3, and the duodenum is transected (Fig. 4b). The gastroduodenal artery is usually visible under the first duodenum after this section.

FIG. 2. Duodenal switch: trocars' positioning.

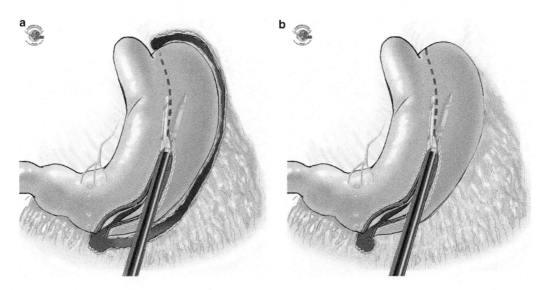

FIG. 3 Sleeve gastrectomy: (**a**) lateral-to-medial and (**b**) medial-to-lateral approaches.

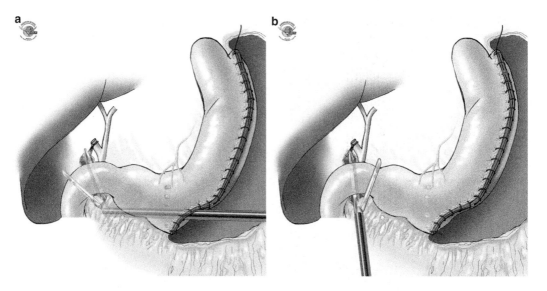

Fɪɢ. 4. Duodenal section: (**a**) posterior and (**b**) anterior approaches.

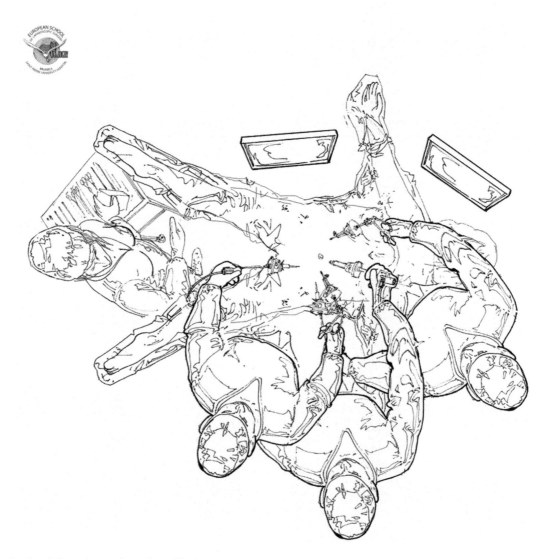

Fɪɢ. 5. Duodenal switch: patient and team's positioning.

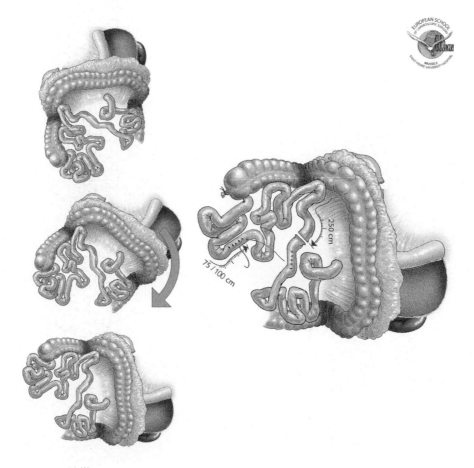

FIG. 6. Common, alimentary and biliopancreatic limbs' measurement.

Common, Alimentary and Biliopancreatic Limbs' Measurement

The patient is positioned in the Trendelenburg position with a right tilt. The surgeon, camera person, and assistant moved to the patient's left (Fig. 5). Appendectomy is performed and retrieved in a plastic bag at the end of the procedure through the T3. The cecum is dissected off the parietal wall by the coagulating hook, in order to facilitate subsequent lifting of the alimentary loop for the duodenoileostomy. From the ileocecal valve, the small bowel is measured for a distance of 75 or 100 cm (common limb) (Fig. 6). The measurements are made by stretching the bowel along a 25 cm cotton tissue tape. A stitch (polydiaxone 2/0) is placed on the small bowel wall at this measured level (Fig. 6) and temporarily parked into the parietal peritoneum. The small bowel distal to the stitch, and going in the direction of the ileocecal valve, is superficially marked by the coagulating hook and constitutes the common limb. From this point, another 175 or 150 cm is measured and constitutes the alimentary limb (Fig. 6). The bowel proximal to the measured segment of 175-150 cm, and going in the direction of the angle of Treitz, is marked by the coagulating hook and constitutes the biliopancreatic limb.

A temporary clip is placed just distal to this point and represents the proximal end of the alimentary limb, which will be used for the duodenoileostomy. A firing of linear stapler (T3) (white/tan load) divides the small bowel between the biliopancreatic limb and the proximal end of the alimentary limb (Fig. 6). The common and alimentary limbs are fashioned and measured at 75–100 and 175–150 cm, respectively.

Jejunoileostomy

This anastomosis can be performed through three different methods:

– *Totally handsewn side-to-side*: the stitch parked into the parietal peritoneum is used to join the common limb to the biliopancreatic limb in a continuous layer (polydiaxone 2/0), which represents the posterior layer of the jejunoileostomy. The running suture is held by a grasper (T2) and the common limb by another grasper (T4) in the opposite direction, in order to place the bowel loops under traction. A new running suture is started (polydiaxone 2/0), and both bowel loops are opened by the coagulating hook (Fig. 7a). The new running suture

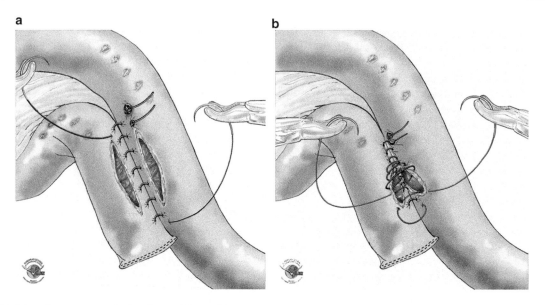

FIG. 7. (**a**, **b**) Jejunoileostomy: totally handsewn side-to-side.

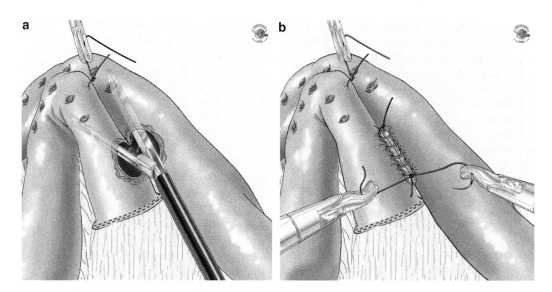

FIG. 8. (**a**, **b**) Jejunoileostomy: linear mechanical side-to-side.

is used for the anterior layer of the jejunoileostomy. The posterior running suture, taken along the inferior angle of the anastomosis, is continued on for a short distance onto the anterior layer of the anastomosis (Fig. 7b). The posterior and the anterior running sutures are finally tied halfway on the anterior layer.

– *Linear mechanical side-to-side*: the small bowel at the 75–100 cm marking (the marks will help to remain oriented) is sutured to the biliopancreatic limb, using the same stitch (polydiaxone 2/0) that was parked into the parietal peritoneum. The stitch is maintained under tension by a grasper (T4), and the common and biliopancreatic limbs are opened with the coagulating hook. A linear stapler

(white/tan load) is introduced through the T3 and fired to join both limbs (Fig. 8a). The enteric openings are closed by two running sutures using absorbable materials (polydiaxone 2/0) (Fig. 8b), and the temporary stitch is removed.

– *Totally mechanical side-to-side*: the common limb is positioned beside the biliopancreatic limb. Both small bowel loops are opened by the coagulating hook. A first firing of linear stapler (white/tan load), introduced through the T4, joins the common limb to the biliopancreatic limb in one direction. A second firing of the linear stapler limb (white/tan load), introduced through the T3, joins the two loops in the opposite direction (Fig. 9a). Finally, the enteric openings are closed by a third firing of the linear

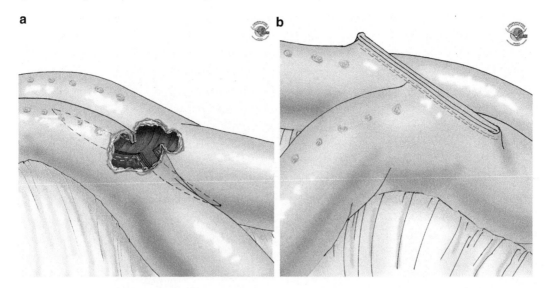

FIG. 9. (**a**, **b**) Jejunoileostomy: totally mechanical side-to-side.

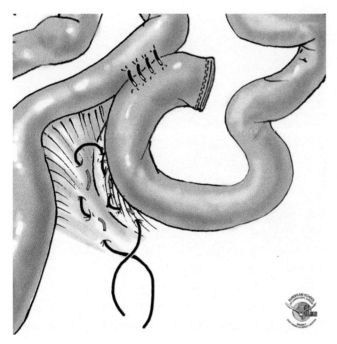

FIG. 10. Mesenteric defect closure.

stapler (white/tan load), introduced through the T3 and positioned perpendicular to the first two firings (Fig. 9b).

Regardless of the type of the jejunoileostomy, the mesenteric defect, between the common and the biliopancreatic limbs, is closed after the anastomosis. A nonabsorbable purse-string suture (polypropylene 1) is used to close this defect in order to prevent internal hernia (Fig. 10). The proximal end of the alimentary limb is taken by a grasper (T6) in the direction of the first duodenum.

Duodenoileostomy

The patient is replaced in the reversed Trendelenburg position. The surgeon returns between the patient's legs, the camera person to the patient's right, and the assistant to the patient's left (Fig. 1). The proximal end of the alimentary limb is maintained cephalic by the grasper (T6).

The duodenoileostomy can be performed through two main methods:

– *Totally handsewn end-to-side*: a running suture (polydiaxone 2/0) is begun on the superior corner of the transected duodenum and successive bites are taken alternatively on the duodenum and on the proximal end of the alimentary limb in order to perform the end-to-side duodenoileostomy (Fig. 11a). This suture, which constitutes the posterior layer of the anastomosis, is continued around the inferior corner and onto the anterior layer for a short distance, and the duodenum and the alimentary limb are opened with the coagulating hook (Fig. 11b). A new running suture (polydiaxone 2/0) starting on the superior corner constitutes the anterior layer of the duodenoileostomy. Finally the two running sutures are tied together halfway on the anterior layer.

– *Linear mechanical end-to-side*: the duodenum is opened at its inferior angle by the coagulating hook, and the alimentary limb at the same level as well. A linear stapler (blue load) is introduced through the T3 and advanced into the duodenum and the alimentary limb and fired (Fig. 12a). The enteric openings are closed using two converting running sutures (polydiaxone 2/0), starting at both angles and tied together halfway (Fig. 12b).

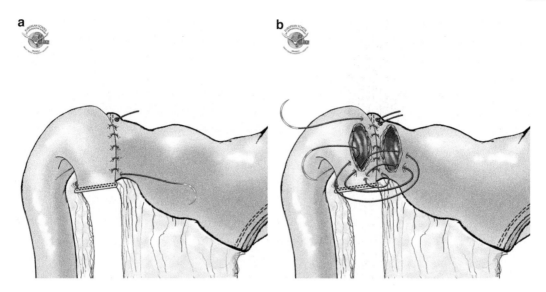

FIG. 11. (**a**, **b**) Duodenoileostomy: totally handsewn end-to-side.

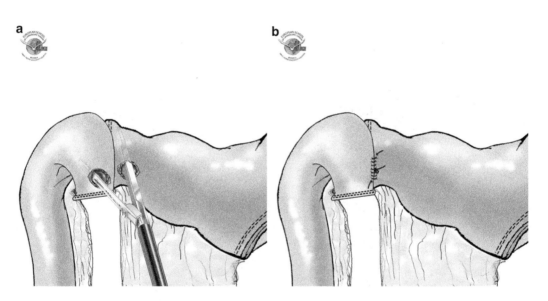

FIG. 12. (**a**, **b**) Duodenoileostomy: linear mechanical end-to-side.

Regardless of the type of duodenoileostomy, Petersen's space, a potential defect formed as a result of the procedure between the mesentery of the alimentary limb and the transverse mesocolon, is closed to prevent an internal hernia. A nonabsorbable purse-string suture (polypropylene 1) is used to close the defect (Fig. 13).

Leak Test

The leak test is performed both to test the sleeve gastrectomy and the duodenoileostomy (Fig. 14). The patient is placed in the Trendelenburg position and the operating field is immersed under saline solution. Compressed air is insufflated into the stomach by the anesthesiologist. The absence of air bubbles is testimony of the integrity of the sleeve gastrectomy and of the duodenoileostomy. This maneuver allows assessing good symmetry of the sleeve. Moreover, the advantage of using compressed air is also to check the jejunoileostomy distally.

Specimens' Removal

The stomach, gallbladder, and appendix are extracted in plastic bags through the enlargement of the T3, which is subsequently closed in layers. The procedure is concluded with the placement of a drain along the sleeve gastrectomy, up to the upper pole of the spleen, and another drain close to the duodenoileostomy.

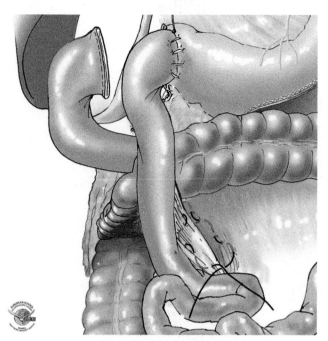

FIG. 13. Petersen's space closure.

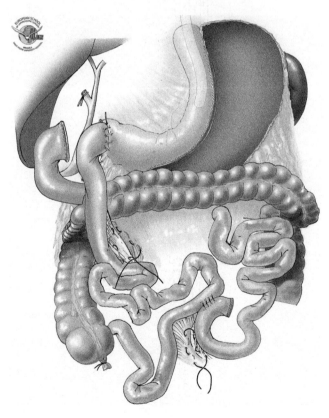

FIG. 14. Leak test.

Postoperative Management

A nasogastric tube is left in place for the first 24 h. A peroral methylene blue test is performed on the second postoperative day, and if negative, the patient is allowed to start a liquid diet on the third postoperative day. The patient is discharged from the hospital on the fifth postoperative day.

The patient is restricted to a liquid diet for the first 4 weeks, then to a semiliquid diet for another 4 weeks, followed by a pureed diet for another 4 weeks. At that time if there are no problems, the patient is advanced to a regular diet. Exercising is encouraged from the second postoperative week onwards. Patients are instructed to take either an H2 blocker or proton-pump inhibitor for at least 3 months.

Patients are followed up by the surgeon, nutritionist, and psychologist. The first follow-up visit is at 1 month after the procedure. Following that, the patient is reviewed at 3-monthly intervals in the first year, followed by two 6-monthly visits in the second year, and by further annual visits for the next 3 years.

References

1. Hess DS, Hess DW. Biliopancreatic diversion with a duodenal switch. Obes Surg. 1998;8:267–82.
2. Marceau P, Hould FS, Simard S, et al. Biliopancreatic diversion with duodenal switch. World J Surg. 1998;22:947–54.
3. Dapri G, Vaz C, Cadière GB, Himpens J. A prospective randomized study comparing two different techniques for laparoscopic sleeve gastrectomy. Obes Surg. 2007;17:1435–41.
4. Dapri G, Cadière GB, Himpens J. Reinforcing the staple line during laparoscopic sleeve gastrectomy: prospective randomized clinical study comparing three different techniques. Obes Surg. 2010;20:462–7.
5. Ren CJ, Patterson E, Gagner M. Early results of laparoscopic biliopancreatic diversion with duodenal switch: a case series of 40 consecutive patients. Obes Surg. 2000;10:514–23.
6. Dapri G, Cadière GB, Himpens J. Superobese and super super-obese patients: 2-step laparoscopic duodenal switch. Surg Obes Relat Dis. 2011;7:703–8.

33

Laparoscopic Malabsorption Procedures: Outcomes

Mitchell S. Roslin and Robert Sung

Introduction

The fantasy for many is to eat what they want, when they want it. Often, this cannot occur without gaining weight or suffering medical consequences from obesity. Thus, it is easy to understand the attraction of malabsorption for weight loss. Superficially, it seems that more can be eaten but less digested. Therefore, food can be consumed in excess, with the short-circuiting of the intestine causing less to be absorbed and resulting in sustained weight loss. Unfortunately, operations designed in this manner had predictable issues with short bowel length.

Bariatric surgery and metabolic surgery have evolved to reverse highly morbid chronic diseases, improve quality of live, and extend live expectancy. However, there is also a history of failed procedures and unanticipated morbidity and mortality. Frequently, severe complications arise years following the procedure.

The purpose of this chapter is to review what we have learned from the past using the jejunoileal bypass as a model and explain the differences in the procedures that are performed today. Although purely malabsorptive procedures have been abandoned, we still evaluate patients that have had recent malabsorptive procedures that are likely to fail. They are performed to offer the weight loss advantages of procedures such as the duodenal switch and biliopancreatic diversion. However, while the goal is to simplify the technical difficulty that is required to perform these procedures minimally invasively, they ignore the subtle differences that make these procedures tolerable for the majority of patients.

As an example, we have recently cared for a middle-aged female that had to work from home secondary to an odor coming from her entire body after conversion to a distal gastric bypass. In 2002, she had an open gastric bypass and went from 250 to 160 lb. Five years later, she began to regain weight and was over 230 lb when she decided to have a conversion to a distal procedure. Her Roux limb was detached and then reattached 50 cm from the terminal ileum. At reoperation performed in June, she had a total bowel length of 175 cm and common channel of 50 cm. She had lost weight and was only 150 lb but required TPN for over a year. She had to consume 5,000–6,000 cal/day to stay off TPN. This caused 20 bowel movements daily and an odor that was transmitted from every bodily surface, including her skin and mouth. Her chief complaint was "I smell and cannot live this way." Her co-workers actually called the Department of Health. The reason we decided to start with this unfortunate case is to highlight the dangers of short bowel length. Sadly in this case, history was forgotten. Thirty-five years since the jejunoileal bypass has been abandoned, operations that cause similar issues are still performed with a surgically induced short bowel syndrome as the consequence.

Our objective in bariatric and weight loss surgery is to achieve meaningful long-term weight loss, which correlates with improved medical and emotional health. Consequently, procedures that cause weight loss but result in loss of muscle mass, bone density, and poor overall function are not satisfactory. Unfortunately, this data is hard to assemble. Outcome studies tend to focus on weight loss, resolution of comorbidities, and early morbidity and mortality. Patients that have lasting weight loss, no sentinel early complication, may seem like they had an outstanding result. However, many of the problems present years after surgery and cause debilitating issues that are difficult to manage.

Short Bowel Syndrome

In essence, the principle of malabsorption for weight loss necessitates the creation of a shortened bowel or a tolerable short bowel syndrome. Therefore before contemplating a malabsorptive bariatric procedure, we should review short bowel syndrome. How much bowel is required, how does it present, and what are the short- and long-term complications?

S.A. Brethauer et al. (eds.), *Minimally Invasive Bariatric Surgery*,
DOI 10.1007/978-1-4939-1637-5_33, © Springer Science+Business Media New York 2015

It is estimated that the average adult has approximately 23 ft of small bowel. Additionally, the compensatory capacity of the bowel is so vast that after resections for inflammatory bowel disease or bowel ischemia, the majority of individuals can tolerate having 6–7 ft of small bowel. These patients also generally have a normal stomach with the pylorus preserved and a competent ileocecal valve. Patients with less than 6 ft of bowel that initially require parenteral nutrition can occasionally be taken off these feeds as villi hypertrophy and the small bowel compensates. Unfortunately, certain patients cannot be weaned and potentially can require small bowel transplant.

What happens when there is too little bowel? The first issue to arise is frequent diarrhea. In order to maintain hydration and any level of nutrition, patients need to eat and drink continuously. This actually increases the passage of caustic items to the colon, stimulating inflammation and exacerbating these already problematic issues.

Obviously, absorption of nutrients is limited. As a result, protein deficiency can occur with all its resultant manifestations. Essential fatty acids and vitamins are missing which can lead to irreversible neurologic conditions. Vitamin A deficiency can lead to blindness. Poor calcium and vitamin D absorption causes bone breakdown and osteoporosis. Iron and B12 deficiencies cause anemia, further weakening the malnourished patient. Oxalate is passed into the colon, leading to its reabsorption and the formation of oxalate stones in the kidney. Poor nutrition leads to deficiencies in immune function.

Clearly short bowel and its manifestations do not meet the objective that most of us have in bariatric surgery.

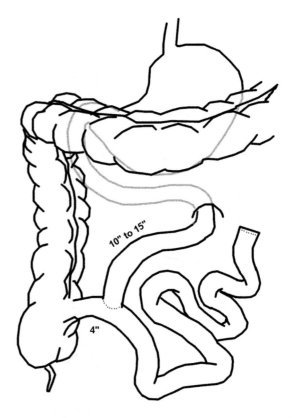

Fig. 1. The Payne jejunal-ileal bypass. Reproduced with permission from Diana McPhee.

The JIB: What Was It and What Were the Problems It Created? Surgical Short Bowel Syndrome

The classic intestinal-only operation or malabsorptive procedure was the jejunoileal bypass or JIB. Introduced in the 1950s, it remained popular until the early 1970s. While there were several variations, the most common divided the small bowel 10–15 in. from the ligament of Treitz. The divided end was anastomosed to the ileum approximately 4 in. proximal to the ileocecal valve in an end-to-side manner. The classic Payne procedure anastomosed the cut end of the proximal jejunum into the side of the terminal ileum (Fig. 1) [1]. A modification by Scott divided the distal bowel as well and anastomosed the proximal jejunum to the distal ileum in an end-to-end fashion (Fig. 2). Then, the proximal end of the divided jejunum was anastomosed to the transverse or descending colon to prevent a closed loop obstruction [2].

In essence, the JIB was a surgically induced short bowel syndrome. It was based on the notion that morbidly obese individuals had excess reserves. Thus, they could sustain the

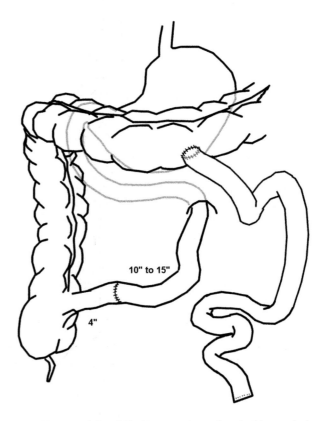

Fig. 2. The Scott jejunal-ileal bypass. Reproduced with permission from Diana McPhee.

early period, eat enough, and have the bowel hypertrophy and compensate. Unfortunately, we have learned that with obesity you have excess fat and increased inflammation, not increased nutritional reserve.

While weight loss was acceptable, there were many issues.

1. Inadequate Bowel Length

   While the stomach was left unchanged, the JIB shortened overall bowel length drastically. There is a wide range of total bowel length in individuals with average ranging from 20 to 23 ft. The JIB reduced total bowel length to approximately 18 in. This led to poor absorption of all classes of food. With an ileal segment of only 12 in., there was often inadequate length to absorb bile salts. The high food content was passed into the colon. The bile salts irritated the colonic mucosa causing colitis adding to water and protein loss.

2. Bacterial Overgrowth

   Whereas in patients with standard short bowel syndrome the bowel is absent, in JIB the majority of the small bowel was present but did not have bile or food coming through. This stagnation led to bacterial overgrowth that entered the portal system and occasionally caused hepatic failure. In addition, immune complexes formed secondary to bacterial overgrowth lodged into joints causing arthritis.

In 1976, Payne reported his experience with 230 jejunal-ileal bypass surgeries since 1962. A total of 19 (8 %) deaths were reported, of which 10 were related to hepatic failure. Electrolyte abnormalities were common, with hypokalemia and hypocalcemia being present in over 20 % of patients. Other reported complications included hypoalbuminemia, metabolic acidosis, arthritis, urinary calculi, cholelithiasis, liver impairment, and major emotional upset. Overall rehospitalization for complications was approximately 50 % [3].

Evolving Dangerous Concepts into Successful Bariatric Procedures

The original bariatric procedures came from the fact that patients who underwent gastric resection subsequently lost weight. Additionally, it was known that the intestine was adaptable, but at a certain level, when shortened, weight loss would occur. Thus, the issue became whether these concepts could be titrated and balanced to offer those with severe obesity procedures that would effectively allow them to lose weight and not become malnourished or symptomatically micronutrient deficient.

Edward Mason, who performed the first gastric bypass for obesity, argued that any manipulation of the bowel would result in an unacceptable rate of anemia and bone loss and only gastric reduction procedures should be performed [4]. The alternative viewpoint was that gastric-only procedures would not allow the majority of patients to reach their weight loss goals. Many would develop a maladaptive eating pattern

that would limit surgical effectiveness. Furthermore, gastric restriction has been plagued by ulcers, strictures, esophageal dysfunction, and decreased satisfaction with eating and choice of food. This debate remains a sentinel issue in bariatric surgery. Whether vertical banded gastroplasty versus gastric bypass or, in the laparoscopic era, gastric bypass versus adjustable banding and now sleeve gastrectomy, gastric-only procedures reduce the risk of the manifestations of short bowel syndrome. The cost is that they also do not offer the intestinal mechanisms that help cause weight loss.

By definition, every bariatric procedure produces an abnormality. The more the anatomy is altered, i.e., the more stomach removed and intestine bypassed, the greater the weight loss. The corollary of this statement is that the more that is altered, the greater the chance of nutritional deficiency. How these factors are balanced in aggressive operations that add an intestinal component is the emphasis of this chapter. We realize that our operations are more than the sum of making the stomach smaller and the intestine shorter. However, while we know that radically shortening bowel length causes weight loss, albeit with unacceptable side effects, we do not know exactly what our shorter bypass lengths do. Additionally, little is known about what the ideal lengths should be for a Roux limb, biliopancreatic limb, or common channel. Few meaningful studies have evaluated these issues. A recent systematic review of short versus long Roux limb length examined a total of eight studies. A trend was identified supporting the early efficacy of longer Roux limbs in the super obese patient category. However, the authors questioned the overall quality of the data due to inconsistent data reporting [5].

What are the most important variables? It would seem that the total intestinal length in contact with food and the common channel length are critical factors. In traditional gastric bypass, both of these values vary between patients and certainly between centers. Despite this, reported results seem to be consistent, thus further adding to our need for knowledge and understanding about what happens when an intestinal bypass is added to a gastric restriction (with or without pyloric preservation).

For the intestinal component there are several points that must be remembered from the knowledge obtained from the JIB and early bariatric procedures:

1. Total bowel length must be adequate. It is generally believed that most individuals require 6 ft or 2 m of small bowel. A competent ileocecal valve may reduce this to some degree. But as a starting point, in young individuals it would seem that all operations should preserve at least a minimum of 2–3 m of intestinal length.
2. There must be adequate length of intestine in the biliopancreatic limb and common channel to absorb enough bile salts and prevent bile-induced colitis.
3. Long segments of small bowel should not be left without flow of food or pancreatic and biliary secretions or stagnation and bacterial overgrowth will occur.

4. The jejunum and ileum are acid sensitive and if exposed to high acid load, marginal ulcers can occur.
5. The reconstruction allows supplementation with vitamins and minerals and protein to mitigate against irreversible deficiencies.
6. Gastrointestinal side effects must be tolerable with an acceptable number of daily bowel movements.

The Development of the Biliopancreatic Diversion or Scopinaro Procedure

Dr Nicolai Scopinaro, an Italian surgeon and pioneer in bariatric surgery, hoped to modify the JIB and develop an operation that would be lasting. Dr Scopinaro believed that a significant amount of intestine needed to be bypassed to allow for weight loss. The window was narrow, and the intestines' ability to hypertrophy and increase its absorptive surface was substantial. Furthermore, he believed that gastric restriction would be fleeting and if there was not an intestinal component causing malabsorption, considerable weight regain was inevitable. After adjustment, meal size would increase and recidivism would occur. Scopinaro hypothesized that significant weight loss would need to be achieved in the first year. During this period of time, consumption would increase and the bowel would hypertrophy. Thus, there would be a narrow window between bypassing too much bowel and enough bowel to have impact as the intestine adapted.

Scopinaro thus decided to combine a gastric resection with an aggressive intestinal bypass (Fig. 3) [6]. There have been different variations and even alterations depending on eating behavior or whether the patient was from Southern or Northern Italy. The operation involved a distal gastrectomy preserving between 250 and 400 cc of gastric volume. The fundus thus was preserved at the angle of His. The small bowel was measured from the terminal ileum for 250 cm then divided. The biliopancreatic limb was reattached 50 cm from the colon. In certain patients, the intestine was divided 300 cm from the ileocecal valve. There were many differences between the Scopinaro procedure and the JIB. Total intestinal length was increased from 0.5 to 2.5 to 3 m. Bile could be absorbed throughout the entire biliopancreatic limb, reducing the impact of bile salts on the colon. The distal gastric resection reduced the amount of food eaten following surgery and reduced acid secretion, allowing attachment of the small bowel to the stomach.

In 1998, Scopinaro reported a 21-year experience with the biliopancreatic diversion in 2,241 patients with a mean BMI of 47 kg/m^2 (range 29–87 kg/m^2) [7]. Mean reduction of initial excess weight was 75 % with a follow-up rate of 98 %. Additional beneficial effects of biliopancreatic diversion included improvement or resolution of hypertension, fatter liver, leg stasis, hypercholesterolemia, diabetes mellitus,

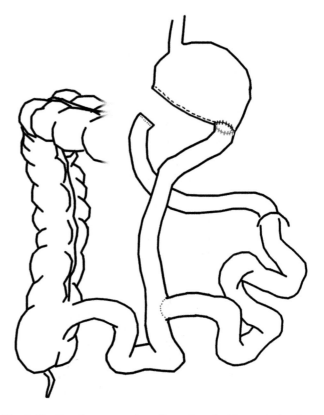

FIG. 3. The Scopinaro procedure. Reproduced with permission from Diana McPhee.

hyperuricemia, and gout. Furthermore, there is an in-depth analysis on the eating behavior and the amount of food that is actually absorbed by patients years from surgery.

According to Scopinaro, weight loss occurs in the first year following surgery, and the intestinal bypass allows that weight loss to be maintained. In the first several months following surgery, intake is a significant challenge, even with what would be considered large gastric pouches. Ghrelin and other gut peptides were not known at the time of this report, but Scopinaro believed that much of the symptomatology came from intestinal distension following eating or postcibal syndrome. Over the course of the first year, this symptom disappeared, and meal size approached preoperative levels.

Therefore the intestinal bypass caused weight loss to last more than 10 years after surgery. Scopinaro measured absorption of different food groups in patients that reached weight stabilization. 57 % of total energy was absorbed. Only 27 % of fat was absorbed. Virtually 100 % of simple sugars would be absorbed and approximately 60 % of total protein. Additionally Scopinaro pointed out that protein, starch, and carbohydrate percentage absorption would be affected by the total length of intestine in contact with food. Only fat absorption would vary with common channel.

Another contribution to the literature from this report was the concept that the intestinal bypass actually increased energy expenditure. Detailed analysis in this report demonstrated that, compared to controls with similar weight loss and size, resting energy expenditure decrease was lower than would be expected in the surgical group. Recently, Kaplan highlighted that this, not malabsorption, is the significant contribution in an experimental model of gastric bypass [8].

Of course the BPD was not without issue. There was a 2 % rate that required reoperation for protein malnutrition. Scopinaro highlights that the likelihood of this increases if patients consume excessive carbohydrates. When that occurs insulin is stimulated which results in an increased amount of endogenous protein breakdown exacerbating the protein deficiency. During the first year frequent bowel movements are common, which are reduced to 2–4 more than a year following surgery. The marginal ulcer rate reported was greater than 8 %. Deficiencies of the fat-soluble vitamins and iron exceed 25 %. Calcium deficiency and bone demineralization can occur. Scopinaro shows that this stabilizes. Countering these adverse effects, there was a 100 % resolution of diabetes and hypercholesterolemia.

In summary, there is much that can be learned from this incredible data set. Obviously, the long-term data was quite impressive. Yet, there are many reasons why this operation did not expand in popularity and become an international standard. The list of side effects was numerous. In the setting of 100 % follow-up, many of these could be simply handled. In the United States and many other places, this level of follow-up cannot be expected. Furthermore, the duodenal switch, which reduced the marginal ulcer rate to near zero, became the preferential method for the performance of a biliopancreatic diversion. Even with this adaption and potential improvement, duodenal switch and other forms of BPD represent a small minority of bariatric procedures currently performed.

Development of the Duodenal Switch

In 1998, Dr Douglas Hess became interested in the research of Dr Thomas DeMeester on duodenal gastric reflux and his concept of attaching a small segment of duodenum to the Roux limb of the small bowel. Hess wanted to utilize a similar approach to Scopinaro on revisions but encountered dense adhesions and, following these challenging revisions, a high rate of marginal ulceration. As a result, Hess developed the concept of combining a vertical gastrectomy of the greater curvature with a duodenal division preserving a small cuff of the duodenum.

Hess calibrated his gastrectomy using a 40 Fr bougie or dilator. The length of the small bowel was determined by measuring the total intestinal length from the stomach to the cecum. Then, 40 % of the total length was used to create the alimentary limb, and 10 % of the total length to create the common channel [9].

Advantages of the duodenal switch include preservation of the pylorus and the reduction of marginal ulcer rates. In a 1998 report, Hess reported an 85 % excess weight loss with 10 of 440 patients requiring revision for either protein malnutrition or diarrhea. The duodenal switch has become the most common version of biliopancreatic diversion. Within North America, Dr Gary Anthone [10] and Drs Marceau and Biron [11] have published extensive series with lengthy follow-up. In contrast, to Hess, they have used fixed bowel length rather than calculating based on total intestinal length.

In the late 1990s and early 2000s, bariatric surgery rapidly increased in popularity. The increasing obesity epidemic, combined with the development of laparoscopy, led to this growth. With the movement to laparoscopy, techniques were developed to perform the duodenal switch in a minimally invasive nature.

Laparoscopic Duodenal Switch

The first major report of laparoscopic duodenal switch came from Ren and Gagner [12] in 2000. This report discussed their technique for laparoscopic bypass and highlighted an increased complication rate for those with a BMI greater than 60. It was the basis of this study that made Dr Gagner postulate that staging the procedure and doing the vertical gastrectomy and then following weight loss proceed to the intestinal bypass. Interestingly, despite the fact that Scopinaro always felt that the gastric aspect caused much of the early weight loss, many trained in North America felt that in BPD the major component was from the intestine. Now with sleeve gastrectomy accepted as a stand-alone weight loss procedure, it is clear that the gastric resection is an important, if not dominant, component.

Following Gagner's report, Baltazar [13] published his series of laparoscopic duodenal switch in 2001. At our center, vertical sleeve gastrectomy and duodenal switch have become our preferential stapling procedures (Fig. 4). Contrary to many reports, a significant proportion of our patients are super morbidly obese, and we do not find this to be a contraindication for surgery.

The technical aspects that need comment are the duodenal dissection, the duodenal enteral anastomosis, and the distal anastomosis. At this point, the majority of bariatric surgeons are comfortable with the vertical gastrectomy. For the duodenal dissection, it is imperative to elevate the pylorus and take the posterior adhesions. A cuff of the duodenum, of at least 2 cm, needs to be dissected. Care must be taken to avoid any dissection of pancreatic attachments. If the pancreas needs to be taken off the duodenum, the surgeon has moved too distal. Trauma to the pancreas can cause prolonged postoperative fluid collections and a duodenal stump leak.

We currently perform our sleeve gastrectomy over a 38 Fr bougie and start the staple line 3–4 cm from the pyloric valve. Our total intestinal length is 3 m with a common channel of 125 cm. With these parameters, our average patient moves their bowels 1–3 times daily. In over 400 cases, we have had to place only 2 patients on TPN; both had other inflammatory bowel conditions and were able to be weaned and maintained adequate protein levels without further support. We have not had to surgically revise any patient for persistent hypoproteinemia.

In our initial duodenal switch procedures more than 5 years ago, we utilized a side-to-side stapling technique with a linear stapler. After several cases where we experienced issues, we have changed to hand-sewn and end-to-end two-layered anastomoses using PDS. With this approach, we have had less than a 1 % leak rate. Additionally, with this technique and preservation of an adequate cuff, we have not encountered either stricture or marginal ulcer.

According to statistics from the BOLD database, weight loss is greater than gastric bypass and is better maintained. Offsetting these results is the technical difficulty of the procedure. Thirty-day reoperation rates are estimated to be from 3 to 5 %. Few surgeons have mastered the technical aspects of laparoscopic duodenal switch. Besides increased perioperative complications, the extended operative times potentially increase the likelihood of venous thrombosis and pulmonary embolism.

Comparing Duodenal Switch to Gastric Bypass

In addition to the BOLD data, several recent studies have compared gastric bypass to duodenal switch. In a randomized trial in patients with a BMI greater or equal to 55, significantly greater weight loss was shown following duodenal switch. There was a tendency for a higher rate of nutritional complications in DS; however this difference was not significant. Alverdy et al. [14] compared the resolution of comorbidities between RYGB and DS. All major comorbidities, except GERD, were more likely to be resolved following DS, including diabetes, hypercholesterolemia, sleep apnea, and hypertension. Potentially, even more important is a report from Germany that studied the DS in patients with insulin-dependent type 2 diabetes, who were on injectable therapy for many years [15]. This subset has been shown to be least likely to have diabetes remission with bariatric surgery. All were able to be weaned from injectable insulin and remained off for 1 year of follow-up. A subgroup in this study had a BMI under 40. Similarly, the Scopinaro BPD was compared to RYGB in a randomized trial conducted by Rubino et al. [16]. This study, published in the *New England Journal of Medicine*, showed a substantial advantage for BPD.

Recently our group has compared glucose regulation in the RYGB, VSG, and DS. The DS group had the greatest weight loss and lowest HgbA1c. RYGB had a reduction in fasting insulin but with glucose challenge had a rapid rise in glucose that corresponded to a 1 h insulin level that was greater than baseline [17]. In comparison, DS patients maintained euglycemia without the abrupt rise in insulin level, and thus less likely to cause hypoglycemia. VSG results were in between, meaning that preservation of the pylorus is not the only reason for this more balanced glucose control. As control of insulin levels is considered an objective in medical efforts to control weight, it is probable this is also true for surgical approaches and may be part of the reason that weight loss is better maintained following duodenal switch.

Increasing Malabsorption for Revision of RYGB

It would seem to be a simple alternative for those with weight regain following RYGB to convert to a similar procedure as BPD, by extending the bypass. Many believe that as the patient has started to regain weight, they can tolerate the needed volume of food to handle a distal bypass. However, there are many things to consider.

Virtually all RYGB gastric pouches are based on the lesser curvature of the stomach and thus remove the fundus. The Scopinaro procedure preserves the fundus which allows food to pool in that area. The duodenal switch preserves the pylorus, which in Latin means gatekeeper. As a result, the pouch of the gastric bypass empties rapidly. Furthermore, if this option is contemplated, adequate intestinal length must be created even if multiple small bowel attachments must be made. Frequently, the Roux limb, which measures 150 cm, is divided proximal to the distal anastomosis and reattached 50–75 cm from the colon. The combination of a rapid emptying pouch and short bowel can be debilitating as the case presented in the beginning of the chapter demonstrated.

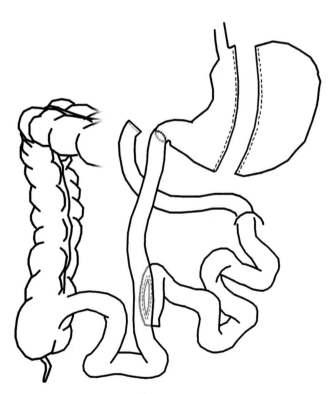

FIG. 4. The modern duodenal switch. Reproduced with permission from Diana McPhee.

Both Sugerman [18] and Fobi [19] have published series that discuss this approach. Both showed an unacceptable risk of protein malnutrition and a substantial number required revision. Additionally, when these cases are revised, there is abrupt weight gain, as they have had to eat supranormal quantities to attempt to handle the malabsorption. As a result, we do not recommend this approach. If selected the surgeon must make sure that the total intestinal length is at least 3 m and/or there is retained fundus. When earlier trials of this procedure were performed, many patients had transverse staple lines that did not exclude the fundus. During this period, many still did not tolerate the distal bypass.

Conversion of Sleeve Gastrectomy to Duodenal Switch

As vertical sleeve gastrectomy grows in frequency, an increasing number of patients will consider revision for either inadequate weight loss or weight regain. For these patients options include redoing the sleeve, conversion to gastric bypass, or conversion to duodenal switch. For many reasons, we believe that conversion to duodenal switch is the most attractive option. A major benefit is that rather than revision, this conversion is really doing a second primary procedure, as the duodenal area should not be affected by the initial operation. Re-sleeving and gastric bypass would involve dissection in the original surgical field. It is also logical to introduce an intestinal operation in a patient that failed a gastric or restrictive procedure. There are many concerns for conversion to gastric bypass. The sleeve pouch has been shown to exist at higher pressure than the gastric bypass pouch. Thus, there is potentially less restriction. Additionally, the exact contribution of the intestinal component of a gastric bypass is unknown. The average bypass has a common channel greater than 4 m and intestinal length longer. It is unlikely that much malabsorption occurs. Thus, there is probably some early weight loss caused by food entering almost immediately into the intestine causing a postprandial reaction. Nominal weight loss and even regain will be seen shortly after. If this option is considered, the bypass will need to be very aggressive, and the patient is at risk for the issues discussed above.

It is our belief that conversion to duodenal switch from sleeve gastrectomy will grow in popularity and cause growth in the popularity of duodenal switch. Once surgeons become comfortable with doing these second-stage procedures, more primary DS will also be performed. Several recent studies support the efficacy and safety of a single-stage procedure [20–22]. However, studies thus far have been limited to case series, and a randomized controlled trial has yet to be performed. While staging is attractive, as the second stage is done after there is loss of adiposity in the abdomen and the patient has already adjusted to gastric volume reduction making nutritional sequelae potentially less likely, it is not known if the effects are additive. It is possible that the combination of gastric reduction and intestinal bypass acts synergistically. Only further study will resolve these issues.

Patient Instructions

It is essential that patients following duodenal switch eat a high-protein diet and require 70–90 g of protein daily. Additionally, fatty foods will lead to malodorous and more frequent stools. Simple carbohydrates will be absorbed and also increase insulin levels and further increasing the amount of protein required. Supplements containing high levels of vitamins A, D, E, and K as well as vitamin B complex and B12 need to be taken. Iron and calcium supplementation are required. We also advise taking two zinc tablets daily. Some of the rules we advise are:

1. Eat protein first and stick to a high-protein low-fat diet.
2. Avoid simple sugar and alcohol. These will be absorbed normally.
3. To avoid malodorous stools, avoid fatty foods, and you can use chlorophyll stool deodorant such as Devrom.
4. Take your vitamins and supplements daily.
5. Have blood work twice in first year and then annually.

Patient complaints of flatulence and diarrhea can usually be handled by adjustment of food intake. At times, patients may benefit from short course of metronidazole. Similarly, low protein levels should be treated by reintroducing high-protein shake or powder. There are a greater variety of high-protein low-fat and low-carbohydrate supplements now available which can potentially improve outcomes.

Future Directions

It seems that since there has been bariatric surgery, the debate of whether to perform a gastric-only procedure or combination gastric and intestinal procedure has existed. Gastric-only operations have a much lower incidence of anemia, bone demineralization, hypoproteinemia, and vitamin deficiency. However, consumption gradually increases, and weight regain commonly occurs. If too tight or overly restrictive, the likelihood of maladaptive eating increases. Healthy choices are replaced by fatty greasy alternatives and simple carbohydrates. Despite removing 70 % of the stomach, at 1 year, Scopinaro reported normal meal size.

Today's gastric sleeve attempts to reduce gastric volume to 100 cc or less. Thus, there is perhaps a more lasting reduction of gastric volume. In addition, the impact of gut peptides such as ghrelin is unknown. However, in all probability, an increasing number of patients will have inadequate weight loss or weight regain.

There are many attractive aspects to adding malabsorption. But certain rules must be remembered. Total intestinal length has to be adequate and be at least 2–3 m. The biliopancreatic limb has to be long enough to allow for the majority of bile salts to be reabsorbed and not irritate the colon. The impact of the gastric pouch must be understood. It should be small enough to cause early weight loss but allow adequate intake of protein supplements. It cannot empty too rapidly, and thus increase the likelihood of diarrhea. Additionally, it must be remembered that total intestinal length determines the amount of protein and total energy absorbed. Common channel length is important in determining the percentage of fat that is absorbed.

Simply stated, by adding malabsorption, there is a greater likelihood that weight loss is maintained. Perhaps, it can be reduced to a fundamental philosophical decision. Is the role of bariatric surgery to provide weight loss and have the patient learn skills that allow for weight stability? Or, to be successful, does bariatric surgery require a physiologically lasting mechanism that reduces caloric consumption, or reduces absorption, or increases resting energy expenditure? Certainly, some patients are capable of making lifetime behavioral changes. For others, it is possible that only procedures that offer substantial malabsorption will have a lasting effect.

Acknowledgments The authors would like to thank Dr Diana J. McPhee for the original artwork created for this book chapter.

Review Questions and Answers

1. Complications of jejunoileal bypass included
    (a) Liver failure
    (b) Oxalate stones
    (c) Protein malnutrition
    (d) Hypoglycemia
    (e) A, B, and C only

    Answer: E

2. To reduce the incidence of hypoproteinemia the surgeon should
    (a) Increase common channel length
    (b) Have adequate pouch size, preserve fundus or pylorus, and have adequate total intestinal length
    (c) Place patients on high-carbohydrate-based diet
    (d) Always remove gallbladder

    Answer: A, B

3. Postoperative instructions following BPD should include all of the following except
    (a) Taking glucose tablets to avoid hypoglycemia
    (b) Requiring approximately 100 g of protein as 1/3 not absorbed
    (c) Supplementing fat-soluble vitamins
    (d) Calcium, iron, and zinc supplementation
    (e) Blood work twice in the first year and then annually

    Answer: A

4. Revision of gastric bypass to distal bypass
    (a) Is an effective procedure with no long-term issue
    (b) Must leave the patient with adequate bowel length to avoid consequences of short bowel syndrome
    (c) Works exactly the same as duodenal switch or Scopinaro procedure
    (d) Is more effective as there is no pylorus or fundus

    Answer: B

References

1. Payne JH, DeWind LT, Commons RR. Metabolic observations in patients with jejunocolic shunts. Am J Surg. 1963;106:273–89.
2. Scott Jr HW, Sandstead HH, Brill AB, Burko H, Younger RK. Experience with a new technic of intestinal bypass in the treatment of morbid obesity. Ann Surg. 1971;174(4):560–72.
3. DeWind LT, Payne JH. Intestinal bypass surgery for morbid obesity. Long-term results. JAMA. 1976;236(20):2298–301.
4. Mason EE, Ito C. Gastric bypass in obesity. Surg Clin North Am. 1967;47(6):1345–51.
5. Orci L, Chilcott M, Huber O. Short versus long Roux-limb length in Roux-en-Y gastric bypass surgery for the treatment of morbid and super obesity: a systematic review of the literature. Obes Surg. 2011;21(6):797–804.
6. Scopinaro N, Gianetta E, Civalleri D, Bonalumi U, Bachi V. Biliopancreatic bypass for obesity: 1. An experimental study in dogs. Br J Surg. 1979;66(9):613–7.
7. Scopinaro N, Adami GF, Marinari GM, Gianetta E, Traverso E, Friedman D, Camerini G, Baschieri G, Simonelli A. Biliopancreatic diversion. World J Surg. 1998;22(9):936–46.
8. Stylopoulos N, Hoppin AG, Kaplan LM. Roux-en-Y gastric bypass enhances energy expenditure and extends lifespan in diet-induced obese rats. Obesity (Silver Spring). 2009;17:1839–47.
9. Hess DS, Hess DW. Biliopancreatic diversion with a duodenal switch. Obes Surg. 1998;8(3):267–82.
10. Anthone G, Lord R, DeMeester T, Crookes P. The duodenal switch operation for the treatment of morbid obesity. Ann Surg. 2003;238(4):618–28.
11. Marceau P, Biron S, Bourque R, Potvin M, Hould F, Simard S. Biliopancreatic diversion with a new type of gastrectomy. Obes Surg. 1993;3(1):29–35.
12. Ren CJ, Patterson E, Gagner M. Early results of laparoscopic biliopancreatic diversion with duodenal switch: a case series of 40 consecutive patients. Obes Surg. 2000;10(6):514–23; discussion 524.
13. Baltasar A, Bou R, Bengochea M, Arlandis F, Escrivá C, Miró J, Martínez R, Pérez N. Duodenal switch: an effective therapy for morbid obesity–intermediate results. Obes Surg. 2001;11(1):54–8.
14. Prachand VN, Ward M, Alverdy JC. Duodenal switch provides superior resolution of metabolic comorbidities independent of weight loss in the super-obese (BMI > or = 50 kg/m2) compared with gastric bypass. J Gastrointest Surg. 2010;14(2):211–20.
15. Frenken M, Cho EY, Karcz WK, Grueneberger J, Kuesters S. Improvement of type 2 diabetes mellitus in obese and non-obese patients after the duodenal switch operation. J Obes. 2011;2011:860169. Epub 2011 Mar 3.
16. Mingrone G, Panunzi S, De Gaetano A, Guidone C, Iaconelli A, Leccesi L, Nanni G, Pomp A, Castagneto M, Ghirlanda G, Rubino F. Bariatric surgery versus conventional medical therapy for type 2 diabetes. N Engl J Med. 2012;366(17):1577–85. Epub 2012 Mar 26.
17. Roslin MS, Oren JH, Polan BN, Damani T, Brauner R, Shah PC. Abnormal glucose tolerance testing after gastric bypass. Surg Obes Relat Dis. 2013;9:26–31.

18. Sugerman HJ, Kellum JM, Engle KM, Wolfe L, Starkey JV, Birkenhauer R, Fletcher P, Sawyer MJ. Gastric bypass for treating severe obesity. Am J Clin Nutr. 1992;55(2 Suppl):560S–6. Review.

19. Fobi MA, Lee H. SILASTIC ring vertical banded gastric bypass for the treatment of obesity: two years of follow-up in 84 patients. J Natl Med Assoc. 1994;86(2):125–8.

20. Iannelli A, Schneck AS, Topart P, Carles M, Hébuterne X, Gugenheim J. Laparoscopic sleeve gastrectomy followed by duodenal switch in selected patients versus single-stage duodenal switch for superobesity: case-control study. J Surg Obes Relat Dis. 2013;9: 531–8.

21. Topart P, Becouarn G, Ritz P. Should biliopancreatic diversion with duodenal switch be done as single-stage procedure in patients with BMI > or = 50 kg/m2? Surg Obes Relat Dis. 2010;6(1):59–63. Epub 2009 May 13.

22. Buchwald H, Kellogg TA, Leslie DB, Ikramuddin S. Duodenal switch operative mortality and morbidity are not impacted by body mass index. Ann Surg. 2008;248(4):541–8.

34

Laparoscopic Malabsorption Procedures: Management of Surgical Complications

Fady Moustarah, Frédéric-Simon Hould, Simon Marceau, and Simon Biron

Introduction

Malabsorptive bariatric procedures are highly effective in inducing substantial weight loss and significant improvements in obesity-related comorbidities, and their effects are sustained over long periods of time [1–3]. Purely malabsorptive procedures, such as the historic jejunoileal bypass and its variants, are rarely if ever practiced today, and they have been rightly abandoned because of their serious side effect profile, especially on long-term follow-up [4, 5]. Contemporary malabsorptive procedures have a mixed restrictive and malabsorptive component and include one of the following three main operations: the biliopancreatic diversion with distal gastrectomy (BPD), the biliopancreatic diversion with duodenal switch and sleeve gastrectomy (BPD-DS), and the distal Roux-en-Y gastric bypass [5–8]. Complications related to malabsorptive procedures are particular and mandate careful follow-up and timely intervention to maintain the surgical benefits and good health of patients postoperatively [9].

Bariatric surgery is elective; thus there is generally a low tolerance for complications. Bariatric surgeons, no doubt, must be closely familiar with the diagnosis and management of specific complications when they do occur. With the increasing number of procedures being offered to morbidly obese patients since the adoption of laparoscopy [10–12], it is also important for physicians of various specialties, particularly general surgeons and primary care providers, to have the requisite knowledge required to effectively evaluate and treat these challenging patients, especially in emergency settings. This chapter reviews the management of *important early and late surgical, non-nutritional* complications specific to the laparoscopic biliopancreatic diversion procedure with and without duodenal switch (BPD±DS).

Biliopancreatic Diversion

To better discuss complications specific to commonly practiced BPD±DS surgery, a brief description of procedure variations is warranted. In principle, biliopancreatic diversion changes a patient's anatomy to reduce fat energy absorption by diverting pancreatic digestive enzymes and bile to the distal segment of the small intestine. The standard BPD was developed and introduced in 1979 by an Italian team led by Scopinaro, who was the first to demonstrate its safety, efficacy, and durability [13, 14]. The Scopinaro BPD consists of a distal gastrectomy, leaving approximately 1/3 of the proximal stomach (300–500 mL capacity), with a long Roux-en-Y gastroileal reconstruction: the alimentary limb is 250 cm (from the gastroileal anastomosis to the ileocecal valve), and the enteroenterostomy connecting the diverted biliopancreatic limb (BPL) (majority of the small bowel) to the alimentary limb is placed 50 cm from the ileocecal valve, resulting in a short 50 cm common channel for incomplete fat digestion and absorption.

The BPD-DS was introduced into clinical practice in North America in 1988 as a modification of the standard BPD with the aim of reducing some of the complications related to marginal ulceration at the gastroileal junction, dumping, and protein-calorie malnutrition [15, 16]. The BPD-DS includes a longitudinal acid-reducing gastrectomy (creating a gastric tube along the lesser curve of the stomach) with pyloric preservation and duodeno-ileal anastomosis, after dividing the first portion of the duodenum [7]. Again, a Roux-en-Y type reconstruction of the small intestine is performed, but the enteroenterostomy is placed 100 cm from the ileocecal valve. However, similar to the Scopinaro BPD, the total alimentary limb length (from the duodenoileostomy to the ileocecal valve) is kept at 250 cm in the standard BPD-DS. Intestinal

S.A. Brethauer et al. (eds.), *Minimally Invasive Bariatric Surgery*,
DOI 10.1007/978-1-4939-1637-5_34, © Springer Science+Business Media New York 2015

limb length variations are practiced in attempts to alter the side effect profile of the operation, but evidence for the added safety and efficacy of such practice is lacking. Surgical, physiologic, and nutritional complications related to the BPD±DS are not simply limited to the approach used for surgical access, the particular anatomic reconfiguration employed, and the perioperative period: they can occur years after surgery and require lifelong attention and follow-up.

General Postoperative Complications Related to Obesity

Diversionary procedures induce weight loss by limiting nutrient absorption, and they are generally recommended to patients whose body mass index (BMI) exceeds 50 kg/m²; yet, they are also performed on patients with lower BMI [17]. Procedural complications can, therefore, be related to the obesity itself and to the complexity of surgical interventions in settings of extreme obesity [18, 19]. Obese patients often have a number of cardiovascular and pulmonary comorbidities. Conditions such as ischemic heart disease, hypertension, hypercoagulability, venous stasis, obstructive sleep apnea, restrictive lung disease, and diabetes are often present; and any one of them alone or together may increase the risk of perioperative cardiopulmonary and/or wound-related complications. Preoperative optimization of these patients from a cardiopulmonary standpoint is, therefore, paramount to reduce perioperative risk during anesthesia and early during postoperative recovery [20].

In addition, the obese abdomen presents substantial technical challenges relating to surgical exposure, retraction, and bowel manipulation [18, 21]. A high BMI (particularly in the form of excessive visceral obesity), male gender, and advanced age have been identified as predictors of increased perioperative morbidity and mortality [22–24]. In a large patient sample from a US national database, independent predictors associated with significantly increased mortality after bariatric surgery included the following: age >45 years, male gender, a BMI of 50 kg/m² or higher, open bariatric procedures, diabetes, functional status of total dependency before surgery, prior coronary intervention, dyspnea at preoperative evaluation, more than 10 % unintentional weight loss in 6 months, and bleeding disorders [24]. These factors should be taken into consideration as surgeons select and counsel patients for complex abdominal weight loss procedures to minimize risk of complications and guide perioperative management.

Regardless of the surgical approach used, postoperative management of the obese patient focuses on aggressive and early mobilization and pulmonary physiotherapy to reduce pulmonary complications. Vigilance in following vital signs and careful attention to symptoms in the early postoperative period can help detect potentially life-threatening complications such as anastomotic leaks, pulmonary embolism, or hemorrhage. These conditions, in themselves, may pose diagnostic challenges in the obese patient after abdominal surgery, and they mandate different and timely management plans as will be reviewed below.

General Complications Related to Laparoscopy in the Obese

Reducing complications of malabsorptive bariatric procedures starts with safely offering these procedures, and laparoscopically when possible, by well trained specialists. Believed to contribute to lower morbidity, laparoscopic techniques were used in bariatric surgery since the early 1990s, and they have been increasing in popularity and scope of application with both surgeons and patients ever since [25–28]. One study estimates that the proportion of laparoscopic bariatric operations in the United States increased from 20.1 % in 2003 to 90.2 % in 2008 [10]. Today all major bariatric procedures are performed laparoscopically, including what is viewed as the most complex weight loss procedure: the laparoscopic BPD±DS. Gagner performed the first laparoscopic BPD-DS in July of 1999 [18]. The procedure was offered to high-risk super-morbidly obese patients, with BMIs >50 kg/m², and complication rates were high [18, 29, 30]. The technical aspects of the procedure have since been refined, reducing complications [31], and concepts of staging the laparoscopic BPD-DS over time to reduce perioperative risk were also introduced [32–34].

The laparoscopic approach offers real benefits to bariatric patients, but it comes with its own set of technical challenges related to access, exposure, and bowel handling, thus influencing both the *intraoperative* and the *early and delayed* postoperative complication profile. The principal benefits of laparoscopy relate to lowering the incidence of wound problems in comparison to procedures performed by laparotomy, where wound infections and delayed incisional hernias contribute to significant morbidity in up to 15 % and 20 % of open cases, respectively [35–37]. A number of small randomized control studies and larger observational series have all pointed to the benefits associated with laparoscopic bariatric surgery [38]. In addition to reducing the physiologic insult related to incision size, laparoscopic surgery offers bariatric patients other advantages: improved postoperative pulmonary function, reduced atelectasis, lower blood loss, lesser postoperative pain, improved early mobility, and possibly shorter hospital stay.

Safe abdominal access is the first surgical challenge in morbidly obese patients undergoing laparoscopy. The goal is to avoid injury to abdominal organs or retroperitoneal vessels. The main ways to access the abdomen for laparoscopic surgery include the closed technique using a Veress needle, the open technique with a blunt Hasson trocar, and the direct trocar insertion technique without pneumoperitoneum [39].

All have been used safely [40], but mortality from access injury has been reported, and certain surgical principles can minimize complications, especially in the obese.

In patients with high BMI undergoing laparoscopic BPD, it is usually difficult to lift the skin at the umbilicus to facilitate safe Veress needle insertion or even perform a cutdown for the Hasson technique. If the Hasson technique is chosen at the umbilicus, care must be taken to avoid excessive gas leakage during the procedure after trocar placement. The weight of the abdominal wall can be a limiting factor in creating a pneumoperitoneum with adequate working space, and gas leakage from poor access technique and port placement can result in poor exposure and, thereby, increase operative risk.

We prefer placing the first port in the midline above the umbilicus (about 15–20 cm from the xiphoid process) using an optical trocar, after having raised a pneumoperitoneum with a Veress needle inserted under the left costal margin (between the midclavicular and anterior axillary lines). The needle is inserted perpendicular to the skin and is then aspirated to ensure that blood, succus, or stool is not present. Then 5 mL of sterile saline can be injected to assess resistance to flow, and finally a water drop test can be performed to observe a drop of saline descend through the hub of the needle without resistance. These signs are reassuring and observable even in the obese with increased abdominal pressures. Finally, the needle is hooked up to the insufflator, and pressure readings are noted. Intra-abdominal pressure may be elevated in bariatric patients, but expected readings are usually between 9 and 13 mmHg. Loss of hepatic dullness on percussion after insufflation of 100 cc of CO_2 is another reassuring sign of intra-abdominal needle placement. The abdominal cavity is then evaluated, and trocars are placed under direct vision to minimize injury.

Because exposure remains a challenge in obese patients, the surgeon should not hesitate to use additional 5 mm ports to improve retraction and tissue handling as needed. An additional insufflator may sometimes help in lifting a heavy abdominal wall and improving the working space. While conversion to laparotomy to deal with complications difficult to address with laparoscopy remains an option every surgeon should be ready to take, we tend not to resort to conversion simply to complete a BPD-DS. If exposure, anatomic, or medical variables are limiting at the time of surgery, we prefer to stage the procedure and perform a primary sleeve gastrectomy first with plans to perform a duodenal switch as needed in about 18 months, after weight loss and improvements in the risk profile have occurred.

Surgical and Acute Postoperative Complications

Some complications after bariatric surgery are procedure specific. Important early and late postoperative complications associated with BPD±DS are summarized in Table 1.

TABLE 1. Important early and late surgical postoperative complications related to BPD

	Early (<30 days)	Late
BPD±DS	Anastomotic leak with peritonitis	Stomal stenosis
	Abdominal abscess	Marginal ulcer
	Pulmonary embolism	Dumping syndrome
	Bleeding	Intestinal obstruction
	Intestinal obstruction	Internal hernia
	Pulmonary complications	Incisional hernia
	Wound infection	Complicated cholelithiasis
	Acute renal failure	Poor weight loss or weight regain
	Cardiovascular events	Liver failure
		Nutritional:
		Anemia
		Hypocalcemia
		Hypoalbuminemia
		Hyperparathyroidism (secondary)
		Fat-soluble vitamin deficiencies
		Vit. A: night blindness
		Vit. D: secondary hyperparathyroidism
		Vit. E: dry skin
		Vit. K: increased prothrombin time
		Vitamin B12 deficiency
		Osteoporosis
		Protein-calorie malnutrition

Anastomotic or suture line leakage, pulmonary embolism, and hemorrhage remain among the most serious and potentially life-threatening early complications and will receive special mention. In general, morbidity rates after BPD±DS range from 2.9 to 16.3 % as reported in large series of greater than 100 patients, some of which also included open cases [3, 15]. Major complications account for ≤8 % in institutions where BPD-DS is the principal procedure performed [17, 31].

Anastomotic Leakage

Leaks occur with a reported incidence of 0–8 % in different series of laparoscopic BPD [31, 41–43]. Leaks are a serious source of morbidity and are a leading cause of mortality after bariatric procedures. Leakage has been implicated in mortality in up to 29 % of deaths after bariatric surgery [23]. Despite advancements in supportive care, mortality after intra-abdominal leakage is often due to delayed diagnosis, so a high index of suspicion allows for early detection and timely intervention.

Leaks at any staple or suture line can result from technical factors at the time of surgery. Such factors may include any or all of the following: division of blood supply during dissection, anastomotic tension, tissue injury from poor handling with laparoscopic instruments, or stapler misuse or malfunction. In a BPD±DS, anastomotic leaks can occur at the following areas: (1) the gastric staple or suture line, (2) the gastroileostomy (Scopinaro procedure) or the duodenoileostomy (BPD-DS), (3) the duodenal stump, or (4) the ileo-ileostomy. Leaks, however, have also resulted from small bowel injuries due to intestinal handling with graspers during laparoscopic surgery, and this source of peritonitis should be considered when evaluating or treating postoperative patients.

The most common and serious site of leakage after a BPD±DS is from the gastroileostomy/duodenoileostomy. The foot anastomosis, or ileoileostomy, leaks infrequently. When leakage occurs at this site, however, it tends to be high in output and associated with rapid deterioration of the patient, leading to potentially higher morbidity and mortality. In the BPD-DS with sleeve gastrectomy, another important (and often difficult to manage) area of leakage is the gastric staple line.

A leak can be immediate or may present up to 1–2 weeks postoperatively. A negative intraoperative leak test and an UGI swallow on the first postoperative day, if performed, offer some reassurance regarding the integrity of the upper anastomosis in a BPD, but these tests can be falsely negative, and a leak from ischemia at an anastomosis may take some time to manifest. We do not routinely perform an UGI swallow postoperatively in our patients after a BPD-DS. In addition, we do not routinely place drains intraoperatively. However, if a functioning drain had been appropriately positioned at the time of surgery, a change in the character of the drainage or an elevated amylase content of the drain fluid may be the first and only sign of anastomotic disruption in an otherwise well appearing patient.

Diagnosing postoperative peritonitis is often difficult in obese patients, and this is more so in the early postoperative state where pain and other cardiopulmonary conditions can cloud the presentation. Although fever, tachycardia, and abdominal pain are common, often the only sign is tachycardia in the absence of classic peritoneal signs such as guarding and rebound tenderness. A heart rate greater than 120 beats/min should alert the evaluating clinician to consider a leak, even if the patient feels and looks well [44]. Tachycardia alone, however, may not be a reliable early indicator of leakage [45]. A proximal gastric leak often results in left shoulder pain on deep inspiration. This is a sign of diaphragm irritation mediated by the phrenic nerve (C3–C5) and referred to the shoulder region (Kehr's sign). Computed tomography (CT) can be very useful in all patients with unexplained tachycardia, fever, or abdominal pain after BPD±DS. If a CT scan is unavailable, emergency re-laparoscopy should be offered for diagnosis and timely management.

Gastric leaks in a BPD-DS procedure tend to occur high on the neo-greater curve of the stomach near the GE junction, resulting in a perigastric collection or subphrenic abscess. Their treatment depends on the timing of presentation and patient stability [46]. Late gastric leaks are often more difficult to resolve than early ones, and to date a generally accepted algorithm for the management of gastric leaks is yet to be described [47]. Surgical or percutaneous drainage of leaks presenting in the early postoperative course is needed. In select stable patients, contained leaks can be managed nonoperatively with adequate percutaneous drainage, bowel rest, total parenteral nutrition, and antibiotics. A nasojejunal gavage tube may be temporarily utilized for nutritional support. When leaks are not contained, diffuse peritonitis results; and if left untreated, sepsis will follow with possible multisystem organ failure. Surgical treatment, on the other hand, involves early reoperation, copious irrigation, and wide drainage, while suture repair is avoided or reserved for cases where tissue is clearly amenable to manipulation without increasing the risk of further damage [48]. Omental patching may be helpful, but the key is effective drainage. For large gastric or upper anastomotic leaks requiring surgical drainage for sepsis, a jejunal feeding tube is best placed at the time surgery in the biliopancreatic limb for nutritional support. The feeding tube allows for outpatient management before complete healing of the leak site is achieved. For early leaks, endoscopically placed covered stents may be utilized to allow early oral intake, reduced hospitalization, and promote tissue healing [49, 50]. Any endoscopic treatment modality must be an adjunct to adequate drainage and broad-spectrum antibiotic therapy, as clinically indicated, along with appropriate nutritional support. For a late leak, which often manifests as a subphrenic abscess, percutaneous drainage is first performed. If the fistula does not heal after a few weeks (which is often the case), endoscopic placement of clips, stents, sutures, and glue products may be appealing options but are often unsuccessful. Eventually, surgical intervention may be required to treat chronic persistent fistulas. Many approaches have been attempted with varying success: (a) placement of a gastrostomy tube through the leak site, (b) a serosal patch with the small intestine pulled up to cover the leak, (c) a Roux-en-Y pull-up of the small bowel anastomosed to the leak site, (d) conversion from sleeve to gastric bypass with resection of the leak area, (e) a gastric seromyotomy, or (f) resection of the gastric sleeve with an esophagojejunostomy [51–53].

Venous Thromboembolism

Pulmonary embolism is another common cause of mortality after bariatric surgery, and death from this condition can occur after discharge from hospital. Because of the type of resection and reconstruction involved in BPD±DS, operative times are longer than other commonly performed bariatric procedures. Long times on the table and prolonged postoperative immobilization, along with the underlying state of obesity, place morbidly obese patients at elevated risk of deep venous thrombosis (DVT). The incidence of pulmonary emboli after bariatric surgery is about 1 %. A recent outcome study from the Michigan collaborative group establishes a baseline for the incidence of venous thromboembolic complications following bariatric surgery in recent years. In their multicenter review, the Michigan group reported that the prevalence of DVT not accompanied by pulmonary embolism (PE) was 6,480 events in 508,230 bariatric cases (1.3 %), and venous thromboembolism (VTE), either PE or DVT, occurred in 10,980 of 508,230 (2.2 %). The prevalence of PE was 0.9 %. The reported in-hospital mortality among patients with PE was 130 of 508,231 (0.03 %) in the same study [54].

Patients with a PE may become hypotensive and tachycardic with signs similar to those of sepsis. Nevertheless, in patients with signs of sepsis and hypoxia, the diagnosis of a PE and leak should be simultaneously considered, and appropriate imaging studies to guide diagnosis and treatment should be ordered promptly. An angio-CT of the thorax and a CT scan of the abdomen with oral contrast are helpful. In patients whose body size precludes them from undergoing diagnostic spiral CT imaging, a pulmonary V/Q scan may be helpful; but serious consideration should be given to immediate exploration in the operating room. If no intra-abdominal pathology is found at surgery, therapeutic anticoagulation can be initiated thereafter on clinical grounds.

Early ambulation is the key element of VTE prophylaxis. Difficult cases expected to require prolonged operative times due to poor exposure and difficult dissection are either better staged laparoscopically or converted to open to avoid unnecessary time on the OR table just to complete the procedure under laparoscopy. Sequential compression devices are used intraoperatively and in the early postoperative period to decrease VTE risk. This is often done in addition to pharmacologic prophylaxis with an appropriate dose of low molecular weight heparin (LMWH). It is our practice to discharge patients on subcutaneous LMWH injections for 20 additional days at a dose of 7,500 units of dalteparin.

To date, there are no high quality data favoring one DVT prophylaxis approach over another. In early 2013, the American Society for Metabolic and Bariatric Surgery (ASMBS) Clinical Issues Committee released its recommendations for VTE prophylaxis [55]. The committee considers all bariatric surgery patients as being at elevated risk for VTE. Factors that increase risk include high BMI, advanced age, immobility, prior VTE, known hypercoagulable condition, hormonal therapy, expected long operative time or open approach, and male gender. In the absence of evidence supporting any one regimen for VTE prophylaxis and recognizing that the risk cannot be completely eliminated, the committee recommended that individual bariatric practices should develop and adhere to a protocol for prophylaxis to reduce the risk of thromboembolic disease. While mechanical compression devices and early postoperative ambulation are encouraged, the combination of mechanical prophylaxis and chemoprophylaxis is to be considered based on clinical judgment and risk of bleeding. Although there is some low-level evidence to support using only mechanical prophylaxis, the weight of the data supports using a combination of chemoprophylaxis and mechanical prophylaxis in bariatric patients to lower overall VTE rates to less than 0.5 %. In the absence of contraindications, extended post-discharge VTE prophylaxis for patients deemed to be at high risk should be considered; evidence to support a dose and duration of therapy remains lacking, however.

Hemorrhage

Bleeding is not an infrequent complication after laparoscopic BPD±DS surgery. It is often self-limited, and life-threatening hemorrhage is rare. In a series of 1,000 patients, gastrointestinal hemorrhage after BPD-DS was reported at a rate of 0.5 % [31]. Higher rates, however, have been reported after laparoscopic bariatric procedures involving anastomoses [56]. Bleeding can occur at port sites, intra-abdominally, or intraluminally in the gastrointestinal tract. Intraoperative and postoperative bleeding can be minimized and prevented with measures that include deliberate port placement and removal techniques, careful dissection, and appropriate utilization of energy sources for controlling blood vessels.

Carefully placed single absorbable stitches are recommended to close laparoscopic port sites greater than 10 mm in size, and all port sites should be removed under vision at the end of the procedure. Postoperatively, any significant port site bleed will either result in discoloration around the port site on the first or second postoperative day or abdominal pain with or without hypotension or a drop in hemoglobin (Hb). If a port site bleeds intra-abdominally, a hematoma requiring surgical evacuation may result. A postoperative drop in Hb associated with bruising around a port site or abdominal pain may indicate a significant bleed, but such bleeds are often self-limited and do not require a transfusion.

The gastrosplenic area can pose a hemostatic challenge, especially in cases where the gastric fundus is large, posterior, and sometimes closely intimate with the spleen near its upper pole. Bleeding from short gastric vessels or the splenic capsule can be difficult to control. It is best to avoid bleeding in this area by carefully using laparoscopic energy sources such as ultrasonic or bipolar devices with the judicious aid of metallic clips.

After performing a sleeve gastrectomy in a BPD-DS, the long staple line on the vascular stomach is prone to bleeding, and this can be exacerbated by subcutaneous heparin. Oozing from the staple line can be controlled with clips or suturing. Some surgeons use suture or biosynthetic strips to reinforce the gastric staple line and reduce hemorrhage [57, 58]. Fortunately, staple-line bleeding is usually self-limited, but any large intra-abdominal hematomas resulting from such bleeds may require evacuation to reduce the risk of gastric obstruction and/or leak formation due to a compressive effect of a large hematoma and to facilitate recovery and discharge from hospital.

Postoperative bleeding may cause tachycardia, hypotension, oliguria, persistent hypothermia, a decrease in hematocrit (late sign), or possibly blood collecting in the drains placed at the time of surgery. Intraluminal gastrointestinal hemorrhage can present with hematemesis or melena. The source can be from the gastric mucosa or the upper or lower anastomosis. Upper endoscopy may enable direct visualization and coagulation of the bleeding point. Managing hemorrhage after bariatric surgery depends on the cause and persistence of bleeding, and sometimes endoscopy or surgical exploration is needed for definitive diagnosis and treatment [59]. Bleeding at the mesentery can occur but is often self-limited. It may, however, contribute to a prolonged postoperative ileus or an early small bowel obstruction.

Delayed Postoperative Complications

BPD±DS can result in surgical complications long after the procedure is performed. With appropriate recognition and management, these potential complications can be resolved without significant morbidity or mortality. Common delayed gastrointestinal complications after BPD±DS include marginal ulcers, anastomotic stenosis, intestinal obstruction, dumping syndrome, cholelithiasis, changes in bowel habits, and intestinal bacterial overgrowth.

Marginal Ulcer

Marginal ulcers represent mucosal erosions on the intestinal side of a gastroileal anastomosis or on the ileal side of a duodeno-ileal anastomosis. Because the alkaline bile is diverted in a BPD, the intestinal mucosa at the gastroileal anastomosis receives the gastric acid without having the protective mechanism of acid neutralization with the alkaline biliopancreatic secretions. Scopinaro initially reported a 12.5 % incidence of marginal ulceration, but this later decreased to 3.2 % after resecting more of the distal stomach and utilizing H2 blockers after surgery [14].

In the BPD-DS, the sleeve gastrectomy results in the removal of most of the parietal cell mass, and, hence, the majority of the acid secreting stomach is resected in this procedure [7]. In addition, preserving the pylorus and first portion of the duodenum allows for more controlled gastric emptying and some buffering of the gastric juice entering the small bowel. As expected, this resulted in a low marginal ulceration rate of about 0–1.6 % [16, 60]. We place the patients on PPI for 3 months after BPD-DS and according to symptoms thereafter.

Marginal ulcers can present any time after surgery but seem to be more common after the first few months. The anastomotic technique is not clearly related to the ulceration rate. Patients usually present with upper epigastric pain. Nausea, vomiting, and food intolerance can also be present. Evaluation includes an upper GI endoscopy or a barium swallow. Treatment often involves conservative measures such as smoking cessation, stopping NSAID use, and starting PPI therapy; revision of the anastomosis is infrequently needed in recalcitrant cases.

Stenosis

Stenosis can occur at the proximal or distal anastomosis in the BPD±DS operation. Stenosis at the foot enteroenterostomy is less common but can occasionally present with bowel obstruction as discussed in the section on "Intestinal Obstruction" below. Proximal stenosis can present with food intolerance, nausea, vomiting, and dehydration. It occurs at a reported rate of 0–11 % in laparoscopic series of BPD±DS and often occurs in the first few months after surgery [31, 42, 61]. Workup includes an UGI endoscopy or an UGI series. Occasionally, the patient may require admission to the hospital for rehydration and definitive treatment. In the case of dehydration due to excessive vomiting, we start intravenous vitamin and mineral repletion, particularly thiamine, prior to administration of intravenous glucose containing rehydration solutions to minimize the risk of neurologic sequelae. Stenoses respond well to endoscopic dilation, although more than one session is often required. Surgery is rarely needed to resolve a stenosis unless the endoscopic dilatation is complicated with perforation at or around the site of stenosis [62, 63].

Dumping

Dumping is a syndrome characterized by diaphoresis, tremulousness, nausea, and a sensation of malaise following food ingestion, particularly of foods containing simple sugars [64]. In bariatric surgery, it is more frequently seen after Roux-en-Y gastric bypass or after a BPD with a gastroileal anastomosis [65]. In the BPD-DS, the presence of the pylorus and first part of the duodenum mitigates dumping and reduces symptoms [7]. Physiologically, dumping syndrome can be described as either early or late [64, 66]. Early dumping is characterized by a sympathetic response after the fast arrival of hyperosmolar food into the small bowel; late dumping is caused by a reactive hypoglycemia secondary to hyperinsulinemia after ingestion of a hypercaloric diet. Although uncomfortable, the dumping phenomena are thought to help certain patients in maintaining their weight by preventing them from consuming large amounts of high-calorie, simple sugar foods; evidence for this remains lacking.

Intestinal Obstruction

Intestinal obstruction after laparoscopic BPD surgery can occur as a result of a number of conditions: (1) internal hernias, (2) adhesions, (3) intestinal anastomotic stenosis, (4) port site hernias, (5) ventral abdominal wall hernias, and (6) incorrect bowel limb anastomosis. Measures can be taken to reduce postoperative intestinal obstruction by understanding the different causes and paying attention to the surgical techniques used to perform the operation. Adhesions can occur after the primary bariatric procedure, and some may be due to subclinical postoperative leaks; they can also be secondary to other prior operations, particularly pelvic or gynecologic surgery, and this must be kept in mind to guide management. No current treatment exists to prevent adhesive bowel obstruction.

A potentially serious complication after bariatric surgery is that of intestinal obstruction secondary to internal hernia formation. In malabsorptive procedures, the creation of mesenteric defects during surgical reconstruction of the gastrointestinal tract with the upper and lower anastomoses predisposes patients to internal hernias through these defects in the short and long term, especially after weight loss. Bowel obstruction in this context, unlike other general surgical conditions, can be devastating due to the tendency of the obstruction to be closed loop and ischemic in nature rather than a simple adhesive intestinal obstruction. Laparoscopic techniques create fewer adhesions postoperatively and decrease the risk of adhesive obstruction to 0.3 % [67]. This, however, has not translated into an overall lower incidence of small bowel obstruction after laparoscopic bariatric procedures compared to open ones (about 3.6 % versus 2 %), and this is explained by the greater tendency of the bowel to move and herniate through surgically created defects [68]. Proper closure of these defects with permanent suture is generally recommended despite data in the Roux-en-Y gastric bypass literature showing low internal hernia rates in some series where defects are left unclosed. The enteroenteric mesenteric defect is usually more amenable to safe closure and should be closed in all instances. The defect between the alimentary limb (or Roux limb) mesentery and the mesocolon (Petersen defect) is usually more challenging to close, but attempts should be made to safely do so. It is believed that antecolic placement of the Roux limb is associated with a lower incidence of internal hernia and bowel obstruction than the retrocolic passage of this Roux limb through the transverse colon mesentery [68]. Champion et al. noted a decrease in the incidence of small bowel obstruction from 4.5 to 0.4 % after changing to the antecolic approach [69]. Internal hernias observed with the retrocolic technique tend to be more related to the mesocolic defect than to the true Petersen defect itself, and closure of mesocolic defects, when created, is preferred. One must keep in mind that hernias can occur even after closure of mesenteric defects due to sutures tearing out of the weak mesenteric peritoneum early after suture placement or due to suture resorption or migration over time.

While antecolic Roux limb placement and closure of surgical defects with suture may decrease internal hernias, it may increase adhesive small bowel obstructions or acute angulation at the ileoileostomy. The technique of mesenteric defect closure can predispose to angulation at the ileoileostomy. Anti-obstructive sutures placed here between the two segments of the small bowel can minimize angulation. Obstruction at the ileoileostomy can occur more often if the enteroenterostomy is closed with a stapler, narrowing the lumen. This complication can be minimized with careful stapler placement or with the use of suture to close the roof of the mechanically created foot anastomosis.

Incorrect bowel limb anastomosis (Roux-en-O) is not often reported, but may occur sporadically. The incorrect limb is anastomosed to the duodenum/stomach. It is important to prevent this complication intraoperatively by systematically labeling and verifying intestinal limbs prior to reconstruction. It is also preferable to recognize this situation and repair it at the time of the initial surgery, as detection in the postoperative period may be delayed and early radiologic images may be nondiagnostic. In our experience of about 5,000 patients, this complication occurred twice. One was recognized intraoperatively and repaired without consequences. Another was recognized 3 months postoperatively in a patient who had excessive weight loss and vomiting in the absence of gastric obstruction or anastomotic stenosis, and reoperation in this patient was associated with lethal complications. A HIDA scan provided the best imaging of the condition as the radioactive label was traced from the BPL back to the stomach.

Because bowel obstruction after bariatric surgery can be a real surgical emergency, timely recognition of clinical signs and symptoms and appropriate utilization of diagnostic tests can reduce morbidity and mortality [70]. The surgeon must have a high index of suspicion for serious conditions (closed-loop obstruction and intestinal strangulation) and a low threshold for surgical exploration of any postoperative BPD±DS patient who presents with persistent or recurrent GI complaints such as abdominal pain, nausea, or vomiting. The small bowel may become ischemic in as little as 6 h after the onset of closed-loop obstruction. Symptoms vary in severity from mild intermittent epigastric abdominal pain and cramping to severe incapacitating pain radiating to the back and associated with persistent nausea and vomiting.

While obstruction of the alimentary limb or common channel presents with the typical symptoms of nausea, vomiting, and/or obstipation, obstruction of the BPL is more difficult to diagnose. It may cause abdominal fullness and bloating and pain from visceral distention or from pancreatitis. Yet, the patient may eat, pass gas, and have bowel movements. One must always be aware of obstructions involving the BPL, leading to duodenal distention with bile and pancreatic enzymes and possible blowout of the duodenal stump. If detected late in its clinical course, closed-loop obstruction from internal hernias can lead to ischemia and necrosis of a significant length of intestine with perforation resulting in peritonitis, short bowel syndrome post resection, or even death. Laboratory test such as serum lipase or amylase and liver enzymes may be elevated with ischemic bowel or BPL obstruction, and this may be confused with pancreatitis or gallstone disease.

Diagnostic imaging is very helpful in the evaluation of stable patients. It is worth noting that obstruction in the BPL segment does not necessarily show on the flat and upright abdominal radiographs routinely used to diagnose small bowel obstruction because air-fluid levels are often absent. Abdominal CT scans are generally more helpful in bariatric patients. However, if the patient is unstable, immediate surgical exploration may be the best diagnostic and therapeutic modality. Spiral helical CT scanning with only small amounts of oral contrast can be the most accurate diagnostic tool outside of the operating room, and it should be performed with the shortest delay possible in relatively stable patients [71]. Radiologic signs on CT include dilated bowel, thickened bowel wall, contrast or fluid in the BPL, increased free intraperitoneal fluid, a preponderance of bowel on one side of the abdomen, and mesenteric vascular congestion or twisting (the "swirl" or "twirl" sign, which may be enhanced with the addition of IV contrast to the study). Bariatric surgeons should ideally review all the abdominal CT scans with radiologists to improve image interpretation at the time of presentation.

Since clinical and radiologic signs can be nonspecific and CT scans may be nondiagnostic or falsely interpreted as negative, surgeons must keep a high index of suspicion for pathology best evaluated in the operating room. Nonoperative management of small bowel obstruction should be utilized with caution. The majority of adhesive small bowel obstructions resolve with conservative management. In contrast, obstruction from internal hernia is a surgical emergency, needing reduction of herniated small bowel and possible revision of the anastomosis, resection of nonviable bowel, and repair of the defect.

Surgical exploration requires a systematic and comprehensive examination of the entire abdomen and pelvis, regardless of the suspected etiology. Having access to the bariatric operative record is helpful in clarifying how the GI tract was reconstructed. Laparoscopic evaluation should include running the small intestine from the cecum to the foot anastomosis identifying the common channel and then to the duodeno-ileal/gastroileal anastomosis and to the ligament of Treitz to evaluate the rest of the alimentary limb and the BPL, respectively. All potential defects should be evaluated and closed. There may be a role for intraoperative endoscopy to examine the proximal anastomosis. In case of internal hernias with significant distortion of the anatomy,

conversion to open surgery may be needed. Adhesions should be lysed and mobilized, especially around the ileoileostomy. Stenosis of this anastomosis may be managed with resection and revision. A feeding jejunostomy placed in the proximal BPL may be required to decompress the small bowel and later provide nutritional support, especially if hypoproteinemia is present preoperatively or if ischemic bowel or perforation with peritonitis is diagnosed and a protracted recovery is expected.

Cholelithiasis

Rapid weight loss, whether surgical or after lifestyle changes, has been associated with gallstone formation [72–74]. Performing a cholecystectomy at the time of a bariatric procedure to prevent cholelithiasis and related complications is not sufficiently addressed in the literature, and surgical practices vary. Many series describe performing a routine cholecystectomy at the time of open BPD±DS surgery [75]. This practice evolved in the absence of a good evidence base and has started to change in the era of laparoscopic surgery without availability of consensus or guidelines [76, 77]. In Scopinaro's early reports on BPD, a high incidence of gallstones was diagnosed in their patients after surgery; simultaneous routine cholecystectomy was, therefore, recommended [78]. We have also adhered to this practice from 1994 to 2008 in open BPD-DS surgery. In 1995, Sugerman et al. described the effectiveness of ursodeoxycholic acid as a prophylactic treatment of gallstone formation after weight loss surgery [79].

Recently a large population-based study from Sweden reviewed a cohort of over 13,000 patients and confirmed the increased occurrence of cholecystectomy after bariatric surgery [80]. It suggested that this might be more related to gallstone detection bias than to an elevated risk of symptomatic gallstones. In this study, an individual's risk of symptomatic cholelithiasis mandating cholecystectomy after bariatric surgery remained low, making prophylactic cholecystectomy during bariatric surgery questionable.

In the setting of BPD-DS surgery, a recent publication described selectively performing a cholecystectomy in patients with gallstones [81]. Patients who did not undergo a cholecystectomy were placed on ursodeoxycholic acid for 6 months. Of these patients, 8.7 % subsequently required a cholecystectomy. This led the investigators to conclude that a routine cholecystectomy in the context of a BPD-DS is unwarranted and that selective gallbladder removal is more appropriate.

When we perform laparoscopic BPD-DS, we are liberal yet selective in our decision to remove the gallbladder. The presence of asymptomatic gallstones on preoperative ultrasound is one indication for removing the gallbladder, especially in younger patients who have a greater lifetime risk of complicated cholelithiasis and in women of childbearing age. In brief, other factors that influence our decision, however, include the following: (1) procedure time, (2) gallbladder size and position, (3) technical difficulty in achieving the critical view for gallbladder dissection, and (4) other advantages of performing a concomitant cholecystectomy. To avoid prolonging surgical time under anesthesia in difficult cases, the gallbladder may be left in situ. The gallbladder is also left in place if the dissection and identification of the cystic duct and common bile duct junction appear problematic. On the other hand, if the gallbladder size and position hinder adequate exposure for dissection and division of the duodenum and subsequent creation of the duodenoileostomy, the gallbladder is removed. If the gallbladder is left in place, our routine is to prescribe ursodeoxycholic acid for 6 months postoperatively. We feel that after weight loss, and if gallstone symptoms develop, the favorable anatomy and better exposure can reduce the risk of bile duct injury. Nevertheless, real advantages of performing a concomitant cholecystectomy at the time of BPD±DS cannot be ignored, even when preoperative ultrasound does not show cholelithiasis: the chances of gallstone formation after a BPD±DS may be higher than with other less malabsorptive bariatric operations because of the reduction in enterohepatic circulation and greater loss of bile salts as well as the greater cholesterol excretion seen with greater weight loss. A subsequent urgent cholecystectomy may also be more difficult in the presence of an inflamed gallbladder and adhesions in the area of the duodeno-ileal anastomosis. Also, if patients develop choledocholithiasis after a BPD±DS, access to the bile duct by endoscopic retrograde cholangiopancreatography is more challenging and impossible in the routine fashion. Management of symptomatic and complicated choledocholithiasis will, therefore, be more involved and often percutaneous or surgical in nature with transintestinal ERCP or direct common bile duct exploration.

Changes in Bowel Habits and Intestinal Bacterial Overgrowth

For patients, increased stool frequency and malodorous stools and gas can be one of the most annoying side effects of malabsorptive procedures. The odor is typical of pancreatic insufficiency, and pancreatic enzymes taken orally with meals can improve this symptom but can be associated with weight regain. These side effects or symptoms are reported by about 1/3 of patients and forces them to decrease fat intake and to avoid certain food altogether; nevertheless, over 90 % consider their eating habits after BPD-DS as normal. The problems with stools and gas subside over the years but can remain intermittent and annoying for some individuals. The number of stools after surgery is about 3 per day [3, 82], and stools were loose more than three times a week in 30 %, while constipation was reported by 12 %

[82]. Symptoms after BPD±DS also include frequent abdominal bloating, often reported in association with excess carbohydrate intake. Bacterial overgrowth is thought to contribute to these gastrointestinal symptoms of abdominal distension, diarrhea, foul stools and gas, and proctitis. Although, there is no blind limb in the standard BPD±DS operations, symptomatic bacterial overgrowth can occur, and this is evidenced by the response of related symptoms to intermittent brief pulses of antibiotic therapy mostly in the form of oral metronidazole [82–84]. When no improvement is reported after such therapy, dietary factors must be evaluated and adjusted.

Weight Recidivism

BPD±DS is a very effective surgical weight loss procedure. It is among the most potent treatments for morbid obesity as far as weight loss and sustained results are concerned [1–3]. Nevertheless, insufficient weight loss can occasionally result, but much less so than with other bariatric procedures, and weight loss failure or recidivism does not pose a frequent problem after BPD±DS surgery [85]. In 2007, Marceau et al. summarized their 15-year experience with BPD±DS as a primary (open) procedure in 1,423 patients [82]. Revision surgery for weight loss failure was needed in only 1.5 % and resulted on average in an additional 14 kg weight loss. When revision surgery was offered in this series, it included shortening of the intestinal channels to the conventional 250/100 cm, as alimentary limb elongation was observed at repeat surgery and was deemed secondary to intestinal adaptation over time. Interestingly, this phenomenon was also observed in a rodent BPD-DS model [86]. In a few of the revised patients, a repeat sleeve gastrectomy was also performed. Re-sleeve alone has been shown to work in the short term [87]. Revisional bariatric surgery for weight loss failure must be considered carefully as it is not clear which patients will benefit from further surgical intervention [88]. In malabsorptive surgery, shortening the common channel to less than 75 cm is generally not recommended as it can result in increased rates of protein-calorie deficiency [8]. In evaluating patients with insufficient weight loss and weight regain, the presence of certain surgical situations or medical conditions should be considered and evaluated with appropriate investigational modalities. These conditions may include (1) a residual large gastric pouch, (2) a long common channel, (3) uncontrolled eating disorder, (4) wrong choice of initial operation for the patient, (5) alcohol addiction, (6) drug side effects, and (7) undiagnosed medical condition leading to secondary obesity. Binge eating behavior, for example, which is common among the morbidly obese, may recur after surgery and is associated with weight regain [89]. Addressing nonsurgical factors contributing to weight loss failure is, therefore, important before subjecting patients to revision surgery, which is known to be associated with higher complication rates than primary operations. Patient education and dietary modifications are essential to good outcomes. Nutritionists are important members of the assessment team at the time of initial evaluation, during follow-up, and when evaluating patients with weight regain.

Conclusion

Malabsorptive bariatric procedures like the BPD±DS offer powerful and sustained weight loss and improvements in obesity-related comorbidities. Offering these procedures laparoscopically improves the complication profile of the operation and accelerates postoperative recovery and discharge from hospital. Early recognition of procedure-related complications and timely intervention depend on a knowledge of the bariatric procedure, the anatomic reconfiguration of the gastrointestinal tract, and the associated physiologic changes after surgery. Intraoperative strategies are employed to minimize surgical complications in hospital, and early postoperative management involves close patient follow-up and prompt investigation when patients stray from the usual postoperative course. Active patient participation in follow-up and adherence to dietary and medical counseling is also essential for success. In this fashion, both surgeons and patients can achieve great satisfaction from the effect these procedures have on improving the medical condition and quality of life of severely obese patients.

Review Questions and Answers

Question 1

Which of the following statements about important factors that influence postoperative morbidity is false?

1. Advanced age and BMI are two factors that predict postoperative morbidity related to bariatric surgical procedures requiring gastrointestinal anastomoses.
2. The more a patient is dependent on others for assistance with activities of daily living in the immediate preoperative period, the higher the risk of postoperative morbidity and mortality.
3. Whether bariatric procedures with a malabsorptive component are performed laparoscopically or via open laparotomy does not influence the risk of postoperative morbidity.
4. In large patient database samples, male gender and diabetes appear to increase the 30-day risk of perioperative complications after laparoscopic bariatric surgery.

Question 2

Which of the following statements about leaks after biliopancreatic diversion with duodenal switch (BPD-DS) is true?

1. Potential sites of gastrointestinal leakage after a laparoscopic BPD-DS are limited to one of the following four areas: the duodenoileostomy, the ileoileostomy, the gastric staple line, and the duodenal stump staple line.
2. Although leaks are a serious source of morbidity and occur with a reported incidence of 0–8 % in different laparoscopic series, they are implicated in less than 2 % of deaths after bariatric surgery.
3. Gastric leaks in a BPD-DS procedure occur most often along the greater curve opposite the gastric incisura.
4. To date, a generally accepted algorithm for the management of gastric staple line leaks in the early postoperative period is yet to be described.

Question 3

Which of the following statements regarding delayed surgical complications following laparoscopic malabsorptive surgery is false?

1. Marginal ulcers are low in incidence after contemporary malabsorptive procedures.
2. Because BPD-DS results in loss of continuity of the foregut making future routine ERCP impossible if needed, a cholecystectomy must be performed at the time of the BPD-DS.
3. Dumping syndrome is more frequently seen after Roux-en-Y gastric bypass than after biliopancreatic diversion with duodenal switch.
4. Bowel obstruction secondary to internal herniation is a surgical emergency requiring a high index of suspicion for timely diagnosis and management.

Answers

Q1: #3
Q2: #4
Q3: #2

References

1. Buchwald H, Avidor Y, Braunwald E, Jensen MD, Pories W, Fahrbach K, et al. Bariatric surgery: a systematic review and meta-analysis. JAMA. 2004;292(14):1724–37.
2. Demaria EJ, Jamal MK. Surgical options for obesity. Gastroenterol Clin North Am. 2005;34(1):127–42.

3. Anthone GJ, Lord RV, DeMeester TR, Crookes PF. The duodenal switch operation for the treatment of morbid obesity. Ann Surg. 2003;238(4):618–27; discussion 627–8. PMCID: 1360120.

4. Buchwald H, Varco RL, Moore RB, Schwartz MZ. Intestinal bypass procedures. Partial ileal bypass for hyperlipidemai and jejunoileal bypass for obesity. Curr Probl Surg. 1975;1–51.

5. Baker MT. The history and evolution of bariatric surgical procedures. Surg Clin North Am. 2011;91(6):1181–201; viii.

6. Fisher BL, Schauer P. Medical and surgical options in the treatment of severe obesity. Am J Surg. 2002;184(6B):9S–16.

7. Marceau P, Biron S, Bourque RA, Potvin M, Hould FS, Simard S. Biliopancreatic diversion with a new type of gastrectomy. Obes Surg. 1993;3(1):29–35.

8. Brolin RE, LaMarca LB, Kenler HA, Cody RP. Malabsorptive gastric bypass in patients with superobesity. J Gastrointest Surg. 2002;6(2):195–203; discussion 204–5.

9. Dumon KR, Murayama KM. Bariatric surgery outcomes. Surg Clin North Am. 2011;91(6):1313–38; x.

10. Nguyen NT, Masoomi H, Magno CP, Nguyen XM, Laugenour K, Lane J. Trends in use of bariatric surgery, 2003-2008. J Am Coll Surg. 2011;213(2):261–6.

11. Nguyen NT, Nguyen B, Gebhart A, Hohmann S. Changes in the makeup of bariatric surgery: a national increase in use of laparoscopic sleeve gastrectomy. J Am Coll Surg. 2013;216(2):252–7.

12. Buchwald H, Oien DM. Metabolic/bariatric surgery worldwide 2011. Obes Surg. 2013;23:427–36.

13. Scopinaro N, Gianetta E, Civalleri D, Bonalumi U, Bachi V. Biliopancreatic bypass for obesity: II. Initial experience in man. Br J Surg. 1979;66(9):618–20.

14. Scopinaro N, Adami GF, Marinari GM, Gianetta E, Traverso E, Friedman D, et al. Biliopancreatic diversion. World J Surg. 1998;22(9):936–46.

15. Marceau P, Hould FS, Simard S, Lebel S, Bourque RA, Potvin M, et al. Biliopancreatic diversion with duodenal switch. World J Surg. 1998;22(9):947–54.

16. Hess DS, Hess DW. Biliopancreatic diversion with a duodenal switch. Obes Surg. 1998;8(3):267–82.

17. Biertho L, Biron S, Hould FS, Lebel S, Marceau S, Marceau P. Is biliopancreatic diversion with duodenal switch indicated for patients with body mass index <50 kg/m2? Surg Obes Relat Dis. 2010;6(5):508–14.

18. Ren CJ, Patterson E, Gagner M. Early results of laparoscopic biliopancreatic diversion with duodenal switch: a case series of 40 consecutive patients. Obes Surg. 2000;10(6):514–23; discussion 524.

19. DeMaria EJ, Schauer P, Patterson E, Nguyen NT, Jacob BP, Inabnet WB, et al. The optimal surgical management of the super-obese patient: the debate. Presented at the annual meeting of the Society of American Gastrointestinal and Endoscopic Surgeons, Hollywood, Florida, USA, April 13–16, 2005. Surg Innov. 2005;12(2):107–21.

20. Chand B, Gugliotti D, Schauer P, Steckner K. Perioperative management of the bariatric surgery patient: focus on cardiac and anesthesia considerations. Cleve Clin J Med. 2006;73 Suppl 1:S51–6.

21. Sekhar N, Gagner M. Complications of laparoscopic biliopancreatic diversion with duodenal switch. Curr Surg. 2003;60(3):279–80; discussion 280–1.

22. DeMaria EJ, Portenier D, Wolfe L. Obesity surgery mortality risk score: proposal for a clinically useful score to predict mortality risk in patients undergoing gastric bypass. Surg Obes Relat Dis. 2007;3(2):134–40.

23. Fernandez Jr AZ, Demaria EJ, Tichansky DS, Kellum JM, Wolfe LG, Meador J, et al. Multivariate analysis of risk factors for death following gastric bypass for treatment of morbid obesity. Ann Surg. 2004;239(5):698–702; discussion–703. PMCID: 1356278.

24. Khan MA, Grinberg R, Johnson S, Afthinos JN, Gibbs KE. Perioperative risk factors for 30-day mortality after bariatric surgery: is functional status important? Surg Endosc. 2013;27: 1772–7.

25. Broadbent R, Tracey M, Harrington P. Laparoscopic gastric banding: a preliminary report. Obes Surg. 1993;3(1):63–7.

26. Catona A, La Manna L, La Manna A, Sampiero C. Swedish adjustable gastric banding: a preliminary experience. Obes Surg. 1997;7(3):203–5; discussion 206.

27. Wittgrove AC, Clark GW. Laparoscopic gastric bypass, Roux-en-Y-500 patients: technique and results, with 3-60 month follow-up. Obes Surg. 2000;10(3):233–9.

28. Gagner M, Matteotti R. Laparoscopic biliopancreatic diversion with duodenal switch. Surg Clin North Am. 2005;85(1): 141–9; x–xi.

29. Paiva D, Bernardes L, Suretti L. Laparoscopic biliopancreatic diversion for the treatment of morbid obesity: initial experience. Obes Surg. 2001;11(5):619–22.

30. Scopinaro N, Marinari GM, Camerini G. Laparoscopic standard biliopancreatic diversion: technique and preliminary results. Obes Surg. 2002;12(3):362–5.

31. Biertho L, Lebel S, Marceau S, Hould FS, Lescelleur O, Moustarah F, et al. Perioperative complications in a consecutive series of 1000 duodenal switches. Surg Obes Relat Dis. 2013;9(1):63–8.

32. Regan JP, Inabnet WB, Gagner M, Pomp A. Early experience with two-stage laparoscopic Roux-en-Y gastric bypass as an alternative in the super-super obese patient. Obes Surg. 2003;13(6):861–4.

33. Silecchia G, Rizzello M, Casella G, Fioriti M, Soricelli E, Basso N. Two-stage laparoscopic biliopancreatic diversion with duodenal switch as treatment of high-risk super-obese patients: analysis of complications. Surg Endosc. 2009;23(5):1032–7.

34. Topart P, Becouarn G, Ritz P. Should biliopancreatic diversion with duodenal switch be done as single-stage procedure in patients with BMI > or = 50 kg/m2? Surg Obes Relat Dis. 2010;6(1):59–63.

35. Pories WJ, Swanson MS, MacDonald KG, Long SB, Morris PG, Brown BM, et al. Who would have thought it? An operation proves to be the most effective therapy for adult-onset diabetes mellitus. Ann Surg. 1995;222(3):339–50; discussion 350–2. PMCID: 1234815.

36. Oh CH, Kim HJ, Oh S. Weight loss following transected gastric bypass with proximal Roux-en-Y. Obes Surg. 1997;7(2):142–7; discussion 148.

37. Kellum JM, DeMaria EJ, Sugerman HJ. The surgical treatment of morbid obesity. Curr Probl Surg. 1998;35(9):791–858.

38. Reoch J, Mottillo S, Shimony A, Filion KB, Christou NV, Joseph L, et al. Safety of laparoscopic vs open bariatric surgery: a systematic review and meta-analysis. Arch Surg. 2011;146(11):1314–22.

39. Vilos GA, Ternamian A, Dempster J, Laberge PY, The Society of Obstetricians and Gynaecologists of Canada. Laparoscopic entry: a review of techniques, technologies, and complications. J Obstet Gynaecol Can. 2007;29(5):433–65.

40. Ahmad G, O'Flynn H, Duffy JM, Phillips K, Watson A. Laparoscopic entry techniques. Cochrane Database Syst Rev. 2012;(2):CD006583.

41. Baltasar A, Bou R, Miro J, Bengochea M, Serra C, Perez N. Laparoscopic biliopancreatic diversion with duodenal switch: technique and initial experience. Obes Surg. 2002;12(2):245–8.

42. Dolan K, Hatzifotis M, Newbury L, Fielding G. A comparison of laparoscopic adjustable gastric banding and biliopancreatic diversion in superobesity. Obes Surg. 2004;14(2):165–9.

43. Sudan R, Puri V, Sudan D. Robotically assisted biliary pancreatic diversion with a duodenal switch: a new technique. Surg Endosc. 2007;21(5):729–33.

44. Hamilton EC, Sims TL, Hamilton TT, Mullican MA, Jones DB, Provost DA. Clinical predictors of leak after laparoscopic

Roux-en-Y gastric bypass for morbid obesity. Surg Endosc. 2003;17(5):679–84.

45. Leslie DB, Dorman RB, Anderson J, Serrot FJ, Kellogg TA, Buchwald H, et al. Routine upper gastrointestinal imaging is superior to clinical signs for detecting gastrojejunal leak after laparoscopic Roux-en-Y gastric bypass. J Am Coll Surg. 2012;214(2): 208–13.

46. Aurora AR, Khaitan L, Saber AA. Sleeve gastrectomy and the risk of leak: a systematic analysis of 4,888 patients. Surg Endosc. 2012;26(6):1509–15.

47. Sakran N, Goitein D, Raziel A, Keidar A, Beglaibter N, Grinbaum R, et al. Gastric leaks after sleeve gastrectomy: a multicenter experience with 2,834 patients. Surg Endosc. 2013;27(1):240–5.

48. Burgos AM, Braghetto I, Csendes A, Maluenda F, Korn O, Yarmuch J, et al. Gastric leak after laparoscopic-sleeve gastrectomy for obesity. Obes Surg. 2009;19(12):1672–7.

49. El Mourad H, Himpens J, Verhofstadt J. Stent treatment for fistula after obesity surgery: results in 47 consecutive patients. Surg Endosc. 2013;27(3):808–16.

50. Simon F, Siciliano I, Gillet A, Castel B, Coffin B, Msika S. Gastric leak after laparoscopic sleeve gastrectomy: early covered self-expandable stent reduces healing time. Obes Surg. 2013;23: 687–92.

51. Court I, Wilson A, Benotti P, Szomstein S, Rosenthal RJ. T-tube gastrostomy as a novel approach for distal staple line disruption after sleeve gastrectomy for morbid obesity: case report and review of the literature. Obes Surg. 2010;20(4):519–22.

52. Baltasar A, Bou R, Bengochea M, Serra C, Cipagauta L. Use of a Roux limb to correct esophagogastric junction fistulas after sleeve gastrectomy. Obes Surg. 2007;17(10):1408–10.

53. Martin-Malagon A, Rodriguez-Ballester L, Arteaga-Gonzalez I. Total gastrectomy for failed treatment with endotherapy of chronic gastrocutaneous fistula after sleeve gastrectomy. Surg Obes Relat Dis. 2011;7(2):240–2.

54. Stein PD, Matta F. Pulmonary embolism and deep venous thrombosis following bariatric surgery. Obes Surg. 2013;23:663–8.

55. Clinical Issues Committee. ASMBS updated position statement on prophylactic measures to reduce the risk of venous thromboembolism in bariatric surgery patients. Surg Obes Relat Dis. 2013;9: 493–7.

56. Podnos YD, Jimenez JC, Wilson SE, Stevens CM, Nguyen NT. Complications after laparoscopic gastric bypass: a review of 3464 cases. Arch Surg. 2003;138(9):957–61.

57. Glaysher M, Khan OA, Mabvuure N, Wan A, Reddy M, Vasilikostas G. Staple line reinforcement during laparoscopic sleeve gastrectomy: does it affect clinical outcomes? Int J Surg. 2013;11:286–9.

58. Sajid MS, Khatri K, Singh K, Sayegh M. Use of staple-line reinforcement in laparoscopic gastric bypass surgery: a meta-analysis. Surg Endosc. 2011;25(9):2884–91.

59. Ferreira LE, Song LM, Baron TH. Management of acute postoperative hemorrhage in the bariatric patient. Gastrointest Endosc Clin N Am. 2011;21(2):287–94.

60. Baltasar A, Bou R, Bengochea M, Arlandis F, Escriva C, Miro J, et al. Duodenal switch: an effective therapy for morbid obesity–intermediate results. Obes Surg. 2001;11(1):54–8.

61. Topart P, Becouarn G, Ritz P. Comparative early outcomes of three laparoscopic bariatric procedures: sleeve gastrectomy, Roux-en-Y gastric bypass, and biliopancreatic diversion with duodenal switch. Surg Obes Relat Dis. 2012;8(3):250–4.

62. Catalano MF, Chua TY, Rudic G. Endoscopic balloon dilation of stomal stenosis following gastric bypass. Obes Surg. 2007;17(3): 298–303.

63. Carrodeguas L, Szomstein S, Zundel N, Lo Menzo E, Rosenthal R. Gastrojejunal anastomotic strictures following laparoscopic

64. Tack J, Arts J, Caenepeel P, De Wulf D, Bisschops R. Pathophysiology, diagnosis and management of postoperative dumping syndrome. Nat Rev Gastroenterol Hepatol. 2009;6(10): 583–90.

65. Lim RB, Blackburn GL, Jones DB. Benchmarking best practices in weight loss surgery. Curr Prob Surg. 2010;47(2):79–174. PMCID: 3134527.

66. Ukleja A. Dumping syndrome: pathophysiology and treatment. Nutr Clin Pract. 2005;20(5):517–25.

67. Schauer PR, Ikramuddin S, Gourash W, Ramanathan R, Luketich J. Outcomes after laparoscopic Roux-en-Y gastric bypass for morbid obesity. Ann Surg. 2000;232(4):515–29. PMCID: 1421184.

68. Koppman JS, Li C, Gandsas A. Small bowel obstruction after laparoscopic Roux-en-Y gastric bypass: a review of 9,527 patients. J Am Coll Surg. 2008;206(3):571–84.

69. Champion JK, Williams M. Small bowel obstruction and internal hernias after laparoscopic Roux-en-Y gastric bypass. Obes Surg. 2003;13(4):596–600.

70. Garza Jr E, Kuhn J, Arnold D, Nicholson W, Reddy S, McCarty T. Internal hernias after laparoscopic Roux-en-Y gastric bypass. Am J Surg. 2004;188(6):796–800.

71. Ahmed AR, Rickards G, Johnson J, Boss T, O'Malley W. Radiological findings in symptomatic internal hernias after laparoscopic gastric bypass. Obes Surg. 2009;19(11):1530–5.

72. Deitel M, Petrov I. Incidence of symptomatic gallstones after bariatric operations. Surg Gynecol Obstet. 1987;164(6):549–52.

73. Worobetz LJ, Inglis FG, Shaffer EA. The effect of ursodeoxycholic acid therapy on gallstone formation in the morbidly obese during rapid weight loss. Am J Gastroenterol. 1993;88(10):1705–10.

74. Yang H, Petersen GM, Roth MP, Schoenfield LJ, Marks JW. Risk factors for gallstone formation during rapid loss of weight. Dig Dis Sci. 1992;37(6):912–8.

75. Sudan R, Jacobs DO. Biliopancreatic diversion with duodenal switch. Surg Clin North Am. 2011;91(6):1281–93; ix.

76. Mason EE, Renquist KE. Gallbladder management in obesity surgery. Obes Surg. 2002;12(2):222–9.

77. Patel JA, Patel NA, Piper GL, Smith III DE, Malhotra G, Colella JJ. Perioperative management of cholelithiasis in patients presenting for laparoscopic Roux-en-Y gastric bypass: have we reached a consensus? Am Surg. 2009;75(6):470–6; discussion 476.

78. Scopinaro N, Gianetta E, Civalleri D, Bonalumi U, Bachi V. Two years of clinical experience with biliopancreatic bypass for obesity. Am J Clin Nutr. 1980;33(2 Suppl):506–14.

79. Sugerman HJ, Brewer WH, Shiffman ML, Brolin RE, Fobi MA, Linner JH, et al. A multicenter, placebo-controlled, randomized, double-blind, prospective trial of prophylactic ursodiol for the prevention of gallstone formation following gastric-bypass-induced rapid weight loss. Am J Surg. 1995;169(1):91–6; discussion 96–7.

80. Plecka Ostlund M, Wenger U, Mattsson F, Ebrahim F, Botha A, Lagergren J. Population-based study of the need for cholecystectomy after obesity surgery. Br J Surg. 2012;99(6):864–9.

81. Bardaro SJ, Gagner M, Consten E, Inabnet WB, Herron D, Dakin G, et al. Routine cholecystectomy during laparoscopic biliopancreatic diversion with duodenal switch is not necessary. Surg Obes Relat Dis. 2007;3(5):549–53.

82. Marceau P, Biron S, Hould FS, Lebel S, Marceau S, Lescelleur O, et al. Duodenal switch: long-term results. Obes Surg. 2007;17(11):1421–30.

83. Marceau P, Hould FS, Lebel S, Marceau S, Biron S. Malabsorptive obesity surgery. Surg Clin North Am. 2001;81(5):1113–27.

84. Michielson D, Van Hee R, Hendrickx L. Complications of biliopancreatic diversion surgery as proposed by scopinaro in the treatment of morbid obesity. Obes Surg. 1996;6(5):416–20.

85. Topart P, Becouarn G, Ritz P. Weight loss is more sustained after biliopancreatic diversion with duodenal switch than Roux-en-Y gastric bypass in superobese patients. Surg Obes Relat Dis. 2013;9:526–30.

86. Nadreau E, Baraboi ED, Samson P, Blouin A, Hould FS, Marceau P, et al. Effects of the biliopancreatic diversion on energy balance in the rat. Int J Obes (Lond). 2006;30(3):419–29.

87. Iannelli A, Schneck AS, Noel P, Ben Amor I, Krawczykowski D, Gugenheim J. Re-sleeve gastrectomy for failed laparoscopic sleeve gastrectomy: a feasibility study. Obes Surg. 2011;21(7):832–5.

88. Kellogg TA. Revisional bariatric surgery. Surg Clin North Am. 2011;91(6):1353–71; x.

89. Hsu LK, Benotti PN, Dwyer J, Roberts SB, Saltzman E, Shikora S, et al. Nonsurgical factors that influence the outcome of bariatric surgery: a review. Psychosom Med. 1998;60(3):338–46.

35

Laparoscopic Malabsorption Procedures: Management of Nutritional Complications After Biliopancreatic Diversion

Fady Moustarah and Frédéric-Simon Hould

Introduction

The biliopancreatic diversion (BPD), with or without duodenal switch (BPD±DS), is the main bariatric procedure practiced today with a significant malabsorptive component. It induces substantial and sustained weight loss, plus remarkable improvements in obesity-related comorbidities compared to other bariatric surgeries [1–3]. Although food malabsorption is the principal mechanism responsible for weight loss maintenance, BPD±DS procedures also have restrictive components. The Scopinaro-type BPD has evolved over time [4], now leaving about 1/3 of the proximal stomach intact (300–500 mL reservoir) proximal to the gastroileostomy; the BPD with duodenal switch (BPDDS) procedure includes a sleeve gastrectomy [5, 6]. Thus, restricted caloric intake can contribute to metabolic changes, weight loss, and nutritional consequences after BPD±DS, especially in the early postoperative period (3–14 days) and in the early weight loss phase (first 12–18 months). Since the number of bariatric procedures performed dramatically increased over the past two decades [7–9], familiarity with clinically important nutritional sequelae that can appear after malabsorptive procedures is paramount to maintaining good postoperative outcomes [10]. This chapter reviews the management of important nutritional complications specific to BPD±DS, highlighting the importance of perioperative evaluation and management, multidisciplinary care, and lifelong follow-up.

Perioperative Nutritional Management

Nutritional management of patients who are being considered for BPD±DS starts before surgery and continues for life. In general, poor dietary habits or maladaptive eating behaviors and vitamin deficiencies are common in bariatric surgery candidates [11–14]. Eating disorders such as binging or emotional eating existing before surgery or poor eating habits and food choices emerging after surgery, for example to alleviate discomfort related to certain foods,

may comprise outcomes. Strong evidence supporting the benefits of addressing these conditions preoperatively remains insufficient, and some studies have showed mixed results [15–17]. Nevertheless, the role of preoperative psychosocial and nutritional assessments cannot be ignored, as it allows identification of areas for therapeutic intervention and helps in assessing patient candidacy for major malabsorptive bariatric procedures. When one considers that the chosen malabsorptive procedure and the length of intestinal bypass can directly affect the type and extent of nutritional deficiencies [18], identifying potential problems preoperatively offers clinicians an opportunity to initiate and focus the therapeutic process. In particular, the multidisciplinary team composed of a surgeon, psychologist, nutritionist, nurse educator, and other medical specialists as required can be engaged to accomplish the following objectives: (a) correct any preoperative medical problems and replace vitamin and mineral deficiencies, (b) address any disordered eating behavior, (c) involve patients with a nutritionist to commence dietary education and follow-up relating to different eating habits and food choices important to acquire and adhere to before and after surgery, (d) identify social and financial factors that may interfere with patients' ability to realize their weight loss objectives or adhere to necessary dietary and vitamin supplement regimens, (e) assess the level of patient compliance and guide the choice for an optimal surgical intervention and its timing, and (f) plan strategies and follow a schedule to minimize complications in patients warranting closer attention.

A multidisciplinary team evaluates candidates for the BPDDS procedure at the authors' institute. We perform bedside medical evaluations, broad blood work panels for nutritional biomarkers and micronutrients, and clinical psychosocial and nutritional assessments to identify modifiable behavior patterns and initiate education and treatment. Patients are taught to improve their food choices and incorporate protein-rich items, adhere to a dietary schedule, and avoid high-calorie-density foods with a low nutritional index that are incompatible with their objective of undergoing a malabsorptive bariatric procedure. Medical conditions, nutritionally related illnesses such as preoperative anemia, or lifestyle habits that may influence surgical outcomes are addressed. Micronutrient replacement is initiated as indicated by results of testing. Low serum 25-hydroxy vitamin D3 levels are commonly encountered, and preoperative replacement is started with a daily oral dose of 10,000 IU of vitamin D for 1 month, followed by a daily dose of 800 IU until surgery. Patients are on a low residue diet up till the day of surgery, and they are allowed oral intake on the first postoperative day. They are quickly advanced from a liquid to a pureed diet within their short 3–5-day hospital stay. During their admission, patients are seen again by a nutritionist to review and reinforce important postoperative dietary education prior to hospital discharge.

One month after BPDDS, patients are started on a daily multivitamin regimen that includes the following: 1 fortified multivitamin complex; 50,000 IU of vitamin D2; 1,000 mg of calcium carbonate; 20,000 IU of vitamin A; and 300 mg of iron sulfate. In addition, patients are advised to consume about 75–90 g of protein per day, and they are followed postoperatively every 4 months during the first year with blood work and then yearly thereafter, unless otherwise indicated. The routine blood work panel is similar to that obtained preoperatively and includes a complete blood count, creatinine, measurements of serum glucose, albumin, calcium, phosphate, magnesium, folate, serum iron panel including transferrin, vitamin B12, 25 (OH) vitamin D3, vitamin A, parathyroid hormone, liver enzyme panel, and INR. On follow-up, patients are carefully evaluated to identify signs and symptoms or risk factors for potential nutritional complications that may develop in the early or late postoperative period. Specific testing is then requested as deemed appropriate. Important clinical concerns after BPD surgery include: protein malnutrition, anemia, neurologic conditions, fat-soluble vitamin deficiencies, and metabolic bone disease.

Protein and Energy Deficiency

Protein-calorie malnutrition is considered one of the more serious complications of malabsorptive procedures and may require hospitalization for nutritional support [19, 20]. The degree of protein malnutrition following bariatric surgery is uncertain because reports vary in procedures performed and defining diagnostic criteria. In Scopinaro's series of 958 patients, an 11.9 % incidence of protein-calorie malnutrition was reported, with 4.1 % requiring surgical revision/restoration between 14 and 63 months postoperatively [19]. Such incidence and associated need for hospitalization or revision surgery seem to have decreased with the duodenal switch-type BPD described by Marceau et al., which has a longer, 100 cm, common intestinal channel [21]. By modifying the Scopinaro procedure since its inception and leaving a larger 300–500 mL gastric reservoir, the Italian team also observed

a decrease in the incidence of protein malnutrition to about 2 % [22]. This points to the importance of limiting the degree of gastric restriction in patients undergoing malabsorptive procedures, like BPD±DS, so as not to interfere with adequate oral nutrient intake. While restriction is desired, the "sleeve" gastrectomy component of a BPDDS should not be the same as in a stand-alone "sleeve gastrectomy" procedure, for it should provide patients with adequate gastric capacity to enable easy eating and sufficient protein intake and digestion, keeping up with increased protein needs after surgery.

Beyond gastric restriction, reduced protein intake can result from decreased consumption of meats, which patients may tolerate poorly in the early period after surgery, or from gastrointestinal problems like anastomotic stenosis or gastric narrowing that may decrease food tolerance and lead to food aversion or poor food choices. Clinically, protein deficiency manifests as fatigue, loss of muscle strength, alopecia, edema, and occasionally greater than expected weight loss. Patients often develop hypoalbuminemia or anemia, and they may have suffered from repeated infections prior to clinical presentation, possibly due to a degree of immunosuppression resulting from a protein deficient state [22].

Diminished visceral protein markers such as albumin and prealbumin are helpful in diagnosing protein malnutrition, keeping in mind that these biomarkers are also acute phase reactants that are suppressed by acute or critical illness [23]. Other signs of malnutrition or protein-calorie deficiency must, therefore, be considered. After BPDDS, lower serum albumin levels are expected; albumin decreases but remains within normal limits and relatively constant over time. Reporting on the long-term results of the duodenal switch in 1,028 patients with pre- and post-op serum albumin levels, the Québec group observed that the prevalence of moderate hypoalbuminemia (30–36 g/L) increased from 4.6 % at baseline to 8.5 % postoperatively at a mean follow-up time of about 7 years. Severe hypoalbuminemia (<30 g/L) was seen in only 0.9 %, and this was similar to the observed preoperative prevalence of this condition [20]. In their same cohort, 70 out of 1,423 patients were reported to require hospitalization for malnutrition and 9 patients in total required revision surgery. A recent report from the same group on BPDDS in patients with BMI < 50 kg/m² suggests that the hospitalization rate for malnutrition (4–5 % of studied cohorts), although not always related to protein-calorie deficiency, remains consistent over time and in different groups undergoing BPDDS [24].

Factors contributing to protein-calorie malnutrition vary and may be related to the time of clinical presentation. If the condition is observed in the first year after surgery, it is often a consequence of poor protein intake due to the restrictive component of surgery at the level of the stomach or proximal anastomosis, exacerbated by poor nutritional choices patients may make in reaction to the restriction they experience. Occasionally, poor patient compliance with nutritional advice may be the culprit. In either case, after anatomic complications such as stenosis or obstruction are ruled out, the problem can usually be successfully corrected with diet modification, nutritional re-education, and oral or enteral nutritional therapy. The restrictive effect of the operation also decreases over time as the stomach and anastomosis stretch, contributing to further ease of eating and overall improvement. Late or recurrent cases may, on the other hand, be related to decreased protein intake, impaired intestinal absorption due to the persistent and excessive effect of the operation, or both; and late cases are more likely to require revision surgery to elongate the common channel or, in exceptional cases, to reverse the procedure completely [19, 21].

After BPD surgery, patients are routinely advised to increase their protein intake and favor protein food sources over carbohydrates. Obligatory protein losses are observed after BPD, and compensating for this with increasing protein intake is thought to be important in avoiding the hypoalbuminemic form of protein-calorie malnutrition; this form can compromise visceral function leading to decreased visceral protein synthesis, low circulating albumin, edema, decreased intestinal absorption, and worsening malnutrition [25]. Good management starts with prevention by increasing the amount of protein consumed in the postoperative state to at least 90 g/day. As consuming sufficient amount of protein from meat sources can be difficult in the early period after surgery, protein supplements in the form of soluble protein food additives or shakes are often provided with or between meals as snacks. Postoperatively, patients are followed at regular intervals with blood testing and are encouraged to see the dietitian if hypoalbuminemia or maladaptive eating patterns are identified. Increasing protein intake to 100–120 g/day should correct most mild to moderate cases of protein deficiency and avoid the need for hospital admission.

Clinicians should be alert to any excessive early and rapid weight loss, as it is an important diagnostic sign for malnourishment that may be missed due to the presence of edema. Fluid retention secondary to hypoalbuminemia must be evaluated at the time of clinical presentation, as it tends to underestimate the true body weight loss. Improving intestinal absorptive function starts with addressing the edematous state. In cases where hypoproteinemia with edema and asthenia are identified, the patient is admitted to the hospital, where IV albumin and diuretic therapy (e.g., furosemide) is started to treat the initial edema. Shortly thereafter, enteral gavage or total parenteral nutrition can be started. Enteral feeding with oligo-protein containing solutions is preferred to parenteral nutrition due to its safety profile and trophic effect promoting intestinal absorptive adaptation. Most patients respond well to this treatment, and enteral gavage can be continued for 6–12 weeks on an outpatient basis. Oral pancreatic enzymes can be used to improve digestion and absorption in the alimentary limb during this phase of treatment. In rare cases where protein-calorie malnutrition recurs, revision surgery is considered.

Revision surgery is also needed in cases of malnutrition and advanced liver failure nonresponsive to corrective nutritional therapies. In general, steatosis and nonalcoholic steatohepatitis improve after malabsorptive surgery as shown by overall improvements in liver histology after weight loss [26, 27]. Nevertheless, a few cases of hepatic failure out of the thousands of BPD±DS surgeries performed over the past 50 years have been reported [28–30], with some being serious enough to receive liver transplants [31, 32]. The frequency of hepatic complications following BPD±DS surgery is difficult to estimate, given the rarity of the condition and possible underreporting; yet the link between contemporary BPD±DS surgery, protein malnutrition, and the development of cirrhosis or liver failure is even more difficult to establish, as confounding factors have often been present in reported cases [33, 34]. Alcoholism, poor diet, drug reactions, and infectious hepatitis are examples of important confounders that may become a problem at any point in life, and bariatric patients are no exception even if these problems did not exist preoperatively. Close follow-up of patients after surgery with liver enzyme panels at regular intervals is recommended. Transient elevations of liver enzymes in the early postoperative period are expected [35], but when observed, they warrant closer follow-up and evaluation of patients' overall nutritional status. Focus is on ensuring compliance with nutritional counseling, avoidance of excessive weight loss due to poor dietary choices or substance abuse, treatment of any gastrointestinal symptoms suggestive of bacterial overgrowth, and achieving normalization of liver enzymes. If specialized transplant teams who evaluate patients with liver failure after BPD±DS commit to liver transplantation, involving bariatric surgeons, or better yet, the patient's bariatric surgical team if possible, is always advisable. Serious consideration should be given to reversing the patient's malabsorptive procedure, or at the very least inserting a feeding jejunostomy tube in the biliopancreatic limb. This serves to (1) remove any unknown underlying bariatric surgical factor that may continue to damage the grafted liver and to (2) improve absorption of immunosuppressive agents needed after transplantation. Concerns regarding weight regain and recurrent hepatic steatosis in this context are valid, but they need to be balanced against the risk of repeat cirrhosis or graft rejection. Weight management issues can be addressed after patient recovery from transplantation. Although quite rare, cases of advanced hepatic failure may be life threatening and can occur anytime after surgery [36]. Therefore, the importance of lifelong follow-up cannot be overemphasized; and even though there is insufficient evidence to etiologically link liver failure to protein malnutrition and the type of BPD±DS surgery practiced today, preoperative informed consent should include a discussion about hepatic improvements seen after surgery as well as the potential for rare, serious liver failure, possibly requiring transplantation and reversal of the bariatric procedure.

Nutritional Anemia

Malabsorptive bariatric procedures can result in multifactorial nutritional anemia. While anemia secondary to iron deficiency is more commonly seen after BPD±DS, deficiencies in protein, vitamin B12, folic acid, zinc, copper, and selenium can also contribute to anemia. In postoperative patients with low hemoglobin, the initial approach for evaluating the anemia is similar to that used in other patients. When the work up for iron deficiency is unyielding, special attention must be paid to protein or micronutrient deficiencies like vitamin B12, folate, copper, and zinc that may need correction. Treating unrecognized copper deficiency anemia as one of iron deficiency and prescribing iron, for example, may lead to iron overload and organ damage without correcting the anemia.

Iron

Because microcytic iron deficiency is prevalent after malabsorptive surgery, especially in menstruating women, postoperative iron supplementation is essential [37]. The incidence of iron deficiency after BPD±DS surgery has been reported to be up to 26 % [38]. Dietary iron requires gastric acid to reduce it to its absorbable ferrous form; it is then absorbed primarily in the duodenum. Factors contributing to iron deficiency after BPD±DS include decreased consumption of heme-containing foods in patients who tend to avoid eating meat after malabsorptive surgery, reduced gastric secretions due to reduced parietal cell mass and/or prolonged postoperative PPI therapy, and exclusion of the duodenum and proximal jejunum from the path of nutrients, depending on the procedure performed. Keeping a couple of centimeters of the first part of the duodenum in continuity with the alimentary tract in a duodenal switch procedure seems to contribute to a lower observed incidence of iron and ferritin deficiency after duodenal switch when compared to BPD with distal gastrectomy and gastroileostomy [6, 21]. With blood tests performed at regular intervals, iron deficiency is often diagnosed before symptoms develop. Symptoms may include fatigue, depression, headaches, glossitis, stomatitis, or brittle nails. Multiple regimens exist for iron supplementation. Vitamin C improves iron absorption and is sometimes included empirically with iron supplementation. BPD±DS patients also take calcium supplements, and attention should be given to taking iron and calcium separately, as calcium in any of its common oral forms (calcium carbonate, calcium citrate, and calcium phosphate) can interfere with the efficiency of iron absorption [39]. This interference may be of short duration, however, due to compensatory mechanisms with time [40]. We prescribe 300 mg of iron sulfate once daily to our patients on discharge after BPD±DS, and this is adjusted over time based on results of blood tests. When there is concern over patient compliance with oral therapy, we use intravenous replacement on an annual basis. Supplementation is provided to correct and maintain hemoglobin levels and regular lifelong surveillance with blood testing is needed. Interestingly, a randomized trial of iron supplementation (65 mg of elemental iron orally twice daily) prevented iron deficiency but did not prevent anemia. This highlights the importance of considering other micronutrient deficiencies that can contribute to anemia [41].

Vitamin B12

Vitamin B12 deficiency is rare after duodenal switch surgery, and in fact, serum levels tend to improve after surgery. Body stores of vitamin B12 are large and daily needs are very small in comparison. Aside from supplements, the only dietary source of vitamin B12 is from animal meat or dairy product. Absorption of food vitamin B12 requires an intact and functioning stomach, exocrine pancreas, intrinsic factor, and small bowel [42]. Roux-en-Y gastric bypass (RYGB) is a milder form of malabsorptive surgery than BPD±DS due to the shorter limb of the bypassed intestine, but the majority of the stomach, duodenum, and proximal jejunum are excluded from the path of nutrients in gastric bypass. Unlike RYGB surgery where deficiencies of Vitamin B12 can be seen in up to 30 % of patients as early as 1 year after surgery in the absence of supplementation [43], reports of significant vitamin B12 deficiencies after BPD surgery are few. After BPDDS, we give a fortified multivitamin complex and supplement this with vitamin B12 if a deficiency develops. The rate of B12 deficiency in a series of 942 patients with pre- and post-op serum levels was 1 % on long-term follow-up; it improved from a 3 % preoperative prevalence [20]. Nevertheless, because of efficient storage and low needs, B12 deficiency can manifest late; and blood levels should be followed annually to allow timely intervention as needed prior to symptom development. Deficiency can lead to megaloblastic anemia and, via demyelination, to potentially irreversible neurologic changes including peripheral neuropathy, subacute combined degeneration of the spinal cord, optic atrophy, and dementia [42].

Folate

Folate is a water-soluble vitamin and less commonly implicated in anemia. In contrast to vitamin B12, which is absorbed in the terminal ilium and with the aid of a gastric parietal cell intrinsic factor, folate is absorbed along the entire length of small intestine. Folate deficiency can result in megaloblastic anemia or a normocytic anemia if there is concomitant iron deficiency anemia. In nonpregnant adults, folate needs can easily be met with one multivitamin a day supplementation. After BPDDS, folate levels actually improved postoperatively with this kind of supplementation [20].

In general, bariatric studies have suggested that biomarker levels of folate are not necessary [44, 45]. Needs increase during pregnancy, and women who express interest in childbearing should have supplementation to ensure normal serum folate levels to minimize the risk for neural tube defects [46].

Copper

Like vitamin B12, copper deficits can lead to hematological abnormalities like normocytic or macrocytic anemia and to neurologic problems. Myelopathy and neuropathy in the lower extremities with spastic ataxic gait, symmetrically brisk reflexes, and loss of pinprick and light touch sensation have been seen after malabsorptive surgery of the RYGB type [47–50]. In patients with neurologic symptoms and whose serum B12 level are normal, copper measurement to confirm the diagnosis is helpful, and administration of IV copper can result in improvement. We do not routinely measure copper in our patients before or after BPDDS, and we have not diagnosed isolated symptomatic hypocupremia. In our patients, copper and other mineral micronutrients are administered postoperatively as part of the daily dose of fortified multivitamin complex taken by patients who comply with the treatment. Recent evidence points to a high prevalence of zinc and copper deficiencies in morbidly obese patients seeking bariatric surgery, and these deficiencies increase on follow-up over the years after BPD even when copper supplements are given intermittently [51, 52]. A rapid review of the literature, however, failed to identify any reported cases of neurologic deficits from copper deficiency after BPD; and others have also recently confirmed this observation [52]. An intriguing finding of one study is that no BPD patient developed hematologic problems or evidence of neurological deficits, even though some patients in their cohort suffered hypocupremia for a long time. Serious cases of hypocupremia related to bariatric surgery reported in the literature have been mostly observed in patients after RYGB [52, 53]. This may be a reflection of the fact that many more RYGB procedures are performed worldwide than are BPD operations [9], but it also adds to the importance of ongoing follow-up after any bariatric procedure with a malabsorptive component to ensure overall patient well-being and prevent prolonged malnourishment. Bariatric patients that have had their clinical follow-up interrupted should undergo a comprehensive evaluation and blood testing for micronutrients and minerals including copper and zinc.

Zinc

Zinc deficiency can cause hair loss, dermatitis, impaired immunity, and delayed wound healing. Plasma zinc levels are poor biomarker for zinc status [54], and they are not routinely measured perioperatively. Conditions causing chronic diarrhea can increase zinc losses [55]. Like copper, low serum zinc levels have been documented and persist over the years after BPD surgery in 10–50 % of patients, although symptomatic cases have not been reported [52, 56, 57]. Zinc as part of a daily multivitamin complex is recommended for patients after malabsorptive surgery. Documented deficiency can be treated with separate zinc supplementation in the form of zinc (30–50 mg of elemental zinc every other day) [58]. Care must be taken not to prescribe high doses of zinc to avoid toxicity and interference with copper transport and metabolism [50]. When ingested in excess, zinc can result in anemia, as it contributes to decreased copper and ceruloplasmin levels.

Vitamin B1 (Thiamine) Deficiency

Thiamine is also essential in neural function as well as carbohydrate metabolism. Being the first B vitamin to be identified, thiamine is also known as vitamin B1. Mild deficiency causes anorexia, irritability, apathy, and generalized weakness. Major deficiency can lead to the recognized beriberi heart or nerve diseases [59]. In both conditions, patients experience pain and neurologic symptoms. Wet beriberi involves the heart and results in an edematous state. Dry beriberi presents with a symmetrical mixed motor and peripheral neuropathy. Involvement of the central nervous system can result in a Wernicke-type encephalopathy, characterized by nystagmus, ophthalmoplegia, cerebellar ataxia, and mental impairment. The presence of memory loss and confabulation is known as the Wernicke-Korsakoff syndrome. This syndrome is classically associated with alcohol-related malnutrition [60], but it is also a serious nutritional complication that has been reported after bariatric surgery [61].

Thiamine is primarily absorbed in the proximal small bowel and is stored in the body in small amounts with its biologic half-life being about 2–3 weeks. Humans cannot make thiamine and must receive it in their diet. Thiamine is also a good substrate for bacteria [62]. Procedures or conditions that exclude the proximal bowel from nutrient exposure or that are associated with intestinal bacterial overgrowth syndromes can, over a short period of time, contribute to thiamine deficiency and occasionally even the Wernicke-Korsakoff encephalopathy (WE) syndrome. This syndrome has been seen after BPD surgery [25]. It must be emphasized that WE can occur after all commonly performed bariatric procedures [61], including restrictive ones; and it has been noted as early as a few weeks after surgery [63]. Poor adherence (involuntary or voluntary) to the recommended postoperative dietary and supplement regimen may result in unusually rapid weight loss seen at the time of diagnosis. Most cases have presented with poor oral intake due to profuse nausea and vomiting preceding the development of neurological symptoms. Prompt recognition and administration of high-dose thiamine can virtually eliminate the development of neurologic symptoms [25].

A complex oral multivitamin, containing thiamine, should prevent thiamine deficiency in bariatric patients. Some have advocated a dose of 25–50 mg/day in addition to the recommended daily allowance [64]. If deficiency is suspected, it can be confirmed by measuring serum transketolase activity before and after administration of vitamin B1, since thiamine is a cofactor for the reaction. Laboratory testing, however, is less important than keeping a low threshold for diagnosis and initiating early parenteral thiamine therapy in the acute postoperative period when patients present with a history of poor eating or gastrointestinal symptoms that interfere with adequate nutrient intake, even before significant weight loss has occurred.

Recognition of the clinical presentation becomes important to avoid serious neurologic problems. Managing medical conditions or surgical complications that contribute to reduced food intake or persistent nausea and vomiting involves aggressively addressing the underlying cause of the problem but without delaying early parenteral vitamin B1 supplementation. Patients often present with weakness and dehydration, and giving them thiamine is recommended prior to the administration of intravenous glucose-containing hydration solutions to minimize worsening of neurologic symptoms and progression towards the Wernicke syndrome [65]. Initiating intravenous thiamine on presentation in the emergency department, regardless of symptom severity, is far more practical than laboratory testing for deficiency. In the acute setting, deficiency is treated with parenteral thiamine at a dose of 300 mg/day for 3 days followed by continuation of oral supplementation at a dose of 10 mg/day until symptoms resolve. Patients with advanced neuropsychiatric beriberi symptoms should be treated as medical emergencies requiring hospital admission. In this context, high-dose IV thiamine of at least 300–500 mg given daily for 3–5 days is recommended as initial therapy [50, 58].

Fat-Soluble Vitamins

Designed to induce fat malabsorption, BPD±DS also leads to decreased absorption of fat-soluble vitamins A, D, E, and K, resulting in deficiencies [25, 56]. There remains a lack of high-quality studies evaluating the true incidence of vitamin deficiencies after malabsorptive surgery and how these deficiencies can best be prevented with optimal supplementation protocols. Reports are also difficult to compare or generalize because of variation in patient populations, lengths and segments of bypassed intestine, and regularity of patient vitamin supplementation and blood testing intervals. What has been documented is that despite regular nutritional counseling and empiric supplementation, the incidence of vitamin deficiency can increase with time after malabsorptive surgery [56]. One randomized study showed that decreased serum vitamin

values are observed as early as the first year after surgery, even with supplementation; this was especially remarkable for deficiencies in fat-soluble vitamins A and D after duodenal switch surgery [18]. It is currently well accepted that lifelong patient compliance with postoperative vitamin supplementation is essential to minimize deficiencies and their potential clinical effects after BPD±DS [20, 25]. Symptomatic fat-soluble vitamin deficiency, however, is either uncommon or underreported, yet it is easily treated with vitamin supplementation when it occurs, highlighting the importance of early recognition before potentially serious complications result.

Vitamin A

Vitamin A is a name for a group of compounds with the biologic activity of retinol and consists of retinoids and some carotenoids (provitamin A). These substances are hydrophobic and depend on micelle formation for efficient intestinal absorption. Vitamin A deficiency has been reported after BPD±DS [20, 25], with increasing incidence and severity of this deficiency observed over time. In a retrospective review, where BPDDS was performed with a 175–200 cm alimentary limb and a 50–75 cm common channel, the prevalence of vitamin A deficiency was found to be 52 % at 1 year after surgery and 69 % for patients 4 years after their operation [56]. The Québec group also reported an increase in the prevalence of vitamin A deficiency on long-term follow-up in BPDDS patients who had a 250 cm total alimentary limb and a 100 cm common channel, but lower rates were observed. Summarizing their 15-year experience, they documented an increase in vitamin A deficiency from 8 % of 807 patients before surgery to 23 % on last follow-up, with their mean follow-up being just over 7 years. In another cohort reviewed by the same group, Marceau et al. reported that 10 years after DS, the proportion of patients with vitamin A levels below 1.2 μmol/L was 10 % [21]. Adjusting levels as needed by changing the oral supplement dose of vitamin A was sufficient, and intramuscular administration was rarely used. Vitamin A deficiency can result in poor night vision, itching, dry hair, and skin lesions. A few cases of impaired vision and skin problems due to vitamin A deficiency after BPD have been reported, and symptoms resolved with treatment [66–68]. Initial treatment is by administering vitamin A in higher doses than those used for routine supplementation. High-dose vitamin A has known toxicities, but daily doses as high as 60,000–90,000 IU have been used in cases of symptomatic deficiencies [66, 69].

Vitamins E

Vitamin E levels have not been very well studied in the context of bariatric surgery, but symptomatic deficiency is quite uncommon, even after malabsorptive procedures. One group documented that vitamin E levels adjusted for serum lipid changes were noted to be increased 1 year after BPDDS, and this is deemed related to routine supplementation [18]. Other series have revealed asymptomatic low serum vitamin E levels more than 2–4 years after BPD±DS with a short common channel [56, 57]. Complaints of ataxia, muscle weakness, and visual symptoms, or findings of anemia or dysarthria are indicative of vitamin E deficiency and should be evaluated and treated appropriately. Again, with anemia after malabsorptive procedures, one should keep in mind the contributory role of other potential micronutrient deficiencies like vitamin B12, copper, and zinc already mentioned. Oral vitamin E at 800–1,200 IU can be given daily as initial therapy in cases of symptomatic deficiency [58]. Some have recommended an additional supplement of 10 mg/day of vitamin E [64], but this has not been universally adopted nor is it our practice.

Vitamin K

Vitamin K is required for blood clotting, bone formation, and other functions [70].

In addition to good absorption in the ileum, vitamin K can be absorbed in the rest of the intestine and depends on biliary secretions and micelle formation [71]. Due to rapid metabolism, vitamin K is not stored in the body. For humans, usable sources are either dietary or products of biosynthesis from intestinal flora. Perhaps this explains why serious cases of symptomatic vitamin K deficiency are rare after malabsorptive surgery, since intestinal bacteria may provide enough of this vitamin for absorption in the colon when dietary sources are low. Low serum levels of vitamin K have been documented in a high proportion of patients after malabsorptive procedures years after their surgery [56, 57]. While symptoms rarely develop, attention is still warranted in pregnant patients who require closer monitoring. A few case reports linking a history of remote BPD to perinatal complications, although non-definitive in establishing causation, do warrant attention given the seriousness of the reported problems. Serious neonatal hemorrhage and long lasting neurologic deficits in children born to mothers after bariatric surgery have been observed [72]. A more recent case report emerged, placing further emphasis on the need to consider vitamin K deficiency and replacement in pregnant mothers after BPD to minimize the rare but serious risk of hemorrhage in the mother and child at the time of delivery [73]. We do not routinely measure vitamin K postoperatively on follow-up, but PT-INR is measured. Prior to any major operation with a high risk for blood loss or where bleeding is not well tolerated, we do recommend that patients take oral vitamin K supplementation for a week before their planned elective procedure, even if a patient's INR is normal or only slightly elevated. Personal experience with patients after BPDDS has also shown that warfarin dosing can be more challenging in those requiring chronic anticoagulation. These implications

of BPD±DS surgery are, therefore, best discussed with patients before surgery as part of the informed consent process.

Vitamin D, Calcium, and Metabolic Bone Disease

Vitamin D is better absorbed in the jejunum and ileum, while calcium is preferentially absorbed in the duodenum and proximal jejunum. Calcium absorption is facilitated by vitamin D in an acid environment [74]. Low vitamin D levels can lead to a decrease in dietary calcium absorption but are not always accompanied by a reduction in serum calcium, as parathyroid hormone is released to maintain serum calcium levels. Chronic insufficiency in calcium, vitamin D, or both can lead to secondary hyperparathyroidism. In addition to increasing intestinal calcium and vitamin D absorption and decreasing calcium loss in the urine, parathyroid hormone maintains serum calcium levels at the cost of bone resorption. This can lead over time to osteoporosis and increased risk of fractures.

Bone, therefore, becomes an important source of calcium in the setting of malabsorptive procedures where the efficiency of intestinal calcium absorption is altered by the operation and affected by the length and region of bypassed intestine, intestinal absorptive capacity, dietary sources of calcium, and patient compliance with supplementation in the long-term. Special attention should also be given to patients with health conditions and taking medications that interfere with calcium absorption such as antiepileptic agents, long-term glucocorticoids or thyroid hormone, methotrexate, heparin, or cholestyramine [75]. Symptoms of metabolic bone disease secondary to hyperparathyroidism in adults are often nonspecific and the diagnosis is commonly delayed. Generalized skeletal pain, muscle weakness, and bony tenderness are usual symptoms; and pathologic fractures may occur. Those who care for patients after bariatric surgery should have a low threshold for the exclusion of metabolic bone disease when vague but suspicious symptoms are present, especially if patient follow-up had been interrupted.

In principle, malabsorptive surgery can increase the risk of bone disease over time, but to date evidence to this effect is poor, difficult to interpret, or nonconclusive, as demonstrated by a recently published review on the link between bariatric surgery, bone loss, and osteoporosis [76]. The extent of reviewed evidence will not be repeated here; but suffice it to say that, although imperfect, available evidence is reassuring and is in fact a testament to the ability of calcium and vitamin D supplementation after surgery to keep parathyroid hormone levels from rising excessively and leading to bone disease. While severe metabolic bone disease has been reported long after bariatric surgery [77], many observational reports have suffered from lack of nonoperated groups, controlled for age and gender. In their review, Scibora et al. report that in evaluated cross-sectional and retrospective studies, age-related bone loss seen in bariatric patients is no greater than what would normally be expected for age and gender. They did note that longitudinal studies, however, showed a relationship between declining bone density (mostly in the hip and spine region in women) and malabsorptive procedures. While mineral density decreased over time in patients who had DEXA scores, osteoporosis was not present at the time of last evaluation [76].

The Québec group reported prevalence of hypocalcemia in 22 %, low vitamin D in 45 %, and elevated parathyroid hormone in 49 % on a mean follow-up of 7.3 years after BPDDS [20]. Increasing oral calcium lowered parathyroid hormone levels and kept bone from excessive exposure to high levels of this hormone. Marceau et al. had also previously reported that a greater increase in bone markers and bone turnover after BPDDS was associated with an increased risk of bone loss, but the overall bone density remained remarkably stable at 10 years in their study [78]. As evidenced by more recent investigations into serum calcium, vitamin D, and parathyroid hormone levels after malabsorptive surgery, bone turnover is an active process, more so early postoperatively and persisting for at least 2–5 years thereafter [79, 80]. It is of interest to note that bone demineralization appears to peak around 4 years after surgery, and that this has not been found to be an increasing clinical problem afterwards in large clinical series of BPD±DS surgery [19, 25].

Although the bone seems to be relatively tolerant to the metabolic changes following malabsorptive procedures, this should not encourage complacency with adequate supplementation of both calcium and vitamin D for life after surgery. Perhaps there is an adaptation process that occurs in bone with time making it more resilient to osteoporosis. This effect has intriguingly been observed after the more drastic, previously practiced jejuno-intestinal bypass procedures, where spontaneous healing of osteomalacia was noted on long-term follow-up [81]. Besides potential adaptation, the confounding effects of vitamin supplementation, improved diet and physical activity, smoking cessation, and overall better health of patients cannot be eliminated as contributing to the relative stability of bone after BPD±DS surgery. Markedly elevated levels of parathyroid hormone levels (>100 ng/L) on follow-up, especially if associated with elevated alkaline phosphatase levels, is a good sign of active bone turnover and provides a good reason for aggressive therapy with oral calcium and vitamin D and close surveillance to ensure compliance and normalization of serum levels [20]. After BPDDS, we increase oral calcium dosing to 1–2 g of calcium carbonate per day as long as there is no renal dysfunction. Calcium citrate can also be used, as it tends to be better absorbed. Plus, if vitamin D deficiency is present, oral vitamin D2 dosing is increased to 50,000 IU BID (max 150,000 IU per day) from our routine supplement dose of 50,000 IU daily. Alternatively, vitamin D3, which tends to have better absorption, can be tried.

Conclusion

The BPD±DS is a potent metabolic and weight loss procedure with durable effects. By design, the procedure is intended to achieve its clinical benefits by inducing caloric malabsorption. The objective is to achieve controlled malabsorption, balancing the desired clinical effects against the risks of complications and potentially serious acute or long-term nutritional problems. Empiric evidence from thousands of patients who have received BPD±DS procedures over the last several decades continues to be reassuring as to the efficacy and safety of this type of malabsorptive surgery. With increasing experience and modification of the BPD procedure since its original introduction, there have been significant reductions in the incidence of serious nutritional complications, even when the procedure is offered to patients with relatively lower body mass indices. Traditional concerns regarding the nutritional risks of the BPD±DS procedures, arising mostly from observations made in patients who underwent other, now obsolete or rarely practiced, malabsorptive procedures should no longer be a hindrance to referring patients for BPD±DS surgery. The great majority of patients now derive metabolic improvements, sustained weight loss, and an improved quality of life, with a high level of global satisfaction after BPD±DS, without suffering significant protein-calorie malnutrition, metabolic bone disease, or irreversible neurological problems secondary to vitamin or mineral deficiencies. Revision surgery for nutritional complications after BPD±DS has also become the exception rather than the rule. Nevertheless, because the surgery sufficiently alters anatomy and physiology, serious problems can result if patients are not well prepared and followed, and if serious signs and symptoms are not recognized early by patients and their healthcare providers. To maintain good outcomes, patients must be committed to participating in their own health maintenance by adhering to good dietary habits, taking lifelong multivitamin and mineral supplements, and keeping their follow-up. The introduction of the multidisciplinary team approach to patient assessment and the commitment to lifelong follow-up strategies are also key to the continued success of BPD±DS surgery in properly selected and well-prepared patients.

Review Questions and Answers

Questions

Question 1: Which of the following statements about perioperative nutritional management of the bariatric patient is true?

1. Malabsorptive procedures are limited to the biliopancreatic diversion, and only patients awaiting this surgery need preoperative assessment with a multidisciplinary team that includes a dietitian.
2. Currently, there is strong conclusive evidence that addressing preexisting conditions such as eating disorders and vitamin deficiencies preoperatively is associated with improved postoperative outcomes after malabsorptive surgery.
3. Initiating the therapeutic process preoperatively for patients seeking biliopancreatic diversion surgery offers many advantages such as an opportunity to address preexisting eating disorders and vitamin deficiencies and assess patient compliance and candidacy for surgery.
4. Multidisciplinary teams have little role in the assessment of patients receiving malabsorptive surgery as long as a dietitian is involved in the preoperative assessment and preparation of patients with the surgeon.

Question 2: Protein energy malnutrition is an important potential complication of malabsorptive procedures. Which of the following regarding protein-calorie malnutrition after biliopancreatic diversion is true?

1. Protein-calorie malnutrition is a rare but serious complication of biliopancreatic diversion surgery and is not encountered in the duodenal switch variant of the procedure.
2. The presence of edema may underestimate the degree of weight loss, clouding the diagnosis and influencing the treatment of protein-calorie malnutrition.
3. Regardless of when protein malabsorption presents in the postoperative period after biliopancreatic diversion surgery, the condition consistently resolves with increasing the administration of enteral protein, without needing to revise the procedure.
4. Protein malnutrition is associated with the intestinal bypass component of malabsorptive surgery and not related to the type of gastrectomy performed.

Question3: The management of nutritional anemia after malabsorptive surgery involves:

1. Giving all patients supplemental folate in addition to the folate present in a single complex multivitamin tablet because folate levels consistently decrease with time after biliopancreatic diversion with duodenal switch.
2. The routine administration of oral vitamin B12 on a daily or monthly basis, since vitamin B12 deficiency is an important cause of anemia after biliopancreatic diversion and prevention involves.
3. Empiric oral iron therapy for patients with low hemoglobin, recognizing that iron deficiency anemia is the only important anemia resulting in clinical symptoms warranting investigation and therapy after bariatric surgery.

4. The routine administration of oral iron supplementation postoperatively to minimize the incidence of iron deficiency anemia, given that it is the most common form of nutritional anemia encountered after bariatric surgery

Answers
Q1: #3
Q2: #2
Q3: #4

References

1. Buchwald H, Avidor Y, Braunwald E, Jensen MD, Pories W, Fahrbach K, et al. Bariatric surgery: a systematic review and meta-analysis. JAMA. 2004;292(14):1724–37.
2. Demaria EJ, Jamal MK. Surgical options for obesity. Gastroenterol Clin North Am. 2005;34(1):127–42.
3. Anthone GJ, Lord RV, DeMeester TR, Crookes PF. The duodenal switch operation for the treatment of morbid obesity. Ann Surg. 2003;238(4):618–27. discussion 27-8.
4. Scopinaro N. Thirty-five years of biliopancreatic diversion: notes on gastrointestinal physiology to complete the published information useful for a better understanding and clinical use of the operation. Obes Surg. 2012;22(3):427–32.
5. Marceau P, Biron S, Bourque RA, Potvin M, Hould FS, Simard S. Biliopancreatic Diversion with a New Type of Gastrectomy. Obes Surg. 1993;3(1):29–35.
6. Marceau P, Hould FS, Simard S, Lebel S, Bourque RA, Potvin M, et al. Biliopancreatic diversion with duodenal switch. World J Surg. 1998;22(9):947–54.
7. Nguyen NT, Masoomi H, Magno CP, Nguyen XM, Laugenour K, Lane J. Trends in use of bariatric surgery, 2003-2008. J Am Coll Surg. 2011;213(2):261–6.
8. Nguyen NT, Nguyen B, Gebhart A, Hohmann S. Changes in the makeup of bariatric surgery: a national increase in use of laparoscopic sleeve gastrectomy. J Am Coll Surg. 2013;216(2):252–7.
9. Buchwald H, Oien DM. Metabolic/Bariatric Surgery Worldwide 2011. Obes Surg. 2013;23(4):427–36.
10. Dumon KR, Murayama KM. Bariatric surgery outcomes. Surg Clin North Am. 2011;91(6):1313–38. x.
11. Colles SL, Dixon JB, O'Brien PE. Grazing and loss of control related to eating: two high-risk factors following bariatric surgery. Obesity (Silver Spring). 2008;16(3):615–22.
12. Kruseman M, Leimgruber A, Zumbach F, Golay A. Dietary, weight, and psychological changes among patients with obesity, 8 years after gastric bypass. J Am Diet Assoc. 2010;110(4):527–34.
13. Ernst B, Thurnheer M, Schmid SM, Schultes B. Evidence for the necessity to systematically assess micronutrient status prior to bariatric surgery. Obes Surg. 2009;19(1):66–73.
14. Botella Romero F, Milla Tobarra M, Alfaro Martinez JJ, Garcia Arce L, Garcia Gomez A, Salas Saiz MA, et al. [Bariatric surgery in duodenal switch procedure: weight changes and associated nutritional deficiencies]. Endocrinol Nutr. 2011;58(5):214–8.
15. Ashton K, Heinberg L, Windover A, Merrell J. Positive response to binge eating intervention enhances postoperative weight loss. Surg Obes Relat Dis. 2011;7(3):315–20.
16. Wadden TA, Faulconbridge LF, Jones-Corneille LR, Sarwer DB, Fabricatore AN, Thomas JG, et al. Binge eating disorder and the outcome of bariatric surgery at one year: a prospective, observational study. Obesity (Silver Spring). 2011;19(6):1220–8.
17. Scholtz S, Bidlake L, Morgan J, Fiennes A, El-Etar A, Lacey JH, et al. Long-term outcomes following laparoscopic adjustable gas-

tric banding: postoperative psychological sequelae predict outcome at 5-year follow-up. Obes Surg. 2007;17(9):1220–5.

18. Aasheim ET, Bjorkman S, Sovik TT, Engstrom M, Hanvold SE, Mala T, et al. Vitamin status after bariatric surgery: a randomized study of gastric bypass and duodenal switch. Am J Clin Nutr. 2009;90(1):15–22.

19. Scopinaro N, Gianetta E, Adami GF, Friedman D, Traverso E, Marinari GM, et al. Biliopancreatic diversion for obesity at eighteen years. Surgery. 1996;119(3):261–8.

20. Marceau P, Biron S, Hould FS, Lebel S, Marceau S, Lescelleur O, et al. Duodenal switch: long-term results. Obes Surg. 2007;17(11): 1421–30.

21. Marceau P, Biron S, Hould FS, Lebel S, Marceau S, Lescelleur O, et al. Duodenal switch improved standard biliopancreatic diversion: a retrospective study. Surg Obes Relat Dis. 2009;5(1):43–7.

22. Scopinaro N, Marinari G, Camerini G, Papadia F. Biliopancreatic diversion for obesity: state of the art. Surg Obes Relat Dis. 2005; 1(3):317–28.

23. Barbosa-Silva MC. Subjective and objective nutritional assessment methods: what do they really assess? Curr Opin Clin Nutr Metab Care. 2008;11(3):248–54.

24. Biertho L, Biron S, Hould FS, Lebel S, Marceau S, Marceau P. Is biliopancreatic diversion with duodenal switch indicated for patients with body mass index <50 kg/m²? Surg Obes Relat Dis. 2010;6(5):508–14.

25. Scopinaro N, Adami GF, Marinari GM, Gianetta E, Traverso E, Friedman D, et al. Biliopancreatic diversion. World J Surg. 1998; 22(9):936–46.

26. Mattar SG, Velcu LM, Rabinovitz M, Demetris AJ, Krasinskas AM, Barinas-Mitchell E, et al. Surgically-induced weight loss significantly improves nonalcoholic fatty liver disease and the metabolic syndrome. Ann Surg. 2005;242(4):610–7. discussion 8-20.

27. Kral JG, Thung SN, Biron S, Hould FS, Lebel S, Marceau S, et al. Effects of surgical treatment of the metabolic syndrome on liver fibrosis and cirrhosis. Surgery. 2004;135(1):48–58.

28. Baltasar A, Serra C, Perez N, Bou R, Bengochea M. Clinical hepatic impairment after the duodenal switch. Obes Surg. 2004;14(1):77–83.

29. Castillo J, Fabrega E, Escalante CF, Sanjuan JC, Herrera L, Hernanz F, et al. Liver transplantation in a case of steatohepatitis and subacute hepatic failure after biliopancreatic diversion for morbid obesity. Obes Surg. 2001;11(5):640–2.

30. Grimm IS, Schindler W, Haluszka O. Steatohepatitis and fatal hepatic failure after biliopancreatic diversion. Am J Gastroenterol. 1992;87(6):775–9.

31. Geerts A, Darius T, Chapelle T, Roeyen G, Francque S, Libbrecht L, et al. The multicenter Belgian survey on liver transplantation for hepatocellular failure after bariatric surgery. Transplant Proc. 2010; 42(10):4395–8.

32. D'Albuquerque LA, Gonzalez AM, Wahle RC, de Oliveira Souza E, Mancero JM, de Oliveira e Silva A. Liver transplantation for subacute hepatocellular failure due to massive steatohepatitis after bariatric surgery. Liver Transpl. 2008; 14(6): 881–5.

33. Scopinaro N. Invited Commentary. Obes Surg. 1994;4(3):291–2.

34. Greco M, De Micheli E, Lonardo A. Multifactorial hepatopathy in a patient with biliopancreatic diversion. Ann Ital Med Int. 2003; 18(2):99–103.

35. Papadia F, Marinari GM, Camerini G, Adami GF, Murelli F, Carlini F, et al. Short-term liver function after biliopancreatic diversion. Obes Surg. 2003;13(5):752–5.

36. van Dongen JL, Michielsen PP, Van den Eynden GG, Pelckmans PA, Francque SM. Rapidly evolving liver decompensation with some remarkable features 14 years after biliopancreatic derivation: a case report and literature review. Acta Gastroenterol Belg. 2010;73(1):46–51.

37. Mechanick JI, Youdim A, Jones DB, Timothy Garvey W, Hurley DL, Molly McMahon M, et al. Clinical practice guidelines for the

perioperative nutritional, metabolic, and nonsurgical support of the bariatric surgery patient–2013 update: cosponsored by American Association of Clinical Endocrinologists, the Obesity Society, and American Society for Metabolic & Bariatric Surgery. Surg Obes Relat Dis. 2013;9(2):159–91.

38. Brolin RE, Leung M. Survey of vitamin and mineral supplementation after gastric bypass and biliopancreatic diversion for morbid obesity. Obes Surg. 1999;9(2):150–4.

39. Cook JD, Dassenko SA, Whittaker P. Calcium supplementation: effect on iron absorption. Am J Clin Nutr. 1991;53(1):106–11.

40. Lonnerdal B. Calcium and iron absorption–mechanisms and public health relevance. Int J Vitam Nutr Res. 2010;80(4–5):293–9.

41. Brolin RE, Gorman JH, Gorman RC, Petschenik AJ, Bradley LB, Kenler HA, et al. Prophylactic iron supplementation after Roux-en-Y gastric bypass: a prospective, double-blind, randomized study. Arch Surg. 1998;133(7):740–4.

42. Stabler SP. Clinical practice. Vitamin B12 deficiency. N Engl J Med. 2013;368(2):149–60.

43. Provenzale D, Reinhold RB, Golner B, Irwin V, Dallal GE, Papathanasopoulos N, et al. Evidence for diminished B12 absorption after gastric bypass: oral supplementation does not prevent low plasma B12 levels in bypass patients. J Am Coll Nutr. 1992;11(1): 29–35.

44. Brolin RE. Gastric bypass. Surg Clin North Am. 2001;81(5): 1077–95.

45. Brolin RE, Gorman JH, Gorman RC, Petschenik AJ, Bradley LJ, Kenler HA, et al. Are vitamin B12 and folate deficiency clinically important after roux-en-Y gastric bypass? J Gastrointest Surg. 1998;2(5):436–42.

46. Berghella V, Buchanan E, Pereira L, Baxter JK. Preconception care. Obstet Gynecol Surv. 2010;65(2):119–31.

47. Kumar N, Ahlskog JE, Gross Jr JB. Acquired hypocupremia after gastric surgery. Clin Gastroenterol Hepatol. 2004;2(12):1074–9.

48. Goldberg ME, Laczek J, Napierkowski JJ. Copper deficiency: a rare cause of ataxia following gastric bypass surgery. Am J Gastroenterol. 2008;103(5):1318–9.

49. Tan JC, Burns DL, Jones HR. Severe ataxia, myelopathy, and peripheral neuropathy due to acquired copper deficiency in a patient with history of gastrectomy. JPEN J Parenter Enteral Nutr. 2006;30(5):446–50.

50. Rudnicki SA. Prevention and treatment of peripheral neuropathy after bariatric surgery. Curr Treat Options Neurol. 2010;12(1): 29–36.

51. de Luis DA, Pacheco D, Izaola O, Terroba MC, Cuellar L, Martin T. Zinc and copper serum levels of morbidly obese patients before and after biliopancreatic diversion: 4 years of follow-up. J Gastrointest Surg. 2011;15(12):2178–81.

52. Balsa JA, Botella-Carretero JI, Gomez-Martin JM, Peromingo R, Arrieta F, Santiuste C, et al. Copper and zinc serum levels after derivative bariatric surgery: differences between Roux-en-Y Gastric bypass and biliopancreatic diversion. Obes Surg. 2011; 21(6):744–50.

53. Juhasz-Pocsine K, Rudnicki SA, Archer RL, Harik SI. Neurologic complications of gastric bypass surgery for morbid obesity. Neurology. 2007;68(21):1843–50.

54. King JC, Shames DM, Woodhouse LR. Zinc homeostasis in humans. J Nutr. 2000;130(5S Suppl):1360S–6S.

55. Hambidge KM. Zinc and diarrhea. Acta Paediatr Suppl. 1992; 381:82–6.

56. Slater GH, Ren CJ, Siegel N, Williams T, Barr D, Wolfe B, et al. Serum fat-soluble vitamin deficiency and abnormal calcium metabolism after malabsorptive bariatric surgery. J Gastrointest Surg. 2004;8(1):48–55. discussion 4-5.

57. Dolan K, Hatzifotis M, Newbury L, Lowe N, Fielding G. A clinical and nutritional comparison of biliopancreatic diversion with and without duodenal switch. Ann Surg. 2004;240(1):51–6.

58. Bal BS, Finelli FC, Shope TR, Koch TR. Nutritional deficiencies after bariatric surgery. Nat Rev Endocrinol. 2012;8(9):544–56.

59. Lonsdale D. A review of the biochemistry, metabolism and clinical benefits of thiamin(e) and its derivatives. Evid Based Complement Alternat Med. 2006;3(1):49–59.

60. Victor M, Adams RD, Collins GH. The Wernicke-Korsakoff syndrome. A clinical and pathological study of 245 patients, 82 with post-mortem examinations. Contemp Neurol Ser. 1971;7:1–206.

61. Aasheim ET. Wernicke encephalopathy after bariatric surgery: a systematic review. Ann Surg. 2008;248(5):714–20.

62. Lakhani SV, Shah HN, Alexander K, Finelli FC, Kirkpatrick JR, Koch TR. Small intestinal bacterial overgrowth and thiamine deficiency after Roux-en-Y gastric bypass surgery in obese patients. Nutr Res. 2008;28(5):293–8.

63. Bozbora A, Coskun H, Ozarmagan S, Erbil Y, Ozbey N, Orham Y. A rare complication of adjustable gastric banding: Wernicke's encephalopathy. Obes Surg. 2000;10(3):274–5.

64. Davies DJ, Baxter JM, Baxter JN. Nutritional deficiencies after bariatric surgery. Obes Surg. 2007;17(9):1150–8.

65. Loh Y, Watson WD, Verma A, Chang ST, Stocker DJ, Labutta RJ. Acute Wernicke's encephalopathy following bariatric surgery: clinical course and MRI correlation. Obes Surg. 2004;14(1):129–32.

66. Smets RM, Waeben M. Unusual combination of night blindness and optic neuropathy after biliopancreatic bypass. Bull Soc Belge Ophtalmol. 1999;271:93–6.

67. Ocon J, Cabrejas C, Altemir J, Moros M. Phrynoderma: a rare dermatologic complication of bariatric surgery. JPEN J Parenter Enteral Nutr. 2012;36(3):361–4.

68. Stroh C, Weiher C, Hohmann U, Meyer F, Lippert H, Manger T. Vitamin A deficiency (VAD) after a duodenal switch procedure: a case report. Obes Surg. 2010;20(3):397–400.

69. Lee WB, Hamilton SM, Harris JP, Schwab IR. Ocular complications of hypovitaminosis a after bariatric surgery. Ophthalmology. 2005;112(6):1031–4.

70. Booth SL. Roles for vitamin K beyond coagulation. Annu Rev Nutr. 2009;29:89–110.

71. Shearer MJ. Vitamin K, metabolism and nutriture. Blood Rev. 1992;6(2):92–104.

72. Eerdekens A, Debeer A, Van Hoey G, De Borger C, Sachar V, Guelinckx I, et al. Maternal bariatric surgery: adverse outcomes in neonates. Eur J Pediatr. 2010;169(2):191–6.

73. Bersani I, De Carolis MP, Salvi S, Zecca E, Romagnoli C, De Carolis S. Maternal-neonatal vitamin K deficiency secondary to maternal biliopancreatic diversion. Blood Coagul Fibrinolysis. 2011;22(4):334–6.

74. Kopic S, Geibel JP. Gastric acid, calcium absorption, and their impact on bone health. Physiol Rev. 2013;93(1):189–268.

75. Gosch M, Jeske M, Kammerlander C, Roth T. Osteoporosis and polypharmacy. Z Gerontol Geriatr. 2012;45(6):450–4.

76. Scibora LM, Ikramuddin S, Buchwald H, Petit MA. Examining the link between bariatric surgery, bone loss, and osteoporosis: a review of bone density studies. Obes Surg. 2012;22(4):654–67.

77. Goldner WS, O'Dorisio TM, Dillon JS, Mason EE. Severe metabolic bone disease as a long-term complication of obesity surgery. Obes Surg. 2002;12(5):685–92.

78. Marceau P, Biron S, Lebel S, Marceau S, Hould FS, Simard S, et al. Does bone change after biliopancreatic diversion? J Gastrointest Surg. 2002;6(5):690–8.

79. Sinha N, Shieh A, Stein EM, Strain G, Schulman A, Pomp A, et al. Increased PTH and 1.25(OH)(2)D levels associated with increased markers of bone turnover following bariatric surgery. Obesity (Silver Spring). 2011;19(12):2388–93.

80. Balsa JA, Botella-Carretero JI, Peromingo R, Caballero C, Munoz-Malo T, Villafruela JJ, et al. Chronic increase of bone turnover markers after biliopancreatic diversion is related to secondary hyperparathyroidism and weight loss. Relation with bone mineral density. Obes Surg. 2010;20(4):468–73.

81. Halverson JD, Haddad JG, Bergfeld M, Teitelbaum SL. Spontaneous healing of jejunoileal bypass-induced osteomalacia. Int J Obes (Lond). 1989;13(4):497–504.

36

Alternative Minimally Invasive Options: Neural Modulation

Sajani Shah, Elizabeth A. Hooper, and Scott A. Shikora

Current estimates are that there are over 300 million obese people worldwide, which is a substantial increase from the estimated 200 million 10 years ago [1]. In the United States, nearly two-thirds of the adult population is overweight or obese, and one-third of the adult population is obese. The most recent US National Health and Nutrition Examination Survey (NHANES) report compared the age-adjusted prevalence of overweight and obese adults in the United States 20–75 years of age. Their figures demonstrated that from 1976 to 2004, the percentage of overweight and obese adults increased from 47.0 to 66.3 %. Alarmingly, obesity more than doubled during this period (from 15.0 to 32.9 %). The increase in obesity was more common in men than in women: Between 1999 and 2004, women's obesity rates did not change significantly (from 33.4 to 33.2 %) [2]. Most significantly, based on standard criteria, over 20 % of the population is likely eligible for bariatric surgery for weight loss and resolution of comorbidities.

More than 177,000 people underwent bariatric surgery in the United States in 2006; however, this is only a fraction (<1 %) of the persons in the United States who currently meet the clinical criteria for surgery [3, 4]. Research efforts to identify factors that limit the utilization of bariatric surgery are needed to ensure that all patients who qualify receive the optimal treatment for their obesity.

Although some potential candidates are denied surgery because of lack of medical insurance coverage or other disqualifying factors, a great number will simply avoid surgery out of fear of potential operative complications and the long-term consequences of these operative procedures. Therefore, there is a critical need to develop effective therapeutic options that are less invasive, less complex, and safer. Such options may be more widely accepted and broadly used. Further understanding of the anatomic and physiologic mechanisms underlying bariatric surgery will facilitate the development of novel therapies that meet these criteria.

Since the 1990s, there has been a growing interest in the concept of neuromodulation for obesity treatment. Research effort began in the mid-1990s with continuous gastric stimulation and has progressed to include meal-activated gastric stimulation and vagal nerve blocking. Currently, all forms of neuromodulation are extremely attractive to both patients and clinicians in that there is no alteration to the anatomy of the gastrointestinal tract and no dietary restrictions. Research efforts thus far have demonstrated impressive safety but inconsistent but improving weight loss. This chapter reviews the current state of the research involving neuromodulation therapies for weight loss and improvements of the associated metabolic disorders.

Gastric Electrophysiology and Motility

Normal motility is crucial to the physiologic preservation of the normal human gut function. With dysmotility, either slowed or hypermotility, absorption of nutrients is altered and may not take place.

Gastric electrical activity (GEA) is a complex phenomenon resulting in gastric motility, which in turn leads to gastric emptying [5]. The stomach is only active intermittently. For this reason, gastric electrical activity is more complex than cardiac electrical activity. The stomach has a component, known as the electrical control activity (ECA), which has a frequency of repetition in humans of only about 0.05 Hz or 3 cycles per minute (cpm) and 5 cpm in dogs. This activity originates somewhere in the proximal stomach, but no dedicated or anatomically modified pacemaker cells have been identified to clearly establish a pacemaker region similar to the sine node in the heart [6, 7]. The electrical control activity is established by opening of the sodium and the potassium channels on smooth muscle cellular level, and the resulting depolarization wave propagates distally with an increasing velocity [8]. The gastric slow wave determines the maximum frequency, propagation velocity, and propagation direction of gastric contractions (Fig. 1). Spike potentials occur on top of the gastric slow wave and function much like an action potential. When superimposed on the gastric slow wave, a strong lumen-occluding contraction occurs.

S.A. Brethauer et al. (eds.), *Minimally Invasive Bariatric Surgery*,
DOI 10.1007/978-1-4939-1637-5_36, © Springer Science+Business Media New York 2015

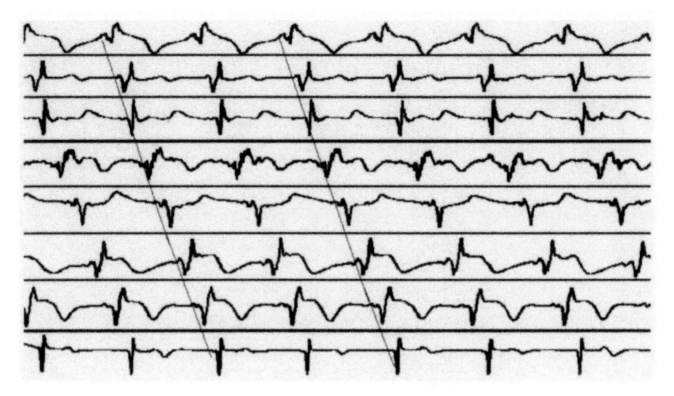

FIG. 1. Normal gastric slow waves. Gastric slow waves recorded from electrodes implanted on the serosal surface of the stomach along the greater curvature in a healthy dog (1.5 min recording). The top tracing was obtained from a pair of electrodes 16 cm above the pylorus, and the bottom one was from the electrodes 2 cm above the pylorus (Courtesy of Jiande Chen, Ph.D).

Similar to the arrhythmias of cardiac electrical function, dysrhythmias are irregularly timed and located and/or ineffective myoelectrical activity. For example (Fig. 2), there can be an ectopic pacemaker in the distal stomach in addition to the normal pacemaker in the proximal stomach. The ectopic pacemaker generates slow-wave potentials at a higher rate than normal, leading to tachygastria along with retrograde propagation toward the proximal stomach. This may interfere with normal waves and lead to disruption of the normal gastric contractions.

The prevalence and origin of various gastric dysrhythmias have been investigated in canine models. Most bradygastric impulses originate in the proximal stomach (80.5±9.4 %) and propagate to the distal antrum. Therefore most bradygastria is attributed to a decrease in the frequency of the normal pacemaker of the myoelectrical activity of the stomach. Tachygastria by contrast originates in the distal antrum (80.6±8.8 %) and propagates in a reverse fashion toward the proximal stomach. In the setting of tachygastria, the normal proximal pacemaker slow waves may or may not be present. This can lead to slow waves in one direction and distal tachygastria, leading to overall dysrhythmia [9].

Gastric motility is different in fed and fasting states. In the fed state, the human stomach contracts at the maximum frequency of 3 cpm as discussed earlier. In the fasting state, there are periodic fluctuations divided into three phases.

Phase I lasts 40–60 min with no contraction activity, phase II lasts 20–40 min with intermittent contractions, and phase III involves regular rhythmic contractions lasting 2–10 min. In the fed state, the contraction begins in the proximal stomach and follows the propagation of the spike potential as it continues toward the pylorus. In healthy subjects 2 h after a meal, 50 % or more of a meal is cleared by the contractions of the stomach, and at 4 h, 95 % of the meal should be cleared. Once emptied the motility pattern of the stomach changes [10].

Gastric emptying plays an important role in food intake regulation. Distension of the stomach acts as a satiety signal [11]. Meanwhile, rapid gastric emptying can be directly linked to some episodes of overeating and obesity. There have been numerous animal studies linking lesions in the hypothalamus to overeating and obesity [12]. There are also multiple studies which report higher rates of gastric emptying in obese subjects without a clear explanation at this point [13].

Innervation of the stomach comes from two sources: parasympathetic fibers via the vagus and sympathetic fibers via the celiac plexus. The vagus nerve has both efferent and afferent fibers, but it has predominately afferent fibers. The efferent fibers originate in the medulla and synapse with neurons located in the myenteric and submucosal plexus of the stomach. This leads to acetylcholine release and increased gastric motor function and gastric secretions. The afferent

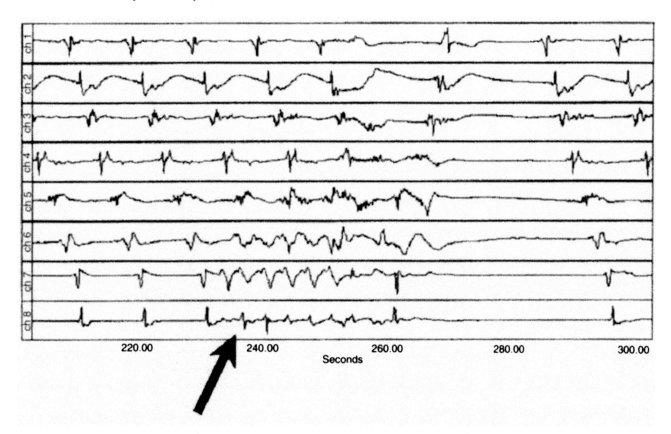

FIG. 2. Tachygastria. Gastric slow waves recorded from electrodes implanted on the serosal surface of the stomach along the greater curvature showing the ectopic tachygastrial activity in the distal stomach (*arrow*). The top tracing was obtained from a pair of electrodes 16 cm above the pylorus, and the bottom one was from the electrodes 2 cm above the pylorus (Courtesy of Jiande Chen, Ph.D).

fibers are predominant, making up approximately 90 % of the fibers. And they carry stimuli signals from the gut back to the brain. Multiple gastric peptides have also been implicated in this pathway including serotonin, substance P, ghrelin, cholecystokinin (CCK), and somatostatin [14].

The true mechanism of action for weight loss from vagotomy is not completely elucidated. This technique was first indicated in epilepsy [15] and severe, therapy-resistant depression [16]. Vagal pacing showed to diminish food intake, fat mass, and weight in pigs [17], rats [18], and obese minipigs [17], suggesting that VNS induces satiety signals. Body weight was found to be reduced mainly at the expense of body fat, whereas metabolic rate remained unaffected [19]. Depressed patients undergoing VNS were also reported to have less sweet cravings [20] and to lose weight [19, 20]. However, discussion remains on both the ideal positioning of the electrode and the frequency of the blocking algorithm.

Animal studies have looked at the effect of destruction of just the afferent fibers of the vagus in comparison to complete vagal interruption for weight loss. The blockade of afferent fibers was previously shown to downregulate the intestinal sodium-glucose cotransporter SGLT-1. Both treatments showed weight reduction in a rat model but a statistically higher rate of weight loss for complete vagal interruption (19 % for total vagotomy, 7 % for selective deafferentation). The study also revealed a significant difference in the decrease in the amount of visceral fat (52 % vagotomy vs. 18 % deafferentation) [21].

Vagal interruption in humans has been shown in a few studies to result in weight loss. This has been demonstrated over the last 35 years including early reported experiences of vagotomy for refractory obesity [22]. The effects of truncal vagotomy include preferential emptying of liquids and early satiety secondary to reduced receptive relaxation. However, dumping syndrome and diarrhea can result.

Aside from a few published studies, the clinical benefits of vagotomy have not been widely appreciated. Many surgeons have included truncal vagotomy with gastric bypass surgery; there are no reports which have shown that vagotomy increased the weight loss achieved with gastric bypass. There are many explanations for this inconsistency. Firstly, gastric bypass is such a robust weight loss procedure that it shadows any potential benefit of vagotomy. Secondly, the physiologic changes after gastric bypass negate the effects of vagotomy. Lastly, ligation of the vagus nerves activates compensatory mechanisms that overcome the benefits of vagotomy. Therefore, permanent ligation of the vagus nerves as a primary or adjuvant treatment for weight loss fell out of favor.

Gastric Stimulation and Pacing

Given the physiologic understanding of how intrinsic gastric pacing changes gastric emptying, one can postulate that manipulation of this physiology could create dysregulated pacing and also change satiety and caloric intake. Unfortunately, these mechanisms are still not completely understood as efforts to induce weight loss this way have had variable results.

A number of papers have described electrical stimulation for gastrointestinal dysmotility. The aim is to normalize the underlying rhythm by entraining the antegrade stimulation of the myoelectrical activity of the stomach. The concept of entraining gastric electrical activity to facilitate "proper" gastric motility is based on the hypothesis that electrical rhythm disturbances are the underlying reason for a variety of gastric motility disorders, including gastroparesis and possibly functional dyspepsia [23]. Capture and control of the electrical signal is dependent on both the width and the frequency of the stimulation pulse [24]. McCallum et al. [25] demonstrated in patients suffering from gastroparesis that antegrade gastric pacing could entrain gastric slow waves in all nine patients. They paced the greater curvature of the stomach at frequencies approximately 10 % higher than the slow-wave frequencies measured. In two patients, it converted tachygastria to normal slow waves.

Based on the physiology of normal gastric propagation leading to stomach clearance, it is postulated that retrograde pacing or disentrainment may slow emptying in patients with rapid gastric emptying, and based on studies suggesting obese patients may have faster gastric emptying, the principle of retrograde pacing may lead to slowed emptying, increased satiety, and lower caloric consumption. An artificial pacemaker is connected to the distal stomach along the lesser curvature, resulting in electrical waves propagating from the distal to the proximal stomach. These waves conflict with the normal and physiologic electrical waves that propagate from the proximal to the distal stomach. Consequently, gastric dysrhythmia is induced, and the regular propagation of gastric electrical waves is impaired. The severity of impairment is determined by the strength of the electrical stimulation [26].

However, to date, there have been no clinical studies to demonstrate the effectiveness of normalizing the antegrade stimulation in treatment of gastroparesis. In fact, only several studies published reports about spontaneously existing intermittent "tachygastria" and "bradygastria" in humans, and their impact on gastric emptying remains unclear [27, 28].

Implantable Gastric Stimulation for Weight Loss

Conceptualized first by Italian surgeon Valerio Cigaina in the late 1980s, the concept of stimulation of the stomach has been shown to be safe and effective. At that time, he hypothesized that exogenous electrical impulses could be used to dysregulate normal gastric electromotor activity in obese patients, resulting in weight loss.

In 1996, Cigaina et al. reported that retrograde gastric electrical stimulation was both safe and effective in moderating weight gain in a porcine model. Three groups were studied, and once beyond 12 weeks, a statistical difference in weight loss appeared. Weight was 10.5 % less than for sham controls [29].

The initial human studies began in 1995. Four women with a BMI of 40 or greater were implanted and followed for up to 40 months. Via laparoscopy, patients had platinum electrodes implanted intramuscularly on the anterior gastric wall, adjacent to the lesser curve and attached to a prototype generator. No dietary instructions were given. At 40 months after implantation, two patients had significant weight loss of 32 and 62 kg. Malfunctions in their stimulator system were discovered in the other two patients with fracture of the lead. Neither lost significant weight, highlighting the importance of bipolar stimulation.

Initiated in 2000, the first US investigation (US O-01) was a multicenter, randomized, controlled, double-blinded trial that was developed to evaluate both the safety and efficacy of the commercially produced implantable gastric stimulator (IGS), a pacemaker-like device (Transcend, Medtronic, Minneapolis, Minnesota). It includes a battery-operated pulse generator and a bipolar lead. It is implanted via laparoscopy. With the subcutaneous generator, it can be interrogated or programmed in the office. 100 devices were placed via laparoscopic means. This trial had difficulty with lead dislodgement (17/41). Despite alterations in technique with improved lead contact, there was still no significant weight loss between the control arm (2.4 %) and the study arm (1.4 %). No dietary or behavioral counseling was included in this study and patients with binge-eating behaviors were admitted potentially confounding the results [30].

The Dual-Lead Implantable Gastric Electrical Stimulation Trial (DIGEST) was designed following the lessons from European experience and the US O-01 trials. This was an open-label study for dual-lead placement. Two clinical sites enrolled seemingly similar populations, but results as measured by weight loss were significantly different. When combined, overall, there was a 15 % excess weight loss at 38 weeks and 23 % excess weight loss at 16 months. The two sites did not have equivalent weight loss, possibly from difference in patient selection [31]. Due to the difference in weight loss between the two sites, the investigators utilized

BaroScreen™ to screen participants as responders and non-responders [30].

In 2004, following the satisfactory results of safety and efficacy in carefully selected patients, a double-blinded multicenter study was undertaken comparing active devices to inactive devices. Potential participants met stringent inclusion criteria as well as prospective BaroScreen™ scores that suggested >15 % weight loss would occur with electrical stimulation. 190 patients were enrolled and all underwent laparoscopic implantation of the Transcend II (Medtronic, Minneapolis, MN) implantable gastric stimulator. There was no statistical difference in percent of excess weight loss between the treatment and control groups at 12 months. The excess weight loss was 11.7 % for the treatment group and 11.9 % for the control group. It appears that low battery life may have contributed to lower weight loss in the active group in addition to positive weight loss in the control group through screening for highly motivated individuals coupled with a reduced-calorie diet [31].

Reflecting on the worldwide clinical experience with implantable gastric stimulation, the data could be interpreted to suggest that this technology is inadequate for achieving significant or reproducible weight loss in severely obese persons. However, a wealth of good animal studies that exists has found that electrical stimulation of the stomach [32] or intestine [33], or a combination of both [34], has consistently resulted in reduced food intake and/or weight loss. Additionally, all the previous studies of an implantable gastric stimulator, as well as a pilot trial with a meal-activated gastric electrical stimulator [35], have reported that some subjects responded extremely well and achieved both meaningful and sustainable weight loss.

TANTALUS™: Meal-Activated Gastric Stimulation

Unlike conventional gastric pacing, where electrical signals are continuously delivered, typically at rates higher than that of the intrinsic pacemaker, the TANTALUS™ (Metacure Ltd. Bermuda) enhances smooth muscle contractions by delivering signals in synchrony with sensed spontaneous electrical activity. Stimulation is applied on demand using a specialized algorithm to detect the onset of a meal by measurements of electromechanical parameters in the gut. By enhancing spontaneous gastric contractions in an early stage of the meal before reaching full gastric distension, early satiety is induced through stimulation of distal stretch receptors, eliciting an increased afferent input to the CNS to convey satiety [32].

In Europe, an open-label, five-center study was undertaken to primarily study the effect of meal-activated gastric stimulation on diabetes with weight loss considered as a secondary outcome [35]. A previous study suggested that the patients with the best potential to benefit were those on oral hypoglycemic agents with a hemoglobin A1c (HgbA1c) averaging between 7.5 and 9.5 % [35]. Thirteen patients were enrolled and underwent laparoscopic placement of the TANTALUS™. At 3 months, the HgbA1c significantly reduced from an average of 8.0–6.9 %. Fasting glucose decreased from 175 to 127 mg/dL. Weight reduction was also significant but modest from a mean weight of 104 kg down to 99.7 kg (−4.1 %). Two mechanisms of action were postulated for the results of meal-activated gastric stimulation. First, the increased vagal afferent stimulation led to the neural signals for early satiety and the resulting weight loss. Second, the gastric electrical stimulation improved glycemic control via direct effects on neurohormonal mechanisms [35].

The US experience was similar. The study was part of a 2-year, open-label trial intended to test the safety and feasibility of the TANTALUS system. Fourteen obese T2DM patients (10 females) participated in the 6-month study. They had a mean age of 42 years (range, 32–54), mean weight of 107.3 ± 20.1 kg, and mean body mass index of 39 ± 1 kg/m^2 (range, 31–45). At enrollment, mean HbA1c was 8.4 %. HgbA1c levels fell from the average of 8.5–7.6 %. Weight decreased on average from 107.7 to 102.4 kg [36]. There was fasting glucose improvement although not clinically significant. In addition, there was no correlation between weight loss and glucose improvement. Though a reduction of mean HbA1c was seen in all studies, HbA1c normalized only in about 50 % of patients in one study, with other studies reporting less impressive outcomes.

Intestinal Electrical Stimulation

Intestinal electrical stimulation (IES) is a novel potential therapy that has been shown to reduce gastric emptying and increase intestinal motility. IES affects intestinal slow waves, contractions, and transit through vagal, and cholinergic, and adrenergic pathways. Duodenal electrical stimulation (DES) is thought to successfully delay gastric emptying and reduces water intake [37]. Kelly and Code [38] demonstrated that duodenal electrical stimulation slowed gastric emptying and increased duodenogastric reflux in dogs. Recently, Liu et al. [39] demonstrated that intestinal pacing decreased absorption of nutrients and accelerated bowel transit in healthy humans.

Khawaled et al. [40] in 2009 studied intestinal electrical stimulation and the effect on postprandial glucose levels in rats. ES applied immediately after the glucose tolerance test caused a significant decrease in the rising phase slope and the maximal serum blood glucose level. Additionally, the area under the curve of the blood glucose levels was reduced by approximately 50 %. Insulin secretion decreased by 21 %. The main reduction in insulin secretion was during the first 30 min after the glucose tolerance test. IES also caused a nearly 80 % decrease of the gastric emptying rate and a 40 % increase in the flow rate of nutrients inside the intestine. The effect was immediate after IES activation and reversible [40].

Preliminary data suggests that modulating intestinal transit time and gastric emptying might play a role in treatment of diabetes and obesity. There still need to be comprehensive, long-term, and placebo-controlled clinical trials on a significant number of patients.

Vagal Blocking for Obesity Control Therapy

Directly targeting the vagal nerves as a means for weight loss has begun to again gather interest. The philosophy of intermittent vagal interruption comes from the knowledge that complete (or permanent) truncal vagotomy has decreased effectiveness over time, presumably as compensatory mechanisms to offset the responses develop. Therefore, intermittent vagal interruption that would allow the return of normal vagal function may prevent the activation of compensatory mechanisms.

An intermittent vagus nerve blocking technology is currently under investigation. VBLOC system (Enteromedics Inc, St. Paul, MN), as it is called, involves the laparoscopic placement of electrodes onto the anterior and posterior vagal nerve trunks at the gastroesophageal junction. The electrodes are connected by wire leads to an electrical pulse generator called a neuromodulator. The neuromodulator is placed in the subcutaneous tissue. In early investigations, the power source was externally imbedded in a belt that was worn around the waist. Patients were instructed to wear the belt 10–14 h daily. When on, the device was charged and the vagus nerves blocked. During the hours that the belt was not worn, the device was inactive and the vagus nerves quickly resumed normal function.

The VBLOC system is currently undergoing extensive human investigations. An open-label, three-center study assessed its safety and weight loss efficacy. Thirty-one patients participated in the trial. Patients were instructed to wear the belt for at least 12 h per day. While activated, the neuromodulator alternated 5 min of blocking with 5 min of inactivity. Excess weight loss was evaluated at multiple time points: 4 weeks (7.5 %), 12 weeks (11.6 %), and 6 months (14.2 %). For one-quarter of participants, excess weight loss was greater than 25 %. The device itself was demonstrated to be safe, and no major complications were recorded. However, one subcutaneous pocket seroma occurred, one patient was admitted for a respiratory infection, and one patient was admitted with *Clostridium difficile* infection, which resolved [41]. Through interpretation of the best weight loss data, an optimal time frame of 120 s of blockade has been utilized to improve excess weight loss to 22.7 % at 6 months [41].

With safety and efficacy established, a double-blind, multicenter study (EMPOWER) was undertaken using VBLOC therapy. Fifteen centers enrolled a total of 294 subjects. The methods of implantation of the Maestro system (EnteroMedics Inc, St Paul MN) were the same as described for the open-label study. All patients had the VBLOC system implanted. Patients were randomized to a study group that received active therapy versus a control group with inactive but implanted devices. Randomization and activation of the external controller occurred one to three weeks post-implantation. Like the open-label trials, the transmit coil and battery pack were housed in a belt apparatus designed to be worn for 9–16 h by the treatment group. The control group received low-dose short-burst activation when wearing the battery pack/transmitter as well.

The active therapy group had 17 % weight loss. Surprisingly, the control group weight loss was 16 % compared to the pretest expected loss of 8 %. The weight loss in the control group was greater than expected based on pretest statistical analysis and raises the question of an unanticipated effect of vagal manipulation alone with low-frequency changes contributing to the effects of vagal blocking [42]. This effect was subsequently demonstrated in a study using a rat sciatic nerve model which demonstrated a decrease of 31 % in the amplitude of the compound amplitude potential of the nerve. This suggests that the safety checks and low-dose frequency and amplitude checks may have altered the function of the vagal nerve stimulation of the stomach in the control group [43].

Therefore, it has been postulated that the control group was possibly a low-energy treatment group instead of a non-treatment group. Further post hoc analysis of the data supported this theory because weight loss seen in both groups was directly dependent on the number of hours that the belt was worn. Analysis also suggests the device is effective because the weight loss is greater for both groups than the expected nonintervention rate of 8 % [42].

To eliminate the effects of patient noncompliance with wearing the belt, the VBLOC system was modified to include a fully programmable and implantable energy source. Human investigation has shown that the fully implantable device was equivalent in function to the first generation device with a belt [44]. It is possible that the overall results of vagal blocking will improve as patients can no longer inadvertently reduce therapy by neglecting to wear the externally applied power source.

The benefits of vagal blocking may go beyond just weight loss. The vagus nerve is also involved with blood pressure regulation and hepatic gluconeogenesis. In 28 type 2 diabetic subjects fitted with the active implanted Maestro rechargeable system, excess weight loss at 12 months was 25 %. In addition, the HgbA1c dropped from 7.8 to 6.6 %, and mean arterial pressure (MAP) fell from a baseline of 98–91. All three categories were statistically significant [45].

Interestingly, the decrease in blood pressure was only noted in the hypertensive patients, and the improvements in blood pressure and HgbA1c occurred early and potentially independent of the weight loss.

A new multicenter double-blinded study (ReCharge Trial) is currently underway using VBLOC therapy. To prevent the potential confounding variables including noncompliance that may have adversely affected the results of the EMPOWER trial, the current study only uses the implantable power source. Additionally, to prevent any possibility that electrical impulses (even ambient electrical activity) could reach the vagus nerves of the patients in the control group, only the subcutaneous neuromodulator was implanted, and no electrodes or leads are placed around the vagus nerves. The trial is ongoing and the preliminary results should be available in the near future.

Conclusion

The battle against the obesity epidemic has given rise to many new interdisciplinary developments and an increasingly important role for more noninvasive treatment modalities. For morbidly obesity, conventional bariatric surgery is considered to be the only effective and best studied therapy. However, the current era also demands effective therapies for the relatively moderate obese population. In addition, partially due to costs and the fear of complications, only a small percentage of the eligible candidates undergo bariatric surgery. Therefore, novel less invasive treatment options are a focus in research. The need for effective minimal invasive treatments will continue to increase, but a sound critical attitude toward these novel techniques. As previously stated by the expert panel on weight loss surgery, the golden standard to investigate the safety and efficacy of interventions for the treatment of obesity and its complications should be by means of randomized, blinded, sham-controlled clinical trials.

Some techniques/devices have been or will be failures, some will be revisited, and some will turn out to be successful in only a specific patient population. Even though short-term results of some of the recently developed techniques and devices are promising, it is important to consider them as experimental until convincing evidence is published.

Neuromodulation, including gastric stimulation and vagal blocking, is an exciting new surgical technology that may offer safe and effective weight loss alternatives. Worldwide investigation is encouraging but still very preliminary. Many questions remain unanswered such as what is the exact mechanisms of action, which patients will respond to it, how to program the device, will the benefits be sustainable, and lastly will it be safe long term?

While there is still much to be learned about this technology, it is clear that less invasive and simpler procedures are desirable, and those proven to be efficacious may introduce a paradigm shift in the surgical management of moderate and severe obesity.

Review Questions and Answers

1. The vagus nerve is the longest cranial nerve. It contains motor and sensory fibers and, because it passes through the neck and thorax to the abdomen, has the widest distribution in the body. It contains somatic and visceral afferent fibers, as well as general and special visceral efferent fibers. Which of the following is not a function of the nerve?
   (a) Swallowing and phonation
   (b) Involuntary muscle and gland control of the digestive tract
   (c) Responsible for taste
   (d) Ocular movement (Answer)

2. Which is true of gastric myoelectrical activity?
   (a) It consists of an uninterrupted sequence of electrical potential variations called "slow waves" that spring out continuously, at a frequency of about 3/min in man, from a small zone of the proximal gastric corpus near the great curvature (pacemaker area).
   (b) The origin of slow waves lies in the interstitial cells of Cajal type I (ICC), a series of highly ramified cells located between the longitudinal and circular muscle coats.
   (c) In gastroparesis, there are more or less severe alterations in gastric myoelectrical activity, which may be recorded with intraluminal, serosal, and cutaneous electrodes.
   (d) All of the above (Answer)

3. Which of the following is not true regarding vagal stimulation/blockage?
   (a) Leads are placed around the vagus nerve that delivers high-frequency, intermittent low-energy electrical signals.
   (b) Increase in transmission of vagal signals has been shown to reduce hunger, increase satiety, and possibly has neuroendocrine effects on the liver and pancreas. (Answer)
   (c) The vagus is responsible for contraction of the stomach pump (the antrum) which grinds up food and mixes it with stomach enzymes, acid secretion, stomach emptying, secretion of digestive enzymes by the pancreas and emptying of the gallbladder, and modulation of sensations of being full (satiation), hunger, nausea, dull pain, and discomfort
   (d) All of the above

References

1. Calle EE, Rodriguez C, Walker-Thurmond K, et al. Overweight, obesity, and mortality from cancer in a prospectively studied cohort of U.S. adults. N Engl J Med. 2003;348(17):1625–38.

2. Mokdad AH, Ford ES, Bowman BA, et al. Prevalence of obesity, diabetes, and obesity-related health risk factors. JAMA. 2003; 289(1):76–9.

3. Surgery ASMBS. Metabolic surgery expected to play bigger role in treating type 2 diabetes and other metabolic diseases [press release]. Gainesville, Florida; August 22, 2007. Available at: http://www. asbs.org/Newsite07/resources/press_release_8202007.pdf. Accessed 4 Dec 2012.

4. Zhao Y, Encinosa W. Bariatric surgery utilization and outcomes in 1998 and 2004: statistical brief no. 23. Rockville (MD): Agency for Healthcare Research and Quality . 2007;(updated 2007). Available at: http://www.hcup-us.ahrq.gov/reports/statbriefs/sb23.pdf

5. Kwong NK, Brown BH, Whittaker GE, Duthie HL. Electrical activity of the gastric antrum in man. Br J Surg. 1970;57(12):913–6.

6. Daniel EE, Chapman KM. Electrical activity of the gastrointestinal tract as an indication of mechanical activity. Am J Dig Dis. 1963;8(1):54–102.

7. Szurszewski JH. Electrical basis for gastrointestinal motility. Physiology of the Gastrointestinal Tract; 2: 383–422. New York: Raven Press; 1987.

8. Pullan A, Cheng L, Yassi R, Buist M. Modelling gastrointestinal bioelectric activity. Prog Biophys Mol Biol. 2004;85(2–3):523–50.

9. Qian LW, Pasricha PJ, Chen JDZ. Origins and patterns of spontaneous and drug-induced canine gastric myoelectrical dysrhythmia. Dig Dis Sci. 2003;48:509–15.

10. Tougas G, Eaker EY, Abell TL, et al. Assessment of gastric emptying using a low fat meal: establishment of international control values. Am J Gastroenterol. 2000;95:1456–62.

11. Phillips RJ, Powley TL. Gastric volume rather than nutrient content inhibits food intake. Am J Physiol. 1996;271:R766–79.

12. Duggan JP, Booth DA. Obesity, overeating, and rapid gastric emptying in rats with ventromedial hypothalamic lesions. Science. 1986;231:609–11.

13. Mahvi DM, Krantz SB. In: Townsend CM, Beauchamp RD, Evers BM, Mattox KL, editors. Sabiston textbook of surgery. 19th ed. Philadelphia: Elselvier Sanders; 2012. p. 1182–226.

14. Wright RA, Krinsky S, Fleeman C, et al. Gastric emptying and obesity. Gastroenterology. 1983;84:747–51.

15. Burneo JG, Faught E, Knowlton R, Morawetz R, Kuzniecky R. Weight loss associated with vagus nerve stimulation. Neurology. 2002;59(3):463–4.

16. Kosel M, Schlaepfer TE. Mechanisms and state of the art of vagus nerve stimulation. J ECT. 2002;18(4):189–92.

17. Matyja A, Thor PJ, Sobocki J, et al. Effects of vagal pacing on food intake and body mass in pigs. Folia Med Cracov. 2004;45(3–4):55–62.

18. Bugajski AJ, Gil K, Ziomber A, Zurowski D, Zaraska W, Thor PJ. Effect of long-term vagal stimulation on food intake and body weight during diet induced obesity in rats. J Physiol Pharmacol. 2007;58(1):5–12.

19. Sobocki J, Fourtanier G, Estany J, Otal P. Does vagal nerve stimulation affect body composition and metabolism? Experimental study of a new potential technique in bariatric surgery. Surgery. 2006;139(2):209–16.

20. Bodenlos JS, Kose S, Borckardt JJ, et al. Vagus nerve stimulation acutely alters food craving in adults with depression. Appetite. 2007;48(2):145–53.

21. Stearns AT, Balakrishnan A, Radmanesh A, Ashley SW, et al. Relative contributions of afferent vagal fibers to resistance to diet-induced obesity. Dig Dis Sci. 2012;57:1281–90.

22. Kral JG. Effects of truncal vagotomy on body weight and hyperinsulinemia in morbid obesity. Am J Clin Nutr. 1980;33:416–9.

23. Zhangand J, Chen JDZ. Pacing the gut in motility disorders. Curr Treat Options Gastroenterol. 2006;9(4):351–60.

24. Lin ZY, McCallum RW, Schirmer BD, et al. Effects of pacing parameters in the entrainment of gastric slow waves in patients with gastroparesis. Am J Physiol Gastrointest Liver Physiol. 1998;27:G186–91.

25. McCallum RW, Chen JDZ, Lin ZY, et al. Gastric pacing improves emptying and symptoms in patients with gastroparesis. Gastroenterology. 1998;114:456–61.

26. Eagon JC, Kelly KA. Effects of gastric pacing on canine gastric motility and emptying. Am J Physiol. 1993;265:G767–74.

27. Dubois A. Gastric dysrhythmias: pathophysiologic and etiologic factors. Mayo Clin Proc. 1989;64(2):246–50.

28. You CH, Chey WY. Study of electromechanical activity of the stomach in humans and in dogs with particular attention to tachygastria. Gastroenterology. 1984;86(6):1460–8.

29. Cigaina V, Saggioro A, Rigo V, et al. Long-term effects of gastric pacing to reduce feed intake in swine. Obes Surg. 1996;6:250–3.

30. Shikora SA, Storch K. Implantable gastric stimulation for the treatment of severe obesity: the American experience. Surg Obes Relat Dis. 2005;1:334–42.

31. Shikora SA, Bergenstal R, Bessler M, et al. Implantable gastric stimulation for the treatment of clinically severe obesity: results of the SHAPE trial. Surg Obes Relat Dis. 2009;5:31–7.

32. Aelen E, Neshev MC, et al. Manipulation of food intake and weight dynamics using retrograde neural gastric electrical stimulation in a chronic canine model. Neurogastroenterol Motil. 2008;20(4):358–68.

33. Arriagada AJ, Jurkov AS, Neshev E, Muench G, Andrews CN, Mintchev MP. Design, implementation and testing of an implantable impedance-based feedback-controlled neural gastric stimulator. Physiol Meas. 2011;32:1103–15.

34. Yin, Chen JDZ. Mechanisms and potential applications of intestinal electrical stimulation. Dig Dis Sci. 2010;55(5):1208–20.

35. Bohdjalian A, Ludvik B, Guerci B, et al. Improvement in glycemic control by gastric electrical stimulation (TANTALUS) in overweight subjects with type 2 diabetes. Surg Endosc. 2009;23:1955–60.

36. Sanmiguel CP, Conklin JL, Cunneen SA, et al. Gastric electrical stimulation with the TANTALUS system in obese type 2 diabetes patients: effect on weight and glycemic control. J Diabetes Sci Technol. 2009;3(4):964–70.

37. Liu S, Hou X, Chen JDZ. Therapeutic potential of duodenal electrical stimulation for obesity: acute effects on gastric emptying and water intake. Am J Gastroenterol. 2005;100(4):792–6.

38. Kelly KA, Code CF. Duodenal-gastric reflux and slowed gastric emptying by electrical pacing of the canine duodenal pacesetter potential. Gastroenterology. 1977;72:429–33.

39. Liu J, Qiao X, Hou X, Chen JD. Effect of intestinal pacing on small bowel transit and nutrient absorption in healthy volunteers. Obes Surg. 2009;19:196–201.

40. Khawaled R, Blumen G, Fabricant G, Ben-Arie J, Shikora S. Intestinal electrical stimulation decreases postprandial blood glucose levels in rats. Surg Obes Relat Dis. 2009;5(6):692–7. doi:10.1016/j.soard.2009.05.013. Epub 2009 Jun 11.

41. Camilleri M, Toouli J, Herrera MF, et al. Intra-abdominal vagal blocking (VBLOC therapy): clinical results with a new implantable medical device. Surgery. 2008;143(6):723–31.

42. Camilleri M, Toouli J, Herrera MF, et al. Selection of electrical algorithms to treat obesity with intermittent vagal block using an implantable medical device. Surg Obes Relat Dis. 2009;5:224–30.

43. Sarr MG, Billington CJ, Brancatisoan R, et al. The EMPOWER study: randomized, prospective double-blind, multicenter trial of vagal blockade to induce weight loss in morbid obesity. Obes Surg. 2012;22:1771–82.

44. Kow L, Herrera M, Kulseng B, et al. Vagal blocking for the treatment of obesity delivered using the fully implantable MAESTRO Rechargeable system: 12 month results. Emerging Technologies Sessions (ET-103). Surg Obes Relat Dis. 2011;7:363–4.

45. Herrera MF, Toouli J, Kulseng B, et al. Treatment of obesity-related co-morbidities with VBLOC therapy. Plenary sessions IFSO 2011. Obes Surg. 2011;21:998.

37
Intragastric Balloon

Manoel Galvao Neto, Josenberg Marins Campos,
and Lyz Bezerra Silva

Introduction

The intragastric balloon (IGB) is considered a temporary and minimally invasive strategy for weight loss. It is the most used endoluminal obesity therapy, with the potential to benefit patients with mild obesity, as a bridge to bariatric surgery, and even for the ones who do not want the permanent modifications of bariatric surgery.

The idea of using this method was introduced in 1982, by Nieben and Harboe, aiming to increase satiety and achieve weight loss [1]. The procedure was developed through clinical observation of the effects caused by bezoars in weight loss, with adaptation of its physiology and anatomy. Basically, it is a space-occupying device that will reduce stomach endoluminal size, preventing the patient to eat the usual amount of food ending in less food intake.

Physiologic data for IGBs are sparse. It is said that it may have an effect in cholecystokinin, increasing its secretion, thus delaying gastric emptying [2]. In patients with morbid obesity, IGB-induced weight loss is associated with a decrease in plasma concentration of leptin and a transitory increase of plasma ghrelin. It is possible that the hormonal changes that regulate the energy balance caused by the IGB can prevent an increase in adiponectin levels [3]. Hormonal changes described are not enough to say they prevail over the restrictive nature of the device.

The first balloon was approved for use by the FDA in the USA as the Garren-Edwards Gastric Bubble (GEGB), a cylindrical device insufflated with 220 ml of air. In the late 1980s, several studies showed no difference between the GEGB and lifestyle and diet modifications, with controversial results concerning safety and efficacy and multiple side effects and complications such as intolerance, damage to gastric mucosa, Mallory-Weiss tears, esophageal laceration

Electronic supplementary material: Supplementary material is available in the online version of this chapter at 10.1007/978-1-4939-1637-5_37. Videos can also be accessed at http://www.springerimages.com/videos/978-1-4939-1636-8.

during balloon placement, and spontaneous deflation leading to small bowel obstruction [4–6]. Due to its poor results and high rate of complications, the GEGB was abandoned and later forbidden to be used in the USA.

These relatively frustrating experiences were probably due to two main aspects. First, some obese subjects overeat for reasons more related to compulsive eating than to actual physiologic hunger. Binge-eating behavior has been related with unsatisfactory weight loss results even when more aggressive techniques are used, such as gastric banding and gastric bypass [7]. The second aspect involves a technical issue: early balloons were air filled, most of them having rough surfaces potentially injurious to the gastric mucosa, and the use of PPIs was not routine.

In 1987, international experts met and defined the necessary characteristics of a safe and effective balloon. These characteristics included a smooth surface to avoid gastric ulceration, a small and flexible deflated structure enabling implant and explant under direct endoscopic visualization, construction with a soft and highly elastic material, and that the device be filled with fluid instead of air [8].

The complications of the first balloons led to a new generation of IGBs adopting the recommendations of the 1987 Tarpon Springs Conference. The BIB® (Apollo Endosurgery, Austin, TX) (Fig. 1) was introduced in 1991, meeting those recommendations. It is approved for use in Europe, several countries in South America, Middle East, and Asia, but not in the USA [9].

The BIB® is made of a transparent silicone elastomer, resistant to corrosion by gastric acid. It has a self-sealing radiopaque valve to which a silicone catheter is attached to fill the balloon. The balloon has an initial cylindrical shape and final oval shape, with a variable filling from 400 to 700 ml, allowing an adequate volumetric adjustment for each patient, designed to float freely inside the stomach, increasing satiety and decreasing gastric reservoir capacity and food intake. It can be kept in the stomach for up to 6 months, after which there is an increased risk of spontaneous deflation and resultant bowel obstruction. Balloon deflation is accomplished

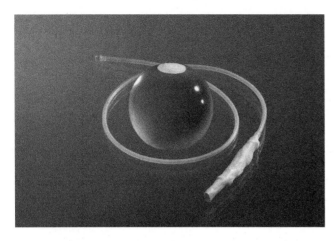

FIG. 1. BIB® (reproduced with permission of Apollo Endosurgery, Austin, TX).

by puncturing the balloon with a needle and simply removing it with a foreign-body grasper or a customized one.

In 2004, an air-filled balloon, the Heliosphere® (Helioscopie, Vienne, France), was approved for use in Europe, Canada, South America, and other countries, but not in the USA [9]. It is a double-bag polymer balloon covered with a smooth external pouch of biocompatible silicone with a radiopaque marker, which must be filled with air to a final volume of 650 to 750 ml. The Heliosphere® is a lighter balloon (30 g), a characteristic that possibly increases patient tolerability.

Indications

The balloon, an endoscopic approach to obesity, is positioned in-between clinical and surgical treatment. It overcomes the results of clinical treatment on inducing more effective and durable weight loss and cannot be compared with the much better and long-term efficacy of the bariatric surgery.

Traditionally, IGBs have been used on morbidly obese patients and as a bridge to surgical procedures. More recently, there is a trend to its use on low-BMI patients even with cosmetic purposes, for example, in Brazil, the BIB® is approved by the FDA-like agency (ANVISA, reg# 80143600103) to be used in patients with BMI of 27 and over. Another trend is the use for specific achievements like effectively lose weight to have a more conservative treatment in orthopedic and spinal surgery or effectively lose weight to get pregnant as it improves fertility, among other benefits. Other interesting indication is on morbidly obese children and teenagers under a strict protocol.

A list of indications follows below:

- Patient with BMI > 35 kg/m², unresponsive to clinical treatment who refuses surgical therapy or has contraindications
- Patient with BMI < 35 kg/m², comorbidities, unresponsive to clinical treatment in a period superior to 3 years
- Super-obese presurgical preparation (bridge procedure)

- Anesthesia risk reduction before major surgeries
- Pre-op weight loss for orthopedic patients, allowing a more conservative approach or decreasing surgical risk
- Clinical risk reduction for severe chronic diseases associated, induced, or worsened by obesity

Contraindications

Relative Contraindications

- Severe reflux esophagitis (higher risk for complications)
- GEJ conditions or diseases
- Chronic use of NSAIDs

Absolute Contraindications

- Previous gastric surgery (especially Nissen fundoplication and gastrectomy)
- Gastric or duodenal active ulcer
- Hiatal hernia > 5 cm
- Collagen diseases
- Hepatic cirrhosis, portal hypertension
- Cancer
- AIDS
- Crohn's disease
- Anticoagulant chronic use
- Drug and alcohol abuse
- Pregnancy and lactation
- Psychiatric disorder (uncontrolled)

Technique

Implant

- Patient under deep sedation with anesthesiologist (can be changed to anesthesia with intubation under anesthesiologist's discretion and patient's clinical condition).
- Endoscopic evaluation of esophagus, stomach, and duodenum for planning of the procedure, measuring the distance until the GEJ.
- Aspirate gastric residues.
- Removal of the endoscope.
- Insertion of the deflated balloon into the stomach, in an orogastric manner until surpassing the previously measured GEJ (Fig. 2).
- Confirm that the balloon is well positioned and if not, reposition it under endoscopic view in an optimal location (between gastric fundus and body).
- Removal of guidewire from insufflation catheter.
- Connect unidirectional valve to the 0.9 % saline + methylene blue solution.

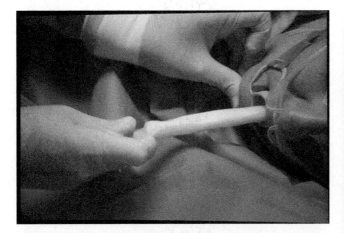

FIG. 2. Insertion of the deflated balloon into the stomach in an orogastric manner until surpassing the previously measured GEJ with the patient under deep sedation with anesthesiologist.

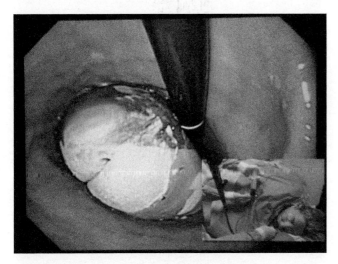

FIG. 3. Injection of 400–700 ml of methylene blue solution keeping visual inspection during balloon filling.

- Inject of 400–700 ml of the solution with "luer-lock" syringes (60 ml syringes, inject each syringe in a 10 s period) (Fig. 3).
- Keep visual inspection during balloon filling.
- After insufflated, the balloon should touch gastric walls.
- After completing the desired volume, close the unidirectional valve and apply gentle negative pressure in the catheter with the syringe (optional).
- Retrieve endoscope to esophagus.
- Pull the balloon against the GEJ, keeping constant pressure until disconnection of the valve.
- Remove insufflation catheter.
- Advance the endoscope to the stomach for inspection of balloon and valve looking for leaks (Fig. 4).
- Aspirate stomach and remove the endoscope.

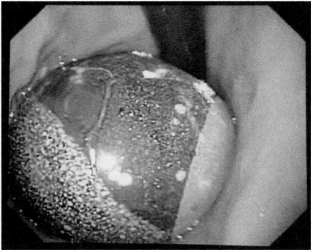

FIG. 4. Balloon at the end of the procedure well positioned on the gastric fundus with no signs of leak observed in a "U-turn" maneuver.

*Air-filled balloon has a security system with a prolene thread that must be sectioned before insufflation. Afterward, the white nylon thread is pulled, opening the safety layer. The balloon is then filled with 650 to 750 ml of air by means of a unidirectional valve system, having the insufflation catheter removed at the end.

Prescription and Post-Implant Recommendations (By the Authors)

- Steroids—continue for 3 days.
- Prokinetics (start during procedure)—continue for 7 days.
- Ondansetron and steroids—continue for 7 days.
- Scopolamine (patch or oral)—continue for 7 days.
- PPI on double dose—continue as long as the patient has the balloon.
- Weekly follow-up during the first 2 weeks with endoscopy team.
- Monthly visits—until explant—multidisciplinary team.
- Remind the patient that he will have mild to severe nausea/vomiting during the first days, and in case of dehydration or uncontrollable pain, he should contact the team.
- Patient must comply with follow-up plan, doing regular physical activities.

Continuous use of PPI is mandatory, not only for protection of the gastric mucosa and to ameliorate gastroesophageal reflux but also to protect the balloon itself from the deleterious action of hydrochloridric acid [10].

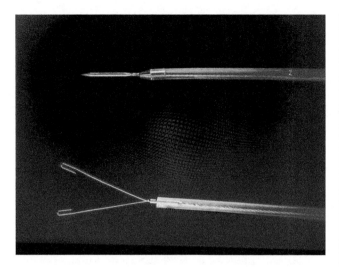

FIG. 5. Customized needle catheter and double-hook grasper (Apollo Endosurgery, Austin, TX).

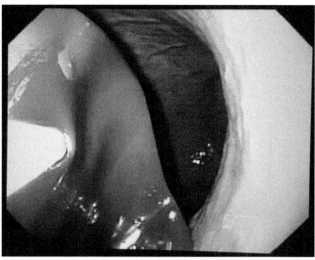

FIG. 7. Visual inspection until complete suction of the liquid, observing the thin edges of the balloon collapsing.

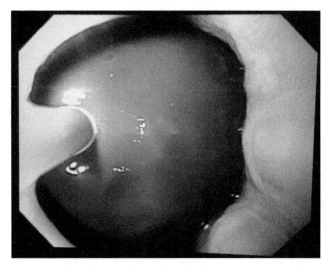

FIG. 6. Balloon puncture with customized needle catheter under direct view, anterograde.

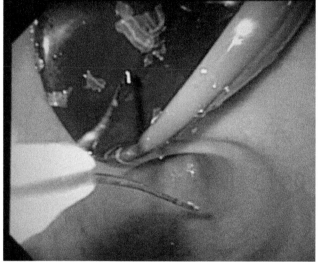

FIG. 8. Customized double-hook grasper opened to capture the balloon.

Explant Recommendations (By the Authors)

- Patient under general anesthesia, intubated.
- Endoscopy for evaluation of stomach and planning of the procedure.
- Aspirate residues as much as possible (mandatory intubation in the presence of residues).
- It is recommended to have two suction sources (one for the endoscope and another for the suction catheter in order to be precise with amount of liquid aspirated from the balloon).
- Balloon puncture with an appropriate customized needle catheter (Fig. 5) always under direct view, anterograde (preferable) (Fig. 6), or in U-turn (alternative), according to endoscopist's choice and stomach conditions.

- After puncture, remove the needle and connect to the suction tube with a separate container for measuring the aspirated content.
- Intermittent aspiration avoiding collapse/bending of the catheter.
- Keep constant visual inspection until complete suction of the liquid, observing the thin edges of the balloon collapsing (Fig. 7).
- Keep track of the amount of liquid aspirated.
- For balloon retrieval, adequate material will be needed: double-hook grasper (Fig. 5), polypectomy snare, foreign-body graspers, based on endoscopist's preference.
- The balloon capture point must be planned in a way that there is a good contact area, avoiding the valve and being sure there is an adequate hold (Fig. 8).

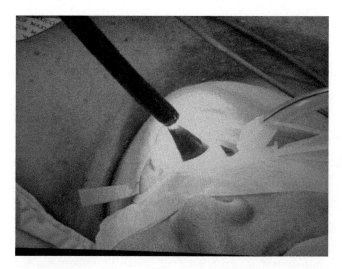

FIG. 9. Balloon removal at the end with the balloon close to the endoscope tip.

- A therapeutic endoscope might be useful in more difficult cases.
- Scopolamine (with intention to relax the EGJ) should be administered after the balloon has been captured and before retrieval.
- Keeping the balloon close to the endoscope tip makes removal easier.
- Traction must be uniform, without bumps or stops, under visual control.
- The GEJ offers certain resistance, demanding more attention.
- In the esophageal body, the passage is easier.
- When the balloon reaches the cervical region, the neck must be hyperextended, deflating the orotracheal tube cuff (optional), increasing sedation as needed (Fig. 9).
- After the balloon has been removed, a second-look endoscopy is mandatory, to assure that the esophagus and the gastric wall have not been harmed.
- In cases of challenging removal, therapeutic scopes and overtube are helpful.

Pre- and Post-explant Prescription and Recommendations

- Pre-explant
  - Prolonged fasting (16–18 h), decreasing solid food residues.
  - Liquid diet for 24–36 h.
  - Prokinetics—start 5–7 days before.
  - Patient must go through a consultation with nutritionist and psychologist to prepare for balloon removal.
- Post-explant
  - Prokinetics—continue for 2 or 3 days
  - Ondansetron (optional)
  - Scopolamine—continue for 2 or 3 days
  - PPI on double dose—continue for 7 days
  - Monthly follow-up with the multidisciplinary team for at least 6 months

Results

In a systematic review, 15 articles (3,608 patients) were evaluated to estimate BIB® effectiveness. The weight loss at balloon removal were 14.7 kg, 12.2 % of initial weight, 5.7 kg/m^2 drop from initial BMI, and 32.1 % of EWL. However, data were scant after balloon removal. Efficacy at balloon removal was estimated with a meta-analysis of two randomized controlled trials (75 patients) comparing balloon versus placebo, indicating the balloon group lost more weight than the placebo group. Regarding BIB® safety, the majority of complications were mild, and early removal rate was 4.2 % [9]. The 12.2 % estimated rate of total weight loss at the end of treatment is an amount considered sufficient to obtain health benefits, according to the knowledge obtained with clinical treatment that a weight loss of 10 % improves morbid conditions associated with obesity (hypertension, diabetes, hyperlipidemia, among others) and also reduces mortality [11].

A Brazilian multicenter study evaluated 483 overweight and obese patients treated with the BIB®. Of these, 323 completed a 6-month follow-up and 85 of them completed a 1-year follow-up. At 6 months, patients showed a global weight reduction from baseline BMI of 38.2±9.4 to a 6-month BMI of 32.9±8.3 kg/m^2. Super-obese patients under preoperative preparation ($n=32$) showed a mean weight loss of 26.1 kg, mean % EWL of 23.5 %. Considering surgical risk, most patients showed a significant improvement from ASA III–IV before placement of balloon to ASA II, with easier control of comorbidities, enabling safer surgical procedures. Patients with BMI<35 kg/m^2 ($n=148$) showed a %EWL of 63.4±28.6 %, with a success rate of 94 %. At 1-year follow-up, a subset of patients had maintained a substantial weight reduction. The 1-year % EWL was 50.9±28.8 [10].

Overall, 85 patients who showed up for the 1-year follow-up maintained more than 90 % of their BMI reduction observed at the 6-month follow-up. 17 patients followed at 2 years after BIB® placement have maintained more than 89 % of their 6-month BMI reduction, but again, results in patients who did not come back remain speculative. Although this follow-up represents less than 50 % of patients, it suggests that when patients agree to multidisciplinary treatment and change their behavior, they can maintain the weight loss more than 1–2 years after BIB® removal [10].

From 76 subjects evaluated under BAROS Qol score, more than 85 % were satisfied with the treatment. However, such results should be viewed with caution because the gratitude for a good result in these patients could render them more motivated to reply to a questionnaire than others who did not have as good an outcome. Binge eaters have a large gastric capacity, less negative feedback, and therefore lose less weight with the intragastric balloon. Identification and treatment of binge-eating disorders are essential to satisfactory results with the BIB [10].

Obese adolescents may be a promising indication for intragastric balloon because the shorter duration of obesity allows a greater possibility for them to change their eating behavior and lifestyle [10].

In a study done by Genco et al., 2,515 patients had a BIB® implanted. Placement was uncomplicated in all, but two cases (0.08 %) with acute gastric dilatation were treated conservatively. The balloon was removed before 1 month after positioning in 11 patients (0.44 %) due to psychological intolerance. Overall complication rate was 2.8 % ($n=70$). Gastric perforation happened in 5 patients (0.19 %), 4 of whom had undergone previous gastric surgery: 2 died and 2 were treated successfully by laparoscopic gastric repair after BIB® removal. Gastric obstruction presented in 19 patients (0.76 %) during the first week after positioning and was treated by device removal. There was balloon rupture in nine patients (0.36 %). In relation to comorbidities, there was improvement (less medication dosage required or shift to other therapy) in 625/1,394 patients (44.8 %). After 6 months, %EWL was 33.9 ± 18.7 (range 0–87) [12].

A small double-blind randomized study compared the fluid-filled BioEnterics BIB® and air-filled Heliosphere® gastric balloons. Eighteen subjects were given the Heliosphere® and 15 the BIB®. Body weight significantly decreased at 6 months after balloon insertion in both groups, with no differences between them. At 6 months, the mean %EWL was 27 ± 16 for the Heliosphere® and 30.2 ± 19 for the BIB®. All 30 patients kept their balloons for 6 months. In relation to safety, endoscopic times were shorter for Heliosphere® balloon at placement and retrieval. However, balloon insertion under conscious sedation was impossible in two Heliosphere® patients due to rigidity of the device at the pharynx, causing severe discomfort, requiring general anesthesia. System failure at positioning was observed in one BIB® due to impossibility of saline injection through the catheter, requiring a new balloon placement. At the time of removal, two Heliosphere® bags had passed in the stool and were not found in the stomach. Balloon removal was more difficult in the Heliosphere® group: one patient required surgical removal of the balloon by laparoscopy, and in other three patients, a rigid esophagoscopy was required following attempted endoscopic extraction. In all these patients, the deflated balloons failed to be pulled out through the cardia, as the hook forceps tore the external pouch of the balloon in every attempt. Altogether, 30 % of Heliosphere® bags had an adverse event at removal. After these results, the study was prematurely stopped for safety reasons. Regarding tolerance, at 1 month after discharge, three patients had intolerance to the BIB® balloon (20 %), requiring early removal. There was no difference between devices for epigastric pain, gastroesophageal reflux, or vomits [13].

These results are similar to those found by Giardiello et al. In this study, 60 patients were randomized to receive either a BIB® or a Heliosphere® bag. In 3 patients of the BIB® group, early balloon removal was performed for intractable nausea and vomiting. At time of removal, weight loss was similar between groups. Significant longer extraction time, with high patient discomfort, was observed in the Heliosphere® group due to difficult passage through the cardia and lower pharynx. In 1 patient in the BIB® group and 10 (33.3 %) patients in the Heliosphere® group, the balloon was found partially deflated at removal time [14]. The self-deflation in the air-filled balloon without a marker like methylene blue makes it an issue because it may not be recognizable, increasing the risk of balloon migration into the intestinal loop.

In the author's experience with the BIB®, 320 patients had the device implanted and were effectively followed up [15]. Mean weight loss was 38.1 % EWL at 6 months for patients with a previous BMI of 35–40 kg/m^2, 42.5 % EWL in a BMI of 40–50 kg/m^2, and 45.3 %EWL in a BMI > 50 kg/m^2. There was nausea and vomiting in 65 %, abdominal pain in 30 %, and dehydration in 9 % during the first week. There was also one early removal due to intolerance and no complications during implant or removal. A small subset of 20 female patients on this group selected among low-BMI (30–35 kg/m^2) patients that gained weight after the second pregnancy were enrolled in a prospective single-arm trial with intensive multidisciplinary follow-up during implant period and after removal up to 6 months, achieved 58.4 ± 13.4 %EWL and 28.7 ± 1.8 (25.2–32.5) BMI from its initial 33.6 ± 2.2 (30–37.9) kg/m^2 with 76.9 % protocol adhesion. At the end of 6-month post-explant period, mean BMI was 29.5 ± 2 (25.3–33.7) kg/m^2, with 68.3 % protocol adhesion [16].

In the long term, intragastric balloon-induced weight loss seems to be maintained in patients who comply with multidisciplinary treatment and undergo behavioral modifications since the beginning of treatment. A 5-year follow-up study concluded that patients who lost 80 % of total weight loss during the first 3 months of treatment succeeded in maintaining a % EWL > 20 long term after BIB® removal [17]. Although it is not a routine, balloon reimplantation in order to extend the weight loss duration is feasible and had been used in some cases, but data are scarce.

Complications

Complications of the BIB® are less frequent than what was seen with earlier balloons. They include intolerance to the balloon (which might result in early removal), gastric erosions and ulcers, esophagitis, spontaneous deflation, persistent vomiting, gastroesophageal reflux, and abdominal pain. There have been reports of several gastric perforations, small bowel obstructions, impaction, and significant gastric dilatation [18].

Methylene blue is used together with saline for balloon filling, minimizing the risk of bowel obstruction. If there is spontaneous balloon deflation, the dye is systemically absorbed, turning patient's urine green. As an observation, propofol (sedative agent commonly used during endoscopic procedures) has a rare side effect of making urine green, and the clinician must be aware of this false-positive marker for balloon deflation [19].

In a systematic review, early removed balloons were 4.2 %, with 43 % of those being voluntary removals, a rate that is much lower in isolated series. The reported adverse events, leading to removal or not, were nausea and vomiting after first week (8.6 %), abdominal pain (5.0 %), deflation and displacement (2.5 %), inflammation (2.1 %), gastro-esophageal reflux (1.8 %), dehydration (1.6 %), deflation without displacement (0.9 %), displacement and obstruction (0.8 %), diarrhea and/or constipation (0.7 %), gastric ulcer (0.4 %), gastric perforation (0.1 %), and mortality related with balloon gastric perforation (0.1 %) [9].

In the Brazilian multicenter trial, the most prevalent side effects were nausea/vomiting (39.9 %) and epigastric pain (20.1 %) during the first week. Dehydration requiring intravenous saline infusion occurred in 4.6 %, and 3.4 % of patients had early intolerance leading to BIB® removal. Minor complications were clinically controlled: reflux esophagitis in 12.4 % and symptomatic gastric stasis in 8.7 % from transient obstruction of the pyloric antrum by the balloon. Major complications were balloon impaction (0.6 %) in the antrum with gastric hyperdistention, requiring removal of gastric content under general anesthesia. There was one case of spontaneous deflation of the balloon and migration into the small bowel, causing intestinal obstruction 5 months after device placement [10].

Balloon placement must be careful, and the esophagus must be evaluated after the procedure. If implant is difficult, there might be esophageal damage, and even esophageal tear, a life-threatening condition [20].

Regarding the transient obstruction of the pyloric antrum by the BIB®, which may occur in up to 9 % of the cases, the mechanical maneuver of putting the patient in left lateral decubitus and progressive massage of epigastrium from the right to left hypochondrium usually results in migration of balloon to the gastric fundus with relief of symptoms [10].

Spontaneous deflation can occur, and when the balloon is fluid filled, there is a change in the color of urine and stools, due to methylene blue [21, 22]. It is essential that the patient is aware of this possibility, decreasing the risk of an intestinal obstruction. The diagnosis is usually straightforward, based on a clinical history and physical exam. The most useful imaging exams are abdominal X-ray and ultrasound [23]. A computerized tomography may also be used. Even though some deflated balloons can be eliminated through the gastrointestinal tract without major problems, surgical therapy might be needed. Balloon removal can be done by a laparotomic, laparoscopic, or a combined way. An enteroscopic or colonoscopic removal can also be attempted.

A rare but serious complication is gastric perforation. Ulcers and gastric erosions in the presence of a balloon may be related to gastric wall irritation and lack of cytoprotection secondary to mucosal prostaglandins production. The presence of food residues impacted between the gastric wall and the balloon and/or the irregular surface of the filling valve can generate a high pressure and ischemia zone, which might culminate in a perforation [24]. Previous gastric surgery is an absolute contraindication to balloon placement, due to possibility of perforation [12, 25]. Intense and sudden abdominal pain, days or months after balloon implant, must raise the possibility of gastric perforation, a complication that can lead to sepsis and death if not treated early. The diagnosis is clinical, with intense epigastric pain and an acute abdomen on physical exam. Imaging exams may reveal pneumoperitoneum and intracavitary collections. The definitive and etiologic diagnosis is made through an endoscopy. The treatment is surgical, preferably laparoscopic, through laceration closure [26].

Multidisciplinary Follow-Up

Before balloon placement, the patient must be evaluated by a psychologist, searching for previous history of mood, anxiety or eating disorders, alcohol or drug abuse, and family history of psychological or neurological diseases that may interfere with the treatment.

Nutritional follow-up is needed in order to make the patient aware of the necessary behavior and eating habit modifications. After IGB implant, there is an adaptation period in which the diet gradually goes from liquid to solid. Usually, only in the 3rd week after implant the patient starts eating solid foods. Also, it is important to know that the balloon only restricts quantity of food ingestion, and awareness of the quality of food is necessary, avoiding hypercaloric diet.

Physical activity should be encouraged, since it is highly important for IGB success. Before starting to exercise, all patients must undergo a physical evaluation, adapting physical activity to each subject, considering age, sex, physical condition, and comorbidities. It is recommended that exercising becomes a habit, going beyond the 6-month balloon period.

Future Perspectives

More recently, new fluid-filled balloons with the same characteristics of the BIB have been designed in Latin America and Asia with scarce literature supporting it [27].

Considering the early intolerance and complications associated with traditional IGBs, an adjustable balloon was developed, the Spatz Adjustable Balloon System (ABS)® (Spatz FGIA, Inc., NY, USA). It is composed of a silicone balloon mounted on a catheter on one surface. This catheter has two loops, one is a non-collapsible loop meant to prevent or delay balloon passage through the pylorus and duodenum in case of a deflation. There is a stretchable inflation tube that can be pulled out of the stomach and snare, enabling volume adjustability, while the balloon remains in the stomach. In a first-in-man study, 18 patients had an Spatz ABS® implanted. Implantation time ranged from 8 to 15 min. Mean % EWL at 24 weeks was 36 % and 48.8 % at 52 weeks, demonstrating that patients safely continue to lose weight beyond 6 months. There was device removal in seven patients during the follow-up, due to leaks, erosive gastritis, Mallory-Weiss tears, gastric perforation, or patient request. There was mild nausea in 20 % of patients and mild vomiting in 50 %, lasting 1–2 days. There was one spontaneous balloon deflation, which was removed endoscopically, since the anchor kept it inside the stomach. Two patients requested downward adjustment of the balloon, to decrease intolerance, which was achieved successfully, allowing patients to remain in the trial. Further studies are needed to confirm the safety of this device and analyze its advantages compared to more traditional IGBs [28]. In contrary of what was reported in this trial, case report shows that it is possible for a deflated Spatz ABS® to migrate into the duodenum, although authors believe that the rigidity of the antimigration system helped to avoid distal intestinal progression of the device, facilitating endoscopic removal [29].

Another perspective for endoluminal treatment of obesity is the use of an ingestible wireless capsule. It aims to reduce the cost and side effects associated with endoscopic procedures required to implant and explant commercially available IGBs. The pill is inserted through natural ingestion, and its volume increases after it enters the stomach. After treatment, the pill will be deflated and removed from the body by natural discharge process. The inflation mechanism consists of a chemical reaction between acetic acid and sodium bicarbonate, generating a gas. This reaction is controlled through a wireless system, also allowing volume control [30]. There are no human trials of this device so far.

In endoscopy there will be restrictive/space-occupying devices and procedures like balloons and endoluminal gastric volume reduction/restriction and bypass or bowel diversion ones, like endoscopic duodenal-jejunal endoluminal bypass [31, 32], a device already approved for clinical use in Latin America and Europe [33, 34].

The nearby perspective for IGBs is the repositioning of its indication from the morbidly obese to the low-BMI obese and overweight patients, due to the efficacy and safety profile of this device, since those large groups of patients are not candidates to bariatric surgery, and the clinical treatments are still far from achieving the same results. The future of intragastric balloons is to become part of the spectrum of endoscopic treatments of obesity, integrated with the new endoscopic devices, which could then have a classification similar to bariatric surgery, as restrictive, malabsorptive/metabolic procedures.

Conclusion

Intragastric balloon is a current endoscopic treatment for obesity with effective temporary weight loss and a very good safety profile that has been used worldwide with exception of few countries like the USA. It may be the best option for overweight and obese patients unresponsive to clinical therapy or who are either not candidates for surgery or who do not wish to undergo surgery and also can serve as a bridge to surgery. On the other hand, a number of patients may not respond to the device, since all obesity treatments have failure rates. Patients who do not comply with conventional therapy and binge eaters are unlikely to respond to balloon placement. The risks of intolerance and complications must be explained to the patients. The device has a good overall safety profile and can now be used in the USA as well as in other countries (Video 1).

Review Questions and Answers

1. How do the risks and benefits of intragastric balloons compare to bariatric surgery?
   A. Higher risk, greater benefits than surgery
   B. Lower risk, lower benefits than surgery
   C. Higher risk, lower benefits than surgery
   D. Lower risk, higher benefits than surgery
   Answer: B

2. What is the expected weight loss with intragastric balloons?
   A. 5 % total weight loss
   B. 12 % total weight loss
   C. 50 % excess weight loss
   D. 30 % total weight loss
   Answer: B

3. What are the most commonly reported adverse events with intragastric balloons?
   A. Perforation, bleeding
   B. Nausea, obstruction
   C. Pain, nausea
   D. Vomiting, balloon rupture
   Answer: C

References

1. Nieben OG, Harboe H. Intragastric balloon as an artificial bezoar for treatment of obesity. Lancet. 1982;1(8265):198–9.
2. Kissileff HR, Carretta JC, Geliebter A, Pi-Sunyer FX. Cholecystokinin and stomach distension combine to reduce food intake in humans. Am J Physiol Regul Integr Comp Physiol. 2003;285(5):R992–8.

3. Konopko-Zubrzycka M, Baniukiewicz A, Wroblewski E, Kowalska I, Zarzycki W, Gorska M, et al. The effect of intragastric balloon on plasma ghrelin, leptin, and adiponectin levels in patients with morbid obesity. J Clin Endocrinol Metab. 2009;94(5):1644–9.

4. Mathus-Vliegen EM, Tytgat GN, Veldhuyzen-Offermans EA. Intragastric balloon in the treatment of super-morbid obesity. Double-blind, sham-controlled, crossover evaluation of 500-milliliter balloon. Gastroenterology. 1990;99(2):362–9.

5. Benjamin SB. Small bowel obstruction and the Garren-Edwards gastric bubble: an iatrogenic bezoar. Gastrointest Endosc. 1988; 34(6):463–7.

6. Ulicny Jr KS, Goldberg SJ, Harper WJ, Korelitz JL, Podore PC, Fegelman RH. Surgical complications of the Garren-Edwards Gastric Bubble. Surg Gynecol Obstet. 1988;166(6):535–40.

7. Hsu LK, Benotti PN, Dwyer J, Roberts SB, Saltzman E, Shikora S, et al. Nonsurgical factors that influence the outcome of bariatric surgery: a review. Psychosom Med. 1998;60(3):338–46.

8. Schapiro M, Benjamin S, Blackburn G, Frank B, Heber D, Kozarek R, et al. Obesity and the gastric balloon: a comprehensive workshop. Tarpon Springs, Florida, March 19-21, 1987. Gastrointest Endosc. 1987;33(4):323–7.

9. Imaz I, Martinez-Cervell C, Garcia-Alvarez EE, Sendra-Gutierrez JM, Gonzalez-Enriquez J. Safety and effectiveness of the intragastric balloon for obesity. A meta-analysis. Obes Surg. 2008;18(7):841–6.

10. Sallet JA, Marchesini JB, Paiva DS, Komoto K, Pizani CE, Ribeiro ML, et al. Brazilian multicenter study of the intragastric balloon. Obes Surg. 2004;14(7):991–8.

11. Goldstein DJ. Beneficial health effects of modest weight loss. Int J Obes Relat Metab Disord. 1992;16(6):397–415.

12. Genco A, Bruni T, Doldi SB, Forestieri P, Marino M, Busetto L, et al. BioEnterics intragastric balloon: The Italian Experience with 2,515 patients. Obes Surg. 2005;15(8):1161–4.

13. De Castro ML, Morales MJ, Del Campo V, Pineda JR, Pena E, Sierra JM, et al. Efficacy, safety, and tolerance of two types of intragastric balloons placed in obese subjects: a double-blind comparative study. Obes Surg. 2010;20(12):1642–6.

14. Giardiello C, Borrelli A, Silvestri E, Antognozzi V, Iodice G, Lorenzo M. Air-filled vs water-filled intragastric balloon: a prospective randomized study. Obes Surg. 2012;9.

15. In press for the Bariatric Endoscopy book of Brazilian Society of Digestive Endoscopy. 2013

16. Presented at Brazilian Congress of Bariatric Surgery in November of 2006; Salvador, Bahia, Brazil.

17. Kotzampassi K, Grosomanidis V, Papakostas P, Penna S, Eleftheriadis E. 500 intragastric balloons: what happens 5 years thereafter? Obes Surg. 2012;22(6):896–903.

18. Ubeda-Iglesias A, Irles-Rocamora JA, Povis-Lopez CD. Antral impaction and cardiorespiratory arrest. Complications of the intragastric balloon. Med Intensiva. 2012;36(4):315–7.

19. Bernante P, Francini F, Zangrandi F, Menegon P, Toniato A, Feltracco P, et al. Green urine after intragastric balloon placement for the treatment of morbid obesity. Obes Surg. 2003;13(6):951–3.

20. Nijhof HW, Steenvoorde P, Tollenaar RA. Perforation of the esophagus caused by the insertion of an intragastric balloon for the treatment of obesity. Obes Surg. 2006;16(5):667–70.

21. Matar ZS, Mohamed AA, Abukhater M, Hussien M, Emran F, Bhat NA. Small bowel obstruction due to air-filled intragastric balloon. Obes Surg. 2009;19(12):1727–30.

22. Vanden Eynden F, Urbain P. Small intestine gastric balloon impaction treated by laparoscopic surgery. Obes Surg. 2001;11(5):646–8.

23. Francica G, Giardiello C, Iodice G, Cristiano S, Scarano F, Delle Cave M, et al. Ultrasound as the imaging method of choice for monitoring the intragastric balloon in obese patients: normal findings, pitfalls and diagnosis of complications. Obes Surg. 2004; 14(6):833–7.

24. Koutelidakis I, Dragoumis D, Papaziogas B, Patsas A, Katsougianopoulos A, Atmatzidis S, et al. Gastric perforation and death after the insertion of an intragastric balloon. Obes Surg. 2009;19(3):393–6.

25. Giardiello C, Cristiano S, Cerbone MR, Troiano E, Iodice G, Sarrantonio G. Gastric perforation in an obese patient with an intragastric balloon, following previous fundoplication. Obes Surg. 2003;13(4):658–60.

26. Sanchez-Perez MA, Munoz-Juarez M, Cordera-Gonzalez de Cosio F, Revilla-Pacheco F, Herrada-Pinedaherrada-Pineda T, Gonzalez Jauregui-Diaz F, et al. Gastric perforation and subarachnoid hemorrhage secondary to intragastric balloon device. Rev Gastroenterol Mex. 2011;76(3):264–9.

27. Carvalho GL, Barros CB, Moraes CE, Okazaki M, Ferreira Mde N, Silva JS, et al. The use of an improved intragastric balloon technique to reduce weight in pre-obese patients–preliminary results. Obes Surg. 2011;21(7):924–7.

28. Machytka E, Klvana P, Kornbluth A, Peikin S, Mathus-Vliegen LE, Gostout C, et al. Adjustable intragastric balloons: a 12-month pilot trial in endoscopic weight loss management. Obes Surg. 2011;21(10):1499–507.

29. de la Riva S, Munoz-Navas M, Rodriguez-Lago I, Silva C. Small-bowel migration: a possible complication of adjustable intragastric balloons. Endoscopy. 2012;44 Suppl 2 UCTN:E224.

30. Kencana AP, Rasouli M, Huynh VA, Ting EK, Lai JC, Huy QD, et al. An ingestible wireless capsule for treatment of obesity. Conf Proc IEEE Eng Med Biol Soc. 2010;2010:963–6.

31. Nanni G, Familiari P, Mor A, Iaconelli A, Perri V, Rubino F, et al. Effectiveness of the Transoral Endoscopic Vertical Gastroplasty (TOGa®): a good balance between weight loss and complications, if compared with gastric bypass and biliopancreatic diversion. Obes Surg. 2012;23.

32. Galvão Neto M, Rodriguez L, Zundel N, Ayala JC, Campos J, Ramos A. Endoscopic revision of Roux-en-Y gastric bypass stomal dilation with a suturing device: preliminary results of a first Out-of-United States series. Bariatric Times. 2011;8(6):32–4.

33. de Moura EG, Orso IR, Martins Bda C, Lopes GS, de Oliveira SL, Galvao-Neto Mdos P, et al. Improvement of insulin resistance and reduction of cardiovascular risk among obese patients with type 2 diabetes with the duodenojejunal bypass liner. Obes Surg. 2011;21(7):941–7.

34. de Moura EG, Martins BC, Lopes GS, Orso IR, de Oliveira SL, Galvao Neto MP, et al. Metabolic improvements in obese type 2 diabetes subjects implanted for 1 year with an endoscopically deployed duodenal-jejunal bypass liner. Diabetes Technol Ther. 2012;14(2):183–9.

38

Alternative Minimally Invasive Options: Endoluminal Bariatric Procedures

Nitin Kumar and Christopher C. Thompson

Introduction

Obesity and its comorbidities, including diabetes, hypertension, hyperlipidemia, and fatty liver disease, are a significant challenge for physicians, patients, and society in the United States and around the world [1]. The cost of obesity is $190 billion annually in the United States [2]. Lifestyle modifications, including diet changes and exercise, have been ineffective in arresting the growth of this epidemic. Medications have been successful in a fraction of patients and are currently an adjunctive therapy. Bariatric surgery, while effectively applied to hundreds of thousands of patients annually, can only be applied to a fraction of eligible patients with the current number of practicing surgeons [3].

Endoscopic bariatric therapies may be used to address obesity in patients with BMI below bariatric surgery criteria, to bridge patients to bariatric surgery, to address metabolic disease, to revise bariatric surgery and, eventually, as an alternative to bariatric surgery. Potential benefits include lower invasiveness, reversibility, and lower cost. These characteristics may allow endoscopic bariatric therapy to be repeated at regular intervals if needed. Currently, primary endoscopic bariatric therapy is restrictive, space occupying, or malabsorptive. Restrictive procedures include endoscopic gastroplasty and restrictive implantation. Space-occupying devices include intragastric balloons. Malabsorptive technologies prevent contact of food with portions of the small intestine.

Primary endoscopic bariatric therapies continue to build records for safety and long-term efficacy in the treatment of obesity and metabolic disease. Endoscopic revision of Roux-en-Y gastric bypass, developed a decade ago, has acquired level 1 evidence for effectiveness [4].

Restrictive Procedures

Restrictive procedures are used to reduce gastric volume. Plications can be made endoscopically using tissue anchors or sutures. These procedures continue to evolve.

The EndoCinch (CR Bard, Murray Hill, NJ), originally used to treat GERD, is a suction-based superficial-thickness suturing device. A hollow capsule at the endoscope tip is used to suction mucosa and trap tissue; a needle is then passed through the tissue. EndoCinch has been used for transoral gastroplasty. Fogel et al. have published multiple studies in adolescents and adults. One study of 64 patients with mean BMI 39.9 kg/m² categorized participants into group 1 (BMI ≥ 40 kg/m², 33 patients); group 2 (BMI 35–40 kg/m², 19 patients); and group 3 (BMI < 35 kg/m², 12 patients) [5]. There were no serious adverse events or need for overnight observation. 1-year follow-up captured 94.1 % of patients. Weight loss was 39.6 ± 11.3 % of EWL at 3 months and 58.1 ± 19.9 % of EWL at 1 year. Notably, this study was not approved by an IRB. A subsequent study of transoral gastroplasty by Fogel included 21 adolescents aged 13–17 with mean BMI of 36.2 kg/m² [6]. Weight loss was 63.8 % of EWL at 6 months, 67.3 % of EWL at 12 months, and 61.5 % of EWL at 18 months.

A newer version of the EndoCinch, called RESTORe Suturing System, allowed suture reloading without endoscope removal. It was capable of full-thickness plication. Brethauer et al. studied the device in transoral gastroplasty in 18 patients at two sites [7]. There were no significant complications. An average of six plications were created (Fig. 1); procedure time was 125 ± 23 min. Mean weight loss was 11.0 ± 10 kg after 1 year, or 27.7 ± 21.9 % of EWL; half of patients lost at least 30 % of EWL. Average decrease in waist

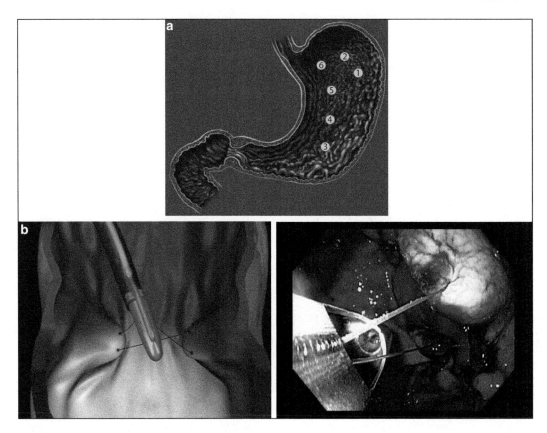

Fɪɢ. 1. (**a**) Pattern of anterior to posterior plications utilized by the RESTORe Suturing System (© 2014 C. R. Bard, Inc; used with permission) for primary endoluminal procedure. (**b**) Plication placement.

circumference was 12.6 ± 9.5 cm. Additionally, a significant decrease in systolic (15.2 mmHg) and diastolic (9.7 mmHg) blood pressure was seen. On follow-up endoscopy, however, partial or complete release of plications was noted in 13 patients.

The TransOral GAstroplasty (TOGA) system (Satiety Inc, Palo Alto, CA) has been studied for endoscopic gastroplasty. The device is a flexible stapler capable of performing full-thickness tissue apposition. Vacuum is used to appose the gastric walls, and a partition is created parallel to the lesser curvature (Fig. 2). The device must be removed for reloading. Deviere et al. reported TOGA in 21 patients with BMI of 43.3 kg/m^2 [8]. No serious adverse events were noted, although vomiting, pain, nausea, and transient dysphagia were reported. All patients had partially or fully intact stapled sleeves at 6 months, although gaps were noted in 13 patients. Average weight loss was 12 kg after 6 months, or 24.4 % of EWL. Moreno et al. reported successful TOGA in 11 patients using a second-generation device and retreatment to create additional distal restrictions if necessary [9]. No serious adverse events were reported. Average weight loss was 17.5 kg at 3 months and 24.0 kg at 6 months. Mean BMI decreased from 41.6 to 33.1 kg/m^2 after 6 months. A multicenter study including 67 patients (53 were available for follow-up) reported EWL of 52.2 % in patients with BMI

≥ 40 and 41.3 % in BMI <40 [10]. Hemoglobin A1c decreased significantly, from 7.0 to 5.7 %; there were also significant improvements in triglyceride levels and HDL. One case of respiratory insufficiency and another of asymptomatic pneumoperitoneum were noted.

The TERIS, or Trans-Oral Endoscopic Restrictive Implant System (BaroSense, Menlo Park, CA), is an implanted diaphragm containing a 10 mm orifice (Fig. 3). The device is stapled into the gastric cardia. De Jong et al. studied 13 patients and reported 12 successful placements [11]. One patient was unsuccessful due to gastric perforation. Two patients developed pneumoperitoneum. After these events, technical adjustments were made to the procedure, and no further complications were seen. Average procedure time was 142 min. Median BMI decreased from 42.1 to 37.9 kg/m^2 after 3 months. Weight loss of 16.9 kg, and EWL of 22.2 %, was reported at 3 months.

Space-Occupying Devices

Space-occupying devices offer a noninvasive option for weight loss. These include balloons and polymers. Space-occupying devices result in volume displacement and gastric distention (Fig. 4). Additionally, changes in gastric motility

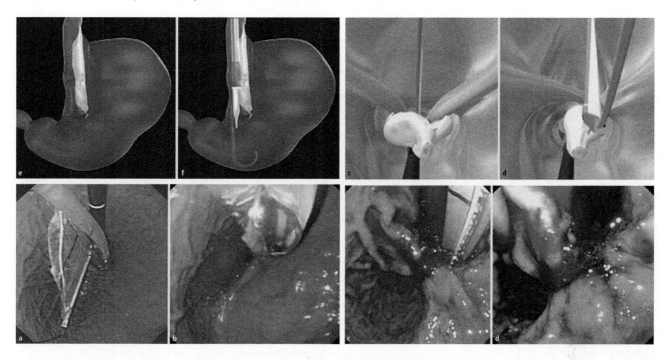

FIG. 2. The TransOral GAstroplasty (TOGA) system was used to create a vertical stapled gastroplasty along the lesser curvature of the stomach. The anterior and posterior walls of the stomach were drawn into the suction chamber and stapled together (Courtesy of Ethicon, Cincinnati, OH, with permission).

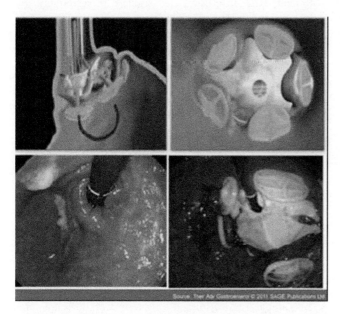

FIG. 3. The TERIS, or Trans-Oral Endoscopic Restrictive Implant System (BaroSense, Menlo Park, CA, with permission), places a restrictive device across the gastric cardia.

and hormones have been noted. Notably, cholecystokinin may be released due to gastric distention, inducing pyloric constriction and delayed gastric emptying. The first intragastric balloon was approved for use in the United States in 1985, inspired by the observation that patients with bezoars lost weight. The technology has not seen widespread adop-tion in the United States over the past three decades. Devices in use to date, primarily in Europe, have been utilized as a bridge to definitive therapy.

The BioEnterics Intragastric Balloon, or BIB (Allergan, Irvine, CA), is a silicone elastomer balloon that can be implanted into the stomach endoscopically [12]. It can be filled with saline and methylene blue dye, which leaks and changes the color of urine if the balloon's integrity is com-promised. The balloon is resistant to gastric acid for approxi-mately 6 months.

The BIB has been studied in a large number of patients compared to other endoscopic bariatric therapies. A meta-analysis of 3,698 patients reported weight loss of 14.7 kg and 32.1 % EWL after 6 months [13]. BMI decreased by 5.7 kg/m^2. Complications included nausea, vomiting, bowel obstruction (0.8 %), and gastric perforation (0.1 %). 4.2 % of patients had early removal. A retrospective study of 2,515 patients with mean BMI of 44.4 kg/m^2 reported that BIB placement resulted in two mortalities in patients with previ-ous gastric surgery. After 6 months, there was decrease in BMI by 9.0 kg/m^2 [14]. There was significant improvement in blood pressure and lipid profile, and fasting glucose. Of 488 diabetics, 87.2 % had significant decrease or normaliza-tion in hemoglobin A1c.

A prospective study of the metabolic changes after BIB placement included 130 patients with BMI of 43.1 kg/m^2 [15]. Ten patients required early balloon removal, 6 of which were due to intolerance, abdominal pain, or vomiting. During the 6-month follow-up period, patients were kept on

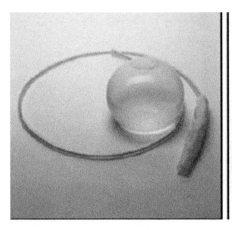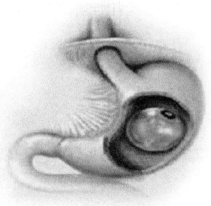

Fɪɢ. 4. Intragastric balloon.

1,000–1,200 kcal per day. Weight loss after 6 months was 13.1 kg, resulting in decrease of class IV obesity from 23 to 8 % in the cohort. Statistically significant metabolic improvements were noted, with decrease in prevalence of hyperglycemia from 50 to 12 %. Hypertriglyceridemia decreased from 58 to 19 %. Prevalence of severe hepatic steatosis decreased from 52 to 4 % in patients who had BMI decrease greater than 3.5 kg/m². Follow-up after balloon removal, for a median 22 months, found that 50 % of patients regained some weight.

The importance of dietitian counseling after balloon placement was studied by Tai et al. [16]. Twenty-eight patients with mean BMI of 32.4±3.7 kg/m² had BIB placement for 6 months, with decrease in BMI to 28.5±3.7 kg/m² at removal. Dietitian follow-up was scheduled at every week for 2 weeks, every 2 weeks for 1 month, and then monthly. Good adherence was defined as appearance for 50 % of scheduled visits. Responders were those who had at least 20 % EWL. Twenty patients were responders and 8 were nonresponders. Of the responders, 85 % had good adherence versus 25 % of nonresponders.

A prospective single-blinded study examined histologic improvement in nonalcoholic steatohepatitis [17]. Patients were randomized to BIB placement (11 patients) or sham endoscopy with gastric instillation of 500 mL of saline (10 patients). All patients were placed on the American Heart Association diet. Three BIB patients had removal due to epigastric discomfort and vomiting. BMI decreased by 1.6 kg/m² in the BIB group versus 0.8 kg/m² in the control group. At the end of treatment, NAFLD activity score was significantly lower in the BIB group (2 versus 4), and there was a trend towards improvement in median steatosis score in the BIB group. There was no change in median lobular inflammation, hepatocellular ballooning, or fibrosis. ALT and AST were not significantly changed in either group.

The effects of balloon placement on depression were studied by Deliopoulou et al. [18]. One hundred consecutive females were classified into depressed (65 patients) and non-depressed (35 patients) groups based on Beck Depression Inventory score. The groups were otherwise similar. Weight loss of 39.3 % EWL in the depressed group was similar to weight loss of 36.1 % EWL in the non-depressed group. The depressed group had decrease in depression score from 20.3±8.5 to 7.9±5.6 at the time of balloon removal. Additionally, 70.8 % of the patients had resolution of depression; the rate of severe depression declined from 27.7 to 1.5 %.

Repeat BIB insertion was studied prospectively by Dumonceau et al. [19]. Of 118 patients, 8 had immediate balloon reinsertion, 11 had placement after a balloon-free interval, and 99 had no balloon replacement. Patients with second balloon after a balloon-free interval regained an average 13.6 kg during that interval. The second balloon placement resulted in significantly less weight loss (9.0 kg versus 14.6 kg) and less EWL (18.2 % versus 49.3 %). The complication rate, including esophagitis and intolerance, was higher with the second balloon (26 % versus 11 %), although this was not significant. There was no difference in weight loss with second balloon placement by the third year of follow-up. Second balloon placement had no effect on the proportion of patients having ≥ 10 % weight loss or bariatric surgery during the 4.9-year follow-up period. Another study reported 112 patients with second balloon placement within 1 month of removing the first balloon [20]. Mean BMI loss was 6.5 kg/m² with the first balloon, versus 2.5 kg/m² with the second balloon.

Kotzampassi et al. studied long-term weight trends after BIB removal in 500 patients with initial BMI of 43.7 kg/m² [21]. At the time of BIB removal, 83 % of patients were classified as successful, with EWL of at least 20 %. This group had mean weight loss of 23.9±9.1 kg and BMI loss of 8.3 kg/m². At 5-year follow-up, including 41 % of the original cohort, mean weight loss was 7.3±5.4 kg and BMI loss was 2.5 kg/m². Twenty-three percent of patients maintained weight loss of at least 20 % of EWL.

BIB has been studied as a bridge to RYGB in super-superobese patients [22]. Sixty consecutive patients with mean BMI of 66.5±3.4 kg/m² had either BIB placement (23 patients) or no BIB (37 patients). BIB was left in place for 155±62 days with BMI loss of 5.5±1.3 kg/m². The BIB group experienced significant decrease in systolic blood pressure and gamma-glutamyl transpeptidase. Operative time for RYGB was significantly shorter in the BIB group (146±47 versus 201±81 min). There were significantly fewer major adverse events, classified as conversion to laparotomy, ICU stay over 2 days, and hospital stay over 2 weeks, in the BIB group (2 versus 13). Weight loss was similar in both groups 1 year after RYGB.

BIB, filled with 500 mL saline, has been compared with Heliosphere BAG, which is filled with 950 mL of air [23]. Thirty patients with mean BMI of 46.3 kg/m² were randomized to each group. Decrease in BMI was 5.7 kg/m² in the BIB group versus 4.2 kg/m² in the Heliosphere group. Patients in the Heliosphere group did experience significantly longer extraction time and significantly more extraction discomfort during passage through the cardia and lower pharynx. A nonrandomized study by Caglar et al. compared the BIB with Heliosphere BAG [24]. Thirty-two patients nonresponsive to 6 months of medical and diet therapy had BIB placement (19 patients, BMI 45.6±9 kg/m²) or Heliosphere BAG placement (13 patients, BMI 45.0±8 kg/m²). After 6 months, weight loss was significantly higher in the BIB group (19.0 kg versus 13.0 kg), as was EWL (38.3 % versus 21.9 %). One patient in the BIB group had early removal due to persistent nausea and vomiting at 1 month. One patient in the BIB group died 13 days after placement due to cardiac arrest related to aspiration of gastric contents.

The silicone TransPyloric Shuttle (BAROnova, Goleta, CA) comprises a large spherical bulb connected to a smaller cylindrical bulb by a flexible tether. The sphere is too large to traverse the pylorus, while the cylinder can pass into the duodenal bulb during peristalsis. The device intermittently blocks the pylorus, reducing gastric emptying rate. The device is delivered via transoral catheter and is removed endoscopically. A prospective single-center open-label study of 20 patients with mean BMI of 36.0 kg/m² reported weight loss of 8.9±5.2 kg and EWL of 31.3±15.7 % after 3 months [24]. Mean weight loss was 14.6±5.7 kg and 50.0±26.4 % EWL after 6 months. Persistent gastric ulcer required early removal in two patients.

The Duo balloon (ReShape, San Clemente, CA) comprises two silicone spheres filled with 900 mL of saline. Deflation of one balloon alone will not result in migration. According to company data, patients have experienced loss of one-third of excess weight after 6 months. A 3-center prospective trial included balloon placements in 21 patients and 9 control patients [25]. Both groups had similar diet and exercise counseling. In the balloon group, 4 patients required readmission for nausea. Two had gastritis at balloon removal. At 48 weeks, 30 % of the balloon group reached the 25 % EWL target versus 25 % of the control group.

The SatiSphere (EndoSphere, Columbus, OH) is a preformed memory wire that self-anchors in the distal stomach and duodenum by conforming to the shape of the duodenum.

The device slows the travel of food through the duodenum, altering satiety hormones and glucose metabolism. An early trial reported that all patients lost weight, with average EWL of 12 % over the first month. Another trial of 31 patients with mean BMI 41.3 kg/m² compared 10 controls with 21 implanted patients. Device migration occurred in 10 of 21 implanted patients, requiring emergency surgery in two patients. Weight loss was 6.7 kg after 3 months in patients completing the trial versus 2.2 kg in controls. The device was found to delay glucose absorption and insulin secretion and to alter GLP-1 kinetics [26].

Malabsorptive Procedures

Small intestinal bypass is a key component of many bariatric surgical procedures. It is postulated to play an especially important role in the improvement of metabolic parameters after bariatric surgery. Endoluminal devices have been developed to bypass absorption of nutrients in the small intestine.

The EndoBarrier duodenal-jejunal bypass liner, or DJBL (GI Dynamics, Lexington, Mass), is a self-expanding nickel-titanium implant attached to a 60 cm tubular polymer sleeve that extends from the duodenal bulb into the jejunum (Fig. 5). It prevents food from contacting the mucosa of the small intestine, but allows biliary and pancreatic secretions to travel along the outside of the sleeve to the jejunum. A multicenter randomized trial of 41 patients assigned 30 patients with BMI 48.9 kg/m² to DJBL placement and 11 patients with BMI 47.4 kg/m² to diet control [27]. Four patients required device removal due to migration, obstruction, pain, and dislocation of the anchor. There were no serious adverse events. After 3 months, BMI decrease was significantly higher in the DJBL group: 5.5 kg/m² versus 1.9 kg/m² in the control group. Of 8 diabetics with DJBL placement, 7 had

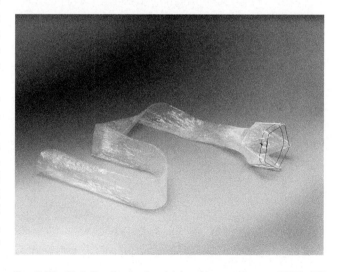

Fig. 5. The EndoBarrier duodenal-jejunal bypass liner, or DJBL (GI Dynamics, Lexington, Mass, with permission), is anchored in the duodenal bulb and extends 60 cm into the duodenum.

improvement in diabetes. Gersin et al. reported an open-label randomized multicenter trial including 25 patients, with successful implantation in 21 patients [28]. Implantation was not successful in patients with a small duodenal bulb. Seven patients required device removal due to adverse events, 3 of which were bleeding presenting as hematemesis. Weight loss after 3 months was significantly higher in the DJBL group: 8.2 ± 1.3 kg versus 2.0 ± 1.1 kg in the sham group. Another randomized trial by Tarnoff et al. included 25 patients implanted with DJBL and 14 control patients [29]. All patients received baseline dietary and lifestyle counseling. After 12 weeks, EWL was 22 % for the device group versus 5 % for the control group. There was an adverse event rate of 20 %, including bleeding, migration, and obstruction.

A modified version of the DJBL with a restrictive (4 mm) proximal opening was studied by Escalona et al. in ten patients with average BMI of 40.8 kg/m^2 [30]. Weight loss after 3 months was 16.7 ± 1.4 kg. Eight patients required balloon dilation of the restrictive orifice after developing abdominal pain, nausea, and vomiting. Gastric emptying was delayed in 84 % of patients at 3 months but generally improved after the device was removed.

Escalona et al. studied 1-year outcomes after DJBL implantation in an open-label prospective trial [30]. Thirty-nine patients with BMI 43.7 ± 5.9 kg/m^2 had implantation of the device; 3 patients could not be implanted due to short duodenal bulb. There were 15 early removals, due to anchor movement (8), device obstruction (3), abdominal pain (2), acute cholecystitis (1), and patient request (1). In the 24 patients with the device in place for 1 year, average weight loss was 22.1 ± 2.1 kg, BMI loss was 9.1 ± 0.9 kg/m^2, and EWL was 47.0 ± 4.4 %. Decrease in waist circumference from 120.5 ± 6.8 to 96.0 ± 2.6 cm was significant. Statistically significant decreases were also seen in blood pressure, hemoglobin A1c, total cholesterol, LDL, triglycerides, and in the prevalence of metabolic syndrome (83.3–41.6 % of patients).

Rodriguez et al. randomly assigned patients with type II diabetes and mean BMI of 38.9 kg/m^2 to DJBL or sham endoscopy [31]. After 6 months, hemoglobin A1c fell by 2.4 ± 0.7 % in the DJBL patients, versus a fall of 0.8 ± 0.4 % in the sham arm. The result did not reach significance.

Weight Regain

Bariatric Surgery

Roux-en-Y gastric bypass (RYGB), sleeve gastrectomy, adjustable gastric band, vertical banded gastroplasty, duodenal switch, and biliopancreatic diversion are the most common bariatric surgeries encountered by physicians treating weight regain [32].

Of these, RYGB is the most prevalent [33]. Additionally, RYGB can be revised endoscopically. RYGB typically results in EWL of 56.7–66.5 % over 24 months after surgery; additionally, there is commonly improvement in or resolution of diabetes in 84 %, hypertension in 68 %, obstructive sleep apnea in 81 %, and improvement in hyperlipidemia in 97 % [32–36]. The mechanisms by which RYGB induces weight loss and improvements in comorbidities are not entirely understood, but restriction induced by small gastric pouch size and stoma aperture likely results in reduced caloric intake. Bypass of portions of the gastrointestinal tract likely results in decreased calorie absorption [37].

Patients typically experience rapid weight loss for 12–18 months after RYGB and then reach a stable weight as energy intake and expenditure reach equilibrium [37, 38]. Approximately 20 % of patients fail to achieve >50 % EWL within 1 year of surgery. Additionally, 30 % of patients have had weight regain at 18–24 months postoperatively; weight regain of a mean 18 kg at 2 years has been reported [39, 40]. Another study reported weight regain in 63.6 % within 48 months [41]. The superobese (BMI >50 kg/m^2) fail to achieve BMI <35 kg/m^2 in 60 % of cases [42, 43]. Weight regain can result in recurrence of comorbidities, decreased quality of life, and adverse effects on mental health.

The mechanisms of weight regain after RYGB are likely multifactorial. Long-term outcomes after RYGB are influenced by preoperative BMI and postoperative dietary adherence [44]. Neuroendocrine-metabolic dysregulation may result in a starvation response, increasing appetite and decreasing metabolic rate [45, 46]. Decreased satiety may also be secondary to loss of restriction; larger pouch size and larger diameter of the gastrojejunal anastomosis (GJA) correlate with increased postoperative weight regain [47–50]. Loss of malabsorptive bypass may be an issue if there is a gastrogastric fistula [51].

Treatment of Weight Regain

There are multiple surgical procedures to address weight regain after RYGB, including reconstruction of the gastrojejunal anastomosis, placement of adjustable gastric band over the gastric pouch, revision of the pouch, and distal gastric bypass [50]. However, none is ideal, and surgical revision is relatively uncommon compared to the number of patients with weight regain [52]. Patients requiring surgical revision are older [53]. Complication rates are high, with patients experiencing greater intraoperative blood loss and longer procedure times [53–55]. Mortality rates are over twice as high as that of the primary surgery [52]. The cost may not be covered by insurance [56].

Less invasive endoluminal revisions that reduce gastric pouches' size and GJA diameter may have a more favorable risk profile in this population, as well as lower cost. Many techniques have been studied; of these, sclerotherapy, endoluminal suturing, and tissue plication will be discussed.

Sclerotherapy

Endoscopic injection of sclerosant, such as sodium morrhuate, around the GJA can be used to reduce GJA aperture and tissue compliance. Endoscopic sclerotherapy can be performed under conscious sedation. The procedure begins with injection of a test dose at the rim of the GJA, followed by monitoring for adverse reactions. The sclerosant is then injected into the submucosa around the circumference of the GJA until a bleb forms. Overinjection can result in bleeding; this is preceded by dark red or black discoloration. Aliquots are usually 2 mL, and the total injection is usually 10–25 mL [57]. Intravenous ciprofloxacin is usually given before the procedure and a 5-day course of liquid ciprofloxacin or trimethoprim-sulfamethoxazole should be provided. The patient should be nil per os for a day after the procedure and advance from liquid to regular diet over the following 4 weeks. Repeat sclerotherapy sessions are scheduled every 3–6 months with a goal GJA diameter of 12 mm; most patients require two or three sessions [58]. GJA measurements should be performed at the beginning of the next sclerotherapy session as the diameter immediately after injection is transiently obscured by edema [57]. Injection may be difficult during repeat procedures as tissue sclerosis can make bleb formation challenging.

Endoscopic sclerotherapy has proven effective in reversing weight regain after RYGB. The initial study reported weight loss in 15/20 patients within 8 weeks [58]. A 2007 study of 28 patients reported weight loss of >75 % of regained weight in 64 % of patients after an average 2.3 sessions; however, patients with GJA diameter >15 mm did not appear to have successful outcome [59]. Another 2007 study including 32 patients reported that endoscopic sclerotherapy arrested or reversed weight regain in 91.6 % of patients after 1 year, and a 2008 study of 71 patients reported weight maintenance or loss in 72 % of patients at 1 year [57, 59].

Sodium morrhuate is not commercially available, and alternative sclerosants are being investigated to measure weight loss outcomes in patients with weight regain.

Endoscopic Suturing

Endoluminal suturing has been studied for endoscopic revision of dilated pouches and GJA. The EndoCinch Suturing System, Incisionless Operating Platform, StomaphyX, and OverStitch will be discussed below.

EndoCinch Suturing System

The Bard EndoCinch Suturing System (CR Bard, Murray Hill, NJ) is a suction-based superficial-thickness suturing device. A hollow capsule at the endoscope tip is used to suc-

tion mucosa and trap tissue; a needle is then passed through the tissue. The EndoCinch has been used for transoral outlet reduction (TORe) by placement of interrupted stitches at the anastomotic margin. The rim of the GJA is pretreated with argon plasma coagulation.

TORe using the EndoCinch was first described in 2004 [60]. The first published study included eight patients with average weight regain of 24 kg and average GJA diameter of 25 mm [61]. An average of 2 interrupted stitches were used to reduce stoma diameter to an average of 10 mm. There were no significant adverse events. Six of 8 patients lost an average of 10 kg at 4 months. Of the 3 patients who had repeat TORe, 2 had weight loss of 19 kg and 20 kg after 5 months. Average BMI decreased from 40.5 to 37.7 kg/m².

RESTORe, a randomized double-blinded sham-controlled multicenter trial, resulted in level 1 evidence for effectiveness of TORe [62]. There were 77 patients with GJA diameter >20 mm and mean BMI of 47.6 kg/m² included. GJA was reduced to <10 mm in 89 % of the TORe group. The rate of adverse events was similar to the sham group, and there were no perforations. Mean weight loss in the TORe group was 3.8 % of body weight versus 0.3 % in the sham group ($p = 0.02$) in intent-to-treat analysis. Of the TORe group, 96 % achieved weight loss or stabilization during the 6-month follow-up period.

Incisionless Operating Platform

The Incisionless Operating Platform (USGI Medical, San Clemente, CA) is a multichannel device that can perform full-thickness plication. A 4.9 mm super-slim endoscope inserted through one of the accessory channels provides endoscopic visualization. Two other channels are used for a tissue grasper and a tissue approximator. The grasper is used to pull tissue in, and the tissue approximator is used to drive a needle through the tissue and then plicate the tissue together with tissue anchors [63].

The IOP has been prospectively studied in reduction of dilated gastric pouch and GJA, called the Revision Obesity Surgery Endoscopic (ROSE) procedure. Mullady et al. studied 20 patients with weight regain. Technical success was achieved in 85 %, reducing GJA aperture by 65 % to a mean 16 mm and gastric pouch length by 36 %. Average weight loss at 3 months was 8.8 kg. The second-generation device is able to function in smaller gastric pouches. A study by Ryou et al. in five patients demonstrated weight loss in all patients, with average weight loss of 7.8 kg [64]. A ROSE prospective multicenter registry of 116 patients with dilated GJA and gastric pouch demonstrated technical success in 97 % [65]. GJA aperture was reduced by 50 %, and gastric pouch length by 44 %. There were no procedural complications. Those patients achieving GJA aperture of less than 10 mm had 24 % EWL. Overall, the group lost 32 % of regained weight during 6-month follow-up.

StomaphyX

The StomaphyX device (EndoGastric Solutions, Redmond, WA) can create full-thickness plications using polypropylene H-fasteners. GJA aperture reduction can be performed by circumferentially applying approximately 20 fasteners around the anastomotic margin. A study of 39 patients with BMI of 39.8 kg/m² revealed average procedure time of 35 min and no significant adverse events [66]. Patients had 13.1 % EWL after 3 months and 19.5 % EWL after 1 year. A subsequent study of 64 patients with mean BMI of 39.5 kg/m² reported use of 23 plications and average reduction of GJA diameter from 22 to 9 mm [67]. Procedures took 50 min on average. One patient had bleeding at the plication site, although transfusion was not necessary; there were no other significant adverse events. Average weight loss was 7.6 kg after 5.8 months.

Apollo OverStitch

The OverStitch (Apollo Endosurgery, Austin, TX) is a full-thickness endoscopic suturing system. It uses a catheter-based needle to place interrupted or running stitches under direct endoscopic visualization (Fig. 6). The endoscope does not need to be removed to reload sutures. A helical tissue retractor accessory can also be used through one channel of the double-channel endoscope.

OverStitch has recently been studied for TORe in 25 patients [68]. GJA aperture was reduced from 26.4 to 6 mm on average. No significant adverse events were noted. During the 6-month follow-up period, patients lost 69.5 % of the regained weight. Six-month average weight loss was 11.7 kg, and 1-year weight loss was 10.8 kg.

Superficial-thickness TORe using EndoCinch and full-thickness TORe using OverStitch were directly compared in a matched cohort study by Kumar and Thompson [69]. There were 118 patients, 59 in each group, who were matched sequentially by pre-TORe GJA aperture, BMI, and age. Six-month weight loss was 4.4 ± 0.8 kg in the EndoCinch group versus 10.6 ± 1.8 kg in the OverStitch group (p < 0.01). One-year weight loss was 2.9 ± 1.0 kg in the EndoCinch group versus 8.6 ± 2.5 kg in the OverStitch group (p < 0.01).

The interrupted stitch suturing method used in these studies has since been modified to a full-thickness purse-string technique, with superior early results; studies are ongoing.

Other Technologies

OTSC Clip

The OTSC clip (Ovesco, Tubingen, Germany) is an over-the-endoscope clip with multiple applications, including perfo-

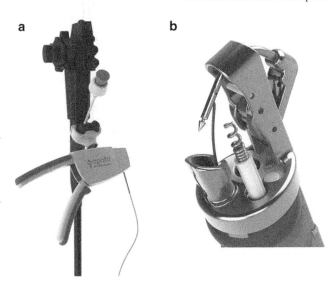

FIG. 6. (**a**) Apollo OverStitch™ device (Apollo Endosurgery, Inc., Austin, TX, with permission). (**b**) Suturing device is placed at the end of a dual-channel endoscope with a catheter-based suture system that is placed through the working channel.

ration and fistula closure. It is a nitinol clip attached to an applicator, which is placed on the endoscope tip. Opposite sides of the GJA can be grasped with endoscopic forceps and pulled into the cap at the tip of the endoscope. Deployment of the clip apposes and secures the tissue. Heylen et al. studied OTSC for reduction of GJA aperture in a study of 94 patients with mean BMI of 32.8 kg/m² [70]. Mean GJA aperture was reduced from 35 to 8 mm. Average procedure time was 35 min, and no major adverse events were reported. After 3 months, BMI had fallen to 29.7 kg/m²; 1 year after the procedure, BMI was 27.4 kg/m².

Olympus T-Tags

T-tags (Olympus, Tokyo, Japan) have been used to reduce GJA aperture [71]. Using a double-channel endoscope, multiple T-tags can be deployed around the anastomotic margin. The T-tag comprises two T-bars, each in a hollow needle. Once the distal tag has been driven through tissue, a proximal tag is advanced over the connecting suture and then secured. The excess suture is cut with an endoscopic loop cutter. A nonsurvival study in pigs demonstrated average GJA aperture reduction of 27 % in a mean time of 61 min [72]

Review Questions and Answers

1. Which of these procedures is supported by level 1 evidence for efficacy?

    A. Sclerotherapy
    B. TORe

C. TOGA

D. TERIS

2. True or false, BIB has been shown to be effective for treatment of NASH:

A. True

B. False

3. The endoscopic bariatric therapy with the largest body of evidence is:

A. BIB

B. TOGA

C. TERIS

References

1. Nguyen NT, Magno CP, Lane KT, et al. Association of hypertension, diabetes, dyslipidemia, and metabolic syndrome with obesity: findings from the National Health and Nutrition Examination Survey, 1999 to 2004. J Am Coll Surg. 2008;207(6):928–34.

2. Cawley J, Meyerhoefer C. The medical care costs of obesity: an instrumental variables approach. J Health Econ. 2012;31:219–30.

3. Buchwald H, Oien DM. Metabolic/bariatric surgery worldwide. Obes Surg. 2009;19:1605–11.

4. Thompson CC, Chand B, Chen YK, et al. Endoscopic Suturing for Transoral Outlet Reduction Increases Weight Loss After Roux-en-Y Gastric Bypass Surgery. Gastroenterology. 2013;145(1):129–37.

5. Fogel R, De Fogel J, Bonilla Y, et al. Clinical experience of transoral suturing for an endoluminal vertical gastroplasty: 1-year follow-up in 64 patients. Gastrointest Endosc. 2008;68:51–8.

6. Fogel R, De Fogel J. Trans-oral vertical gastroplasty as a viable treatment for childhood obesity—a study of 21 adolescents with up to 18 months of follow-up. Gastrointest Endosc. 2009;69(5):AB169–70.

7. Brethauer SA, Chand B, Schauer PR, Thompson CC. Transoral gastric volume reduction as intervention for weight management: 12-month follow-up of TRIM trial. Surg Obes Relat Dis. 2012;8(3):296–303.

8. Deviere J, Ojeda Valdes G, et al. Safety, feasibility and weight loss after transoral gastroplasty: first human multicenter study. Surg Endosc. 2008;22:589–98.

9. Moreno C, Closset J, Dugardeyn S, et al. Transoral gastroplasty is safe, feasible, and induces significant weight loss in morbidly obese patients: results of the second human pilot study. Endoscopy. 2008;40:406–13.

10. Familiari P, Costamagna G, Blero D, et al. Transoral gastroplasty for morbid obesity: a multicenter trial with a 1-year outcome. Gastrointest Endosc. 2011;74(6):1248–58.

11. de Jong K, Mathus-Vliegen EM, Veldhuyzen EA, et al. Short-term safety and efficacy of the trans-oral endoscopic restrictive implant system for the treatment of obesity. Gastrointest Endosc. 2010;72(3):497–504.

12. Evans JT, DeLegge MH. Intragastric balloon therapy in the management of obesity: why the bad wrap? JPEN J Parenter Enteral Nutr. 2011;35:25–31.

13. Imaz I, Martínez-Cervell C, García-Alvarez EE, Sendra-Gutiérrez JM, González-Enríquez J. Safety and effectiveness of the intragastric balloon for obesity. A meta-analysis. Obes Surg. 2008;18(7):841–6.

14. Genco T, Bruni B, Doldi SB, et al. BioEnterics intragastric balloon: The Italian Experience with 2515 patients. Obes Surg. 2005;15(8):1161–4.

15. Forlano R, Ippolito AM, Iacobellis A, et al. Effect of the BioEnterics intragastric balloon on weight, insulin resistance, and liver steatosis in obese patients. Gastrointest Endosc. 2010;71(6):927–33.

16. Tai CM, Lin HY, Yen YC, et al. Effectiveness of intragastric balloon treatment for obese patients: one-year follow-up after balloon removal. Obes Surg. 2013;23(12):2068–74.

17. Lee YM, Low HC, Lim LG, et al. Intragastric balloon significantly improves nonalcoholic fatty liver disease activity score in obese patients with nonalcoholic steatohepatitis: a pilot study. Gastrointest Endosc. 2012;76(4):756–60.

18. Deliopoulou K, Konsta A, Penna S, et al. The impact of weight loss on depression status in obese individuals subjected to intragastric balloon treatment. Obes Surg. 2013;23(5):669–75.

19. Dumonceau JM, François E, Hittelet A, et al. Single vs repeated treatment with the intragastric balloon: a 5-year weight loss study. Obes Surg. 2010;20(6):692–7.

20. Lopez-Nava G, Rubio MA, Prados S, et al. BioEnterics intragastric balloon (BIB). Single ambulatory center Spanish experience with 714 consecutive patients treated with one or two consecutive balloons. Obes Surg. 2011;21(1):5–9.

21. Kotzampassi K, Grosomanidis V, Papakostas P, et al. 500 intragastric balloons: what happens 5 years thereafter? Obes Surg. 2012;22(6):896–903.

22. Zerrweck C, Maunoury V, Caiazzo R, et al. Preoperative weight loss with intragastric balloon decreases the risk of significant adverse outcomes of laparoscopic gastric bypass in super-super obese patients. Obes Surg. 2012;22(5):777–82.

23. Giardiello C, Borrelli A, Silvestri E, et al. Air-filled vs water-filled intragastric balloon: a prospective randomized study. Obes Surg. 2012;22(12):1916–9.

24. Caglar E, Dobrucali A, Bal K. Gastric balloon to treat obesity: filled with air or fluid? Dig Endosc. 2013;25(5):502–7.

25. Marinos G, Eliades C, Muthusamy V, et al. First clinical experience with the TransPyloric shuttle (TPS(r)) device, a non-surgical endoscopic treatment for obesity: results from a 3-month and 6-month study. SAGES. 2013 [abstract].

26. Ponce J, Quebbemann BB, Patterson EJ. Prospective, randomized, multicenter study evaluating safety and efficacy of intragastric dual-balloon in obesity. Surg Obes Relat Dis. 2013;9(2):290–5.

27. Sauer N, Rösch T, Pezold J, et al. A new endoscopically implantable device (SatiSphere) for treatment of obesity-efficacy, safety, and metabolic effects on glucose, insulin, and GLP-1 levels. Obes Surg. 2013;23(11):1727–33.

28. Schouten R, Rijs CS, Bouvy ND, et al. A multicenter, randomized efficacy study of the EndoBarrier gastrointestinal liner for presurgical weight loss prior to bariatric surgery. Ann Surg. 2010;251(2):236–43.

29. Gersin KS, Rothstein RI, Rosenthal RJ, et al. Open-label, sham-controlled trial of an endoscopic duodenojejunal bypass liner for preoperative weight loss in bariatric surgery candidates. Gastrointest Endosc. 2010;71(6):976–82.

30. Tarnoff M, Rodriguez L, Escalona A, et al. Open label, prospective, randomized controlled trial of an endoscopic duodenal-jejunal bypass sleeve versus low calorie diet for pre-operative weight loss in bariatric surgery. Surg Endosc. 2009;23(3):650–6.

31. Escalona A, Yáñez R, Pimentel F, Galvao M, et al. Initial human experience with restrictive duodenal-jejunal bypass liner for treatment of morbid obesity. Surg Obes Relat Dis. 2010;6(2):126–31.

32. Rodriguez L, Reyes E, Fagalde P, et al. Pilot clinical study of an endoscopic, removable duodenal-jejunal bypass liner for the treatment of type 2 diabetes. Diabetes Technol Ther. 2009;11(11):725–32.

33. Pratt GM, Learn CA, Hughes GD, et al. Demographics and outcomes at American Society for Metabolic and Bariatric Surgery Centers of Excellence. Surg Endosc. 2009;23:795–9.

34. Buchwald H, Avidor Y, Braunwald E, et al. Bariatric surgery: A systematic review and meta-analysis. JAMA. 2004;292(14):1724–37.

35. Schauer PR, Burguera B, Ikramuddin S, et al. Effect of laparoscopic Roux-en Y gastric bypass on type 2 diabetes mellitus. Ann Surg. 2003;238:467–85.

36. Maggard MA, Shugarman LR, Suttorp M, et al. Meta-analysis: surgical treatment of obesity. Ann Intern Med. 2005;142:547–59.

37. Elder KA, Wolfe BM. Bariatric surgery: a review of procedures and outcomes. Gastroenterology. 2007;132:2253–71.

38. Mitchell JE, Lancaster KL, Burgard MA, et al. Long-term follow-up of patients' status after gastric bypass. Obes Surg. 2001;11:464–8.

39. Sjostrom L, Lindroos AK, Peltonen M, et al. Lifestyle, diabetes, and cardiovascular risk factors 10 years after bariatric surgery. N Engl J Med. 2004;351:2683–93.

40. Powers PS, Rosemurgy A, Boyd F, et al. Outcome of gastric restriction procedures: weight, psychiatric diagnoses, and satisfaction. Obes Surg. 1997;7:471–7.

41. Hsu LK, Benotti PN, Dwyer J, et al. Nonsurgical factors that influence the outcome of bariatric surgery: a review. Psychosom Med. 1998;60:338–46.

42. Magro DO, Gelonese B, Delfini R, et al. Long-term weight regain after gastric bypass: a 5-year prospective study. Obes Surg. 2008;18(6):648–51.

43. Christou NV, Look D, MacLean LD. Weight gain after short- and long-limb gastric bypass in patients followed for longer than 10 years. Ann Surg. 2006;244(5):734–40.

44. Prachand V, DaVee R, Alverdy J. Duodenal switch provides superior weight loss in the super-obese (BMI > 50 kg/m²) compared with gastric bypass. Ann Surg. 2006;244:611–9.

45. Malone M, Alger-Mayer S. Binge status and quality of life after gastric bypass surgery: a one-year study. Obes Res. 2004;12:473–81.

46. Flier JS. Clinical review 94: what's in a name? In search of leptin's physiologic role. J Clin Endocrinol Metab. 1998;83:1407–13.

47. Ahima RS, Prabakaran D, Mantzoros C, et al. Role of leptin in the neuroendocrine response to fasting. Nature. 1996;382:250–2.

48. Muller MK, Wildi S, Scholz T, et al. Laparoscopic pouch resizing and redo of gastro-jejunal anastomosis for pouch dilatation following gastric bypass. Obes Surg. 2005;15:1089–95.

49. Gagner M, Gentileschi P, de Csepel J, et al. Laparoscopic reoperative bariatric surgery: experience from 27 consecutive patients. Obes Surg. 2002;12:254–60.

50. Dayyeh BK, Lautz DB, Thompson CC. Gastrojejunal stoma diameter predicts weight regain after Roux-en-Y gastric bypass. Clin Gastroenterol Hepatol. 2011;9(3):228–33.

51. Gumbs AA, Pomp A, Gagner M. Revisional bariatric surgery for inadequate weight loss. Obes Surg. 2007;17:1137–45.

52. Carrodeguas L, Szomstein S, Soto F, et al. Management of gastrogastric fistulas after divided Roux-en-Y gastric bypass surgery for morbid obesity: analysis of 1,292 consecutive patients and review of literature. Surg Obes Relat Dis. 2005;1(5):467–74.

53. Behrns K, Smith C, Kelly K, et al. Reoperative bariatric surgery—lessons learned to improve patient selection and results. Ann Surg. 1993;218:646–53.

54. Ryou M, Ryan MB, Thompson CC. Current status of endoluminal bariatric procedures for primary and revision indications. Gastrointest Endosc Clin N Am. 2011;21(2):315–33.

55. Dapri G, Cadiere GB, Himpens J. Laparoscopic conversion of adjustable gastric banding and vertical banded gastroplasty to duodenal switch. Surg Obes Relat Dis. 2009;5:678–83.

56. Coakley BA, Deveney CW, Spight DH, et al. Revisional bariatric surgery for failed restrictive procedures. Surg Obes Relat Dis. 2008;4:581–6.

57. Livingston EH. Hospital costs associated with bariatric procedures in the United States. Am J Surg. 2005;190(5):816–20.

58. Spaulding L, Osler T, Patlak J. Long-term results of sclerotherapy for dilated gastrojejunostomy after gastric bypass. Surg Obes Relat Dis. 2007;3:623–6.

59. Catalano MF, Rudic G, Anderson AJ, et al. Weight gain after bariatric surgery as a result of a large gastric stoma: endotherapy with sodium morrhuate may prevent the need for surgical revision. Gastrointest Endosc. 2007;66:240–5.

60. Loewen M, Barba C. Endoscopic sclerotherapy for dilated gastrojejunostomy of failed gastric bypass. Surg Obes Relat Dis. 2008;4:539–42.

61. Thompson CC, Carr-Locke DL, Saltzman J, et al. Peroral endoscopic repair of staple-line dehiscence in Roux-en-Y gastric bypass: a less invasive approach [abstract]. Gastroenterology. 2004;126 (Suppl 2):A.

62. Thompson CT, Slattery J, Bundga ME, et al. Peroral endoscopic reduction of dilated gastrojejunal anastomosis after Roux-en-Y gastric bypass: a possible new option for patients with weight regain. Surg Endosc. 2006;20:1744–8.

63. Thompson CC, Roslin MS, Bipan C, et al. RESTORE: Randomized Evaluation of Endoscopic Suturing Transorally for Anastomotic Outlet Reduction: A double-blind, sham-controlled multicenter study for treatment of inadequate weight loss or weight regain following Roux-en-Y gastric bypass. Gastroenterology. 2010;138(5, Suppl 1):S-388.

64. Seaman DL, Gostout CJ, de la Mora Levy JG, Knipschield MA. Tissue anchors for transmural gut-wall apposition. Gastrointest Endosc. 2006;64:577–81.

65. Ryou MK, Mullady DK, Lautz DB, Thompson CC. Pilot study evaluating technical feasibility and early outcomes of second-generation endosurgical platform for treatment of weight regain after gastric bypass surgery. Surg Obes Relat Dis. 2009;5(4):450–4.

66. Horgan S, Jacobsen G, Weiss GD, et al. Incisionless revision of post-Roux-en-Y bypass stomal and pouch dilation: multicenter registry results. Surg Obes Relat Dis. 2010;6:290–5.

67. Mikami D, Needleman B, Narula V, et al. Natural orifice surgery: Initial US experience utilizing the StomaphyX device to reduce gastric pouches after Roux-en-Y gastric bypass. Surg Endosc. 2010;24:223–8.

68. Letiman IM, Virk CS, Avgerinos DV, Patel R, Lavarias V, Surick B, Holup JL, Goodman ER, Karpeh Jr MS. Early results of trans-oral endoscopic placation and revision of the gastric pouch and stoma following Roux-en-Y gastric bypass surgery. JSLS. 2010;14:217–20.

69. Jirapinyo P, Slattery J, Ryan MB, et al. Evaluation of an endoscopic suturing device for transoral outlet reduction in patients with weight regain following Roux-en-Y gastric bypass. Endoscopy. 2013;45(7):532–6.

70. Kumar N, Lautz DB, Thompson CC. Comparison of a suction-based superficial suturing device with a full-thickness suturing device for transoral outlet reduction: a matched cohort study [abstract]. Gastrointest Endosc. 2013;77(5):AB203–4.

71. Heylen AM, Jacobs A, Lybeer M, Prosst RL. The OTSC(R)-Clip in revisional endoscopy against weight regain after bariatric gastric bypass surgery. Obes Surg. 2011;21(10):1629–33.

72. Herron DM, Birkett DH, Thompson CC, et al. Gastric bypass pouch and stoma reduction using a transoral endoscopic anchor placement system: A feasibility study. Surg Endosc. 2008;22:1093–9.

73. Tang SJ, Olukoga CO, Provost DA, et al. Gastrojejunal stomal reduction with the T-tag device in porcine models (with videos). Gastrointest Endosc. 2008;68:132–8.

39

Innovative Metabolic Operations

Ricardo Cohen, Pedro Paulo Caravatto, and Tarissa Petry

Abbreviations

BMI	Body mass index
DJB	Duodenal-jejunal bypass
DJBL	Duodenal-jejunal bypass liner
DPP4	Dipeptidyl-peptidase-4
FPG	Fasting plasma glucose
GLP-1	Glucagon-like peptide-1
IT	Ileal transposition
LDL cholesterol	Low-density-lipoprotein cholesterol
T2DM	Type 2 diabetes mellitus

Introduction

The latest epidemiological data regarding type 2 diabetes (T2DM) show that we are in the midst of an epidemic. Approximately 26 million Americans were diabetic in 2011 (11.3 % of the population), and by 2025, almost 30 % of the US population will have T2DM. Furthermore, T2DM is the leading cause of kidney failure, nontraumatic lower limb amputations, coronary heart disease, stroke, and visual impairments among adults in the USA [1].

Several clinical trials (the Diabetes Control and Complications Trial [DCCT], the United Kingdom Prospective Diabetes Study [UKPDS], and others) [2] established that glycemic control is the most important step in the control and prevention of microvascular problems, while broader management focusing on lipids, blood pressure, and a glycemic approach showed better performance in patients with macrovascular disease [3].

New types of drugs were recently made available to diabetologists, such as glucagon-like peptide-1 (GLP-1) analogues and dipeptidyl-peptidase-4 (DPP4) inhibitors. Nonetheless, the average glucose control in US patients with diabetes remains suboptimal [4, 5]. Although the 10-year mortality rate has decreased, it is still too high [6]. In addition, the overall risk of death among people with diabetes is at least double that of their peers without diabetes [7]. Therefore, strategies must be developed to reduce the development of this devastating disease so that chronic complications may be minimized.

Medications and lifestyle interventions in patients with diabetes may delay cardiovascular events and other major complications but require patient compliance, frequent medical consultation, and lifelong medications that are not exempt from major side effects. However, even with such major advances, T2DM control remains elusive [4], with less than 20 % of the North American population being able to achieve the three end points of metabolic control (glycemic, blood pressure, and lipid control).

On the other hand, gastrointestinal surgery has been shown to be effective in the treatment and even prevention of T2DM, reducing the mortality rate in the long term when compared with clinical treatment in morbidly obese patients in major longitudinal prospective studies [8].

Metabolic surgery involves any intervention that alters the food passage through the gastrointestinal tract, resulting in improved metabolic control in patients with T2DM. Such a result does not solely depend on weight loss. In some cases, the effects can be observed some days or weeks after the surgical procedure, long before considerable weight loss, precluding a direct antidiabetic effect. The term "bariatric" is gradually being replaced by "metabolic" because the operations previously recommended for the treatment of morbidly obese individuals (defined by a BMI of >40 kg/m^2 or >35 kg/m^2 when associated with comorbidities that are difficult to control) have demonstrated excellent results in terms of diabetes remission, even in patients with a BMI of <35 kg/m^2 based at least initially on several weight loss-independent mechanisms [9–16].

S.A. Brethauer et al. (eds.), *Minimally Invasive Bariatric Surgery*,
DOI 10.1007/978-1-4939-1637-5_39, © Springer Science+Business Media New York 2015

Surgery for T2DM and Metabolic Syndrome

Innumerous data obtained from observational, nonrandomized, and randomized trials have demonstrated the safety and efficacy of "traditional" gastrointestinal operations (Roux-en-Y gastric bypass, sleeve gastrectomy, biliopancreatic diversion, and adjustable gastric banding) in treating T2DM in both morbidly obese and less obese patients [17–25]. However, the medical community is still skeptical when it comes to accepting surgery as a treatment modality for T2DM, particularly in less obese individuals. Efforts have been concentrated on treating sicker patients with uncontrolled disease, regardless of BMI, because this parameter alone should not be the only criterion with which to determine adequate therapy, either medical or surgical. BMI alone discriminates patients by gender, age, sex, and fitness status but does not predict body composition, outcomes, or cardiovascular risk.

Why Innovative Procedures?

Based on the metabolic results following "traditional" operations and after gaining an understanding that gastrointestinal interventions may have a direct antidiabetic effect not initially related to weight loss, efforts were directed toward operations that reroute the food through the gastrointestinal tract. These operations led to no or mild weight loss and followed some anatomical and pathophysiological patterns to achieve metabolic control in a population that in theory does not need massive weight loss. Procedures that preserve the pylorus were designed [26–28], thus decreasing gastric emptying and hypothetically leading to an easier restoration of the impaired first-phase insulin secretion. These procedures include ileal transposition and its variations, duodenal-jejunal bypass with or without sleeve gastrectomy, and others discussed below [29].

Ileal Transposition and Its Variants

Ileal transposition (IT) was first described in 1926 [30], and its application to obesity treatment began several decades later [31–33]. Several IT techniques were developed: IT alone, IT with sleeve gastrectomy, and IT with sleeve gastrectomy and duodenal exclusion (IT with diverted sleeve gastrectomy) [34, 35] (Figs. 1 and 2).

The rationale for the mechanisms of action behind IT is the introduction of a segment of terminal ileum into the proximal jejunum, allowing premature exposure of nutrients to the interposed ileum. This results in stimulation of GLP-1 and peptide tyrosine-tyrosine–producing L cells, in theory without disruption of intestinal transit or absorption [36–38].

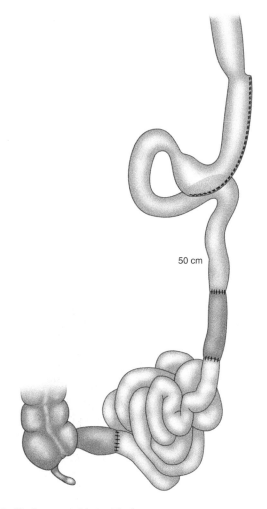

50 cm

Fig. 1. Ileal transposition with sleeve gastrectomy.

The increased level of anorectic peptides and the delay in gastric emptying reduce hunger and provide a longer sensation of satiety, both of which contribute to weight loss. The effects associated with the increased levels of GLP-1 induced by procedures involving intestinal derivation could be the basis of metabolic surgery because this hormone inhibits acid secretion by the stomach, increases the sensation of satiety, and reduces appetite and gastric motility [39–43]. In addition, augmentation of GLP-1 leads to increased secretion of insulin and postprandial suppression of glucagon secretion together with preservation, and possible hypertrophy, of the β-cell mass. Moreover, it is believed that GLP-1 is involved in the differentiation of progenitor duct cells into β-cells, thus limiting apoptosis of these cells [44–46].

In 2006, De Paula et al. [47] reported the first description of laparoscopic IT plus sleeve gastrectomy in 19 severely obese patients with comorbidities. The surgical technique involved transposing a 100-cm-long ileal segment to the jejunum, approximately 50 cm from the ligament of Treitz. The addition of sleeve gastrectomy provided additional restriction, leading to less caloric intake, faster gastric

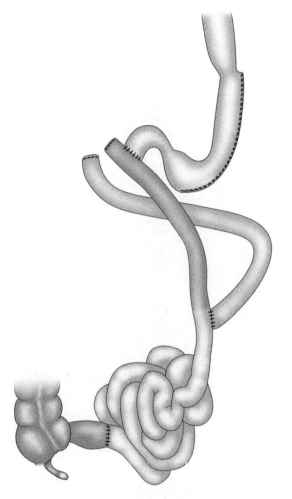

FIG. 2. Ileal transposition with sleeve gastrectomy and duodenal exclusion.

emptying, reduced undesired side effects such as persistent nausea, and decreased serum levels of ghrelin. They reported a short follow-up (11.6 months) with two major complications, good weight loss (38.4 % of body weight), and resolution (without a clear definition) in five of five patients with T2DM.

Aiming to further improve glycemic control, the same authors added a duodenal exclusion by transecting the duodenum and closing it distally about 1 to 2 cm below the pylorus and transposing an ileal segment. This created a pyloroileostomy to reroute nutrient flow and allow for an early delivery of nutrients to the ileum (hindgut and foregut mechanisms combined) [48, 49].

Evidence of superior outcomes of IT + sleeve gastrectomy + duodenal exclusion was reported; nearly 95 % of patients achieved adequate glycemic control (HbA1c < 7 %) with no antidiabetic medications [50].

More recently, the same author published the outcomes of 202 diabetic patients submitted to IT + sleeve gastrectomy vs. IT + sleeve gastrectomy + duodenal exclusion. The mean

HbA1c decreased from 9.7 to 6.2 %, and 90 % of patients showed an HbA1c of <7 % at 39 months, an impressive outcome. There was a trend toward lower HbA1c in the IT + sleeve gastrectomy + duodenal exclusion group, showing that foregut exclusion plays an important role in T2DM control because duodenal exclusion was the only variable between the two studied groups [51].

A few other authors worldwide have reported favorable outcomes following IT and its variants, as described in Table 1 [43, 52–55].

It seems that IT is effective for T2DM, but it is a very complex procedure. Significant improvement in metabolic diseases has been reported; however, the complication rates are higher than those of other procedures (major complications occur in approximately 10 % of cases). Moreover, some complications are specific to this type of procedure, such as ischemia of the transposed ileum and higher incidences of intestinal obstruction due to internal hernias. Such complications lead to a higher mortality rate compared with standard bariatric procedures (3.6 % vs. 0.15 %). More studies involving independent analysis of the two technique variables and longer follow-up are needed.

Duodenal-Jejunal Bypass and Its Variant (Figs. 3 and 4)

Rubino et al. [56] demonstrated that by excluding the duodenum and proximal jejunum without restriction of gastric volume, good glycemic control was achieved in nonobese diabetic rats in the absence of weight loss or decreased caloric intake.

One of the possible mechanisms that underlie this glucose-lowering effect is jejunal nutrient sensing. Breen et al. [57] reported that intrajejunal nutrient administration lowered endogenous glucose production in normal and streptozotocin-induced uncontrolled diabetic rats through a gut-brain-liver network without changes in insulin concentration. Moreover, when these rats were submitted to duodenal-jejunal bypass (DJB), higher concentrations of nutrients were delivered to the jejunum, causing a more profound reduction in glucose concentrations 2 days after surgery, independently of changes in plasma insulin concentrations, food intake, and body weight.

Another potential mechanism reported by Salinari et al. [58] is the action of jejunal hormones inducing insulin resistance. In this study, the authors were able to isolate jejunal conditioned medium proteins from insulin-resistant diabetic animals and insulin-resistant humans. The authors found that these proteins impaired insulin signaling, reducing glucose uptake by skeletal muscle cell cultures. A similar effect was obtained with human serum from insulin-resistant subjects, suggesting that there are circulating duodenal factors that induce insulin resistance by impairing insulin signaling.

TABLE 1. Outcomes of ileal transposition and its variants

	Type of procedure	Number of patients	Mean preop BMI (kg/m^2)	TBWL (%)	T2DM remission (%)	Mean follow-up (months)
Tinoco [43]	SGIT	30	30.8	14	80[a]	18
Kota [52]	DSGIT	17	29.2	20	70[a]	9.7
Kota [53]	SGIT	43	33.2	25	47[a]	20.2
De Paula [54]	SGIT+DSGIT	38	28.9	25	90.9[b]	25.6
De Paula [55]	SGIT	120	43.4	BMI to 25.7	84.2[a]	38.4

Mean preop BMI mean preoperative body mass index (kg/m^2), *TBWL* total body weight loss, *T2DM remission* type 2 diabetes mellitus remission ([a]HbA1c<6.5 %, [b]HbA1c<7 %), *SGIT* sleeve gastrectomy+ileal transposition, *DSGIT* diverted sleeve gastrectomy+ileal transposition

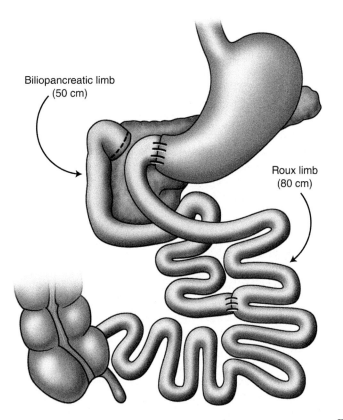

FIG. 3. "Classic" duodenal-jejunal bypass.

Biliopancreatic limb
(50 cm)

Roux limb
(80 cm)

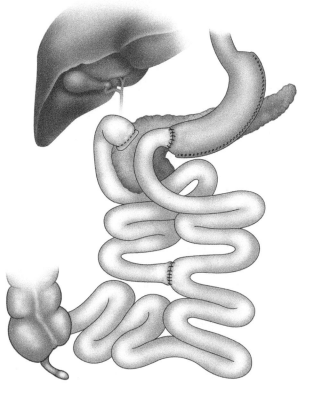

FIG. 4. Duodenal-jejunal bypass with sleeve gastrectomy.

The implication of such findings is that by rerouting the food passage (e.g., after DJB), endocrine factors present in the duodenum and proximal jejunum that induce insulin resistance may halt, causing an immediate and long-standing metabolic response.

We reported the first two patients to undergo DJB with no gastric manipulation ("classic DJB") [59]. The surgical technique involved Roux-en-Y duodenojejunostomy with a 50-cm biliopancreatic limb and 80-cm Roux limb. Both patients showed a decrease in HbA1c with no correlation to weight variation.

Later, we published our experience with 36 non-morbidly obese diabetic patients who underwent classic DJB [60]. Diabetes remission (HbA1c<7 % and fasting plasma glucose FPG<126 mg/dL) was achieved in 40 % of patients at 1 year

of follow-up. Remission was not related to weight change in this study. We further assessed glucose and β-cell response to an oral glucose load before and at 6, 9, and 12 months after surgery [61] and compared the results with subjects with normal glucose tolerance. DJB improved β-cell function and glycemic control in overweight and class I obese subjects with T2DM. It did not normalize β-cell function when compared with the subjects with normal glucose tolerance but increased it two- to threefold compared with baseline.

Geloneze et al. [62] published their results on DJB in 12 overweight diabetic patients. Remission (HbA1c<6.5 %, no medications) occurred in two (16.7 %) patients. This result was due to the selection of patients with a long history of diabetes and/or established macrovascular disease, slightly worsening their results regarding T2DM control. In their

TABLE 2. Outcomes of duodenal-jejunal bypass and its variants

	Type of procedure	Number of patients	Mean preop BMI (kg/m²)	TBWL (%)	T2DM remission (%)	Mean follow-up (months)
Cohen [60]	DJB	36	28.4	4.5	40	12
Geloneze [62]	DJB	12	26.1	BMI to 25.6	16.7	6
Ramos [66]	DJB	20	27.1	7.8	90	6
Kasama [67]	DJB+SG	21	41	34.2	92.9	18
Praveen Raj [68]	DJB+SG	38	42.3	BMI to 29.4	92.3	17

Mean preop BMI mean preoperative body mass index (kg/m²), *TBWL* total body weight loss, *T2DM remission* type 2 diabetes mellitus remission (HbA1c < 7 %, with or without medication), *DJB* duodenal-jejunal bypass, *DJB+SG* duodenal-jejunal bypass + sleeve gastrectomy

study, although all patients were undergoing insulin therapy before surgery, 10 (83 %) patients began taking only oral medications 24 weeks after surgery and experienced a significant decrease in HbA1c levels (8.78 to 7.84 %).

Seeking better outcomes and attempting to reproduce the results found in class 1 or morbidly obese patients, we moved forward with some technical and pathophysiological modifications as follows. We conducted our second protocol and performed a "sleeved duodenal exclusion" or "short duodenal switch" by adding sleeve gastrectomy with a 50/60-F bougie in 47 patients. The primary end points were fasting and postprandial glycemic control, and the secondary end points were lipid and hypertension control and carotid intima-media thickness, an important surrogate marker for atherosclerosis progression. In addition, based on our own studies on better metabolic/diabetes outcomes with longer limb lengths in the morbidly obese population [63], we have increased the biliary limb to 100 cm and the alimentary limb to 150 cm. We believe that resecting the gastric fundus longitudinally, thus removing part of the major ghrelin production site, may lead to slower gastric emptying, decreasing the glucose load to the intestine. Preserving the pylorus may be key in decreasing the glycemic peaks after food ingestion, leading to an improved first-phase insulin response and better glycemic outcomes. Ghrelin has the capability to decrease pancreatic insulin secretion through direct and counter-regulatory mechanisms [64, 65]. Thus, removing the main ghrelin production site would allow for better control of diabetes. With an average follow-up of 1 year, we found that adding sleeve gastrectomy and increasing the limb lengths does not add any excessive weight loss to this leaner group (total body weight loss of 6 %). In addition, so far we have seen diabetes resolution in approximately 71 % of patients, and 100 % if we include patients from remission to improvement (unpublished data). As secondary end points, we achieved control of hypertension in 67 % of patients at 12 months (≤130/80 mmHg, no or minimal medications), normalization of triglycerides in 77 % of patients, and normalization of low-density-lipoprotein (LDL) cholesterol in 81 % of patients. The carotid intima-media thickness was significantly reduced from baseline in 12 months.

Several other authors have reported their experience with DJB, as described in Table 2 [60, 62, 66–68].

DJB Liner

Finally, a new tool for T2DM control was introduced. The DJB liner (DJBL) is an endoscopically placed device that prevents contact between partially digested nutrients and the proximal intestine, mimicking the exclusion of the proximal bowel, which is a component of several effective metabolic surgeries [69]. Escalona et al. [70] implanted the DJBL in 39 morbidly obese patients, and after 12 months, all achieved good loss of excess body weight (47.0±4.4 %). The patients also showed significant improvements in waist circumference, blood pressure, total and LDL cholesterol, triglycerides, and fasting glucose.

The only report in the literature regarding low-BMI T2DM was recently published by Cohen et al. [71]. Sixteen of 20 subjects implanted with the DJBL completed the 1-year study (mean BMI of 30 kg/m²). Ten of 16 subjects (62.5 %) who completed the study demonstrated HbA1c levels of <7 % at week 52, and statistically significant lipid control was achieved (LDL and triglycerides). No significant correlations between changes in body weight and changes in FPG or HbA1c were observed. Based on the results of that study, the DJBL appears to reproduce some aspects of metabolic surgery in terms of its ability to improve HbA1c, FPG, and lipid parameters without a direct relation to weight modification. Interestingly, after some mathematical modeling of data extracted from the oral test after a mixed meal challenge glucose excursions, C-peptide deconvolution, and insulin curves, we found almost immediate, weight loss-independent improved insulin sensitivity after the placement of the DJBL. Moreover, this effect was maintained throughout the year that the device was kept in place. No improvement in insulin secretion was seen. This finding supports the animal studies of Breen and Jiao [57, 72]. The DJBL seems to be an effective tool for metabolic control, allowing some potential associations with GLP-1 analogues and DPP4 inhibitors because the device itself possibly does not change insulin secretion. It is an outpatient-based endoscopic procedure that is associated with virtually no major complications, but the main drawback is that its design is only safe for 1 year of implantation. It may be a good screening tool for the effectiveness of duodenal exclusion before a surgical procedure or an excellent way to quickly improve glycemic and metabolic control in individuals with glucotoxicity and lipotoxicity who may need prompt, effective, and safe intervention.

Sleeve Gastrectomy with Transit Bipartition

Laparoscopic sleeve gastrectomy with transit bipartition was proposed by Santoro et al. [73] in an observational study of 1,020 morbidly obese patients. The surgical procedure involves gastroileal anastomosis added to sleeve gastrectomy, without exclusion of the duodenum and proximal jejunum. The mean BMI was 42.2 kg/m^2, and excess BMI loss was 91 % and 74 % in the first and fifth postoperative years, respectively. T2DM was diagnosed in 32.6 % of patients, and 86 % went into complete remission (HbA1c < 6.5 % without medication).

Although the authors emphasize the enterohormonal pathways of metabolic surgery and the mechanisms involved in metabolic syndrome amelioration, this paper was not a diabetes treatment study. Rather, it was a study on the treatment of morbid obesity (BMI of 33–72 kg/m^2) and the improvement observed in glycemic control and other comorbidities which was the result of diminished food intake and weight loss. Furthermore, the follow-up period was relatively short, and a high proportion of patients were lost to follow-up. Allowing two routes for food passage (ileal and duodenal) associated with sleeve gastrectomy makes the exact rationale behind this proposed operation unclear.

Final Considerations: Is Metabolic Surgery Ready for Prime Time?

Every new T2DM treatment must be safe and effective. It must not only correct hyperglycemia but also prevent or mitigate the complications of this chronic disease. The continuing morbidity and mortality in individuals with T2DM diabetes and the lack of control even with new medications are a sign that the best management in terms of maximizing metabolic control remains elusive. Given this scenario, the option of metabolic surgery must be considered in appropriately selected individuals.

A growing number of metabolic interventions are being performed every year worldwide, and they are expected to be part of the algorithm for diabetes therapy in combination with changes in lifestyle and drug therapy. However, we still need well-designed, long-term clinical trials addressing issues such as the proper time for surgery, best selection criteria, and optimal procedure [74].

Some accomplishments have been made, such as at the Diabetes Surgery Summit held in Rome in 2007 [75], where surgery was recognized as a beneficial tool for select patients with diabetes and bariatric surgery was mentioned in T2DM treatment guidelines for the first time [76]. More recently, the 2011 IDF statement is a landmark in the future role of metabolic surgery as an alternative therapy in patients with a BMI of 30 to 35 kg/m^2 and uncontrolled, higher-cardiovascular-risk T2DM [77].

In the context of an uncontrolled epidemic, gastrointestinal interventions for metabolic control are here to stay pending better definition of their place in the T2DM treatment algorithm. Whereas bariatric surgery was conceived as a mere weight loss intervention, the results of several studies mentioned in this chapter demonstrate that gastrointestinal surgery can also control and prevent T2DM, thereby reducing the incidence of cardiovascular disease and death. Accordingly, metabolic surgery is a more appropriate physiological approach to treat disease rather than behavioral issues [16].

References

1. Lebovitz HE. Science, clinical outcomes and the popularization of diabetes surgery. Curr Opin Endocrinol Diabetes Obes. 2012; 19(5):359–66.
2. Murray P, Chune GW, Raghavan VA. Legacy effects from DCCT and UKPDS: what they mean and implications for future diabetes trials. Curr Atheroscler Rep. 2010;12(6):432–9.
3. Gaede P, Lund-Andersen H, Parving H-H, Pedersen O. Effect of a multifactorial intervention on mortality in type 2 diabetes. N Engl J Med. 2008;358(6):580–91.
4. Stark Casagrande S, Fradkin JE, Saydah SH, Rust KF, Cowie CC. The prevalence of meeting A1C, blood pressure, and LDL goals among people with diabetes, 1988-2010. Diabetes Care. 2013;36(8):2271–9.
5. Grant RW, Buse JB, Meigs JB. University Health System Consortium (UHC) Diabetes Benchmarking Project Team. Quality of diabetes care in U.S. academic medical centers: low rates of medical regimen change. Diabetes Care. 2005;28(2):337–442.
6. Gregg EWE, Cheng YJY, Saydah SS, Cowie CC, Garfield SS, Geiss LL, et al. Trends in death rates among U.S. Adults with and without diabetes between 1997 and 2006: findings from the national health interview survey. Diabetes Care. 2013;35(6):1252–7.
7. Arterburn DE, OÇonnnor PJ. A look ahead at the future of diabetes prevention and treatment. JAMA. 2012;308:2517–1519.
8. Carlsson LMS, Peltonen M, Ahlin S, Anveden Å, Bouchard C, Carlsson B, et al. Bariatric surgery and prevention of type 2 diabetes in swedish obese subjects. N Engl J Med. 2012;367(8): 695–704.
9. Shah SS, Todkar JS, Shah PS, Cummings DE. Diabetes remission and reduced cardiovascular risk after gastric bypass in Asian Indians with body mass index. Surg Obes Relat Dis. 2010; 6(4):332–8.
10. Cohen RV, Rubino F, Schiavon C, Cummings DE. Diabetes remission without weight loss after duodenal bypass surgery. SOARD. 2011;8(5):e66–8.

11. Cohen RV, Schiavon CA, Pinheiro Filho JC, Correa JLL. Laparoscopic bariatric surgery: new technologies, trends and perspectives. Rev Hosp Clin Fac Med Sao Paulo. 2003;58(5):1–8.

12. Geloneze B, Geloneze SR, Chaim E, Hirsch FF, Felici AC, Lambert G, et al. Metabolic surgery for non-obese type 2 diabetes: incretins, adipocytokines, and insulin secretion/resistance changes in a 1-year interventional clinical controlled study. Ann Surg. 2012;256(1):72–8.

13. DePaula AL, Macedo ALV, Rassi N, Machado CA, Schraibman V, Silva LQ, et al. Laparoscopic treatment of type 2 diabetes mellitus for patients with a body mass index less than 35. Surg Endosc. 2007;22(3):706–16.

14. Cummings DE, Flum DR. Gastrointestinal surgery as a treatment for diabetes. JAMA. 2008;299(3):341–3.

15. Rubino F. Is type 2 diabetes an operable intestinal disease? A provocative yet reasonable hypothesis. Diabetes Care. 2008;31 Suppl 2:S290–6.

16. Rubino F, Cummings DE. Surgery: the coming of age of metabolic surgery. Nat Rev Endocrinol. 2012;8(12):702–4.

17. Sjöström L, Lindroos A-K, Peltonen M, Torgerson J, Bouchard C, Carlsson B, et al. Lifestyle, diabetes, and cardiovascular risk factors 10 years after bariatric surgery. N Engl J Med. 2004;351(26): 2683–93.

18. Sjöström L, Narbro K, Sjöström CD, Karason K, Larsson B, Wedel H, et al. Effects of bariatric surgery on mortality in Swedish obese subjects. N Engl J Med. 2007;357(8):741–52.

19. Schauer PR, Burguera B, Ikramuddin S, Cottam D, Gourash W, Hamad G, et al. Effect of laparoscopic Roux-en Y gastric bypass on type 2 diabetes mellitus. Ann Surg. 2003;238(4):467–84. discussion 84–5.

20. Pories WJ, Swanson MS, MacDonald KG, Long SB, Morris PG, Brown BM, et al. Who would have thought it? An operation proves to be the most effective therapy for adult-onset diabetes mellitus. Ann Surg. 1995;222(3):339–50. discussion 350–2.

21. Schauer PR, Kashyap SR, Wolski K, Brethauer SA, Kirwan JP, Pothier CE, et al. Bariatric surgery versus intensive medical therapy in obese patients with diabetes. N Engl J Med. 2012;366(17): 1567–76.

22. Mingrone G, Panunzi S, De Gaetano A, Guidone C, Iaconelli A, Leccesi L, et al. Bariatric surgery versus conventional medical therapy for type 2 diabetes. N Engl J Med. 2012;366(17):1577–85.

23. Cohen RV, Pinheiro JC, Schiavon CA, Salles JE, Wajchenberg BL, Cummings DE. Effects of gastric bypass surgery in patients with type 2 diabetes and only mild obesity. Diabetes Care. 2012;35(7): 1420–8.

24. Gill RS, Birch DW, Shi X, Sharma AM, Karmali S. Sleeve gastrectomy and type 2 diabetes mellitus: a systematic review. SOARD. 2011;6(6):707–13.

25. Dixon JB, O'Brien PE, Playfair J, Chapman L, Schachter LM, Skinner S, et al. Adjustable gastric banding and conventional therapy for type 2 diabetes: a randomized controlled trial. JAMA. 2008;299(3):316–23.

26. Bagger JI, Knop FK, Lund A, Vestergaard H, Holst JJ, Vilsboll T. Impaired regulation of the incretin effect in patients with type 2 diabetes. J Clin Endocrinol Metab. 2011;96(3):737–45.

27. Dirksen C, Hansen DL, Madsbad S, Hvolris LE, Naver LS, Holst JJ, et al. Postprandial diabetic glucose tolerance is normalized by gastric bypass feeding as opposed to gastric feeding and is associated with exaggerated GLP-1 secretion: a case report. Diabetes Care. 2010;33(2):375–7.

28. Pilichiewicz AN, Chaikomin R, Brennan IM, Wishart JM, Rayner CK, Jones KL, et al. Load-dependent effects of duodenal glucose on glycemia, gastrointestinal hormones, antropyloroduodenal motility, and energy intake in healthy men. Am J Physiol Endocrinol Metab. 2007;293(3):E743–53.

29. Halperin F, Goldfine AB. Metabolic surgery for type 2 diabetes: efficacy and risks. Curr Opin Endocrinol Diabetes Obes. 2013; 20(2):98–105.

30. Spies JW, Johnson CE, Wilson CS. Reconstruction of the ureter by means of bladder flaps. Exp Biol Med. 1933;30(4):425–6.

31. Koopmans HS, Sclafani A. Control of body weight by lower gut signals. Int J Obes (Lond). 1981;5(5):491–5.

32. Koopmans HS, Sclafani A, Fichtner C, Aravich PF. The effects of ileal transposition on food intake and body weight loss in VMH-obese rats. Am J Clin Nutr. 1982;35(2):284–93.

33. Sclafani A, Koopmans HS, Vasselli JR, Reichman M. Effects of intestinal bypass surgery on appetite, food intake, and body weight in obese and lean rats. Am J Physiol. 1978;234(4):E389–98.

34. De Paula AL, Stival AR, Macedo A, Ribamar J, Mancini M, Halpern A, et al. Prospective randomized controlled trial comparing 2 versions of laparoscopic ileal interposition associated with sleeve gastrectomy for patients with type 2 diabetes with BMI 21–34 kg/m2. SOARD. 2011;6(3):296–304.

35. DePaula AL, Macedo ALV, Schraibman V, Mota BR, Vencio S. Hormonal evaluation following laparoscopic treatment of type 2 diabetes mellitus patients with BMI 20–34. Surg Endosc. 2008; 23(8):1724–32.

36. Mason EE. Ileal transposition and enteroglucagon/GLP-1 in obesity (and diabetic?) surgery. Obes Surg. 2003;9(3):223–8.

37. Strader AD. Ileal transposition provides insight into the effectiveness of gastric bypass surgery. Physiol Behav. 2006;88(3):277–82.

38. Strader AD. Weight loss through ileal transposition is accompanied by increased ileal hormone secretion and synthesis in rats. Am J Physiol Endocrinol Metab. 2005;288(2):E447–53.

39. Flint A, Raben A, Astrup A, Holst JJ. Glucagon-like peptide 1 promotes satiety and suppresses energy intake in humans. J Clin Invest. 1998;101:515–20.

40. Scrocchi LA, Brown TJ, MaClusky N, Brubaker PL. Glucose intolerance but normal satiety in mice with a null mutation in the glucagon-like peptide 1 receptor gene. Nat Med. 1996;2(11): 1254–8.

41. Turton MD, O'shea D, Gunn I, Beak SA, Edwards C. A role for glucagon-like peptide-1 in the central regulation of feeding. Nature. 1996;379(6560):69–72.

42. Yeğen BÇ, Bozkurt A, Coşkun T. Glucagon-like peptide-1 inhibits gastric emptying via vagal afferent-mediated central mechanisms. Am J Physiol. 1997;273(4 Pt 1):G92–7.

43. Tinoco A, El-Kadre L, Aquiar L, Tinoco R, Savassi-Rocha P. Short-term and mid-term control of type 2 diabetes mellitus by laparoscopic sleeve gastrectomy with ileal interposition. World J Surg. 2011;35(10):2238–44.

44. Vilsboll T, Holst JJ. Incretins, insulin secretion and Type 2 diabetes mellitus. Diabetologia. 2004;47(3):357–66.

45. Baggio LL, Drucker DJ. Biology of incretins: GLP-1 and GIP. Gastroenterology. 2007;132(6):2131–57.

46. Ahrén B, Holst JJ, Mari A. Characterization of GLP-1 effects on beta-cell function after meal ingestion in humans. Diabetes Care. 2003;26(10):2860–4.

47. de Paula AL, Macedo ALV, Prudente AS, Queiroz L, Schraibman V, Pinus J. Laparoscopic sleeve gastrectomy with ileal interposition ("neuroendocrine brake")—pilot study of a new operation. SOARD. 2006;2(4):464–7.

48. Donglei Z, Liesheng L, Xun J, Chenzhu Z, Weixing D. Effects and mechanism of duodenal-jejunal bypass and sleeve gastrectomy on GLUT2 and glucokinase in diabetic Goto-Kakizaki rats. Eur J Med Res. 2012;17:15.

49. Stefater MA, Wilson-Perez HE, Chambers AP, Sandoval DA, Seeley RJ. All bariatric surgeries are not created equal: insights from mechanistic comparisons. Endocr Rev. 2012;33(4):595–622.

50. DePaula AL, Macedo ALV, Rassi N, Vencio S, Machado CA, Mota BR, et al. Laparoscopic treatment of metabolic syndrome in patients with type 2 diabetes mellitus. Surg Endosc. 2008;22(12):2670–8.

51. DePaula AL, Stival AR, DePaula CCL, Halpern A, Vencio S. Surgical treatment of type 2 diabetes in patients with BMI below 35: mid-term outcomes of the laparoscopic ileal interposition associated with a sleeve gastrectomy in 202 consecutive cases. J Gastrointest Surg. 2012;16(5):967–76.

52. Kota SK, Ugale S, Gupta N, Naik V, Kumar KVSH, Modi KD. Ileal interposition with sleeve gastrectomy for treatment of type 2 diabetes mellitus. Indian J Endocrinol Metab. 2012;16(4):589–98.

53. Kota SK, Ugale S, Gupta N, Modi KD. Laparoscopic ileal interposition with diverted sleeve gastrectomy for treatment of type 2 diabetes. Diabetes Metab Syndr. 2012;6(3):125–31.

54. DePaula AL, Stival AR, Halpern A, Vencio S. Surgical treatment of morbid obesity: mid-term outcomes of the laparoscopic ileal interposition associated to a sleeve gastrectomy in 120 patients. Obes Surg. 2010;21(5):668–75.

55. Paula AL, Stival AR, Halpern A, DePaula CCL, Mari A, Muscelli E, et al. Improvement in insulin sensitivity and B-cell function following ileal interposition with sleeve gastrectomy in type 2 diabetic patients: potential mechanisms. J Gastrointest Surg. 2011;15(8):1344–53.

56. Rubino F, Marescaux J. Effect of duodenal–jejunal exclusion in a non-obese animal model of type 2 diabetes: a new perspective for an old disease. Ann Surg. 2004;239(1):1–11.

57. Breen DM, Rasmussen BA, Kokorovic A, Wang R, Cheung GWC, Lam TKT. Jejunal nutrient sensing is required for duodenal-jejunal bypass surgery to rapidly lower glucose concentrations in uncontrolled diabetes. Nat Med. 2012;18(6):950–5.

58. Salinari S, Debard C, Bertuzzi A, Durand C, Zimmet P, Vidal H, et al. Jejunal proteins secreted by db/db mice or insulin-resistant humans impair the insulin signaling and determine insulin resistance. PLoS One. 2013;8(2):e56258.

59. Cohen RV, Schiavon CA, Pinheiro JS, Correa JL, Rubino F. Duodenal-jejunal bypass for the treatment of type 2 diabetes in patients with body mass index of 22-34 kg/m^2: a report of 2 cases. SOARD. 2007;3(2):195–7.

60. Cohen R, Caravatto PP, Correa JL, Noujaim P, Petry TZ, Salles JE, et al. Glycemic control after stomach-sparing duodenal-jejunal bypass surgery in diabetic patients with low body mass index. SOARD. 2012;8(4):375–80.

61. Klein S, Fabbrini E, Patterson BW, Polonsky KS, Schiavon CA, Correa JL, et al. Moderate effect of duodenal-jejunal bypass surgery on glucose homeostasis in patients with type 2 diabetes. Obesity (Silver Spring). 2009;20(6):1266–72.

62. Geloneze B, Geloneze SR, Fiori C, Stabe C, Tambascia MA, Chaim EA, et al. Surgery for nonobese type 2 diabetic patients: an interventional study with duodenal-jejunal exclusion. Obes Surg. 2009;19(8):1077–83.

63. Pinheiro JS, Schiavon CA, Pereira PB, Correa JL, Noujaim P, Cohen R. Long-long limb Roux-en-Y gastric bypass is more efficacious in treatment of type 2 diabetes and lipid disorders in superobese patients. SOARD. 2008;4(4):521–5. Discussion 526–7.

64. Cummings DE, Shannon MH. Ghrelin and gastric bypass: is there a hormonal contribution to surgical weight loss? J Clin Endocrinol Metab. 2003;88(7):2999–3002.

65. Chopin LK, Seim I, Walpole CM, Herington AC. The ghrelin axis–does it have an appetite for cancer progression? Endocr Rev. 2012;33(6):849–91.

66. Ramos AC, Neto MG, de Souza YM, Galvão M. Laparoscopic duodenal–jejunal exclusion in the treatment of type 2 diabetes mellitus in patients with BMI. Obes Surg. 2009;19(3):307–12.

67. Kasama K, Tagaya N, Kanehira E, Oshiro T, Seki Y, Kinouchi M, et al. Laparoscopic sleeve gastrectomy with duodenojejunal bypass: technique and preliminary results. Obes Surg. 2009;19(10):1341–5.

68. Praveen Raj P, Kumaravel R, Chandramaliteeswaran C, Vaithiswaran V, Palanivelu C. Laparoscopic duodenojejunal bypass with sleeve gastrectomy: preliminary results of a prospective series from India. Surg Endosc. 2011;26(3):688–92.

69. Escalona A, Yáñez R, Pimentel F, Galvão M, Ramos AC, Turiel D, et al. Initial human experience with restrictive duodenal-jejunal bypass liner for treatment of morbid obesity. SOARD. 2010;6(2):126–31.

70. Escalona A, Pimentel F, Sharp A, Becerra P, Slako M, Turiel D, et al. Weight loss and metabolic improvement in morbidly obese subjects implanted for 1 year with an endoscopic duodenal-jejunal bypass liner. Ann Surg. 2012;255(6):1080–5.

71. Cohen RV, Neto MG, Correa JL, Sakai P, Martins B, Schiavon CA, et al. A pilot study of the duodenal-jejunal bypass liner in low body mass index type 2 diabetes. J Clin Endocrinol Metab. 2013;98(2):E279–82.

72. Jiao J, Bae EJ, Bandyopadhyay G, Oliver J, Marathe C, Chen M, et al. Restoration of euglycemia after duodenal bypass surgery is reliant on central and peripheral inputs in Zucker fa/fa rats. Diabetes. 2013;62(4):1074–83.

73. Santoro S, Castro LC, Velhote MCP, Malzoni CE, Klajner S, Castro LP, et al. Sleeve gastrectomy with transit bipartition: a potent intervention for metabolic syndrome and obesity. Ann Surg. 2012;256(1):104–10.

74. Shukla AP, Moreira M, Dakin G, Pomp A, Brillon D, Sinha N, et al. Medical versus surgical treatment of type 2 diabetes: the search for level 1 evidence. Soard. 2012;8(4):476–82.

75. Rubino F, Kaplan LM, Schauer PR, Cummings DE. The diabetes surgery summit consensus conference. Ann Surg. 2010;251(3):399–405.

76. ADA. Summary of revisions for the 2009 clinical practice recommendations. Diabetes Care. 2009;32 Suppl 1:S3–5.

77. Dixon JB, Zimmet P, Alberti KG, Rubino F. Bariatric surgery: an IDF statement for obese Type 2 diabetes. Diabet Med. 2011;28(6):628–42.

40

Venous Thrombosis and Pulmonary Embolism in the Bariatric Surgery Patient

Brandon T. Grover and Shanu N. Kothari

Introduction

As obesity rates continue to escalate throughout the world, our understanding of its effects on various body systems has similarly increased. Surgery has become one of the few successful long-term treatment options for the morbidly obese patient. One of several potential major complications of bariatric surgery is venous thromboembolic (VTE) disease. VTE in this patient population is typically defined as deep vein thrombosis (DVT) and/or pulmonary embolism (PE).

Pathophysiology

A well-recognized theory in describing the pathogenesis of venous thrombosis is Virchow's Triad. Interestingly, not wholly proposed by Rudolf Virchow, but rather named after him, it includes: hypercoagulability, alterations in blood flow (stasis/turbulence), and vascular endothelial injury.

At least one risk factor can be found in over 90 % of patients who develop a venous thrombotic event, and commonly multiple risk factors are identified [1]. Morbid obesity itself has been suggested to be an independent risk of VTE [2–6].

There are multiple factors that place the morbidly obese patient at risk for VTE events. Physical changes of increased body weight can lead to increased intra-abdominal pressure with potential decreased venous return to the heart. There is potential increased blood viscosity in the femoral veins, lower extremity venous stasis disease, patient physical inactivity, and difficulty with ambulation seen in this patient population.

Multiple biochemical changes related to obesity have also been shown to create an increased risk of venous thrombotic complications. Several abnormalities of fibrinolysis and hemostasis occur in the obese patient. Recently recognized are increased circulating levels of plasminogen activator inhibitor-1 (PAI-1) due to its origins from visceral and subcutaneous fat cells [7–9]. PAI-1 decreases fibrinolytic activity by blocking the conversion of plasminogen to plasmin via the inhibition of plasminogen activators, thus creating a pro-thrombotic state. There is evidence that increased production of PAI-1 is mediated through the inflammatory cytokines interleukin-1, tumor necrosis factor-α (TNF-α), and transforming growth factor-β (TGF-β) [10]. These cytokines produced in adipose tissues are more prevalent in the obese patient [11, 12]. Additionally, the adipokine leptin is elevated in this patient population. Leptin has been shown to act on the hypothalamus to decrease appetite and increase energy expenditure [13, 14]. As the central nervous system becomes resistant to its effects, in the obese patient, circulating levels increase. Leptin has been shown to upregulate the expression of PAI-1 in coronary artery endothelial cells [15].

Increased levels of fibrinogen are well documented in the obese population. Fibrinogen is a glycoprotein synthesized by hepatocytes and is the precursor to fibrin. It acts as the major protein for thrombosis and can form bridges between aggregating platelets. Thus, hyperfibrinogenemia has been strongly associated with an increased risk of VTE.

Other factors from the coagulation cascade have been shown to be elevated with increasing body mass index (BMI) and waist-to-hip ratio. These include factors VII, VIII, and von Willebrand factor [16]. It has been theorized that hyperinsulinemia and/or a chronic inflammatory state observed in the obese patient are the reasons for these elevations. Many of these prothrombotic factors have been shown to decrease in concentration after significant weight loss [17, 18].

In addition to the intrinsic risk obesity plays on VTE disease, bariatric surgery further increases the thrombotic risk profile. Major abdominal surgery carries an increased risk of VTE complications. As the majority of bariatric surgery is now performed laparoscopically, reverse Trendelenburg positioning and the pneumoperitoneum decrease venous return to the heart and contribute to a prothrombotic state. Poor mobility after surgery related to potential underlying ambulation difficulties, postoperative pain, or somnolence from recent anesthesia may also play a role in increasing VTE risk.

Fortunately, despite most bariatric patients being considered a moderate to high risk for thrombotic complications,

S.A. Brethauer et al. (eds.), *Minimally Invasive Bariatric Surgery*,
DOI 10.1007/978-1-4939-1637-5_40, © Springer Science+Business Media New York 2015

clinically detected DVTs and PEs are fairly uncommon in the bariatric surgical patient. A survey of bariatric surgeons in North America conducted in 1998 revealed that 86 % considered their patients to be at high risk for VTE complications [19]. A follow-up survey conducted in 2007, by one of the same lead authors, found that 95 % of bariatric surgeons are using some form of chemoprophylaxis to prevent VTE complications [20].

In the modern era of bariatric surgery with a majority of programs having VTE prophylaxis protocols in place, the incidence of symptomatic DVT and PE ranges from 0 to 5.4 % [21, 22] and 0 to 6.4 % [23, 24], respectively. Although overall incidence is low, VTE events remain a leading cause of mortality after bariatric surgery [1, 25, 26]. A review of 10 autopsies performed after bariatric surgery revealed PE was the direct cause of death in 30 % of patients; however, 80 % were found to have PEs [27]. Additionally, studies have shown that the risk of VTE complications continues to be elevated for several weeks after surgery, long after the patient has been discharged home from the hospital [28–30]. In his 2007 survey, Barba reported that 60 % of surgeons would consider discharging higher-risk patients home with chemical prophylaxis.

Prevention and Prophylaxis

The ideal method of prophylaxis for VTE complications in bariatric surgery has yet to be elucidated. Patients undergoing bariatric surgery are considered to be at moderate to high risk for having thrombotic complications. Published literature varies widely on optimal guidelines for the prevention of perioperative VTE events. The major accepted forms of prophylaxis range from mechanical compression devices with early ambulation alone to the addition of chemoprophylaxis and finally to the use of inferior vena cava (IVC) filters.

Mechanical Prophylaxis Alone

Due to concerns for bleeding after bariatric surgery, there have been studies looking at the efficacy of preventing perioperative venous thrombotic complications by mechanical means alone. Significant postoperative bleeding may require blood transfusions, endoscopic treatment, re-operative treatment, and significantly increased hospital stay and cost. The use of pharmacologic anticoagulation agents has been associated with an increased risk of postoperative hemorrhage [31, 32].

Several retrospective studies have looked at rates of DVT, PE, and bleeding complications following bariatric surgery with the routine use of mechanical prophylaxis alone.

Frantzides et al. retrospectively reviewed their experience of 1,692 patients undergoing bariatric surgery [33]. They divided their patient population into two groups based on a change in their protocol for the prevention of VTE complications. Group A included 435 patients who were treated postoperatively with 40 mg enoxaparin subcutaneously twice daily and sequential compression devices (SCDs). Group B consisted of 1,257 patients who had SCDs placed, but did not receive routine anticoagulation. This group of patients was required to ambulate within 2 h of arrival to their inpatient bed. Several patients from each group were excluded due to being considered high risk and receiving preoperative IVC filters. Other than Group A having a higher BMI, 51.6 ± 4 kg/m^2 vs. 45.3 ± 3 kg/m^2, other demographics were similar. On average, Group B had 18 min shorter operative times. Findings of their study revealed a DVT rate of 1.6 % in Group A and 0.4 % in Group B with a PE rate of 1.1 and 0 %, respectively. Their intraluminal bleeding rate defined as melena or hematemesis was 4.8 % in Group A and 0.4 % in Group B. They reported two non-VTE mortalities, both in Group A. Their conclusion was that VTE prophylaxis can adequately be achieved with the routine use of SCDs, early ambulation, appropriate hydration, and shorter operative times. They recommended not using pharmacologic agents except in the highest-risk population—those with a personal or family history of hypercoagulable state or prior VTE event.

Clements et al. reported a retrospective analysis of their prospective database comprised of 957 consecutive patients undergoing laparoscopic Roux-en-Y gastric bypass surgery who received no pharmacologic treatment for VTE prevention [34]. They placed calf-length SCDs before surgery, which the patients kept on during their hospitalization, unless they were ambulating. Additionally they educated and encouraged all patients to ambulate the day of surgery. Patients were excluded if they had a personal or strong family history of VTE events, or known hypercoagulable state. The mean BMI of their patients was 49.1 with a 30-day follow-up of 99.9 %. They reported DVT and PE rates of 0.31 % and 0.10 %, respectively, with one non-VTE-related postoperative death. Bleeding complications occurred in 0.73 % of patients.

The conclusions drawn from their experience were that pharmacologic anticoagulation is not mandatory in patients undergoing bariatric surgery who have no prior history of VTE events. Adequate prophylaxis can be obtained with the use of SCDs, early ambulation, and short operative times.

Both of these studies excluded patients who were considered among the highest risk for VTE complications due to either personal or family history of thrombotic complications. According to the authors of these two studies, these higher-risk patients were treated with chemoprophylactic measures and/or IVC filters. Additionally, as with most studies published on this topic, rates of VTE complications did not include potential asymptomatic patients. Imaging studies to evaluate for VTE events were only performed in patients in whom there was a clinical suspicion.

The Use of Chemoprophylaxis

Due to the suspected moderate to high risk of VTE events in the bariatric patient, a majority of bariatric surgeons routinely use pharmacologic agents, typically in adjunct to mechanical methods, to prevent potentially lethal VTE complications. There is no set standard agent, dose, or timing of these medications. The most commonly used agents include unfractionated heparin (UFH) and low-molecular-weight heparins (LMWHs), either enoxaparin (Lovenox) or dalteparin (Fragmin).

Heparin. The properties of heparin as an effective anticoagulant have been known since the mid-1930s. Heparin has its major effect by binding to the enzyme inhibitor antithrombin III (AT III). This activates the AT III which in turn inactivates thrombin (factor IIa) and other coagulation factors, particularly factor Xa. Several advantages of using heparin as a prophylactic agent are that it is inexpensive, is reversible, and has a short-half life (1–2 h). The major concerning side effects include the potential for bleeding and heparin-induced thrombocytopenia (HIT), both of which can typically be treated with discontinuation of the medication. Prophylactic dosing for UFH is typically 5,000 U three times daily (TID), but larger dosing has been used, 7,500 U TID [35].

Low-Molecular-Weight Heparin (LMWH). The low-molecular-weight heparins have a similar mechanism of action to heparin, but they have less of an impact on thrombin with a similar effect on factor Xa. They have excellent bioavailability when injected subcutaneously and pharmacokinetics of a stable dose–response curve. When used as a prophylactic agent, they require less frequent administration. Additionally they have a significantly lower risk of causing HIT. Disadvantages include significant variations among the LMWHs in their antithrombotic and anticoagulant activities. In comparison to UFH, the LMWHs tend to be more expensive, are not reversible with protamine, and have a longer half-life (4–6 h). Serum levels cannot be evaluated by measuring the aPTT, but can be followed using anti-factor Xa (anti-FXa) activity. The ability to measure anti-FXa activity is not as readily available as aPTT levels. These agents are cleared by the kidneys, so they must be used with caution in patients with significant renal dysfunction (estimated creatinine clearance < 30 min/mL). The most common side effect of the LMWHs is bleeding. The use of these agents in the pre- and postoperative setting has led to bleeding rates as high as 5.9 % [32].

Higher doses of LMWH may be required in the morbidly obese patients as the vascular composition of adipose tissue is different than that of lean body mass. Manufacturer recommendations state that at prophylactic doses, levels do not require monitoring. Several studies have looked at different dosing regimens and measured anti-FXa levels, in the bariatric surgery patient, to ensure appropriate prophylactic doses are being achieved.

A retrospective study by Simoneau et al. sought to identify the effects of LMWH on anti-FXa levels after bariatric surgery [36]. They administered 7,500 IU of dalteparin subcutaneously daily starting on the second postoperative day. They found an inverse linear relationship between body weight and anti-FXa levels. Also reported was a statistically significant difference on not achieving a goal anti-FXa target level of at least 0.2 IU/mL in the heaviest group of patients, those weighing 181 kg or more. Even though the administered dose was 50 % more than the typical prophylactic dose of 5,000 IU, it was still associated with subtherapeutic anti-FXa levels in the heaviest group of patients. Despite this finding, they reported no clinical VTE events and a 2.2 % hemorrhagic complication rate.

Enoxaparin has been administered with doses ranging from 30 to 60 mg either as daily or twice daily frequency. Scholten published his retrospective review of their bariatric patients after a change in protocol where their first 92 patients received Lovenox 30 mg every 12 h and compared them to 389 subsequent patients who received the same medication at 40 mg every 12 h [22]. All patients were additionally treated with early ambulation, compression stockings, and SCDs. They found a 5.4 % DVT complication rate in the first set of patients and 0.6 % in the second group. Operative times and length of hospital stay were longer in the first group at 213 min vs. 175 min and 5.67 days vs. 3.8 days, respectively. They had one patient in each group with postoperative bleeding. The conclusion from their study was that a multimodality treatment regimen is important in this patient population in order to achieve a low thrombotic complication rate and that the higher dose of enoxaparin, 40 mg every 12 h, may reduce the incidence of VTE complications without increasing the risk of hemorrhagic complications.

Simone et al. reported their comparison of administering enoxaparin 40 mg ($n=24$) or 60 mg ($n=16$) every 12 h in their patients undergoing laparoscopic bariatric surgery [37]. They measured anti-FXa levels 4 h after the first and third dose. After the third dose, 44 % of patients in the 40 mg group were subtherapeutic vs. 0 % in the 60 mg group. There were however 57 % of patients in the 60 mg group that were supratherapeutic vs. 0 % in the 40 mg group. They had one postoperative bleeding event in the 40 mg group and none in the 60 mg group. Conclusions from their study were that the higher dose of enoxaparin achieved superior therapeutic anti-FXa concentrations avoiding subtherapeutic levels. Their small population of 40 patients was too small to detect any significance in clinical outcomes between the two groups. They did not report on VTE events.

Although it appears that consideration could be made to use higher doses of LMWH to achieve proper therapeutic levels, the true clinical significance of this has yet to be proven. It is not well defined if this practice may lead to a decreased risk of VTE complications and/or if an increased rate of major bleeding complications will occur.

While there is a recognized risk of potential major bleeding with the use of pharmacologic chemoprophylaxis in the perioperative period, it is commonly believed that it is easier to manage bleeding than a major thrombotic event. Bleeding will frequently stop with the cessation of anticoagulants. If continued bleeding occurs, there are several treatment options available to include angiographic embolization, endoscopic treatment, and/or operative control of the hemorrhage. Significant postoperative bleeding defined as either requiring blood transfusions or an intervention occurs in 0.9–5.9 % of patients [28, 32]. Alternatively, patient mortality has been well described due to major bleeding after bariatric surgery and cannot be taken lightly [28, 38].

Inferior Vena Cava Filters

With the introduction of retrievable IVC filters, there has been an increase use of these devices. In Barba's 2007 survey of ASMBS members, 55 % of bariatric surgeons reported using IVC filters in their high-risk patients [20]. This was a significant increase from their previously reported usage rate of 7 % in 1998 [19]. IVC filters act as a mechanical device to trap venous thromboemboli that originate in the lower extremities or pelvis, with the intent of preventing PEs. They are typically placed through the femoral or internal jugular vein into the inferior vena cava. Multiple complications can occur with the placement of these devices including: bleeding, pneumothorax, filter migration, erosion through the IVC, vena cava thrombosis, insertion site thrombosis, breakthrough PEs, and increased long-term rate of DVT [39–41].

Several case studies and single center case series have reported on the safety and efficacy of these devices in the high-risk bariatric patient [42–45]. To date, there are no randomized controlled trials evaluating the efficacy of IVC filters in bariatric surgery patients. What is deemed high risk is variable; however some common factors include: known hypercoagulable state, prior VTE event, strong family history of VTE events, and immobility. Additional conditions used to classify patients as high risk include: venous stasis disease, obstructive sleep apnea, pulmonary hypertension, use of oral contraceptives, and a BMI > 55–60 kg/m^2.

Rajasekhar and colleagues performed a systematic review of the literature and reported results of an exhaustive search [46]. After filtering out low-quality publications, they identified 11 (level 2B) articles [24, 42–45, 47–52] that evaluated the use of IVC filters for VTE prophylaxis in the bariatric patient (Table 1). Only four of these studies compared an IVC filter group to a non-IVC filter group. One of these compared two groups of high-risk bariatric patients and found a significantly decreased incidence of PE and fatal PE between the cohort of patients who received an IVC filter and the patients who did not have an IVC filter placed (PE rate of 0 % vs. 28 % and fatal PE of 0 % vs. 11 %, respectively) [48]. All patients were given preoperative heparin

and placed on UFH postoperatively until they were ambulating. Another study looked at their 15 high-risk patients, some of whom had an IVC filter placed and the other group who were treated with continuous IV heparin intraoperatively [47]. Postoperatively all patients were treated with weight-based enoxaparin for 15 days followed by warfarin for ≥3 months. They reported no clinically evident DVT or PE. Two of the studies showed no significant difference in the incidence of PE between their two groups of patients, IVC filter vs. no IVC filter [43, 50]. However, both of these studies compared high-risk patients who had an IVC filter placed with low-risk patients without IVC filters. It appears that by placing an IVC filter in the high-risk patients, the risk of VTE became similar to the low-risk patient. In evaluating the additional seven studies cited and performing a summation of their patients with outcomes, out of 227 high-risk patients who received preoperative IVC filters, the DVT and PE rates were 5.7 % and 1.3 %, respectively. This excludes one patient who developed a PE after IVC filter removal. The indications for what was considered high risk and additional VTE prophylactic measures differed among each of these studies. All 11 authors recommended the use of IVC filters in the high-risk patient. Reported IVC filter complication rates ranged from 0 to 2.47 %. Despite the unanimous agreement on the safety and benefit of IVC filters in the high-risk patient, Rajasekhar and colleagues concluded that there is insufficient evidence to support the use of IVC filters at the time of surgery and recommended against their routine use.

Several studies have shown an increased risk of perioperative morbidity in bariatric patients who had a preoperative IVC filter placed, raising the concern for these devices causing more harm than good. Birkmeyer et al. performed a retrospective review of the Michigan Bariatric Surgery Collaborative database between 2006 and 2008 [53]. Out of 6,376 patients undergoing gastric bypass surgery, 542 patients (8.5 %) had a preoperative IVC filter placed. They used propensity scores in an attempt to control for selection bias related to IVC filter placement in higher-risk patients. In their review, patients receiving IVC filters were in fact higher risk with significantly higher rates of multiple comorbidities to include: history of VTE, age > 50 years, BMI > 50 kg/m^2, male gender, mobility problems, lung disease, cardiovascular disease, diabetes, and sleep apnea. Additionally these patients were more likely to undergo open gastric bypass and have operative times > 3 h. Without risk adjustment, the IVC filter group experienced significantly higher complication rates including postoperative VTE events 2.03 % vs. 0.53 %, serious complications 7.56 % vs. 3.62 % (not specifically defined in the study), and permanent disability/death 1.85 % vs. 0.51 %. After applying risk-adjusted propensity scores, the statistical significance of these adverse outcomes was no longer present, but there was a trend towards worse outcomes in the IVC filter group. There were two reported complications directly

TABLE 1. Review of observational studies reporting venous thromboembolism with prophylactic inferior vena cava filter use after bariatric surgery

References	Definitions of high risk	Bariatric patient groups	Pharmacologic prophylaxis	Outcomes
Frezza et al. [47]	BMI 50 kg/m^2, prior DVT or PE, prior pelvic surgery, cardiac failure	High risk + IVCF, $n=15$	Preop—LV 2 mg/kg SQ×1 or UFH 7,000 U SQ×1	No PE or DVT
		High risk + intraop UFH, $n=9$	POD#1—LV 1.5–2 mg/kg SQ BID×15 days then Coumadin ≥3 months	
Gargiulo et al. [48]	BMI >55 kg/m^2, prior DVT/PE, pulm HTN	1. High risk + IVCF $n=17$	Preop—UFH 50 U/kg SQ×1	Decreased PE (28 % vs. 0 %) and fatal PE (11 % vs. 0 %) favoring IVCF
		2. High risk, no IVCF, $n=18$	Postop—UFH 50 U/kg SQ q12 h until ambulatory	
Halmi et al. [49]	Prior DVT/PE, hypercoag state, severe OSA, pulm HTN, immobility, BMI >65 kg/m^2	High risk, $n=27$	Preop—UFH 5,000 U×1 or LV 40 mg SQ×1	No DVT or PE
			Postop—UFH 5,000 U SQ q 8 h or LV 40 mg SQ q12 h×3 weeks	
Kardys et al. [24]	BMI >50 kg/m^2, venous insuff, hypercoag state, immobility, or prior VTE	High risk, $n=31$	Preop—UFH 5,000 U SQ×1 POD#1—LV 40 mg SQ BID If BMI >60 LV×2 weeks	DVT 1/31, PE 2/31
Keeling et al. [42]	Prior PE/DVT, venous stasis	High risk, $n=14$	Periop—LV 40 mg SQ BID If BMI >60—LV 30 mg SQ BID	No PE
Obeid et al. [43]	Immobility, prior DVT/PE, venous disease, BMI >60 kg/m^2, prior IVCF	1. High risk + IVCF $n=248$	Postop—LV dose not specified IVCF group—LV + Coumadin 1 mg/d	No difference in PE (0.81 % vs. 0.59 %), DVT (1.21 % vs. 0.65 %), or death (0.81 % vs. 0.22 %)
		2. Low risk, no IVCF $n=1,851$		
Overby et al. [50]	Thrombophilia, immobility, h/o venous stasis, pulm HTN, severe OSA, BMI >60 kg/m^2, Prior DVT/PE	1. High risk + IVCF, $n=160$	Preop—UFH 5,000–75,000 U SQ q8 h	No difference in PE (3 % vs. 2 %) or DVT (0.6 % vs. 3 %)
		2. Low risk, no IVCF $n=170$	Postop—UFH 5,000–7,500 U Q q8 h	
Piano et al. [51]	BMI >55 kg/m^2, hypercoagulable state, immobility, venous stasis, prior DVT/PE	High risk $n=60$	Preop—none Intraop—IV UFH max 750 U/h Postop—LV BID at discharge (goal LMW level 0.3–0.5)	PE 1/60 (received no pharmacologic prophylaxis)
Schuster et al. [44]	Prior DVT/PE, severe venous stasis, sleep apnea, wt >400 lbs	High risk, $n=24$	Preop—SQ UFH	DVT 5/24, PE 1/24 (after IVCF retrieval)
Trigilio-Black et al. [45]	Prior DVT/PE, venous stasis, pulmonary compromise, immobility	High risk $n=41$	Preop—LV 30 mg SQ×1 Postop—LV 30 mg SQ BID	DVT 1/41, no PE
Vaziri et al. [52]	Prior VTE	High risk $n=30$	Preop—UFH 5,000 U SQ×1 Postop—UFH 5,000 U SQ q8 h	DVT 6/30, no PE

Adapted with permission from: Rajasekhar A, Crowther M. Inferior vena cava filter insertion prior to bariatric surgery: a systematic review of the literature. J Thromb Haemost. 2010;8(6):1266–70

PE pulmonary embolism, *DVT* deep vein thrombosis, *VTE* venous thromboembolism, *OSA* obstructive sleep apnea, *BMI* body mass index, *UFH* unfractionated heparin, *LV* enoxaparin, *NR* not reported, *HTN* hypertension

related to the IVC filter to include a fatal IVC thrombosis and an IVC filter migration to the heart. They concluded that prophylactic IVC filters in gastric bypass patients do not decrease the risk of PEs and may lead to additional complications.

Despite the rare complications directly related to the IVC filter, it is difficult to quantify the potential benefit in this high-risk group of patients who were perhaps protected from major PEs and possible subsequent mortality.

Another concern with using IVC filters is the potential for delayed mechanical and/or pharmacologic prophylaxis due to the perception of the patient being protected from a PE. Caution must be taken to avoid this misconception as an IVC filter alone is not sufficient to safeguard against VTE events including a significant and potentially fatal PE. The American Society of Hematology consensus statements concluded that there is insufficient evidence to support the use of IVC filters at the time of bariatric surgery [54].

Systematic Reviews

There have been two key review articles evaluating the published literature of VTE prophylaxis in the bariatric patient. Rocha et al. performed a systemic review of the risk of VTE complications and efficacy of prophylaxis in both obese medical and bariatric surgery patients [25]. Their review found eight studies, six-level 2B and two-level 2C, published between 2001 and 2005 looking at VTE prophylaxis in the bariatric patient. They were unable to find any level 1A recommendations for prophylaxis for either the medical or surgical patients. A lack of high-quality prospective studies prevented identifying the most effective and/or safest prophylactic regimen. However, they concluded that the use of some form of chemoprophylaxis is needed. They also determined that obesity was an independent risk factor for VTE events in the medical patients.

Agarwal et al. updated the systemic review by Rocha, looking at the literature between 2006 and 2009 (Table 2) [55]. The goal was to examine the best, most current evidence for VTE prophylaxis in bariatric surgery patients. They reviewed two evidence-based guidelines which will be discussed later and discovered 30 primary studies, including the 8 cited by Rocha. Only one of these was a randomized controlled trial (RCT), and 22 studies did not have a control cohort. There was a wide range of prophylactic methods used which included: mechanical prophylaxis alone (1 study) [56], LMWH alone (3 studies) [28, 31, 57], LMWH and mechanical prophylaxis (4 studies) [22, 32, 58, 59], subcutaneous UFH and mechanical prophylaxis (2 studies) [35, 60], IV UFH and mechanical prophylaxis (2 studies) [61–63], IVC filters combined with mechanical and/or pharmacologic prophylaxis (11 studies) [23, 24, 42–45, 48, 49, 51, 64, 65], and variable methods (5 studies). They discovered a lack of RCTs and case-controlled studies in the published literature. There were several important findings from their systemic review. In most studies both mechanical and pharmacologic prophylaxis were used in both the preoperative and postoperative settings, including the encouragement of early ambulation. Patients who were considered to be higher risk (i.e., history of hypercoagulable disorder, prior DVT or PE, immobile, pulmonary hypertension, obstructive sleep apnea, venous stasis disease, BMI > 55 kg/m²) were commonly treated with the addition of IVC filters. The studies also identified that VTE events frequently occurred after hospital discharge. Conclusions drawn from their review that can provide treatment guidelines are:

1. Bariatric surgery patients have a significant risk of VTE complications.
2. It is reasonable to use UFH 5,000 IU subcutaneously every 8 h or enoxaparin 30–40 mg subcutaneously every 12 h for VTE prophylaxis. Higher doses could be justified.
3. Pharmacologic prophylaxis should be started preoperatively and combined with SCDs and early ambulation.
4. Preoperative placement of IVC filters should be considered in the highest-risk patients.
5. Extended pharmacologic prophylaxis with enoxaparin 40 mg/day for 3–4 weeks postoperatively may be considered in higher-risk patients.

These recommendations are largely derived from uncontrolled studies where the use of these prophylactic measures has shown a low incidence of VTE events.

Current Guidelines

Evidence-based guidelines have been established based on the available literature by the American College of Chest Physicians (ACCP) and by the American Association of Clinical Endocrinologists, The Obesity Society, and the American Society for Metabolic and Bariatric Surgery (AACE/TOS/ASMBS).

In February 2012 the 9th edition of the guidelines on Antithrombotic Therapy and Prevention of Thrombosis was published by the ACCP [66]. They reported that virtually all bariatric surgery patients are at least at a moderate risk of VTE with many patients at high risk for VTE complications. Due to the paucity of randomized controlled trials in the bariatric literature, the recommendations established for the bariatric patient were based on relative risks from randomized controlled trials in patients who underwent abdominal and pelvic surgery. For the patient at moderate risk of VTE who are not at high risk of having a major bleeding complication, they recommend prophylaxis with LMWH, UFH, or mechanical prophylaxis ideally with SCDs, compared to no prophylaxis. For the high-risk VTE patient who is not at high risk of having a major bleeding complication, they recommend prophylaxis with LMWH or UFH compared to no prophylaxis. They also suggest the added use of mechanical prophylaxis with either SCDs or elastic compression stockings. They give no direct recommendation for IVC filter use but state, "… although placement of an IVC filter probably reduces the risk of PE over the short term, complications appear to be frequent, and long-term, benefits are unclear."

AACE/TOS/ASMBS guidelines recommend the use of UFH 5,000 U or LMWH subcutaneously, shortly before bariatric surgery and administered every 8–12 h postoperatively until the patient is completely mobile [67]. They remark that the use of higher doses of these medications does not have a proven benefit. They mention that most facilities also use mechanical prophylactic devices. They also suggest considering the use of IVC filters in patients with a personal history of VTE.

TABLE 2. Systematic review of prophylactic regimens to prevent venous thromboembolism after bariatric surgery

Category	Year of publication	Investigator	Study design	Patients (n)	Procedure	Intervention	DVT, %	PE, %	Bleeding, %	Mortality, %
LMWH	2001	Kalifarentzos et al. [31]	RCT	60	Roux-en-Y (unspecified)	Nadroparin 5,700 IU/d	0	NR	0	NR
LMWH/mechanical prophylaxis	2002	Scholten et al. [22]	Prospective, controlled	481	Various	Enoxaparin 30 mg BID; mechanical prophylaxis/enoxaparin 40 mg BID; mechanical prophylaxis	5.4/0.5 combined DVT/PE	NR	1.1/0.3	NR
Intravenous heparin/mechanical prophylaxis	2003	Shepherd et al. [61]	Prospective, uncontrolled	700	Laparoscopic Roux-en-Y	IV heparin continuous, target anti-factor Xa. 11–25 U/mL; mechanical prophylaxis	0	0.4	2.3	0
Mechanical prophylaxis	2004	Gonzalez et al. [56]	Prospective, uncontrolled	380	Laparoscopic Roux-en-Y	Mechanical prophylaxis	0.26	0	NR	NR
Subcutaneous heparin/mechanical prophylaxis	2004	Miller et al. [35]	Retrospective, uncontrolled	250	Laparoscopic Roux-en-Y	SQ heparin TID 5,000 U if BMI <50 kg/m², 7,500 U if BMI >50 kg/m²; mechanical prophylaxis	0.4	1.2	2.4	NR
Intravenous heparin/mechanical prophylaxis	2004	Shepherd et al. [62]	Prospective, uncontrolled	19	Laparoscopic Roux-en-Y	IV heparin continuous, target anti-factor Xa 0.15–0.20 U/mL; mechanical prophylaxis	0	0	0	NR
Subcutaneous heparin/mechanical prophylaxis	2005	Cotter et al. [60]	Retrospective, uncontrolled	107	Open or laparoscopic Roux-en-Y	SQ heparin 5,000 U BID; mechanical prophylaxis	0.9	NR	NR	NR
LMWH	2005	Hamad et al. [28]	Retrospective, uncontrolled	668	Various	Enoxaparin (various doses)	0.1	0.9	1	0.3
IVC filter/pharmacologic prophylaxis/mechanical prophylaxis	2005	Keeling et al. [42]	Retrospective, uncontrolled	14	Unspecified gastric bypass	IVC filter; SQ heparin (dose NR); enoxaparin if BMI 40–60 kg/m², 40 U/d; if BMI >60 kg/m², 30 U BID; mechanical prophylaxis	0	0	NR	NR
IVC filter/pharmacologic prophylaxis/mechanical prophylaxis	2005	Prystowsky et al. [64]	Prospective, uncontrolled	106	Unspecified Roux-en-Y	IVC filter; SQ heparin 5,000 U BID; mechanical prophylaxis	3.8	0	1.9	0
Intravenous heparin/mechanical prophylaxis	2005	Quebbemann et al. [21]	Prospective, uncontrolled	822	Various	IV heparin, continuous, 400 U/h; mechanical prophylaxis	0	0.1	1.3	NR
LMWH/mechanical prophylaxis	2006	Abou-Nukta et al. [58]	Retrospective, uncontrolled	1,225	Open Roux-en-Y	Enoxaparin 40 mg BID; mechanical prophylaxis	NR	0.9	NR	NR
IVC filter/pharmacologic prophylaxis/mechanical prophylaxis	2006	Gargiulo et al. [48]	Prospective, controlled	571	Open Roux-en-Y	IVC filter indicated for h/o DVT, PE, or pulmonary HTN; SQ heparin 50 U/kg BID; mechanical prophylaxis/IVC filter indicated for h/o DVT, PE, or pulmonary HTN or BMI >55 kg/m²; SQ heparin 50 U/kg BID; mechanical prophylaxis/IVC filter offered to patients with BMI >55 kg/m²; SQ heparin 50 U/kg BID; mechanical prophylaxis	NR	2.1/0/NR	NR	2.1/0.6/NR

(continued)

TABLE 2. (CONTINUED)

Category	Year of publication	Investigator	Study design	Patients (n)	Procedure	Intervention	DVT, %	PE, %	Bleeding, %	Mortality, %
IVC filter/pharmacologic prophylaxis/mechanical prophylaxis	2006	Gonzalez et al. [65]	Prospective, uncontrolled	660	Laparoscopic Roux-en-Y	IVC filter; SQ heparin (dose NR); enoxaparin 40 mg/d for BMI <50 kg/m² and 30 mg BID for BMI ≥50 kg/m²; mechanical prophylaxis; extended prophylaxis for high-risk factors	1.4	0.9	NR	0.5
Intravenous heparin/mechanical prophylaxis	2007	Cossu et al. [63]	Pre–post comparison study	151	Biliopancreatic diversion or vertical banded gastroplasty	IV heparin 2,500–5,000 U, single dose; mechanical prophylaxis/SQ heparin aPTT adjusted; mechanical prophylaxis	NR	3.1/1.2	0/0	4.6/0
LMWH/mechanical prophylaxis	2007	Forestieri et al. [59]	Prospective, uncontrolled	10	Biliointestinal bypass	Parnaparin 3,200–6,400 IU/d; mechanical prophylaxis	0	10	0	NR
IVC filter/pharmacologic prophylaxis/mechanical prophylaxis	2007	Halmi et al. [49]	Prospective, controlled	652	Open Roux-en-Y	IVC filter; SQ heparin 5,000 U TID or enoxaparin 40 mg BID; mechanical prophylaxis; enoxaparin 40 mg/d for 3-week postoperative/SQ heparin 5,000 U tid or enoxaparin 40 mg BID; mechanical prophylaxis; enoxaparin 40 mg/d for 3-week postoperative	0/1	0/0.3	NR	NR
LMWH/mechanical prophylaxis	2007	Kothari et al. [32]	Retrospective, uncontrolled	476	Laparoscopic Roux-en-Y gastric bypass	Enoxaparin 40 mg BID; mechanical prophylaxis/SQ heparin 5,000 U TID; mechanical prophylaxis	0/0	0/0	1.7/0	0/0
IVC filter/pharmacologic prophylaxis/mechanical prophylaxis	2007	Obeid et al. [43]	Retrospective, controlled	2,009	Open or laparoscopic Roux-en-Y	IVC filter; warfarin; enoxaparin (dose NR); mechanical prophylaxis/enoxaparin (dose NR); mechanical prophylaxis	1.21/0.65	0.81/0.59	NR	0.81/0.22
IVC filter/pharmacologic prophylaxis/mechanical prophylaxis	2007	Piano et al. [51]	Prospective, uncontrolled	59	Laparoscopic Roux-en-Y	IVC filter; IV heparin continuous 500–750 U/h; mechanical prophylaxis; patients discharged with enoxaparin (dose NR)	NR	1.7	NR	0
IVC filter/pharmacologic prophylaxis/mechanical prophylaxis	2007	Schuster et al. [44]	Prospective, uncontrolled	24	Laparoscopic gastric bypass	IVC filter; SQ heparin (dose NR); mechanical prophylaxis	21 (combined DVT and PE)		NR	0
IVC filter/pharmacologic prophylaxis/mechanical prophylaxis	2007	Trigilio-Black et al. [45]	Prospective, uncontrolled	41	Various	IVC filter; enoxaparin 30 mg BID; mechanical prophylaxis	2.4	0	NR	2.4
LMWH	2008	Brasileiro et al. [57]	Prospective, uncontrolled	126	Open or laparoscopic Roux-en-Y	Nadroparin 9,500 IU/d/enoxaparin 40 mg/d	0/0.8	NR/0	6.7/3.2	NR/0.8
IVC filter/pharmacologic prophylaxis/mechanical prophylaxis	2008	Escalante-Tattersfield et al. [23]	Retrospective, uncontrolled	618	Laparoscopic Roux-en-Y	IVC filter; SQ heparin 5,000 U TID for first 24 h; enoxaparin 40 mg BID; mechanical prophylaxis	0.16	0	1.6	0
IVC filter/pharmacologic prophylaxis/mechanical prophylaxis	2008	Kardys et al. [24]	Retrospective, uncontrolled	31	Unspecified Roux-en-Y	IVC filter; SQ heparin (dose NR); enoxaparin 40 mg BID; mechanical prophylaxis; enoxaparin for 2 weeks postoperative if BMI >60 kg/m²	3.1	6.4	NR	6.5

Adapted with permission from: Agarwal R, Hecht TE, Lazo MC, Umscheid CA. Venous thromboembolism prophylaxis for patients undergoing bariatric surgery: a systematic review. Surg Obes Relat Dis. 2010;6:213–20

Diagnosis of Deep Vein Thrombosis and Pulmonary Embolism

The evaluation of a patient suspected of having a DVT is typically initiated based on symptoms. The most common complaint is pain or swelling of the lower extremity. Physical exam findings may include swelling, tenderness, skin discoloration, a palpable cord, and/or increased warmth. The morbidly obese patient is more difficult to examine secondary to body habitus. They commonly have what appears to be lower extremity swelling/edema; however, this may be due to increased deposition of fatty tissue in the extremities. As physical exam findings can be relatively nonspecific and potential complications of anticoagulation may exist, further testing is indicated to confirm the diagnosis.

Multiple diagnostic studies have been used to diagnose DVTs including: contrast venography, compression ultrasonography, impedance plethysmography, computed tomography, and magnetic resonance venography. The most common modality used is compression ultrasonography (Fig. 1). Findings suggestive of DVT with this modality include non-compressibility of the vein (Fig. 2), abnormal Doppler color flow, abnormal change in vein diameter with Valsalva, and the presence of an echogenic band. Ultrasound has the advantage of being noninvasive and has been shown to have greater than 95 % sensitivity and specificity for proximal DVTs if venous non-compressibility is demonstrated [68]. If the initial examination is negative, repeat compression ultrasonography can be performed at a future date. A repeat negative study performed 5–7 days after the initial study has been shown to have a less than 1 % incidence of DVT over several months of follow-up [69]. Limitations of this modality include difficulty in detecting thrombus in the iliac veins and the distal femoral vein within the adductor canal. Increased fatty tissue in the morbidly obese patient may also contribute to poor visualization of the venous anatomy.

Signs and symptoms of acute pulmonary embolism can be nonspecific. The most common symptoms are dyspnea at rest and/or with exertion, pleuritic chest pain, cough, hemop-

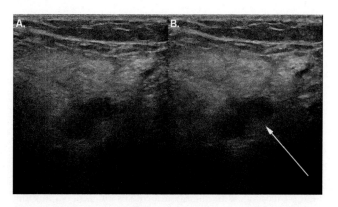

Fig. 2. Abnormal lower extremity ultrasound illustrating (**a**) popliteal artery and vein and (**b**) non-compressed popliteal vein indicating a deep vein thrombosis (*arrow*).

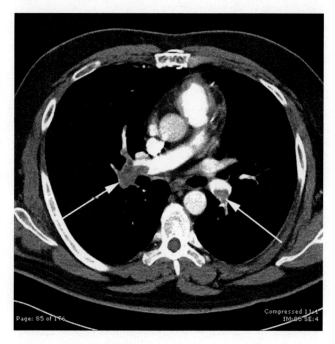

Fig. 3. Computed tomography with contrast illustrating thrombus in the pulmonary arteries (*arrows*).

tysis, orthopnea, calf or thigh pain and swelling, and respiratory wheezing. Signs include tachypnea, tachycardia, decreased breath sounds, jugular venous distension, accentuated pulmonic component of the second heart sound, and signs of DVT as discussed above. Hypotension is typically a late sign and is concerning for a massive PE. In this setting acute right ventricular heart failure may be present with findings of jugular venous distension, parasternal shift, and the presence of a right-sided S3 heart sound.

Confirmatory studies should be performed in hemodynamically stable patients who are suspected of having a PE. The most commonly used modalities include spiral CT pulmonary angiography (CTPA) (Fig. 3), ventilation-perfusion (V/Q) scan, pulmonary angiography, and ultrasound to evaluate for DVTs. The use of CTPA has become the preferred modality for evaluating the patient who is

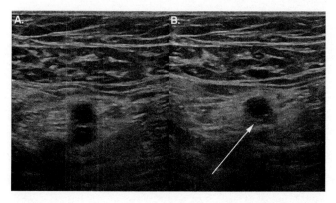

Fig. 1. Normal lower extremity ultrasound illustrating (**a**) femoral artery and vein and (**b**) femoral artery with a compressed femoral vein (*arrow*).

suspected of having a PE. It has the advantage of being readily available, relatively rapid, moderately to highly sensitive and specific, able to diagnose other pathology, and can be performed through a peripheral IV. Contraindications to the use of CTPA include contrast allergy and non-dialysis-dependent renal failure. Other modalities such as the V/Q scan can be used in these situations, but may not provide the diagnostic accuracy of the CTPA.

The mainstay of treatment for both DVTs and PEs is anticoagulation. Challenges in instituting treatment in the recent postoperative bariatric patient stem around the concerns for major bleeding with therapeutic doses of anticoagulation. Initial treatment should focus on respiratory and cardiovascular support. Hypoxia should be treated with supplemental oxygen and endotracheal intubation performed if the patient is experiencing respiratory distress. The initial treatment of hypotension should be IV fluid administration. Vasopressor support (e.g., norepinephrine, dopamine, epinephrine) should be considered early if there is no rapid return of normal blood pressure.

If there is a high clinical suspicion for PE and the patient is not stable, empiric administration of anticoagulation may be necessary prior to confirmatory studies. As recent surgery significantly increases the risk of bleeding, obtaining a confirmatory study expeditiously is preferred. Clinical judgment weighing the risks and benefits of anticoagulation is critical. If anticoagulation is felt to be contraindicated, IVC filter placement and embolectomy using catheters or surgery are potential treatment options, but may carry a high mortality rate [70].

Initial pharmacologic treatment options for DVTs and PEs include UFH, LMWHs, and fondaparinux. In the postoperative patient UFH has the advantage of having a shorter half-life and being reversible. Documented VTE should be treated with long-term anticoagulation, 3–6 months if transient risk factors are present, and longer if there have been prior episodes or if significant risk factors persist. The oral anticoagulant warfarin is most commonly used, and therapeutic levels of INR between 2.0 and 3.0 can easily be followed. Newer oral anticoagulant medications like dabigatran and rivaroxaban currently have not been approved for the long-term treatment of VTE events. These medications have a direct anti-FXA activity and do not require monitoring for therapeutic levels. Unlike warfarin, they carry a major drawback of not being reversible even with the administration of vitamin K and/or transfusion of blood products.

Indications for the use of IVC filters in patients known to have a PE include: high risk of bleeding, complication from pharmacologic treatment, PE despite receiving therapeutic anticoagulation, or thromboembolic burden sufficient to cause concern that further clot propagation would be lethal.

Conclusions

Despite a plethora of published data on VTE prophylaxis, in the bariatric surgery patient, there remains a lack of level 1A evidence to provide best practice guidelines. Multiple retrospective reviews have shown successful prophylaxis with varying methods. In the properly selected patient, mechanical treatment with SCDs, early ambulation, and short operating room times without the use of pharmacologic agents has shown acceptable low VTE rates. The most common prophylactic measures involve these same treatments with the addition of UFH or LMWH used in the pre- and postoperative period. Although there is a lack of strong evidence to support the use of IVC filters, these devices have been used in the high-risk bariatric patient with success in decreasing the incidence of PEs. Until such a time that well-designed randomized controlled trials are performed, instituting a protocol that results in a low incidence of DVTs and PEs combined with low bleeding and treatment complication rates is critical in the care of this complex population of patients.

Review Questions and Answers

1. What two proteins have been found to be elevated in the morbidly obese patient that contribute to an increased risk of thromboembolic events?

   A. Plasminogen activator inhibitor-1 (PAI-1)
   B. Adiponectin
   C. Fibrinogen
   D. Interleukin-6
   Answer: A, C

2. If chemoprophylaxis is not used in the perioperative bariatric surgery setting, what other strategies can be employed to decrease VTE risk?

   A. Early ambulation after surgery
   B. Mechanical prophylaxis
   C. Extended operative times
   D. Adequate hydration
   Answer: A, B, D

3. Which of the following are potential complications of IVC filter placement?

   A. Increased long-term rate of DVT
   B. Filter migration
   C. Vena cava thrombosis
   D. Pneumothorax
   E. All of the above
   Answer: E

References

1. Sapala JA, Wood MH, Schuhknecht MP, Sapala MA. Fatal pulmonary embolism after bariatric operations for morbid obesity: a 24-year retrospective analysis. Obes Surg. 2003;13(6):819–25.
2. Stein PD, Beemath A, Olson RE. Obesity as a risk factor in venous thromboembolism. Am J Med. 2005;118(9):978–80.
3. Goldhaber SZ, Savage DD, Garrison RJ, Castelli WP, Kannel WB, McNamara PM, et al. Risk factors for pulmonary embolism. The Framingham study. Am J Med. 1983;74(6):1023–8.
4. Ageno W, Becattini C, Brighton T, Selby R, Kamphuisen PW. Cardiovascular risk factors and venous thromboembolism: a meta-analysis. Circulation. 2008;117(1):93–102.
5. Snell AM. The relation of obesity to fatal post-operative pulmonary embolism. Arch Surg. 1927;15:237–44.
6. Hansson PO, Eriksson H, Welin L, Svardsudd K, Wilhelmsen L. Smoking and abdominal obesity: risk factors for venous thromboembolism among middle-aged men: "the study of men born in 1913". Arch Intern Med. 1999;159(16):1886–90.
7. Pannacciulli N, De Mitrio V, Marino R, Giorgino R, De Pergola G. Effect of glucose tolerance status on PAI-1 plasma levels in overweight and obese subjects. Obes Res. 2002;10(8):717–25.
8. Juhan-Vague I, Alessi MC, Mavri A, Morange PE. Plasminogen activator inhibitor-1, inflammation, obesity, insulin resistance and vascular risk. J Thromb Haemost. 2003;1(7):1575–9.
9. Alessi MC, Peiretti F, Morange P, Henry M, Nalbone G, Juhan-Vague I. Production of plasminogen activator inhibitor 1 by human adipose tissue: possible link between visceral fat accumulation and vascular disease. Diabetes. 1997;46(5):860–7.
10. Zoccali C, Mallamaci F, Tripepi G. Adipose tissue as a source of inflammatory cytokines in health and disease: focus on end-stage renal disease. Kidney Int Suppl. 2003;63(84):S65–8.
11. Bara L, Nicaud V, Tiret L, Cambien F, Samama MM. Expression of a paternal history of premature myocardial infarction on fibrinogen, factor VIIC and PAI-1 in European offspring—the EARS study. European Atherosclerosis Research Study Group. Thromb Haemost. 1994;71(4):434–40.
12. Duncan BB, Schmidt MI, Chambless LE, Folsom AR, Carpenter M, Heiss G. Fibrinogen, other putative markers of inflammation, and weight gain in middle-aged adults—the ARIC study. Atherosclerosis Risk in Communities. Obes Res. 2000;8(4):279–86.
13. Friedman JM, Halaas JL. Leptin and the regulation of body weight in mammals. Nature. 1998;395(6704):763–70.
14. Caro JF, Sinha MK, Kolaczynski JW, Zhang PL, Considine RV. Leptin: the tale of an obesity gene. Diabetes. 1996;45(11):1455–62.
15. Singh P, Peterson TE, Barber KR, Kuniyoshi FS, Jensen A, Hoffmann M, et al. Leptin upregulates the expression of plasminogen activator inhibitor-1 in human vascular endothelial cells. Biochem Biophys Res Commun. 2010;392(1):47–52.
16. Mertens I, Van Gaal LF. Obesity, haemostasis and the fibrinolytic system. Obes Rev. 2002;3(2):85–101.
17. Folsom AR, Qamhieh HT, Wing RR, Jeffery RW, Stinson VL, Kuller LH, et al. Impact of weight loss on plasminogen activator inhibitor (PAI-1), factor VII, and other hemostatic factors in moderately overweight adults. Arterioscler Thromb. 1993;13(2):162–9.
18. Rissanen P, Vahtera E, Krusius T, Uusitupa M, Rissanen A. Weight change and blood coagulability and fibrinolysis in healthy obese women. Int J Obes Relat Metab Disord. 2001;25(2):212–8.
19. Wu EC, Barba CA. Current practices in the prophylaxis of venous thromboembolism in bariatric surgery. Obes Surg. 2000;10(1):7–13; discussion 14.
20. Barba CA, Harrington C, Loewen M. Status of venous thromboembolism prophylaxis among bariatric surgeons: have we changed our practice during the past decade? Surg Obes Relat Dis. 2009;5(3):352–6.
21. Quebbemann B, Akhondzadeh M, Dallal R. Continuous intravenous heparin infusion prevents peri-operative thromboembolic events in bariatric surgery patients. Obes Surg. 2005;15(9):1221–4.
22. Scholten DJ, Hoedema RM, Scholten SE. A comparison of two different prophylactic dose regimens of low molecular weight heparin in bariatric surgery. Obes Surg. 2002;12(1):19–24.
23. Escalante-Tattersfield T, Tucker O, Fajnwaks P, Szomstein S, Rosenthal RJ. Incidence of deep vein thrombosis in morbidly obese patients undergoing laparoscopic Roux-en-Y gastric bypass. Surg Obes Relat Dis. 2008;4(2):126–30.
24. Kardys CM, Stoner MC, Manwaring ML, Barker M, Macdonald KG, Pender JR, et al. Safety and efficacy of intravascular ultrasound-guided inferior vena cava filter in super obese bariatric patients. Surg Obes Relat Dis. 2008;4(1):50–4.
25. Rocha AT, de Vasconcellos AG, da Luz Neto ER, Araujo DM, Alves ES, Lopes AA. Risk of venous thromboembolism and efficacy of thromboprophylaxis in hospitalized obese medical patients and in obese patients undergoing bariatric surgery. Obes Surg. 2006;16(12):1645–55.
26. Andersen T, Juhl E, Quaade F. Fatal outcome after jejunoileal bypass for obesity. Am J Surg. 1981;142(5):619–21.
27. Melinek J, Livingston E, Cortina G, Fishbein MC. Autopsy findings following gastric bypass surgery for morbid obesity. Arch Pathol Lab Med. 2002;126(9):1091–5.
28. Hamad GG, Choban PS. Enoxaparin for thromboprophylaxis in morbidly obese patients undergoing bariatric surgery: findings of the prophylaxis against VTE outcomes in bariatric surgery patients receiving enoxaparin (PROBE) study. Obes Surg. 2005;15(10):1368–74.
29. Huber O, Bounameaux H, Borst F, Rohner A. Postoperative pulmonary embolism after hospital discharge. An underestimated risk. Arch Surg. 1992;127(3):310–3.
30. Scurr JH, Coleridge-Smith PD, Hasty JH. Deep venous thrombosis: a continuing problem. BMJ. 1988;297(6640):28.
31. Kalfarentzos F, Stavropoulou F, Yarmenitis S, Kehagias I, Karamesini M, Dimitrakopoulos A, et al. Prophylaxis of venous thromboembolism using two different doses of low-molecular-weight heparin (nadroparin) in bariatric surgery: a prospective randomized trial. Obes Surg. 2001;11(6):670–6.
32. Kothari SN, Lambert PJ, Mathiason MA. Best Poster Award. A comparison of thromboembolic and bleeding events following laparoscopic gastric bypass in patients treated with prophylactic regimens of unfractionated heparin or enoxaparin. Am J Surg. 2007;194(6):709–11.
33. Frantzides CT, Welle SN, Ruff TM, Frantzides AT. Routine anticoagulation for venous thromboembolism prevention following laparoscopic gastric bypass. JSLS. 2012;16(1):33–7.
34. Clements RH, Yellumahanthi K, Ballem N, Wesley M, Bland KI. Pharmacologic prophylaxis against venous thromboembolic complications is not mandatory for all laparoscopic Roux-en-Y gastric bypass procedures. J Am Coll Surg. 2009;208(5):917–21; discussion 921-3.

35. Miller MT, Rovito PF. An approach to venous thromboembolism prophylaxis in laparoscopic Roux-en-Y gastric bypass surgery. Obes Surg. 2004;14(6):731–7.

36. Simoneau MD, Vachon A, Picard F. Effect of prophylactic dalteparin on anti-factor Xa levels in morbidly obese patients after bariatric surgery. Obes Surg. 2010;20(4):487–91.

37. Simone EP, Madan AK, Tichansky DS, Kuhl DA, Lee MD. Comparison of two low-molecular-weight heparin dosing regimens for patients undergoing laparoscopic bariatric surgery. Surg Endosc. 2008;22(11):2392–5.

38. Omalu BI, Ives DG, Buhari AM, Lindner JL, Schauer PR, Wecht CH, et al. Death rates and causes of death after bariatric surgery for Pennsylvania residents, 1995 to 2004. Arch Surg. 2007;142(10):923–8; discussion 929.

39. Linsenmaier U, Rieger J, Schenk F, Rock C, Mangel E, Pfeifer KJ. Indications, management, and complications of temporary inferior vena cava filters. Cardiovasc Intervent Radiol. 1998;21(6):464–9.

40. Decousus H, Leizorovicz A, Parent F, Page Y, Tardy B, Girard P, et al. A clinical trial of vena caval filters in the prevention of pulmonary embolism in patients with proximal deep-vein thrombosis. Prevention du Risque d'Embolie Pulmonaire par Interruption Cave Study Group. N Engl J Med. 1998;338(7):409–15.

41. PREPIC Study Group. Eight-year follow-up of patients with permanent vena cava filters in the prevention of pulmonary embolism: the PREPIC (Prevention du Risque d'Embolie Pulmonaire par Interruption Cave) randomized study. Circulation. 2005;112(3):416–22.

42. Keeling WB, Haines K, Stone PA, Armstrong PA, Murr MM, Shames ML. Current indications for preoperative inferior vena cava filter insertion in patients undergoing surgery for morbid obesity. Obes Surg. 2005;15(7):1009–12.

43. Obeid FN, Bowling WM, Fike JS, Durant JA. Efficacy of prophylactic inferior vena cava filter placement in bariatric surgery. Surg Obes Relat Dis. 2007;3(6):606–8; discussion 609–10.

44. Schuster R, Hagedorn JC, Curet MJ, Morton JM. Retrievable inferior vena cava filters may be safely applied in gastric bypass surgery. Surg Endosc. 2007;21(12):2277–9.

45. Trigilio-Black CM, Ringley CD, McBride CL, Sorensen VJ, Thompson JS, Longo GM, et al. Inferior vena cava filter placement for pulmonary embolism risk reduction in super morbidly obese undergoing bariatric surgery. Surg Obes Relat Dis. 2007;3(4):461–4.

46. Rajasekhar A, Crowther M. Inferior vena caval filter insertion prior to bariatric surgery: a systematic review of the literature. J Thromb Haemost. 2010;8(6):1266–70.

47. Frezza EE, Wachtel MS. A simple venous thromboembolism prophylaxis protocol for patients undergoing bariatric surgery. Obesity (Silver Spring). 2006;14(11):1961–5.

48. Gargiulo 3rd NJ, O'Connor DJ, Veith FJ, Lipsitz EC, Vemulapalli P, Gibbs K, et al. Long-term outcome of inferior vena cava filter placement in patients undergoing gastric bypass. Ann Vasc Surg. 2010;24(7):946–9.

49. Halmi D, Kolesnikov E. Preoperative placement of retreivable inferior vena cava filters in bariatric surgery. Surg Obes Relat Dis. 2007;3(6):602–5.

50. Overby DW, Kohn GP, Cahan MA, Dixon RG, Stavas JM, Moll S, et al. Risk-group targeted inferior vena cava filter placement in gastric bypass patients. Obes Surg. 2009;19(4):451–5.

51. Piano G, Ketteler ER, Prachand V, Devalk E, Van Ha TG, Gewertz BL, et al. Safety, feasibility, and outcome of retrievable vena cava filters in high-risk surgical patients. J Vasc Surg. 2007;45(4):784–8; discussion 788.

52. Vaziri K, Bhanot P, Hungness ES, Morasch MD, Prystowsky JB, Nagle AP. Retrievable inferior vena cava filters in high-risk patients undergoing bariatric surgery. Surg Endosc. 2009;23(10):2203–7.

53. Birkmeyer NJ, Share D, Baser O, Carlin AM, Finks JF, Pesta CM, et al. Preoperative placement of inferior vena cava filters and outcomes after gastric bypass surgery. Ann Surg. 2010;252(2):313–8.

54. Rajasekhar A, Crowther MA. ASH evidence-based guidelines: what is the role of inferior vena cava filters in the perioperative prevention of venous thromboembolism in bariatric surgery patients? Hematology Am Soc Hematol Educ Program. 2009;302–304.

55. Agarwal R, Hecht TE, Lazo MC, Umscheid CA. Venous thromboembolism prophylaxis for patients undergoing bariatric surgery: a systematic review. Surg Obes Relat Dis. 2010;6(2):213–20.

56. Gonzalez QH, Tishler DS, Plata-Munoz JJ, Bondora A, Vickers SM, Leath T, et al. Incidence of clinically evident deep venous thrombosis after laparoscopic Roux-en-Y gastric bypass. Surg Endosc. 2004;18(7):1082–4.

57. Brasileiro AL, Miranda Jr F, Ettinger JE, Castro AA, Pitta GB, de Moura LK, et al. Incidence of lower limbs deep vein thrombosis after open and laparoscopic gastric bypass: a prospective study. Obes Surg. 2008;18(1):52–7.

58. Abou-Nukta F, Alkhoury F, Arroyo K, Bakhos C, Gutweiler J, Reinhold R, et al. Clinical pulmonary embolus after gastric bypass surgery. Surg Obes Relat Dis. 2006;2(1):24–8; discussion 29.

59. Forestieri P, Quarto G, De Caterina M, Cuocolo A, Pilone V, Formato A, et al. Prophylaxis of thromboembolism in bariatric surgery with parnaparin. Obes Surg. 2007;17(12):1558–62.

60. Cotter SA, Cantrell W, Fisher B, Shopnick R. Efficacy of venous thromboembolism prophylaxis in morbidly obese patients undergoing gastric bypass surgery. Obes Surg. 2005;15(9):1316–20.

61. Shepherd MF, Rosborough TK, Schwartz ML. Heparin thromboprophylaxis in gastric bypass surgery. Obes Surg. 2003;13(2):249–53.

62. Shepherd MF, Rosborough TK, Schwartz ML. Unfractionated heparin infusion for thromboprophylaxis in highest risk gastric bypass surgery. Obes Surg. 2004;14(5):601–5.

63. Cossu ML, Pilo L, Piseddu G, Tilocca PL, Cossu F, Noya G. Prophylaxis of venous thromboembolism in bariatric surgery. Chir Ital. 2007;59(3):331–5.

64. Prystowsky JB, Morasch MD, Eskandari MK, Hungness ES, Nagle AP. Prospective analysis of the incidence of deep venous thrombosis in bariatric surgery patients. Surgery. 2005;138(4):759–63; discussion 763–5.

65. Gonzalez R, Haines K, Nelson LG, Gallagher SF, Murr MM. Predictive factors of thromboembolic events in patients undergoing Roux-en-Y gastric bypass. Surg Obes Relat Dis. 2006;2(1):30–5; discussion 35–6.

66. Gould MK, Garcia DA, Wren SM, Karanicolas PJ, Arcelus JI, Heit JA, Samama CM. American college of chest physicians. Prevention of VTE in nonorthopedic surgical patients. Antithrombotic therapy and prevention of thrombosis, 9th ed: American college of chest physicians evidence-based clinical practice guidelines. Chest. 2012;141(2 Suppl):e227S–77S.

67. Clinical Issues Committee of the American Society for Metabolic and Bariatric Surgery. Prophylactic measures to reduce the risk of venous thromboembolism in bariatric surgery patients. Surg Obes Relat Dis. 2007;3(5):494–5.

68. Lensing AW, Prandoni P, Brandjes D, Huisman PM, Vigo M, Tomasella G, et al. Detection of deep-vein thrombosis by real-time B-mode ultrasonography. N Engl J Med. 1989;320(6):342–5.

69. Birdwell BG, Raskob GE, Whitsett TL, Durica SS, Comp PC, George JN, et al. The clinical validity of normal compression ultrasonography in outpatients suspected of having deep venous thrombosis. Ann Intern Med. 1998;128(1):1–7.

70. Meyer G, Tamisier D, Sors H, Stern M, Vouhe P, Makowski S, et al. Pulmonary embolectomy: a 20-year experience at one center. Ann Thorac Surg. 1991;51(2):232–6.

41
Role of Flexible Endoscopy in the Practice of Bariatric Surgery

Andrea Zelisko and Matthew Kroh

Abbreviations

AGB   Adjustable gastric banding
BMI   Body mass index
BPD/DS   Biliopancreatic diversion with and without duodenal switch
CT   Computed tomography
EEA   End-to-end anastomosis
ERCP   Endoscopic retrograde cholangiopancreatography
GERD   Gastroesophageal reflux disease
GI   Gastrointestinal
GP   Gastric plication
IOP   Incisionless Operating Platform
PEG   Percutaneous endoscopic gastrostomy
RYGB   Roux-en-Y gastric bypass
SG   Sleeve gastrectomy
TTS   Through-the-scope
VBG   Vertical banded gastroplasty

Introduction

The burden of obesity continues to increase in the United States and worldwide. Surgical intervention has been demonstrated as an effective long-term treatment for obesity and obesity-related health comorbidities. Due to this, the number of bariatric procedures performed in the last decade has increased significantly and there has also been a shift in the type of procedures performed. Currently, the most commonly performed bariatric procedures include Roux-en-Y gastric bypass (RYGB), sleeve gastrectomy (SG), and adjustable gastric banding (AGB) [1, 2]. Other procedures less commonly performed include biliopancreatic diversion with and without duodenal switch (BPD/DS), vertical banded

gastroplasty (VBG), and gastric plication (GP). Other historical bariatric surgical procedures, such as a jejunoileal bypass and horizontal gastroplasty, are no longer performed due to complications and lack of efficacy, respectively, but patients that have previously undergone these operations may present for evaluation. Consideration of the types of procedures performed, both anatomically and physiologically, is critical in evaluating patients pre- and postoperatively. Surgeons and physicians caring for bariatric surgery patients need to understand the anatomical changes as a result of such operations and how these changes relate to the mechanisms of weight loss. Furthermore, it is imperative to recognize the expected complications and long-term out comes for these patients.

Flexible endoscopy is an increasingly valuable tool in managing bariatric surgery patients. Flexible upper endoscopy has roles in the evaluation, management, and treatment of patients undergoing all types of bariatric surgical procedures. Endoscopists that evaluate bariatric patients may include bariatric surgeons, general surgeons, gastroenterologists, and other physicians that incorporate these procedures into their practices. However, as a bariatric surgeon, one should give strong consideration to being adept with flexible upper endoscopy for use in the work-up and management of patients. Bariatric surgeons have the advantage of knowing the specific surgical details of each bariatric operation, and often they are the practitioners performing the procedure on the patient they are evaluating or treating.

The evolution of flexible endoscopy has allowed for both diagnostic and therapeutic procedures. Newer endoscopic technologies have been developed to enhance medical care, reduce costs, and also improve patient satisfaction. Such examples include: disposable endoscopy, capsule endoscopy, 3D endoscopy, and advanced endoluminal procedures including clipping, stent placement, and suturing devices.

The following chapter addresses applications of flexible upper endoscopy in bariatric surgery patients during the pre-, intra-, and postoperative periods and the unique clinical and technical considerations during these periods.

Electronic supplementary material: Supplementary material is available in the online version of this chapter at 10.1007/978-1-4939-1637-5_41. Videos can also be accessed at http://www.springerimages.com/videos/978-1-4939-1636-8.

Preoperative Assessment and Management

The preoperative use of flexible upper endoscopy to evaluate a patient prior to bariatric surgery is typically based on the presence of foregut gastrointestinal (GI) symptoms. The most common symptoms are reflux, dyspepsia, dysphagia, and abdominal pain. In non-bariatric patients who present with upper GI symptoms, the guidelines for the utilization of upper endoscopy are well described [3, 4], and these recommendations can similarly be applied to the preoperative bariatric surgery patient. However, as many of the bariatric operations either alter the anatomy of patients or alter the physiologic mechanisms of the GI tract, there may be benefit to a more frequent use of preoperative endoscopy in bariatric patients. The anatomic alterations caused by an RYGB or BPD/DS create challenges in postoperative endoscopic evaluation of the distal stomach, duodenum, and biliary tree, as these areas are difficult to assess with standard endoscopic techniques after surgery. Utilizing endoscopy prior to surgery may eliminate or reduce the need to access these difficult anatomic locations. Early identification of patients at higher risk for postoperative complications may alter their treatment plan and possibly modify the choice of bariatric operation.

Though not widely implemented, there is evidence to support routine use of endoscopy before bariatric surgery in asymptomatic patients. Many obese individuals with esophageal dysmotility, reflux, or other upper GI pathology are asymptomatic or have atypical symptoms. These patients may present with chest pain, cough, or asthma. A recent study demonstrated that 71 % of patients with documented manometric esophageal motility disorders prior to bariatric surgery were asymptomatic [5]. Kuper and associates reported that 80 % of patients who underwent routine preoperative endoscopy had pathologic findings, and only 20 % of these patients had any symptoms [6]. Furthermore, there is a high prevalence of GI pathology in obese individuals. In support of this finding, a meta-analysis revealed that obesity alone was associated with a significantly increased risk of gastroesophageal reflux disease (GERD), erosive esophagitis, and esophageal adenocarcinoma [7]. Through the use of routine endoscopy in all preoperative patients, multiple studies confirm the high prevalence of GI disorders in obese patients (Table 1) [6, 8–12].

Identification of anatomic defects or upper GI pathology in both asymptomatic and symptomatic patients can alter the course of treatment and also the surgical operation. Recommendations for upper endoscopy in all patients prior to bariatric surgery, regardless of the presence of symptoms, have already been suggested by guidelines outside of the United States [13]. A study conducted at the University of Virginia examined 667 patients with routine endoscopy prior to surgery; as a result, 4.6 % of patients had their operations altered by the findings from endoscopy [14]. The most common alteration in this cohort was the addition of a remnant gastrostomy tube based on preoperative endoscopic findings of the distal stomach. Another study of 447 patients demonstrated that preoperative endoscopy changed medical management prior to surgery in 18 % of patients but only altered or postponed surgery in <1 % [8]. Common findings by upper endoscopy that may impact the choice of operation or preoperative management include: esophagitis, GERD, ulcers, *Helicobacter pylori*, hiatal hernia, cancer, and polyps. Sharaf and colleagues retrospectively reviewed records of patients that were endoscopically evaluated prior to surgery and demonstrated that out of 195 patients, 89.7 % had one or more lesions, and of these, 61.5 % were clinically significant [15]. Biopsies for *H. pylori* should be obtained during endoscopy, especially in the presence of gastritis, and treated if positive. Studies have demonstrated a lower rate of marginal ulcers and foregut symptoms after bariatric surgery in patients that were either *H. pylori* negative or had been tested and treated [14, 16].

The utilization of preoperative flexible endoscopy is essential in the evaluation of patients prior to revisional bariatric surgery. Operative records should be reviewed before intervention, but specific anatomic constructs may not be accurately described in the report or the original operative reports may not be available. The indications for reoperation vary, and they often involve poor or failed weight loss, acute symptoms, or complications from the primary operation. This type of patient can present with complex problems and variable anatomy. Determination of the anatomy, assessment of the anastomoses and staple lines, and identification of any upper GI pathology will dictate the appropriate surgical intervention.

TABLE 1. Prevalence of pathologic findings during preoperative upper endoscopy in bariatric patients

Source	Year	No. of patients	Mean BMI (kg/m^2)	Prevalence of pathologic findings on endoscopy (%)
Madan et al. [10]	2004	102	48.2	91.0
Loewen et al. [8]	2008	448	48.6	29.2
de Moura Almeida et al. [9]	2008	162	44.1	77.2
Munoz et al. [12]	2009	626	42.0	46.0
Kuper et al. [6]	2010	69	47.6	79.7
Dietz et al. [11]	2012	126	51.2	57.9

BMI body mass index

Flexible upper endoscopy traditionally examines the mucosa of the upper GI tract and allows biopsies for histologic diagnosis. Supplemental techniques, such as the use of a pH probe and manometry, can provide further objective measures to evaluate a patient and determine treatment. In addition, radiographic studies may enhance medical decisions when used in combination with endoscopy. An upper GI series and a barium esophagram are two such examples. In a retrospective series of patients presenting for weight regain after previous bariatric surgery, Brethauer et al. demonstrated that the use of both endoscopy and upper GI series allowed for the detection of abnormalities in 90 % of patients [17].

Intraoperative Management and Techniques

Applications of endoscopy during bariatric surgery vary depending on the operation and technique. It has been described in the literature for many intraoperative applications, including identification of anatomy and inspection of surgical technique, and is also widely practiced.

For RYGB, different techniques have been described for the creation of the gastrojejunostomy, some utilizing endoscopy. Wittgrove and Clark described the use of endoscopy to pass the anvil of an end-to-end anastomosis (EEA) stapler into the gastric pouch during an RYGB [18]. Initial concerns for perforation with transoral passage of the anvil led to modifications in this technique, including manipulating the anvil to facilitate passage and also the development of a pre-tilted anvil [19]. Endoscopy also has a role in SG, and although sizing of the gastric tube is often done by means of a bougie, Diamantis and colleagues reported their experience of using an endoscope to perform a laparoscopic SG safely and effectively [20].

Anastomotic integrity is vital for a successful outcome and is often evaluated endoscopically at the time of operation. Failure to identify anastomotic leaks imposes significant morbidity [21]. Methylene blue dye injected near the gastrojejunal anastomosis via a nasogastric tube can identify leaks intraoperatively, and it has been used successfully in clinical practice. Unfortunately, positive leak tests stain the operative field, prohibit repeat exams, and may not precisely identify the area of leakage. Intraoperative endoscopy may circumvent these pitfalls. Endoscopy allows for visualization of the GI tract, for direct placement of the endoscope near the anastomosis or staple line, and for multiple leak tests since it does not utilize methylene blue dye. It also provides additional information about the pouch size and mucosal perfusion and allows for treatment of bleeding that may occur at staple lines. Intraoperative endoscopy can be used to evaluate both the gastrojejunostomy as well as the jejunojejunostomy. Schauer and colleagues described the use of

endoscopy to evaluate the staple line of all gastrojejunostomies during RYGB as well as to perform a leak test [22]. A leak test is performed by clamping the Roux limb and submerging the gastrojejunal anastomosis and pouch in saline, while the lumen is inflated endoscopically. Leaks may be evidenced as bubbles emanating from a staple line. If a leak is present, it can be directly repaired at that time. The utilization of intraoperative endoscopy identified a 3.7 % anastomotic leak rate in 290 patients in one study [23] and a 4.1 % incidence of intraoperative technical errors in another, including 29 suture and staple line leaks, 2 bougie perforations, 2 inadvertent stoma closures secondary to the suture line, and 1 mucosal perforation in a gastric pacemaker, during 825 bariatric procedures [24]. Alaedeen and colleagues performed a retrospective review of 400 bariatric cases that included intraoperative endoscopy or methylene blue to identify leaks [25]. Postoperatively, all the patients underwent an upper GI series to evaluate for missed leaks, and the reported anastomotic leak rate was significantly lower after the use of endoscopy instead of methylene blue, at 0.4 % vs. 4 %, respectively. Similar techniques can be applied to SG to assess the staple line construction with a leak test, to check for bleeding, and to identify any technical errors such as narrowing at the esophageal–hiatal junction or incisura or endoluminal twisting of the sleeve. A leak test in an SG is performed by clamping proximally to the pylorus and submerging the stomach and staple line in saline while the lumen is inflated.

Endoscopy also serves as a valuable technique when facing challenging surgical cases or when treating complicated patients. Intraoperative endoscopy can be used to control bleeding and to deliver instruments. It can also be used for direct, percutaneous placement of feeding or decompression tubes into the Roux limb if needed.

Intraoperative endoscopy during revisional surgery is often helpful as an adjunct to external, surgical views. Even after extensive preoperative evaluation, intraoperative endoscopy is important to verify the distorted anatomy as well to determine the placement of new anastomoses. Similarly to an initial bariatric operation, endoscopy can be used to assess the integrity of anastomoses and to inspect for bleeding [26]. In reoperative bariatric surgery, a leak test may be performed on the newly revised or created pouch prior to anastomosis creation, evaluating the staple line integrity before committing to an anastomosis, thus allowing for immediate revision if needed. Intraoperative endoscopy during revisional bariatric surgery can also decrease operating times by helping to locate and identify gastrogastric fistulas, stenotic lesions, and gastrojejunal stoma locations [27].

Intraoperative endoscopy can also advance the training of future gastrointestinal and bariatric surgeons. It allows for the development and mastery of endoscopic skills under a structured and supervised setting [28, 29].

Postoperative Management and Techniques

Experience and skill in flexible endoscopy are important to bariatric surgeons in the postoperative period as well. Patients may present with varying symptoms suggestive of postoperative GI pathology or complications that require evaluation. Flexible endoscopy allows visualization of anatomy, identification of pathology, and potential intervention. Furthermore, the utilization of endoscopy by the surgeon who performed the primary operation establishes a unique firsthand knowledge when treating a patient; however, this is not always possible. Physicians unfamiliar with the anatomic changes as a result of bariatric surgery may potentially misinterpret findings on upper endoscopy.

Indications for Endoscopy

Symptoms frequently direct the clinical evaluation of postoperative bariatric surgery patients. Common symptoms include nausea, emesis, abdominal or retrosternal pain, dysphagia, and inadequate weight loss or weight regain [30, 31]. In general, the two most common indications for endoscopy in these patients are the evaluation of symptoms and the treatment of complications. The etiology of symptoms is often multifactorial; however, symptoms are frequently associated with dietary noncompliance and insufficient mastication. Patients with persistent symptoms should be further evaluated as these symptoms may indicate the development of complications after surgery. Patient history may be helpful in differentiating the etiology of pain and may guide patient work-up. Endoscopy is often the preferred diagnostic strategy and can effectively assess mucosal integrity, detect stenosis, and/or exclude other pathologic abnormalities in the surgically altered GI tract. Nausea, emesis, and bloating, with or without abdominal pain, can suggest an obstructive cause (strictures, internal hernias, or bezoars), a marginal ulcer, and band erosion or slippage or be indicative of dumping syndrome [26]. Dysphagia can be caused by esophageal dysmotility or anastomotic stenosis. In a study by Wilson and colleagues, 62 % of patients who were seen with persistent nausea and emesis after RYGB had significant findings of upper endoscopy (ulcers, stomal stenosis, staple line dehiscence) [32]. Retrosternal or abdominal pain may be caused by acid reflux, bile reflux, ulceration, or band erosion and should be evaluated by endoscopy. In addition to endoscopic evaluation, an upper GI contrast series or computed tomography (CT) scan with oral contrast should be considered.

Endoscopic Findings in Normal Postsurgical Anatomy

Roux-en-Y Gastric Bypass—The esophagus and esophagogastric junction should appear normal after an RYGB (Fig. 1a). It is important to limit the amount of air insufflation when evaluating the gastric pouch as it is of variable size. Further, special care should be made to examine the pouch and suture line for fistulas and ulcerations. The gastrojejunostomy will normally have a stoma measuring 10–20 mm in diameter. When an endoscopy is not performed by the surgeon who operated on the patient, variation in surgical technique must be determined and thoroughly identified. There can be variations in the anastomosis of the gastrojejunostomy and also in the length of the Roux limb. The gastrojejunostomy anastomosis is dependent on surgical technique, handsewn or stapled, and also the type of stapler used, circular or linear. Distal to the gastrojejunostomy, a short, blind limb is often seen alongside the efferent jejunal limb, often referred to as a candy cane. The Roux limb length typically ranges from 75 to 150 cm. The jejunojejunostomy may or may not be able to be reached with a standard upper endoscope.

Adjustable Gastric Banding and Vertical Banded Gastroplasty—Endoscopy is relatively straightforward after AGB and VBG. Dependent on the fluid volume in the band, AGB can produce a variable amount of extrinsic circumferential compression on the stomach that can be seen with the endoscope (Fig. 1b). At the time of endoscopy, it is important to determine the length of the pouch above the compression of the band to the gastroesophageal junction in order to assess for pouch dilatation or band slippage. The endoscopist should also evaluate for possible band erosion into the gastric wall. This may best be seen on retroflexion. In a VBG, the lesser curvature channel allows endoscopic visualization of the pouch, and the stoma is typically located 7–8 cm distal to the gastroesophageal junction. The banded portion in a VBG is variable in diameter, and once this area is traversed, the distal stomach and duodenum are accessible. In both procedures, retroflexion of the endoscope within the antrum will reveal the greater curvature and gastric fundus.

Sleeve Gastrectomy—The SG creates a long tubular stomach limited in expansion by a staple line that parallels the lesser curvature. During endoscopy, the staple line should be examined for defects and ulcerations (Fig. 1c). Specific attention should also be paid to patency at the incisura, located approximately midway to 2/3 of the distance to the pylorus from the esophagogastric junction, as well as to twisting of the lumen of the sleeve.

Biliopancreatic Diversion/Duodenal Switch—This procedure is often performed in conjunction with a partial gastrectomy, but it also involves a duodeno-ileal anastomosis that can be visible just distal to an intact gastric pylorus. The ampulla is not available for visualization or for endoscopic retrograde cholangiopancreatography (ERCP) in a standard fashion.

Bariatric Surgery Complications

Complications after bariatric surgery may present early or late in the postoperative course. Studies have reported varying rates of postoperative complications (Table 2) [22, 33–36];

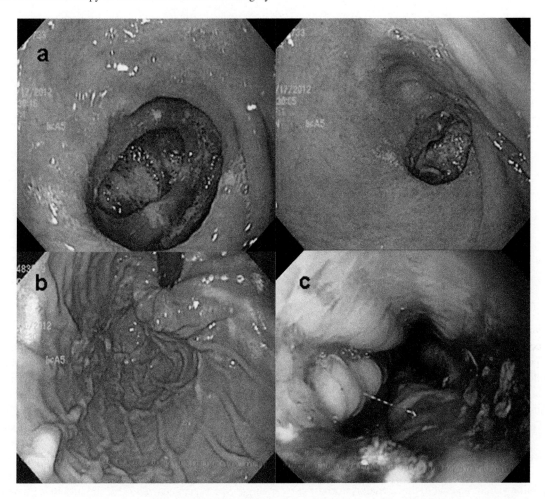

FIG. 1. Endoscopic appearance of (**a**) normal gastrojejunostomy and gastric pouch after gastric bypass, (**b**) normal compression from band seen on retroflexed view after adjustable gastric banding, and (**c**) normal staple line after sleeve gastrectomy.

TABLE 2 Complication rates after bariatric surgery

Source	Year	No. of patients	Late complication rate (%)	Early complication rate (≤30 days) (%)
Schauer et al. [22]	2000	275	47.3	30.5
Weller et al. [34]	2008	19,156	NR[a]	5.0
Encinosa et al. [33][b]	2009	2,522/7,060	41.7/32.8	33.7/25.5
Flum et al. [35]	2009	4,610	NR	4.1
Masoomi et al. [36]	2012	226,043	NR	4.9

[a]*NR* not reported
[b]Two time frames: 2001–2002 and 2005–2006

however, the rate of major adverse postoperative complications has been demonstrated between 4 and 6 % [35, 37]. Early complications such as bleeding, infection, and anastomotic leaks often require surgical intervention [37–39]. Furthermore, if a leak is suspected shortly after surgery, a contrast radiologic study can serve as the initial diagnostic test and is helpful to delineate anatomy. Complications can also develop later in the postoperative period. Late complications, such as ulcers, stenosis, gastrogastric fistulas, obstruction, band slippage or erosion, pouch dilation, and primary weight loss failure or weight regain, can occur with varying rates after any operation;

however, some are more procedure specific (e.g., erosion after adjustable gastric banding). Several of these complications can be managed successfully endoscopically.

Endoscopic Management of Postoperative Complications

Marginal Ulcers—Defined as ulcers that occur at the gastrojejunal anastomosis, they can occur in 1–16 % of patients following RYGB [40–43]. Marginal ulcers typically present with

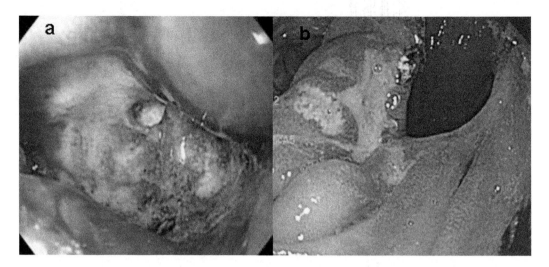

Fig. 2. (**a**) Endoscopic view of large marginal ulcer and (**b**) retroflexed view of marginal ulcer.

epigastric or abdominal pain, bleeding, or nausea, although they may be asymptomatic [32]. Ulceration can occur at any time postoperatively, but most ulcers occur in the first several months following surgery [44]. In a study conducted on all patients who underwent bariatric surgery, postoperative endoscopic examination 1 month after surgery demonstrated ulcers in 4.1 % of patients after open RYGB and in 12.3 % of patients after laparoscopic RYGB. 28 % of the demonstrated ulcers occurred in the absence of symptoms [45]. Marginal ulcers are frequently located on the jejunal side of the anastomosis, so careful attention should be paid to this area during endoscopy (Fig. 2). When possible, a retroflexed view can identify a potentially missed location of an ulcer. Even though the exact etiology is unknown, ulcers may result from gastric acidity (due to staple line dehiscence or gastrogastric fistula), pouch orientation and size (that may incorporate a greater parietal cell mass), *H. pylori* infection, the presence of staples and suture material (inciting a localized inflammatory reaction), and local ischemia and tension at the anastomosis [41, 44, 46]. Smoking and nonsteroidal anti-inflammatory drug use increase the risk of marginal ulcers, and the use of proton pump inhibitors appears to decrease risk [1].

The role of endoscopy for marginal ulcers is primarily diagnostic with limited therapeutic use. When identified during endoscopy, the pouch must be carefully examined for a fistula. Staple line dehiscence and the formation of a gastrogastric fistula can result in an increase in acid exposure in the pouch, stoma, and jejunum and make the mucosa more vulnerable to damage [26]. One study reported that stomal ulcers were associated with gastrogastric fistula in as many as 65 % of cases [46]. Ulcers may also represent foreign body reactions to sutures or staples, and judicious removal of foreign material with endoscopic tools may cause ulcer resolution [30]. If marginal ulcerations are not associated with staple line dehiscence or foreign body reaction, the management includes evaluation of the pouch for *H. pylori* status, proton

pump inhibitor therapy, and liquid sucralfate and the elimination of ulcerogenic medication [38]. If marginal ulcers are severe and persist despite these measures, surgical revision may be required to prevent complications such as perforation, recurrent bleeding, and anastomotic strictures.

Stenosis—Luminal stenosis or stricture is an important complication of bariatric surgery. After RYGB, postoperative stricture formation is around 3 % [28]. The gastrojejunal anastomosis is the most common site of stenosis after bariatric surgery and has been reported in 5.1–6.8 % of patients after laparoscopic RYGB, typically within the first year [30]. Other locations where stenosis can develop include the gastric band, site of passage through the mesocolon, jejunojejunal anastomosis, and at adhesions. Anastomotic strictures are defined as anastomoses that are smaller than 10 mm in diameter [1]. Stenosis may arise from ischemia or ulceration, but the rates of stenosis are also somewhat technique dependent; the use of circular staplers has a higher rate of stricture than hand-sewn or linear staplers. Also, the use of 25 mm circular stapler reduced the rates of stricture when compared to the use of a 21 mm circular stapler [47]. Patients may present postoperatively with nausea, emesis, dysphagia, malnourishment, or unhealthy weight loss. Stenosis can be diagnosed by contrast radiography, but direct endoscopic visualization is preferable because it has high sensitivity and therapeutic measures can be performed (Fig. 3) [48]. Typical findings on endoscopy include a narrowed orifice precluding the passage of the endoscope; however, other potential findings include gastric pouch dilatation, undigested food, or foreign material [49].

Endoscopic treatment of strictures can be safely and effectively performed by using through-the-scope (TTS) balloon dilators or wire-guided bougie dilators [30, 50, 51]. Although initial success rates of up to 93 % have been reported, management may require multiple dilations. The length of time from surgery to stricture formation and the diameter achieved

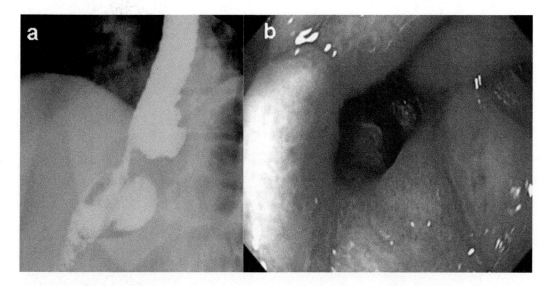

Fig. 3. (a) Radiographic evidence of a stricture and (b) endoscopic appearance of stenosis after gastric bypass.

with the first dilation procedure are significant predictors of the need for further dilations [52]. Repeat dilation with progressively larger balloons may also be required to achieve more durable results, and gradual dilations over multiple sessions may reduce the risk of perforation [53, 54]. Even still, some stenoses cannot be sufficiently dilated, and these patients will require surgical revision. Overaggressive dilation should be avoided, not only to reduce perforation risk, but also because dumping symptoms and weight regain can occur [49]. There have been reports of successful dilation up to 20 mm [55] without weight regain, but data is controversial on dilation greater than 15 mm, and many authors recommend against it [49]. When standard dilation is unsuccessful, additional strategies can be utilized such as the removal of exposed sutures with endoscopic scissors, injection at the anastomosis with saline or steroids after dilation, needle-knife electrocautery of scar tissue, or even argon plasma coagulation combined with diathermy [26, 30, 56].

Stenosis following AGB may be due to fibrosis of gastric tissue in the region of the band, formation of adhesions, or band angulation or slippage. Endoscopic dilation may be effective when the cause is fibrosis or adhesions but is rarely useful in the setting of band angulation or rotation [26]. Such patients should not have repeated dilations but instead treated surgically with either band removal, removal and replacement, or conversion to another procedure. After a VBG, stenosis is usually the result of stricturing and scarring of the outflow tract in the proximal stomach and thus the creation of a hypertrophic scar or frank erosion. The incidence of stricture has been reported at 13 % [57]. Endoscopic balloon dilation is not durable in the long term but may transiently alleviate symptoms [58]. Operative revision is typically required due to the fixed nature of the mesh band or for erosion into the lumen.

Stenosis can occur after SG with an incidence that ranges from 0.2 to 4 % [59]. Strictures have a higher occurrence with the use of a smaller bougie size and a tighter sleeve. They are generally seen in the proximal to mid stomach, at the incisura, or at the esophagogastric junction. The incisura is a common spot of narrowing resulting from stapling too close to the lesser curvature. Management options of strictures and stenosis after SG include: observation, endoscopic dilation with or without stent placement, seromyotomy, and conversion to RYGB. If endoscopic dilation has failed for 6 weeks, reoperation is typically recommended [60]. After SG, torsion or rotation of the remnant sleeve may present similarly to a stenosis with obstructive symptomatology and can be managed with dilation, myotomy, or revisional surgery.

Gastrointestinal Bleeding—Bleeding in patients after bariatric surgery may be acute or chronic or present as an iron deficiency anemia [61]. Bleeding can occur anywhere in the GI tract, including in the biliopancreatic limb and remnant stomach after an RYGB. Significant upper GI bleeding occurs in about 1–4 % of patients after RYGB [62], about 0.1 % after AGB [63, 64], and between 1 and 2 % after a sleeve gastrectomy [65, 66]. Patients with signs or symptoms of acute or chronic bleeding should be evaluated with endoscopy, preferably in close consultation with a surgeon, should complications arise or endoscopic interventions fail [62, 67]. The benefit of endoscopy is the ability to provide diagnosis and treatment simultaneously. However, endoscopy in the early postoperative period may be challenging, especially after RYGB and BPD because of the inaccessibility of the biliopancreatic limb, remnant stomach, and the jejunojejunostomy and the potential risks associated with early postoperative endoscopy such as perforation at the surgical anastomoses [68]. If more advanced endoscopic techniques, such as double-balloon enteroscopy, are unsuccessful at

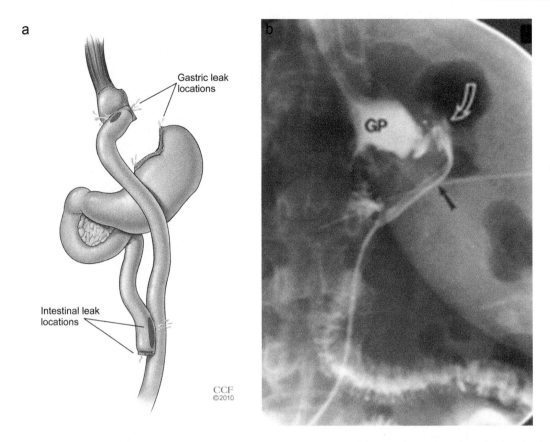

Fig. 4. (**a**) Illustration of common leak locations after Roux-en-Y gastric bypass (RYGB). (**b**) Upper gastrointestinal study showing leak at gastrojejunal anastomosis after RYGB (*white arrow* pointing at leak). Reprinted with permission, Cleveland Clinic Center for Medical Art & Photography © 2010–2013. All Rights Reserved.

accessing the bypassed anatomy, access may be gained through a surgically created gastrostomy [69]. Endoscopy after an SG, VBG, and AGB is relatively straightforward, and standard flexible upper endoscopy is usually sufficient for the management of endoluminal bleeding in this situation.

Numerous approaches for treating active upper GI bleeds have been described in the literature. Techniques that involve the use of thermal energy (electrocoagulation, heater probe, and argon plasma coagulation), mechanical application of clips, and local injections with epinephrine, sclerosants, and thrombin/fibrin glue have all been successfully reported [70]. A retrospective review of 933 patients after RYGB reported a 3.2 % incidence of postoperative hemorrhage and an 80 % rate of successful endoscopic intervention [71]. Bleeding after an SG tends to occur at the staple line and is usually self-limited. Rarely, the use of endoscopy to suction out or push out a blood clot may be necessary [66].

Leaks and Fistulas—Gastric leaks and fistulas are potentially serious complications of bariatric surgery and cause significant morbidity. Overall, the occurrence of leaks is between 0.4 and 6 % in gastric bypass patients [24, 50, 72] and is 2.4 % in SG patients [73]. High-volume centers tend

to report anastomotic leak rates of less than 2 % [24, 74, 75]. Identification of a leak in the immediate postoperative period suggests that either an intraoperative leak test with endoscopy missed the defect or that the leak developed after the completion of the operation. Staple line disruption can result in extraluminal leaks or eventually gastrogastric fistulas (most common type). Extraluminal leaks tend to present early in the postoperative period and can result in peritonitis, abscess, sepsis, organ failure, and even death [30, 76]. After RYGB, most leaks occur at the gastrojejunal anastomosis followed by the remnant stomach; leaks at the jejunojejunal anastomosis are rare but do occur and usually need reoperation (Fig. 4a). After SG, leaks are typically found in the proximal third of the stomach and specifically at the areas of the esophagogastric junction [73]. Upper GI studies are typically used to diagnose extraluminal leaks (Fig. 4b). CT scans are another common imaging modality used to examine the anatomy of the anastomoses and staple lines. Typically, leaks with clinical signs of sepsis require operative repair, drainage of infection, and establishment of enteral access. Endoscopy has an adjunct role in the operating room, for example, to define the precise location of the leak and, increasingly, to be used as a therapeutic measure. There have

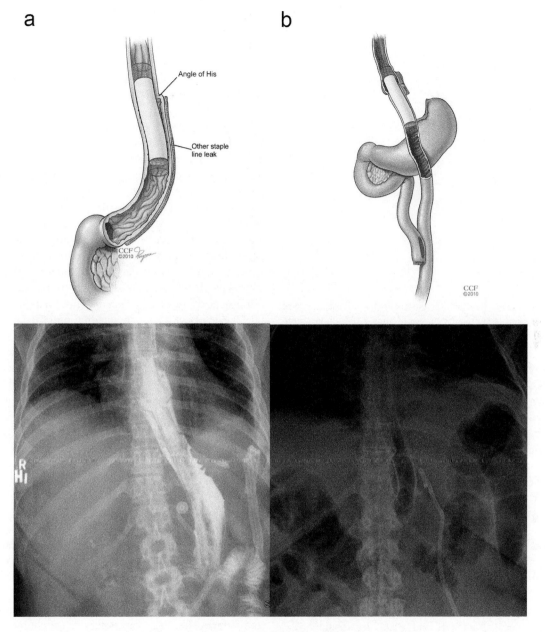

FIG. 5. (**a**) Sleeve gastrectomy with stent and radiographic appearance of stent after placement. (**b**) Roux-en-Y gastric bypass with stent and radiographic appearance of stent. Reprinted with permission, Cleveland Clinic Center for Medical Art & Photography © 2010–2013. All Rights Reserved.

been small series that have described endoscopic management of leaks using partially covered self-expanding metal stents, Polyflex stents, argon plasma coagulation, endoscopic clips, and fibrin glue [77, 78]. Merrifield and colleagues reported successfully treating three patients with leaks endoscopically and concluded that endoscopy may be a feasible, less invasive alternative to surgical repair [77]. A study at the Cleveland Clinic, which used three different types of stents for the management of anastomotic complications after bariatric surgery (a prototype salivary stent, a partially or fully covered self-expanding metal stent, and a silicone-coated

polyester stent), demonstrated that endoscopic stent placement successfully resolved anastomotic leaks in 85 % of patients (Fig. 5) [79]. Such novel methods are still currently investigational, and further research is needed to define the role of endoscopy to treat postoperative anastomotic leaks.

Chronic fistulas may be found in the presence of marginal ulcers or as a result of staple line disruption. Staple line dehiscence after SG has been reported at rates ranging from 0.3 to 5 % [80]. Patients with a chronic fistula may present with nausea, emesis, epigastric pain, and weight gain. However, many fistulas may remain subclinical, and the true

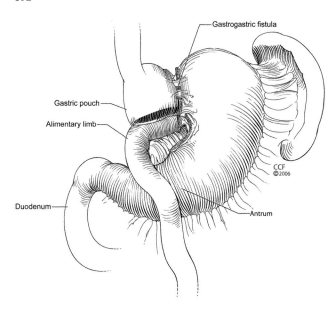

Gastrogastric fistula

Gastric pouch

Alimentary limb

Duodenum

Antrum

CCF
©2006

FIG. 6. Gastrogastric fistula after gastric bypass. Reprinted with permission, Cleveland Clinic Center for Medical Art & Photography © 2010–2013. All Rights Reserved.

incidence is not entirely known [41]. Fistulas, similar to acute leaks, are typically diagnosed with upper GI series. A large fistula may also be visualized by endoscopy. A gastrogastric fistula is the most common type and is depicted in Fig. 6. Surgery is the mainstay of treatment, but techniques of endoscopic management are being actively investigated [81]. For example, endoscopic treatment of postoperative fistulas has been accomplished with self-expanding stents and endoscopic suturing and clipping [82–85]. Successful closure of gastrocutaneous fistulas after VBG and BPD using endoscopic fibrin sealant injection has also been reported [86]. Although these techniques are feasible, long-term durability is dependent on fistula size, with large fistulas yielding suboptimal results [87].

Band Erosion and Slippage—Band erosion into the gastric lumen can occur after AGB and VBG. Band slippage is another complication that can occur after AGB. The incidence of band erosion after VBG and AGB is uncommon and has been reported at 1–3 % after VBG and 0.9–3.8 % after AGB [88–90]. Band erosion can be asymptomatic or can cause abdominal pain, nausea, emesis, access port site infection, fistula, increased food intake, and GI bleeding. Band slippage may present with weight gain, worsening reflux symptoms, or obstruction. Erosion is best diagnosed endoscopically. Endoscopy can allow for direct visualization of a band eroding through gastric mucosa (Fig. 7), and endoscopic removal techniques for near completely eroded bands have been described [89, 91]. However, surgical repair is usually recommended with excision and replacement or conversion. While band slippage can be demonstrated with endoscopy, it may be best diagnosed with contrast radiography, since findings on

upper endoscopy are variable and dependent on the degree and type of slippage encountered. Findings may include an enlarged pouch size, reflux esophagitis, gastritis, or ulcers. Severe cases are potentially life-threatening as they can lead to gastric necrosis [92, 93]; this may be demonstrated endoscopically as mucosal ischemia.

Acid Reflux and Gastroesophageal Reflux Disease (GERD)—Symptomatic GERD is frequent in bariatric patients, and obesity itself is a risk factor for GERD. Studies have reported a prevalence of 30–60 % in the severely obese population [94–97]. The effect of bariatric surgery on GERD appears to be variable and is likely dependent on the type of bariatric operation performed. Most studies agree that RYGB has a positive effect on GERD, resulting in a decrease in prevalence, symptoms, and medication use [94, 98–100]. Research has indicated that VBG is either unassociated with any change in reflux postoperatively [101] or associated with a transient decrease and later increase in reflux symptoms [102]. The effect of gastric banding on GERD is inconclusive; some studies report an increase in reflux [101, 103], while others report a decrease [104]. Due to limited data on pre- and postoperative reflux in SG, there is a lack of consensus in regard to the effect this operation has on GERD [65, 105]. Symptoms of GERD after bariatric surgery should be managed like those in patients who did not have bariatric surgery [4]. Flexible upper endoscopy should be reserved for the evaluation of symptoms refractory to medical therapy and to rule out complications and diagnose causes of GERD. Reflux symptoms after AGB can be the result of an excessively tight band or slippage [106]. A contrast study may be helpful to assess the degree of constriction, and endoscopy should be performed if symptoms persist after deflation of the band. Further, for patients who report symptoms of GERD after gastric banding, conversion to RYGB is often recommended as it treats both reflux and weight [107, 108].

Weight Regain or Inadequate Weight Loss—Initial weight loss failures after bariatric surgery or weight regain after an initial postoperative weight loss may be the result of a technical failure. These may include gastrogastric fistula from a staple line dehiscence, a large patulous gastrojejunal anastomosis that fails to restrict food intake, dilatation of the gastric pouch, or band slippage. However, often the cause is related to dietary noncompliance, and thus, preoperative counseling is needed to establish realistic weight loss goals. Endoscopy remains the best way to assess postoperative anatomy [30], and it can also provide a method for management. Endoscopic therapies for weight regain are evolving. Large gastrojejunal anastomoses can be treated with four-quadrant endoscopic injection of sodium morrhuate into the stoma to cause scarring and reduction in stomal size [109]. Novel techniques utilizing endoscopic suturing devices can allow for nonoperative revision of the gastrojejunal anasto-

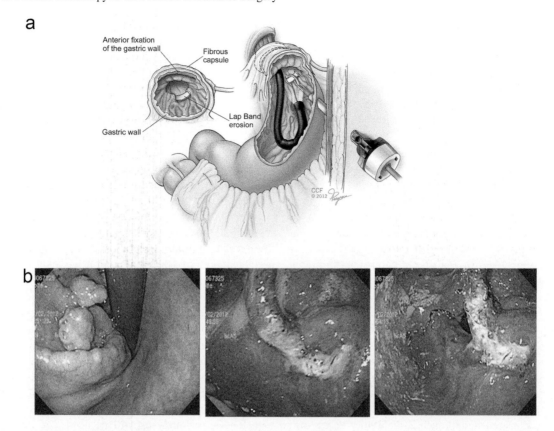

FIG. 7. (**a**) Illustration and (**b**) endoscopic views of band erosion. Reprinted with permission, Cleveland Clinic Center for Medical Art & Photography © 2010–2013. All Rights Reserved.

mosis and reduction of pouch size after RYGB. The long-term durability of these endoscopic techniques remains to be demonstrated [110].

Bezoars—Food bezoars can occur in patients after bariatric surgery and are most common after AGB [111, 112]. They form within the first postoperative month, and patients typically present with nausea, emesis, and dysphagia. Bezoars can be diagnosed and effectively treated with upper endoscopy by fragmentation and removal [113]. If an anastomotic stricture or stenosis is discovered with the bezoar, then it should be treated with endoscopic dilation.

Special Considerations—Endoscopic Retrograde Cholangiopancreatography (ERCP) and Transgastric Endoscopy

Pancreaticobiliary disease and specifically gallstone disease are common after bariatric surgery. Studies showed postoperative rates of gallstone detection from 22 to 71 % and cholecystectomy rates from 7 to 41 % in patients who had a prior gastric bypass [114, 115]. The occurrence of choledocholithiasis has not been determined for this patient group. ERCP after AGB, VBG, and SG is relatively straightforward. On the

other hand, exclusion of the ampulla after RYGB makes access technically more difficult. Successful biliary cannulation after RYGB depends on factors including the skill of the endoscopist and the lengths of the biliopancreatic and/or Roux limbs. Using varying techniques, both side-viewing and forward-viewing endoscopes have been used successfully. Wright et al. reported on a series of 15 patients in which the papilla was reached and successfully cannulated in 66 %; this was accomplished through the use of various techniques including advancing a duodenoscope over a stiff guide wire that was previously placed with a forward-viewing scope and pulling up a duodenoscope with a wire-guided biliary balloon anchored at the pylorus. Therapeutic maneuvers including sphincterotomy, sphincter of Oddi manometry, stone extraction, and stent placement were also successfully accomplished in this study [116]. Other techniques that may be used to cannulate the biliary system include single- and double-balloon-assisted enteroscopy. These enteroscopes more effectively pleat the small bowel and improve the advancement of the scope through the small intestine. Medical centers with experience in balloon-assisted enteroscopy report an 80 % success rate [117]. The double-balloon enteroscope may also be used to place a retrograde percutaneous endoscopic gastrostomy (PEG) tube in the remnant stomach and then perform an ERCP through the PEG tube [118, 119]. Similar to the factors associated with successful biliary cannulation mentioned above, the success of reaching the gastric remnant is largely dependent on the length of the Roux limb. Schreiner and associates reviewed the records of post-RYGB bariatric patients who underwent an ERCP and reported that patients with a Roux limb less than 150 cm have a significantly higher rate of therapeutic success. For patients with a Roux limb greater than 150 cm, a laparoscopically assisted ERCP was a better initial option [120].

Although the previously mentioned techniques to access the biliary system and gastric remnant after bariatric surgery have been shown to be effective, they may not be widely replicated due to lack of equipment or expertise. Further, methods such as balloon and overtube endoscopy require the use of front-viewing endoscopes instead of the side-viewing endoscopes typically used for ERCP. Transgastric endoscopy can access the gastric remnant or duodenum through a laparoscopic approach or by placement of a percutaneous gastrostomy tube with radiologic guidance [121–123]. These techniques have been associated with high success rates and low postoperative morbidity [124]. Laparoscopic-assisted transgastric ERCP has been demonstrated to be an effective technique in the treatment of biliary pathology including stone disease, sphincter of Oddi dysfunction, ampullary stenosis, and the diagnosis of and treatment of both benign and malignant strictures [125, 126]. An additional benefit of the laparoscopic transgastric approach is the ability to perform an abdominal exploration to evaluate for any other causes of abdominal pain, such as an internal hernia. The use of laparoscopic transgastric endoscopy through the gastric remnant is safe, reliable, and associated with a high success rate and low complication rate.

Future Considerations

Flexible upper endoscopy in bariatric patients currently also includes revisional procedures as well as primary weight loss therapies, in both experimental models and in patients. Such endoscopic interventions require advanced skill sets with novel equipment and methods.

Obesity is a multifactorial disease and the changes that occur after bariatric surgery are numerous. Specifically, mechanical changes in the postbariatric anatomy, such as dilation of an anastomosis or pouch, are thought to contribute to weight regain. Several endoscopic revisional procedures have presented potential solutions. Sclerotherapy is a procedure that uses a traditional endoscope with an injection needle to inject sodium morrhuate around the gastric outlet. About 2 cm^3 per injection (a total of 20 cm^3 per procedure) and about 2–3 sessions are needed to achieve a desired outlet size. Initial studies reported a 75 % weight loss in patients over 6 months compared to 50 % in matched controls [127]. The EndoCinch is another endoscopic technique that was originally developed for fistula repair and gastric pouch reduction. This device guides a needle through a piece of vacuum-acquired

tissue within a metal cap and thereby places a stitch. Stoma reduction using the EndoCinch was investigated using a randomized sham control trial; using an average of four sutures per patient, the results of this study demonstrated a 4.7 % weight loss compared to 1.9 % in the sham group [128]. The invention of Incisionless Operating Platform (IOP) allowed the ability to perform serosal tissue plications under direct visualization to adjust dilated pouches and gastric outlets. Plications were made using specialized jaws and nitinol tissue anchors that were deployed through a curved hollow needle. Only initial feasibility studies have been performed for this device [129, 130].

There is significant interest in the development of successful and effective endoscopic techniques and alternatives to surgery for primary weight loss. No such method has been perfected, but three different approaches stand out in the literature—endoscopic gastroplasty, intragastric balloons, and endoluminal sleeves. Endoscopic gastroplasty has been performed using stapling and suturing devices. Suturing devices achieve volume reduction by anterior and posterior gastric wall approximation. Devices that have been used and described in the literature include the EndoCinch, the Endo Stitch, and the OverStitch. Alternatively, with the TOGA system (Satiety Inc.), staples are used to form a gastric sleeve similar to an unsupported VBG [131]. Well-designed studies with long-term follow-up will be needed to determine the outcomes of these techniques. Since the 1980s, intragastric balloons have been used as space-occupying devices for weight loss. They may have value in select high-risk patient groups as a bridge to surgery in those individuals who may have otherwise been nonoperative candidates [132]. There are two available models of the intragastric balloon, the BioEnterics balloon and the Heliosphere BAG, both of which were used in a prospective randomized study that resulted in 27–30 % excess weight loss at 6 months [133]. Long-term studies are lacking, and complications including esophagitis, nausea, emesis, abdominal pain, rupture, and obstruction have been associated with placement of these devices. Placement of these devices is relatively uncomplicated, but knowledge of proper removal is important to minimize the risk to the patient [131]. Currently, these devices remain unapproved by the Food and Drug Administration for use in the United States [134]. Similar to the surgical interventions that alter anatomy and exclude the proximal small bowel, endoscopic insertion of a barrier in the small bowel may replicate this intestinal bypass. Two unique, novel devices are currently under study: the ValenTx endoluminal bypass and the EndoBarrier (GI Dynamics) (Fig. 8). The ValenTx endoluminal bypass is anchored at the esophagogastric junction with a specialized device, and the sleeve extends 120 cm through the stomach and into the mid-jejunum. The impermeable sleeve allows nutrients to bypass the proximal bowel and entice metabolic effects through stimulation of the distal small bowel [131]. The EndoBarrier is similar in concept to the ValenTx endoluminal bypass, but it is a duodenojejunal

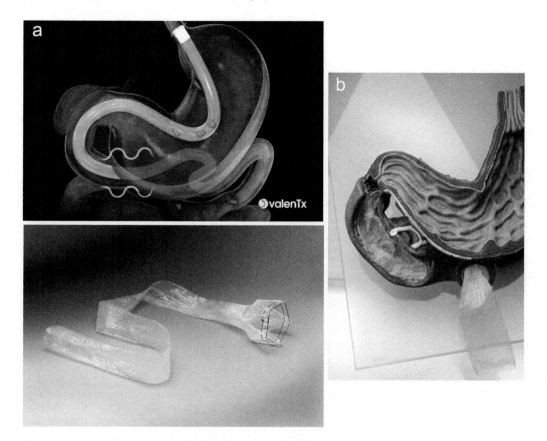

FIG. 8. (**a**) ValenTx endoluminal bypass (courtesy of ValenTx, with permission). (**b**) GI Dynamics EndoBarrier (courtesy of GI Dynamics, with permission).

bypass sleeve that anchors in the duodenal bulb by a self-expanding cuff and extends a polyethylene sleeve 60 cm into the small bowel. It does not need additional equipment for anchoring at the proximal end and is easily removable with a removal loop. A short-term study by Schouten et al. evaluated 26 patients after the placement of the EndoBarrier and demonstrated a 19 % excess weight loss in 3 months along with a reduction in hemoglobin A1C and glucose control medications [135]. However, complications of migration, stent obstruction, and upper GI bleeding have been reported with these novel devices [136], and further studies are presently underway to clarify their safety and efficacy. As was the case with the intragastric balloons, the endoluminal sleeves are not approved for use within the United States at this time.

Conclusions

As bariatric surgery evolves and new techniques are developed, perioperative management of such patients becomes very important. Flexible upper endoscopy can be a helpful tool in the armamentarium for the diagnosis and treatment of bariatric patients in all stages of their care. It has wide applications in the preoperative setting, but routine use is not yet observed. On the other hand, the routine use of intraoperative

endoscopy is well documented in the medical literature. In addition, the use of flexible upper endoscopy has been validated throughout medical literature for the evaluation of postoperative patients and has both diagnostic and therapeutic potential. Such widespread advantages of flexible endoscopy should encourage bariatric surgeons to develop and refine their endoscopic skills and proficiencies (Video 1).

References

1. ASGE STANDARDS OF PRACTICE COMMITTEE, Anderson MA, Gan SI, Fanelli RD, Baron TH, Banerjee S, et al. Role of endoscopy in the bariatric surgery patient. Gastrointest Endosc. 2008;68(1):1–10.
2. Glatt D, Sorenson T. Metabolic and bariatric surgery for obesity: a review. S D Med. 2011; Spec No: 57–62.
3. Ikenberry SO, Harrison ME, Lichtenstein D, Dominitz JA, Anderson MA, Jagannath SB, et al. The role of endoscopy in dyspepsia. Gastrointest Endosc. 2007;66(6):1071–5.
4. Standards of Practice Committee, Lichtenstein DR, Cash BD, Davila R, Baron TH, Adler DG, et al. Role of endoscopy in the management of GERD. Gastrointest Endosc. 2007;66(2):219–24.
5. Jaffin BW, Knoepflmacher P, Greenstein R. High prevalence of asymptomatic esophageal motility disorders among morbidly obese patients. Obes Surg. 1999;9(4):390–5.
6. Kuper MA, Kratt T, Kramer KM, Zdichavsky M, Schneider JH, Glatzle J, et al. Effort, safety, and findings of routine preoperative

endoscopic evaluation of morbidly obese patients undergoing bariatric surgery. Surg Endosc. 2010;24(8):1996–2001.

7. Hampel H, Abraham NS, El-Serag HB. Meta-analysis: obesity and the risk for gastroesophageal reflux disease and its complications. Ann Intern Med. 2005;143(3):199–211.

8. Loewen M, Giovanni J, Barba C. Screening endoscopy before bariatric surgery: a series of 448 patients. Surg Obes Relat Dis. 2008;4(6):709–12.

9. de Moura AA, Cotrim HP, Santos AS, Bitencourt AG, Barbosa DB, Lobo AP, et al. Preoperative upper gastrointestinal endoscopy in obese patients undergoing bariatric surgery: is it necessary? Surg Obes Relat Dis. 2008;4(2):144–9; discussion 150–1.

10. Madan AK, Speck KE, Hiler ML. Routine preoperative upper endoscopy for laparoscopic gastric bypass: is it necessary? Am Surg. 2004;70(8):684–6.

11. Dietz J, Ulbrich-Kulcynski JM, Souto KE, Meinhardt NG. Prevalence of upper digestive endoscopy and gastric histopathology findings in morbidly obese patients. Arq Gastroenterol. 2012;49(1):52–5.

12. Munoz R, Ibanez L, Salinas J, Escalona A, Perez G, Pimentel F, et al. Importance of routine preoperative upper GI endoscopy: why all patients should be evaluated? Obes Surg. 2009;19(4):427–31.

13. Sauerland S, Angrisani L, Belachew M, Chevallier JM, Favretti F, Finer N, et al. Obesity surgery: evidence-based guidelines of the European Association for Endoscopic Surgery (EAES). Surg Endosc. 2005;19(2):200–21.

14. Schirmer B, Erenoglu C, Miller A. Flexible endoscopy in the management of patients undergoing Roux-en-Y gastric bypass. Obes Surg. 2002;12(5):634–8.

15. Sharaf RN, Weinshel EH, Bini EJ, Rosenberg J, Sherman A, Ren CJ. Endoscopy plays an important preoperative role in bariatric surgery. Obes Surg. 2004;14(10):1367–72.

16. Ramaswamy A, Lin E, Ramshaw BJ, Smith CD. Early effects of Helicobacter pylori infection in patients undergoing bariatric surgery. Arch Surg. 2004;139(10):1094–6.

17. Brethauer SA, Nfonsam V, Sherman V, Udomsawaengsup S, Schauer PR, Chand B. Endoscopy and upper gastrointestinal contrast studies are complementary in evaluation of weight regain after bariatric surgery. Surg Obes Relat Dis. 2006;2(6):643–8; discussion 649–50.

18. Wittgrove AC, Clark GW. Laparoscopic gastric bypass, Roux-en-Y- 500 patients: technique and results, with 3–60 month follow-up. Obes Surg. 2000;10(3):233–9.

19. Nguyen NT, Nguyen XM, Masoomi H. Minimally invasive intrathoracic esophagogastric anastomosis: circular stapler technique with transoral placement of the anvil. Semin Thorac Cardiovasc Surg. 2010;22(3):253–5.

20. Diamantis T, Alexandrou A, Pikoulis E, Diamantis D, Griniatsos J, Felekouras E, et al. Laparoscopic sleeve gastrectomy for morbid obesity with intra-operative endoscopic guidance. Immediate peri-operative and 1-year results after 25 patients. Obes Surg. 2010;20(8):1164–70.

21. Buckwalter JA, Herbst Jr CA. Complications of gastric bypass for morbid obesity. Am J Surg. 1980;139(1):55–60.

22. Schauer PR, Ikramuddin S, Gourash W, Ramanathan R, Luketich J. Outcomes after laparoscopic Roux-en-Y gastric bypass for morbid obesity. Ann Surg. 2000;232(4):515–29.

23. Alasfar F, Chand B. Intraoperative endoscopy for laparoscopic Roux-en-Y gastric bypass: leak test and beyond. Surg Laparosc Endosc Percutan Tech. 2010;20(6):424–7.

24. Champion JK, Hunt T, DeLisle N. Role of routine intraoperative endoscopy in laparoscopic bariatric surgery. Surg Endosc. 2002; 16(12):1663–5.

25. Alaedeen D, Madan AK, Ro CY, Khan KA, Martinez JM, Tichansky DS. Intraoperative endoscopy and leaks after laparoscopic Roux-en-Y gastric bypass. Am Surg. 2009;75(6):485–8; discussion 488.

26. Obstein KL, Thompson CC. Endoscopy after bariatric surgery (with videos). Gastrointest Endosc. 2009;70(6):1161–6.

27. Morales MP, Wheeler AA, Ramaswamy A, Scott JS, de la Torre RA. Laparoscopic revisional surgery after Roux-en-Y gastric bypass and sleeve gastrectomy. Surg Obes Relat Dis. 2010;6(5):485–90.

28. Gill RS, Whitlock KA, Mohamed R, Sarkhosh K, Birch DW, Karmali S. The role of upper gastrointestinal endoscopy in treating postoperative complications in bariatric surgery. J Interv Gastroenterol. 2012;2(1):37–41.

29. Mittendorf EA, Brandt CP. Utility of intraoperative endoscopy: implications for surgical education. Surg Endosc. 2002;16(4):703–6.

30. Schreiner MA, Fennerty MB. Endoscopy in the obese patient. Gastroenterol Clin North Am. 2010;39(1):87–97.

31. Eslick GD. Prevalence and epidemiology of gastrointestinal symptoms among normal weight, overweight, obese and extremely obese individuals. Gastroenterol Clin North Am. 2010;39(1):9–22.

32. Wilson JA, Romagnuolo J, Byrne TK, Morgan K, Wilson FA. Predictors of endoscopic findings after Roux-en-Y gastric bypass. Am J Gastroenterol. 2006;101(10):2194–9.

33. Encinosa WE, Bernard DM, Du D, Steiner CA. Recent improvements in bariatric surgery outcomes. Med Care. 2009;47(5):531–5.

34. Weller WE, Rosati C. Comparing outcomes of laparoscopic versus open bariatric surgery. Ann Surg. 2008;248(1):10–5.

35. Longitudinal Assessment of Bariatric Surgery (LABS) Consortium, Flum DR, Belle SH, King WC, Wahed AS, Berk P, et al. Perioperative safety in the longitudinal assessment of bariatric surgery. N Engl J Med. 2009;361(5):445–54.

36. Masoomi H, Nguyen NT, Stamos MJ, Smith BR. Overview of outcomes of laparoscopic and open Roux-en-Y gastric bypass in the United States. Surg Technol Int. 2012;XXII:sti22/15.

37. Benotti PN, Wood GC, Rodriguez H, Carnevale N, Liriano E. Perioperative outcomes and risk factors in gastric surgery for morbid obesity: a 9-year experience. Surgery. 2006;139(3):340–6.

38. Bal B, Koch TR, Finelli FC, Sarr MG. Managing medical and surgical disorders after divided Roux-en-Y gastric bypass surgery. Nat Rev Gastroenterol Hepatol. 2010;7(6):320–34.

39. Podnos YD, Jimenez JC, Wilson SE, Stevens CM, Nguyen NT. Complications after laparoscopic gastric bypass: a review of 3464 cases. Arch Surg. 2003;138(9):957–61.

40. Rasmussen JJ, Fuller W, Ali MR. Marginal ulceration after laparoscopic gastric bypass: an analysis of predisposing factors in 260 patients. Surg Endosc. 2007;21(7):1090–4.

41. MacLean LD, Rhode BM, Nohr C, Katz S, McLean AP. Stomal ulcer after gastric bypass. J Am Coll Surg. 1997;185(1):1–7.

42. Capella JF, Capella RF. Gastro-gastric fistulas and marginal ulcers in gastric bypass procedures for weight reduction. Obes Surg. 1999;9(1):22–7; discussion 28.

43. Capella JF, Capella RF. Staple disruption and marginal ulceration in gastric bypass procedures for weight reduction. Obes Surg. 1996;6(1):44–9.

44. Pope GD, Goodney PP, Burchard KW, Proia RR, Olafsson A, Lacy BE, et al. Peptic ulcer/stricture after gastric bypass: a comparison of technique and acid suppression variables. Obes Surg. 2002;12(1):30–3.

45. Csendes A, Burgos AM, Altuve J, Bonacic S. Incidence of marginal ulcer 1 month and 1 to 2 years after gastric bypass: a prospective consecutive endoscopic evaluation of 442 patients with morbid obesity. Obes Surg. 2009;19(2):135–8.

46. Jordan JH, Hocking MP, Rout WR, Woodward ER. Marginal ulcer following gastric bypass for morbid obesity. Am Surg. 1991; 57(5):286–8.

47. Takata MC, Ciovica R, Cello JP, Posselt AM, Rogers SJ, Campos GM. Predictors, treatment, and outcomes of gastrojejunostomy stricture after gastric bypass for morbid obesity. Obes Surg. 2007;17(7):878–84.

48. Messmer JM, Wolper JC, Sugerman HJ. Stomal disruption in gastric partition in morbid obesity (comparison of radiographic and endoscopic diagnosis). Am J Gastroenterol. 1984;79(8):603–5.

49. Huang CS, Farraye FA. Endoscopy in the bariatric surgical patient. Gastroenterol Clin North Am. 2005;34(1):151–66.

50. Carrodeguas L, Szomstein S, Soto F, Whipple O, Simpfendorfer C, Gonzalvo JP, et al. Management of gastrogastric fistulas after divided Roux-en-Y gastric bypass surgery for morbid obesity: analysis of 1,292 consecutive patients and review of literature. Surg Obes Relat Dis. 2005;1(5):467–74.

51. Peifer KJ, Shiels AJ, Azar R, Rivera RE, Eagon JC, Jonnalagadda S. Successful endoscopic management of gastrojejunal anastomotic strictures after Roux-en-Y gastric bypass. Gastrointest Endosc. 2007;66(2):248–52.

52. Da Costa M, Mata A, Espinos J, Vila V, Roca JM, Turro J, et al. Endoscopic dilation of gastrojejunal anastomotic strictures after laparoscopic gastric bypass. Predictors of initial failure. Obes Surg. 2011;21(1):36–41.

53. Schwartz ML, Drew RL, Chazin-Caldie M. Factors determining conversion from laparoscopic to open Roux-en-Y gastric bypass. Obes Surg. 2004;14(9):1193–7.

54. Go MR, Muscarella 2nd P, Needleman BJ, Cook CH, Melvin WS. Endoscopic management of stomal stenosis after Roux-en-Y gastric bypass. Surg Endosc. 2004;18(1):56–9.

55. Ahmad J, Martin J, Ikramuddin S, Schauer P, Slivka A. Endoscopic balloon dilation of gastroenteric anastomotic stricture after laparoscopic gastric bypass. Endoscopy. 2003;35(9):725–8.

56. Schubert D, Kuhn R, Lippert H, Pross M. Endoscopic treatment of benign gastrointestinal anastomotic strictures using argon plasma coagulation in combination with diathermy. Surg Endosc. 2003;17(10):1579–82.

57. Papavramidis ST, Theocharidis AJ, Zaraboukas TG, Christoforidou BP, Kessissoglou II, Aidonopoulos AP. Upper gastrointestinal endoscopic and histologic findings before and after vertical banded gastroplasty. Surg Endosc. 1996;10(8):825–30.

58. Wayman CS, Nord JH, Combs WM, Rosemurgy AS. The role of endoscopy after vertical banded gastroplasty. Gastrointest Endosc. 1992;38(1):44–6.

59. Parikh A, Alley JB, Peterson RM, Harnisch MC, Pfluke JM, Tapper DM, et al. Management options for symptomatic stenosis after laparoscopic vertical sleeve gastrectomy in the morbidly obese. Surg Endosc. 2012;26(3):738–46.

60. Rosenthal RJ, International Sleeve Gastrectomy Expert Panel, Diaz AA, Arvidsson D, Baker RS, Basso N, et al. International Sleeve Gastrectomy Expert Panel Consensus Statement: best practice guidelines based on experience of >12,000 cases. Surg Obes Relat Dis. 2012;8(1):8–19.

61. Buchwald H, Avidor Y, Braunwald E, Jensen MD, Pories W, Fahrbach K, et al. Bariatric surgery: a systematic review and meta-analysis. JAMA. 2004;292(14):1724–37.

62. Huang CS. The role of the endoscopist in a multidisciplinary obesity center. Gastrointest Endosc. 2009;70(4):763–7.

63. Biertho L, Steffen R, Ricklin T, Horber FF, Pomp A, Inabnet WB, et al. Laparoscopic gastric bypass versus laparoscopic adjustable gastric banding: a comparative study of 1,200 cases. J Am Coll Surg. 2003;197(4):536–44; discussion 544–5.

64. Rao AD, Ramalingam G. Exsanguinating hemorrhage following gastric erosion after laparoscopic adjustable gastric banding. Obes Surg. 2006;16(12):1675–8.

65. Deitel M, Gagner M, Erickson AL, Crosby RD. Third International Summit: current status of sleeve gastrectomy. Surg Obes Relat Dis. 2011;7(6):749–59.

66. Jossart GH. Complications of sleeve gastrectomy: bleeding and prevention. Surg Laparosc Endosc Percutan Tech. 2010;20(3): 146–7.

67. Jamil LH, Krause KR, Chengelis DL, Jury RP, Jackson CM, Cannon ME, et al. Endoscopic management of early upper gastrointestinal hemorrhage following laparoscopic Roux-en-Y gastric bypass. Am J Gastroenterol. 2008;103(1):86–91.

68. Nguyen NT, Rivers R, Wolfe BM. Early gastrointestinal hemorrhage after laparoscopic gastric bypass. Obes Surg. 2003;13(1): 62–5.

69. Sundbom M, Nyman R, Hedenstrom H, Gustavsson S. Investigation of the excluded stomach after Roux-en-Y gastric bypass. Obes Surg. 2001;11(1):25–7.

70. Laine L, McQuaid KR. Endoscopic therapy for bleeding ulcers: an evidence-based approach based on meta-analyses of randomized controlled trials. Clin Gastroenterol Hepatol. 2009;7(1):33–47; quiz 1-2.

71. Rabl C, Peeva S, Prado K, James AW, Rogers SJ, Posselt A, et al. Early and late abdominal bleeding after Roux-en-Y gastric bypass: sources and tailored therapeutic strategies. Obes Surg. 2011;21(4):413–20.

72. Filho AJ, Kondo W, Nassif LS, Garcia MJ, Tirapelle Rde A, Dotti CM. Gastrogastric fistula: a possible complication of Roux-en-Y gastric bypass. JSLS. 2006;10(3):326–31.

73. Aurora AR, Khaitan L, Saber AA. Sleeve gastrectomy and the risk of leak: a systematic analysis of 4,888 patients. Surg Endosc. 2012;26(6):1509–15.

74. Carrasquilla C, English WJ, Esposito P, Gianos J. Total stapled, total intra-abdominal (TSTI) laparoscopic Roux-en-Y gastric bypass: one leak in 1000 cases. Obes Surg. 2004;14(5):613–7.

75. Higa KD, Ho T, Boone KB. Laparoscopic Roux-en-Y gastric bypass: technique and 3-year follow-up. J Laparoendosc Adv Surg Tech A. 2001;11(6):377–82.

76. Carucci LR, Conklin RC, Turner MA. Roux-en-Y gastric bypass surgery for morbid obesity: evaluation of leak into excluded stomach with upper gastrointestinal examination. Radiology. 2008;248(2):504–10.

77. Merrifield BF, Lautz D, Thompson CC. Endoscopic repair of gastric leaks after Roux-en-Y gastric bypass: a less invasive approach. Gastrointest Endosc. 2006;63(4):710–4.

78. Eisendrath P, Cremer M, Himpens J, Cadiere GB, Le Moine O, Deviere J. Endotherapy including temporary stenting of fistulas of the upper gastrointestinal tract after laparoscopic bariatric surgery. Endoscopy. 2007;39(7):625–30.

79. Yimcharoen P, Heneghan HM, Tariq N, Brethauer SA, Kroh M, Chand B. Endoscopic stent management of leaks and anastomotic strictures after foregut surgery. Surg Obes Relat Dis. 2011; 7(5):628–36.

80. Brethauer SA, Hammel JP, Schauer PR. Systematic review of sleeve gastrectomy as staging and primary bariatric procedure. Surg Obes Relat Dis. 2009;5(4):469–75.

81. Bhardwaj A, Cooney RN, Wehrman A, Rogers AM, Mathew A. Endoscopic repair of small symptomatic gastrogastric fistulas after gastric bypass surgery: a single center experience. Obes Surg. 2010;20(8):1090–5.

82. Gonzalez R, Sarr MG, Smith CD, Baghai M, Kendrick M, Szomstein S, et al. Diagnosis and contemporary management of anastomotic leaks after gastric bypass for obesity. J Am Coll Surg. 2007;204(1):47–55.

83. Kriwanek S, Ott N, Ali-Abdullah S, Pulgram T, Tscherney R, Reiter M, et al. Treatment of gastro-jejunal leakage and fistulization after gastric bypass with coated self-expanding stents. Obes Surg. 2006;16(12):1669–74.

84. Salinas A, Baptista A, Santiago E, Antor M, Salinas H. Self-expandable metal stents to treat gastric leaks. Surg Obes Relat Dis. 2006;2(5):570–2.

85. Fukumoto R, Orlina J, McGinty J, Teixeira J. Use of Polyflex stents in treatment of acute esophageal and gastric leaks after bariatric surgery. Surg Obes Relat Dis. 2007;3(1):68–71; discussion 71–2.

86. Papavramidis ST, Eleftheriadis EE, Papavramidis TS, Kotzampassi KE, Gamvros OG. Endoscopic management of gastrocutaneous fistula after bariatric surgery by using a fibrin sealant. Gastrointest Endosc. 2004;59(2):296–300.

87. Spaun GO, Martinec DV, Kennedy TJ, Swanstrom LL. Endoscopic closure of gastrogastric fistulas by using a tissue apposition system (with videos). Gastrointest Endosc. 2010;71(3):606–11.

88. Greve JW. Surgical treatment of morbid obesity: role of the gastroenterologist. Scand J Gastroenterol Suppl. 2000;232:60–4.

89. Evans JA, Williams NN, Chan EP, Kochman ML. Endoscopic removal of eroded bands in vertical banded gastroplasty: a novel use of endoscopic scissors (with video). Gastrointest Endosc. 2006;64(5):801–4.

90. Chisholm J, Kitan N, Toouli J, Kow L. Gastric band erosion in 63 cases: endoscopic removal and rebanding evaluated. Obes Surg. 2011;21(11):1676–81.

91. Adam LA, Silva Jr RG, Rizk M, Gerke H. Endoscopic argon plasma coagulation of Marlex mesh erosion after vertical-banded gastroplasty. Gastrointest Endosc. 2007;65(2):337–40.

92. Iannelli A, Facchiano E, Sejor E, Baque P, Piche T, Gugenheim J. Gastric necrosis: a rare complication of gastric banding. Obes Surg. 2005;15(8):1211–4.

93. Foletto M, De Marchi F, Bernante P, Busetto L, Pomerri F. Late gastric pouch necrosis after Lap-Band, treated by an individualized conservative approach. Obes Surg. 2005;15(10):1487–90.

94. Nelson LG, Gonzalez R, Haines K, Gallagher SF, Murr MM. Amelioration of gastroesophageal reflux symptoms following Roux-en-Y gastric bypass for clinically significant obesity. Am Surg. 2005;71(11):950–3; discussion 953–4.

95. Klaus A, Gruber I, Wetscher G, Nehoda H, Aigner F, Peer R, et al. Prevalent esophageal body motility disorders underlie aggravation of GERD symptoms in morbidly obese patients following adjustable gastric banding. Arch Surg. 2006;141(3):247–51.

96. Foster A, Richards WO, McDowell J, Laws HL, Clements RH. Gastrointestinal symptoms are more intense in morbidly obese patients. Surg Endosc. 2003;17(11):1766–8.

97. Di Francesco V, Baggio E, Mastromauro M, Zoico E, Stefenelli N, Zamboni M, et al. Obesity and gastro-esophageal acid reflux: physiopathological mechanisms and role of gastric bariatric surgery. Obes Surg. 2004;14(8):1095–102.

98. Perry Y, Courcoulas AP, Fernando HC, Buenaventura PO, McCaughan JS, Luketich JD. Laparoscopic Roux-en-Y gastric bypass for recalcitrant gastroesophageal reflux disease in morbidly obese patients. JSLS. 2004;8(1):19–23.

99. Raftopoulos I, Awais O, Courcoulas AP, Luketich JD. Laparoscopic gastric bypass after antireflux surgery for the treatment of gastroesophageal reflux in morbidly obese patients: initial experience. Obes Surg. 2004;14(10):1373–80.

100. Nguyen T, Lau DC. The obesity epidemic and its impact on hypertension. Can J Cardiol. 2012;28(3):326–33.

101. Ovrebo KK, Hatlebakk JG, Viste A, Bassoe HH, Svanes K. Gastroesophageal reflux in morbidly obese patients treated with gastric banding or vertical banded gastroplasty. Ann Surg. 1998;228(1):51–8.

102. Ortega J, Escudero MD, Mora F, Sala C, Flor B, Martinez-Valls J, et al. Outcome of esophageal function and 24-hour esophageal pH monitoring after vertical banded gastroplasty and Roux-en-Y gastric bypass. Obes Surg. 2004;14(8):1086–94.

103. Suter M, Dorta G, Giusti V, Calmes JM. Gastric banding interferes with esophageal motility and gastroesophageal reflux. Arch Surg. 2005;140(7):639–43.

104. Lundell L, Ruth M, Olbe L. Vertical banded gastroplasty or gastric banding for morbid obesity: effects on gastro-oesophageal reflux. Eur J Surg. 1997;163(7):525–31.

105. Chiu S, Birch DW, Shi X, Sharma AM, Karmali S. Effect of sleeve gastrectomy on gastroesophageal reflux disease: a systematic review. Surg Obes Relat Dis. 2011;7(4):510–5.

106. de Jong JR, van Ramshorst B, Timmer R, Gooszen HG, Smout AJ. The influence of laparoscopic adjustable gastric banding on gastroesophageal reflux. Obes Surg. 2004;14(3):399–406.

107. Gulkarov I, Wetterau M, Ren CJ, Fielding GA. Hiatal hernia repair at the initial laparoscopic adjustable gastric band operation reduces the need for reoperation. Surg Endosc. 2008;22(4):1035–41.

108. Dolan K, Finch R, Fielding G. Laparoscopic gastric banding and crural repair in the obese patient with a hiatal hernia. Obes Surg. 2003;13(5):772–5.

109. Catalano MF, Chua TY, Rudic G. Endoscopic balloon dilation of stomal stenosis following gastric bypass. Obes Surg. 2007;17(3):298–303.

110. Thompson CC, Slattery J, Bundga ME, Lautz DB. Peroral endoscopic reduction of dilated gastrojejunal anastomosis after Roux-en-Y gastric bypass: a possible new option for patients with weight regain. Surg Endosc. 2006;20(11):1744–8.

111. Parameswaran R, Ferrando J, Sigurdsson A. Gastric bezoar complicating laparoscopic adjustable gastric banding with band slippage. Obes Surg. 2006;16(12):1683–4.

112. Veronelli A, Ranieri R, Laneri M, Montorsi M, Bianchi P, Cosentino F, et al. Gastric bezoars after adjustable gastric banding. Obes Surg. 2004;14(6):796–7.

113. Pinto D, Carrodeguas L, Soto F, Lascano C, Cho M, Szomstein S, et al. Gastric bezoar after laparoscopic Roux-en-Y gastric bypass. Obes Surg. 2006;16(3):365–8.

114. Wudel Jr LJ, Wright JK, Debelak JP, Allos TM, Shyr Y, Chapman WC. Prevention of gallstone formation in morbidly obese patients undergoing rapid weight loss: results of a randomized controlled pilot study. J Surg Res. 2002;102(1):50–6.

115. Puzziferri N, Austrheim-Smith IT, Wolfe BM, Wilson SE, Nguyen NT. Three-year follow-up of a prospective randomized trial comparing laparoscopic versus open gastric bypass. Ann Surg. 2006;243(2):181–8.

116. Wright BE, Cass OW, Freeman ML. ERCP in patients with long-limb Roux-en-Y gastrojejunostomy and intact papilla. Gastrointest Endosc. 2002;56(2):225–32.

117. Lopes TL, Wilcox CM. Endoscopic retrograde cholangiopancreatography in patients with Roux-en-Y anatomy. Gastroenterol Clin North Am. 2010;39(1):99–107.

118. Baron TH. Double-balloon enteroscopy to facilitate retrograde PEG placement as access for therapeutic ERCP in patients with long-limb gastric bypass. Gastrointest Endosc. 2006;64(6):973–4.

119. Ross AS, Semrad C, Alverdy J, Waxman I, Dye C. Use of double-balloon enteroscopy to perform PEG in the excluded stomach after Roux-en-Y gastric bypass. Gastrointest Endosc. 2006;64(5):797–800.

120. Schreiner MA, Chang L, Gluck M, Irani S, Gan SI, Brandabur JJ, et al. Laparoscopy-assisted versus balloon enteroscopy-assisted ERCP in bariatric post-Roux-en-Y gastric bypass patients. Gastrointest Endosc. 2012;75(4):748–56.

121. Pimentel RR, Mehran A, Szomstein S, Rosenthal R. Laparoscopy-assisted transgastrostomy ERCP after bariatric surgery: case report of a novel approach. Gastrointest Endosc. 2004;59(2):325–8.

122. Peters M, Papasavas PK, Caushaj PF, Kania RJ, Gagne DJ. Laparoscopic transgastric endoscopic retrograde cholangio-

pancreatography for benign common bile duct stricture after Roux-en-Y gastric bypass. Surg Endosc. 2002;16(7):1106.

123. Martinez J, Guerrero L, Byers P, Lopez P, Scagnelli T, Azuaje R, et al. Endoscopic retrograde cholangiopancreatography and gastroduodenoscopy after Roux-en-Y gastric bypass. Surg Endosc. 2006;20(10):1548–50.

124. Richardson JF, Lee JG, Smith BR, Nguyen B, Pham KP, Nguyen NT. Laparoscopic transgastric endoscopy after Roux-en-Y Gastric bypass: case series and review of the literature. Am Surg. 2012;78(10):1182–6.

125. Lopes TL, Clements RH, Wilcox CM. Laparoscopy-assisted ERCP: experience of a high-volume bariatric surgery center (with video). Gastrointest Endosc. 2009;70(6):1254–9.

126. Falcao M, Campos JM, Galvao Neto M, Ramos A, Secchi T, Alves E, et al. Transgastric endoscopic retrograde cholangiopancreatography for the management of biliary tract disease after Roux-en-Y gastric bypass treatment for obesity. Obes Surg. 2012;22(6):872–6.

127. Ryou M, Dayyeh B, Yu S. M1356 endoscopic revision of dilated gastrojejunostomy in gastric bypass patients experiencing weight regain: a matched cohort comparison of transoral sutured revision versus sclerotherapy versus controls. Gastroenterology. 2010;138(5):S-387.

128. Thompson C, Roslin M, Chand B, et al. M1359 restore: randomized evaluation of endoscopic suturing transorally for anastomotic outlet reduction; a double-blind, sham-controlled multicenter study for treatment of inadequate weight loss or weight regain following Roux-en-Y gastric bypass. Gastroenterology. 2010;138(5):S-388.

129. Mullady DK, Lautz DB, Thompson CC. Treatment of weight regain after gastric bypass surgery when using a new endoscopic platform: initial experience and early outcomes (with video). Gastrointest Endosc. 2009;70(3):440–4.

130. Ryou M, Mullady DK, Lautz DB, Thompson CC. Pilot study evaluating technical feasibility and early outcomes of second-generation endosurgical platform for treatment of weight regain after gastric bypass surgery. Surg Obes Relat Dis. 2009;5(4):450–4.

131. Shaikh S, Ryou M, Thompson C. Bariatric endoscopy. In: Cohen J, editor. Successful training in gastrointestinal endoscopy. 1st ed. Oxford: Blackwell Publishing Ltd; 2011. p. 270–81.

132. Cote GA, Edmundowicz SA. Emerging technology: endoluminal treatment of obesity. Gastrointest Endosc. 2009;70(5):991–9.

133. De Castro ML, Morales MJ, Del Campo V, Pineda JR, Pena E, Sierra JM, et al. Efficacy, safety, and tolerance of two types of intragastric balloons placed in obese subjects: a double-blind comparative study. Obes Surg. 2010;20(12):1642–6.

134. Levitzky BE, Wassef WY. Endoscopic management in the bariatric surgical patient. Curr Opin Gastroenterol. 2010;26(6):632–9.

135. Schouten R, Rijs CS, Bouvy ND, Hameeteman W, Koek GH, Janssen IM, et al. A multicenter, randomized efficacy study of the EndoBarrier Gastrointestinal Liner for presurgical weight loss prior to bariatric surgery. Ann Surg. 2010;251(2):236–43.

136. Tarnoff M, Rodriguez L, Escalona A, Ramos A, Neto M, Alamo M, et al. Open label, prospective, randomized controlled trial of an endoscopic duodenal-jejunal bypass sleeve versus low calorie diet for pre-operative weight loss in bariatric surgery. Surg Endosc. 2009;23(3):650–6.

42

Bariatric Surgery in Adolescents

Sean J. Barnett, Marc P. Michalsky, and Thomas H. Inge

Paralleling the epidemic of adult obesity are the increasing trends in prevalence and incidence of childhood obesity. Recent data from the National Health and Nutrition Examination Survey (NHANES) reports that approximately 69 % of adults in the United States are overweight and 36 % obese [1], while 17 % of children and adolescents are overweight or obese [2]. Furthermore, approximately 4 % (over two million children and adolescents) may be considered extremely obese (body mass index (BMI) > 99th percentile) [3]. The immediate and long-term health consequences of childhood obesity as well as the psychosocial and economic effects continue to provide compelling arguments to perform bariatric surgery on adolescents to achieve aggressive weight loss. Clinical trials show that behavioral weight management may have long-lasting effects in younger children compared with adults, but durable weight loss is rare. Furthermore, such conventional treatment approaches are not effective for those who suffer from severe obesity [4–7], leading to the consideration of weight loss surgical options for select adolescents. In order to provide a framework for considering and/ or performing adolescent bariatric surgery, this section discusses the basic concepts of severe pediatric obesity, including definitions, risk factors, and consequences of obesity unique to the adolescent population. In addition, we review the available evidence for the efficacy of bariatric procedures in the adolescent population and provide suggested guidelines and pathways for the application of bariatric surgery among adolescents.

Definition of Pediatric Obesity

Body mass index (BMI, kg/m^2) is a relatively simple means to define the term overweight in adults who have attained full growth. Adults with a BMI > 25 kg/m^2 are considered overweight, while those with BMI ≥ 30 kg/m^2 are considered obese. In children and adolescents, we expect physiologic increases in adiposity, height, and weight during growth; thus we cannot simply use a single BMI value to make accurate predictions about adiposity. Instead, for the vast majority of children and adolescents, growth charts are used to assign cutoffs for obesity that are actually age, race, and sex specific [8]. In this context, some authors have defined pediatric obesity as BMI greater than the 95th percentile for age and sex. Overweight, or *at risk* for overweight, has been defined as a BMI > 85th percentile [9–11]. It is important to first recognize that these percentile definitions of obesity and overweight become unreliable at the extreme categories of obesity. In essence, for the very severe categories of obesity, which might prompt consideration for bariatric surgery in adolescence, there are currently no strong, reliable population-based data by which one can calculate percentile boundaries. This is due to children and adolescents with BMI values in the >40 kg/m^2 range being very poorly represented in the National Health and Nutrition Examination Survey (NHANES)—the dataset that provides the weight and height information used to create the commonly used pediatric growth charts. Alternatively, most have used BMI ≥ 40 kg/m^2 as a conservative threshold for defining morbid obesity in youth, which is congruent with the World Health Organization definition for adults.

Adopting a BMI threshold as a *general guideline* for considering adolescent bariatric surgery is done with the understanding that an obese adolescent with an advanced, severe, and incontrovertibly weight-related comorbidity also should be considered for weight loss surgery without strictest regard to level of BMI.

Risk Factors for Adolescent Obesity

When considering bariatric surgery among adolescents, it may be useful to identify those groups of patients who are at highest risk of persistent obesity and its sequelae. The risk of a child carrying obesity into adulthood is influenced by genetic, biological, psychological, cultural, and environmental factors [12]. There are critical phases in the development of adolescent obesity within the period between preconception and

S.A. Brethauer et al. (eds.), *Minimally Invasive Bariatric Surgery*,
DOI 10.1007/978-1-4939-1637-5_42, © Springer Science+Business Media New York 2015

adolescence [13, 14]. In neonates, lower birth weight has been linked to higher BMI in childhood and adulthood [15–19]. Childhood obesity risks are also higher for offspring of mothers with diabetes mellitus [20, 21]. Through a recent critical review of the literature, it seems that the most critical early markers for obesity during the neonatal period are related most to maternal BMI, smoking, and weight gain during pregnancy [22]. Extended duration of breast-feeding in the postnatal period reduces the risk of adolescent overweight [23–27]. In fact, early bottle-feeding accelerates the age of obesity rebound, which predicts obesity in later life [23]. It should also be noted that those infants who grow more rapidly during the first 3 months to 2 years of life are more likely to be obese as adults [28].

Due in part to the rapid hormonal changes, puberty is also considered to be a critical period for the development of both insulin resistance [29] and obesity [30]. Interestingly, earlier menarche is seen in obese children, suggesting that the obese experience an earlier onset of physiologic maturation compared with children of normal weight [31].

Obesity in family members is an additional and important risk factor for adolescent obesity. As an example, recent evidence demonstrates that the risk for persistence of childhood obesity into adulthood is elevated threefold and tenfold if one or both parents are obese, respectively [32–35]. The risk of obesity persisting into adulthood is far higher among obese adolescents than among overweight younger children [36]. Finally, there is a preexisting racial-ethnic disparity in the risk of obesity, with lower socioeconomic groups being especially vulnerable because of poor diet and limited opportunity for physical activity [37, 38].

In summary, important risk factors for childhood and adolescent obesity include (1) low birth weight; (2) bottle-feeding; (3) maternal factors including weight, smoking habits, and diabetes; (4) rapid growth at a young age; and (5) parental obesity. Knowledge of these important risk factors for adolescent obesity and its persistence into adulthood gives some insight into the phenotypes of those individuals who may be least likely to succeed with nonsurgical management of obesity and, by inference, those who may benefit most from early application of surgical therapy.

Consequences of Obesity in Adolescence

In association with the remarkable increase in the prevalence of pediatric obesity is a parallel increase in the severity of obesity and in obesity-related chronic diseases. Important complications of obesity commonly encountered in adolescents include increased risk of cardiovascular disease (especially hypertension and left ventricular hypertrophy), nonalcoholic fatty liver disease (NAFLD), type 2 diabetes mellitus and insulin resistance, sleep apnea, pseudotumor cerebri, and psychosocial impairment [39–42]. These diseases have an onset at a younger age and carry an increased risk for adult morbidity and mortality [43–45]. This serves to heighten awareness about the significance of medical consequences of obesity among adolescents.

Cardiovascular Disease

There is a relative paucity of data focusing on the cardiac health of severely obese adolescents, likely due to the general belief that associated sequelae (i.e., atherosclerosis, peripheral vascular disease, etc.) become more clinically relevant later in life. However, a mounting body of evidence has demonstrated that the pathogenesis of various cardiovascular disease states can find their development and subsequent progression in early childhood and adolescence. Recent evidence demonstrates the presence of these cardiovascular risk factors, namely, hypertension, hypertriglyceridemia, elevated fasting serum glucose, and cholesterol abnormalities, as well as cardiac structural and functional abnormalities in the obese adolescent population [41, 42, 46, 47]. Almost 60 % of obese children in the Bogalusa Heart Study had one risk factor for cardiovascular disease, with 20 % having two or more risk factors [48]. Of note, following gastric bypass and significant weight loss in obese adolescents, recent data demonstrates significant improvement in left ventricular hypertrophy and overall cardiac function [41]. Gastric bypass in adolescents has also been shown to significantly improve the major cardiovascular risk, hypertension, and hyperlipidemia in those patients at 1-year follow-up [46, 49]. Large, prospective trials are currently ongoing to better investigate the cardiac health of this patient population.

Glucose Impairment

Given the current increases in childhood diabetes and obesity prevalence, epidemiologists at the Centers for Disease Control and Prevention (CDC) have made a sobering prediction: type 2 diabetes is expected to develop in 33–50 % of all Americans born in the year 2000 [50]. There have also been recent reports linking the development of abnormalities related to normal glucose regulation, including hyperinsulinemia (60–80 %), impaired glucose tolerance (12–15 %), and type 2 diabetes mellitus (1–6 %) to childhood obesity [40]. The prevailing thought is that the generalized state of low-grade chronic inflammation could be a significant factor leading to insulin resistance and subsequent dysregulation (i.e., metabolic syndrome). Of note, there is not only a relationship between severely obese adolescent patients and insulin resistance (elevated hemoglobin A1c and C-reactive protein (CRP) levels), but there is significant improvement seen in most markers of metabolic dysfunction within the first year following gastric bypass and significant weight loss [46, 49].

Obstructive Sleep Apnea

Sleep deprivation and excessive daytime sleepiness are more common in obese children, and poor school performance has been associated with disordered sleep patterns in these children [51, 52]. Alarmingly, recently studies have documented obstructive sleep apnea (OSA) rates as high as 46 % in obese children [53]. Of particular concern is the fact that children with chronic OSA also exhibit the development and progression of early cardiac abnormalities such as right and left ventricular hypertrophy and dysfunction associated with cardiac remodeling [42]. Despite the prevalence of this chronic disease, reversal of cardiovascular abnormalities [42] as well as improvement in school performance has been documented among affected adolescents following surgical weight loss [52].

Polycystic Ovarian Syndrome (PCOS)

A consequence of the epidemic of adolescent obesity is the increasing incidence of polycystic ovarian syndrome (PCOS) and hyperandrogenism related to insulin resistance and hyperinsulinism, which affect ovarian function [54]. Obesity is present in over 50 % of adolescents with PCOS; thus sustained weight loss can ameliorate the clinical manifestations of acne and hirsutism as well as favorably impact insulin resistance [55].

Nonalcoholic Fatty Liver Disease (NAFLD)

NAFLD and steatohepatitis occur more frequently in obese children and adolescents, present in up to 83 % of liver biopsies obtained from severely obese adolescents undergoing gastric bypass [56]. The most serious consequence of liver injury associated with obesity is fibrosis and accelerated cirrhosis, which can lead to end-stage liver disease. Studies in the adult population demonstrate improvement or complete resolution of steatosis, steatohepatitis, and subsequent fibrosis following bariatric surgery [57] with similar studies in adolescents ongoing.

Psychological and Quality of Life Issues

Psychosocial and quality of life issues are among the most prevalent in obese adolescents. The patterns of discrimination against obese children are established early in life and become ingrained in a culture in which thinness is admired [58]. Recent evidence has demonstrated a link between obesity in adolescents and an increased risk for the development of depression [59]. Further studies have predicted a significant increased risk for adult depression in those children that

identify themselves as overweight [60]. Data does suggest that following significant weight loss after gastric bypass, adolescents experience significant improvement in psychosocial and health-related quality of life scores [61].

Best Practice Guidelines for Adolescent Bariatric Surgery

The application of surgical weight loss procedures in the severely obese adolescent population has been an ongoing and evolutionary process over the past decade and continues to gain attention within the medical community as an effective treatment strategy. The increased interest in the use of surgical weight loss surgery in the adolescent population comes on the heels of a significant body of literature demonstrating the safety and efficacy of bariatric intervention for the treatment of severely obese adults [62, 63], as well as the disappointing results associated with attempts to lower pediatric and adolescent BMI through diet, exercise, and behavior modification [64, 65]. The increasing use of this treatment modality is further supported by an increasing body of literature reporting encouraging longitudinal outcomes for adolescents undergoing surgical weight reduction. As a result of these factors, the reported volume of adolescent bariatric procedures in the United States has risen three to fivefold between the late 1990s to 2005 [66, 67] with more recent reports demonstrating a surprisingly high number of adolescent cases being performed supporting the consensus that the rising trend continues into the current decade [68, 69]. Although an accurate accounting of the number of adolescent bariatric procedures being performed in the United States annually is uncertain at the present time, several trends have emerged with regard to the general environment in which adolescent bariatric procedures have been undertaken during the previous decade that lend support for the need to establish specific guidelines and standardization of adolescent bariatric care [67]. Schilling et al. reported that 87 % of hospitals performing adolescent bariatric surgical operations from 1997 to 2003 performed four or fewer on an annual basis and that the majority (85 %) were carried out within an adult facility. A similar pattern of adolescent bariatric care within adult facilities is seen in a more recent review of 890 adolescent bariatric procedures performed between 2004 and 2010 at 360 adult facilities in the United States [69]. Although no specific inferences can be drawn regarding the associated level of adolescent-specific resources from these reports, including whether or not an adolescent-specific multidisciplinary team was involved in the patient management process, the recent rise in the number of centers focusing strictly on the surgical weight reduction for severely obese adolescents underscores the need for standardized patient selection criteria as well as recommendations for the development of bariatric surgical centers that take into account the specific needs of this emerging population.

Early guidelines addressing the specific use of bariatric surgery in the adolescent population, first presented in 2004 [70], have been updated several times and should be referred to for in-depth consideration [71–73]. Since no national consensus conference pertaining to the surgical treatment of severe adolescent obesity has been convened as yet, the previous and more current recommendations for adolescent bariatric care have been based on modification of the 1991 National Institutes of Health (NIH) consensus guidelines for adult bariatric surgery, which offer little to no substantive recommendations for the surgical care of the severely obese pediatric population. In contrast to the initial report by Inge et al. [70], current recommendations have undergone a shift toward a less conservative approach that has become more consistent with the widely accepted adult eligibility criteria and appear to reflect a general consensus among centers providing adolescent bariatric surgery at this time. Although several of the initial recommendations have been modified based on nearly a decade's worth of experience since the original publication, the most significant departure relates to the assessment of preoperative BMI with regard to surgical eligibility (i.e., originally recommended to be BMI $\geq$ 40 kg/m^2 with serious comorbid conditions and BMI $\geq$ 50 kg/m^2 with less severe comorbid conditions). In addition to an expanding body of literature demonstrating safe and efficacious outcomes that support the shift toward a lower than previously recommended BMI range, recent observations demonstrating a potentially fixed "ceiling" effect (i.e., maximal expected reduction in BMI) among adolescent bariatric patients suggest that the earlier timing of bariatric intervention (i.e., at a lower BMI) may result in a high propensity to achieve an optimal postoperative result (i.e., BMI $\leq$ 35 kg/m^2) [49]. As the number of healthcare institutions providing bariatric surgical care for the severely obese adolescent population has increased, a parallel consensus has developed regarding a number of key elements that serve as the foundation for an adolescent-specific multidisciplinary team approach, which are briefly reviewed herein.

In a recent effort to establish a more uniform approach to adolescent bariatric surgical care in the United States, national accreditation guidelines for adolescent bariatric care are presently under development and are expected to be fully incorporated within the newly developed Metabolic and Bariatric Surgery Accreditation and Quality Improvement Program (MBSAQIP) which is expected to replace the previous independent bariatric standards and accreditation programs separately administered by the American College of Surgeons (ACS) and the American Society for Metabolic and Bariatric Surgery (ASMBS) in the near future. The fundamental components representing previously published best practice recommendations will be included and are presented below [72–74]. The effort to provide widely accepted standards for the treatment of the severely obese adolescent population will most likely occur in one of several programmatic models (i.e., an adult facility vs. a pediatric facility under the direction of an adult bariatric surgeon, a pediatric surgeon specializing in bariatric care, or a combination of the two). The following key items are presented for consideration herein as a general overview and do not take into consideration institutional-specific logistics and available clinical resources at the local level:

1. *Surgical specialist*: A surgeon performing adolescent bariatric surgery must demonstrate certification by the American Board of Surgery, American Osteopathic Board of Surgery, and/or the Royal College of Physicians and Surgeons of Canada. In addition, he or she must have appropriate training and experience performing bariatric procedures and be institutionally credentialed to perform such procedures.

2. *Medical specialist*: A physician with specialty training in pediatrics (including possible subspecialty training in endocrinology, gastroenterology, cardiology, nutrition, etc.), adolescent medicine, or family practice experience. The medical specialist should have or obtain experience screening adolescents for bariatric surgery and be willing to assume responsibility for the management of obesity-related comorbid conditions in coordination with the patient's primary care provided (i.e., medical home).

3. *Behavioral health specialist*: A behavioral health specialist may include a psychologist, psychiatrist, or other qualified and independently licensed mental health provider with specific experience treating children, adolescents, and families. In addition, the individual should have experience treating obesity and eating disorders as well as specific experience regarding pre-bariatric evaluation.

4. *Bariatric program coordinator*: A bariatric surgical coordinator may consist of a registered nurse or social worker or any other member of the bariatric team who has the responsibility of coordinating the care of the adolescent patient and helping to facilitate patient compliance and clinical follow-up.

5. *Registered dietician*: A dietician with experience treating children and families with obesity. Experience with bariatric surgical patients is ideal but not mandatory. Nutritional recommendations and structured educational content should be provided to the patient and associated caregivers (e.g., parents, grandparents, siblings) in an effort to establish an understanding of age-appropriate healthy nutritional guidelines by multiple family members in the home prior to undergoing a bariatric procedure.

6. *Exercise physiologist/physical therapist*: An exercise physiologist, physical therapist, or other licensed provider with specialty training to provide safe physical activity education for the severely obese adolescent population.

7. *Social worker*: A dedicated social worker is not mandatory but highly recommended and may serve to assist in the evaluation of the patient's psychosocial needs as well as perioperative logistics including transportation, access to community resources, insurance coverage, etc.

In addition to the recommended adolescent-specific resources outlined above and in keeping with the multidisciplinary care model, the development of an adolescent bariatric surgery program should include the establishment of a formal multidisciplinary adolescent bariatric committee designed to review individual cases that are being considered for surgical intervention. The committee, consisting of core members (i.e., surgical and medical director, dietician, behavioral specialist, and program coordinator), should meet on a regular basis to review patient-specific information. In addition, ad hoc members of the review committee may include subspecialists such as experts in adolescent pulmonary medicine, hematology, cardiology, endocrinology, and medical ethics (including formal involvement of the institutional ethics committee when considered necessary).

As mentioned earlier, the development of criteria for adolescent bariatric patient selection has been an ongoing and evolutionary process which, since its earliest recommendation, has been based on a modification of the adult surgical patient selection guidelines defined by the 1991 National Institutes of Health (NIH) consensus panel on bariatric surgery [70–72, 74]. Because all adolescent boys and most adolescent girls <18 years of age with a BMI of 35 kg/m^2 correspond to BMI percentile of 99th percentile for age, the application of adult selection criterion based on BMI appears to be appropriate [40], with a more conservative approach regarding the incorporation of associated comorbid disease thresholds [72, 73]. Currently, recommendations for selection criteria for adolescent bariatric surgery based on preoperative BMI and examples of associated obesity-related comorbid diseases are seen below:

- BMI ≥ 35 kg/m^2 with major comorbid disease

Type 2 diabetes mellitus
Pseudotumor cerebri
Severe NASH
Moderate to severe obstructive sleep apnea [apnea-hypopnea index >15]
- BMI ≥ 40 kg/m^2 with less severe comorbid disease

Glucose intolerance
Hypertension
Dyslipidemia
Impaired weight-related quality of life
Mild to moderate obstructive sleep apnea [apnea-hypopnea index >5]

Since adolescence represents an extensive period of substantial growth and maturation, both physically and emotionally, special attention to developmental issues in adolescents is critical when considering bariatric procedures that will have marked impact on future growth and development. For adolescents who have attained the vast majority (>95 %) of linear growth, there is clearly little reason to believe that growth would be impaired by a bariatric procedure. Based on peak height velocity measurements in normal-weight girls

(8–9 cm/year) and boys (9–10 cm/year), girls should achieve >95 % linear growth by 13 years of age and boys by 15 years of age [75]. The onset of menarche is also a marker for physiologic maturity in girls, and growth is generally completed within 2 years after menarche. Bone age can also be assessed by plain radiography of the hand and wrist if there is uncertainty about status of physiologic maturation. Nomograms are used by radiologists to accurately predict the percentile of adult stature that a child has attained.

While overall physiological assessment is an important foundation during the patient selection process leading up a weight reduction surgery, additional factors are equally important and include several that distinguish themselves from the routine preoperative evaluation process in the corresponding adult bariatric population. In addition to individual BMI and comorbid disease status, as the basis of eligibility criteria, assessment of the adolescent patient's psychosocial maturity level, including the ability to demonstrate a general understanding of the benefits and risks of bariatric surgery, has been shown to be an important factor in determining eligibility. Although the factors related to maturity and general comprehension regarding bariatric surgery among adolescents are only now beginning to emerge, preoperative evaluation should attempt to determine an adolescents patient's ability to demonstrate the ability to comply with nutritional guidelines prior to surgical intervention. Despite the paucity of data regarding the advisability of mandatory preoperative weight loss and its ability to offer predictive value regarding postoperative dietary compliance, it is currently recommended that the adolescent be able to successfully demonstrate stabilization of preoperative weight (i.e., avoid significant weight gain) prior to surgical intervention. In addition, it is considered extremely important to assess the quality of the patient's "support mechanisms" (i.e., home environment, parental/caregiver status, etc.) in an effort to determine the likelihood of postoperative nutritional and behavioral compliance as well as the ability to comply with required postoperative follow-up. Finally, adolescent bariatric surgical intervention should take into consideration the overall risk-benefit ratio related to the progression of untreated or poorly treated comorbid diseases (i.e., type 2 diabetes, hyperlipidemia, hypertension, etc.) if left untreated. As mentioned earlier, this may include the decision to seek input from an institutional medical ethics committee in certain cases when needed.

Outcomes of Bariatric Surgery in Adolescents

Currently, the most commonly performed bariatric procedures in the adolescent population are the Roux-en-Y gastric bypass (RYGB), the adjustable gastric band (AGB), and the more recently introduced vertical sleeve gastrectomy (VSG). The successful use of the duodenal switch has been reported in this population [76], but is generally considered more complex and with its associated significant malabsorption and nutritional complications is not commonly performed. In general, published literature suggests that overall weight loss, resolution of comorbidities, and safety are comparable to or better in adolescents when compared to adults [49, 77, 78].

Roux-en-Y Gastric Bypass (RYGB)

The use of RYGB for weight loss in the United States can trace its origins back to the 1960s for adults and the 1970s for adolescents [79]. Multiple small studies have been published looking at long-term outcomes following RYGB in adolescents [42, 49, 80–85] with a recent meta-analysis reporting the outcomes of adolescents undergoing RYGB demonstrating sustained reduction in excess body weight and improvement in associated comorbidities [86]. Multiple studies demonstrate improvements or complete resolution of comorbidities related to obesity including type 2 diabetes mellitus [46], obstructive sleep apnea [87], depression and psychosocial function [61], and hypertension [46]. A recent publication from Cincinnati Children's Hospital demonstrated significant weight loss (decrease in BMI by 37 % at 1 year) in patients following gastric bypass. Interestingly, the study demonstrated a "fixed ceiling" with regard to expected reduction in BMI regardless of preoperative BMI. Specifically, such results highlight the potential timeliness of bariatric surgical intervention within the spectrum of preoperative BMI in that subjects noted to have the highest BMI values (i.e., >50 kg/m^2) have a lower probability of achieving a nonobese nadir weight despite significant reduction in excess body weight and in comparison to subjects who were noted to have a lower initial BMI (i.e., <50 kg/m^2) [49]. Given the concern over long-term metabolic and nutritional deficiencies as a result of RYGB in this young population, adequate nutritional and vitamin supplementation is of the utmost importance. Reasonable protocols have been established to meet the needs of this growing patient population [88].

Adjustable Gastric Band (AGB)

Though not approved in the United States for patients under the age of 18 years of age by the Food and Drug Administration (FDA), there have been a number of short-term studies published for the use of AGB in adolescents. These studies do show a modest amount of weight loss at 1 year, but long-term follow-up is lacking [82, 89, 90]. Over a period of 2 years (2007 to 2009), their use had dramatically increased in the state of California [68], but their current usage is unclear across the country. In addition, a recent randomized control trial comparing the use of the AGB versus medical weight loss among two groups of severely obese adolescents has demonstrated a significant amount of weight loss at 2 years when compared to lifestyle intervention alone (BMI reduction of 28 % vs. 3 %) but noted a significantly high reoperation rate (33 %) [91]. Finally, the results of a nearly completed multi-institutional industry-sponsored FDA trial designed to investigate longitudinal outcomes among a cohort of 200 severely obese adolescent (less than 18 years of age) are still pending.

Vertical Sleeve Gastrectomy (VSG)

The VSG, historically utilized as a key anatomic component of the highly complex duodenal switch operation, has recently gained popularity as a primary weight loss procedure in the United States and abroad. Given the propensity for less complications, particularly metabolic and vitamin deficiency when compared to RYGB, it has quickly gained acceptance in the treatment of obesity in adolescents. Although initial reports have been encouraging, only a few long-term and large-scale reports are currently available examining the use of the sleeve gastrectomy in the adolescent population. The largest study to date, consisting of 108 patients from Saudi Arabia, has demonstrated a significant weight loss (excess weight loss of 61.8 %) at 1 year with no serious postoperative complications and significant resolution of the expected comorbidities [92]. When compared to adult counterparts, VSG in the pediatric patient was noted to be similar in its effectiveness and safety with fewer major complications [93]. Given the paucity of long-term data coupled with the durability of weight loss and the potential for significant gastroesophageal reflux induced by VSG, there remains cautious optimism for its widespread use in adolescents.

Summary

Surgical approaches for clinically severely obese adolescents may be reasonable for individuals who have obesity-related comorbidities and have been unsuccessful in achieving sustained weight loss following organized attempts. Suggested indications and contraindications for operative intervention should not be inflexibly applied to every patient but rather should be considered guidelines for use of bariatric surgery in adolescents. Individuals should be considered based on the degree of obesity, the severity of comorbid conditions, physical and emotional maturity level, and the stability of family support. The benefits of a multidisciplinary approach in adolescent weight management and bariatric surgery cannot be overemphasized. Families and patients alike must participate fully in all aspects of preoperative decision making given the level of comprehension about potential complications that must exist before bariatric interventions are made. Families and patients must understand bariatric surgery to be a valuable weight loss tool as opposed to a *cure* for obesity to promote continued compliance with lifestyle and dietary changes postoperatively. Adolescent bariatric surgery should be conducted only in institutions capable of managing adolescents with complications of severe obesity and where detailed clinical data collection and outcome studies can be accomplished. Finally, highly trained and skilled bariatric surgeons must have an integral role within the multidisciplinary team to guarantee safe and appropriate application of bariatric surgical procedures in adolescents.

Review Questions and Answers

1. Current recommendations allow for the use of bariatric surgery in adolescents with a BMI ≥ 35 kg/m^2 and one of the following comorbidities *except*:

A. Type 2 diabetes mellitus
B. Hypertension
C. Severe nonalcoholic steatohepatitis (NASH)
D. Severe obstructive sleep apnea
E. Pseudotumor cerebri

The answer is B, hypertension. Surgery is indicated in those individuals with hypertension only if their BMI ≥ 40 kg/m^2. The remaining comorbidities are considered serious and warrant consideration for surgery with a BMI ≥ 35 kg/m^2

2. All of the following are considered acceptable bariatric surgical options for an adolescent of 18 years of age *except*:

A. Duodenal switch
B. Adjustable gastric band
C. Sleeve gastrectomy
D. Roux-en-Y gastric bypass

The answer is A, duodenal switch. Given significant nutritional deficiencies associated with the duodenal switch operation and limited data, it is not generally used in the adolescent population. The band is approved by the FDA for use in those 18 years of age or older. Sleeve gastrectomy and gastric bypass are the most commonly performed operations for weight loss currently

3. The age at which most girls have attained the vast majority (>95 %) of linear growth and should therefore be considered reasonable candidates for bariatric surgery is:

A. 11
B. 12
C. 13
D. 14
E. 15

The correct answer is C, 13 years of age

References

1. Flegal KM, Carroll MD, Kit BK, Ogden CL. Prevalence of obesity and trends in the distribution of body mass index among US adults, 1999–2010. JAMA. 2012;307:491–7.
2. Ogden CL, Carroll MD, Curtin LR, McDowell MA, Tabak CJ, Flegal KM. Prevalence of overweight and obesity in the United States, 1999–2004. JAMA. 2006;295:1549–55.
3. Freedman DS, Mei Z, Srinivasan SR, Berenson GS, Dietz WH. Cardiovascular risk factors and excess adiposity among overweight children and adolescents: the Bogalusa Heart Study. J Pediatr. 2007;150:12–7; e12.
4. Epstein LH, Valoski A, Wing RR, McCurley J. Ten-year follow-up of behavioral, family-based treatment for obese children. JAMA. 1990;264:2519–23.
5. Yanovski JA. Intensive therapies for pediatric obesity. Pediatr Clin North Am. 2001;48:1041–53.
6. Spear BA, Barlow SE, Ervin C, Ludwig DS, Saelens BE, Schetzina KE, Taveras EM. Recommendations for treatment of child and adolescent overweight and obesity. Pediatrics. 2007;120 Suppl 4:S254–88.
7. Hearnshaw C, Matyka K. Managing childhood obesity: when lifestyle change is not enough. Diabetes Obes Metab. 2010;12:947–57.
8. Himes JH, Dietz WH. Guidelines for overweight in adolescent preventive services: recommendations from an expert committee. The Expert Committee on Clinical Guidelines for Overweight in Adolescent Preventive Services. Am J Clin Nutr. 1994;59:307–16.
9. Flegal KM, Wei R, Ogden CL, Freedman DS, Johnson CL, Curtin LR. Characterizing extreme values of body mass index-for-age by using the 2000 Centers for Disease Control and Prevention growth charts. Am J Clin Nutr. 2009;90:1314–20.
10. Strauss RS, Pollack HA. Epidemic increase in childhood overweight, 1986–1998. JAMA. 2001;286:2845–8.
11. Ogden CL, Flegal KM, Carroll MD, Johnson CL. Prevalence and trends in overweight among US children and adolescents, 1999–2000. JAMA. 2002;288:1728–32.
12. Cameron N, Demerath EW. Critical periods in human growth and their relationship to diseases of aging. Am J Phys Anthropol. 2002;35(Suppl):159–84.
13. Michels KB. Early life predictors of chronic disease. J Womens Health (Larchmt). 2003;12:157–61.
14. Wahlqvist ML. Chronic disease prevention: a life-cycle approach which takes account of the environmental impact and opportunities of food, nutrition and public health policies—the rationale for an eco-nutritional disease nomenclature. Asia Pac J Clin Nutr. 2002;11 Suppl 9:S759–62.
15. Ravelli AC, van Der Meulen JH, Osmond C, Barker DJ, Bleker OP. Obesity at the age of 50 y in men and women exposed to famine prenatally. Am J Clin Nutr. 1999;70:811–6.
16. Parsons TJ, Power C, Logan S, Summerbell CD. Childhood predictors of adult obesity: a systematic review. Int J Obes Relat Metab Disord. 1999;23 Suppl 8:S1–107.
17. Sorensen HT, Sabroe S, Rothman KJ, Gillman M, Fischer P, Sorensen TI. Relation between weight and length at birth and body mass index in young adulthood: cohort study. BMJ. 1997;315:1137.
18. Li H, Stein AD, Barnhart HX, Ramakrishnan U, Martorell R. Associations between prenatal and postnatal growth and adult body size and composition. Am J Clin Nutr. 2003;77:1498–505.
19. Wei JN, Li HY, Sung FC, Lin CC, Chiang CC, Li CY, Chuang LM. Birth weight correlates differently with cardiovascular risk factors in youth. Obesity (Silver Spring). 2007;15:1609–16.
20. Dabelea D, Hanson RL, Lindsay RS, Pettitt DJ, Imperatore G, Gabir MM, Roumain J, Bennett PH, Knowler WC. Intrauterine exposure to diabetes conveys risks for type 2 diabetes and obesity: a study of discordant sibships. Diabetes. 2000;49:2208–11.

21. Jouret B, Ahluwalia N, Cristini C, Dupuy M, Negre-Pages L, Grandjean H, Tauber M. Factors associated with overweight in preschool-age children in southwestern France. Am J Clin Nutr. 2007;85:1643–9.

22. Brisbois TD, Farmer AP, McCargar LJ. Early markers of adult obesity: a review. Obes Rev. 2012;13:347–67.

23. Bergmann KE, Bergmann RL, Von Kries R, Bohm O, Richter R, Dudenhausen JW, Wahn U. Early determinants of childhood overweight and adiposity in a birth cohort study: role of breast-feeding. Int J Obes Relat Metab Disord. 2003;27:162–72.

24. Michels KB, Willett WC, Graubard BI, Vaidya RL, Cantwell MM, Sansbury LB, Forman MR. A longitudinal study of infant feeding and obesity throughout life course. Int J Obes (Lond). 2007;31:1078–85.

25. Gillman MW, Rifas-Shiman SL, Camargo Jr CA, Berkey CS, Frazier AL, Rockett HR, Field AE, Colditz GA. Risk of overweight among adolescents who were breastfed as infants. JAMA. 2001;285:2461–7.

26. Gillman MW. Breast-feeding and obesity. J Pediatr. 2002;141:749–50.

27. Rudnicka AR, Owen CG, Strachan DP. The effect of breastfeeding on cardiorespiratory risk factors in adult life. Pediatrics. 2007;119:e1107–15.

28. Baird J, Fisher D, Lucas P, Kleijnen J, Roberts H, Law C. Being big or growing fast: systematic review of size and growth in infancy and later obesity. BMJ. 2005;331:929.

29. Caprio S. Insulin resistance in childhood obesity. J Pediatr Endocrinol Metab. 2002;15 Suppl 1:487–92.

30. Heald FP, Khan MA. Teenage obesity. Pediatr Clin North Am. 1973;20:807–17.

31. Wattigney WA, Srinivasan SR, Chen W, Greenlund KJ, Berenson GS. Secular trend of earlier onset of menarche with increasing obesity in black and white girls: the Bogalusa Heart Study. Ethn Dis. 1999;9:181–9.

32. Whitaker RC, Wright JA, Pepe MS, Seidel KD, Dietz WH. Predicting obesity in young adulthood from childhood and parental obesity. N Engl J Med. 1997;337:869–73.

33. Pi-Sunyer FX. The obesity epidemic: pathophysiology and consequences of obesity. Obes Res. 2002;10 Suppl 2:97S–104.

34. Durand EF, Logan C, Carruth A. Association of maternal obesity and childhood obesity: implications for healthcare providers. J Community Health Nurs. 2007;24:167–76.

35. Santiago S, Zazpe I, Cuervo M, Martinez JA. Perinatal and parental determinants of childhood overweight in 6–12 years old children. Nutr Hosp. 2012;27:599–605.

36. Whitaker RC. Understanding the complex journey to obesity in early adulthood. Ann Intern Med. 2002;136:923–5.

37. Gordon-Larsen P, Adair LS, Popkin BM. Ethnic differences in physical activity and inactivity patterns and overweight status. Obes Res. 2002;10:141–9.

38. Baum 2nd CL, Ruhm CJ. Age, socioeconomic status and obesity growth. J Health Econ. 2009;28:635–48.

39. Freedman DS, Dietz WH, Srinivasan SR, Berenson GS. The relation of overweight to cardiovascular risk factors among children and adolescents: the Bogalusa Heart Study. Pediatrics. 1999;103:1175–82.

40. Brandt ML, Harmon CM, Helmrath MA, Inge TH, McKay SV, Michalsky MP. Morbid obesity in pediatric diabetes mellitus: surgical options and outcomes. Nat Rev Endocrinol. 2010;6:637–45.

41. Ippisch HM, Inge TH, Daniels SR, Wang B, Khoury PR, Witt SA, Glascock BJ, Garcia VF, Kimball TR. Reversibility of cardiac abnormalities in morbidly obese adolescents. J Am Coll Cardiol. 2008;51:1342–8.

42. Teeple EA, Teich S, Schuster DP, Michalsky MP. Early metabolic improvement following bariatric surgery in morbidly obese adolescents. Pediatr Blood Cancer. 2012;58:112–6.

43. Biro FM, Wien M. Childhood obesity and adult morbidities. Am J Clin Nutr. 2010;91:1499S–505.

44. The NS, Suchindran C, North KE, Popkin BM, Gordon-Larsen P. Association of adolescent obesity with risk of severe obesity in adulthood. JAMA. 2010;304:2042–7.

45. Reilly JJ, Kelly J. Long-term impact of overweight and obesity in childhood and adolescence on morbidity and premature mortality in adulthood: systematic review. Int J Obes (Lond). 2010;35:891–8.

46. Inge TH, Miyano G, Bean J, Helmrath M, Courcoulas A, Harmon CM, Chen MK, Wilson K, Daniels SR, Garcia VF, et al. Reversal of type 2 diabetes mellitus and improvements in cardiovascular risk factors after surgical weight loss in adolescents. Pediatrics. 2009;123:214–22.

47. Michalsky M, Rama S, Teich S, Schuster DP, Bauer J. Cardiovascular recovery following bariatric surgery in extremely obese adolescents: preliminary results using cardiac magnetic resonance (CMR) imaging. J Pediatr Surg. 2013;48:170–7.

48. Freedman DS, Khan LK, Dietz WH, Srinivasan SR, Berenson GS. Relationship of childhood obesity to coronary heart disease risk factors in adulthood: the Bogalusa Heart Study. Pediatrics. 2001;108:712–8.

49. Inge TH, Jenkins TM, Zeller M, Dolan L, Daniels SR, Garcia VF, Brandt ML, Bean J, Gamm K, Xanthakos SA. Baseline BMI is a strong predictor of nadir BMI after adolescent gastric bypass. J Pediatr. 2010;156:103–8; e101.

50. Narayan KM, Boyle JP, Thompson TJ, Sorensen SW, Williamson DF. Lifetime risk for diabetes mellitus in the United States. JAMA. 2003;290:1884–90.

51. Gozal D, Wang M, Pope Jr DW. Objective sleepiness measures in pediatric obstructive sleep apnea. Pediatrics. 2001;108:693–7.

52. Gozal D. Sleep-disordered breathing and school performance in children. Pediatrics. 1998;102:616–20.

53. Ahrens W, Bammann K, de Henauw S, Halford J, Palou A, Pigeot I, Siani A, Sjostrom M. Understanding and preventing childhood obesity and related disorders—IDEFICS: a European multilevel epidemiological approach. Nutr Metab Cardiovasc Dis. 2006;16:302–8.

54. Gordon CM. Menstrual disorders in adolescents. Excess androgens and the polycystic ovary syndrome. Pediatr Clin North Am. 1999;46:519–43.

55. Rahmanpour H, Jamal L, Mousavinasab SN, Esmailzadeh A, Azarkhish K. Association between polycystic ovarian syndrome, overweight, and metabolic syndrome in adolescents. J Pediatr Adolesc Gynecol. 2012;25:208–12.

56. Xanthakos S, Miles L, Bucuvalas J, Daniels S, Garcia V, Inge T. Histologic spectrum of nonalcoholic fatty liver disease in morbidly obese adolescents. Clin Gastroenterol Hepatol. 2006;4:226–32.

57. Mummadi RR, Kasturi KS, Chennareddygari S, Sood GK. Effect of bariatric surgery on nonalcoholic fatty liver disease: systematic review and meta-analysis. Clin Gastroenterol Hepatol. 2008;6:1396–402.

58. Richardson SA, Goodman N, Hastorf AN, et al. Cultural uniformity in reaction to physical disabilities. Am Soc Rev. 1961;26:241–7.

59. Sanchez-Villegas A, Pimenta AM, Beunza JJ, Guillen-Grima F, Toledo E, Martinez-Gonzalez MA. Childhood and young adult overweight/obesity and incidence of depression in the SUN project. Obesity. 2010;18:1443–8.

60. Wang F, Wild TC, Kipp W, Kuhle S, Veugelers PJ. The influence of childhood obesity on the development of self-esteem. Health Rep. 2009;20:21–7.

61. Zeller MH, Reiter-Purtill J, Ratcliff MB, Inge TH, Noll JG. Two-year trends in psychosocial functioning after adolescent Roux-en-Y gastric bypass. Surg Obes Relat Dis. 2011;7:727–32.

62. Buchwald H, Estok R, Fahrbach K, Banel D, Jensen MD, Pories WJ, Bantle JP, Sledge I. Weight and type 2 diabetes after bariatric

surgery: systematic review and meta-analysis. Am J Med. 2009;122:248–56; e245.

63. Aggarwal R, Hodgson L, Rao C, Ashrafian H, Chow A, Zacharakis E, Athanasiou T, Darzi A, Johnston D. Surgical management of morbid obesity. Br J Hosp Med (Lond). 2008;69:95–100.

64. McGovern L, Johnson JN, Paulo R, Hettinger A, Singhal V, Kamath C, Erwin PJ, Montori VM. Clinical review: treatment of pediatric obesity: a systematic review and meta-analysis of randomized trials. J Clin Endocrinol Metab. 2008;93:4600–5.

65. Savoye M, Nowicka P, Shaw M, Yu S, Dziura J, Chavent G, O'Malley G, Serrecchia JB, Tamborlane WV, Caprio S. Long-term results of an obesity program in an ethnically diverse pediatric population. Pediatrics. 2011;127:402–10.

66. Tsai WS, Inge TH, Burd RS. Bariatric surgery in adolescents: recent national trends in use and in-hospital outcome. Arch Pediatr Adolesc Med. 2007;161:217–21.

67. Schilling PL, Davis MM, Albanese CT, Dutta S, Morton J. National trends in adolescent bariatric surgical procedures and implications for surgical centers of excellence. J Am Coll Surg. 2008;206:1–12.

68. Jen HC, Rickard DG, Shew SB, Maggard MA, Slusser WM, Dutson EP, DeUgarte DA. Trends and outcomes of adolescent bariatric surgery in California, 2005–2007. Pediatrics. 2010;126:e746–53.

69. Messiah SE, Lopez-Mitnik G, Winegar D, Sherif B, Arheart KL, Reichard KW, Michalsky MP, Lipshultz SE, Miller TL, Livingstone AS, et al. Changes in weight and co-morbidities among adolescents undergoing bariatric surgery: 1-year results from the Bariatric Outcomes Longitudinal Database. Surg Obes Relat Dis. 2013; 9:503–13.

70. Inge TH, Krebs NF, Garcia VF, Skelton JA, Guice KS, Strauss RS, Albanese CT, Brandt ML, Hammer LD, Harmon CM, et al. Bariatric surgery for severely overweight adolescents: concerns and recommendations. Pediatrics. 2004;114:217–23.

71. Apovian CM, Baker C, Ludwig DS, Hoppin AG, Hsu G, Lenders C, Pratt JS, Forse RA, O'Brien A, Tarnoff M. Best practice guidelines in pediatric/adolescent weight loss surgery. Obes Res. 2005; 13:274–82.

72. Pratt JS, Lenders CM, Dionne EA, Hoppin AG, Hsu GL, Inge TH, Lawlor DF, Marino MF, Meyers AF, Rosenblum JL, et al. Best practice updates for pediatric/adolescent weight loss surgery. Obesity (Silver Spring). 2009;17:901–10.

73. Michalsky M, Reichard K, Inge T, Pratt J, Lenders C. ASMBS pediatric committee best practice guidelines. Surg Obes Relat Dis. 2012;8:1–7.

74. Michalsky M, Kramer RE, Fullmer MA, Polfuss M, Porter R, Ward-Begnoche W, Getzoff EA, Dreyer M, Stolzman S, Reichard KW. Developing criteria for pediatric/adolescent bariatric surgery programs. Pediatrics. 2011;128 Suppl 2:S65–70.

75. Tanner JM, Davies PS. Clinical longitudinal standards for height and height velocity for North American children. J Pediatr. 1985;107:317–29.

76. Marceau P, Marceau S, Biron S, Hould FS, Lebel S, Lescelleur O, Biertho L, Kral JG. Long-term experience with duodenal switch in adolescents. Obes Surg. 2010;20:1609–16.

77. Varela JE, Hinojosa MW, Nguyen NT. Perioperative outcomes of bariatric surgery in adolescents compared with adults at academic medical centers. Surg Obes Relat Dis. 2007;3:537–40; discussion 541-532.

78. Al-Qahtani AR. Laparoscopic adjustable gastric banding in adolescent: safety and efficacy. J Pediatr Surg. 2007;42:894–7.

79. Inge TH, Xanthakos SA, Zeller MH. Bariatric surgery for pediatric extreme obesity: now or later? Int J Obes (Lond). 2007;31:1–14.

80. Barnett SJ, Stanley C, Hanlon M, Acton R, Saltzman DA, Ikramuddin S, Buchwald H. Long-term follow-up and the role of surgery in adolescents with morbid obesity. Surg Obes Relat Dis. 2005;1:394–8.

81. Capella JF, Capella RF. Bariatric surgery in adolescence. is this the best age to operate? Obes Surg. 2003;13:826–32.

82. de la Cruz-Munoz N, Messiah SE, Cabrera JC, Torres C, Cuesta M, Lopez-Mitnik G, Arheart KL. Four-year weight outcomes of laparoscopic gastric bypass surgery and adjustable gastric banding among multiethnic adolescents. Surg Obes Relat Dis. 2010;6:542–7.

83. Fatima J, Houghton SG, Iqbal CW, Thompson GB, Que FL, Kendrick ML, Mai JL, Collazo-Clavel ML, Sarr MG. Bariatric surgery at the extremes of age. J Gastrointest Surg. 2006;10:1392–6.

84. Sugerman HJ, Sugerman EL, DeMaria EJ, Kellum JM, Kennedy C, Mowery Y, Wolfe LG. Bariatric surgery for severely obese adolescents. J Gastrointest Surg. 2003;7:102–7; discussion 107-108.

85. Papadia FS, Adami GF, Marinari GM, Camerini G, Scopinaro N. Bariatric surgery in adolescents: a long-term follow-up study. Surg Obes Relat Dis. 2007;3:465–8.

86. Treadwell JR, Sun F, Schoelles K. Systematic review and meta-analysis of bariatric surgery for pediatric obesity. Ann Surg. 2008;248:763–76.

87. Kalra M, Inge T, Garcia V, Daniels S, Lawson L, Curti R, Cohen A, Amin R. Obstructive sleep apnea in extremely overweight adolescents undergoing bariatric surgery. Obes Res. 2005;13:1175–9.

88. Xanthakos SA. Nutritional deficiencies in obesity and after bariatric surgery. Pediatr Clin North Am. 2009;56:1105–21.

89. Ananthapavan J, Moodie M, Haby M, Carter R. Assessing cost-effectiveness in obesity: laparoscopic adjustable gastric banding for severely obese adolescents. Surg Obes Relat Dis. 2010;6:377–85.

90. Holterman AX, Browne A, Tussing L, Gomez S, Phipps A, Browne N, Stahl C, Holterman MJ. A prospective trial for laparoscopic adjustable gastric banding in morbidly obese adolescents: an interim report of weight loss, metabolic and quality of life outcomes. J Pediatr Surg. 2010;45:74–8; discussion 78-79.

91. O'Brien PE, Sawyer SM, Laurie C, Brown WA, Skinner S, Veit F, Paul E, Burton PR, McGrice M, Anderson M, et al. Laparoscopic adjustable gastric banding in severely obese adolescents: a randomized trial. JAMA. 2010;303:519–26.

92. Alqahtani AR, Antonisamy B, Alamri H, Elahmedi M, Zimmerman VA. Laparoscopic sleeve gastrectomy in 108 obese children and adolescents aged 5 to 21 years. Ann Surg. 2012;256:266–73.

93. Alqahtani A, Alamri H, Elahmedi M, Mohammed R. Laparoscopic sleeve gastrectomy in adult and pediatric obese patients: a comparative study. Surg Endosc. 2012;26:3094–100.

43

Bariatric Surgery in the Elderly

Elizabeth A. Hooper, Bamdad Farhad, and Julie J. Kim

Introduction

Advances in health care have continued to enable people to live longer and healthier lives than ever before. In 2008 the overall life expectancy in the United States was 78 years and is projected to reach 79.5 or nearly 80 years by 2020, a number already achieved in the female subset since 2006 [1]. This is a dramatic increase since Roman times, when the average life span was only 25–30 years.

Although there is no clear consensus or standard definition, the use of the term "elderly" is generally reserved for individuals that are at least 60–65 or more years of age. In the bariatric literature, however, age >50–55 years has also been used to define "elderly." In 2010 there were 40.3 million people age 65 in the United States, reflecting an increase of five million people since 2000. The first baby boomer (those individuals born between 1946 and 1964) turned 65 years old on Jan 1, 2011. With 77 million baby boomers, it is estimated that more than 10,000 people will turn 65 every day for the next 19 years, making the elderly one of the fastest-growing subsets and projected to comprise 20 % of the population by the year 2030 [1]. Individuals above the age of 65 currently undergo more surgical procedures than any other age group; the incidence of which is expected to increase over the next several decades [2]. Surgical utilization is not equally distributed, however, with the highest volume projected in the areas of ophthalmology, cardiothoracic surgery, and to a lesser extent orthopedics, urology, and neurosurgery [3]. Also anticipated to increase is the prevalence of obesity. Overall, 34.6 % of adults aged 65 and over, representing 13 million adults, were obese in 2007–2010, with a lower prevalence of obesity among those aged 75 and over (27.8 %) than the 65–74 age group (40.8 %) [4]. It is projected that nearly 50 % of the elderly will be obese by 2030, raising numerous policy issues regarding coverage of healthcare costs, the allocation of available resources at both the state and federal level [5], as well as increasing numbers of elderly patients likely seeking bariatric surgery.

Despite numerous increases in the understanding of obesity as a disease, bariatric and metabolic surgery remains the only safe, effective, and durable treatment of morbid obesity for the far majority of individuals. The advancement of laparoscopic and minimally invasive techniques has revolutionized the field of metabolic and bariatric surgery. Quality improvement initiatives in the form of accreditation processes and national database collection have resulted in significant reduction of morbidity and mortality over the past decade.

Assessing the effect of chronologic age on operative risk is difficult given the wide heterogeneity of operations in question and the lack of randomized controlled trials evaluating bariatric surgery in the elderly. Most analyses of perioperative care in the elderly have been extrapolated from the literature on younger patients, making them prone to error. Bariatric surgery in the elderly, however, may entail a risk profile that is inherently different from that of orthopedic, cancer, or cardiac surgery. As the percentage of obese elderly continues to rise, it will be important that standard guidelines are created to help facilitate the process of patient selection, procedure selection, and perioperative care for this group of bariatric patients. Until sufficient evidence is obtained from prospective studies, the ultimate decision to operate on the elderly will be left to the discretion of each individual bariatric surgeon or practice.

How Does Obesity Impact the Elderly?

Most research on obesity is derived from young and middle-aged patients. There is limited data regarding the prognostic importance of overweight and obesity in the elderly. Surprisingly, overweight and mild obesity do not seem to be associated with any significant increase in cardiovascular mortality in individuals 65 years of age or older, as compared with younger cohorts. The data, in fact, suggest that individuals 65 and older may require a higher optimum

S.A. Brethauer et al. (eds.), *Minimally Invasive Bariatric Surgery*,
DOI 10.1007/978-1-4939-1637-5_43, © Springer Science+Business Media New York 2015

body mass index (BMI) than the ideal weight currently defined in federal guidelines for all individuals as a BMI between 18.7 and 24.9 [6]. Longitudinal studies looking at the effects of aging on body composition suggest that aging is associated with a decrease in lean muscle mass and increase in fat mass regardless of changes in overall body weight [7, 8]. This loss of muscle mass that occurs with aging is a process called sarcopenia, which may not be as clearly identified by BMI alone [9]. In addition, the natural loss of height seen with increases in age is more significant in females and may also arbitrarily elevate BMI [10]. Several studies have shown that the excess mortality associated with obesity actually declines with age [11]. In addition, there have been conflicting data from observational studies associating weight loss with increased mortality in the elderly [12–14]; however, the far majority of studies do not make the distinction between intentional and unintentional weight loss, the latter of which may be a reflection of other confounding conditions such as cancer, failure to thrive, or worsening of chronic comorbid conditions, which would increase mortality risk and may explain some of the discrepancy. A recent RCT, however, found no significant difference in all-cause mortality between older (mean age 65.5±4.5 years) overweight and obese (mean BMI 31.1±2.3) adults who were randomized to intentional dietary weight loss (mean weight loss of 4.4 kg) over a 12-year period [15]. Given the increased incidence of sarcopenic obesity in the elderly population, future prospective studies will need to continue to separate and make the clear distinction between intentional and unintentional weight loss when determining the risk of mortality.

Therefore, until age-specific recommendations are made, elderly patients who are being considered for weight reduction surgery should continue to meet whatever the currently accepted weight criteria or other criteria for defining morbid obesity and clinically severe obesity exist, whether this be the NIH consensus guidelines or other new emerging guidelines. There are also very few studies involving medical weight loss in the elderly. Most studies on supervised diets or medications have been performed in younger patients. Thus, it is recommended that elderly patients have attempted a serious effort at documented medical weight loss before undergoing surgical treatment, particularly since moderate dietary reduction and exercise have been shown to be safe in preserving lean muscle mass. Studies looking at physical activity in the elderly have shown that increased physical activity is associated with decreased mortality. In an observational study by Lee et al., it was shown that there was a higher all-cause and cardiovascular mortality in lean unfit subject than in obese fit subjects, once again emphasizing the importance of physical activity and muscle mass preservation over the amount of body fat alone, in predicting the risk of mortality [16].

Patient Selection and Preoperative Assessment of Surgical Risk in the Elderly

Due to the lack of any uniform consensus, the onus of patient selection falls on the bariatric surgeon. Chronologic age alone is a poor predictor of the outcome as the elderly patient may have limited ability for recovery. Preoperative evaluation necessitates further investigations compared to the general population [17]. Emphasis should be placed on the evaluation of the functional status of the individual. The impact of age on surgical risk arises from a decrease in vital organ function. This is attributable to the normal aging process in conjunction with any preexisting disease, resulting in a decreased ability to respond optimally to operative stress [18]. The decline in physiologic capacity to respond to surgical stress, independent of specific individual organ system dysfunction, is referred to as frailty [17].

Frailty takes into account multiple factors that may place the geriatric patient at a distinct physiologic disadvantage. It is important to note that a patient does not simply fall into one of the two categories: for an elderly with or without frailty rather, one needs to carry out a quantitative analysis for measurement of frailty index [19]. There are multiple tools that can be used for preoperative frailty assessment, one of which is the Katz ADL score which examines the patients' level of independence on daily activities. The patient is given a point for each of six activities: grooming, bathing, feeding, dressing, toiletry, and dressing [20]. In addition to independence in daily life and medical comorbidites, an assessment for mobility, nutritional, and cognitive status (the mini-mental test) has been recommended for preoperative evaluation of patients in general surgery literature [21].

In addition to age, one should consider other independent patient risk characteristics associated with increased morbidity and mortality, which include male gender [22]. Patients should be stratified into a high- or low-risk category based on the number of associated diseases. The literature suggests that the preoperative condition of the patient is more important than intraoperative events in predicting adverse outcomes after surgery. A dramatic increase in perioperative deaths has been seen in elderly patients with multisystem disease. Premorbid conditions that may increase perioperative risk include congestive heart failure (CHF) and coronary artery disease [23]. Nguyen et al. published data from the National Inpatient Sample which reviewed >300,000 inpatients undergoing lap and open gastric bypass over a 3-year period (2006–2008) and identified peripheral vascular disease and chronic renal failure as comorbid conditions associated with increased risk of inpatient mortality. The goal of any bariatric operation should be to improve the quality of postoperative life, or at minimum, not impair it. Therefore, preoperative optimization of the elderly patient's overall condition, without undue delay in surgery, is advocated.

There are several normal age-related physiologic changes that may or may not have any overt clinical findings. These age-related changes result in altered end organ function, most importantly cardiac, pulmonary, and renal function. Cardiac output can be decreased from a blunted response to catecholamines, which can lead to increased ectopy that may not be seen in the resting state. Hypertrophy of the left ventricular mass can add to any underlying diastolic dysfunction already present. It may be prudent in elderly patients to evaluate the functional cardiac status under stressed conditions (using a treadmill stress test or a Persantine thallium scan), even in the presence of a normal electrocardiogram. A transthoracic echocardiogram should also be considered in any patient with history of CHF.

The changes in the respiratory system include decreased chest wall compliance, decreased lung volumes, and decreased strength of the respiratory musculature, resulting in an overall decline of pulmonary function. Elderly patients, therefore, may be more susceptible to postoperative respiratory complications. Pulmonary function tests are not normally required in the workup of a routine bariatric candidate but may be informative, particularly if there is a question regarding pulmonary reserve in a patient with baseline chronic lung disease (previous episodes of pneumonia, long smoking history, pulmonary embolus, asthma) or obesity hypoventilation syndrome.

Normal renal changes include decreased renal blood flow with resultant decreased glomerular filtration rate and decreased creatinine clearance. Patients who present with marginal renal function should have close attention to their perioperative fluid status. Gentle hydration without large volume shifts is generally better tolerated. Any potentially nephrotoxic drugs should be discontinued prior to surgery [18].

One postoperative complication that is relatively unique to the elderly population is delirium. Delirium is defined as a "clinical syndrome in which there is an acute disruption of attention and cognition" [24]. Delirium has been associated most commonly with cardiac and orthopedic procedures but has been reported in all types of surgery. When delirium occurs postoperatively, it has been associated with increased morbidity and mortality [25]. Preoperative risk factors include age, history of or current alcohol abuse, history of depression, dementia, and the presence of any metabolic derangements [25]. Recent studies have suggested preoperative variables associated with an increased risk of postoperative delirium to include: age, low serum albumin, impaired functional status, medical comorbidities, and presence of dementia. The strongest single risk factor for the development of delirium was preexisting dementia [26]. Screening for these risk factors and correction preoperatively as necessary should be attempted.

Immobility is a problem associated with morbid obesity that can become aggravated in elderly patients. The incidence of degenerative joint disease increases with age, and many obese elderly patients may be denied corrective joint repair due to their excess weight. Their immobility, however, may limit their ability to lose weight through more conservative measures such as diet and exercise, leaving surgery as one of the few options for effective treatment. Immobility can also result in wound care issues, with the formation of decubitus ulcers. Elderly bariatric patients requiring long-term intensive care are at high risk for the development of such ulcers. For the uncomplicated postoperative patient, early ambulation is essential, which in the elderly may require assistance from physiotherapists or the nursing staff. In addition, consideration for extended DVT chemoprophylaxis and/or placement in acute rehab postoperatively should be discussed as part of informed consent and preoperative planning for patients with poor mobility.

Outcomes of Bariatric Surgery in the Elderly

There are several studies in the literature that suggest an increased risk of mortality in the elderly after surgery. In general, most of these studies, however, have small sample size, include patients in their eighth and ninth decades of life, as well as those undergoing cancer operations, cardiac procedures, or semi-emergent operations [27–30]. It is on the basis of such a wide range of operations that much of our early outcomes data on the elderly had been gathered. Although we are still gaining insight on the safest way to manage elderly patients, certain trends have been established. Emergency surgery is associated with higher morbidity and mortality in all age groups, but particularly in the elderly. Elderly patients often present with more advanced disease, forcing surgical therapy once complications have already occurred. Elderly patients have a higher percentage of preexisting comorbid conditions, making them less likely to tolerate complications, if they occur; therefore, prevention remains essential [23].

Historically, many bariatric centers refused surgery to patients over 50. In 1977, Printen et al. [31] reported a greater than twofold increase in mortality after gastric bypass in patients older than 50 compared with those younger than 50 (8 % vs. 2.8 %). This, however, was an evaluation of only 36 patients during a time when the overall mortality for gastric bypass was significantly higher than what is seen today. In contrast, MacGregor and Rand [32] in 1993 did not find a statistical difference in mortality (1.1 % vs. 0.6 %) in those patients aged 50 or older as compared with younger patients undergoing a variety of obesity operations. Similar findings were shown by Murr et al. [33] in 1995. A later study by Livingston et al. [34] suggested that increasing age was not associated with increased morbidity after gastric bypass. However, if a complication were to occur in this population, the incidence of mortality associated with an adverse event was threefold in older patients, reinforcing the concept that elderly patients may have less physiologic reserve than younger patients to overcome an adverse event [35].

National databases have been utilized to examine morbidity trends in older populations with some variability. In 2005, Flum et al. reported on a large retrospective database of Medicare recipients undergoing bariatric surgery from 1998 to 2002. This study found higher 30-day, 90-day, and 1-year mortality for those greater than 65 with low-volume surgeons and/or hospitals. It also showed that those over age 75 had the most significant increase in mortality risks, when compared to the under 65 population. Notably, in those 65 or older undergoing surgery with high-volume surgeons, there was no significant increase in mortality 1.8 % vs. 1.1 %. Despite a sample size of over 16,000 patients, only 10 % of those included were over age 65. At the time of the study, there were no formal CPT codes for laparoscopic bariatric procedures. This led to inclusion of all open operations but possible undersampling of laparoscopic bariatric procedures [35]. Livingston and Langert reviewed data from 2001 to 2002 NIS database which also included open procedures and found a threefold increase in mortality when compared to under 55 group [34].

In the last 10 years, there have been significant advances in patient selection, preoperative preparation of patients, perioperative care, ICU care when required, and long-term follow-up of patients in multidisciplinary settings. Although there is no longer a paucity of literature about obesity surgery in the 60 and older population, the quality of the data remains variable. Many studies continue to include patient cohorts from the pre-laparoscopic era or retrospective evaluations of single institution experiences.

The 2006 CMS National Coverage Determination (NCD) for bariatric surgery has allowed increasing numbers of patients 65 and older access to bariatric surgery and better data collection. The post-NCD addition of the LAGB, increasing utilization of laparoscopic over open techniques particularly for the gastric bypass, and mandating centers of excellence have all resulted in significant decrease in the risk of death, complications, readmissions, and per patient payments. In 2011 a study by Flum et al., utilizing pre- and post-NCD Medicare data from 2004 to 2008, found the 90-day mortality pre-NCD was 1.5 % (1.8 % ORYGB, 1.1 % LRYGB) and post-NCD was 0.7 % (1.7 % ORYGB, 0.8 % LRYGB, 0.3 % LAGB; $P < 0.001$) [36] consistent with other comparisons [37].

The current literature for bariatric surgery reports mortality rates of 0.5 % or less for all comers [38] with emerging data supporting a much lower mortality risk for patients 60 years and above [39]. Wittgrove reported a single institution experience of 120 patients over age 60 with a 0 % mortality rate and 19 % morbidity for laparoscopic Roux-en-Y gastric bypass. Ten percent of the morbidity was attributed to stenosis at the GJ anastomosis, which is more likely a function of technical considerations than the age of the patient. Associated

comorbid conditions, however, showed dramatic resolution: 75 % DM, 88 % HTN, and 94 % sleep apnea [39]. Similar findings have also been reported by Hallowell et al., comparing patients undergoing gastric bypass looking at Medicare and non-Medicare cohorts as well as age less than 60 versus over 60 with no difference in morbidity or mortality [10].

In 2011, Leivonen et al. found equivalent safety profile for laparoscopic sleeve gastrectomy in >55 compared to under 55 populations. Excess weight loss in the two age groups was equivalent with 0 % mortality rates They did find a higher incidence of vitamin irregularities in the elderly group highlighting the continued importance of routine follow-up care [40].

In 2009, utilizing the ACS NSQIP database, Dorman et al. analyzed a data set that included laparoscopic procedures and pooled data from a wide range of care settings. Patients were separated into age groups and evaluated for significant morbidity or mortality differences. The overall 30-day mortality was 0.15 % with the 65–69 subset = 0.4 % and >70 year age = 0.5 %. Although there was an increasing trend with age, statistical significance was not determined. Major adverse events were also reported and were less than 5 % in all age groups. Predicted length of stay more than 3 days was, however, significantly higher in the 65–69 and >70 subset group [41].

In 2012, Lynch et al. published a meta-analysis of the available literature and found 18 studies which included 1,200 patients over the age of 55 who underwent bariatric surgery. 30-day mortality was 0.25 % for the population again in line with the longitudinal Assessment of Bariatric Consortium mortality rate of 0.30 % for a younger patient population. There continued to be significant improvement in comorbidity resolution [42].

Several other studies of nonbariatric laparoscopic procedures have been shown to be safe and effective in the elderly, including laparoscopic cholecystectomies, laparoscopic Nissen fundoplications, and laparoscopic colectomies [43–46]. In 2012, the ACS NSQIP group collaborated with the American Geriatrics Society (AGS) to review the literature on the presurgical assessment in patients. After an exhaustive search of the literature, 117 articles were reviewed to create a consensus approved checklist for preoperative assessment. Interestingly, this article did not suggest that more testing is better for all patients. It instead suggests thorough screening for all patients with a detailed history and physical and lab tests only as warranted. The exceptions to that would be that measurement of hemoglobin, renal function, and albumin should be obtained for all geriatric patients, but other tests may be obtained for higher-risk patients based on the presence of comorbid conditions [47].

One argument against performing bariatric surgery on the elderly is that it may offer limited benefits with respect to prolongation of life and provision of quality-of-life years compared to the younger severely obese population. At a time when fewer than 1 % of individuals eligible to undergo bariatric surgery with its expected benefits are actually receiving surgical treatment, one could pose an argument in favor of continuing to target these procedures to younger patients or to elderly patients who by physiologic assessment are low risk for surgery.

Conclusion

The elderly comprise the fastest-growing segment of the population in the United States. The proportion of elderly patients who will consider weight reduction surgery is likely to increase over the next several decades. Performing bariatric surgery in the elderly today is less controversial and is supported by retrospective publications as being safe and feasible, in patients over the age of 65 and even 70. Given the limitations found in current studies looking at the effect of obesity on mortality outcomes in the elderly, the decision to offer bariatric surgery should still be made with consideration of current weight guidelines and failure of conservative efforts. Careful preoperative screening is advocated in elderly patients in hopes of optimizing functional status and improving outcome or improving morbidity. Chronologic age will continue to be less clinically significant than previously thought; however, better understanding of natural changes that occur with aging and emphasis of maintaining cardiovascular fitness in addition to weight loss (reduction of body fat) will be important.

Review Questions and Answers

1. Which of the following patients has the lowest frailty index?

   A. Fifty-nine years old female with a history of HTN, CHF, and DM that lives by herself but is unable to cook for herself and requires monthly financial assistance from her daughter.

   B. Sixty-seven years old male with a history of anxiety and depression that lives at a nursing home and does not require assistance with any of his daily activities but uses a walker.

   C. Fifty-three years old well-nourished male with normal affect and good sense of humor that lives with his family and requires assistance with bathing, toileting, and getting dressed.

   D. Fifty-nine years old male with h/o bipolar disorder. He is stable on medications and lives in a group home and requires assistance with feeding and bathing.

The answer is A.
Using the Katz ADL scoring patient A received 6 out of a possible 6 points and therefore has the lowest frailty index. Although patient B can perform all essential daily activities

independently, his mobility (transferring) is somewhat restricted as he has to use a walker so would receive 5 points. Patient C and D both require assistance with multiple daily activities and received 3 and 4 points respectively, giving each a higher frailty score than patient A.

2. Unintentional weight loss in the elderly is:
   A. Associated with decreased risk of mortality
   B. May represent confounding conditions such as cancer, failure to thrive or worsening of underlying comorbid conditions
   C. Associated with decreased fat mass
   D. Has a similar benefit as intentional weight loss

The answer is B.
Unintentional weight loss in the elderly may represent confounding conditions such as cancer, failure to thrive or worsening of underlying comorbid conditions and can be associated with a higher risk of mortality.

References

1. U.S. Census Bureau, Statistical Abstract of the United States. 2012
2. Ergina P, Gold S, Meakin J. Perioperative care of the elderly patient. World J Surg. 1993;17:192–8.
3. Etzoni DA, Liu JH, Maggard MH, et al. The aging population and its impact on the surgery workforce. Ann Surg. 2003;238:170–7.
4. Fakhouri THI, Ogden CL, Carroll MD, et al. Prevalence of obesity among older adults in the united states 2007–2010. NCHS Data Brief. No. 106. Sept 2012.
5. Sommers AR. Obesity among older Americans. Congressional Research Service. Feb 2009.
6. Heiat A, Vaccarino V, Krunholz HM. An evidence-based assessment of federal guidelines for overweight and obesity as they apply to elderly persons. Arch Intern Med. 2001;161:1194–203.
7. Forbes GB. Longitudinal changes in adult fat-free mass: influence of body weight. Am J Clin Nutr. 1999;70:1025–31.
8. Hughes VA, Frontera WR, Roubenoff R, et al. Longitudinal changes in body composition in older men and women: role of body weight change and physical activity. Am J Clin Nutr. 2002;76:473–81.
9. Janssen I, Heymsfield SB, Ross R. Low relative skeletal muscle mass (Sarcopenia) in older persons is associated with functional impairment and physical disability. J Am Geriatr Soc. 2002;50:889–96.
10. Hallowell PT, Stellato TA, Schuster M, et al. Avoidance of complications in older patients and Medicare recipients undergoing gastric bypass. Arch Surg. 2007;142:506–12.
11. Bender R, Jockel KH, Trautner C, et al. Effect of age on excess mortality in obesity. JAMA. 1999;281:1498–504.
12. Knudtson MD, Klein BE, Klein R, et al. Associations with weight loss and subsequent mortality risk. Ann Epidemiol. 2005;15:483–91.
13. Sorensen TI, Rissanen A, Korkeila M, et al. Intention to lose weight, weight changes, and 18-y mortality in overweight individuals without co-morbidities. PLoS Med. 2005;2:e171.
14. Yaari S, Goldbourt U. Voluntary and involuntary weight loss: associations with long term mortality in 9,228 middle-age. Am J Epidemiol. 1998;148:546–55.
15. Shea MK, Nicklas BJ, Houston DK, Miller ME, et al. The effect of intentional weight loss on all-cause mortality in older adults: results of a randomized controlled weight-loss trial. Am J Clin Nutr. 2011;94:839–46.

16. Lee CD, Blair SN, Jackson AS. Cardiorespiratory fitness, body composition, and all-cause and cardiovascular disease mortality in men. Am J Clin Nutr. 1999;69:373–80.

17. Robinson TN, Eiseman B, Wallace JI, et al. Redefining geriatric pre-operative assessment using frailty, disability and co-morbidity. Ann Surg. 2009;250:449.

18. Beliveau MM, Multach M. Perioperative care for the elderly patient. Med Clin North Am. 2003;87:273–89.

19. Rockwood K, Song X, MacKnight C, et al. A global clinical measure of fitness and frailty in elderly people. CMAJ. 2005;173:489.

20. Katz S, Ford AB, Moskowitz RW. Studies of illness in the aged. The Index of ADL: a standardized measure of biological and psychosocial function. JAMA. 1963;185(12):914–9.

21. McGory ML, Sekelle PG, Rubenstein LZ, et al. Developing quality indicators for elderly patients undergoing abdominal operations. J Am Coll Surg. 2005;201:870.

22. Ninh T, Nguyen MD, Hossein Masoomi MD, Kelly Laugenour BS. Predictive factors of mortality in bariatric surgery: data from the nationwide inpatient sample. Surgery. 2011;150:347–51.

23. Liu L, Leung JM. Predicting adverse postoperative outcomes in patients aged 80 years or older. J Am Geriatr Soc. 2000;48: 405–12.

24. Marcantonio ER, Goldman L, Mangione CM, et al. A clinical prediction rule for delirium after elective non-cardiac surgery. JAMA. 1994;271:134–9.

25. Marcantonio ER, Goldman L, Ovar EJ, et al. The association of intraoperative factors with the development of postoperative delirium. Am J Med. 1998;105:380–4.

26. Robinson TN, Raeburn CD, Tran ZV. Postoperative delirium in the elderly, risk factors and outcomes. Ann Surg. 2009;1:173–8.

27. Bender J, Magnunsun T, Zenilman M, et al. Outcome following colon surgery in the octogenarian. Am Surg. 1996;62:276–9.

28. Keating III J. Major surgery in nursing home patients: procedures, morbidity and mortality in the frailest of the frail elderly. J Am Geriatr Soc. 1992;40:8–11.

29. Adkins RJ, Scott HI. Surgical procedures in patients aged 90 years and older. South Med J. 1984;77:1357–64.

30. Osaki T, Shirakusa T, Kodate M, et al. Surgical treatment of lung cancer in the octogenarian. Ann Thorac Surg. 1994;57:188–93.

31. Printen KJ, Mason EE. Gastric bypass for morbid obesity in patients more than fifty years of age. Surg Gynecol Obstet. 1977;144:192–4.

32. MacGregor AMC, Rand CS. Gastric surgery in morbid obesity. Outcome in patients aged 55 and older. Arch Surg. 1993;128: 1153–7.

33. Murr MM, Siadati MR, Sarr MG. Results of bariatric surgery for morbid obesity in patients older than 50 years. Obes Surg. 1995;5: 399–402.

34. Livingston EH, Langert J. The impact of age and medicare status on bariatric surgical outcomes. Arch Surg. 2006;141:1115–20.

35. Flum D, Salem L, Elrod JA, et al. Early mortality among medicare beneficiaries undergoing bariatric surgical procedures. JAMA. 2005;15:1903–8.

36. Flum DR, Kwon S, MacLeod K, et al. The use, safety and cost of bariatric surgery before and after Medicare's national coverage decision. Ann Surg. 2011;254:860–5.

37. Nguyen NT, Hohmann S, Slone J, et al. Improved bariatric surgery outcomes for Medicare beneficiaries after implementation of the medicare national coverage determination. Arch Surg. 2010;145:72–8.

38. Buchwald H, Avidor Y, Braunwald E, et al. Bariatric surgery. A systematic review and meta-analysis. JAMA. 2004;292:1724–37.

39. Wittgrove A, Martinez T. Laparoscopic gastric bypass in patients 60 years and older: early postoperative morbidity and resolution of comorbidities. Obes Surg. 2009;19:1472–6.

40. Leivonen M, Juuti A, Jaser N, Mustonen H. Laparoscopic sleeve gastrectomy in patients over 59 years: early recovery and 12-month follow-up. Obes Surg. 2011;21:1180–7.

41. Dorman R, Abraham A, Al-Refaie W, et al. Bariatric surgery outcomes in the elderly: an ACS NSQIP study. J Gastrointest Surg. 2012;16:33–44.

42. Lynch J, Belgaumkar A. Bariatric surgery is effective and safe in patients over 55: a systematic review and meta-analysis. Obes Surg. 2012;22:1507–16.

43. Trus TL, Laycock WS, Wo JM, et al. Laparoscopic antireflux surgery in the elderly. Am J Gastroenterol. 1998;93:351–3.

44. Bammer T, Hinder RA, Klaus A, et al. Safety and long-term outcome of laparoscopic antireflux surgery in patients in their eighties and older. Surg Endosc. 2002;16:40–2.

45. Law WL, Chu KW, Tung PH. Laparoscopic colorectal resection: a safe option for elderly patients. J Am Coll Surg. 2002;195:768–73.

46. Bingener J, Richards ML, Schwesinger WH. Laparoscopic cholecystectomy for elderly patients: gold standard for golden years? Arch Surg. 2003;138:535–6.

47. Chow WB, Rosenthal RA, Merkow RP, et al. Optimal preoperative assessment of the geriatric surgical patient: a best practices guideline from the American College of Surgeons National Surgical Quality Improvement Program and the American Geriatrics Society. J Am Coll Surg. 2012;4:453–63.

48. Livingston EH, Huerta S, Arthur D, et al. Male gender is a predictor of morbidity and age a predictor of mortality in patients undergoing gastric bypass surgery. Ann Surg. 2002;236:576–82.

49. Frutos M, Lujan J, Hernandez Q, et al. Results of laparoscopic gastric bypass in patients >55 years old. Obes Surg. 2006;16:461–4.

44

The High-Risk Bariatric Patient

Eric Ahnfeldt, Monica Dua, and Derrick Cetin

Over the past decade, the number of patients undergoing weight loss surgery has increased exponentially with approximately 13,000 patients undergoing weight loss surgery in 1998 to 200,000 patients in 2009 [1]. During that time, advances in technique and approach to bariatric surgery have decreased the morbidity of these procedures, thus allowing patients that were previously at unacceptably high risk to now be candidates for weight loss surgery. Oftentimes the very comorbidities that placed these patients at high risk (namely, cardiopulmonary disease) are the same comorbidities that effective long-term weight loss could improve.

Careful identification and perioperative management of these higher-risk patients is crucial in decreasing morbidity after weight loss surgery. Recognizing that these patients needed to be specifically identified, the American Heart Association issued "A Science Advisory" in 2009 concerning the evaluation and management of severely obese patients undergoing surgery [1]. Obesity is associated with many comorbidities either known or unknown. Overall risk of developing anyone of a number of comorbidities rises with an increasing BMI. It has been noted that the number of individuals with a BMI > 50 kg/m² has quintupled between 1986 and 2000. For this reason, the scientific advisory was developed to provide recommendations concerning preoperative cardiopulmonary evaluation of severely obese patients undergoing surgery [1]. These recommendations included risk factors such as age, BMI, gender, hypertension, and history of venous thromboembolic events. These risk factors were drawn from the Obesity Surgery Mortality Risk Scoring system developed by DeMaria in 2007 and validated by several other studies since that time [2–4].

However, in addition to these risk factors, there are other factors that place certain patients at higher risk when undergoing weight loss surgery. When considering weight loss surgery on these patients, careful preoperative preparation and perioperative multidisciplinary management can lead to successful outcomes and durable comorbidity resolution or reduction.

This chapter evaluates the evidence behind each of these risk factors and suggests strategies for perioperative planning and risk reduction to aid in the identification and surgical care of the high-risk bariatric patient.

Estimating Risk

Who is the high-risk patient? Every patient undergoing a procedure requiring anesthesia is given an American Society of Anesthesiologist's (ASA) classification category. This category system was developed in 1941 and revised in 1963. Since that time, the ASA classification has been extensively evaluated and correlates well as a predictor of postoperative morbidity and mortality [5]. However, the majority of patients undergoing weight loss surgery have an ASA classification of three or higher based on the BOLD database, making them all high risk by conventional standards [3]. This created a need to further define risk categories within the bariatric population that would guide the perioperative work-up and management.

In 2007 DeMaria and colleagues evaluated 2,075 patients undergoing gastric bypass surgery seeking to define which variables could be used to predict postoperative mortality [2]. They found that BMI, male gender, hypertension, history of venous thromboembolic event, and age greater than 45 were significant independent predictors of mortality. They further developed the Obesity Surgery Mortality Risk Score (OS-MRS). This scoring system is divided into three classes A, B, and C, where each of the five variables is assigned one point. Patients with 0–1 point are included in category A, 2–3 points category B, and 4–5 points category C. Categories A, B, and C were associated with a 0.3 %, 1.90 %, and 7.56 % mortality risk, respectively (Table 1).

That same year, Buchwald and colleagues conducted a meta-analysis to evaluate a 30-day mortality based on type (gastric banding, gastroplasty, gastric bypass, or BPD/DS, or revisional surgery) and approach (laparoscopic vs open) of weight loss surgery [4]. They found significant differences in

S.A. Brethauer et al. (eds.), *Minimally Invasive Bariatric Surgery*,
DOI 10.1007/978-1-4939-1637-5_44, © Springer Science+Business Media New York 2015

TABLE 1. Obesity surgery mortality risk score

Class	No. of points	Mortality rate (%)
A	0–1	0.31
B	2–3	1.90
C	4–5	7.56

One point assigned for each of the following: BMI > 50 kg/m^2, male gender, HTN, PE risk, Age >45 years

TABLE 2. Thirty-day mortality for bariatric surgery by procedure

Surgery type	Death ≤30 days, mean (95 % CI)
Gastric banding	
Open	0.18 (0.00–0.49)
Laparoscopic	0.06 (0.01–0.11)
Gastroplasty	
Open	0.33 (0.15–0.51)
Laparoscopic	021 (0.00–0.48)
Gastric bypass	
Open	0.44 (0.25–0.64)
Laparoscopic	0.16 (0.09–0.23)
Biliopancreatic diversion/duodenal switch	
Open	0.76 (0.29–1.23)
Laparoscopic	1.11 (0.00–2.70)
Revisional surgery	
Open	0.96 (0.09–1.82)
Laparoscopic	0.00 (0.00–1.47)

Adapted from Buchwald et al.

mortality between the various types and approaches to weight loss surgery (Table 2).

Given the evolving definition of the high-risk patient within the bariatric population, the American Heart Association sought to clarify at least the clinical work-up for such patients, thus giving further definition to the high-risk bariatric patient. The 2009 Science advisory from the American Heart Association delineated numerous obesity-related comorbidities that influence the preoperative cardiac assessment and ultimately the management of the severely obese patient. These risk factors included atherosclerotic cardiovascular disease, heart failure, systemic hypertension, pulmonary hypertension related to sleep apnea and obesity hypoventilation, cardiac arrhythmias, deep vein thrombosis, history of pulmonary embolism, and poor exercise capacity [1]. In addition to these factors, the AHA included data from the Women's Health Initiative Observational Study suggesting that diabetes mellitus, elevated serum triglyceride levels, reduced serum high-density lipoprotein cholesterol levels, chronic inflammation, and prothrombotic state associated with obesity contribute to these patients' overall cardiovascular risk. This science advisory also incorporated the Buchwald data in the discussion of assessing preoperative risk.

Additional studies have sought to evaluate other independent risk factors for morbidity and mortality after weight loss surgery. One of the more surprising significant risk factors for increased morbidity and mortality was published in Archives of Surgery in 2006 by Livingston [6]. He evaluated 25,428 patients having undergone bariatric surgery and

found several factors that increased mortality with bariatric surgery: increasing age, male gender, electrolyte abnormalities, and congestive heart failure. He also found that the patients that had Medicare had greater disease burden and thus had higher morbidity.

Finally in 2011, Nguyen proposed a revised bariatric mortality risk classification system for patients undergoing bariatric surgery [7]. This updated, but more complicated, classification system encompassed those factors in DeMaria's classification system and added other risk factors such as presence of diabetes, Medicare status, and type of operation and approach. The significance of this system is the acknowledgement of the differences in the risk profiles of the different types and approaches (open vs laparoscopic) to weight loss surgery.

By using these classification systems and the considerations presented by the American Heart Association, patients that have multiple risk factors can be identified early in the preparation period. They can then be medically optimized for a risk-appropriate weight loss surgery. These patients can more appropriately be counseled as to their increased risk for complications after surgery. However, using a multidisciplinary approach, the perioperative management can help effectively decrease overall morbidity and mortality.

Risk Factors

Age

It has been well demonstrated that advanced age increases postoperative morbidity and mortality for any surgery. Specifically in a study by Livingston in 2006 published in the Archives of Surgery, advanced age (≥65 years) was seen as an independent risk factor for adverse outcomes as defined as length of hospital stay >95th percentile, being discharged to a long-term care facility or having died during the hospital admission for weight loss surgery [6]. Interestingly, they found that there was steady increase in rate of adverse events as age increased. However, there was a sharp increase in rate of adverse events at age 60. Beyond the age of 65, there was a 32 % rate of adverse events and a 3.2 % mortality rate.

Nguyen et al. evaluated more than 105,000 patients between 2002 and 2009. They found that age greater than 60 was a significant factor for in-hospital mortality from the multiple logistic regression analysis [7].

Gender

There are several well-performed studies that demonstrate that male gender is an independent risk factor for perioperative complications after weight loss surgery. In fact when DeMaria was developing the Obesity Surgery Mortality Risk

Score, his evaluation of the >2,000 gastric bypass patients demonstrated that male gender was an independent risk factor for mortality [2]. Livingston came to similar conclusions in his study in 2006 [6]. However, more recently (2011), Nguyen et al. suggested that even more than advanced age, male gender was associated with greater mortality after bariatric surgery [7]. Because of this, he gave male gender a greater contribution to his bariatric mortality risk classification.

Body Mass Index

Elevated weight or body mass index has been evaluated in many studies [8–10]. It seems intuitive that there would be a direct relationship between increasing BMI and risk of perioperative morbidity. Frequently as BMI increases, the physiology of the patient deteriorates. Patients with elevated BMIs typically have a higher incidence of cardiopulmonary insufficiency including right heart failure, pulmonary hypertension, obstructive sleep apnea, and obesity-related hypoventilation syndrome [8–10]. In addition to the physiologic consequences of morbid obesity, there are also mechanical challenges that these patients present. Their thickened abdominal wall, large liver, increased intraperitoneal fat, and limited working space after insufflation add to the technical difficulty of the procedure and may lengthen the duration of surgery [11, 12]. Acute presurgical weight loss may help ameliorate some of these technical difficulties and possibly decrease overall complications [13, 14]. All of these factors probably contribute to the fact that elevated BMI has been found in multiple studies, such as DeMaria's evaluation of 2,075 gastric bypass patients, to be an independent risk factor for perioperative mortality especially in BMI >50 [2].

Thromboembolic Disease

Darvall et al. did an extensive review of the relationship between obesity and venous thrombosis [15]. Within this review which included a medline review and Cochrane data base search from 1966 to 2005, a number of mechanisms were identified which connected obesity and venous thrombotic events.

In fact, the adipose tissue itself acts as an endocrine, paracrine, and autocrine organ, regulating among other processes, vascular homeostasis. The substances that are secreted by the adipose tissue that are potentially involved with venous thrombosis include leptin, adiponectin, resistin, plasminogen activator inhibitor-1 (PAI-1), tissue factor, angiotensin II, and other substances of the renin-angiotensin system, non-esterified free fatty acids (NEFAs), tumor necrosis factor-a (TNF-a), transforming growth factor-b (TGF-b), and interleukin-6 (IL-6) [15].

Leptin has been found to potentiate the aggregation of platelets by enhancing ADP's and thrombin's pro-aggretory effect on platelets. It also increases the synthesis of C-reactive protein contributing to the chronic inflammatory state of obesity. Tissue factor, also secreted from adipose tissue, initiates the coagulation cascade when exposed to blood and bound to factor VIIa. Obese individuals demonstrate higher levels of TF-mediated coagulation. Finally IL-6, a proinflammatory cytokine, secreted from adipose tissue has direct effect on inflammation in the human body. IL-6 overproduction has been implicated in the pathogenesis for inflammatory conditions such as rheumatoid arthritis, Crohn's disease, and juvenile idiopathic arthritis. Approximately one third of circulating IL-6 is produced from adipose tissue, and patients that are morbidly obese have higher circulating levels of IL-6. IL-6 inhibits gene expression and secretion of adiponectin, a powerful anti-inflammatory mediator. This may contribute to increased platelet aggregation and endothelial adhesion.

Furthermore, obese individuals have chronically elevated intra-abdominal pressure and decreased blood velocity in the common femoral vein resulting in venous stasis and ultimately contributing to increased risk for deep venous thrombus formation.

DeMaria recognized the elevated risk of these patients and included "PE risk" in his mortality risk score [2]. He found that the combination or presence of any of the following findings—previous VTE event, previous IVC filter placement, a history of right heart failure or pulmonary hypertension, history of physical findings of venous stasis including brawny edema or typical ulcerations—was highly statistically significant as a predictor of postoperative mortality. As such, he included "PE risk" in his mortality risk score system, underscoring the fact that pulmonary embolism is the leading cause of mortality in bariatric surgery centers, where the incidence of pulmonary embolism in patients who have undergone surgical procedures has been reported as high as 2 % [16].

Risk reduction strategies for decreasing thromboembolic events in patients that are at high risk include preoperative placement of vena cava filters, heparin windows, preoperative subcutaneous heparin administration, postoperative home administration of Lovenox, etc. In an analysis of the BOLD data base by Li, it was found that surgeons more typically put vena cava filters in patients with higher BMIs, that are African-American, who have had previous surgeries, who have prior history of venous thromboembolism, impaired functional status, lower extremity edema, obstructive sleep apnea, and pulmonary hypertension [17]. Interestingly, the patients that had the vena cava filters placed also had a higher incidence of DVTs and higher mortality rate. It is presumed that selection bias is responsible for the association between the filters and higher DVT/mortality rate. However, any decision to place a filter should consider the technical difficulty in placement and retrieval in the super-obese.

At our institution, Lovenox is typically given the day of surgery and a prophylaxis dose is given based on BMI.

(BMI > 60 = 60 mg Lovenox BID; BMI <60 = Lovenox 40 mg BID). Also patients with a BMI >55 are given a prescription for home Lovenox for 2 weeks after hospital discharge for extended prophylaxis. Patients with previous DVT/PE, known hypercoagulable state, or other risk factors (immobility) are also given 2–4 weeks of extended prophylaxis after hospital discharge. However, the optimal strategy for prevention of venous thromboembolism in the setting of bariatric surgery is uncertain [18].

Obstructive Sleep Apnea

Obstructive sleep apnea is discussed in detail in Chap. 51. However, in relationship to risk assessment in the high-risk patient, many studies have demonstrated the association with obstructive sleep apnea and perioperative complications. Memtsoudis et al. performed a case control study that evaluated 58,358 orthopedic patients and 45,547 general surgery patients in the journal Anesthesia and Analgesia in 2011. They found that patients undergoing orthopedic and general surgeries were at statistically significant higher risk for aspiration pneumonia, reintubation, ARDS, and mechanical ventilation [19]. That same year in the journal CHEST, Kaw et al. performed a cohort study evaluating 471 patients undergoing noncardiac surgery within 3 years of polysomnography and found that these patients had higher risks of hypoxemia, transfer to the ICU, and an increased length of hospital stay [20].

Vasu et al. included these two studies as well as nine others in their review of the association between obstructive sleep apnea syndrome and perioperative complications in the Journal of Clinical Sleep Medicine in 2012. They pointed out that beyond the risk association between OSA and perioperative complications, many people that have OSA are undiagnosed at the time of surgery. This makes them at higher risk for these complications since they are not being treated for their OSA in the perioperative period [21].

Cardiovascular Disease

In Livingston's population-based study of patients undergoing bariatric surgery, he found the event rate for cardiac complications to be as high as 15.3 per 1,000 patients. And the Women's Health Initiative Observational Study [22] found that the prevalence of myocardial infarction, angina pectoris, percutaneous coronary intervention, and coronary artery bypass graft to be as high as 11.5 % in morbidly obese women (BMI > 40). Thus, it is easy to understand that patients with higher BMIs are at a higher risk for perioperative events.

However, with minimally invasive techniques and shorter operative times, skilled bariatric surgeons are able to safely perform weight loss surgery on patients that have very poor cardiac performance. In fact there are many case reports of patients undergoing weight loss surgery in order to meet criteria for heart transplantation [23, 24]. Oftentimes these patients have left ventricular ejection fractions as low as 15 %. Ramani et al. demonstrated safety and efficacy of bariatric surgery in morbidly obese patients with severe systolic heart failure, improving their New York Heart Association score and left ventricular ejection fraction some of whom then became candidates for transplantation after lowering their BMI while others improved to the point of not requiring transplantation [25]. These types of patients are all cared for by a multidisciplinary team including experienced bariatric surgeons, cardiologists with fellowship training in heart failure, and cardiac anesthesia teams. The conduct in the OR is to minimize operative time while ensuring integrity of the anastomoses. Oftentimes these heart failure patients or heart transplant patients have either internal cardiac defibrillators or pacemakers. Prior to surgery, it is important to identify the type and model of the patient's device, who controls it, what the patient's underlying rhythm is, what the "magnet mode" default is, and if the institution has a programmer on site. Knowing these details will prevent any delay of care if patients should have device malfunctions.

Surgical Factors

Prior Upper Abdominal Surgery

Prior upper abdominal surgery can cause adhesions that can make exposure difficult. Often the stomach and the liver can be fused via adhesions making formation of the pouch very difficult. If the patient has had a midline laparotomy or even lower abdominal surgery, adhesional disease may require tedious and often lengthy lysis of adhesions before enough small bowel is released to measure and create the jejunojejunostomy. When performing weight loss surgery in a patient that has had multiple prior abdominal surgeries, obtaining previous operative notes can help prepare the surgeon for the environment that he is about to discover. Furthermore, having the requisite skill set to laparoscopically repair any surgical misadventures that may be encountered will spare the patient of the short and long-term complications of having to convert to an open procedure.

Occasionally weight loss surgery is required in patients that have received transplanted organs. Obesity with its associated comorbid conditions may lead to early graft failure and poor outcome including death after transplantation [26]. There are several studies that demonstrate that bariatric surgery can be a safe and effective means of weight loss after organ transplantation [27, 28]. In this patient population, active comanagement with the transplant team is essential for good patient outcomes. Immunosuppressive medication levels need to be followed closely in the perioperative period. And to ensure consistent immunosuppressive medication dosing despite variable oral intake, a gastrostomy tube should strongly be considered at the time of the bariatric surgery.

Revisional Surgery

Revisional bariatric surgery is discussed in depth in previous chapters. However, in analyzing revisional surgery with regard to risk, Sarr et al. from Mayo Clinic performed the largest analysis of revisional bariatric surgery outcomes [29]. They evaluated 218 patients that underwent revisional bariatric surgery (open revisions) and they reported a 0.9 % mortality rate and a 26 % serious operative morbidity rate. As expected, this is much higher than the traditionally quoted rates for primary (non-revisional) bariatric surgery [3]. These rates are consistent with other similar studies [30]. In the series presented by Mayo Clinic, it is important to note that all the revisional surgery was performed by experienced bariatric surgeons. Because of the distorted anatomy and extensive scarring that is present in revisional surgery, the risk factor is indirectly related to surgeons' experience performing such complicated surgeries.

Psychiatric Disorders

One of the contraindications for bariatric surgery is uncontrolled psychiatric disorders that would preclude the patient from having coping skills necessary or support structures in place to handle the psychologic stressors of bariatric surgery (ASMBS position statement on presurgical psychologic testing 2004). However, for patients that have psychologic disorders that are controlled, there are some studies that suggest that even these patients have suboptimal weight loss when compared to patients that do not have an Axis I or II diagnosis (according to the Diagnostic and Statistical Manual of Mental Disorders). When offering surgery to these patients, it is important to have active engagement with the patient's psychiatric team for smooth transition and medication monitoring during the perioperative period.

Life Style Risk Factors

There are many modifiable lifestyle factors that can increase a patients risk for perioperative events. Smoking and sedentary lifestyle have been found to be the most directly related to adverse outcomes after surgery [31]. Preoperative education and postoperative follow-up targeted toward addressing these risk factors can mitigate these risks.

Conclusion

Given these risk factors, surgeons should be prepared to evaluate patients not only in regard to the type of surgery offered but also to each patient's individual risk profile. This allows the surgeon to more comprehensively and realistically estimate the amount of risk that each patient is incurring. In addition, the surgical team can be better prepared for complications, should they arise, and have the appropriate consultants involved with the perioperative care of the patient. True risk seems to be a dynamic interaction between the patient's physical health, medical history, surgeon's skill, type of surgery, operative team's experience, and medical assets available at the medical institution that the surgery is being performed. The very high-risk patients should not necessarily be denied surgery, as long as they can have their surgery at institutions with the capabilities to address the specific factors that make the patient high risk. Further innovations in the surgical treatment for obesity will continue to focus on procedures that decrease risk to patients, while providing excellent long-term weight loss.

Review Questions and Answer

1. Which of the following is not included in the Obesity Mortality Risk Scoring System:

(a) BMI
(b) Age
(c) HTN
(d) Gender
(e) PE risk
(f) Serum creatinine

Answer: f

2. True or False: In published studies, gender has not been found to contribute to increased risk for adverse outcomes
Answer: false

3. Obstructive sleep apnea has been found to be associated with all of the following, except:
(a) Reintubation
(b) Need for mechanical ventilation
(c) Hypoxemia
(d) Transfer to ICU
(e) Prolonged hospital stay
(f) Death
Answer: h

References

1. Poirier P, Alpert MA, Fleisher LA, Thompson PD, Sugerman HJ, Burke LE, et al. Cardiovascular evaluation and management of severely obese patients undergoing surgery: a science advisory from the American Heart Association. Circulation. 2009;120(1):86–95.
2. DeMaria EJ, Portenier D, Wolfe L. Obesity surgery mortality risk score: proposal for a clinically useful score to predict mortality risk in patients undergoing gastric bypass. Surg Obes Relat Dis. 2007;3(2):134–40.

3. Maciejewski ML, Winegar DA, Farley JF, Wolfe BM, Demaria EJ. Risk stratification of serious adverse events after gastric bypass in the bariatric outcomes longitudinal database. Surg Obes Relat Dis. 2012;8:671–7.

4. Buchwald H, Estok R, Fahrbach K, Banel D, Sledge I. Trends in mortality in bariatric surgery: a systematic review and meta-analysis. Surgery. 2007;142(4):621–32; discussion 632-5.

5. Davenport DL, Bowe EA, Henderson WG, Khuri SF, Mentzer Jr RM. National surgical quality improvement program (NSQIP) risk factors can be used to validate american society of anesthesiologists physical status classification (ASA PS) levels. Ann Surg. 2006;243(5):636–41; discussion 641-4.

6. Livingston EH, Langert J. The impact of age and medicare status on bariatric surgical outcomes. Arch Surg. 2006;141(11):1115–20; discussion 1121.

7. Nguyen NT, Nguyen B, Smith B, Reavis KM, Elliott C, Hohmann S. Proposal for a bariatric mortality risk classification system for patients undergoing bariatric surgery. Surg Obes Relat Dis. 2013;9:239–46.

8. Lauer MS, Anderson KM, Kannel WB, Levy D. The impact of obesity on left ventricular mass and geometry: the Framingham heart study. JAMA. 1991;266(2):231–6.

9. Gabrielsen AM, Lund MB, Kongerud J, Viken KE, Roislien J, Hjelmesaeth J. The relationship between anthropometric measures, blood gases, and lung function in morbidly obese white subjects. Obes Surg. 2011;21(4):485–91.

10. Nordstrand N, Gjevestad E, Dinh KN, Hofso D, Roislien J, Saltvedt E, et al. The relationship between various measures of obesity and arterial stiffness in morbidly obese patients. BMC Cardiovasc Disord. 2011;11:7.

11. Silecchia G, Boru C, Pecchia A, Rizzello M, Casella G, Leonetti F, et al. Effectiveness of laparoscopic sleeve gastrectomy (first stage of biliopancreatic diversion with duodenal switch) on co-morbidities in super-obese high-risk patients. Obes Surg. 2006; 16(9):1138–44.

12. Dominguez-Escrig JL, Vasdev N, O'Riordon A, Soomro N. Laparoscopic partial nephrectomy: technical considerations and an update. J Minim Access Surg. 2011;7(4):205–21.

13. Riess KP, Baker MT, Lambert PJ, Mathiason MA, Kothari SN. Effect of preoperative weight loss on laparoscopic gastric bypass outcomes. Surg Obes Relat Dis. 2008;4(6):704–8.

14. Collins J, McCloskey C, Titchner R, Goodpaster B, Hoffman M, Hauser D, et al. Preoperative weight loss in high-risk super obese bariatric patients: a computed tomography-based analysis. Surg Obes Relat Dis. 2011;7(4):480–5.

15. Darvall KA, Sam RC, Silverman SH, Bradbury AW, Adam DJ. Obesity and thrombosis. Eur J Vasc Endovasc Surg. 2007;33(2): 223–3.

16. Mechanick JI, Kushner RF, Sugerman HJ, Gonzalez-Campoy JM, Collazo-Clavell ML, Guven S, et al. American Association of Clinical Endocrinologists, the obesity society, and American Society for Metabolic & Bariatric Surgery medical guidelines for clinical practice for the perioperative nutritional, metabolic, and nonsurgical support of the bariatric surgery patient. Endocr Pract. 2008;14 Suppl 1:1–83.

17. Li W, Gorecki P, Semaan E, Briggs W, Tortolani AJ, D'Ayala M. Concurrent prophylactic placement of inferior vena cava filter in gastric bypass and adjustable banding operations in the bariatric outcomes longitudinal database. J Vasc Surg. 2012;55(6):1690–5.

18. Geerts WH, Bergqvist D, Pineo GF, Heit JA, Samama CM, Lassen MR, et al. Prevention of venous thromboembolism: American college of chest physicians evidence-based clinical practice guidelines (8th edition). Chest. 2008;133(6 Suppl):381S–453.

19. Memtsoudis S, Liu SS, Ma Y, Chiu YL, Walz JM, Gaber-Baylis LK, et al. Perioperative pulmonary outcomes in patients with sleep apnea after noncardiac surgery. Anesth Analg. 2011;112(1): 113–21.

20. Kaw R, Pasupuleti V, Walker E, Ramaswamy A, Foldvary-Schafer N. Postoperative complications in patients with obstructive sleep apnea. Chest. 2012;141(2):436–41.

21. Vasu TS, Grewal R, Doghramji K. Obstructive sleep apnea syndrome and perioperative complications: a systematic review of the literature. J Clin Sleep Med. 2012;8(2):199–207.

22. McTigue K, Larson JC, Valoski A, Burke G, Kotchen J, Lewis CE, et al. Mortality and cardiac and vascular outcomes in extremely obese women. JAMA. 2006;296(1):79–86.

23. Saeed D, Meehan K, McGee Jr EC. Bariatric surgery at the time of ventricular assist device implantation for morbidly obese patients prior to heart transplantation. Artif Organs. 2012;36(4):450–1.

24. Samaras K, Connolly SM, Lord RV, Macdonald P, Hayward CS. Take heart: Bariatric surgery in obese patients with severe heart failure. two case reports. Heart Lung Circ. 2012;21:847–9.

25. Ramani GV, McCloskey C, Ramanathan RC, Mathier MA. Safety and efficacy of bariatric surgery in morbidly obese patients with severe systolic heart failure. Clin Cardiol. 2008;31(11):516–20.

26. Udgiri NR, Kashyap R, Minz M. The impact of body mass index on renal transplant outcomes: a significant independent risk factor for graft failure and patient death. Transplantation. 2003;75(2):249.

27. Al-Sabah S, Christou NV. Laparoscopic gastric bypass after cardiac transplantation. Surg Obes Relat Dis. 2008;4(5):668–70.

28. Szomstein S, Rojas R, Rosenthal RJ. Outcomes of laparoscopic bariatric surgery after renal transplant. Obes Surg. 2010;20(3): 383–5.

29. Nesset EM, Kendrick ML, Houghton SG, Mai JL, Thompson GB, Que FG, et al. A two-decade spectrum of revisional bariatric surgery at a tertiary referral center. Surg Obes Relat Dis. 2007;3(1): 25–30; discussion 30.

30. Coakley BA, Deveney CW, Spight DH, Thompson SK, Le D, Jobe BA, et al. Revisional bariatric surgery for failed restrictive procedures. Surg Obes Relat Dis. 2008;4(5):581–6.

31. Azagury DE, Abu Dayyeh BK, Greenwalt IT, Thompson CC. Marginal ulceration after roux-en-Y gastric bypass surgery: characteristics, risk factors, treatment, and outcomes. Endoscopy. 2011;43(11):950–4.

45

Long-Term Mortality After Bariatric Surgery

Aaron D. Carr and Mohamed R. Ali

Abbreviations

AGB   Adjustable gastric banding
BMI   Body mass index
CVD   Cardiovascular disease
DM   Type II diabetes mellitus
DYS   Dyslipidemia
HTN   Hypertension
RYGB   Roux-en-Y gastric bypass
VBG   Vertical banded gastroplasty
VSG   Vertical sleeve gastrectomy

"Corpulence is not only a disease itself, but the harbinger of others." @ How true are the words of fourth-century BC physician Hippocrates, which have been illuminated by the statistics of modern man. Worldwide obesity rates have doubled since 1980, and excess body weight has surpassed malnutrition as a major cause of mortality in over 65 % of the world's countries [1]. According to the 2008 World Health Organization (WHO) fact sheet, more than 1.4 billion adults age 20 and older were overweight [1].

Health and Financial Burden of Obesity

In the United States, the rate of obesity (defined by a body mass index (BMI) of 30 kg/m^2 or greater) has doubled since 1980, has increased by 50 % since 1994, and has only recently shown signs of leveling for specific subpopulations [2]. As of 2010, obesity affected more than 84 million American adults, corresponding to an overall incidence of 35.5 % in men and 35.8 % in women [3]. Furthermore, class II obesity (BMI 35–39.9 kg/m^2) has an incidence of 11.4 % (32 million individuals), and class III obesity (BMI ≥40 kg/m^2) has an incidence of 6.3 % (17 million individuals) [3]. The current model estimates that, by 2030, 42 % of the US population will be obese and that over 11 % will exhibit class III obesity [2]. This represents a predicted 33 % increase in overall obesity and a 2.2 factor increase in class III obesity over the next 20 years [2].

Obesity continues to place a significant financial burden on American healthcare. In 2009, healthcare expenditure related to obesity was estimated at $139 billion and corresponded to direct costs of $75 billion and indirect costs of $64 billion [4]. This estimate represents approximately 5 % of the total US healthcare expenditure [4]. If current trends continue, this cost is expected to top $344 billion by 2018 [5]. This would represent an average increase of $395 per person per year in costs for inpatient and ambulatory care, surpassing healthcare cost increases associated with smoking ($230), aging ($225), and excessive alcohol intake ($150) [6]. Obese individuals have annual medical care costs that are almost $1,500 higher than patients with normal weight [7].

The cost impact of obesity is due, to a significant extent, to the cost associated with its many comorbidities. Obesity increases the incidence of known metabolic conditions such as dyslipidemia (DYS), type 2 diabetes (DM), and related metabolic syndrome with its cardiovascular consequences. Additional conditions such as hypertension (HTN), sleep apnea syndrome, nonalcoholic steatohepatitis, major depression, and osteoarthritis also contribute to the increased mortality related to obesity. There are more than 40 medical diseases which have been linked to severe obesity [8]. A recent study of the German population indicated that obese men have a 4.5 times higher incidence of HTN, a threefold increase in cardiovascular disease (CVD) and DM, and an equal incidence of cancer [9]. Obese women exhibited an incidence of HTN that was five times higher, a risk of CVD that was increased 3.6 times, significantly higher incidence of DM (6.5 times), and a 1.3-fold increase in the incidence of cancer [9].

Studies also support the notion that obesity poses a significant risk for developing malignancy. The additional cancer risk in obese individuals ranges from 25 to 120 % [10]. The relative risk (RR) of cancer in obese patients is higher for esophageal adenocarcinoma (RR 2.10) as well as endometrial (RR 2.20), renal (RR 1.61), colorectal (RR 1.36), pancreatic (RR 1.28), and postmenopausal breast cancer (RR 1.25) [10]. Other studies have shown a 10 % increase in cancer-related deaths in obese patients [11].

S.A. Brethauer et al. (eds.), *Minimally Invasive Bariatric Surgery*,
DOI 10.1007/978-1-4939-1637-5_45, © Springer Science+Business Media New York 2015

According to the 2009 US Centers for Disease Control and Prevention vital data report, a total of 2,437,163 deaths occurred in the United States. Of those deaths, 24.6 % were related to heart disease, 23.3 % to malignant neoplasm, 5.6 % to respiratory disease, 4.8 % to accidents, 2.8 % to diabetes, 1.5 % to suicide, 1.3 % to liver disease, and 1.1 % to hypertension [12]. As indicated, a number of these leading causes of mortality are associated with severe obesity and are more prevalent among obese individuals than among non-obese individuals. It is inherently difficult to ascertain a singular risk of mortality for a given comorbidity, because all-cause mortality is multifactorial and likely results from the interaction of various comorbidities. Furthermore, mortality is not only a function of the incidence and prevalence of disease, but of the severity of illness at diagnosis and the effectiveness of treatment.

Therefore, the relationship between body mass and mortality is not always readily discernable. This is well-illustrated by CVD, the primary disease-related cause of death in the United States. The major risk factors for CVD are DM, HTN, DYS, and renal impairment. DM is one of the more significant risk factors for CVD and, alone, increases the morbidity and mortality of CVD as much as 29 times compared to non-diabetics with CVD [13]. In addition, metabolic syndrome marks the "perfect storm" of comorbidities for CVD and is defined by increased serum triglycerides (TG), low serum high-density lipoprotein cholesterol (HDL-C), elevated blood pressure, increased fasting plasma glucose, and increased waist circumference [14]. Clearly, the obese patient is at significant risk for metabolic syndrome and CVD.

Furthermore, body mass, as an individual factor, can significantly impact mortality. According to recent estimates, life expectancy may be reduced by 7.1 years in nonsmoking obese women and by 5.8 years in nonsmoking obese men as compared to their normal-weight counterparts [4]. Individuals with BMI ≥ 30 kg/m^2 have a 20–179 % increase in premature death compared to a healthy-weight cohort [15, 16]. Obesity accounts for a 40 % increase in mortality attributable to CVD, a 60 % increase in mortality from DM, and a 10 % increase in cancer-related deaths [17]. Thus, obesity increases the incidence of most major causes of death [12].

Comorbidity Response to Bariatric Surgery

Currently bariatric surgery is the only effective treatment for obesity class II or greater. The annual number of bariatric operations increased exponentially from 12,775 cases in 1998 to over 220,000 cases in 2008 [18, 19]. During this time period, the proportion of operations performed laparoscopically has increased, and overall morbidity and mortality have decreased [20]. Patients who undergo bariatric surgery can experience resolution of the major comorbidities related to obesity [21]. Bariatric surgery results in individual remission

of HTN in 61.7 %, DYS in 83.6 %, DM in 76.8 %, and obstructive sleep apnea in 61.7 % of patients [22]. In the specific context of patients with metabolic syndrome, Roux-en-Y gastric bypass (RYGB) has been shown to reduce the severity of DM in 75 % of patients, HTN in 69.4 %, and DYS in 76.4 % of patients as early as 2 months postoperatively [23]. Complete remission, among these patients, was observed in 65.3 % with DM, 51.4 % with HTN, and 73.6 % with DYS up to 1 year postoperatively [23]. Bariatric surgery has also been shown to reduce the prevalence of metabolic syndrome from 87 to 29 % compared to medical management, which can only achieve a minor reduction from 85 to 75 % [14]. The dramatic improvement in obesity-related comorbidities is the primary driving force behind the decrease in disease-related mortality experienced by patients who undergo bariatric surgery.

Mortality After Bariatric Surgery

The case for mortality benefit following bariatric surgery has been historically based on the hypothesis that significant improvement in obesity-related comorbidities would translate into reduced end-organ injury and, ultimately, improved health and increased survival. Despite widespread acceptance, the premise that weight loss and associated comorbidity improvements following bariatric surgery would decrease long-term mortality (5 or more years after surgery) in obese individuals had, until recently, been subjected to surprisingly little specific scientific evaluation. Long-term mortality can be viewed within the context of specific procedures, namely, adjustable gastric banding (AGB), vertical sleeve gastrectomy (VSG), biliopancreatic diversion (BPD) with or without duodenal switch (DS), and RYGB, or in terms of the effects of bariatric surgery overall.

Adjustable Gastric Banding

AGB is a safe and effective weight loss operation with very low perioperative mortality [24]. While the long-term outcomes of AGB can be confounded by a number of variables, several of these issues deserve specific mention. First, there are a variety of bands made by a number of manufacturers. Second, the technology of AGB has changed, such that current bands are technologically quite different than previous generations. Third, the technical aspects of AGB placement have evolved over the years, most notably illustrated by the change from perigastric to pars flaccida technique and more deliberate diagnosis and treatment of concurrent hiatal hernia [25, 26]. Finally, the weight loss success and health improvement following AGB is highly dependent on postoperative management [27]. Although these limitations increase the heterogeneity of study conditions in this literature, there is strong evidence that AGB is safe and can lead to a survival benefit in morbidly obese patients. The Australian experience of O'Brien et al. has contributed significantly to the current literature regarding AGB. In an early report contrasting 996 AGB patients to 2,119 obese individuals, AGB reduced mortality risk by 72 % (10.6–0.4 %) at 4 years [28]. A recent update to this experience revealed that the survival benefit with AGB continued to 10 years [29]. The authors affirmed the safety of AGB by reporting 0 % perioperative mortality among 3,227 cases. This chapter also provided longer follow-up on the original cohort of 996 AGB patients and reported the same 0.4 % mortality at 10 years with 98 % follow-up for deaths. The four deaths in 10 years occurred from cancer ($n = 2$), suicide ($n = 1$), and CVD ($n = 1$) [29].

Similar low mortality rates following AGB have been reported. At 5 years post-surgery, a significantly lower mortality rate was identified in AGB patients (0.97 %) than matched nonoperative controls (4.38 %) [30]. At the same 5-year follow-up interval, another group identified a mortality risk of 0 % among surgical patients and 2.5 % among matched controls [31]. The same study also reported a non-controlled mortality rate of 0 % in 1,791 AGB patients up to 12 years after surgery [31]. Additional data without control groups revealed long-term mortality at a mean of 7 years post-AGB to range from 0.2 to 2 % [32, 33].

Even studies which report a high reoperation rate corroborate the low long-term mortality risk associated with AGB. At 13 years of follow-up (54.3 % of eligible patients), a significant proportion of patients (59.8 %) required reoperation following AGB while the mortality was only 3.7 %. Furthermore, the three deaths were not directly related to health risks of obesity or operative factors (melanoma, lung cancer, and suicide) [34]. As a consensus statistic, a review of seven studies, with adequate long-term follow-up after AGB, revealed only one death in 6,177 patients (mortality of 0.02 %) over 10 years [29].

Vertical Sleeve Gastrectomy

VSG has only recently gained significant traction as a primary bariatric procedure. The original case for VSG was made as the first stage of two-stage RYGB in high-risk bariatric patients [35]. In the relatively short period since the original reports, data have been amassed to support the safety and efficacy of VSG. However, there are currently no long-term case-controlled mortality data on VSG.

Existing studies which evaluate long-term outcomes following VSG are largely retrospective. The largest study compared 811 VSG patients to 786 RYGB patients for complications and mortality at 1, 2, and 3 years [36]. Although patients who underwent VSG had a relatively low mean BMI (37.9 ± 4.6 kg/m^2), VSG was associated with low operative time (76.6 ± 28 min), short hospital stay (2.8 ± 0.8 days), and low complication rates (early = 2.9 % and late = 3.3 %) [36]. Specifically, leaks occurred in only

0.5 % of cases and only one patient had to be converted to RYGB for stenosis. VSG patients were also able to achieve sustained excess weight loss of 86.8 % ± 27.1 % at 3 years and had significant improvement in metabolic biochemical parameters. This profile of safety and efficacy of LVSG resulted in 0 % mortality during adequate postoperative follow-up at 1 (81.8 %), 2 (74.7 %), and 3 (71.7 %) years [36]. A much smaller study followed only 20 patients who underwent LVSG but was able to achieve 100 % follow-up at 3 years with 0 % mortality [37]. The low power of this study clearly compromises its generalizability to the general population of bariatric surgery patients [37].

The excellent mortality results for VSG have also been shown in high-risk patients. In a recent study, VSG was designed as a first-stage therapy in class V obese patients (mean BMI = 66 kg/m^2) [38]. Although the original intention was to proceed with second-stage conversion to RYGB, 75 patients (60 %) were able to achieve 48 % excess weight loss with VSG as a single procedure [38]. With 93 % follow-up at a mean of 6 years postoperatively, this study also demonstrated 0 % mortality [38].

Biliopancreatic Diversion

No case-controlled studies of long-term mortality following BPD with or without DS have been performed. In a case series of 74 patients undergoing BPD, with excellent follow-up of 93.7 % between 4 and 8 years postoperatively, data were collected for weight loss, changes in comorbidities, nutritional deficiencies, morbidity, and mortality [39]. This study demonstrated 0 % perioperative deaths and 1.35 % long-term mortality. The single death during the study period was unrelated to bariatric surgery and occurred as a consequence of breast cancer [39].

A large series of 1,423 patients evaluated the outcomes of BPD-DS in terms of change in body mass, improvement in medical conditions, nutritional issues, complications, and mortality [40]. BPD-DS was performed via the open technique early in the study and subsequently switched to laparoscopy. The authors were able to achieve follow-up on 93 % of patients at a mean of 7.3 years and reported specific causes of mortality. The patient population, which had a mean age of 40.1 ± 10.5 years and mean BMI of 51.5 ± 9.9 kg/m^2, experienced a mortality rate of 8 % [40]. However, the authors only attributed 20 % of the deaths to surgery (malnourishment, delayed operative death, reoperation, intestinal obstruction, and gastrointestinal hemorrhage). Long-term mortality unrelated to surgery resulted from cancer, trauma, suicide, pulmonary insufficiency, pulmonary embolus, and sudden death [40].

Several other non-case-controlled studies have examined the mortality after BPD-DS at several years follow-up. The largest study had a group of 1,300 BPD-DS patients that were followed from 1 to 15 years and reported mortality of

0.57 % [41]. A similarly low mortality rate of 0.74 % was identified in 540 patients, half of whom underwent BPD while the other half underwent BPD-DS, followed for a mean of 7.4 years [42]. Large surgical experiences seem to corroborate these low mortality rates. A study of 1,000 patients with BPD-DS reported mortality of 0.2 % with a 90 % follow-up at a mean of 2 years [43]. Another multicenter report of 874 patients found a mortality rate of 0.8 % at a mean follow-up of 11.9 years [44]. Smaller series have reported higher rates of mortality, such as 3.9 % in 51 patients who underwent BPD-DS with 92 % follow-up for 5 years [45]. Although somewhat larger with 190 patients, another investigation reported 2.8 % mortality at 3.7 years with 93.7 % follow-up [46].

Roux-en-Y Gastric Bypass

RYGB enjoys a robust body of literature that has examined the outcomes of this procedure over five decades. Numerous studies have elucidated the efficacy of RYGB in achieving and maintaining meaningful weight loss. Additionally, the beneficial effects of RYGB on obesity-related medical conditions have become well established. Mortality following RYGB has been primarily studied from the perspective of surgical safety and has focused heavily on early postoperative results. Thus, sufficiently powered randomized controlled data that address long-term mortality and are specific to RYGB are virtually nonexistent. Furthermore, studies with case-matched controls involve primarily open RYGB, while one case series with exclusively laparoscopic RYGB comments on long-term mortality.

One of the earlier studies followed 154 patients who underwent RYGB and found a mortality rate of 9 % up to 9 years postoperatively. This represented a significant improvement when compared with the control group of 78 morbidly obese patients who did not have surgery and exhibited a mortality rate of 28 % up to 6.2 years of follow-up [47]. An identical mortality rate of 9 % was reported by another study of 233 patients who underwent RYGB and were followed for 10 years postoperatively [48]. This investigation benchmarked surgery patients against a large group of 11,132 morbidly obese individuals in the general population followed for the same 10-year interval and determined a significant reduction in long-term mortality as compared to the approximately 12 % mortality rate observed in the control group [48]. Similar results have been identified by noncomparative descriptive data, illustrated by a report of 8 % all-cause mortality among 1,025 RYGB patients followed for 2–12 years [49].

More recent data corroborate the significant reduction in long-term mortality (40 %) for morbidly obese individuals who undergo RYGB [50]. These data are based on a large experience with RYGB in 7,925 patients operated during an 18-year experience. Surgical patients and an identical number of control patients (matched for age, gender, and BMI) were evaluated over 7 years. While the reduction in mortality following RYGB was significantly lower, mortality in both groups was lower than other studies (2.7 % in the surgery group vs. 4.1 % in the control group) [50]. Another recent report identified a 5-year mortality of 1.8 % following LRYGB [51].

These overall mortality data are most notable in that the reduced rates for surgical patients also inherently contain all mortality-associated surgery and related complications. When specifically investigated, mortality within the first year following surgery was essentially identical between RYGB patients (0.53 %) and matched obese individuals (0.52 %), underscoring the safety of current bariatric surgical practice [50]. In this vein, the transition from open RYGB to laparoscopic RYGB has fundamentally changed the safety profile of this operation. In a review of nine studies which reported a mortality rate of 0.8 % at 10 years among 2,684 RYGB patient, all deaths occurred during the open bypass era [29].

The positive impact of RYGB on mortality is most prominent in patients with significant comorbidities related to obesity. Death attributable to CVD is reduced by 56 % in patients who undergo RYGB [50]. Similarly, mortality related to DM decreases by 92 %, and mortality related to cancer diminishes by 60 % [50]. Men also seem to derive a greater mortality benefit than women (56 % reduction vs. 32 % reduction) [50]. It is hypothesized that this difference may be due to a higher prevalence of medical conditions responsive to RYGB, such as CVD, in morbidly obese male patients. However, the rate of death from accidents and suicide has been reported to be 58 % higher in RYGB patients [50].

These affirmative data certainly seem to point to a distinct survival advantage as a response to RYGB in morbidly obese patients. However, a number of potential confounding issues exist. Most prominent among these is the lack of data on comorbidity severity among RYGB patients or among the control groups of obese individuals. Similarly, there are no indications as to whether or not surgical patients may have received more aggressive treatment of comorbidities. Additionally, patients who undergo surgery may be more predisposed to seeking and adhering to medical care. Finally, the demonstrable increase in deaths not related to disease among RYGB patients has not been fully evaluated. While it is unclear whether such factors would appreciably impact the survival benefit observed following RYGB, they certainly warrant consideration and further study. Variability in mortality reduction has been reported in high-risk patients undergoing RYGB. Advanced age, high BMI, and male gender have been identified as risk factors for poor surgical outcomes, including complications and perioperative mortality [52, 53]. High-risk patients who undergo RYGB experience a 36 % reduction in mortality over 7 years [54]. After adjustment for covariates, this benefit drops to 20 % but remains statistically significant. However, the mortality improvement loses statistical significance when compared to a matched cohort (17 %) and when corrected for follow-up interval (6 %) [54]. It should be noted that within these data lie a relatively high perioperative mortality rate of 1.5 %. This accounts for 86.6 % of deaths at 1 year, 59 % of deaths at 2 years, and 19.4 % of deaths at 6 years. Furthermore, while the hazard ratios may not have been significant, RYGB patients exhibited decreased mortality rates at 1 year (1.5 % vs. 2.2 %), 2 years (2.2 % vs. 4.6 %), and 6 years (6.8 % vs. 15.2 %) when compared to unmatched obese patients [54]. Although early survival was not statistically different when benchmarked against matched obese individuals at 1 and 2 years, a significant reduction was identified at 6 years (6.7 % vs. 12.8 %) [54]. Thus, the interpretation of survival benefit following RYGB in high-risk patients must include three critical variables: optimization of physiologic status to reduce higher than average perioperative mortality risk, potential quality of life gains associated with weight loss, and comorbidity improvement and evidence that a significant survival advantage may not be realized until a long postoperative interval.

As further illustration, 908 patients underwent RYGB and were followed for a mean of 4.4 years [55]. When contrasted to a control group of 112 obese individuals followed for a mean of 3.6 years, surgical patients exhibited significantly reduced overall mortality rate of 2.9 % as compared with 14.3 % in the control group. These investigators reported that the mortality curves diverged more greatly with increasing length of follow-up [55].

Another notable obstacle to determining long-term mortality following RYGB (and bariatric surgery in general) is the inconsistent and often low rate of long-term patient follow-up. Few studies can document excellent patient follow-up at many years postoperatively. Furthermore, many studies of bariatric surgical outcomes do not specifically address the adequacy of patient follow-up. When patient follow-up has been reported, it has frequently been quite low in the long term as exemplified by a study which found an overall mortality rate of 3.3 % but only had follow-up of 33 % at 2 years and 26 % at 10 years [56].

Overall Effect of Bariatric Surgery on Mortality

It is undeniable that bariatric operations have varying mechanisms of achieving weight loss and effects on obesity-related comorbidities. Yet, bariatric surgery has been repeatedly shown to improve overall health in morbidly obese patients regardless of the specific operation [57, 58]. Within this context, the generalized effects of bariatric surgery on overall and disease-specific mortality have been evaluated. In a large series of RYGB and vertical banded gastroplasty (VBG) with case-matched controls, the reported mortality was 0.68 % for the surgical cohort compared to 6.17 % for the control group at 5 years [57].

Perhaps the most robust data set regarding bariatric surgery comes from the Swedish Obese Subjects (SOS) study. The SOS has addressed mortality in a long-term prospective case-controlled fashion. In a report that contrasted 2,010 patients who underwent bariatric surgery (RYGB 13 %, VBG 68 %, and AGB 19 %) to 2,037 patients who received conventional treatment for obesity and related comorbidities, the overall mortality was 5.0 % in the surgery group and 6.3 % in the control group [58]. The corresponding 24 % reduction in mortality was observed at a mean follow-up of 10.9 years [58].

In addition to its breadth, the SOS data collection was also specific and detailed. The patients in both groups were well-matched for anthropomorphic and demographic characteristics. All patients were evaluated at regular intervals, up to 15 years, indexed to the timing of operation of patients in the surgery group. Evaluation consisted of anthropomorphic, physiologic, comorbidity, and biochemical assessments. The investigators were able to achieve excellent follow-up at 2, 10, and 15 years of 94, 84, and 66 % for the surgical arm and 83, 75, and 87 % for the control group [58].

Although the 90-day mortality following bariatric surgery was low (0.25 %), it was higher than mortality in the control group (0.10 %) [58]. However, surgical patients gained survival benefit as the duration of follow-up increased. In terms of cause-specific mortality, surgical patients had less death due to CVD (2.14 % vs. 2.6 %) and noncardiovascular causes (2.88 % vs. 3.7 %) [58]. Cancer-related mortality dropped from 2.36 % in control patients to 1.44 % in surgical patients [58]. The greatest predictor of overall mortality was history of myocardial infarction or stroke, which corresponded to mortality risk of 19.6 % in the surgical group and 24.5 % in the control group [58]. Other factors shown to increase risk of death among all patients included advanced age, smoking, increased plasma triglycerides, and increased blood glucose. Body mass also affected mortality in that more severely obese patients (BMI $\geq$ 40 kg/m^2) realized a greater reduction in mortality (30 %) in response to bariatric surgery than patients with BMI below 40 kg/m^2 (20 %) [58].

Taken together, AGB and RYGB are quite effective at reducing mortality associated with obesity. A recent meta-analysis identified eight case-controlled clinical trials that compared 44,022 bariatric surgery (RYGB or AGB) patients to a control cohort of 29,970 obese individuals to an average follow-up of 7 years [59]. The type of operation (RYGB or AGB) did not statistically affect global mortality or all-cause mortality. Surgical patients exhibited reduced global mortality (50 %), cardiovascular mortality (42 %), and all-cause mortality (30 %) [59]. RYGB more significantly reduced CVD mortality than AGB (52 % vs. 29 %), presumably related to its metabolic effects on DM [59]. In terms of absolute rates, overall mortality was 2.84 % in the surgical group and 9.73 % in the control group [59].

TABLE 1. Mortality following restrictive procedures

Study	N	Mortality (%)	Follow-up (years)	Procedure
Busetto et al. (2004)				
Surgery	821	0.97	5	AGB
Control	821	4.4	5	
Peeters et al. (2007)				
Surgery	996	0.4	4	AGB
Control	2,119	10.6	4	
Miller et al. (2007)				
Surgery	554	0.2	7.6	AGB
Control	N/A			
Favretti et al. (2007)				
Surgery	821	0	5	AGB
Control	821	2.5	5	
Stroh et al. (2011)				
Surgery	200	2	7.8	AGB
Control	N/A			
Himpens, et al. (2011)				
Surgery	82	3.7	13	AGB
Control	N/A			
Boza et al. (2012)				
Surgery	811	0	3	VSG
Control	N/A			
Sarela et al. (2012)				
Surgery	20	0	3	VSG
Control	N/A			
Eid et al. (2012)				
Surgery	75	0	6	VSG
Control	N/A			

AGB adjustable gastric band, *VSG* vertical sleeve gastrectomy

TABLE 2. Mortality following biliopancreatic diversion

Study	N	Mortality (%)	Follow-up (years)	Procedure
Guedea et al. (2004)	74	1.4	4–8	BPD
Hess et al. (2005)	1,300	0.6	1–15	BPD-DS
Marceau et al. (2007)	1,423	8	7.3	BPD-DS
Crea et al. (2011)	540	0.7	7.4	BPD/BPD-DS
Biertho et al. (2011)	1,000	0.2	2	BPD-DS
Topart et al. (2011)	51	3.9	5	BPD-DS
Pata et al. (2012)	874	0.8	11.9	BPD-DS
Dorman et al. (2012)	190	2.8	3.7	BPD-DS

BPD biliopancreatic diversion, *DS* duodenal switch

TABLE 3. Mortality following Roux-en-Y gastric bypass

Study	N	Mortality (%)	Follow-up (years)
McDonald et al. (1997)			
Surgery	154	9	9
Control	78	28	6.2
Sugerman et al. (2003)			
Surgery	1,025	8	2–12
Control	N/A		
Flum et al. (2004)			
Surgery	233	9	10
Control	1,131	16	15
Sowemimo et al. (2006)			
Surgery	908	2.9	4.4
Control	112	14.3	3.6
Adams et al. (2007)			
Surgery	7,925	2.7	7
Control	7,925	4.1	7
Maciejewski et al. (2011)			
Surgery	847	6.8	6
Control	847	15.2	6
Suter et al. (2011)			
Surgery	379	1.8	5
Control	N/A		
Higa et al. (2011)			
Surgery	242	3.3	10
Control	N/A		

Summary

Obese individuals often suffer from associated comorbidities. Left untreated, these medical consequences of obesity can cause end-organ injury and resultant mortality. Bariatric surgery is the best current means of achieving and maintaining significant weight loss [18, 19]. Surgery also effectively treats many of the medical conditions associated with obesity as a consequence of weight loss and by weight-loss-independent mechanisms. Thus, bariatric surgery is hypothesized to significantly reduce mortality, in large part, by improving comorbidities of obesity. The mortality benefit derived from the various bariatric operations is likely related to the comorbidity severity of the individual patients as well as the metabolic effects of each procedure.

The restrictive procedures (AGB and VSG) exert their comorbidity effects primarily as a function of weight loss, and their mortality reduction data are summarized in Table 1. The long-term mortality for AGB ranged from 0 to 3.7 % with a range of mean follow-up of 5–13 years, while the respective controls had mortality of 2.5–10.6 % [28–34]. VSG also demonstrated a low long-term mortality at mean follow-up of 3–6 years, although the data were much less established, not case controlled, and relatively shorter term [36–38]. As observed in the SOS, VBG is associated with 10-year mortality of 5 % compared to 6.3 % in the control group [58].

The procedures that include intestinal bypass (BPD and RYGB) have metabolic effects that act synergistically with weight loss to improve medical comorbidities. The mortality reduction data for these operations are summarized in Tables 2 and Table 3. BPD with or without DS has a reported a mortality of 0.2–8 % at mean follow-up of 2–12 years (Table 2) [36–43]. RYBG had the most data available. The long-term mortality ranged from 1.8 to 9 % at a mean follow-up of 4.4–10 years compared to a control mortality rate of 4.1–28 % during a similar follow-up period (Table 3) [29, 46–51, 54].

Studies that reviewed aggregated mortality of bariatric surgery across multiple procedures are summarized in Table 4. The overall long-term mortality rate for bariatric surgery ranged from 0.68 to 5 % and was significantly lower

TABLE 4. Mortality In mixed studies

Study	N	Mortality (%)	Follow-up (years)	Procedure (%)
Christou et al. (2004)				
Surgery	1,035	0.68	5	RYGB (81.3)
Control	5,746	6.17	5	VBG (18.7)
Sjostrom et al. (2007)				
Surgery	2,010	5.00	10.9	AGB (19)
Control	2,037	6.30	10.9	VBG (68)
				RYGB (13)

RYGB Roux-en-Y gastric bypass, *VBG* vertical banded gastroplasty, *AGB* adjustable gastric band

than control mortality of 6.17–6.3 % at 5–11 years after surgery [57, 58].

Accurate determination of long-term mortality following bariatric surgery can be hindered by several limitations that pervade the current body of literature. First, most of the studies are not case controlled, while randomized trials are even rarer. Many outcome reports do not specifically address long-term mortality as an outcome variable. Also, long-term follow-up is frequently poor in studies of bariatric surgery, such that it is difficult to interpret outcomes in light of diminishing sample sizes. Another inherent issue is the lack of homogeneity of study control groups, which most commonly consist of patients from clinical programs or individuals from the general population. Control groups of patients in clinical programs tend to more closely resemble the comorbidity profiles of surgical patients when contrasted to control groups from the general population. Despite these limitations, the current state of knowledge in bariatric surgery seems to clearly support a reduction in obesity-related mortality in response to bariatric surgery.

Review Questions and Answers

1. According to the World Health Organization, what chronic condition is now a major cause of mortality in the majority of countries?

A. Malnutrition
B. Tuberculosis
C. Obesity
D. Pesticides

Answer: C

2. Which of the following causes of mortality is MOST reduced by Roux-en-Y gastric bypass?

A. Diabetes
B. Cancer
C. Cardiovascular
D. All-cause mortality

Answer: A

3. What is the proposed mechanism by which bariatric surgery reduces long-term mortality?

A. Weight loss
B. Improvement in comorbidities
C. Decrease in cancer incidence
D. Multifactorial
E. All of the above

Answer: E

4. Which of the following is the greatest predictor of overall mortality following bariatric surgery?

A. Previous surgery
B. History of myocardial infarction
C. BMI > 50 kg/m^2
D. Type II diabetes mellitus

Answer: B

References

1. Fact Sheet N 311. Obesity and overweight, World Health Organization May 2012. http://www.who.int/mediacentre/fact-sheets/fs311/en/index.html
2. Finkelstein EA, Khavjou OA, Thompson H, Trogdon JG, Pan L, Sherry B, et al. Obesity and severe obesity forecasts through 2030. Am J Prev Med. 2012;42(6):563–70.
3. Flegal KM, Carroll MD, Kit BK, Ogden CL. Prevalence of obesity and trends in the distribution of body mass index among US adults, 1999–2010. JAMA. 2012;307(5):491–7.
4. Terranova L, Busetto L, Vestri A, Zappa MA. Bariatric surgery: cost-effectiveness and budget impact. Obes Surg. 2012;22(4):646–53.
5. Thorpe KE. The future cost of obesity: national and state estimates of the impact of obesity on direct health care expenses. 2009.
6. Sturm R. The effects of obesity, smoking, and drinking on medical problems and costs. Health Aff (Millwood). 2002;21(2):245–53.
7. Weiss AJ, Elixhauser A. Obesity-related hospitalizations, 2004 versus 2009: statistical brief #137. Healthcare cost and utilization project (HCUP) statistical briefs. Rockville. 2006.
8. Kaplan LM. Body weight regulation and obesity. J Gastrointest Surg. 2003;7(4):443–51.
9. Schienkiewitz A, Mensink GB, Scheidt-Nave C. Comorbidity of overweight and obesity in a nationally representative sample of German adults aged 18–79 years. BMC Public Health. 2012;12(1):658.
10. Eheman C, Henley SJ, Ballard-Barbash R, Jacobs EJ, Schymura MJ, Noone AM, et al. Annual Report to the Nation on the status of cancer, 1975–2008, featuring cancers associated with excess weight and lack of sufficient physical activity. Cancer. 2012;118(9):2338–66.
11. Haslam DW, James WP. Obesity. Lancet. 2005;366(9492):1197–209.
12. Kockanek K, Xu J, Murphy S, Minino A, Kung H. National vital statistics report: deaths: final data for 2009. In: Services U.S.D.o.H.a.H., editor. December 2011.
13. Barkoudah E, Skali H, Uno H, Solomon SD, Pfeffer MA. Mortality rates in trials of subjects with type 2 diabetes. J Am Heart Assoc. 2012;1(1):8–15.
14. Batsis JA, Romero-Corral A, Collazo-Clavell ML, Sarr MG, Somers VK, Lopez-Jimenez F. Effect of bariatric surgery on the metabolic syndrome: a population-based, long-term controlled study. Mayo Clin Proc. 2008;83(8):897–907.
15. Allison DB, Fontaine KR, Manson JE, Stevens J, VanItallie TB. Annual deaths attributable to obesity in the United States. JAMA. 1999;282(16):1530–8.

16. Flegal KM, Graubard BI, Williamson DF, Gail MH. Excess deaths associated with underweight, overweight, and obesity. JAMA. 2005;293(15):1861–7.

17. Whitlock G, Lewington S, Sherliker P, Clarke R, Emberson J, Halsey J, et al. Body-mass index and cause-specific mortality in 900 000 adults: collaborative analyses of 57 prospective studies. Lancet. 2009;373(9669):1083–96.

18. Nguyen NT, Root J, Zainabadi K, Sabio A, Chalifoux S, Stevens CM, et al. Accelerated growth of bariatric surgery with the introduction of minimally invasive surgery. Arch Surg. 2005;140(12):1198–202; discussion 203.

19. Garb J, Welch G, Zagarins S, Kuhn J, Romanelli J. Bariatric surgery for the treatment of morbid obesity: a meta-analysis of weight loss outcomes for laparoscopic adjustable gastric banding and laparoscopic gastric bypass. Obes Surg. 2009;19(10):1447–55.

20. Weller WE, Rosati C. Comparing outcomes of laparoscopic versus open bariatric surgery. Ann Surg. 2008;248(1):10–5.

21. Dumon KR, Murayama KM. Bariatric surgery outcomes. Surg Clin North Am. 2011;91(6):1313–38.

22. Buchwald H, Avidor Y, Braunwald E, Jensen MD, Pories W, Fahrbach K, et al. Bariatric surgery: a systematic review and meta-analysis. JAMA. 2004;292(14):1724–37.

23. Ali MR, Maguire MB, Wolfe BM. Assessment of obesity-related comorbidities: a novel scheme for evaluating bariatric surgical patients. J Am Coll Surg. 2006;202(1):70–7.

24. Smith MD, Patterson E, Wahed AS, Belle SH, Berk PD, Courcoulas AP, et al. Thirty-day mortality after bariatric surgery: independently adjudicated causes of death in the longitudinal assessment of bariatric surgery. Obes Surg. 2011;21(11):1687–92.

25. Dolan K, Finch R, Fielding G. Laparoscopic gastric banding and crural repair in the obese patient with a hiatal hernia. Obes Surg. 2003;13(5):772–5.

26. Dargent J. Pouch dilatation and slippage after adjustable gastric banding: is it still an issue? Obes Surg. 2003;13(1):111–5.

27. Sivagnanam P, Rhodes M. The importance of follow-up and distance from centre in weight loss after laparoscopic adjustable gastric banding. Surg Endosc. 2010;24(10):2432–8.

28. Peeters A, O'Brien PE, Laurie C, Anderson M, Wolfe R, Flum D, et al. Substantial intentional weight loss and mortality in the severely obese. Ann Surg. 2007;246(6):1028–33.

29. O'Brien PE, Macdonald L, Anderson M, Brennan L, Brown WA. Long-term outcomes after bariatric surgery: fifteen-year follow-up of adjustable gastric banding and a systematic review of the bariatric surgical literature. Ann Surg. 2013;257(1):87–94.

30. Busetto L, Mirabelli D, Petroni ML, Mazza M, Favretti F, Segato G, et al. Comparative long-term mortality after laparoscopic adjustable gastric banding versus nonsurgical controls. Surg Obes Relat Dis. 2007;3(5):496–502.

31. Favretti F, Segato G, Ashton D, Busetto L, De Luca M, Mazza M, et al. Laparoscopic adjustable gastric banding in 1,791 consecutive obese patients: 12-year results. Obes Surg. 2007;17(2):168–75.

32. Miller K, Pump A, Hell E. Vertical banded gastroplasty versus adjustable gastric banding: prospective long-term follow-up study. Surg Obes Relat Dis. 2007;3(1):84–90.

33. Stroh C, Hohmann U, Schramm H, Meyer F, Manger T. Fourteen-year long-term results after gastric banding. J Obes. 2011;2011: 128451.

34. Himpens J, Cadiere GB, Bazi M, Vouche M, Cadiere B, Dapri G. Long-term outcomes of laparoscopic adjustable gastric banding. Arch Surg. 2011;146(7):802–7.

35. Cottam D, Qureshi FG, Mattar SG, Sharma S, Holover S, Bonanomi G, et al. Laparoscopic sleeve gastrectomy as an initial weight-loss procedure for high-risk patients with morbid obesity. Surg Endosc. 2006;20(6):859–63.

36. Boza C, Gamboa C, Salinas J, Achurra P, Vega A, Perez G. Laparoscopic Roux-en-Y gastric bypass versus laparoscopic sleeve gastrectomy: a case-control study and 3 years of follow-up. Surg Obes Relat Dis. 2012;8(3):243–9.

37. Sarela AI, Dexter SP, O'Kane M, Menon A, McMahon MJ. Long-term follow-up after laparoscopic sleeve gastrectomy: 8–9-year results. Surg Obes Relat Dis. 2012;8(6):679–84.

38. Eid GM, Brethauer S, Mattar SG, Titchner RL, Gourash W, Schauer PR. Laparoscopic sleeve gastrectomy for super obese patients: forty-eight percent excess weight loss after 6 to 8 years with 93 % follow-up. Ann Surg. 2012;256(2):262–5.

39. Guedea ME, Arribas del Amo D, Solanas JA, Marco CA, Bernado AJ, Rodrigo MA, et al. Results of biliopancreatic diversion after five years. Obes Surg. 2004;14(6):766–72.

40. Marceau P, Biron S, Hould FS, Lebel S, Marceau S, Lescelleur O, et al. Duodenal switch: long-term results. Obes Surg. 2007;17(11): 1421–30.

41. Hess D, Hess D, Oakley R. The biliopancreatic diversion with the duodenal switch: results beyond 10 years. Obes Surg. 2005;15(3): 408–16.

42. Crea N, Pata G, Di Betta E, Greco F, Casella C, Vilardi A, et al. Long-term results of biliopancreatic diversion with or without gastric preservation for morbid obesity. Obes Surg. 2011;21(2): 139–45.

43. Biertho L, Lebel S, Marceau S, Hould FS, Lescelleur O, Moustarah F, et al. Perioperative complications in a consecutive series of 1000 duodenal switches. Surg Obes Relat Dis. 2013;9:63–8.

44. Pata G, Crea N, Di Betta E, Bruni O, Vassallo C, Mittempergher F. Biliopancreatic diversion with transient gastroplasty and duodenal switch: long-term results of a multicentric study. Surgery. 2013;153:413–22.

45. Topart P, Becouarn G, Salle A. Five-year follow-up after biliopancreatic diversion with duodenal switch. Surg Obes Relat Dis. 2011;7(2):199–205.

46. Dorman RB, Rasmus NF, Al-Haddad BJ, Serrot FJ, Slusarek BM, Sampson BK, et al. Benefits and complications of the duodenal switch/biliopancreatic diversion compared to the Roux-en-Y gastric bypass. Surgery. 2012;152(4):758–65; discussion 65-7.

47. MacDonald Jr KG, Long SD, Swanson MS, Brown BM, Morris P, Dohm GL, et al. The gastric bypass operation reduces the progression and mortality of non-insulin-dependent diabetes mellitus. J Gastrointest Surg. 1997;1(3):213–20; discussion 20.

48. Flum DR, Dellinger EP. Impact of gastric bypass operation on survival: a population-based analysis. J Am Coll Surg. 2004;199(4): 543–51.

49. Sugerman HJ, Wolfe LG, Sica DA, Clore JN. Diabetes and hypertension in severe obesity and effects of gastric bypass-induced weight loss. Ann Surg. 2003;237(6):751–6. discussion 7-8.

50. Adams TD, Gress RE, Smith SC, Halverson RC, Simper SC, Rosamond WD, et al. Long-term mortality after gastric bypass surgery. N Engl J Med. 2007;357(8):753–61.

51. Suter M, Donadini A, Romy S, Demartines N, Giusti V. Laparoscopic Roux-en-Y gastric bypass: significant long-term weight loss, improvement of obesity-related comorbidities and quality of life. Ann Surg. 2011;254(2):267–73.

52. Mason EE, Renquist KE, Jiang D. Perioperative risks and safety of surgery for severe obesity. Am J Clin Nutr. 1992;55(2 Suppl): 573S–6.

53. Livingston EH, Huerta S, Arthur D, Lee S, De Shields S, Heber D. Male gender is a predictor of morbidity and age a predictor of mortality for patients undergoing gastric bypass surgery. Ann Surg. 2002;236(5):576–82.

54. Maciejewski ML, Livingston EH, Smith VA, Kavee AL, Kahwati LC, Henderson WG, et al. Survival among high-risk patients after bariatric surgery. JAMA. 2011;305(23):2419–26.

55. Sowemimo OA, Yood SM, Courtney J, Moore J, Huang M, Ross R, et al. Natural history of morbid obesity without surgical intervention. Surg Obes Relat Dis. 2007;3(1):73–7; discussion 7.

56. Higa K, Ho T, Tercero F, Yunus T, Boone KB. Laparoscopic Roux-en-Y gastric bypass: 10-year follow-up. Surg Obes Relat Dis. 2011;7(4):516–25.

57. Christou NV, Sampalis JS, Liberman M, Look D, Auger S, McLean AP, et al. Surgery decreases long-term mortality, morbidity, and health care use in morbidly obese patients. Ann Surg. 2004;240(3):416–23; discussion 23-4.

58. Sjostrom L, Narbro K, Sjostrom CD, Karason K, Larsson B, Wedel H, et al. Effects of bariatric surgery on mortality in Swedish obese subjects. N Engl J Med. 2007;357(8):741–52.

59. Pontiroli AE, Morabito A. Long-term prevention of mortality in morbid obesity through bariatric surgery: a systematic review and meta-analysis of trials performed with gastric banding and gastric bypass. Ann Surg. 2011;253(3):484–7.

46

Gastroesophageal Reflux Disease in the Bariatric Surgery Patient

Maria Altieri and Aurora Pryor

Gastroesophageal Reflux Disease

Gastroesophageal reflux disease, GERD, is a chronic condition that is defined as "a condition that develops when the reflux of stomach contents causes troublesome symptoms and/or complications." It is the most common gastrointestinal diagnosis recorded during visits to outpatient clinics in the United States and affects approximately 19 million Americans (1). Symptoms include heartburn, regurgitation, dysphagia, and chest pain and can range from mild to severe. Those patients with severe symptoms usually seek medical attention.

GERD-related complications include erosive esophagitis, aspiration, Barrett's esophagus, and esophageal adenocarcinoma. In the United States, these conditions have been increasing, as the incidence of esophageal adenocarcinoma has increased fourfold over the past several years (2, 3). The exact reason for the increase in GERD and these conditions is not fully understood, but changes in diet, smoking, alcohol use, and prescription medications have been implicated. Interestingly, with a recently observed increase in obesity, there is a parallel increase in the development of esophageal adenocarcinoma, and a relationship has been hypothesized (4).

GERD is a multifactorial disease in which both functional and anatomical factors play a role. The main mechanism implicated is attributed to transient lower esophageal sphincter relaxation (TLESR) (5). The lower esophageal sphincter (LES) provides the barrier between the esophagus and the stomach, and it prevents gastric contents from entering the esophagus. Three characteristics of the LES are attributed to keep its function: pressure, overall length, and position. The LES is associated with a high-pressure zone to prevent the regurgitation of gastric contents, except in two cases: after swallowing to allow the passage of food and when the fundus is distended with gas, to allow the elimination of gas. The pathology of GERD is associated with abnormal relaxation of the LES, thus allowing contents to enter the esophagus. The resistance of the LES is a combination of both its pressure and the length over which the pressure is exerted, and in GERD both of these mechanisms of protection will be impaired.

The position is also important, since this determines what length is exposed to the positive intra-abdominal pressure. If the intra-abdominal length of the esophagus is decreased, as in cases such as the presence of a hiatal hernia, then there will be less pressure exerted on the LES, which can lead to reflux.

Association Between GERD and Obesity

Obesity is a serious health problem in the United States. Two-thirds of adults are overweight (BMI > 25 kg/m^2) or obese (BMI > 30 kg/m^2) (6). While obesity has been implicated as a cause for a lot of serious diseases, it is strongly associated with the development of GERD. Studies looking at the prevalence of GERD in the obese population have found a combined incidence of between 39 % in a large study at the Houston VA Medical Center and 53 or 61 % in two smaller studies (7–9).

Other studies have looked into the odds ratio (OR) for the development of GERD in the obese population, which has a range between 2.6 and 6.3 (10–12). Nocon et al. studied 7,124 subjects in Germany and confirmed the relationship between reflux symptoms and being overweight or obese (odds ratio 1.8, 95 % confidence interval; odds ratio 2.6, 95 % confidence interval, respectively) (10). The Bristol helicobacter project similarly showed that patients with BMI > 30 kg/m^2 have an adjusted odds ratio of 1.8 of experiencing weekly symptoms of reflux. The group studied 10,537 subjects, age 20–59 in Southwest England (11).

A variety of pathophysiological mechanisms have been proposed to explain the association between GERD and obesity. These can be divided into abnormalities associated with the esophagus, gastroesophageal (GE) junction, or stomach, and they include esophageal and gastric motility disorders (13–16), increased abdominal pressure, diminished LES pressure (13, 17), increased frequency of TLESRs (18), and the presence of hiatal hernia (9, 17).

S.A. Brethauer et al. (eds.), *Minimally Invasive Bariatric Surgery*,
DOI 10.1007/978-1-4939-1637-5_46, © Springer Science+Business Media New York 2015

Transient Relaxations of the Lower Esophageal Sphincter in Obesity

As in nonobese individuals, the most important reflux mechanism in obese individuals appears to be the presence of TLESR (2, 19). Gastric distension is the main stimulus for causing TLESRs, by causing stimulation of both stretch and tension mechanoreceptors in the proximal stomach. In a study done by Wu et al., the researchers compared three groups of study subjects—normal-weight, overweight, and obese individuals—by comparing BMI measurements, upper endoscopy, manometry, and pH recordings for both the fasting and postprandial periods. At the 2-h mark after a meal, both overweight and obese subjects had a higher rate of TLESR episodes ($P < 0.001$). In this study, a direct correlation between increasing BMI and the number of TLESR episodes was identified. It was hypothesized the postprandial TLESR episodes are due to the higher postprandial intragastric pressure (19).

Esophageal Body Motor Disorders in the Obese

An association between esophageal body motor abnormalities and the bariatric patient has been established. In a study done in 2004, which included 345 patients who were selected to undergo bariatric surgery, esophageal manometry revealed that 25.6 % of the patients had abnormal esophageal findings. These included, in decreasing frequency, hypotensive LES pressure (<10 mmHg) (69 %), nutcracker esophagus (19 %), and nonspecific motility disorders (16 %) (13). Koppman et al. also demonstrated motility disorders in 40 % of 116 obese bariatric. Nonspecific motility disorders were the most common presentation, comprising 57 %, followed by nutcracker esophagus, 26 %, and hypotensive LES (7 %) (14).

Hiatal Hernia in Obesity

Hiatal hernia is associated with an increased incidence of GERD due to diminished intra-abdominal esophageal length, diminished angulation at the angle of His, and decreased pressure at the LES. Hiatal hernias are frequently found in obese patients. Several studies have looked into hiatal hernia in obesity and its relation to GERD. The presence of a hiatal hernia was thought to be the strongest predictor of esophagitis in the general population (20). Suter et al. studied 345 morbidly obese patients. One hundred eighty-one (52.6 %) had a diagnosis of hiatal hernia. In the patients with hiatal hernia, compared to the group without hiatal hernia, 47.5 % had esophagitis (vs. 15.8 %) and 7.4 % had low distal esophageal pH (vs. 5.1 %) (13). Similar results were also reported by Iovino et al. and Pandolfino et al. (9, 21).

Lower Esophageal Sphincter Abnormalities

Normal LES pressure is considered between 10 and 35 mmHg. Hypotensive LES (<10 mmHg) is a risk factor for the development of GERD. Several studies have looked into the connection between LES pressure and obesity and have shown an inverse relationship: as the BMI increases, the LES pressure decreases. Two studies done by Iovino et al. and Kouklakis et al. have supported this inverse relationship. Iovino et al. studied 43 obese patients, who were monitored by questionnaires, stationary manometry, and a 24-h ambulatory pH-metry, and compared these patients to control subjects. The group concluded that LES pressures were significantly lower in obese patients (17). Kouklakis et al. studied 64 subjects, who were divided into three groups based on BMI. The group concluded that there is a strong inverse relationship between BMI and LES pressures (22).

In contrast, Fisher et al. showed no correlation between weight and LES pressures. The group showed a correlation between weight and BMI with gastroesophageal reflux; however, no relationship was found between BMI and LES pressures ($P = 0.068$). LES pressures were higher in patients with normal esophageal acid exposure than in those with abnormal findings ($P < 0.05$) (8).

Presentation of GERD

In a study including a large cohort of 10,545 women, there was a significant dose-dependent relationship between increasing BMI and GERD symptoms. Jacobson et al. concluded that BMI is associated with symptoms of GERD in both normal-weight and overweight women, as even moderate weight gain may exacerbate these symptoms (23). GERD symptoms are present in about 55 % of morbidly obese patients, as those include heartburn (87 %), wheezing (40 %), water brash (18 %), laryngitis (17 %), and aspiration (14 %) (24).

Treatment

Medical Treatment in Obese Patients

As with the general population, initial treatment should include diet and lifestyle modifications and medical treatment. Patients should be advised to elevate the head of the bed; eat small, frequent meals; lose weight; and avoid certain foods, such as coffee, alcohol, spicy foods, and others, that may aggravate their symptoms. The core of the medical therapy is acid suppression. Initially patients should attempt antacids, but if symptoms persist, patients should try H2-inhibitors or proton pump inhibitors (PPIs). If patients do not respond to medication, further evaluation is required.

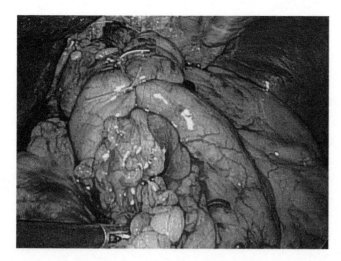

Fig. 1. Laparoscopic Nissen fundoplication.

A 24-h pH study should be obtained, as it is able to confirm the diagnosis of GERD. Endoscopic evaluation is needed to evaluate the esophageal mucosa, during which mucosal biopsies can be obtained to evaluate for any histologic changes. A video esophagogram can identify the presence of hiatal hernia. This is important as medical management is less successful with anatomic abnormality such as hiatal hernia, and hence, these patients ultimately require surgical treatment.

Surgical Treatment

In the general population, indications for surgery include anatomic abnormality, relatively severe GERD, patients who are dependent on PPIs without mucosal injury, presence of erosive esophagitis or Barrett's esophagus, failure of medical management, aspiration, or presence of stricture. The surgical strategies aim to restore the cardioesophageal competence. The standard treatment consists of hiatal reconstruction and fundoplication. Examples of fundoplication include: Toupet, Dor, or Belsey (partial) and Nissen (full wrap) (Fig. 1). Other surgical techniques attempt to reduce the contributors of GERD, such as pyloroplasty, which in principle is used to widen the pylorus and increase gastric emptying; vagotomy, which is used to reduce acid secretion; Hill repair (i.e., Hill posterior gastropexy); and finally vagotomy with antrectomy. In the general population, total fundoplication has a 93 % success rate at 3 years (25) and is considered standard therapy. However, in the obese and severely obese population, there is a controversy regarding the long-term efficacy and durability of these surgeries, with the main concern being herniation of the wrap (26).

In a study done by Perez et al., 224 patients who underwent either Nissen fundoplication or Belsey Mark IV (BM4) procedure were followed for 37 months. Subjects were divided into three groups: normal weight (BMI < 25), overweight (BMI 25–29.9), and obese (BMI > 30).

The overall recurrence of symptoms was identified as 31.3 % in obese patients (22.9 % Nissen, 53.8 % BM4), which was significantly higher than in the normal-weight individuals (4.5 %). The study concluded that obesity adversely affects the long-term success of these operations. Furthermore, there was no difference in rate of recurrence by procedure, i.e., Nissen procedure was no more durable than the BM4 procedure (27).

Similar results were reported by Morgenthal et al., who reported that morbid obesity (BMI > 35 kg/m^2) is a risk factor for failure of laparoscopic Nissen fundoplication for the treatment of GERD. Failure in this study was defined as the need for reoperation, lack of satisfaction, or any severe symptoms at follow-up. The group studied 312 patients who underwent laparoscopic Nissen fundoplication between 1992 and 1995. Preoperative morbid obesity (BMI > 35 kg/m^2) was associated with failure ($P = 0.036$), whereas obesity (BMI 30–34.9 kg/m^2) was not (28).

Smaller studies have shown contradicting results. D'Alessio et al. studied 257 patients who underwent laparoscopic Nissen fundoplication. Patients were stratified by preoperative BMI: normal (BMI < 25), overweight (BMI 25–30), and obese (BMI > 30). Following surgery, mean heartburn and dysphagia symptoms improved for patients in all BMI categories, and there were no statistical differences between different BMI groups (29). Another study, done by Anvari and Bamehriz, showed similar results. The study included 70 patients with proven diagnosis of GERD and mean BMI of 38.4 (range 35–51). Patients underwent laparoscopic Nissen fundoplication. Surgical outcomes were compared to a group containing 70 patients who had BMI < 30. The GERD symptom score improved, and percent acid reflux in 24-h testing decreased in both groups. The authors concluded that morbid obesity does not adversely affect the outcomes of laparoscopic Nissen fundoplication (30).

Even though the standard for surgical treatment for GERD in the general population is fundoplication, there are conflicting data in terms of efficacy of the current treatment in the overweight and obese population. Thus, weight loss procedures have been evaluated as an alternative surgical intervention in the treatment of GERD.

Weight Loss Procedures and Effects on GERD

Bariatric surgeries, which are intended to reduce weight, can also play a role in the treatment of GERD, as they can result in weight loss, restore the cardioesophageal competence, and minimize the gastric reservoir and/or other mechanisms. These can be divided into gastric-specific procedures and gastric with additional malabsorption procedures. Gastric-specific procedures include vertical sleeve gastrectomy and the adjustable gastric band, mostly done laparoscopically. The gastric plus malabsorptive procedures include biliopancreatic diversion with or without duodenal switch and Roux-en-Y gastric bypass (RYGB).

Roux-en-Y Gastric Bypass and GERD

The underlying mechanism for RYGB has been used as a stand-alone reflux procedure: gastric volume reduction and rapid emptying into the small bowel. Several studies have shown that GERD either improves or completely disappears after RYGB. Frezza et al., in a study of 435 patients undergoing laparoscopic Roux-en-Y gastric bypass (LRYGB), in which 55 % had evidence of chronic GERD, showed that there was a significant decrease in GERD-related symptoms, including heartburn (from 87 to 22 %, $P<0.001$), water brash (from 18 to 7 %, $P<0.05$), wheezing (from 40 to 5 %, $P<0.001$), laryngitis (from 17 to 7 %, $P<0.05$), and aspiration (from 14 to 2 %m $P<0.01$). The researchers concluded that this procedure provides a very good control of GERD in morbidly obese patients during the 3-year study. The authors proposed that in addition to volume reduction and rapid egress, the mechanism of how LRYGB affects symptoms of GERD is through weight loss and elimination of acid production in the gastric pouch. The gastric pouch lacks parietal cells; thus, there is no acid production, and also, due to its small size, it minimizes any reservoir capacity to promote regurgitation (24).

Similar results have been reported in other studies. Smith et al. found a significant reduction in reflux symptoms after RYGB with or without distal gastrectomy and gastropexy. In their study of 188 patients who were followed up to 4 years, there was a significant decrease in symptoms, as only 14 patients reported the need for medication postoperatively (31).

Jones compared Nissen fundoplication to RYGB in reflux patients with BMI under 35. RYGB was done primarily as an antireflux procedure in 332 patients from 1987 to 1996. Postoperatively only one patient was symptomatic (32). Varela et al. compared laparoscopic fundoplication with laparoscopic gastric bypass in morbidly obese patients in terms of mean length of stay, observed mortality, risk-adjusted mortality, and hospital costs and concluded that LRYGB is as safe as laparoscopic fundoplication in the treatment of GERD in this group of patients (33) and it may provide additional health-related benefits.

Gastric Banding and GERD

Since its FDA approval in 2001, the gastric band has rapidly become a popular bariatric procedure for obese patients due to its simplicity, lack of reconstruction, and perceived safety profile. However, conflicting results have been published about the effect of gastric banding on GERD. A few studies have shown that the incidence of GERD is still increased after gastric banding; however, the majority of the literature suggests that in fact symptoms and pH improve after the procedure. In fact an overly tightened band can induce reflux. One study, done by Gutschow et al., reported worsening of reflux symptoms. In the study, 31 patients were followed from

1997 to 2003, mean BMI of 46.5 kg/m^2. Upper endoscopy was performed in 18 patients after 30 months showing a high prevalence of esophagitis. Postoperative esophageal pH-manometry was performed in 16 patients and was pathologic in 43.8 % of the cases. The group concluded that the incidence of gastroesophageal reflux and esophagitis remains increased after laparoscopic gastric banding (34). These results were similar to those by Ovrebo et al., Westling et al., and Suter et al. Overall, the mechanism by which this procedure may lead to poorer outcomes in reducing the incidence of GERD is not well understood. However, it is thought that postoperative reflux may be attributed to an unrecognized hernia at the time of procedure or inappropriate (overly tight) adjustment regimens.

Other studies have shown that laparoscopic adjustable gastric banding improves pH and symptoms. De Jong et al. studied 26 patients who underwent gastric banding. The patients were assessed by 24-h pH monitoring, endoscopy, and barium swallow, preoperatively, at 6 weeks, and at 6 months. The group concluded that this procedure generally decreases GERD symptoms, as they claimed that the antireflux effect of a proximally placed gastric band is due to creating a longer intra-abdominal pressure zone or by pulling the stomach more in the abdomen in the presence of a hiatal hernia. They also hypothesized that the pouch formation is a crucial determining factor in the occurrence of symptoms after the procedure, as newer techniques advocate for a "virtually-no-pouch" procedure with placement of the band at or near the gastroesophageal junction. This high placement can still lead to pouch formation and possible dilatation of the esophagus, which can lead to concomitant esophageal motility disorders. They showed that the presence of a pouch leads to esophagitis (35).

Tolonen et al. also studied the relationship between gastric banding and GERD. The study included 31 patients who underwent gastric banding. The patients were monitored using 24-h pH tests, symptom assessment, and upper GI endoscopy. The number of reflux episodes significantly decreased postoperatively (44.6 ± 23.7 SD to 22.9 ± 17.1 SD, $P=0.0006$) after 19 months, symptoms decreased from 48.3 to 16.1 % ($P=0.01$), and the diagnosis of GERD on 24-h pH recordings decreased from 77.4 to 37.4 % ($P=0.01$). No pouch enlargement was noted on upper GI endoscopy. The researchers concluded that a gastric band that is correctly placed is associated with the effective treatment of GERD symptoms. They also hypothesized that these results were due to incomplete relaxation of the LES. No correlation between gastric band and esophageal motility was discovered. The group also felt that the antireflux effect may be mechanical, as the band may provide a narrowing at the region of the gastroesophageal junction similar to the historical Angelchik prosthesis (36).

Due to the conflicting results of studies looking into laparoscopic adjustable gastric banding and GERD, many surgeons would not recommend this procedure for the treatment of GERD in bariatric patients.

Sleeve Gastrectomy and GERD

Laparoscopic sleeve gastrectomy has become a new option for the surgical treatment of morbid obesity. It is a gastric-specific operation, but unlike the gastric band, it does not require adjustments nor does it carry the complications of having a foreign object in the body. When compared to laparoscopic Roux-en-Y, it does not have any of the complications such as malnutrition, dumping syndrome, or marginal ulcers. It has been argued that laparoscopic sleeve gastrectomy is a superior procedure in terms of weight loss compared to the gastric band and it has similar low complications and mortality rates compared to the RYGB (37). Although sleeve gastrectomy is emerging as a favorable procedure, there have been conflicting results, as some have hypothesized that this procedure can promote the development of or exacerbate GERD symptoms.

A study by Himpens et al. showed that the de novo appearance of GERD occurred in 21.8 % of patients a year after sleeve gastrectomy. However, the group also noted that after 3 years, GERD symptoms were present in only 3.1 % of the study population. They hypothesized that these results were most likely due to restoration of the angle of His. Also, symptoms in 75 % of patients who were affected before surgery disappeared by 3 years after surgery (38). Another group with similar results contributed the de novo symptoms to too-radical resection of the gastric antrum (39).

A study done by Soricelli et al. showed that sleeve gastrectomy and crural repair in the obese patients are safe techniques. The group studied 378 patients; 60 patients (15.8 %) had symptomatic GERD, and hiatal hernia alone was diagnosed in 42 patients (11.1 %). 73.3 % of these patients had complete remission of GERD symptoms following sleeve gastrectomy, whereas the rest of the patients had decreased use of antireflux medications. In addition, GERD symptoms developed in 22.9 % of patients undergoing sleeve gastrectomy, but none if hiatal hernia repair was performed (40).

Bariatric Surgery Versus Fundoplication in the Treatment of GERD

As previously mentioned there are conflicting data about the surgical approach for the treatment of GERD in cases of obese patients. Interestingly, there are very few studies that have compared traditional GERD surgeries in this population to bariatric surgery techniques. As laparoscopic gastric bypass is successful in treating both obesity and related disease plus GERD, some surgeons are advocating this surgical procedure as the procedure of choice for morbidly obese patients who also have GERD (41, 42).

Patterson et al. presented one of the few studies that directly compared standard treatment versus bariatric surgery. The group studied 12 patients, 6 undergoing LRYGB (mean BMI 55) and 6 laparoscopic Nissen fundoplication (mean BMI 29.8). The patients underwent preoperative and postoperative esophageal physiologic testing. Both groups experienced a significant improvement in heartburn symptoms postoperatively, as the mean preoperative symptom score improved from 3.5 to 0.5 in the laparoscopic Nissen group ($P=0.01$) and from 2.2 to 0.2 in the gastric bypass group ($P=0.003$). The group concluded that the two procedures are both effective in treating heartburn symptoms and objective acid reflux in the morbidly obese population (43).

Similar results were reported by Varela et al. The group looked into all patients who underwent either laparoscopic fundoplication or laparoscopic gastric bypass from October 2004 to December 2007 ($n=27,264$). The authors compared safety between the two procedures in terms of length of stay, in-hospital overall complications, mortality, risk-adjusted mortality radio, and hospital costs. They concluded that the two procedures were comparably safe in terms of treatment of GERD and recommended that in patients with morbid obesity, laparoscopic gastric bypass should be the preferred procedure of choice due to the favorable effect on other comorbid conditions (44).

Other groups looked into the outcomes of conversion of a failed fundoplication procedure to a gastric bypass. Ibele et al. looked into the impact of takedown of previous fundoplication and conversion to laparoscopic gastric bypass. In their study population, 36 % of patients had recurrent GERD at the time of revision, due to anatomic failure of the original fundoplication, and another 36 %, although with intact fundoplication, had recurrent GERD symptoms. After surgery, all of the patients in this group reported complete resolution of symptoms following surgery (45). Similar results were also reported in a study of 7 patients who originally had a laparoscopic Nissen fundoplication that was converted to a LRYGB, as the study showed significant reduction in symptoms postoperatively (16.7 % vs. 4.4 %) (46).

Kellogg et al. looked into the anatomic findings and outcomes in patients with failed Nissen fundoplication and subsequent conversion to RYGB. The group retrospectively reviewed a database of 1,435 patients who underwent RYGB between 2001 and 2006 and identified 11 patients who had previously undergone fundoplication. The mean BMI prior to gastric bypass procedure was 44 kg/m². Nine of these patients had GERD preoperatively. All patients had 100 % improvement in symptoms, with complete resolution in 78 %. Wrap disruption was present in 45 % of the patients, whereas herniation of an intact wrap occurred in 1 patient (47). Based on these results, many surgeons advocate primary bariatric surgery to avoid the risk of revision to RYGB in the event of wrap failure.

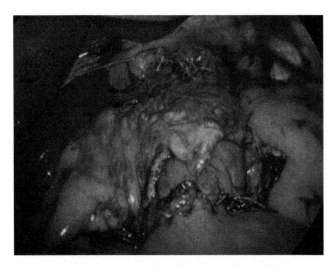

FIG. 2. Paraesophageal hernia repair and Roux-en-Y gastric bypass.

Treatment of GERD in Patients Post-Bariatric Procedures

In the postoperative bariatric patient, the development of GERD is treated in a similar way as in the general population. Initially, medical treatment should be undertaken, including a trial of PPIs and/or Carafate. If medical treatment fails, further studies can be undertaken to evaluate for hiatal hernia (Fig. 2), esophagitis, or Barrett's esophagus, such as upper gastrointestinal endoscopy. If endoscopy is considered, the person performing the procedure should be aware of the exact procedure performed and should understand the anatomy (extent of resection and length of created limbs). Information about preoperative findings would also be helpful (48). Other studies may be done, such as upper GI series, manometry, and pH studies.

In this patient population, GERD can represent several complications depending on the bariatric procedure initially performed. Vertical banded gastroplasty is now a historical procedure in which a ring or a mesh is placed about 4–6 cm down from the GE junction, and staple line is done in order to construct a small pouch. It is known that this procedure can result in severe GERD. It is hypothesized that the introduction of a band can lead to symptoms of GERD by either introduction of a stricture in the upper GI tract or by pouch distension, which may in turn distend the LES and cause symptoms of GERD. Medical management would comprise the initial steps in trying to control symptoms of GERD. In terms of GERD refractory to these interventions, conversion to gastric bypass had been used in several studies (49, 50).

In the case of laparoscopic adjustable gastric banding (LABG), symptoms of GERD are thought to be decreased by weight loss in addition to the introduction of the band as a mechanical barrier to reflux. However, postoperative complications of this procedure can manifest as GERD, such as a high or over-tight band, leading to pseudoachalasia, band slippage, or herniation. Depending on the mechanism, the management of GERD after LAGB can include medical management, including high-dose PPIs, band adjustment, or repair of slippage or hiatal hernia by laparoscopic technique. If symptoms do not resolve, conversion of laparoscopic gastric banding to RYGB has been used as well and deemed a safe procedure with good results.

The development of GERD can be due to stenosis of the gastrojejunal anastomosis in the case of Roux-en-Y bypass. Further, previous undiagnosed motility disorders may worsen after bariatric procedures (51). It is imperative to evaluate for motility disorder in the post-bariatric patient who complains of reflux, particularly after RYGB. There are not many studies done in terms of treatment of GERD after a successful RYGB. One report described the conversion to BM4 fundoplication as a successful treatment of GERD after gastric bypass (52).

In summary, there is a spectrum of considerations for the management of gastroesophageal reflux in the bariatric surgical patient. A full evaluation for anatomic abnormalities is helpful for planning subsequent therapies, either before or after a bariatric procedure. When selecting a weight loss operation, RYGB is generally preferred for the patient with significant reflux disease.

Review Questions and Answers

1. What is the main mechanism of gastroesophageal reflux disease?

(a) The presence of hiatal hernia
(b) Increased frequency of TLESRs
(c) Esophageal motility disorder
(d) All of the above

Answer: b

2. Which of the following are pathophysiological mechanisms associated with GERD in obesity?

(a) The presence of hiatal hernia
(b) Increased frequency of TLESRs
(c) Esophageal motility disorder
(d) All of the above

Answer: d

3. An obese patient presents with symptoms of GERD. What would you recommend as the initial treatment?

(a) 24-h pH study
(b) Trial of antacids, followed by H2-inhibitors or proton pump inhibitors
(c) Laparoscopic Nissen fundoplication
(d) Roux-en-Y Gastric Bypass

Answer: b

4. Which of the following weight loss procedures has the most positive impact on GERD in obese patients?

(a) Vertical band gastroplasty

(b) Laparoscopic gastric band

(c) Roux-en-Y gastric bypass

(d) Sleeve gastrectomy

(e) All of them have the same effect on GERD

Answer: c

References

1. Shaheen NJ, Hansen RA, Morgan DR, et al. The burden of gastrointestinal and liver diseases. Am J Gastroenterol. 2006;101:2128–38.

2. Blot WJ, McIAughlin JK. The changing epidemiology of esophageal cancer. Semin Oncol. 1999;26:2–8.

3. Polednak AP. Trends in incidence rates for obesity-associated cancers in the US. Cancer Detect Prev. 2003;27:415–21.

4. El-Serag HB. The epidemic of esophageal adenocarcinoma. Gastroenterol Clin North Am. 2002;31:421–40.

5. El-Serag H. Role of obesity in GERD-related disorders. Gut. 2008;57:281–4.

6. Flegal KM, et al. Prevalence of obesity and trends in the distribution of body mass index among US adults, 1999-2010. JAMA. 2012;307(5):491–7.

7. El-Serag HB, Graham DY, Satia JA. Obesity is an independent risk factor for GERD symptom and erosive esophagitis. Am J Gastroenterol. 2005;100:1243–50.

8. Fisher BL, Pannathur A, Mutnick JL, et al. Obesity correlates with gastroesophageal reflux. Dig Dis Sci. 1999;44:2290–4.

9. Iovino P, Angrisani L, Galloro G, et al. Proximal stomach function in obesity with normal or abnormal oesophageal acid exposure. Neurogastroenterol Motil. 2006;18:425–32.

10. Nocon M, Labenz J, Willich SN. Lifestyle factors and symptoms of gastro-oesophageal reflux- a population-based study. Aliment Pharmacol Ther. 2006;23:169–74.

11. Murray L, Johnstone B, Lane A, et al. Relationship between body mass and gastroesophageal reflux symptoms: a Bristol helicobacter project. Int J Epidemiol. 2003;32:645–50.

12. Nilsson M, Johnsen R, Ye W, et al. Obesity and estrogen as risk factors for gastroesophageal reflux symptoms. JAMA. 2003;290:66–72.

13. Suter M, Dorta G, Giusti V, et al. Gastro-esophageal reflux and esophageal motility disorders in morbidly obese patients. Obes Surg. 2004;14:959–66.

14. Koppman JS, Poggi L, Szomstein S, et al. Esophageal motility disorders in the morbidly obese population. Surg Endosc. 2007;21:761–4.

15. Jaffin BW, Knoepglmacher P, Greenstein R. High prevalence of asymptomatic esophageal motility disorders among morbidly obese patients. Obes Surg. 1999;9:390–5.

16. Richter JE, Wu WC, Johns DN, et al. Esophageal manometry in 95 healthy adult volunteers. Dig Dis Sci. 1987;32:583–92.

17. Iovino P, Angrisani L, Tremolaterra F, et al. Abnormal esophageal acid exposure is common in morbidly obese patients and improves after a successful lap-band system implantation. Surg Endosc. 2002;16:1631–5.

18. Wu JC, Mui LM, Cheung C. Obesity is associated with increased transient lower esophageal sphincter relaxation. Gastroenterology. 2007;132:883–9.

19. Wu JC, Mui LM, Cheung CM. Obesity is associated with increased transient lower esophageal sphincter relaxation. Gastroenterology. 2007;132:883–9.

20. Jones MP, et al. Hiatal hernia size is the dominant determinant of esophagitis presence and severity in gastroesophageal reflux disease. Am J Gastroenterol. 2001;96:1711–7.

21. Pandolfino JE, et al. Obesity: a challenge to esophagogastric junction integrity. Gastroenterology. 2006;130:639–49.

22. Kouklakis G, et al. Relationship between obesity and gastroesophageal reflux disease as recorded by 3-hour esophageal pH monitoring. Rom J Gastroenterol. 2005;14:117–21.

23. Jacobson BC, et al. Body-mass index and symptoms of gastroesophageal reflux in women. N Engl J Med. 2006;354:2340–8.

24. Frezza EE, et al. Symptomatic improvement in gastroesophageal reflux disease (GERD) following laparoscopic Roux-en-Y gastric bypass. Surg Endosc. 2002;16:1027–31.

25. Bremner RM, et al. The effects of symptoms and nonspecific motility abnormalities on outcomes of surgical therapy for gastroesophageal reflux disease. J Thorac Cadiovasc Surg. 1994;107:1244–9. discussion 1249-1250.

26. Patti MG, Alverdy JC. Gastroesophageal reflux disease and severe obesity: fundoplication or bariatric surgery? World J Gastroenterol. 2010;16(30):3757–61.

27. Perez AR, et al. Obesity adversely affects the outcome of antireflux operations. Surg Endosc. 2001;15(9):986–9.

28. Morgenthal CB, et al. Who will fail laparoscopic Nissen Fundoplication? Preoperative prediction of long-term outcomes. Surg Endosc. 2007;21(11):1978–84.

29. D'Alessio MJ, et al. Obesity is not a contraindication to laparoscopic Nissen fundoplication. J Gastrointest Surg. 2005;9:949–54.

30. Anvari M, Barmehriz F. Outcome of laparoscopic Nissen fundoplication in patients with body mass index >or =35. Surg Endosc. 2006;20:230–4.

31. Smith SC, et al. Symptomatic and clinical improvement in morbidly obese patients with gastroesophageal reflux disease following Roux-en-Y gastric bypass. Obes Surg. 1997;7:479–84.

32. Jones KB. Roux en Y gastric bypass: an effective antireflux procedure. Obes Surg. 1998;1:35–8.

33. Varela JE, et al. Laparoscopic fundoplication compared with laparoscopic gastric bypass in morbidly obese patients with gastroesophageal efflux disease. Surg Obes Relat Dis. 2009;5:139–43.

34. Gutschow CA, et al. Long-term results and gastroesophageal reflux in a series of laparoscopic adjustable gastric banding. J Gastrointerst Surg. 2005;9:941–8.

35. deJong JR, et al. The influence of laparoscopic adjustable gastric banding on gastroesophageal reflux. Obes Surg. 2004;14:399–406.

36. Tolonen P, et al. Does gastric banding for morbid obesity reduce or increase gastroesophageal reflux? Obes Surg. 2006;16:1469–74.

37. Brethauer SA. Systematic review of sleeve gastrectomy as staging and primary bariatric procedure. Surg Obes Relat Dis. 2009;5:469–75.

38. Himpens J, et al. A prospective randomized study between laparoscopic banding and laparoscopic isolated sleeve gastrectomy: results after 1 and 3 years. Obes Surg. 2006;16:1450–6.

39. Nocca D, et al. A prospective multicenter study of 163 sleeve gastrectomies: results at 1 and 2 years. Obes Surg. 2008;18:560–5.

40. Soricelli E, et al. Sleeve gastrectomy and crural repair in obese patient with gastroesophageal reflux disease and/or hiatal hernia. Surg Obes Relat Dis. 2013;9:356–61.

41. Jones JB. Roux-en-Y gastric bypass: an effective antireflux procedure in the less than morbidly obese. Obes Surg. 1998;8:35–8.

42. Smith SC, et al. Symptomatic and clinical improvement in morbidly obese patients with gastroesophageal reflux disease following Roux-en-Y gastric bypass. Obes Surg. 1997;7:479–84.

43. Patterson EJ, et al. Comparison of objective outcomes following laparoscopic Nissen fundoplication vs laparoscopic gastric bypass in the morbidly obese with heartburn. Surg Endosc. 2003;17:1561–5.

44. Varela JE, et al. Laparoscopic fundoplication compared with laparoscopic gastric bypass in morbidly obese patients with gastroesophageal reflux disease. Surg Obes Relat Dis. 2009;5: 139–43.

45. Ibele A, et al. The impact of previous fundoplication on laparoscopic gastric bypass outcomes: a case-control evaluation. Surg Endosc. 2012;26:177–81.

46. Zainabadi K, et al. Laparoscopic revision of Nissen fundoplication to Roux-en-Y gastric bypass in morbidly obese patients. Surg Endosc. 2008;22:2737–40.

47. Kellogg TA, et al. Anatomic findings and outcomes after antireflux procedures in morbidly obese patients undergoing laparoscopic conversion to Roux-en-Y gastric bypass. Surg Obes Relat Dis. 2007;3(1):58–9.

48. ASGE Standards of Practice Committee. Role of endoscopy in the bariatric surgery patient. Gastrointest Endosc. 2008;68(1):1–10.

49. Balsiger BM, et al. Gastroesophageal reflux after intact vertical banded gastroplasty: correction by conversion to Roux-en-Y gastric bypass. J Gastrointest Surg. 2000;4:276–81.

50. Bloomberg RD, Urbach DR. Laparoscopic Roux-en-Y gastric bypass for severe gastroesophageal reflux after vertical banded gastroplasty. Obes Surg. 2002;12:408–11.

51. Klaus A. Prevalent esophageal body motility disorders underlie aggravation of GERD symptoms in morbidly obese patients following adjustable gastric banding. Arch Surg. 2006;141:247–51.

52. Chen RH, et al. Antireflux operation for gastroesophageal reflux after Roux-en-Y gastric bypass for obesity. Ann Thorac Surg. 2005;80:1938–40.

47

Gallbladder and Biliary Disease in Bariatric Surgery Patients

Mohammad H. Jamal and Manish Singh

Introduction

The prevalence of obesity (BMI > 30) in the United States in 2009–2010 was 35.5 % among adult men and 35.8 % among adult women [1]. Bariatric surgery is on the rise given the high prevalence of obesity in developed countries as it proved to be the most effective treatment modality in its management. Gallstones are highly prevalent in the morbidly obese population at rates as high as 45 % which is four to five times higher than the general population [2]. Rapid weight loss is also known to be a risk factor for gallstone formation whether by bariatric surgery or by very low calorie diets. In fact, the speed at which weight loss occurs seems to be proportional to the incidence of gallstone formation [3]; also the more weight a subject loses postoperatively and the higher the body mass index (BMI), the higher the chance of forming cholesterol gallstones. The incidence of newly diagnosed gallstones after laparoscopic Roux-en-Y gastric bypass surgery (LRYGB) varies between 27 and 45 % [4], with some studies finding an incidence as high as 50 % if patients are followed for 1 year after an LRYGB [5].

However, a recent single-center study found an incidence of only 6.9 % of symptomatic cholelithiasis requiring surgery after LRYGB [3]. A similar incidence rate was also found in a recent meta-analysis that evaluated 6,048 subjects who had an LRYGB; the rate of cholecystectomy postoperatively was only 6.8 % [6].

The formation of cholesterol gallstones is attributed to changes in gallbladder motility and bile composition which becomes supersaturated with cholesterol leading to enhanced cholesterol nucleation and crystallization. Also, there is an inflammatory state caused by the increased secretion of mucin gel. The gallbladder is slow to empty in obese subjects giving more time for the cholesterol to crystallize and nucleate along with more mucin gel secretion. Obese subjects are therefore prone to acute and chronic cholecystitis [7].

Obesity itself is associated with biliary cholesterol hypersecretion which is enhanced by insulin resistance. Insulin is known to increase cholesterol production in hyperinsulinemic subjects. Postprandial emptying of the gallbladder is dependent on cholecystokinin (CCK) release and the CCK receptors in the smooth muscle cells of the gallbladder. The motility of the gallbladder is impaired probably due to the cholesterol deposition in the muscularis propria making it less sensitive to CCK release [8].

The pathogenesis of gallstone formation in patients after bariatric surgery is similar. Biliary cholesterol concentration is increased due to weight loss, and the lack of dietary fat reduces CCK release causing delayed gallbladder emptying. This, as well as the increased mucin production during weight loss, leads to increased cholesterol crystallization and nucleation, thus increasing the formation of cholesterol gallstones. Mucosal abnormalities are seen in obese patients' gallbladders in high proportion even in the absence of stones sonographically. The most frequent abnormality is cholesterolosis (37 %), followed by chronic cholecystitis with cholesterolosis (18 %) [9].

In another study, Amaral et al. [10] found that 46 % of patients had cholesterolosis and, of those, 18.2 % had gallstones. The frequency of cholesterolosis in patients with gallstones was 50 %. Weight loss is associated with a reduction in the bile salt pool. However, cholesterol secretion is reduced to a lesser degree than bile salt secretion, possibly due to increased mobilization of adipose tissue. This results in a bile composition that favors cholesterolosis and stone formation.

This change in bile composition was studied by Gustafsson et al. [11] who collected bile samples from the gallbladder of patients at the time of bariatric surgery (vertical banded gastroplasty) and at 1.1–7.3 months postoperatively via ultrasound-guided transhepatic puncture of the gallbladder. They found a 100 % increase in mucin in 6/7 patients who had the bile sampled postoperatively, and gallstones were found in 3 out of those 6 patients.

Gallbladder contractility is also decreased, possibly secondary to diminished sensitivity to cholecystokinin, and this impaired emptying also predisposes these patients to gallstone formation [12]. A study by Bastouly et al. [13]

S.A. Brethauer et al. (eds.), *Minimally Invasive Bariatric Surgery*,
DOI 10.1007/978-1-4939-1637-5_47, © Springer Science+Business Media New York 2015

examined gallbladder emptying before and after LRYGB, by determining the volume of gallbladder pre- and post-liquid meal, as well as measuring the fasting volume, the maximum ejection fraction, and the residual gallbladder volume. Postoperatively, the meal was administered via a gastrostomy tube. Biliary sludge was detected in 65 % of subjects at 1 month post LRYGB, and gallstones were detected in 30 % of subjects subsequently. The study also showed significant reduction in gallbladder motility post-operatively which was independent of duodenal exclusion.

Given the reported incidence of symptomatic gallstone disease requiring cholecystectomy post-bariatric surgery (6–15 %), three different strategies have been suggested and developed. One approach is to perform a simultaneous cho-lecystectomy at the time of bariatric surgery. This was espe-cially popular in the era prior to the use of laparoscopy, as it did not require modifications in the access incision. This would also prevent complications such as gallstone pancre-atitis and common bile duct stones that will become more challenging to treat after bypassing the duodenum in some bariatric procedures including RYGB. A second approach is to perform simultaneous cholecystectomy only in those with abnormal pre-bariatric surgery ultrasound or in those who have biliary symptoms. A third approach is a wait-and-see approach in which cholecystectomy is performed in those who develop symptoms post-bariatric surgery. The last approach, which is utilized by most centers currently, is to wait and see and prophylax with bile salts.

Fobi et al. [14] reviewed 761 patients who underwent an open RYGB (ORYGB) and simultaneous cholecystectomy. 23 % of their patient cohort had a prior cholecystectomy. Of the 76 % who had a simultaneous cholecystectomy at the time of ORYGB, they found that 86.2 % of patients had gall-bladder pathological findings. Gallbladder ultrasound was done preoperatively in all patients, but gallstones were found in only 20 % of patients. Only 14 % of their cohort had nor-mal gallbladder at cholecystectomy. The performance of cholecystectomy added only 15 min to the ORYGB without added morbidity. Therefore the authors recommended rou-tine simultaneous cholecystectomy at the time of ORYGB given the high incidence of gallbladder pathology. Dittrick et al. [15] in a similar study examined 478 obese patients who underwent simultaneous bariatric surgery and cholecys-tectomy and found that only 30 % of these patients had nor-mal gallbladder pathology and that in patients with a BMI above 50, only 14 % had a normal gallbladder pathology.

Hamad et al. [16] studied all patients who had a prophy-lactic cholecystectomy at the time of LRYGB. At their insti-tution a prophylactic cholecystectomy was only offered to those who had gallstone disease prior to the LRYGB. Ninety-four patients underwent a simultaneous cholecystectomy and LRYGB from 556 patients who underwent LARYGB. They found that adding a secondary procedure lengthened the LRYGB significantly but did not require altered port place-ment, and it nearly doubled patients' hospital stay. Kim et al.

[17] found that adding cholecystectomy to LRYGB increased the procedure by an average of 20 min.

In programs where cholecystectomy was not combined with bariatric surgery, the rate of gallbladder symptomatol-ogy requiring surgery varies. D'Hondt et al. studied 625 patients who had LRYGB and found that 43 (6.9 %) of the patients developed symptoms related to gallbladder disease and required cholecystectomy [3]. A study from Duke University Medical Center examined 1,391 patients who had an LRYGB, and 334 (24 %) of this cohort had a cholecystec-tomy prior to the LRYGB. Of the remaining 1,057 patients, 73 6.9 % underwent a simultaneous cholecystectomy at the time of gastric bypass. Of the remaining cohort of 984 patients who did not undergo a cholecystectomy at the time of gastric bypass, only 80 patients (8.1 %) needed a cholecystectomy for symptomatic gallstone disease. All their patients were fol-lowed for more than 6 months, and none received prophylaxis with bile salts. Some of their patients underwent an ORYGB, but the majority had an LRYGB [18].

Benarroch-Gampel et al. [19] studied the cost of the dif-ferent strategies of gallbladder management in patients undergoing bariatric surgery by developing a decision model. The strategies examined were LRYGB without cholecystec-tomy with ursodiol therapy and without, routine simultane-ous cholecystectomy, and selective cholecystectomy based on the presence of gallstones on a preoperative ultrasound. That study found that the most cost-effective strategy is to perform an LRYGB without preoperative ultrasound and without simultaneous cholecystectomy. They concluded that a simultaneous cholecystectomy should not be performed at the time of LRYGB and that ursodiol use postoperatively increases cost without much justification.

A metanalysis by Warschow et al. [6] examined 13 stud-ies that included 6,048 patients who did not have a cholecys-tectomy at the time of gastric bypass and had more than 3 months of follow-up post-bariatric surgery. In six of those studies, bile salts were not used postoperatively as prophy-laxis. The rate of subsequent cholecystectomy was 6.8 % (398 patients from the total cohort of 6,048). The cholecys-tectomy rate correlated with years of follow-up in the ran-dom effect model, whereby the rate increased by 3.1 % for every year of follow-up. The reasons for the subsequent cho-lecystectomies were biliary colic or dyskinesia in 5.3 % of cases, cholecystitis in 1 % of cases, biliary pancreatitis in 0.2 % of cases, and choledocholithiasis in 0.2 % of cases. No mortality was reported in any of the studies. The complica-tion rate of the subsequent cholecystectomy was 1.8 %, and 95.6 % of the procedures were performed laparoscopically. They concluded that cholecystectomy is not necessary at the time of LRYGB.

Worni et al. [20] used the Nationwide Inpatient Sample (NIS) data to identify trends in patients undergoing simulta-neous cholecystectomy at the time of gastric bypass surgery between 2001 and 2008. They found that out of 70,287 patients, simultaneous cholecystectomy was performed in

6,402 (9.1 %) of the patients. This decreased from 26.3 % in 2001 to 3.7 % in 2008. From this study we observe a decline in simultaneous cholecystectomies performed in the United States in favor of the wait-and-see approach. Not all the centers favoring the wait-and-see approach are using prophylaxis with ursodiol, a bile salt which is shown to reduce the formation of gallstones by increasing cholesterol solubility in a period of rapid weight loss.

In a multicenter randomized trial by Sugerman et al. [21], 233 patients who had a negative preoperative gallbladder ultrasound and an RYGB were randomized to a placebo group, a group receiving 300 mg of ursodiol, a group receiving 600 mg of ursodiol, and the fourth group receiving 1,200 mg of ursodiol. All patients received treatment for 6 months or until formation of gallstones, and a gallbladder ultrasound was performed at 2, 4, and 6 months. The rate of gallstones formation was 2 % in those receiving 600 mg of daily ursodiol and 6 % in those receiving 1,200 mg. The placebo group had a rate of 32 % of gallstone formation, while the group receiving 300 mg of daily ursodiol had a 13 % rate. The study concluded that prophylaxis with a daily dose of 600 mg of ursodiol for 6 months is sufficient to reduce gallstone formation in a period of rapid weight loss following RYGB, and hence this will reduce gallbladder disease requiring surgery post RYGB.

Another randomized single-center study by Wudel et al. [22] randomized patients into 3 groups, one receiving 600 mg of ursodiol daily, one receiving 600 mg of ibuprofen daily, and one group receiving a placebo. All patients had a negative gallbladder ultrasound prior to an open RYGB. Ultrasound to check for stone formation was done in subjects enrolled in the study at 3, 6, 9, and 12 months, and gallbladder emptying was assessed at 3 and 6 months. Of the 60 patients enrolled at the beginning of the study, 41 patients completed the study. The investigators found no difference in gallstone formation between the different groups; however, the completion rate for the study was only 28 % (17/60). Therefore, the compliance of patients with this treatment is an issue that needs to be considered.

A single-center randomized trial by Miller et al. [23] examined the role of ursodiol in preventing gallstone formation in patients post-bariatric restrictive procedures vertical banded gastroplasty (VBG) and gastric banding (GB). 152 patients were enrolled in the study that randomized 76 patients to a placebo group and 76 to a group receiving a daily dose of 500 mg of ursodiol. Only 3 % of the ursodiol group had gallstones at 1 year compared to 22 % of the placebo group.

A similar rate of gallstone formation and disease is found following gastric restrictive procedures, and therefore, the management is similar to that following RYGB. Li and Rosenthal compared 496 patients who had an RYGB (group A) to 52 patients who had a sleeve gastrectomy (group B) after excluding revision cases, patients with previous cholecystectomy, and patients with gallstones. The main outcome measure was the number of patients who experienced symptomatic and complicated gallstones disease. They found no significant difference in symptomatic or complicated gallstones between the two groups, despite patients in group A having a significantly higher preoperative BMI than group B and more patients in group A having more than a BMI of 45 preoperatively and more than 25 % weight loss after bariatric surgery [24].

At the Cleveland Clinic, our approach is to perform a combined cholecystectomy and bariatric procedure only if the patient has symptomatic cholelithiasis. Ursodiol is given to all other patients for 6 months after bariatric surgery.

Biliary Disease in Bariatric Patients

With the rise in bariatric surgery, in particular RYGB, the management of bariatric patients with choledocholithiasis or other causes of obstructions at the ampulla of Vater is complicated in those who have undergone a procedure that bypasses the duodenum (Roux-en-Y gastric bypass and duodenal switch). Minimally invasive methods of access to the ampulla involve either the use of laparoscopy, enteroscopy, or interventional radiology to gain entrance to the excluded stomach or the biliopancreatic limb. In most elective cases at our institution, the preferred approach is laparoscopic-assisted transgastric ERCP.

The indications for accessing the biliary tree post-bariatric surgery include sphincter of Oddi dysfunction, biliary pancreatitis, common bile duct stones, pancreatic mass evaluation, and treatment of bile leak postcholecystectomy as reported by Gutierrez et al. [25], who performed surgical gastrostomy to facilitate ERCP in patients post RYGB. Their study included 30 RYGB patients, and the most common indication for biliary access was sphincter of Oddi dysfunction. Surgical gastrostomy was performed laparoscopically in 28 patients and was planned as an open procedure in two patients. The success rate of biliary cannulation and treatment was 100 % in their study.

Sphincter of Oddi dysfunction (SOD) is also discussed in several other reports as a major indication for biliary tree access after RYGB. Without the use of endoscopic transampullary manometry, the diagnosis of SOD is challenging, however. A study by Morgan et al. [26] identified 16 patients who had SOD requiring therapeutic ERCP after RYGB. The median presentation after RYGB was 2 years, and all of these patients had a previous cholecystectomy. The diagnosis of SOD was supported by magnetic resonance cholangiopancreatography with secretin stimulation (ssMRCP) in 11 patients; 7 had a dilated common bile duct, 2 had main pancreatic duct dilation, and 3 had evidence of chronic pancreatitis. Of the 16 patients, 2 did not undergo MRCP, and 3 had normal findings.

All patients underwent open transduodenal sphincteroplasty with biliary sphincteroplasty and pancreatic ductal septoplasty.

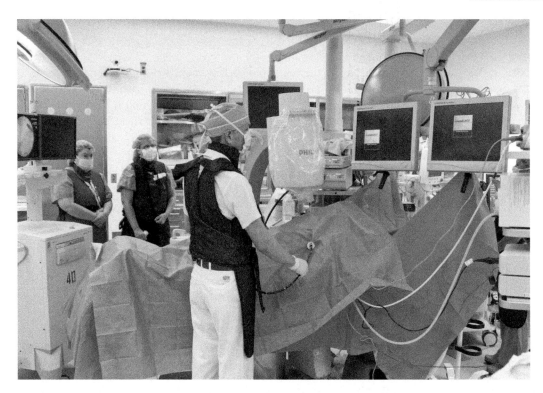

Fɪɢ. 1. A gastrostomy is created and a 15 mm trocar is then inserted in the left upper quadrant and advanced into the gastrostomy. The enteroscope is advanced through the gastrostomy and used as in standard ERCP procedures.

In all patients ampullary stenosis was confirmed by intraoperative examination. At follow-up (median 25 months), 11 patients (85 %) reported improvement of pain with 9 patients reporting discontinuing narcotic pain medications.

Laparoscopic-Assisted ERCP Technique

With the patient supine in the operating table, we use three trocars between 5 and 10 mm in size to perform diagnostic laparoscopy and lysis of adhesions if needed. After identifying the remnant stomach, a purse-string suture is placed at the suitable site in the anterior greater curvature of the remnant stomach. Cautery is then used to create the gastrostomy in the stomach. A 15 mm trocar is then inserted in the left upper quadrant and advanced into the gastrostomy (Fig. 1). The purse-string suture is then tied around the trocar to maintain insufflation. After the surgical field is appropriately draped off, the enteroscope is passed through the 15 mm trocar, and a standard ERCP procedure is completed (Fig. 2). We typically close the gastrostomy and all fascial defects equal or larger than 10 mm. If a stent is placed or there is an expected need to repeat the ERCP, a gastrostomy tube (24Fr or larger) is placed in the gastric remnant, and gastropexy sutures are placed to bring the stomach to the anterior abdominal wall. After the gastrostomy tube tract has matured (3–4 weeks), the site can be

accessed, dilated, and a repeat ERCP performed without laparoscopic assistance.

Retrograde Endoscopy

In order to reach the ampulla of Vater in patients who underwent a Roux-en-Y gastric bypass, the endoscope must travel the length of the alimentary limb which is 100–150 cm and then travels retrograde through the biliopancreatic (BP) limb. The angulation between the BP limb and the anastomosis can be difficult to negotiate. The technical challenges of this procedure are mainly related to the length of the bypassed segment and the angulation at the Roux-en-Y anastomosis. The use of side-viewing scopes that are utilized for ERCP is difficult due to their short lengths. Therefore, a traditional push enteroscopy is used, and more recently single- and double-balloon enteroscopy has been reported. This comes at the cost of losing the side view which makes cannulation of the ampulla more difficult. Choi et al. [27] summarize the limitations of double-balloon enteroscopy which has the potential to be the most successful endoscopic technique due to the length of the scope. These limitations are (1) the lack of an elevator, (2) the absence of the side view, (3) the long time of the procedure and the fact that it is time-consuming (40–180 min), (4) the limited accessories for therapeutic maneuvers, and (5) the presence of a learning curve.

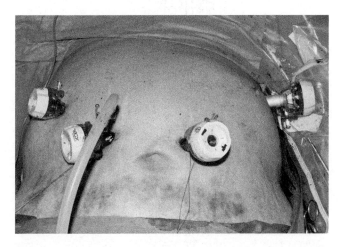

FIG. 2. The distribution and sizes of the trocars used in a standard laparoscopic ERCP.

In their study, Choi et al. examined the indications and outcomes of ERCP via laparoscopy and double-balloon enteroscopy. They included 72 patients with a prior RYGB; 44 of these patients underwent an open or laparoscopic-assisted ERCP via a gastrostomy (GERCP), while 28 patients had a double-balloon enteroscopy-assisted ERCP (DERCP). The most common indication for cholangiography in the GERCP group was sphincter of Oddi dysfunction (77 %), while for the DERCP group (57 %) common bile duct stones were suspected. In the GERCP group ERCP was performed at 4–6 weeks once the gastrostomy tract is matured. The mean total duration of GERCP was 45.9±26.6 min. The mean endoscopic procedure time in the DERCP group was 101.2±36.8 min; this was statistically significantly longer than the GERCP group. The diagnostic and interventional success for the GERCP technique was 100 %. In the DERCP group the ampulla was reached in 78 % of cases, and cannulation was achieved in 63 % of cases with successful intervention in only 56 % of cases.

The complication rate was higher in the GERCP group (14.5 %) when compared to the DERCP group (3.1 %).

In a study from Virginia Mason [28], 56 patients who had a Roux-en-Y gastric bypass underwent assisted ERCP. Twenty-four patients underwent laparoscopic-assisted ERCP, while 32 patients had balloon enteroscopy-assisted ERCP. Despite reaching the major papilla in 72 % of cases of balloon enteroscopy, the therapeutic success of balloon enteroscopy-assisted ERCP was 59 %, while the therapeutic success of laparoscopic-assisted ERCP was 100 %. Laparoscopic-assisted ERCP following a failed balloon enteroscopy saved $1,015 when compared with laparoscopic-assisted ERCP. The only factor associated with successful balloon enteroscopy-assisted ERCP was a Roux limb less than 150 cm in length.

In conclusion, gallstone disease is prevalent in the bariatric population when compared to the general population.

The trend in the United States is to perform a cholecystectomy only if patients are symptomatic at the time of the bariatric operation. Prevention of gallstones formation can be achieved using ursodiol, but compliance may be an issue. Surgically assisted ERCP is the most effective technique in managing diseases of the CBD in patients who have a bypass operation.

Questions

1. Obesity is associated with formation of gallstones because:
   (a) Supersaturation of buying with cholesterol leading to enhanced nucleation and crystallization.
   (b) Increased secretion of Mason General due to inflammatory state.
   (c) Alteration in gallbladder motility.
   (d) All of the above

2. True or false
   (a) The incidence of normal gallbladder in morbidly obese patient undergoing bariatric surgery is 50 %.
   (b) The most frequent abnormality in the gallbladder of morbidly obese patient is cholesterolosis (37 %).
   (c) Gallbladder contractility is increased and is highly sensitive to cholecystokinin after bariatric surgery.
   (d) The most cost-effective strategy for gallstones is to perform LRYGB without preoperative ultrasound and without simultaneous cholecystectomy followed by postoperative ursodiol.
   (e) The only factor associated with successful balloon enteroscopy-assisted ERCP is Roux limb less than 150 cm in length.

3. In the multicenter randomized trial by Sugerman et al., the most effective dose to prevent formation of gallstones was:
   (a) 300 mg of ursodiol daily.
   (b) 600 mg of ursodiol daily.
   (c) 1,200 mg of ursodiol daily.

4. Which of the following is not true:
   (a) The indication for accessing the biliary tree post-bariatric surgery includes sphincter of Oddi dysfunction, biliary pancreatitis, choledocholithiasis, pancreatic mass evaluation, and treatment of by a leak postcholecystectomy.
   (b) The side-viewing scopes (traditional ERCP) are effective for both laparoscopic-assisted ERCP technique and retrograde endoscopy to access the biliary tree.
   (c) Although double-balloon enteroscopy has the potential to be a successful endoscopic technique due to the length of the scope, it has several limitations.
   (d) None of the above.

References

1. Flegal KM, Carroll MD, Kit BK, Ogden CL. Prevalence of obesity and trends in the distribution of body mass index among US adults, 1999-2010. JAMA. 2012;307(5):491–7.

2. Tucker O, Soriano I, Szomstein S, Rosenthal R. Management of choledocholithiasis after laparoscopic Roux-en-Y gastric bypass. Surg Obes Relat Dis. 2008;4(5):674–8.

3. D'Hondt M, Sergeant G, Deylgat B, Devriendt D, Van Rooy F, Vansteenkiste F. Prophylactic cholecystectomy, a mandatory step in morbidly obese patients undergoing laparoscopic Roux-en-Y gastric bypass? J Gastrointest Surg. 2011;15(9):1532–6.

4. Zapata R, Severín C, Manríquez M, Valdivieso V. Gallbladder motility and lithogenesis in obese patients during diet-induced weight loss. Dig Dis Sci. 2000;45(2):421–8.

5. De Oliveira CIB, Adami Chaim E, da Silva BB. Impact of rapid weight reduction on risk of cholelithiasis after bariatric surgery. Obes Surg. 2003;13(4):625–8.

6. Warschkow R, Tarantino I, Ukegjini K, Beutner U, Guller U, Schmied BM, et al. Concomitant cholecystectomy during laparoscopic Roux-en-Y gastric bypass in obese patients is not justified: a meta-analysis. Obes Surg. 2013;23(3):397–407.

7. Rizzello M, Casella G, Abbatini F, Silecchia G, Basso N. Biliary lithiasis and obesity. Biliary Lithiasis: Springer; 2008. p. 415–24.

8. Biancani P. Gallbladder contraction in patients with pigment and cholesterol stones. Gastroenterology. 1989;97(6):1479–84.

9. Smok G, Csendes P, Burgos A, Recio M. Histologic findings of gallbladder mucosa in 87 patients with morbid obesity without gallstones compared to 87 control subjects. J Gastrointest Surg. 2003;7(4):547–51.

10. Amaral JF, Thompson WR. Gallbladder disease in the morbidly obese. Am J Surg. 1985;149(4):551–7.

11. Gustafsson U, Benthin L, Granstrom L, Groen AK, Sahlin S, Einarsson C. Changes in gallbladder bile composition and crystal detection time in morbidly obese subjects after bariatric surgery. Hepatology. 2005;41(6):1322–8.

12. Liddle RA, Goldstein RB, Saxton J. Gallstone formation during weight-reduction dieting. Arch Intern Med. 1989;149(8):1750.

13. Bastouly M, Arasaki CH, Ferreira JB, Zanoto A, Borges FG, Del Grande JC. Early changes in postprandial gallbladder emptying in morbidly obese patients undergoing Roux-en-Y gastric bypass: correlation with the occurrence of biliary sludge and gallstones. Obes Surg. 2009;19(1):22–8.

14. Fobi M, Lee H, Igwe D, Felahy B, James E, Stanczyk M, et al. Prophylactic cholecystectomy with gastric bypass operation: incidence of gallbladder disease. Obes Surg. 2002;12(3):350–3.

15. Dittrick GW, Thompson JS, Campos D, Bremers D, Sudan D. Gallbladder pathology in morbid obesity. Obes Surg. 2005;15(2):238–42.

16. Hamad GG, Ikramuddin S, Schauer PR. Elective cholecystectomy during laparoscopic Roux-en-Y gastric bypass: is it worth the wait? Obes Surg. 2003;13(1):76–81.

17. Kim J-J, Schirmer B. Safety and efficacy of simultaneous cholecystectomy at Roux-en-Y gastric bypass. Surg Obes Relat Dis. 2009;5(1):48–53.

18. Portenier DD, Grant JP, Blackwood HS, Pryor A, McMahon RL, DeMaria E. Expectant management of the asymptomatic gallbladder at Roux-en-Y gastric bypass. Surg Obes Relat Dis. 2007;3(4):476–9.

19. Benarroch-Gampel J, Lairson DR, Boyd CA, Sheffield KM, Ho V, Riall TS. Cost-effectiveness analysis of cholecystectomy during Roux-en-Y gastric bypass for morbid obesity. Surgery. 2012;152(3):363–75.

20. Worni M, Guller U, Shah A, Gandhi M, Shah J, Rajgor D, et al. Cholecystectomy concomitant with laparoscopic gastric bypass: a trend analysis of the nationwide inpatient sample from 2001 to 2008. Obes Surg. 2012;22(2):220–9.

21. Sugerman HJ, Brewer WH, Shiffman ML, Brolin RE, Fobi MA, Linner JH, et al. A multicenter, placebo-controlled, randomized, double-blind, prospective trial of prophylactic ursodiol for the prevention of gallstone formation following gastric-bypass-induced rapid weight loss. Am J Surg. 1995;169(1):91–7.

22. Wudel Jr LJ, Wright JK, Debelak JP, Allos TM, Shyr Y, Chapman WC. Prevention of gallstone formation in morbidly obese patients undergoing rapid weight loss: results of a randomized controlled pilot study. J Surg Res. 2002;102(1):50–6.

23. Miller K, Hell E, Lang B, Lengauer E. Gallstone formation prophylaxis after gastric restrictive procedures for weight loss: a randomized double-blind placebo-controlled trial. Ann Surg. 2003;238(5):697–702.

24. Li VK, Pulido N, Martinez-Suartez P, Fajnwaks P, Jin HY, Szomstein S, et al. Symptomatic gallstones after sleeve gastrectomy. Surg Endosc. 2009;23(11):2488–92.

25. Gutierrez JM, Lederer H, Krook JC, Kinney TP, Freeman ML, Jensen EH. Surgical gastrostomy for pancreatobiliary and duodenal access following Roux en Y gastric bypass. J Gastrointest Surg. 2009;13(12):2170–5.

26. Morgan KA, Glenn JB, Byrne TK, Adams DB. Sphincter of Oddi dysfunction after Roux-en-Y gastric bypass. Surg Obes Relat Dis. 2009;5(5):571–5.

27. Choi EK, Chiorean MV, Cote GA, El Hajj I, Ballard D, Fogel EL, et al. ERCP via gastrostomy vs. double balloon enteroscopy in patients with prior bariatric Roux-en-Y gastric bypass surgery. Surg Endosc. 2013;27(8):2894–9.

28. Schreiner MA, Chang L, Gluck M, Irani S, Gan SI, Brandabur JJ, et al. Laparoscopy-assisted versus balloon enteroscopy-assisted ERCP in bariatric post-Roux-en-Y gastric bypass patients. Gastrointest Endosc. 2012;75(4):748–56.

48

Effects of Bariatric Surgery on Diabetes

Ashwin Soni, Alpana Shukla, and Francesco Rubino

Introduction

The concept that gastrointestinal surgery may be intentionally used to treat T2DM was formalized by a multidisciplinary international group of experts at the Diabetes Surgery Summit in Rome, 2007 [3]. In consideration of the abundant data now available to attest to the efficacy and safety of bariatric surgery to treat T2DM in obese patients, the International Diabetes Federation (IDF) more recently issued its position statement [4], recommending the use of bariatric surgery in patients with diabetes and BMI > 35 kg/m² and as an alternative treatment option in patients with BMI 30–35 kg/m² inadequately controlled with optimal medical regimens.

Experimental data from rodent studies [5, 6] and subsequent observational studies in humans [7, 8] have demonstrated that less obese individuals may benefit similarly to morbidly obese subjects. There are currently several small- to medium-sized randomized controlled trials (RCTs) investigating the efficacy of different bariatric procedures versus optimal medical management to treat T2DM in mild to moderately obese subjects. The outcomes of published RCTs and observational studies and the putative mechanisms of effects of bariatric surgery on diabetes are discussed in this chapter.

Physiological Mechanisms of Diabetes Remission Following Bariatric Surgery

Improvement in glucose homeostasis and insulin sensitivity is an expected outcome of weight loss in obese individuals due to any intervention, whether it is medical or surgical. Concomitant with the profound weight loss following gastrointestinal surgery, there is improvement in insulin sensitivity with elevation in the levels of the insulin-sensitizing hormone adiponectin. The concentration of insulin receptors and markers of insulin signaling increase, and the lipid content within the muscle and liver also decreases after bariatric surgery [9].

It is now abundantly clear, however, that the improvement of glycemia is not determined by weight loss alone. Studies have shown that glycemic control improves within days after Roux-en-Y gastric bypass (RYGB) or biliopancreatic diversion (BPD) prior to any significant weight loss. In addition, glycemic control after equivalent weight loss is superior after RYGB as compared to that after laparoscopic adjustable gastric banding (LAGB) or caloric restriction [2, 7, 8]. Experimental evidence in favor of weight-independent mechanisms is derived from animal investigations using the duodenojejunal bypass (DJB) model developed by Rubino in rodents to study the effects of gastric bypass on glucose homeostasis [5]. In lean diabetic Goto-Kakizaki (GK) rats, Rubino and colleagues found that DJB (a bypass of the proximal intestine by the same amount as RYGB but without gastric restriction) rapidly and durably improved fasting glucose and postprandial hyperglycemia. These effects were not observed in sham-operated animals that had undergone equivalent weight loss by caloric restriction. Other investigators have subsequently made similar observations in nonobese diabetic GK rats and obese diabetic Zucker rats.

The gut is the largest endocrine organ secreting numerous hormones and factors involved not only in digestion but also regulation of body weight and glucose homeostasis. It is now recognized that surgical manipulation of the gut results in a change in the levels of various gut hormones including glucagon-like peptide-1 (GLP-1), peptide-YY (PYY), and ghrelin, which can significantly impact glycemic control and body weight.

GLP-1 is an incretin hormone that increases glucose tolerance by enhancing glucose-dependent insulin secretion, suppressing glucagon secretion, inhibiting gastric emptying, increasing β-cell mass, and possibly improving insulin insensitivity [10]. GLP-1 is produced primarily in the ileum and colon by nutrient-stimulated L cells. The postprandial GLP-1 response is consistently observed to be augmented during an oral glucose tolerance test or mixed meal test after the RYGB or BPD in obese nondiabetic and diabetic patients [9, 11]. The rise in GLP-1 level occurs as early as 2 days after surgery and

S.A. Brethauer et al. (eds.), *Minimally Invasive Bariatric Surgery*,
DOI 10.1007/978-1-4939-1637-5_48, © Springer Science+Business Media New York 2015

has been shown to persist at 6 months and 1 year postoperatively [12]. Restrictive procedures, such as vertical banded gastroplasty (VBG) and LAGB, have not shown to be associated with any changes in the levels of GLP-1 postoperatively [13].

Ghrelin is an orexigenic hormone produced primarily bVBy the stomach, and administration of ghrelin and its analogs stimulates food intake. Ghrelin levels have an inverse relationship with body weight, and consequently obese individuals have lower ghrelin levels. Weight loss induced by caloric restriction results in an increase in the levels of ghrelin, which subsequently may contribute to the resistance to lifestyle interventions for obesity. Ghrelin may play a role in glucose homeostasis and has been shown to inhibit insulin secretion and suppress the insulin-sensitizing hormone adiponectin [14]. Ghrelin deletion in diabetic obese mice models has shown to reduce fasting glucose and insulin and thus improve glucose tolerance [15]. Several groups have reported a decrease in the levels of ghrelin after RYGB, which may partly account for the improved glycemia [12, 16]. This has not been consistently reported with other studies showing either unchanged or increased ghrelin levels [9, 17]. As expected, ghrelin levels are markedly suppressed following resection of the ghrelin-rich gastric fundus as with a sleeve gastrectomy. However, ghrelin levels show the normal physiological rise with weight loss after LAGB and VBG.

PYY is an anorexigenic hormone co-secreted with GLP-1 from intestinal L cells in response to food intake. PYY has been shown to decrease food intake in humans when injected. Experimental studies in rodents suggest that PYY may directly ameliorate insulin resistance [18]. Several studies have reported elevated PYY levels after RYGB. In a prospective, nonrandomized controlled study comparing the effects of medical and surgical treatment on PYY levels after similar weight loss, it was observed that PYY's area under the curve increased following RYGB and sleeve gastrectomy, but remained unchanged in the medical arm [19].

Korner et al. [7] conducted a prospective study of gut hormone and metabolic changes after LAGB and RYGB and suggested that the changes in hormone secretion may contribute to the efficacy of the particular procedure in improving obesity-related comorbidities. It is established that PYY and GLP-1 are secreted shortly after food intake from L cells in the distal small bowel and colon. Both decrease appetite, increase satiety, slow gut motility, and improve insulin sensitivity. GLP-1 also functions as an incretin to potentiate glucose-stimulated insulin release. In contrast, ghrelin stimulates appetite, profoundly promotes food intake and gut motility, and decreases insulin sensitivity [20]. Korner et al. [7] found that in LAGB patients, the postprandial rise of GLP-1 measured at 30 min did not change after surgery, whereas in contrast, postprandial GLP-1 levels after RYGB were significantly greater compared with 30-min values before surgery and threefold higher compared with the same time points after LAGB. Fasting glucose, insulin, and homeostasis model assessment of insulin resistance

(HOMA-IR) were also shown to decrease to a greater extent after RYGB. The degree of suppression of ghrelin levels post-meal did not differ significantly presurgery to week 52 in either the LAGB or RYGB and did not differ between groups. Laferrère et al. [8] suggested that the markedly increased incretin levels and effect observed after the RYGB may well be one of the mediators of the antidiabetic effects of the surgery, and they set out to determine whether the magnitude of change of the incretin levels is greater after the RYGB compared to a hypocaloric diet at an equivalent weight loss. Their results showed a markedly increased GLP-1 response to oral glucose after the RYGB, but GLP-1 levels tended to decrease after diet intervention, although this decrease was not significant. The incretin effect markedly increased after an RYGB, but not with diet, and suggests that this effect was not likely to be weight loss related. Therefore, this could play a key role in the remission and resolution of T2DM after an RYGB. Data from various studies has shown that beneficial changes of incretin levels occur rapidly after the RYGB, which is secondary to the bypass procedure, thus resulting in an improved insulin secretion profile and decreased postprandial glucose [21].

Another mechanism proposed in recent years is the effect of bariatric surgery on the alteration of taste. This novel weight loss mechanism involves alterations in food preferences, which may be secondary to changes in taste detection and reward. Miras et al. [22] have shown that after RYGB, patients' eating behavior changes, and they start to adopt healthier food preferences by avoiding high-calorie and high-fat foods. Patients find sweet and fatty meals less pleasant than preoperatively, and this may be attributed to changes in the sense of taste. A putative mechanism to explain this is that RYGB may reverse the higher activation of brain taste reward and addiction centers in response to high calorie and fat tasting.

Two hypotheses have been proposed to explain improved glycemia following gastrointestinal surgery. The "hindgut hypothesis" posits that the expedited delivery of ingested nutrients to the lower bowel, due to an intestinal bypass, stimulates L cells, which results in an increased secretion of incretin hormones and an improved glucose homeostasis [5]. Consistent with the hindgut hypothesis, the bariatric operations most noted for rapid T2DM remission, RYGB and BPD, create GI shortcuts for food to access the distal bowel. However, a significant improvement in glycemia and remission of diabetes with elevated incretin levels is also noted to occur after a sleeve gastrectomy, which does not involve an intestinal bypass. It must be noted that GLP-1 secretion is stimulated not only by direct nutrient contact with distal intestinal L cells but also by proximal nutrient-related signals that are transmitted from the duodenum to the distal bowel by neural pathways and other unknown mechanisms [9]. The alternative hypothesis is the "foregut hypothesis," which depends on the exclusion of the duodenum and proximal jejunum from the transit of nutrients, possibly preventing secretion of a putative signal that promotes insulin resistance and T2DM [6]. Rubino et al. conducted a study to investigate these mechanisms by testing both hypotheses and found that the exclusion of the proximal small intestine from contact with ingested nutrients is a critical component in the mechanism improving glucose tolerance after the DJB in GK rats, thus supporting the foregut hypothesis [6].

Other hypothesized antidiabetic mechanisms after bariatric surgery include changes in intestinal nutrient-sensing mechanisms regulating insulin sensitivity, disruption of vagal afferent and efferent innervations, bile acid perturbations, changes in gut microbiota, and alterations in undiscovered gut factors.

The Effects and Outcomes of Bariatric Surgery on Diabetes in Patients with a BMI > 35 kg/m^2

The outcomes of bariatric surgery on diabetes and the metabolic profile in patients with a BMI of >35 kg/m^2 have been well documented over many years.

Buchwald et al. [23] conducted a meta-analysis including 22,094 patients with T2DM reported an overall 77 % remission rate of T2DM (defined as persistent normoglycemia without diabetes medication after bariatric surgery). The mean procedure-specific resolution of T2DM was 48 % for LAGB, 68 % for VBG, 84 % for RYGB, and 98 % for BPD. The drawback of this study is that the majority of these studies included was retrospective and had a short follow-up duration of 1–3 years. The multicenter Swedish Obese Subjects (SOS) study, a large prospective observational study [24], compared bariatric surgery (LAGB $n=156$, VBG $n=451$, RYGB $n=34$) with conservative medical management in a group of well-matched obese patients. At 2 years, 72 % of diabetic subjects in the surgical group achieved remission of T2DM compared to 21 % in the medically treated arm. At 10 years, the relative risk of incident T2DM was three times lower, and the rates of recovery from T2DM were three times greater, for patients who underwent surgery than for individuals in the control group. The proportion of subjects in whom the remission was sustained at 10 years declined to 36 % in the surgical group and 13 % in the medical group. It must be noted, however, that approximately 95 % of patients in the SOS study underwent gastric restrictive procedures rather than RYGB.

Recently, Schauer et al. [25] published results from their randomized, non-blinded, single-center trial and compared intensive medical therapy alone versus medical therapy plus RYGB or sleeve gastrectomy (SG) in 150 obese patients (BMI 27–43 kg/m^2) with uncontrolled T2DM. The primary end point was the proportion of patients with a glycated hemoglobin (HbA1c) level of 6.0 % or less 12 months after treatment. The proportion of patients who reached the primary

end point was 12 % for the medical group, 42 % in the RYGB group, and 37 % in the SG group. Glycemic control was demonstrated to improve in all three groups with a mean HbA1c level of 7.5±1.8 % in the medical therapy group, 6.4±0.9 % in the gastric bypass group, and 6.6±1.0 % in the sleeve gastrectomy group. It was demonstrated that many patients in the surgical groups, particularly in the RYGB group, achieved glycemic control without the use of diabetes medications after 1-year follow-up. Secondary end points, including BMI, body weight, waist circumference, and the HOMA-IR, improved more significantly in the surgical groups than the medical therapy group. It was also shown that the reduction in the use of glycemic pharmacotherapy occurred before achievement of maximal weight loss, thus supporting the weight-independent mechanisms of surgery. This trial also supported the notion that bariatric surgery represents a useful management strategy for uncontrolled T2DM.

Mingrone et al. [26] published results from an RCT conducted including 60 patients (BMI ≥ 35 kg/m^2) with a history of at least 5 years of T2DM, and an HbA1c level of 7.0 % or more. They compared conventional medical therapy to the RYGB or BPD. The primary end point was the rate of diabetes remission at 2 years (defined as a fasting glucose level of <100 mg/dL and an HbA1c level of <6.5 % in the absence of pharmacological therapy). At 2 years follow-up, diabetes remission had occurred in no patients in the medical therapy group versus 75 % in the RYGB group, and 95 % in the BPD group. All patients in the surgical groups had discontinued their pharmacotherapy (oral hypoglycemic agents and insulin) within 15 days after the operation. At 2 years, the average baseline HbA1c level (8.65±1.45 %) had decreased in all groups, but patients in the two surgical groups had the greatest degree of improvement (average HbA1c levels, 7.69±0.57 % in the medical therapy group, 6.35±1.42 % in the RYGB group, and 4.95±0.49 % in the BPD group). The findings support the conclusion that bariatric surgery may be more effective than conventional medical therapy in controlling hyperglycemia in severely obese patients with T2DM.

The Effects and Outcomes of Bariatric Surgery on Diabetes in Patients with a BMI > 35 kg/m^2

The effects of bariatric surgery in the morbidly obese population (>35 kg/m^2) are well documented. The field of metabolic surgery has become increasingly researched in recent years, investigating the effects and benefits of operating on those patients with a BMI of less than 35 kg/m^2. The aims of metabolic surgery differ slightly from bariatric surgery; in that, there is a shift in goals of surgery from weight reduction to the control of metabolic disease, with the aim of "curing" T2DM or putting this prevalent condition into remission. Recently, prospective RCTs have been conducted in lower

BMI patients (<35 kg/m^2) in order to compare various gastrointestinal surgical procedures versus intensive medical management, to identify the differences between conventional treatment and metabolic surgery.

Dixon et al. [27] conducted an RCT comparing the LAGB versus conventional therapy in 60 obese patients (BMI > 30 and <40 kg/m^2) with recently diagnosed (<2 years) T2DM. The primary outcome measure was the remission of T2DM (defined as fasting plasma glucose < 126 mg/dL and an HbA1c level of <6.2 % while taking no glycemic therapy). After a 2-year follow-up, remission of T2DM was achieved in 73 % in the surgical group and 13 % in the conventional therapy group, and it was found to be related to weight loss. Mean levels of fasting plasma glucose and HbA1c were significantly lower in the LAGB group at 2 years. There was also a significant reduction in the use of pharmacotherapy for glycemic control in the LAGB group at 2 years. Secondary outcome measures, such as insulin sensitivity and levels of triglycerides and HDL, were also improved in the surgical group. It was concluded that this trial presents evidence to support the early consideration of surgery in the treatment of obese patients with T2DM.

Lee et al. designed a randomized, double-blind trial [28] in order to compare the RYGB versus SG on T2DM resolution (remission defined as fasting plasma glucose < 126 mg/dL, HbA1c < 6.5 % without the use of oral hypoglycemics or insulin) in non-morbidly obese patients (BMI < 35 kg/m^2) who had T2DM that was inadequately controlled. The resolution rate was 93 % in the RYGB group compared with 47 % in the SG group. These results are consistent with the RYGB being more effective than restrictive-type procedures. The RYGB group also achieved a lower waist circumference, fasting plasma glucose level, HbA1c level, and blood lipid level. Therefore, the RYGB group had a higher remission rate for the metabolic syndrome than the SG group. This study concluded that RYGB is more effective than SG for surgical treatment of inadequately controlled T2DM, suggesting that duodenal exclusion plays a role in the mechanism behind the remission of T2DM.

Cohen et al. published results from a prospective study [29] following 66 diabetic patients (BMI 30–35 kg/m^2) up to 6 years who elected to have the RYGB. The percentage of patients experiencing diabetes remission (defined as an HbA1c < 6.5 % without the use of hypoglycemic medication) was identified. The mean HbA1c fell progressively throughout the duration of the study from 9.7 ± 1.5 to 5.9 ± 0.1 %, and fasting plasma glucose fell from 156 ± 11 to 97 ± 5 mg/dL. HOMA-IR also fell dramatically within the first 6 months. Remission of diabetes occurred in 88 % of patients, whose diabetes medications were discontinued 3–26 weeks after surgery. Improvement of diabetes without full remission was seen in 11 % of patients, which lead to a decrease in the usage of pharmacotherapy and withdrawal of insulin when previous used. There was found to be no correlation between the change in body weight and change in HbA1c at any postoperative time point. There was also no association between the amount of weight lost and magnitude of improvement in β-cell sensitivity to glucose.

Despite these prospective RCTs being conducted at various institutions, it is clear that longer-term follow-up of these patients is required. Larger and perhaps multicenter trials are necessary to evaluate the potential benefits of bariatric surgery for the treatment of T2DM in less obese patients. Studies are consistent in showing the efficacy of surgery with regard to the improvement in glycemic indexes as well as improving other aspects of the metabolic syndrome. The impact of surgery on microvascular and macrovascular complications of diabetes needs to be assessed with long-term follow-up.

Improvement in Cardiovascular Outcomes and Mortality in Type 2 Diabetic Patients

It is now evident that apart from its glycemic effects, bariatric surgery confers non-glycemic benefits including improvement of cardiovascular risk factors such as dyslipidemia and hypertension. More importantly, it has been established that there is a reduction in mortality. The meta-analysis by Buchwald et al. [23] showed a marked decrease in levels of total cholesterol, LDL cholesterol, and triglycerides after gastrointestinal surgery. An improvement in hyperlipidemia was shown in approximately 70 % of patients, and hypertension was shown to improve or resolve in 79 % of patients. Lee et al. have demonstrated these beneficial effects of gastrointestinal surgery in patients with a BMI < 35 kg/m^2 [30]. Follow-up of participants in the SOS study after an average of 11 years found that bariatric surgery was associated with a 29 % reduction in all-cause mortality after adjusting for age, sex, and risk factors in this severely obese group [31].

In a recent study, Cohen et al. [29] prospectively followed up type 2 diabetic patients who had an RYGB, and it was demonstrated that the predicted 10-year risk of cardiovascular disease, calculated by the UKPDS risk engine, fell substantially after surgery. There was a decrease in the risk of events: 71 % decrease in coronary heart disease, 84 % decrease in fatal, 50 % decrease in stroke, and 57 % decrease in fatal stroke.

Romeo et al. recently published on the prospective, controlled SOS study, looking at the effects of bariatric surgery on cardiovascular events on participants with T2DM [32]. The mean follow-up was 13.3 years for all cardiovascular events. Bariatric surgery was associated with a reduction in the incidence of fatal and nonfatal cardiovascular events, and importantly, the benefit of surgery was present after adjusting for baseline parameters. Bariatric surgery was associated with a lower incidence of myocardial infarction. A total of 38 of the 345 individuals in the surgery group compared with 43 of the 262 individuals in the control group had myocardial infarction during follow-up. Interestingly, no significant differences in the incidence of myocardial infarction were found between the different surgical procedures (RYGB, LAGB, vertical gastroplasty). However, bariatric surgery was not found to be associated with changes in the incidence of cerebral stroke in these type 2 diabetic patients.

Adams et al. conducted a retrospective cohort study including 7,925 severely obese patients and 7,925 similarly obese matched controls [33]. After a mean follow-up of 8.4 years, it was demonstrated that surgery reduced overall mortality by 40 %, cardiovascular mortality by 56 %, cancer mortality by 60 %, and diabetes-related mortality by 92 %.

Comparative Efficacy of Different Bariatric Procedures to Treat Diabetes

Bariatric procedures differ in their ability to ameliorate T2DM, with intestinal bypass procedures (i.e., RYGB, BPD) generally associated with greater glycemic control and remission rates than purely restrictive procedures (i.e., LAGB). As indicated in the meta-analysis by Buchwald et al. [23], BPD appears to be the most efficacious closely followed by RYGB and then LAGB. A systematic review by Tice et al. [34] of 14 comparative studies, albeit of low quality (mostly retrospective and unmatched), testified to the superior efficacy of RYGB over LAGB in treating T2DM. There has been until now a paucity of data from RCTs comparing the efficacy of various bariatric procedures to treat diabetes. There are currently several ongoing small- to medium-sized RCTs comparing the efficacy of medical versus surgical treatment of type 2 diabetes including some that have more than one bariatric procedure as the surgical comparator. The results of some of these have recently been published. Lee et al. [28] have reported the results of their RCT comparing gastric bypass to sleeve gastrectomy in patients with BMI 25–35 kg/m^2; the remission rate for T2DM was 93 % for patients who underwent RYGB compared to 47 % for those who underwent sleeve gastrectomy. The recently published RCT by Schauer et al. [25] also indicates superior efficacy of RYGB over sleeve gastrectomy in the treatment of diabetes in obese individuals. On the other hand, BPD produced greater remission of diabetes in morbidly obese patients compared to RYGB (95 % versus 75 %) in the RCT reported by Mingrone et al. [26].

Predictors of Remission of Type 2 Diabetes Following Bariatric Surgery

As discussed above, the choice of procedure is an important determinant of outcome with a decreasing gradient of efficacy predicted from BPD, RYGB to SG and then LAGB. Other factors that have been positively correlated with diabetes remission are percentage of excess weight loss (% EWL), younger age, lower preop HbA1c, and shorter duration of diabetes (less than 5 years) [35]. Severity of diabetes, as judged by preop treatment modality, has also been noted to be a significant factor. Schauer et al. [36] have reported in their series of 191 obese diabetic patients (the majority of whom were on oral agents or insulin) a diabetes remission rate of 97 % in diet-controlled, 87 % in oral agent-treated, and 62 % in insulin-treated subjects. This was also confirmed by a recent retrospective analysis of 505 morbidly obese diabetic patients who underwent RYGB [37]. In this study, a more recent diagnosis of T2DM and the absence of preoperative insulin therapy were significant predictors of remission, independent of the percentage of EWL. Dixon et al. [38] have recently identified diabetes duration < 4 years, BMI > 35 kg/m^2, and fasting c-peptide concentration > 2.9 ng/mL as three clinically useful cutoffs and independent preoperative predictors of remission after analyzing the outcomes of 154 ethnic Chinese subjects after gastric bypass. C-peptide > 3 ng/mL has also previously been shown to be an important predictor of diabetes resolution after sleeve gastrectomy in non-morbidly obese diabetic subjects by Lee et al. [39].

The Future of Metabolic Surgery

In recent years, there has been an increasing amount of research conducted to look at minimally invasive methods with the aim of mimicking the effects of gastrointestinal surgery but providing a safer and reversible alternative to conventional surgery. Endoluminal and transgastric procedures are evolving concepts that combine the skills and techniques of flexible endoscopy with minimally invasive surgery. This is the future of bariatric and metabolic surgery in order to develop less morbid and less costly treatment options [40].

The endoluminal sleeve (ELS) was an idea, which stemmed from an experimental model in rats performed by Rubino et al. They developed an (ELS) to prevent contact between nutrients and the duodenal mucosa in rats [2], therefore producing a functional duodenal bypass without creating a rapid delivery of nutrient to the distal bowel. Rats undergoing the ELS demonstrated a dramatic improvement of glucose tolerance compared to matched controls in which the ELS had been fenestrated to allow nutrients to come into contact with the duodenal mucosa. The antidiabetic effect of ELS was also shown by Aguirre et al. [41] in a diet-induced rat model of insulin resistance. A prospective randomized trial comparing ELS to sham endoscopy plus a low-fat diet and exercise showed a dramatic decrease in HbA1c of 2.9 % in the ELS group compared to the conventional therapy group [42].

Gut hormones and the enteric nervous system are involved in the regulation of satiety signals, GI motility, and insulin sensitivity. Electrophysiologic devices interfere with vagal signals between the brain and gastrointestinal tract, through a variety of mechanisms including gastric stimulation or pacing, neuromodulation, vagal resection, and intermittent vagal nerve blockage as a means of controlling satiety [42]. The TANTALUS system is a laparoscopically implantable system, which is a gastric electrical stimulator. Bohdjalian et al. [43] conducted a multicenter open-label European feasibility trial involving 24 obese diabetic patients treated with insulin and/or oral hyperglycemic agents with a BMI between 33.3 and 49.7 kg/m². In those subjects that reached the 1-year visit, weight was reduced by 4.5 ± 2.7 kg ($p < 0.05$) and HbA1c by 0.5 ± 0.3 % ($p < 0.05$). In a subgroup of patients on oral medications, weight was reduced by 6.3 ± 3.4 kg ($p < 0.05$), and HbA1c was reduced by 0.9 ± 0.4 % ($p < 0.05$). The group on insulin had no significant changes in either weight or the HbA1c. The study concluded that the TANTALUS system and gastric electrical stimulation can potentially lead to improvement in glucose metabolism and the lipid profile, as well as inducing weight loss and favorable changes in eating behavior, in obese diabetic individuals. Consistent results were published by Sanmiguel et al. [44] in a study involving 14 obese type 2 diabetic patients. They demonstrated that short-term therapy with the TANTALUS system improves glucose control, induces weight loss, and improves blood pressure and the lipid profile in these subjects on oral antidiabetes therapy and found that the improvement in glucose control did not correlate with weight loss.

These endoluminal procedures and other novel minimally invasive procedures offer a lot of potential for the future of bariatric and metabolic surgery. However, an extensive amount of research is required in order to take it from the experimental trial settings and actually incorporate it into standard practice. Prospective randomized trials are necessary in order to investigate these procedures further, but it certainly offers a lot of scope for the future of interventional diabetology, potentially revolutionizing this newly emerging field.

Conclusion

The incorporation of bariatric surgery into the treatment options for type 2 diabetes is currently being researched quite extensively. Type 2 diabetes is a worldwide epidemic, and current conventional methods of treatment have their limitations. Despite advancements in medical therapy, many patients still fail to achieve optimal glycemic control, and thus surgery may provide a suitable alternative for those who fail conventional methods. Continued research must be conducted in this field in order to understand the mechanisms of surgery with regard to the remission of type 2 diabetes and to further our understanding of the role of the gut. Novel procedures may also introduce minimally invasive surgery into metabolic surgery offering patients a

safer and less risky procedure to treat their diabetes. Further research and prospective studies offer the potential to advance pharmacotherapy in order to develop and uncover new therapeutic targets in order to manage type 2 diabetes more effectively.

Financial Support/Conflict of Interest None.

Review Questions and Answers

1. *Factors that are positively correlated with the remission of T2DM after surgery include all except:*
   A. Increasing age
   B. Lower preoperative HbA1c
   C. Shorter duration of diabetes
   D. Percentage of excess weight loss

   Answer is **A**. Patients who have a lower preoperative HbA1c and a shorter duration of T2DM, and those who have a higher percentage of excess weight loss, have a greater chance of remission of T2DM after surgery.

2. *Improvement in insulin sensitivity following bariatric surgery is accompanied by all of the following mechanisms except:*
   A. Decrease in the lipid content of the liver and muscle
   B. Reduction in the levels of adiponectin
   C. Increase in the concentration of insulin receptors
   D. Increase in the markers of insulin signaling

   Answer is **B**. There is an elevation in the levels of adiponectin following bariatric surgery, as adiponectin is an insulin-sensitizing hormone.

3. *The Swedish Obese Subjects (SOS) study demonstrated the following effects of bariatric surgery on cardiovascular events on participants with T2DM except:*
   A. Reduction in the incidence of fatal and nonfatal cardiovascular events
   B. Lower incidence of myocardial infarction
   C. Lower incidence of cerebral stroke
   D. Similar incidence of myocardial infarction following different surgical procedures

   Answer is **C**. Bariatric surgery was not found to be associated with changes in the incidence of cerebral stroke in type 2 diabetic patients in the SOS study.

References

1. Shaw JE, Sicree RA, Zimmet PZ. Global estimates of the prevalence of diabetes for 2010 and 2030. Diabetes Res Clin Pract. 2010;87(1):4–14.
2. Rubino F, Schauer PR, Kaplan LM, et al. Metabolic surgery to treat type 2 diabetes: clinical outcomes and mechanisms of action. Annu Rev Med. 2010;61:393–411.

3. Rubino F, Kaplan LM, Schauer PR, et al. The Diabetes Surgery Summit consensus conference: recommendations for the evaluation and use of gastrointestinal surgery to treat type 2 diabetes mellitus. Ann Surg. 2010;251(3):399–405.

4. Zimmet P, Alberti KG, Rubino F, et al. IDF's view of bariatric surgery in type 2 diabetes. Lancet. 2011;378(9786):108–10.

5. Rubino F, Marescaux J. Effect of duodenal-jejunal exclusion in a nonobese animal model of type 2 diabetes: a new perspective for an old disease. Ann Surg. 2004;239:1–11.

6. Rubino F, Forgione A, Cummings DE, et al. The mechanism of diabetes control after gastrointestinal bypass surgery reveals a role of the proximal small intestine in the pathophysiology of type 2 diabetes. Ann Surg. 2006;244(5):741–9.

7. Korner J, Inabnet W, Febres G, et al. Prospective study of gut hormone and metabolic changes after adjustable gastric banding and Roux-en-Y gastric bypass. Int J Obes (Lond). 2009;33(7):786–95.

8. Laferrère B, Teixeira J, McGinty J, et al. Effect of weight loss by gastric bypass surgery versus hypocaloric diet on glucose and incretin levels in patients with type 2 diabetes. J Clin Endocrinol Metab. 2008;93:2479–85.

9. Thaler JP, Cummings DE. Minireview: hormonal and metabolic mechanisms of diabetes remission after gastrointestinal surgery. Endocrinology. 2009;150(6):2518–25.

10. Shukla AP, Rubino F. Secretion and function of gastrointestinal hormones after bariatric surgery: their role in type 2 diabetes. Can J Diabetes. 2011;35(2):115–22.

11. Laferrère B, Heshka S, Wang K, et al. Incretin levels and effect are markedly enhanced 1 month after Roux-en-Y gastric bypass surgery in obese patients with type 2 diabetes. Diabetes Care. 2007; 30(7):1709–16.

12. Bose M, Oliván B, Teixeira J, et al. Do incretins play a role in the remission of type 2 diabetes after gastric bypass surgery: what are the evidence? Obes Surg. 2009;19(2):217–29.

13. Korner J, Inabnet W, Conwell IM, et al. Differential effects of gastric bypass and banding on circulating gut hormone and leptin levels. Obesity (Silver Spring). 2006;14(9):1553–61.

14. Cummings DE, Foster-Schubert KE, Overduin J. Ghrelin and energy balance: focus on current controversies. Curr Drug Targets. 2005;6(2):153–69.

15. Sun Y, Asnicar M, Saha PK, et al. Ablation of ghrelin improves the diabetic but not obese phenotype of ob/ob mice. Cell Metab. 2006;3(5):379–86.

16. Cummings DE, Weigle DS, Frayo RS, et al. Plasma ghrelin levels after diet-induced weight loss or gastric bypass surgery. N Engl J Med. 2002;346(21):1623–30.

17. Ybarra J, Bobbioni-Harsch E, Chassot G, et al. Persistent correlation of ghrelin plasma levels with body mass index both in stable weight conditions and during gastric-bypass-induced weight loss. Obes Surg. 2009;19(3):327–31.

18. Boey D, Lin S, Karl T, et al. Peptide YY ablation in mice leads to the development of hyperinsulinaemia and obesity. Diabetologia. 2006;49(6):1360–70.

19. Valderas JP, Irribarra V, Boza C, et al. Medical and surgical treatments for obesity have opposite effects on peptide YY and appetite: a prospective study controlled for weight loss. J Clin Endocrinol Metab. 2010;95(3):1069–75.

20. Wiedmer P, Noguerias R, Broglio F, et al. Ghrelin, obesity and diabetes. Nat Clin Pract Endocrinol Metab. 2007;3(10):705–12.

21. Laferrère B. Diabetes remission after bariatric surgery: is it just the incretins? Int J Obes (Lond). 2011;35 Suppl 3:S22–5.

22. Miras AD, Le Roux CW. Bariatric surgery and taste: novel mechanisms of weight loss. Curr Opin Gastroenterol. 2010;26(2):140–5.

23. Buchwald H, Avidor Y, Braunwald E, et al. Bariatric surgery: a systematic review and meta-analysis. JAMA. 2004;292(14):1724–37.

24. Sjöström L, Lindroos AK, Peltonen M, et al. Lifestyle, diabetes and cardiovascular risk factors 10 years after bariatric surgery. N Engl J Med. 2004;351(26):2683–93.

25. Schauer PR, Kashyap SR, Wolski K, et al. Bariatric surgery versus intensive medical therapy in obese patients with diabetes. N Engl J Med. 2012;366(17):1567–76.

26. Mingrone G, Panunzi S, De Gaetano A, et al. Bariatric surgery versus conventional medical therapy for type 2 diabetes. N Engl J Med. 2012;366(17):1577–85.

27. Dixon JB, O'Brien PE, Playfair J, et al. Adjustable gastric banding and conventional therapy for type 2 diabetes: a randomized controlled trial. JAMA. 2008;299(3):316–23.

28. Lee WJ, Chong K, Ser KH, et al. Gastric bypass vs sleeve gastrectomy for type 2 diabetes mellitus: a randomized controlled trial. Arch Surg. 2011;146(2):143–8.

29. Cohen RV, Pinheiro JC, Schiavon CA, et al. Effects of gastric bypass surgery in patients with type 2 diabetes and only mild obesity. Diabetes Care. 2012;35(7):1420–8.

30. Lee WJ, Wang W, Lee C. Effect of laparoscopic mini-gastric bypass for type 2 diabetes mellitus: comparison of BMI > 35 and < 35 kg/m². J Gastrointest Surg. 2008;12(5):945–52.

31. Sjöström L, Narbro K, Sjöström CD, et al. Effects of bariatric surgery on mortality in Swedish obese subjects. N Engl J Med. 2007;357(8):741–52.

32. Romeo S, Maglio C, Burza MA, et al. Cardiovascular events after bariatric surgery in obese subjects with type 2 diabetes. Diabetes Care. 2012;35(12):2613–7.

33. Adams TD, Gress RE, Smith SC, et al. Long-term mortality after gastric bypass surgery. N Engl J Med. 2007;357(8):753–61.

34. Tice JA, Karliner L, Walsh J, et al. Gastric banding or bypass? A systematic review comparing the two most popular bariatric procedures. Am J Med. 2008;121(10):885–93.

35. Shukla AP, Ahn SM, Patel RT, et al. Surgical treatment of type 2 diabetes: the surgeon perspective. Endocrine. 2011;40(2):151–61.

36. Schauer PR, Burguera B, Ikramuddin S, et al. Effect of laparoscopic Roux-en Y gastric bypass on type 2 diabetes mellitus. Ann Surg. 2003;238(4):467–84.

37. Blackstone R, Bunt JC, Cortés MC, et al. Type 2 diabetes after gastric bypass: remission in five models using HbA1c, fasting blood glucose, and medication status. Surg Obes Relat Dis. 2012;8(5):548–55.

38. Dixon JB, Chuang LM, Chong K, et al. Predicting the glycemic response to gastric bypass surgery in patients with type 2 diabetes. Diabetes Care. 2012;36(1):20–6.

39. Lee WJ, Ser KH, Chong K, et al. Laparoscopic sleeve gastrectomy for diabetes treatment in nonmorbidly obese patients: efficacy and change of insulin secretion. Surgery. 2010;147(5):664–9.

40. Schauer P, Chand B, Brethauer S. New applications for endoscopy: the emerging field of endoluminal and transgastric bariatric surgery. Surg Endosc. 2007;21(3):347–56.

41. Aguirre V, Stylopoulos N, Grinbaum R, et al. An endoluminal sleeve induces substantial weight loss and normalizes glucose homeostasis in rats with diet-induced obesity. Obesity. 2008;16: 2585–92.

42. Soni A, Shukla AP, Rubino F. Interventional diabetology: the evolution of diabetes care in the XXI century. Curr Atheroscler Rep. 2012;14(6):631–6.

43. Bohdjalian A, Prager G, Rosak C, et al. Improvement in glycemic control in morbidly obese type 2 diabetic subjects by gastric stimulation. Obes Surg. 2009;19(9):1221–7.

44. Sanmiguel CP, Conklin JL, Cunneen SA, et al. Gastric electrical stimulation with the TANTALUS® system in obese type 2 diabetes patients: effect on weight and glycemic control. J Diabetes Sci Technol. 2009;3(4):964–70.

49

Cardiovascular Disease in the Bariatric Surgery Patient

Amanda R. Vest and James B. Young

Introduction

By 2015, it is estimated that the number of adults who are overweight (body mass index, BMI, 25.0–29.9 kg/m²) or obese (BMI ≥ 30 kg/m²) will surpass 1.5 billion [1]. One of the greatest healthcare concerns associated with this obesity epidemic is the associated escalation in diabetes mellitus and cardiovascular disease (CVD) prevalence. Obesity, diabetes, and CVD are challenging to treat in isolation and significantly increase the obese patient's mortality risk [2]. Hence, weight loss is a cornerstone of cardiovascular health management for patients with obesity and has the potential to modulate future CVD event rates [3, 4]. The marked superiority of bariatric surgery over pharmacological and lifestyle interventions in addressing excess weight, hyperglycemia, and hypertriglyceridemia has been demonstrated by meta-analysis [5]. The importance of incorporating bariatric surgery into a wider-reaching health promotion strategy including strict pre- and postoperative dietary and physical activity modifications is paramount when using this surgical strategy to optimize future cardiovascular health [6].

As the field has evolved over the past 50 years, the bariatric procedures have graduated from the sphere of cosmetic procedures to a health management strategy with the potential to significantly impact on long-term outcomes [7–10]. Bariatric surgeons have also moved towards offering surgical weight management to more medically comorbid individuals, including patients with preexisting CVD. This chapter will outline the optimization of cardiac patients prior to bariatric surgery, the postoperative outcomes observed in patients with and without preexisting cardiac conditions, and also the pathophysiological basis underlying the beneficial cardiovascular effects of surgical weight loss.

Preoperative Optimization of the Patient with Existing Cardiac Disease

Preoperative screening for coronary artery disease (CAD) before bariatric surgery remains an area of variable practice and is discussed in detail in Chap. 44. Furthermore, it remains unclear how to best manage patients who have a positive cardiac screening test result prior to a planned bariatric procedure. The existing guidance comes from ACC/AHA noncardiac surgery preoperative cardiovascular screening guidelines and also their guidelines specific to preoperative cardiovascular management of severely obese patients [11, 12].

The AHA/ACC recommends that no pre-bariatric surgery cardiac testing is indicated for patients who have one CVD risk factor or known asymptomatic CAD. In individuals with chest pain or dyspnea on exertion, or those with two or more risk factors and who are unable to demonstrate a functional capacity of four or more METS, stress testing should be considered. The optimal testing strategy is unclear because both nuclear stress testing with single-photon emission computed tomography (SPECT) imaging and stress echocardiogram have reduced accuracy in the obese population. False-positive tests are common with SPECT in obese patients, due to soft tissue artifacts, and images can be very limited in patients with excess adiposity, making stress echocardiogram vulnerable to false-negative results [13]. In addition, pre-bariatric surgery patients are often deconditioned and unable to complete an exercise stress protocol. Hence, pharmacological stress agents must be employed, which further decrease the sensitivity of testing because a proportion of pharmacological tests achieve submaximal stresses and are nondiagnostic. However, attenuation correction and combined supine/prone protocols are now more widely available and have the potential to minimize the frequency of false-positive SPECTs in obese patients. Therefore, SPECT, or the related nuclear technique of cardiac position emission tomography (PET) which has the added benefit of superior spatial resolution [14], is usually the preferable modality. Alternate strategies are stress transesophageal echocardiograms [15] or proceeding directly to cardiac catheterization in high-risk individuals, such as those with multiple risk factors.

Coronary revascularization prior to noncardiac surgery has not been shown to enhance survival, and due to the requirement for dual antiplatelet medications for a minimum of 6–8 weeks after percutaneous coronary intervention (the exact time interval is dependent on the stent type and location), revascularization will necessitate postponement of bariatric surgery. Due to these management considerations, preoperative cardiac stress test testing should be restricted to patients in whom the results will actually change outcomes [11]. There remains an absence of consensus among cardiologists as to how an asymptomatic obese patient presenting for bariatric surgery with a positive stress test should be managed [16]. Perioperative beta-blockade is commonly prescribed for patients with a known CAD history or a positive stress, although the risk-benefit ratio has never been studied in the bariatric population [12]. Blood pressure should be kept to target preoperatively, statin therapy should be resumed as soon as possible postoperatively, and any period of time off baseline antiplatelet medications perioperatively should be kept to the minimum duration that is acceptable to the bariatric surgeon. As further discussed below, limited data suggest that patients with compensated, stable heart failure can reasonably be considered for bariatric surgery candidacy [11].

Cardiologists are increasingly considering bariatric surgery as a useful component of comprehensive cardiac management for severely obese patients with established CAD. There is some data, albeit limited, that patients with a diagnosis of CAD show improvements in vascular function and symptoms after surgical weight loss [17–19]. Bariatric procedures with a malabsorptive component may be superior in their impact on coronary atherosclerosis, as there is evidence for a reduction in angina symptoms after gastric bypass but not with gastric volume reduction procedures (HR for angina from 3.8 to 2.04 in men, 3.9 to 0.98 in women) [20]. The pathological process of atherosclerosis within arteries may also be favorably influenced by bariatric surgery. In 136 consecutive subjects returning for 5-year follow-up after gastric bypass, coronary computed tomography (CT) calcium scores were lower in postsurgical subjects than in a nonsurgical obese control cohort, independent of traditional CVD risk factors [21]. Another marker for cardiovascular atherosclerosis burden is carotid intima-media thickness. One group measured intima-media thickness at baseline and 3–4 years post-gastroplasty. The surgical

subjects demonstrated a rate of progression that was more similar to lean controls than the threefold higher progression of patients who continued to be obese [22]. The findings from these two subclinical atherosclerosis assessment modalities generate the hypothesis that bariatric surgery may slow the progression of CAD. Although this is a novel proposition in the cardiology field, there are several lines of basic science and experimental evidence that support potential anti-atherosclerotic and anti-inflammatory actions of bariatric procedures.

Metabolic Effects of Adiposity and Bariatric Surgery on the Heart and Vasculature

The proposed mechanisms linking obesity to adverse cardiovascular outcomes largely center on the signaling proteins known as adipokines and gut hormones. It has been observed that although BMI is an important epidemiological predictor of CVD [23], the location of the excess adipose tissue and its degree of metabolic dysfunction may be the more relevant cardiac risk factor. The degree of "central" or "visceral" adiposity more closely correlates with insulin resistance than overall BMI, and visceral—but not peripheral—adiposity is a significant contributor to asymptomatic atherosclerosis as detected by coronary CT [24]. Similarly the presence of the metabolic syndrome (of which insulin resistance and central adiposity is a central feature) has been independently associated with an increased risk of incident heart failure in cohort without diabetes or baseline CAD, whereas overall adiposity was not an independent predictor [25]. The recognition of this subgroup of overweight and obese patients with the most insulin-resistant state and highest CVD risk has led to a deeper appreciation of dysfunctional adipose tissue and the new concept of "adiposopathy" [26]. Adipokines are proteins that are synthesized and released by adipose tissue, which is now acknowledged as an active endocrine and paracrine organ and not just a passive lipid repository. Adiponectin, resistin, leptin, tumor necrosis factor-α (TNF-α), and interleukin-6 (IL-6) are of particular relevance to cardiovascular health.

Adiponectin, a 244-amino-acid protein, is markedly reduced in obesity. This hormone promotes insulin sensitivity and fatty acid catabolism and exerts anti-inflammatory and antiatherogenic effects [27]. Adiponectin inhibits TNF-α-induced expression of adhesion molecules on the endothelium [28] and suppresses the generation of foam cells [29]. Endothelial dysfunction and transmigration of lipid-laden macrophages into the intima are key inflammatory components of atherosclerotic plaque formation. Lower adiponectin concentrations are associated with an increased risk of coronary events [28], although it is suggested that adiponectin levels do not contribute to cardiac risk prediction once other CVD risk factors have been considered [30]. The Framingham Study group recently demonstrated an inverse relationship between adiponectin and left ventricular mass, adjusted for key covariates including BMI [31]. Levels are reported to be elevated in established heart failure [32–34].

In contrast, resistin, a cysteine-rich protein secreted primarily by adipose tissue, reduces insulin sensitivity and stimulates glycogenolysis and gluconeogenesis [35] and is pro-inflammatory. Circulating levels are increased in obesity. There is a strong association between elevated levels of resistin, obesity, and type 2 diabetes (T2DM) and in vitro evidence of a role in promoting smooth muscle cell proliferation [36]. Increasing serum resistin levels correlate with the degree of heart failure decompensation and are also predictive of rehospitalization or cardiac mortality in individuals with advanced heart failure [37].

Leptin is a pleiotropic adipokine with structural and functional similarities to pro-inflammatory cytokines. It is a 167-amino-acid protein and is a principal stimulant of satiety through its actions on the hypothalamus. It is also an insulin-sensitizing hormone and deficiency due to rare leptin gene mutations causes insulin resistance and obesity. However, in obese states other than that due to leptin gene mutation, leptin levels are markedly increased but the protein's action is reduced due to leptin resistance, thereby abolishing their satiety signal [38, 39]. Leptin is widely expressed in monocytes and atherosclerotic plaques and has been suggested to stimulate macrophage foam cells and platelet aggregation [40, 41]. Leptin is increased in patients with heart failure and is predictive of incident heart failure [42, 43]. The reduction in left ventricular mass with bariatric weight loss has been correlated with reduced circulating leptin concentrations in both animal models and humans [44–46]. Additionally, leptin receptor isoforms are expressed in myocardium, and leptin induces myocyte hypertrophy in culture [47, 48].

TNF-α and IL-6 are also secreted by adipose tissue and hence show higher concentrations in obese individuals. C-reactive protein (CRP), the acute-phase reactant released in response to circulating IL-6, IL-1, and TNF-α, is elevated in obesity. The liver is the predominant site of CRP release, although adipose tissue also appears to be a direct source of CRP [49]. CRP is an independent predictor of coronary events and is also chronically elevated in heart failure [50, 51]. It stimulates endothelial dysfunction by multiple pathways including increasing the expression of circulating adhesion molecules and endothelial PAI-1 [52], upregulating angiotensin type 1 receptors on cell surfaces, and attenuating endothelial nitric oxide release [53, 54]. Adipocytes have also been observed to directly produce PAI-1 and monocyte chemoattractant protein-1 (MCP-1) [55, 56], a substance that is instrumental in leukocyte transmigration into the intima. Adipocytes also release angiotensinogen, a precursor of the pro-atherogenic vasoconstrictor angiotensin, which has roles in promoting both endothelial dysfunction and insulin resistance [57]. The contribution of visceral adipose tissue to the inflammatory milieu probably has a role in the relationship between obesity, insulin resistance, and CVD.

Dramatic changes in these inflammatory markers, adipokines, and gut hormones are seen in the weeks and months after bariatric surgery. CRP and IL-6 levels fall by as much as 81 % and 23 % respectively postoperatively, paralleling the improvement in insulin sensitivity that emerges almost immediately after procedures with a malabsorptive function [58]. These inflammatory and glycemic changes long precede the nadir of weight loss. Both Roux-en-Y gastric bypass (RYGB) and sleeve gastrectomy are also associated with reductions in circulating leptin concentrations by almost half as early as 1 week postoperatively, with ongoing decreases until 12 months postoperatively. Adiponectin progressively rises over this time frame [59]. Circulating resistin levels decrease after gastric bypass or sleeve gastrectomy [60].

Additional contributors to the relationship between obesity and CVD may be the gut hormones. Key gut molecules that are dysregulated in obesity and appear to have cardiac effects are ghrelin, peptide YY (PYY), glucose-dependent insulinotropic peptide (GIP), and glucagon-like peptide 1 (GLP-1). Ghrelin is produced preprandially by the stomach and stimulates appetite via increased expression of neuropeptide Y (NPY) in the hypothalamus; conversely PYY is released postprandially from the distal gastrointestinal tract and inhibits NPY release, which promotes satiety. In obese individuals, total circulating ghrelin levels are lower and not suppressed by food intake, in comparison to normal-weight-matched controls. Peripheral administration of ghrelin induces weight gain in rodents by increasing carbohydrate utilization [61]. Circulating levels of PYY also tend to be reduced in obesity with a blunted postprandial PYY rise. There are potential mechanisms by which reduced circulating levels of ghrelin in obesity could contribute to myocardial dysfunction, because effects of this peptide include anti-inflammatory activity, peripheral vasodilation, enhanced cardiomyocyte contractility, and inhibition of myocyte apoptosis. In a rat model of HF, ghrelin administration improves left ventricular dysfunction and deters development of cardiac cachexia, possibly due to its promotion of growth hormone secretion [62].

The incretins, including GLP-1 and GIP, are a family of gut hormones that stimulate postprandial insulin release, inhibit glucagon, slow gastric empting, and promote weight loss. They are found at subnormal levels in patients with T2DM, and obese subjects show a blunted postprandial GLP-1 response compared to lean subjects. GLP-1 analogs such as exenatide and liraglutide and sitagliptin, a dipeptidyl-peptidase-4 inhibitor that deters the degradation of GLP-1 and GIP, are new pharmacological agents for T2DM that have attracted attention regarding potentially favorable cardiovascular effects. GLP-1 receptors are found on cardiomyocytes, and animal models of heart failure have shown positive responses to GLP-1. GLP-1 agonists appear to have a host of favorable cardiovascular effects, including cholesterol lowering [63], protection from post-myocardial infarction complications in a mouse model [64], and improvements in endothelial dysfunction in stable CAD patients [65].

RYGB patients demonstrate a brisk three- to fivefold increase in postprandial GLP-1 and PYY levels postoperatively, which precedes significant weight loss and is independent of caloric restriction [66]. The sharp increases in postprandial GLP-1 and PYY levels that occur post-RYBG also precede significant weight loss and are independent of caloric restriction [67]. Restored GLP-1 levels may be a mechanism for the recovery of early-phase insulin secretion in response to oral carbohydrates. Ghrelin responses after RYGB are more heterogeneous and are therefore less likely to explain reduced appetite and improved glucose homeostasis postoperatively [60].

The Impact of Bariatric Surgery on Cardiovascular Risk Factors

The impact of bariatric procedures on the key "traditional" cardiovascular risk factors of hypertension, diabetes, and hyperlipidemia is not a new observation—in fact, the first jejunoileal bypass in 1953 was specifically performed to induce weight loss from malabsorption and improve the lipid profiles of severely hyperlipidemic obese patients [68]. Among 114 patients who underwent RYGB (74 % females), total cholesterol change was −23.6 %, −22.3 %, and −18.4 % at 6, 12, and 18 months, respectively [69]. The nadir for total cholesterol was reached at 6 months postoperatively and then remained constant. LDL dropped by −24.1 %, −29.8 %, and −26.7 % at 6, 12, and 18 months, respectively. The nadir for LDL was achieved at 12 months postoperatively, with a small nonsignificant rise 6 months later. HDL, for which higher levels confer cardiovascular risk benefits, initially dropped by 13.0 % at 6 months and then steadily increasing by 3.8 % at 12 months and 19.3 % at 18 months. Triglycerides, a prominent component of the metabolic syndrome, progressively fell by −27.4 %, −37.8 %, and −47.3 % at 6, 12, and 18 months, respectively.

Bariatric surgery also has a significant impact on hypertension. In one study of 347 RYGB and vertical banded gastroplasty patients, systolic blood pressure declined modestly by 5–6 mmHg (mean change to nadir value) and diastolic blood pressure by 4–5 mmHg (mean change to nadir value) [70].

Half of the cohort has a hypertension diagnosis preoperatively. The initial mean systolic blood pressure in the hypertensive group was 145 mmHg; among these subjects, systolic blood pressure declined by approximately 16 mmHg in the first 6–9 months postoperatively. The initial mean diastolic blood pressure in the hypertensive group was 87 mmHg; this declined by approximately 9 mmHg in the first 6–9 months after surgery. A patient's blood pressure was considered to have returned into the normal range if, on 2 of the last 3 clinic visits, systolic blood pressure was less than 140 mmHg and diastolic pressure was less than 90 mmHg. The blood pressures of 65 (73 %) of the 89 unmediated hypertensive patients had decreased into the normal range by the end of the follow-up period. Thirty-four percent of the cohort ceased antihypertensive medication during the follow-up period. The blood pressure of medication cessation group at their final visit was 137 ± 15 mmHg systolic and 80 ± 1 mmHg diastolic.

Approximately three-quarters of patients with diabetes also experience resolution of this CVD risk factor. Two-year data from SOS demonstrated 72 % resolution of preexisting diabetes in the surgical group, compared to 21 % of controls ($p<0.001$) [8]. At 10 years, diabetes remained in remission in 36 % of the surgical group and 13 % of controls ($p=0.001$). These findings were mirrored in Buchwald's 135,246-patient meta-analysis that demonstrated complete resolution of diabetes (defined as cessation of diabetes therapy with fasting blood glucose <100 mg/dL or HgA1c <6 %) for 74.6 % with more than 2 years' follow-up [71]. Adams et al. recently described 75 % diabetes remission at 2 years and 62 % remission at 6 years among 418 RYGB patients, with an odds ratio for remission of 16.5 (95 % CI, 4.7–57.6; $p<0.001$) [72].

The overall impact of bariatric surgery on hypertension, diabetes, and hyperlipidemia prevalence is summarized in Table 1. In a systematic review of 73 cardiovascular risk factor studies involving 19,543 bariatric surgery subjects (mean age 42 years, 76 % female), baseline prevalence of hypertension, diabetes, and hyperlipidemia were 44 %, 24 %, and 44 %, respectively. Postoperative resolution or improvement of hypertension occurred in 63 % of subjects, of diabetes in 73 %, and of hyperlipidemia in 65 % at a mean follow-up of 57.8 months and an average excess weight loss of 54 % [73]. Biomarkers of cardiovascular risk also improve post-bariatric surgery, including a 73 % CRP reduction from 9.1 mg/L preoperatively to 2.5 mg/L across 8 studies (1,157 subjects)

TABLE 1. Rates of comorbidity reduction after bariatric surgery

Disease or symptom	% improvement or remission at 2 years, or less if specified	% improvement or remission at 5–7 years	% improvement or remission at 10 years
Diabetes	72 % Sjöstrom [8]	54 % Sultan [119]	36 % Sjöstrom [8]
Hypertension	24 % Sjöstrom [8]	66 % Sugerman [120]	41 % Sjöstrom [8]
Hypertriglyceridemia	62 % Sjöstrom [8]	82 % Steffen [121]	46 % Sjöstrom [8]
Hypercholesterolemia	22 % Sjöstrom [8]	53 % Bolen [122]	21 % Sjöstrom [8]

Reproduced from Circulation (not yet published)

in this systematic review. Five studies (938 subjects) gave a pooled reduction in Framingham 10-year global coronary heart risk score from 5.9 to 3.3 %.

The Impact of Bariatric Surgery on Cardiovascular Outcomes

To date, the majority of trials seeking to evaluate the cardiovascular impact of bariatric surgery have only presented the cardiovascular risk endpoints of hypertension, diabetes, hyperlipidemia, inflammatory markers, and risk prediction scores, with far fewer reporting actual cardiovascular events or mortality. Among cardiologists, reliance on cardiovascular risk markers as indicators of reduced clinical risk after bariatric surgery is regarded with suspicion, because of prior instances where CVD risk surrogates have not translated into an actual survival benefit. Hence, there is now interest in designing bariatric surgery trials focused on the collection of longer-term data on actual cardiovascular events, cardiovascular mortality, and all-cause mortality. Ideally, such studies should randomize subjects to surgical vs. nonsurgical management of obesity. As all the existing cardiovascular outcomes data is from nonrandomized, matched cohorts, it remains possible that features specific to obese patients who pursue a surgical intervention, as compared to those who do not opt for surgery, are currently confounding the relationship between bariatric surgery and CV outcomes.

There is limited data examining the outcomes of bariatric surgery in cohorts of obese patients with preexisting cardiac disease. The safety of RYGB with preexisting CAD was assessed in a cohort of 52 patients (with prior coronary revascularization, >30 % angiographic coronary stenosis, prior myocardial infarction, or a positive stress test). There were no in-hospital deaths among the 52 CAD patients or 507 surgical patients without CAD. Three CAD patients (5.8 %, 95 % CI, 0–12.2 %) and 7 without CAD (1.4 %, 95 % CI, 0.4–2.4 %) had perioperative cardiac complications ($p=0.06$). Postoperative cardiovascular event data is more abundant for the full population of patients undergoing bariatric surgery. One study of 575 high-risk VA bariatric surgery patients, 42 % with BMI $\geq$50 kg/m², revealed 1.6 % and 0.5 % rates for perioperative cardiac arrest and myocardial infarction, respectively. The overall mortality in this group was 1.4 %, slightly exceeding the national published rates which are under 1 % [74]. Torquati et al. reported a rate of 1 % for CV events in the 5 years after bariatric surgery within a cohort of 500 RYGB patients [75]. SOS investigators have reported cardiovascular outcomes for their 2010 surgical patients and matched nonoperative controls, up to a median follow-up of 14.7 years [3]. Despite an excess of smoking and higher baseline weights and blood pressures in the surgical cohort, bariatric surgery was associated with a lower number of total first-time cardiovascular events (9.9 % vs.

11.5 % adjusted HR, 0.67; 95 % CI, 0.54–0.83; $p<0.001$), fatal myocardial infarctions, and total myocardial infarctions than controls. Cardiovascular deaths were also reduced, with 1.4 % cardiovascular mortality in subjects vs. 2.4 % in controls, adjusted hazard ratio 0.47 (95 % CI, 0.29–0.76, $p=0.002$). The baseline degree of insulin resistance was far more predictive of cardiovascular benefit than baseline BMI in this study, supporting the hypothesis of the importance of metabolic dysfunction in the relationship between adipose tissue and cardiac outcomes. Cardiovascular outcomes have also been investigated specific to patients with diabetes. An adjusted hazard ratio of 0.56 (95 % CI, 0.34–0.93, $p=0.025$) for myocardial infarction was seen at 2 years for 345 SOS surgical subjects compared to 262 nonsurgical controls, all with diabetes [76].

Mortality outcomes after bariatric surgery are considered in greater detail in Chap. 45, but as cardiovascular mortality findings are relevant to the consideration of cardiac benefit from surgical weight loss, they are also outlined here. The favorable mortality rate over 9 years in 154 RYGB patients vs. 78 controls (who were referred for surgery but did not undergo the procedure) was primarily due to a lower rate of CV death [77]. An observational study of 1,035 predominantly open RYGB patients and 5,746 matched controls demonstrated that the surgical subjects had 50 % fewer hospitalizations during the 5-year follow-up and developed significantly fewer cardiovascular diagnoses (4.73 % vs. 26.79 %, RR 0.18, 95 % CI, 0.12–0.22) [78]. At 5 years, the same cohort also showed significantly decreased incidences of new pulmonary edema (RR 0.42, 95 % CI, 0.18–0.96), angina (RR 0.53, 95 % CI, 0.40–0.70), coronary artery bypass grafting (RR 0.28, 95 % CI, 0.14–0.61), and coronary angioplasty (RR 0.36, 95 % CI, 0.19–0.66) in the postsurgical subjects compared to controls, although the decrease in myocardial infarctions (RR 0.71, 95 % CI, 0.50–1.00) did not reach significance ($p=0.05$) [79]. There was favorable all-cause mortality, and also a specific reduction in death from CAD (59 % risk reduction, $p=0.006$), observed among 7,925 RYGB patients vs. 7,925 severely obese matched control subjects [10]. Further details of the patient characteristics and major results from the 14 largest studies reporting cardiovascular outcomes after bariatric surgery are presented in Table 2.

Effects of Adiposity and Bariatric Surgery on Myocardial Structure and Function

The cardiac effects of excess weight and surgical weight loss have been predominantly considered in terms of the impact on atherosclerotic CAD progression and rates of myocardial infarction or other cardiovascular events. However, the direct impact of obesity on the structure and function of the myocardium is also becoming increasingly evident. Obesity is

Table 2. Major studies of bariatric surgery with cardiovascular event or mortality endpoints

First author	Year, country	Surgical subjects, N	Nonsurgical controls, N	Follow-up period	Outcomes	Comments
MacDonald [77]	1997, USA	154 obese patients with non-insulin-dependent diabetes who underwent RYGB (referred 1979–1994)	78 obese patients with non-insulin-dependent diabetes who were referred for, but did not receive, surgery (patient choice/insurance)	9 years mean for subjects, 6.2 years for	9 % mortality in subjects (including perioperative) vs. 28 % in controls, $p<0.0003$; annualized mortality rate of 1.0 % in subjects vs. 4.5 % in controls	Lower CV mortality in the surgical group was the primary driver of the overall survival benefit
Christou [78]	2004, Canada	1035 predominantly open RYGB patients	5,746 age-/gender-matched controls extracted from a health insurance database, baseline BMIs unknown	5 years	0.68 % mortality in surgical group (including 0.4 % perioperative mortality) vs. 6.17 % for controls (relative risk, 0.11, 95 % CI, 0.04–0.27)	50 % fewer hospitalizations in surgical subjects and significantly fewer CV diagnoses (4.73 % vs. 26.79 %, relative risk)
Flum and Dellinger [123]	2004, USA	3,328 gastric bypass patients	62,781 nonsurgical obese subjects matched for age, gender, and comorbidities	4.4 years median; 15.5 years maximum	At 15 years 11.8 % mortality in subjects vs. 16.3 % in controls; after propensity matching, odds of survival at 5 years 59 % higher in surgical group (OR 1.59, 95 % CI, 1.49–1.72)	30-day surgical mortality 1.9 %; postoperative mortality associated with surgeon inexperience
Sampalis [79]	2006, Canada	1,035 predominantly open RYGB patients—morbidity outcomes for the same cohort as Christiou et al.	5,746 age-/gender-matched controls extracted from a health insurance database, baseline BMIs unknown	5 years	Decreased incidences of new pulmonary edema (RR 0.42, 95 % CI, 0.18–0.96), angina (RR 0.53, 95 % CI, 0.40–0.70), coronary artery bypass grafting (RR 0.28, 95 % CI, 0.14–0.61), and coronary angioplasty (RR 0.36, 95 % CI, 0.19–0.66)	The decrease in myocardial infarctions (RR 0.71, 95 % CI, 0.50–1.00) did not reach significance ($p=0.05$)
Livingston [74]	2006, USA	575 veterans affairs patients, 42 % with BMI≥50 kg/m², 87 % open bariatric procedures	None	Maximum 2 years	30-day cardiac arrest rate 1.6 % and 30-day myocardial infarction rate 0.5 %; overall 30-day mortality 1.4 % and 2-year mortality 3.1 %	Adverse postoperative event risk increased in patients >350 lb and smokers
Adams [10]	2007, USA	7,925 RYGB patients (1984–2002)	7,925 age-/gender-/BMI-matched obese controls drawn from driver's license applicants	Mean 7.1 years	All-cause mortality 40 % lower in surgical group (adjusted HR 0.60, 95 % CI, 0.45–0.67, $p<0.001$); lower surgical mortality for all diseases combined (52 %, $p<0.001$), CAD (59 %, $p=0.006$), diabetes (92 %, $p=0.005$), and cancer (60 %, $p=0.001$)	Rates of death not caused by disease, such as accidents and suicide, were 58 % higher in the surgery group ($p=0.04$)
Torquati [75]	2007, USA	500 RYGB patients, mean 45 years, 81 % female	None	5 years	1 % for CV event rate at 5 years	Study primarily reported improvement in Framingham risk scores postoperatively
Sowemimo [124]	2007, USA	908, majority open RYGB (mean age 43.2 vs. 47.9 years in controls; BMI 54 kg/m² vs. 51 kg/m² in controls, both $p<0.0001$)	112 evaluated for surgery but did not proceed for a variety of reasons	9 years	2.9 % mortality in subjects vs. 14.3 % in controls; adjusted mortality 82 % lower in surgical subjects (HR 0.18, 95 % CI, 0.09–0.35, $p<0.0001$)	Greatest surgical benefit seen in patients <55 years and with a BMI >50 kg/m²

Author [Ref]	Year, Country	Surgical group	Controls	Follow-up	Results	Comments
Busetto [125]	2007, Italy	821 LAGB patients with BMI>40 kg/m²	821 gender-, age-, and BMI-matched controls	5 years	Survival was 60 % higher in surgical group, $p=0.0004$; on multivariate Cox, adjusted mortality risk 0.36 (95 % CI, 0.16–0.80) in surgical group	Other factors correlating with death on univariate analysis included male gender, greater age, and higher BMI
Peeters [126]	2007, Australia	966 LAGB patients, mean age 47 years, mean BMI 45 kg/m²	2,119 matched community controls, mean age 55 years, mean BMI 38 kg/m²	Median 4 years for surgical subjects, mean 12 months for controls	Surgical patients had a 72 % lower risk of mortality, adjusted for gender/age/BMI than controls (HR 0.28, 95 % CI, 0.10–0.85)	No perioperative deaths. Gender, age, and degree of obesity did not significantly affect mortality risk
Maciejewski [127]	2011, USA	850 veterans who underwent bariatric surgery, mean age 49.5 years, mean BMI 47.4 kg/m²	41,244 matched controls (mean age 54.7 years, mean BMI 42.0 kg/m²) from the same 12 veterans integrated service networks untreated for obesity	Mean 6.7 years	2-year and 6-year crude mortality significantly lower for surgical patients (2.2 % vs. 4.6 %, $p<0.001$, and 6.8 % vs. 15.3 %, $p<0.001$, respectively); significance of mortality benefit lost with propensity matching of 1,694 patients (HR 0.83, 95 % CI, 0.61–1.14)	Comprehensive claims data permitted adjustment for factors including ethnicity, BMI, comorbidity burden, and marital status
Adams [72]	2012, USA	418 RYGB (2000–2011)	418 obese patients who sought but did not undergo surgery (group 1) and 321 controls from a population sample (group 2)	6 years	2.9 % mortality (12/418) in the surgical cohort vs. 3.3 % mortality in control group 1 and 0.9 % mortality in control group 2	All 4 suicides occurred in the surgical cohort (4 of 12 mortalities)
Sjöström [3]	2012, Sweden	2,010 SOS patients, 68 % with vertical banded gastroplasty (significantly greater prevalence of smoking and higher baseline weights and blood pressures in subjects compared to controls)	2,037 matched controls	Median 14.7 years	Lower CV mortality rate in surgery group (adjusted HR 0.47, 95 % CI, 0.29–0.76, $p=0.002$); first-time CV events also lower in surgical group (adjusted HR 0.67, 95 % CI, 0.54–0.83, $p<0.001$)	The baseline degree of insulin resistance, rather than initial BMI, was the most predictive of CV benefits
Romeo [76]	2012, Sweden	345 SOS surgical subjects with diabetes	262 controls with diabetes	Mean 13.3 years	Adjusted hazard ratio for myocardial infarction 0.56 (95 % CI, 0.34–0.93, $p=0.025$); adjusted HR for first-time cardiovascular event 0.53 (95 % CI, 0.35–0.79, $p=0.002$)	Benefit of bariatric surgery was unrelated to baseline age, gender, or BMI; number of obese diabetics needed to treat with bariatric surgery to prevent one myocardial infarction over 15 years = 16

Reproduced from *Circulation* (not yet published)

strongly associated with left ventricular hypertrophy (thickening of the walls of the main pumping chamber) and diastolic dysfunction (abnormal relaxation of the left ventricle during chamber filling) [80–82]. It has been established, in cohort sizes of 16–60 patients, that obese individuals without overt cardiac disease can show improvements in left ventricular mass and the echocardiographic markers of diastolic function in the 3 months to 3.6 years after bariatric surgery [83–87]. Furthermore, there is evidence that the regression of left ventricular mass is independent of changes in blood pressure post-bariatric surgery [83]. Prolongation of the isovolumic relaxation time is probably the most consistent diastolic abnormality seen in obesity, with left atrial volume, tissue Doppler velocities, and mitral inflow patterns also showing derangement in obese subjects [88, 89].

Most of the current data is from echocardiography studies, but cardiac magnetic resonance imaging (MRI) also has a developing role in defining structural and functional changes after bariatric surgery and can provide superior volumetric assessments. Thirty obese subjects without cardiac risk factors underwent MRIs at baseline and 1-year post-weight loss (bariatric surgery or diet) [90]. There was a 10 % mean reduction in left ventricular mass and a 40 % reduction in right ventricular mass. Left ventricular end-systolic volume, stroke volume, and cardiac output also fell with weight loss. An early echocardiographic study of left ventricular systolic, as well as diastolic, function was published with 38 SOS surgical subjects who underwent echocardiography pre- and post-gastroplasty. An improvement in left ventricular ejection fraction (LVEF) was reported at 1 year postoperatively, but the mean baseline and follow-up LVEFs in both groups were >50 %, so any statistical differences after surgery were not clinically meaningful. Similarly, there was a statistically significant improvement in LVEF at 3 years post-bariatric surgery in another 23-patient cohort, but the baseline LVEF mean was already supranormal at 71 % [88].

More sensitive echocardiographic techniques than LVEF are now available for detecting subtle changes in systolic function, particularly in the setting of left ventricular hypertrophy [91]. Two-dimensional speckle tracking-derived strain and strain rate imaging have highlighted the subclinical systolic dysfunction that can be associated with obesity [92, 93]. Barbosa and colleagues demonstrated slight differences in left ventricular global strain (22.5 %±3.5 vs. 24.4 %±2.5, $p<0.005$) between 92 patients with class III obesity and 31 healthy controls, despite no differences in LVEF between subjects and controls, suggesting incipient systolic dysfunction with obesity. Of note, these authors reported that only 9 patients (9 % of the cohort) had a technically inadequate echocardiogram that was not amendable to strain analysis. Thirteen obese patients with LVEFs above 40 % demonstrated regression of these subclinical abnormalities of myocardial deformability in the 6–24 months after bariatric surgery [94].

The Impact of Bariatric Surgery on Patients with Heart Failure

Several cross-sectional and prospective studies have demonstrated that increasing BMI or waist circumference is independently associated with development of incident heart failure (HF) [95–97]. A prospective Framingham study of 5,881 participants, stratified by BMI at enrollment, found that the risk of clinically symptomatic HF increased by 5 % for men and 7 % for women per unit BMI increase, despite adjustments for demographics and known CAD risk factors [98]. In a prospective study of 4,080 men age 60–79 years without baseline HF followed for a mean period of 9 years, the adjusted hazard ratios associated with a 1-standard deviation (SD) increase in BMI were 1.37 (95 % CI, 1.09–1.72) and 1.18 (95 % CI, 1.00–1.39) in men with and without CHD, respectively. Increased leptin was significantly associated with an increased risk of HF in men without preexisting CHD, independent of BMI and potential mediators (adjusted HR for a 1-SD increase in log leptin 1.30, 95 % CI, 1.06–1.61, $p=0.01$) [43].

The evidence suggesting improvements in obesity-associated diastolic and systolic dysfunction after bariatric surgery raises the possibility of echocardiographic and clinical improvements in obese patients who have a preoperative clinical diagnosis of heart failure. Indeed, there are a handful of early case reports describing HF recovery after surgical weight loss [99–101]. Such reports do, however, feature very obese individuals who were young and predominantly affected by systolic HF, and so the results may not be generalizable.

Beyond case reports, the published evidence in favor of improvements in HF after bariatric surgery is limited to three small studies. The first is a prospective analysis of fractional shortening performed pre- and post-vertical band gastroplasty that incorporated 13 subjects with low preoperative systolic function [102]. There were modest improvements in fractional shortening (22±2 % to 31±2 % $p<0.01$) at a mean of 4.3 months after weight loss plateaued, accompanied by reductions in left ventricular end-diastolic diameter and mean arterial blood pressure. The same group published a study of fractional shortening pre- and post-vertical band gastroplasty in 14 subjects with clinical diagnoses of HF and an average fractional shorting that lies just below the lower limit of normal [103]. This cohort showed improvements in New York Heart Association functional class from III to II in four patients, III to I in three patients, and II to I in five patients but no statistically significant improvements in systolic function. However, these postoperative echocardiograms occurred at only 4.5±1.2 months postoperatively, and the older procedure of vertical band gastroplasty is not associated with the same degree of metabolic recovery as malabsorptive bariatric surgery.

An overlapping cohort of HF patients that underwent bariatric surgery generated two publications [104, 105]. The Ramani study utilized an independent echocardiogram reader. Twelve patients with a mean age of 41 years, BMI of 53 kg/m^2, and LVEF of 22±7 % were retrospectively reviewed. Nine underwent RYGB, two received sleeve gastrectomies, and one underwent gastric banding. Subjects were matched to ten controls who received diet and exercise counseling only. At 1 year, hospital readmission in bariatric patients was significantly lower than controls (0.4±0.8 vs. 2.5±2.6, p=0.04). There was a significant improvement in mean LVEF for the bariatric group (35±15 %, p=0.005) but not for controls, and the NYHA class improved in bariatric patients (2.3±0.5, p=0.02) but deteriorated in controls. The third cohort was a subset of 9 patients with LVEF≤50 %, within a 57-patient cohort of obese subjects with mean BMI of 49 kg/m^2, who underwent RYGB. Although there did appear to be a trend towards increased LVEF in these 9 patients (preoperative LVEF 44.8±7 to postoperative LVEF 59.5±10.1, no p value presented), there was a similar rise in mean LVEF in the nonsurgical controls with initial LVEF≤50 % (44.9±7.9 to 58.6±14.1) [83].

The Obesity Survival Paradox

Despite the suggestions of improvements in symptoms and systolic function after bariatric surgery for patients with HF, HF patients with higher BMIs actually show more favorable survival rates than their leaner counterparts [106–108]. Each incremental 5 kg/m^2 BMI increase was associated with 10 % lower in-hospital mortality among 108,927 decompensated HF patients [109]. A cohort of 2,271 chronic systolic heart failure patients (mean age 71.9±11.3 years, 74.6 % male) was followed for a median of 1,785 days, during which time 912 patients died. Measures of body mass were strong univariable predictors of outcome, and body surface area ($\chi^2=71.3$) was the strongest predictor followed by height ($\chi^2=68.6$), weight ($\chi^2=57.4$), then BMI ($\chi^2=15.2$). The greater the patient's overall size, the greater the likelihood of survival. Body surface area was the single strongest predictor of outcome in a multivariable model including 14 variables [110]. However, the survival advantage of obesity may be lost in individuals with diabetes. Of 2,153 chronic mild to moderate systolic HF patients with diabetes, of whom 798 (37 %) were obese, all-cause mortality occurred in 38 % of obese patients and 39 % of nonobese patients (hazard ratio, 0.99; 95 % CI, 0.80–1.22; p=0.915) [111].

The paradoxical survival relationship noted in HF populations has also been observed in patients with CAD but may disappear when survival is correlated to waist circumference, rather than the cruder parameter of BMI [112]. Conversely, the paradox persists with anthropometric measurements of obesity in HF and was recently demonstrated in advanced systolic HF patients stratified by BMI and waist circumference (WC) [113]. Both high WC and the combination of high WC/high BMI were associated with improved mortality, or freedom from urgent heart transplant, in this cohort.

Analysis of chronic systolic HF subjects in the SOLVD and V-HeFT II trials revealed that the loss of more than 6 % of body weight during the study duration was an independent predictor of mortality [114]. Lower BMIs may simply be a marker of cardiac cachexia and more advanced HF, but the possibility remains that weight loss may be detrimental to survival in obese patients with HF. Heart failure with preserved ejection fraction is also more frequently seen in obese patients than their lean counterparts and is also associated with a survival paradox with increasing BMI (hazard ratio for mortality 0.67, 95 % CI, 0.56–0.81) [115]. These survival observations have sparked interest in a hypothesis that although some of the adipokine and gut hormone changes associated with obesity may promote cardiac dysfunction, others may potentially become protective once HF is established.

The Impact of Bariatric Surgery on Arrhythmias

Atherosclerosis and myocardial dysfunction are not the only cardiac effect of obesity; obese individuals also have an increased risk of arrhythmias and sudden death. It is postulated that the myocardial of obese patients is vulnerable to ventricular repolarization abnormalities. Russo et al. reported a significant postoperative decrease in the heterogeneity of ventricular repolarization among 100 bariatric surgery patients with pre- and postoperative electrocardiograms [116]. Decreased QT interval and QT dispersion have also been observed in 85 patients post-biliopancreatic diversion [117]. Such electrophysiological modulation may reduce the substrate for ventricular arrhythmias in this high-risk patient population. Obesity also increases the risk for atrial arrhythmias such as atrial fibrillation. Significant regression of P-wave dispersion, a marker of atrial refractoriness heterogeneity and a risk factor for atrial fibrillation, has been reported after bariatric surgery [118]. This suggests that surgical weight loss may hold potential for reducing incident atrial fibrillation, or the incidence of new atrial fibrillation, after bariatric surgery.

Conclusion

Although bariatric surgery was initially conceived as a weight loss procedure, the impact of these operations on cardiovascular risk factors and CAD outcomes has now been demonstrated to be substantial. The procedures that incorporate a malabsorptive function appear to have the most significant cardiovascular impact, in line with the known effects of malabsorptive procedures on adipokines and gut hormones, which may even directly mediate the cardiovascular benefits of bariatric surgery. This has elevated bariatric surgery to the spectrum of interventions that may prove useful in minimizing future cardiac morbidity, and perhaps also mortality, in patients who are obese. There is also data to suggest improved biventricular hypertrophy and diastolic dysfunction after bariatric surgery and a possible role in improving symptoms and systolic function in obese heart failure patients. There has been a consequent recent surge in interest in bariatric surgery in the cardiology literature.

The next step for outcomes investigators is to study long-term cardiovascular events for obese patients who undergo bariatric surgery, especially among patients with preexisting cardiac diagnoses. Large randomized controlled trials would yield the most robust data, but large sample sizes would be required to provide adequate power within this population of relatively young and predominantly female subjects who seek bariatric surgery, as their actual cardiovascular and mortality event rates are low. Ongoing refinement of patient selection criteria to select out the cohort of patients who derive the most benefit from surgical weight loss remain a challenge and will require ongoing input from cardiologists and internists. However, the available literature already provides a solid platform from which physicians can initiate discussions with their obese patients regarding the role of bariatric surgery in promoting future cardiovascular health.

Review Questions and Answers

1. Which of the following statements regarding coronary artery disease epidemiological risk factors is correct?

   (a) LDL serum concentration is inversely associated with cardiovascular mortality.
   (b) Systolic blood pressure is an independent coronary artery disease risk factor.
   (c) The strongest predictor of cardiovascular risk in the Framingham equation is body mass index (BMI).
   (d) Obesity is not an independent predictor of coronary artery disease risk.
   (e) HDL serum concentration has been observed to rise significantly within the first postoperative week of Roux-en-Y gastric bypass (RYGB).

Correct answer: (b) Systolic blood pressure is one of the six major epidemiological risk factors for coronary artery disease development and cardiovascular events. The other major risk factors are advancing age, smoking, family history, elevated serum LDL or total cholesterol, low serum HDL, and diabetes. Diabetes is usually considered as a "coronary artery disease equivalent" in terms of risk prevention, because patients with diabetes and no known coronary artery disease have a similar risk of cardiovascular events as patients without diabetes who have a known coronary artery disease diagnosis. Obesity is also

an independent predictor of coronary artery disease development, although it is a weaker association than the six major risk factors. The strongest predictor of cardiovascular risk in any risk equation, including the Framingham Risk Score, is patient age. Serum HDL, for which higher levels confer cardiovascular risk benefits, was observed by Garcia-Marirrodriga et al. [69] to decrease by 13.0 % at 6 months and then steadily increase by 3.8 % at 12 months and 19.3 % at 18 months.

2. Which of the following statements regarding adipokines and gut hormones is correct?

   (a) Circulating leptin levels are consistently low in obese individuals, compared to normal-weight controls.
   (b) Resistin, a cysteine-rich protein secreted primarily by adipose tissue, promotes insulin sensitivity and is anti-inflammatory.
   (c) CRP is an independent predictor of future cardiovascular risk in asymptomatic women and has been observed to fall significantly in the months after bariatric surgery.
   (d) GLP-1 agonists are a group of new diabetes medications that show significant reductions in glycemic parameters but with the adverse effect of weight gain in many patients.
   (e) Ghrelin is the gut hormone with the strongest evidence for mediation of the post-RYGB effects on glycemia.

Correct answer: (c) Ridker et al. [51] described the relationships between CRP, the metabolic syndrome, and incident cardiovascular events among 14,719 apparently healthy women who were followed up for an 8-year period for myocardial infarction, stroke, coronary revascularization, or cardiovascular death. At all levels of severity of the metabolic syndrome, CRP added prognostic information on subsequent risk. Circulating leptin levels are elevated in obese states other than that due to leptin gene mutation, due to leptin resistance. Resistin is an adipokine that promotes insulin resistance, gluconeogenesis, and a pro-inflammatory state. The GLP-1 agonists are subcutaneously injected diabetes medications that also promote small but significant decreases in body weight during treatment duration. Ghrelin responses after RYGB are quite heterogeneous and are therefore less likely to explain reduced appetite and improved glucose homeostasis postoperatively than some of the other gut hormones and adipokines.

3. An asymptomatic 50-year-old patient with a BMI of 45 kg/m^2 and diagnoses of coronary artery disease and diabetes presents for bariatric surgery evaluation. Which of the following statements are *incorrect*?

   (a) Compensated systolic heart failure is not a contraindication to bariatric surgery.
   (b) Markers of inflammation and endothelial function improve in the weeks and months after bariatric surgery.

(c) He must undergo cardiac catheterization, with angioplasty of any significant coronary stenosis, before proceeding to the surgery.

(d) Existing data suggests a lower rate of future cardiovascular events for patients who undergo bariatric surgery, compared to obese matched controls.

(e) Large trials have demonstrated decreases in long-term cardiovascular events in patients who undergo bariatric surgery, compared to patients who receive optimal medical therapy, but none of these studies to date have been randomized.

Correct answer: (c) Preoperative noninvasive cardiac stress testing or cardiac catheterization is only indicated in a select group of high-risk surgical candidates and not in patients with stable chronic coronary artery disease. Answers (a) and (b) are true statements. Although several studies have performed robust matching techniques in the selection of non-surgical control groups, none of the studies of cardiovascular event or mortality studies has been randomized controlled trials. Therefore, (d) and (e) are also true statements.

4. Which of the following statements regarding myocardial structure and function is correct?

(a) Left ventricular hypertrophy reduces more than right ventricular hypertrophy after surgical weight loss.

(b) Obesity is a strong risk factor for diastolic dysfunction, and significant improvements in parameters of myocardial relaxation have been seen within the first postoperative year of bariatric surgery.

(c) Reductions in left ventricular hypertrophy after RYGB are solely dependent on the postoperative reduction in systolic blood pressure.

d) The left ventricular ejection fraction consistently increases postoperatively, both in patients with preexisting heart failure and in patients without prior cardiomyopathies.

(e) Left ventricular ejection fraction is the most sensitive and widely used method of measuring mild reductions in systolic function.

Correct answer: (b) Obesity, diabetes, and hypertension all increase the risk of diastolic dysfunction, in which ventricular filling during diastole is abnormal. Improvements in left ventricular hypertrophy and echocardiographic parameters of diastolic dysfunction have been seen as early as 3 months postoperatively. In an MRI study by Rider et al. [90], right ventricular wall thickening was seen to regress by a much greater degree than left ventricular wall thickening. Several authors have demonstrated that post-bariatric surgery improvements in left ventricular hypertrophy are independent of systolic blood pressure. In patients without preexisting systolic heart failure, stroke volume and left ventricular ejection fraction tend to decrease slightly with weight loss. There is limited data to suggest that some patients with systolic heart failure may experience a postoperative improvement in their left ventricular ejection faction. The ejection fraction is a relatively crude assessment of systolic function, and echocardiographic techniques such as strain and strain rate measurement offer much more sensitive assessments of subclinical abnormalities of systolic function.

References

1. World Health Organization. World Health Statistics 2011. W.H.O.; 2011. p. 1–171.
2. Adams KF, Schatzkin A, Harris TB, Kipnis V, Mouw T, Ballard-Barbash R, et al. Overweight, obesity, and mortality in a large prospective cohort of persons 50 to 71 years old. N Engl J Med. 2006;355(8):763–78.
3. Sjöström L, Peltonen M, Jacobson P, Sjöström CD, Karason K, Wedel H, et al. Bariatric surgery and long-term cardiovascular events. J Am Med Assoc. 2012;307(1):56–65.
4. Caterson ID, Finer N, Coutinho W, Van Gaal LF, Maggioni AP, Torp-Pedersen C, et al. Maintained intentional weight loss reduces cardiovascular outcomes: results from the Sibutramine Cardiovascular OUTcomes (SCOUT) trial. Diabetes Obes Metab. 2012;14(6):523–30.
5. Ashrafian H, Le Roux CW, Darzi A, Athanasiou T. Effects of bariatric surgery on cardiovascular function. Circulation. 2008;118(20):2091–102.
6. Poirier P, Cornier MA, Mazzone T, Stiles S, Cummings S, Klein S, et al. Bariatric surgery and cardiovascular risk factors: a scientific statement from the American Heart Association. Circulation. 2011;123(15):1683–701.
7. Buchwald H, Avidor Y, Braunwald E, Jensen MD, Pories W, Fahrbach K, et al. Bariatric surgery. J Am Med Assoc. 2004; 292(14):1724–37.
8. Sjöström L, Lindroos A-K, Peltonen M, Torgerson J, Bouchard C, Carlsson B, et al. Lifestyle, diabetes, and cardiovascular risk factors 10 years after bariatric surgery. N Engl J Med. 2004;351(26):2683–93.
9. Sjöström L, Narbro K, Sjöström CD, Karason K, Larsson B, Wedel H, et al. Effects of bariatric surgery on mortality in Swedish obese subjects. N Engl J Med. 2007;357(8):741–52.
10. Adams TD, Gress RE, Smith SC, Halverson RC, Simper SC, Rosamond WD, et al. Long-term mortality after gastric bypass surgery. N Engl J Med. 2007;357(8):753–61.
11. Fleisher LA, Beckman JA, Brown KA, Calkins H, Chaikof EL, Chaikof E, et al. ACC/AHA 2007 guidelines on perioperative cardiovascular evaluation and care for noncardiac surgery. J Am Coll Cardiol. 2007;50:1707–32.
12. Poirier P, Alpert MA, Fleisher LA, Thompson PD, Sugerman HJ, Burke LE, et al. Cardiovascular evaluation and management of severely obese patients undergoing surgery: a science advisory from the American Heart Association. Circulation. 2009;120(1):86–95.
13. Lerakis S, Kalogeropoulos AP, El-Chami MF, Georgiopoulou VV, Abraham A, Lynch SA, et al. Transthoracic dobutamine stress echocardiography in patients undergoing bariatric surgery. Obes Surg. 2007;17(11):1475–81.
14. Freedman N, Schechter D, Klein M, Marciano R, Rozenman Y, Chisin R. SPECT attenuation artifacts in normal and overweight persons: insights from a retrospective comparison of Rb-82 positron emission tomography and TI-201 SPECT myocardial perfusion imaging. Clin Nucl Med. 2000;25(12):1019–23.
15. Legault S, Sénéchal M, Bergeron S, Arsenault M, Tessier M, Guimond J, et al. Usefulness of an accelerated transoesophageal

stress echocardiography in the preoperative evaluation of high risk severely obese subjects awaiting bariatric surgery. Cardiovasc Ultrasound. 2010;8:30.

16. Gugliotti D, Grant P, Jaber W, Aboussouan L, Bae C, Sessler D, et al. Challenges in cardiac risk assessment in bariatric surgery patients. Obes Surg. 2008;18(1):129–33.

17. Brethauer SA, Heneghan HM, Eldar S, Gatmaitan P, Huang H, Kashyap S, et al. Early effects of gastric bypass on endothelial function, inflammation, and cardiovascular risk in obese patients. Surg Endosc. 2011;25(8):2650–9.

18. Batsis JA, Sarr MG, Collazo-Clavell ML, Thomas RJ, Romero-Corral A, Somers VK, et al. Cardiovascular risk after bariatric surgery for obesity. Am J Cardiol. 2008;102(7):930–7.

19. Haskell WL, Alderman EL, Fair JM, Maron DJ, Mackey SF, Superko HR, et al. Effects of intensive multiple risk factor reduction on coronary atherosclerosis and clinical cardiac events in men and women with coronary artery disease. The Stanford Coronary Risk Intervention Project (SCRIP). Circulation. 1994;89(3):975–90.

20. Plecka Östlund M, Marsk R, Rasmussen F, Lagergren J, Näslund E. Morbidity and mortality before and after bariatric surgery for morbid obesity compared with the general population. Br J Surg. 2011;98(6):811–6.

21. Priester T, Ault T, Adams T, Hunt S. Coronary calcium scores are lower 5 years after bariatric surgery: evidence for slowed progression of atherosclerosis? Circulation [abstract]. 2009;120:S341–2.

22. Karason K, Wikstrand J, Sjöström L, Wendelhag I. Weight loss and progression of early atherosclerosis in the carotid artery: a four-year controlled study of obese subjects. Int J Obes Relat Metab Disord. 1999;23(9):948–56.

23. Hubert HB, Feinleib M, McNamara PM, Castelli WP. Obesity as an independent risk factor for cardiovascular disease: a 26-year follow-up of participants in the Framingham Heart Study. Circulation. 1983;67(5):968–77.

24. Arad Y, Newstein D, Cadet F, Roth M, Guerci AD. Association of multiple risk factors and insulin resistance with increased prevalence of asymptomatic coronary artery disease by an electron-beam computed tomographic study. Arterioscler Thromb Vasc. 2001;21(12):2051–8.

25. Voulgari C, Tentolouris N, Dilaveris P, Tousoulis D, Katsilambros N, Stefanadis C. Increased heart failure risk in normal-weight people with metabolic syndrome compared with metabolically healthy obese individuals. J Am Coll Cardiol. 2011;58(13):1343–50.

26. Bays HE. Adiposopathy. J Am Coll Cardiol. 2011;57(25):2461–73.

27. Yokota T, Oritani K, Takahashi I, Ishikawa J, Matsuyama A, Ouchi N, et al. Adiponectin, a new member of the family of soluble defense collagens, negatively regulates the growth of myelomonocytic progenitors and the functions of macrophages. Blood. 2000;96(5):1723–32.

28. Ouchi N, Kihara S, Arita Y, Maeda K, Kuriyama H, Okamoto Y, et al. Novel modulator for endothelial adhesion molecules: adipocyte-derived plasma protein adiponectin. Circulation. 1999;100(25):2473–6.

29. Ouchi N, Kihara S, Arita Y, Nishida M, Matsuyama A, Okamoto Y, et al. Adipocyte-derived plasma protein, adiponectin, suppresses lipid accumulation and class A scavenger receptor expression in human monocyte-derived macrophages. Circulation. 2001;103(8):1057–63.

30. Côté M, Cartier A, Reuwer AQ, Arsenault BJ, Lemieux I, Després J-P, et al. Adiponectin and risk of coronary heart disease in apparently healthy men and women (from the EPIC-Norfolk Prospective Population Study). Am J Cardiol. 2011;108(3):367–73.

31. McManus DD, Lyass A, Ingelsson E, Massaro JM, Meigs JB, Aragam J, et al. Relations of circulating resistin and adiponectin and cardiac structure and function: the Framingham offspring study. Obesity. 2012;20(9):1882–6.

32. George J, Patal S, Wexler D, Sharabi Y, Peleg E, Kamari Y, et al. Circulating adiponectin concentrations in patients with congestive heart failure. Heart. 2006;92(10):1420–4.

33. Nakamura T, Funayama H, Kubo N, Yasu T, Kawakami M, Saito M, et al. Association of hyperadiponectinemia with severity of ventricular dysfunction in congestive heart failure. Circ J. 2006;70(12):1557–62.

34. Hong SJ, Park CG, Seo HS, Oh DJ, Ro YM. Associations among plasma adiponectin, hypertension, left ventricular diastolic function and left ventricular mass index. Blood Press. 2004;13(4):236–42.

35. Lazar M. Resistin- and obesity-associated metabolic diseases. Horm Metab Res. 2007;39(10):710–6.

36. Calabro P, Samudio I, Willerson JT, Yeh ETH. Resistin promotes smooth muscle cell proliferation through activation of extracellular signal-regulated kinase 1/2 and phosphatidylinositol 3-kinase pathways. Circulation. 2004;110(21):3335–40.

37. Takeishi Y, Niizeki T, Arimoto T, Nozaki N, Hirono O, Nitobe J, et al. Serum resistin is associated with high risk in patients with congestive heart failure–a novel link between metabolic signals and heart failure. Circ J. 2007;71(4):460.

38. Considine R, Sinha M, Heiman M. Serum immunoreactive-leptin concentrations in normal-weight and obese humans. N Engl J Med. 1996;334:292–5.

39. Tretjakovs P, Jurka A, Bormane I, Mackevics V, Mikelsone I, Balode L, et al. Relation of inflammatory chemokines to insulin resistance and hypoadiponectinemia in coronary artery disease patients. Eur J Intern Med. 2009;20(7):712–7.

40. O'Rourke L, Gronning LM, Yeaman SJ, Shepherd PR. Glucose-dependent regulation of cholesterol ester metabolism in macrophages by insulin and leptin. J Biol Chem. 2002;277(45):42557–62.

41. Konstantinides S, Schafer K, Loskutoff DJ. The prothrombotic effects of leptin possible implications for the risk of cardiovascular disease in obesity. Ann N Y Acad Sci. 2001;947:134–41; discussion 141–2.

42. Schulze PC, Kratzsch J, Linke A, Schoene N, Adams V, Gielen S, et al. Elevated serum levels of leptin and soluble leptin receptor in patients with advanced chronic heart failure. Eur J Heart Fail. 2003;5(1):33–40.

43. Wannamethee SG, Shaper AG, Whincup PH, Lennon L, Sattar N. Obesity and risk of incident heart failure in older men with and without pre-existing coronary heart disease: does leptin have a role? J Am Coll Cardiol. 2011;58(18):1870–7.

44. Rajapurohitam V, Gan XT, Kirshenbaum LA, Karmazyn M. The obesity-associated peptide leptin induces hypertrophy in neonatal rat ventricular myocytes. Circ Res. 2003;93(4):277–9.

45. Perego L, Pizzocri P, Corradi D, Maisano F, Paganelli M, Fiorina P, et al. Circulating leptin correlates with left ventricular mass in morbid (grade III) obesity before and after weight loss induced by bariatric surgery: a potential role for leptin in mediating human left ventricular hypertrophy. J Clin Endocrinol Metab. 2005;90(7):4087–93.

46. Leichman J, Wilson E, Scarborough T, Aguilar D, Miller C, Yu S, et al. Dramatic reversal of derangements in muscle metabolism and left ventricular function after bariatric surgery. Am J Med. 2008;121(11):966–73.

47. Purdham DM, Zou M-X, Rajapurohitam V, Karmazyn M. Rat heart is a site of leptin production and action. Am J Physiol Heart Circ Physiol. 2004;287(6):H2877–84.

48. Madani S, De Girolamo S, Muñoz DM, Li RK, Sweeney G. Direct effects of leptin on size and extracellular matrix components of human pediatric ventricular myocytes. Cardiovasc Res. 2006;69(3):716–25.

49. Ouchi N, Kihara S, Funahashi T, Nakamura T, Nishida M, Kumada M, et al. Reciprocal association of C-reactive protein with adiponectin in blood stream and adipose tissue. Circulation. 2003;107(5):671–4.

50. Ridker PM. Clinical application of C-reactive protein for cardiovascular disease detection and prevention. Circulation. 2003;107(3):363–9.

51. Ridker PM, Buring JE, Cook NR, Rifai N. C-reactive protein, the metabolic syndrome, and risk of incident cardiovascular events: an 8-year follow-up of 14 719 initially healthy American women. Circulation. 2003;107(3):391–7.

52. Devaraj S, Xu DY, Jialal I. C-reactive protein increases plasminogen activator inhibitor-1 expression and activity in human aortic endothelial cells: implications for the metabolic syndrome and atherothrombosis. Circulation. 2003;107(3):398–404.

53. Wang C-H, Li S-H, Weisel RD, Fedak PWM, Dumont AS, Szmitko P, et al. C-reactive protein upregulates angiotensin type 1 receptors in vascular smooth muscle. Circulation. 2003;107(13): 1783–90.

54. Verma S, Wang C-H, Li S-H, Dumont AS, Fedak PWM, Badiwala MV, et al. A self-fulfilling prophecy: C-reactive protein attenuates nitric oxide production and inhibits angiogenesis. Circulation. 2002;106(8):913–9.

55. Loskutoff DJ, Samad F. The adipocyte and hemostatic balance in obesity: studies of PAI-1. Arterioscler Thromb Vasc Biol. 1998;18(1):1–6.

56. Christiansen T, Richelsen B, Bruun JM. Monocyte chemoattractant protein-1 is produced in isolated adipocytes, associated with adiposity and reduced after weight loss in morbid obese subjects. Int J Obes Relat Metab Disord. 2005;29(1):146–50.

57. Kalupahana NS, Massiera F, Quignard-Boulange A, Ailhaud G, Voy BH, Wasserman DH, et al. Overproduction of angiotensinogen from adipose tissue induces adipose inflammation, glucose intolerance, and insulin resistance. Obesity (Silver Spring). 2012;20(1):48–56.

58. Kopp HP. Impact of weight loss on inflammatory proteins and their association with the insulin resistance syndrome in morbidly obese patients. Arterioscler Thromb Vasc. 2003;23(6):1042 7.

59. Woelnerhanssen B, Peterli R, Steinert RE, Peters T, Borbély Y, Beglinger C. Effects of postbariatric surgery weight loss on adipokines and metabolic parameters: comparison of laparoscopic Roux-en-Y gastric bypass and laparoscopic sleeve gastrectomy—a prospective randomized trial. Surg Obes Relat Dis. 2011; 7(5):561–8.

60. Roux CWL, Aylwin SJB, Batterham RL, Borg CM, Coyle F, Prasad V, et al. Gut hormone profiles following bariatric surgery favor an anorectic state, facilitate weight loss, and improve metabolic parameters. Ann Surg. 2006;243(1):108–14.

61. Tschöp M, Smiley DL, Heiman ML. Ghrelin induces adiposity in rodents. Nature. 2000;407(6806):908–13.

62. Nagaya N, Uematsu M, Kojima M, Ikeda Y, Yoshihara F, Shimizu W, et al. Chronic administration of ghrelin improves left ventricular dysfunction and attenuates development of cardiac cachexia in rats with heart failure. Circulation. 2001;104(12):1430–5.

63. Vilsbøll T, Christensen M, Junker AE, Knop FK, Gluud LL. Effects of glucagon-like peptide-1 receptor agonists on weight loss: systematic review and meta-analyses of randomised controlled trials. Br Med J. 2012;344:d7771.

64. Noyan-Ashraf MH, Momen MA, Ban K, Sadi A-M, Zhou Y-Q, Riazi AM, et al. GLP-1R agonist liraglutide activates cytoprotective pathways and improves outcomes after experimental myocardial infarction in mice. Diabetes. 2009;58(4):975–83.

65. Nyström T, Gutniak MK, Zhang Q, Zhang F, Holst JJ, Ahrén B, et al. Effects of glucagon-like peptide-1 on endothelial function in type 2 diabetes patients with stable coronary artery disease. Am J Physiol Endocrinol Metab. 2004;287(6):E1209–15.

66. Rubino F, Gagner M, Gentileschi P, Kini S, Fukuyama S, Feng J, et al. The early effect of the Roux-en-Y gastric bypass on hormones involved in body weight regulation and glucose metabolism. Ann Surg. 2004;240(2):236–42.

67. Le Roux CW, Patterson M, Vincent RP, Hunt C, Ghatei MA, Bloom SR. Postprandial plasma ghrelin is suppressed proportional to meal calorie content in normal-weight but not obese subjects. J Clin Endocrinol Metab. 2005;90(2):1068–71.

68. Buchwald H, Varco RL. A bypass operation for obese hyperlipidemic patients. Surgery. 1971;70(1):62–70.

69. Garcia-Marirrodriga I, Amaya-Romero C, Ruiz-Diaz GP, Férnandez S, Ballesta-López C, Pou JM, et al. Evolution of lipid profiles after bariatric surgery. Obes Surg. 2012;22(4):609–16.

70. Fernstrom JD, Courcoulas AP, Houck PR, Fernstrom MH. Long-term changes in blood pressure in extremely obese patients who have undergone bariatric surgery. Arch Surg. 2006;141(3):276–83.

71. Buchwald H, Estok R, Fahrbach K, Banel D, Jensen MD, Pories WJ, et al. Weight and type 2 diabetes after bariatric surgery: systematic review and meta-analysis. Am J Med. 2009;122(3):248–256.e5.

72. Adams TD, Davidson LE, Litwin SE, Kolotkin RL, LaMonte MJ, Pendleton RC, et al. Health benefits of gastric bypass surgery after 6 years. J Am Med Assoc. 2012;308(11):1122–31.

73. Vest AR, Heneghan HM, Agarwal S, Schauer PR, Young JB. Bariatric surgery and cardiovascular outcomes: a systematic review. Heart. 2012;98(24):1763–77.

74. Livingston EH, Arterburn D, Schifftner TL, Henderson WG, DePalma RG. National Surgical Quality Improvement Program analysis of bariatric operations: modifiable risk factors contribute to bariatric surgical adverse outcomes. J Am Coll Surg. 2006;203(5):625–33.

75. Torquati A, Wright K, Melvin W, Richards W. Effect of gastric bypass operation on Framingham and actual risk of cardiovascular events in class II to III obesity. J Am Coll Surg. 2007;204(5): 776–82.

76. Romeo S, Maglio C, Burza MA, Pirazzi C, Sjoholm K, Jacobson P, et al. Cardiovascular events after bariatric surgery in obese subjects with type 2 diabetes. Diabetes Care. 2012;35(12):2613–7; published online August 1, 2012.

77. MacDonald KG, Long SD, Swanson MS, Brown BM, Morris P, Dohm GL, et al. The gastric bypass operation reduces the progression and mortality of non-insulin-dependent diabetes mellitus. J Gastrointest Surg. 1997;1(3):213–20; discussion 220.

78. Christou NV, Sampalis JS, Liberman M, Look D, Auger S, McLean APH, et al. Surgery decreases long-term mortality, morbidity, and health care use in morbidly obese patients. Ann Surg. 2004;240(3):416–23; discussion 423–4.

79. Sampalis JS, Sampalis F, Christou N. Impact of bariatric surgery on cardiovascular and musculoskeletal morbidity. Surg Obes Relat Dis. 2006;2(6):587–91.

80. Abel ED, Litwin SE, Sweeney G. Cardiac remodeling in obesity. Physiol Rev. 2008;88(2):389–419.

81. Morricone L, Malavazos AE, Coman C, Donati C, Hassan T, Caviezel F. Echocardiographic abnormalities in normotensive obese patients: relationship with visceral fat. Obes Res. 2002; 10(6):489–98.

82. Turkbey EB, McClelland RL, Kronmal RA, Burke GL, Bild DE, Tracy RP, et al. The impact of obesity on the left ventricle: the multi-ethnic study of atherosclerosis (MESA). JACC Cardiovasc Imaging. 2010;3(3):266–74.

83. Garza CA, Pellikka PA, Somers VK, Sarr MG, Collazo-Clavell ML, Korenfeld Y, et al. Structural and functional changes in left and right ventricles after major weight loss following bariatric surgery for morbid obesity. Am J Cardiol. 2010;105(4):550–6.

84. Pontiroli AE, Laneri M, Veronelli A, Frigè F, Micheletto G, Folli F, et al. Biliary pancreatic diversion and laparoscopic adjustable gastric banding in morbid obesity: their long-term effects on metabolic syndrome and on cardiovascular parameters. Cardiovasc Diabetol. 2009;8:37–43.

85. Leichman JG, Aguilar D, King TM, Mehta S, Majka C, Scarborough T, et al. Improvements in systemic metabolism, anthropometrics, and left ventricular geometry 3 months after bariatric surgery. Surg Obes Relat Dis. 2006;2(6):592–9.

86. Ikonomidis I, Mazarakis A, Papadopoulos C, Patsouras N, Kalfarentzos F, Lekakis J, et al. Weight loss after bariatric surgery improves aortic elastic properties and left ventricular function in individuals with morbid obesity: a 3-year follow-up study. J Hypertens. 2007;25(2):439–47.

87. Willens HJ, Chakko SC, Byers P, Chirinos JA, Labrador E, Castrillon JC, et al. Effects of weight loss after gastric bypass on right and left ventricular function assessed by tissue Doppler imaging. Am J Cardiol. 2005;95(12):1521–4.

88. de Cunha L, da Cunha CL, de Souza AM, Chiminacio Neto N, Pereira RS, Suplicy HL. Evolutive echocardiographic study of the structural and functional heart alterations in obese individuals after bariatric surgery. Arq Bras Cardiol. 2006;87(5):615–22.

89. Wong CY, O'Moore-Sullivan T, Leano R, Byrne N, Beller E, Marwick TH. Alterations of left ventricular myocardial characteristics associated with obesity. Circulation. 2004;110(19):3081–7.

90. Rider OJ, Francis JM, Ali MK, Petersen SE, Robinson M, Robson MD, et al. Beneficial cardiovascular effects of bariatric surgical and dietary weight loss in obesity. J Am Coll Cardiol. 2009; 54(8):718–26.

91. Dandel M, Lehmkuhl H, Knosalla C, Suramelashvili N, Hetzer R. Strain and strain rate imaging by echocardiography—basic concepts and clinical applicability. Curr Cardiol Rev. 2009;5(2): 133–48.

92. Barbosa MM, Beleigoli AM, de Fatima DM, Freire CV, Ribeiro AL, Nunes MCP. Strain imaging in morbid obesity: insights into subclinical ventricular dysfunction. Clin Cardiol. 2011;34(5):288–93.

93. Orhan AL, Uslu N, Dayi SU, Nurkalem Z, Uzun F, Erer HB, et al. Effects of isolated obesity on left and right ventricular function: a Tissue Doppler and Strain Rate Imaging Study. Echocardiography. 2010;27(3):236–43.

94. Di Bello V, Santini F, Di Cori A, Pucci A, Talini E, Palagi C, et al. Effects of bariatric surgery on early myocardial alterations in adult severely obese subjects. Cardiology. 2008;109(4):241–8.

95. Chen Y, Vaccarino V, Williams C, Butler J, Berkman L, Krumholz H. Risk factors for heart failure in the elderly: a prospective community-based study. Am J Med. 1999;106(6):605–12.

96. Kenchaiah S, Sesso HD, Gaziano JM. Body mass index and vigorous physical activity and the risk of heart failure among men. Circulation. 2009;119(1):44–52.

97. Djoussé L, Bartz TM, Ix JH, Zieman SJ, Delaney JA, Mukamal KJ, et al. Adiposity and incident heart failure in older adults: the Cardiovascular Health Study. Obesity (Silver Spring). 2012; 20(9):1936–41.

98. Kenchaiah S, Evans JC, Levy D, Wilson PWF, Benjamin EJ, Larson MG, et al. Obesity and the risk of heart failure. N Engl J Med. 2002;347(5):305–13.

99. Zuber M, Kaeslin T, Studer T, Erne P. Weight loss of 146 kg with diet and reversal of severe congestive heart failure in a young, morbidly obese patient. Am J Cardiol. 1999;84(8):955–6.

100. Iyengar S, Leier C. Rescue bariatric surgery for obesity-induced cardiomyopathy. Am J Med. 2006;119(12):e5–6.

101. Ristow B, Rabkin J, Haeusslein E. Improvement in dilated cardiomyopathy after bariatric surgery. J Card Fail. 2008;14(3): 198–202.

102. Alpert MA, Terry BE, Kelly DL. Effect of weight loss on cardiac chamber size, wall thickness and left ventricular function in morbid obesity. Am J Cardiol. 1985;55(6):783–6.

103. Alpert MA, Terry BE, Mulekar M, Cohen MV, Massey CV, Fan TM. Cardiac morphology and left ventricular function in normotensive morbidly obese patients with and without congestive heart failure, and effect of weight loss. Am J Cardiol. 1997;80(6): 736–40.

104. McCloskey CA, Ramani GV, Mathier MA, Schauer PR, Eid GM, Mattar SG, et al. Bariatric surgery improves cardiac function in morbidly obese patients with severe cardiomyopathy. Surg Obes Relat Dis. 2007;3(5):503–7.

105. Ramani GV, McCloskey C, Ramanathan RC, Mathier MA. Safety and efficacy of bariatric surgery in morbidly obese patients with severe systolic heart failure. Clin Cardiol. 2008;31(11):516–20.

106. Horwich TB, Fonarow GC, Hamilton MA, MacLellan WR, Woo MA, Tillisch JH. The relationship between obesity and mortality in patients with heart failure. J Am Coll Cardiol. 2001;38(3): 789–95.

107. Lavie CJ, Osman AF, Milani RV, Mehra MR. Body composition and prognosis in chronic systolic heart failure: the obesity paradox. Am J Cardiol. 2003;91(7):891–4.

108. Curtis JP, Selter JG, Wang Y, Rathore SS, Jovin IS, Jadbabaie F, et al. The obesity paradox: body mass index and outcomes in patients with heart failure. Arch Intern Med. 2005;165(1):55–61.

109. Fonarow GC, Srikanthan P, Costanzo MR, Cintron GB, Lopatin M, ADHERE Scientific Advisory Committee and Investigators. An obesity paradox in acute heart failure: analysis of body mass index and inhospital mortality for 108,927 patients in the Acute Decompensated Heart Failure National Registry. Am Heart J. 2007;153(1):74–81.

110. Futter JE, Cleland JGF, Clark AL. Body mass indices and outcome in patients with chronic heart failure. Eur J Heart Fail. 2011;13(2):207–13.

111. Adamopoulos C, Meyer P, Desai RV, Karatzidou K, Ovalle F, White M, et al. Absence of obesity paradox in patients with chronic heart failure and diabetes mellitus: a propensity-matched study. Eur J Heart Fail. 2011;13(2):200–6.

112. Coutinho T, Goel K, Corrêa de Sá D, Kragelund C, Kanaya AM, Zeller M, et al. Central obesity and survival in subjects with coronary artery disease: a systematic review of the literature and collaborative analysis with individual subject data. J Am Coll Cardiol. 2011;57(19):1877–86.

113. Clark AL, Fonarow GC, Horwich TB. Waist circumference, body mass index, and survival in systolic heart failure: the obesity paradox revisited. J Card Fail. 2011;17(5):374–80.

114. Anker SD, Negassa A, Coats AJ, Afzal R, Poole-Wilson PA, Cohn JN, et al. Prognostic importance of weight loss in chronic heart failure and the effect of treatment with angiotensin-converting-enzyme inhibitors: an observational study. Lancet. 2003;361(9363): 1077–83.

115. Ather S, Chan W, Bozkurt B, Aguilar D, Ramasubbu K, Zachariah AA, et al. Impact of noncardiac comorbidities on morbidity and mortality in a predominantly male population with heart failure and preserved versus reduced ejection fraction. J Am Coll Cardiol. 2012;59(11):998–1005.

116. Russo V, Ammendola E, Crescenzo I, Ricciardi D, Capuano P, Topatino A, et al. Effect of weight loss following bariatric surgery on myocardial dispersion of repolarization in morbidly obese patients. Obes Surg. 2007;17(7):857–65.

117. Bezante GP, Scopinaro A, Papadia F, Campostano A, Camerini G, Marinari G, et al. Biliopancreatic diversion reduces QT interval and dispersion in severely obese patients. Obesity. 2007;15(6): 1448–54.

118. Russo V, Ammendola E, De Crescenzo I, Docimo L, Santangelo L, Calabrò R. Severe obesity and P-wave dispersion: the effect of surgically induced weight loss. Obes Surg. 2008;18(1):90–6.

119. Sultan S, Gupta D, Parikh M, Youn H, Kurian M, Fielding G, et al. Five-year outcomes of patients with type 2 diabetes who underwent laparoscopic adjustable gastric banding. Surg Obes Relat Dis. 2010;6(4):373–6.

120. Sugerman HJ, Wolfe LG, Sica DA, Clore JN. Diabetes and hypertension in severe obesity and effects of gastric bypass-induced weight loss. Ann Surg. 2003;237(6):751–6; discussion 757–8.

121. Steffen R, Potoczna N, Bieri N, Horber FF. Successful multi-intervention treatment of severe obesity: a 7-year prospective study with 96% follow-up. Obes Surg. 2009;19(1):3–12.

122. Bolen SD, Chang H-Y, Weiner JP, Richards TM, Shore AD, Goodwin SM, et al. Clinical outcomes after bariatric surgery: a five-year matched cohort analysis in seven US states. Obes Surg. 2012;22(5):749–63.

123. Flum DR, Dellinger EP. Impact of gastric bypass operation on survival: a population-based analysis. J Am Coll Surg. 2004; 199(4):543–51.

124. Sowemimo OA, Yood SM, Courtney J, Moore J, Huang M, Ross R, et al. Natural history of morbid obesity without surgical intervention. Surg Obes Relat Dis. 2007;3(1):73–7; discussion 77.

125. Busetto L, Mirabelli D, Petroni ML, Mazza M, Favretti F, Segato G, et al. Comparative long-term mortality after laparoscopic adjustable gastric banding versus nonsurgical controls. Surg Obes Relat Dis. 2007;3(5):496–502; discussion 502.

126. Peeters A, O'Brien PE, Laurie C, Anderson M, Wolfe R, Flum D, et al. Substantial intentional weight loss and mortality in the severely obese. Ann Surg. 2007;246(6):1028–33.

127. Maciejewski ML, Livingston EH, Smith VA, Kavee AL, Kahwati LC, Henderson WG, et al. Survival among high-risk patients after bariatric surgery. J Am Med Assoc. 2011;305(23):2419–26.

50

Obesity and Cancer with Emphasis on Bariatric Surgery

Ted D. Adams, Steven C. Hunt, Lance E. Davidson, and Mia Hashibe

Introduction

Reported increases in the prevalence of overweight and obesity in the United States and in many countries of the world have resulted in speculation regarding the clinical impact overweight and obesity may have upon associated comorbidities such as diabetes and cardiovascular disease [1]. Contributing to this concern is the finding that in the United States, the prevalence of extreme obesity is increasing at rates greater than moderate obesity [2, 3]. In fact, some reports have proposed that a consequence of increasing obesity rates may be the reversal of the decline in cardiovascular disease [4, 5] and a future generation whose life expectancy may be lower than that of their parents [6, 7]. An equally significant concern related to increasing obesity rates is the associated link between obesity and cancer development [8, 9]. In fact, the topic of obesity and cancer risk has gained increased clinical interest, with greater than 2,000 scientific papers published on the topic [9]. The aim of this chapter is to identify cancers that to date have been associated with obesity and to briefly highlight the leading physiologic theories linking obesity and cancer. The chapter will then explore the validity of national and international recommendations to reduce adiposity, when appropriate, for the purpose of lowering cancer incidence as well as risk for cancer recurrence. Finally, as a result of bariatric surgery the opportunity has been advanced to investigate whether or not long-term voluntary weight loss for overweight or obesity is associated with reduced cancer risk and lower cancer-related mortality. Therefore, the remaining chapter content will review cancer risk and cancer mortality subsequent to bariatric surgery, with brief mention of cancer diagnosis incidental to weight loss surgery.

Obesity and Cancer Risk

Body mass index (BMI; kilograms of body weight divided by height in meters squared) is generally used in cancer studies to categorize normal weight, overweight, and obesity. Adult overweight is defined as a BMI equal to or greater than 25 kg/m^2, and adult obesity is defined as a measured BMI equal to or greater than 30 kg/m^2, with obesity subcategories: class 1 obesity, 30–34.9 kg/m^2; class 2 obesity, 35–39.9 kg/m^2; and class 3 obesity (extreme obesity) $\geq$40 kg/m^2 [10, 11]. Multiple large population studies, prospective observational studies, and extensive reviews have demonstrated the positive association between increased body fatness and obesity and the risk for specific cancer types [8, 12–27]. An extensive review conducted by the World Cancer Research Fund and American Institute for Cancer Research reported that convincing evidence supports increased body fatness as a cause of adenocarcinoma of the esophagus, and cancers of the pancreas, colorectum, breast (postmenopause), endometrium, and kidney. They also reported greater body fatness to be a probable cause of gallbladder cancer, with limited evidence linking greater body fatness with liver cancer [8]. Accumulating evidence linking obesity with risk of non-Hodgkin lymphoma and ovarian and aggressive prostate cancers was also described. Further, this comprehensive review highlighted convincing evidence linking greater abdominal (central) fatness as a cause of colorectal cancer, with probable evidence demonstrating increased abdominal fatness as a cause of cancers of the pancreas, breast (postmenopause), and endometrium. In contrast, greater body fatness "probably protects" against premenopausal breast cancer [8].

Renehan et al. performed a systematic literature review and meta-analysis for the purpose of evaluating the association between BMI and 20 cancer types with inclusion of sex and ethnic groups [17]. From 221 datasets representing 141 prospective observational studies and over 282,000 incident cases, Renehan et al. reported that a 5 kg/m^2 increase in BMI for men was significantly associated with esophageal adenocarcinoma (RR 1.52, 95 % CI 1.33–1.74; $p < 0.0001$) and renal (RR 1.24, 95 % CI 1.15–1.34; $p < 0.0001$), thyroid (RR 1.33, 95 % CI 1.04–1.70; $P = 0.02$), and colon (RR 1.24, 95 % CI 1.20–1.28; $p < 0.0001$) cancers. In women, a 5 kg/m^2 increase in BMI was significantly associated with esophageal adenocarcinoma (RR 1.51, 95 % CI 1.34–1.74;

S.A. Brethauer et al. (eds.), *Minimally Invasive Bariatric Surgery*,
DOI 10.1007/978-1-4939-1637-5_50, © Springer Science+Business Media New York 2015

$p<0.0001$) and renal (RR 1.34, 95 % CI 1.25–1.43; $p<0.0001$), endometrial (RR 1.59, 95 % CI 1.50–1.68; $p<0.0001$), and gallbladder (RR 1.59, 95 % CI 1.02–2.47; $p=0.04$) cancers [17]. Further, Renehan et al. found "weaker positive associations (RR<1.20)" for increased BMI and rectal and malignant melanoma cancer for men and, for women, postmenopausal breast, pancreatic, thyroid, and colon cancers [17]. For both sexes, an increasing BMI was associated with a greater risk for leukemia, multiple myeloma, and non-Hodgkin lymphoma [17].

Nonsurgical change in weight status and subsequent cancer mortality has also been reported in large population studies [13, 28, 29]. The most recent of these studies examined cancer mortality of 1.2 million UK women (Million Women Study), recruited between 1996 and 2001 and then followed 7.0 years for cancer mortality [13]. The primary predictor measure was BMI, adjusted for a number of factors such as alcohol intake, physical activity, menopausal status, and hormone replacement status. During the follow-up period, a total of 17,203 cancer deaths were reported. The trend of increasing BMI beyond the reference group (BMI=22.5–24.9 kg/m^2) was significantly correlated with an increased mortality for the following cancers: adenocarcinoma of the esophagus (RR 2.24, 95 % CI 1.40–3.58), pancreas (RR 1.21, 95 % CI 1.04–1.41), postmenopausal breast (RR 1.36, 95 % CI 1.12–1.66), endometrium (RR 2,46, 95 % CI 1.78–3.39), kidney (RR 1.65, 95 % CI 1.28–2.13), and ovary (RR 1.17, 95 % CI 1.03–1.33); multiple myeloma (RR 1.56, 95 % CI 1.15–2.10); leukemia (RR 1.34, 95 % CI 1.05–1.71); brain cancer (RR 1.17, 95 % 0.95–1.43); and all cancers (RR 1.06, 95 % CI 1.02–1.10) [13]. Although not significant, Reeves et al. reported a decreased premenopausal cancer-related mortality associated with a trend for increasing BMI (RR 0.68, 95 % CI 0.37–1.24) [13].

Potential Mechanisms: Obesity and Cancer Risk

Considerable research effort regarding how obesity influences cancer has generated several published studies and review articles that have postulated biological mechanisms [8, 9, 30, 31]. A recently published book details possible molecular mechanisms relating adipose tissue and cancer, with specific reference to mechanistic links between obesity and specific cancer types [32]. These scientific reports all point to the presence of multiple mechanisms, suggesting "a web of interacting hormones, growth factors, cytokines, and inflammation mediators that promote tumor initiation and growth." [9] In brief, these mechanisms have been classified into three general areas which focus on: chronic inflammation associated with increased release of inflammatory promoters in obese individuals; over-release of steroid-related hormones such as estrogens, androgens

and progesterone; and tumor growth promotion, a result of hyperinsulinemia (associated with insulin resistance subsequent to increased body fatness, in particular, abdominal or central obesity) [8, 30, 33]. A perspective/opinion paper of the molecular mechanisms or links of how obesity might cause an increased risk for cancer has recently been published by Khandekar et al. [31].

Efforts have been undertaken to further identify bioenergetics (i.e., food, nutrition, and physical activity) associated with overweight and obesity risk and subsequent risk of cancer as well as "tumor behavior." [8] These findings have illustrated the potential protective or promoting influences that food, nutrition, physical activity, and obesity can have upon cancer development [8]. Noting that the timeline for these influences begin with and incorporates the fetal exposure period and subsequent developmental years, careful consideration should be given to the prevention and screening of overweight and obesity among children and adolescents [34–36] in relation to their lifetime cancer risk. Estimates are that obesity among children and adolescents (defined as BMI ≥95th percentile, age and gender specific) in the United States have increased three- to sixfold [37] and suggest that 12–18 % of children and adolescents are obese [36, 38, 39]. Further, children and adolescents who are obese have a greater risk of type 2 diabetes, asthma, and nonalcoholic fatty liver disease [36, 40, 41] and are much more likely to have adult obesity, hypertension, hyperlipidemia, and metabolic syndrome [42, 43]. These data may suggest that obese children and adolescents have a greater lifetime cancer risk. For example, overweight and obesity have been associated with an earlier age onset of puberty [43], and as a result of earlier menarche, breast cancer risk may be significantly greater in adulthood [43–46]. Editors of the World Cancer Research Fund and American Institute for Cancer Research review document (2007) summarize the importance of taking the "whole life course approach" with regard to prevention of overweight and obesity [8]. They state: "Some of the most persuasive evidence in the whole field of food, nutrition, and physical activity indicates that the basis for prevention of cancer should be a whole life course approach, starting at the beginning of life, or even in maternal preparation for pregnancy." [8]

Lifestyle-Based Guidelines for Cancer Prevention

In view of the multiple studies linking obesity with increased cancer risk, one would naturally reason that individuals who are overweight or obese should be advised to reduce their body weight in order to lessen their risk for developing cancer. Following this reasoning, two specific national and international documents have provided lifestyle-related recommendations for the prevention of cancer: the *American*

Cancer Society Guidelines on Nutrition and Physical Activity for Cancer Prevention (American Cancer Society) [47] and *Food, Nutrition, Physical Activity and the Prevention of Cancer: A Global Perspective* (World Cancer Fund and American Institute for Cancer Research) [8]. These two documents focus on the relevance of following a healthy diet and participating in consistent physical activity for the purpose of both preventing and treating overweight and obesity. These recommendations are in concert with prevention-oriented guidelines published by other international organizations (the European Code Against Cancer for cancer prevention [48], the American Heart Association for coronary heart disease prevention [49], and the American Diabetes Association for diabetes prevention) [50] and guidelines aimed at promoting overall good health (the 2010 *Dietary Guidelines for Americans* [51] and the 2008 *Physical Activity Guidelines for Americans*) [47, 52].

Of particular interest, the World Cancer Research Fund and the American Institute for Cancer Research has recommended that for cancer prevention, individuals should "be as lean as possible within the normal range of body weight." In addition, the guidelines identified for people who have gained weight, but remain within the normal weight range, are that they work toward returning to their original weight, and that individuals lose enough weight to approach the normal weight range if they are above the normal weight range [8]. Following an approach similar to the World Cancer Research Fund and the American Institute for Cancer Research regarding the recommendation for body weight and cancer prevention, the American Cancer Society's (ACS) guidelines encourage individuals: "Achieve and maintain weight throughout life; be as lean as possible throughout life without being underweight; and avoid excess weight gain at all ages." [47] Finally, the recommendation of the ACS for individuals who are currently overweight or obese is that they reduce body weight and keep in mind that losing even a small amount of weight is associated with health benefits. The ACS guidelines do not specifically include in their "health benefits" a reduced cancer risk, but this positive health outcome could certainly be implied. In summary, these national and international documents which contain recommendations for lifestyle intervention to prevent cancer include strong implication that individuals who participate in voluntary weight loss can reduce their risk for subsequent cancer development.

Nonsurgical Weight Loss, Cancer Prevention, and Cancer Recurrence

Although convincing evidence has linked obesity and certain cancer types, whether or not intentional weight loss reduces the risk of cancer incidence and cancer recurrence is uncertain [30, 47, 53–56]. Identified research limitations inherent in population-based studies attempting to demonstrate an association of nonsurgical weight loss and subsequent cancer risk have included the inability to maintain sustained weight loss and the limited amount of weight lost [53, 54, 56]. Although multiple studies have demonstrated short-term weight loss success when subjects engage in traditional therapy (i.e., dietary, physical activity, and behavioral interventions), the proportion of participants who achieve long-term weight loss maintenance is estimated to be as minimal as 5–10 % [56, 57]. Additional limitations of weight loss and cancer risk association studies are the failure to identify weight loss intentionality (i.e., was weight loss voluntary or not) within the reported research methods, and the absence of studies whose initial primary outcome is identified as weight loss intention [56]. For these reasons, in meaningful sized weight loss population studies with lifestyle-focused intervention (i.e., physical activity, diet and behavioral modification), successful long-term weight loss outcomes have been difficult to attain [53, 56, 57].

There are, however, a limited number of large population multicenter randomized clinical trials that have demonstrated successful weight loss through intensive lifestyle therapy and inclusion of medication. Examples of such studies are the Diabetes Prevention Program (DPP) study in which all recruited participants were prediabetic [58] and the Action for Health in Diabetes (Look AHEAD) study, where all subjects were overweight and diagnosed with type 2 diabetes [59]. Participants of the DPP who were randomized to the intensive lifestyle therapy had a 1-year reported weight loss of 7 kg (approximately 7.5 % loss from their initial weight) and gradual regain of 5 kg over the approximately next 4 years, resulting in 5-year maintenance of about 2 kg less than their initial weight [60]. Results of the Look AHEAD study, the first randomized control trial to explore whether or not weight loss, in combination with physical activity, results in a reduction of cardiovascular morbidity and mortality [61, 62], showed that participants randomized to the intensive lifestyle group had lost on average 8.6 % of their initial weight at the end of year one. At 4 years, this group had an average weight loss of 6.2 %. The intense lifestyle group also demonstrated a significant improvement in diabetes status (hemoglobin A1c level (-0.36 % versus -0.09 %; $p < 0.001$)) [25].

Based upon the results of these two large population trials, the opportunity to achieve both meaningful and sustained nonsurgical weight loss appears to require intensive lifestyle intervention. Even with this in-depth therapeutic approach, the expected achieved weight loss at 1 year is 7–9 %, with weight regain after year 1. One might hypothesize that in order to sufficiently evaluate the outcome of voluntary weight loss upon subsequent cancer risk, a meaningful follow-up period (i.e., perhaps many years) coupled with a substantial degree of sustained weight loss (i.e., perhaps at least 7–10 % of initial weight) may be required. However, whether or not these weight loss criteria are essential for reducing cancer incidence and/or cancer recurrence is not known. For example, research has demonstrated that even modest weight loss can result in improvements in insulin sensitivity, sex- and metabolic-related hormones, and inflammatory markers, all of which have been proposed to be associated with mechanisms linking obesity and cancer risk [47, 55, 63].

Keeping in mind the potential limitations of intentional weight loss and subsequent cancer risk (i.e., limited degree of weight loss, resistance to long-term weight loss maintenance, and unknown intentionality), several large population studies have explored the question of whether or not weight loss results in reduced cancer risk, cancer recurrence, and cancer mortality [20, 21, 28, 29, 64–72]. Rodriguez et al. examined BMI change (BMI self-reported in 1982 and again measured in 1992 at study enrollment) and incident prostate cancer in 69,991 men participating in the Cancer Prevention Study II Nutrition Cohort [21]. A total of 5,252 incident prostate cancers were detected through the follow-up period (from enrollment through mid-2003) [21]. Results suggested obesity increased the risk of "more aggressive prostate cancer" and "may decrease" incidence of less aggressive tumors [21]. With reference to the men who lost weight (weight loss categories were 6–10, 11–20, or ≥21 lb), the authors reported a reduction in risk of the more aggressive prostate cancer (RR 0.58, 95 % CI 0.42–0.79) [21]. In a study examining weight change (weight gain and weight loss) and cancer risk among a cohort of 64,649 Austrian adults (28,711 men; 96, 938 women), Rapp et al. reported that although the incidence of all cancers combined was not "clearly associated" with weight loss or weight gain, weight loss (>0.10 kg/m^2/year) was inversely associated with colon cancer in men (HR 0.50, 95 % CI 0.29–0.87) [64]. In a prospective study (National Institutes of Health-AARP Diet and Health Study) of adult weight change and breast cancer risk of 99,039 postmenopausal women, Ahn et al. reported that weight gain during adulthood was associated with increased breast cancer risk, but adult weight loss was "unrelated to breast cancer compared with stable weight." [65] In contrast to the study of Ahn et al., Parker and Folsom reported the results of questionnaire data regarding intentional and unintentional weight loss activity of ≥20 lb during adulthood [66]. Of the 21,707 postmenopausal women who participated, those women who "ever experienced" an intentional weight loss of ≥20 lb without a reported unintentional weight loss had an 11 % lower incidence rate for any cancer type (RR 0.89, 95 % CI 0.79–1.00) and 19 % lower for breast cancer (RR 0.81, 95 % CI 0.66–1.00), when compared with women who reported no ≥20 lb weight loss episodes [66].

The association of weight gain and weight loss (in excess of 5 % of body weight) both before and after menopause in relation to postmenopausal breast cancer risk was studied as part of the Iowa Women's Health Study [68]. A total of 33,660 postmenopausal women were followed for over 15 years, in which 1,987 incident cases of breast cancer were reported. Although study analyses were stratified by changes in weight in relation to pre- and postmenopausal time periods, the general conclusion of the results suggested that "weight loss and maintenance during these years (between age 18 years and menopause) reduces the risk of postmenopausal breast cancer." [68] Other examples of weight loss associated with subsequent cancer risk include two population-based case-control studies [67, 73]. Trentham-Dietz et al. analyzed weight change and risk of endometrial cancer in 790 newly diagnosed endometrial cases and 2,342 controls free of cancer [67]. Participants were interviewed regarding whether or not they had ever lost at least 20 lb and then gained at least half of the weight back within a 6-month period. Following adjustment for variables such as tobacco use, menopause status, and diabetes, the authors reported that women reporting a "sustained weight loss" had a reduced endometrial cancer risk (OR, 0.7; 95 % CI 0.6–0.9) [67]. As part of the Long Island Breast Cancer Study Project, Eng et al. studied 990 cases of women diagnosed with postmenopausal breast cancer compared with 1,006 controls and found that in contrast to increased postmenopausal breast cancer risk with weight gain, "weight loss over the lifetime was associated with decreased risk of postmenopausal breast cancer" (OR, 0.55; 95 % CI 0.32–0.96) [73].

More recently, review articles not specifically focused on weight loss through bariatric surgery have focused on weight loss and subsequent risk for cancer incidence and cancer recurrence risk [9, 53, 55, 56]. Wolin and Colditz reviewed the relationship between weight loss and weight gain to cancer incidence, with a specific focus on colon, breast, prostate, esophageal, pancreatic, endometrial, and kidney and renal cell cancers [53]. While their review identified multiple studies demonstrating a positive association between weight gain and some cancers, the research linking weight loss to a reduction in cancer risk was limited. With reference to weight loss and subsequent cancer risk, the authors cited studies that demonstrated reduced risk in postmenopausal breast cancer following weight loss and limited evidence linking reduced prostate cancer risk to weight loss. Further, the authors speculated that weight loss may reduce cancer adenocarcinoma of the esophagus because weight loss has been shown to lower the risk for gastroesophageal reflux, a potential partner in the mechanistic development of this cancer [53]. Wolin and Colditz emphasize that there are limited data on weight loss linked to cancer risk, likely due to "small numbers of individuals able to achieve sustained weight loss," but do conclude:If individuals achieve and maintain weight loss, we could prevent substantial cancer burden. This is most evident for postmenopausal breast cancer. The time frame for the benefits of reduced cancer risk after successful weight loss remains unclear for most cancers [53].

In a review of intentional weight loss and subsequent cancer risk, Byers and Sedjo identified three cohort studies and three dietary randomized trials where intentional weight loss was linked to a reduction in cancer risk [55]. The three cohort studies highlighted in this review have been previously discussed in this report [66, 68, 71]. While the primary design of the three dietary randomized control trial studies focused on breast cancer risk reduction (new incidence or recurrence) following dietary intervention and not on intentional weight loss [74–76], Byers and Sedjo theorized that because the dietary interventions had the potential to achieve differences in weight loss between the randomized groups, the studies could "be taken as indirect evidence about the potential impact of intentional weight loss on cancer risk." [55] In the Women's Healthy Eating and Living (WHEL) randomized trial, Pierce et al. explored the influence of a diet high in vegetables and fruit and low in fat on women who previously had been treated from early-stage breast cancer [74]. The intervention group ($n=1,537$) received telephone-based dietary counseling and cooking classes, and the comparison group ($n=1,551$) was given print material describing the 5-A-Day program. Over a mean follow-up period of 7.3 years, there were no significant differences in invasive breast cancer events or mortality between the intervention and the comparison groups. There were also no significant differences in change in body weight between groups with each group losing less than 1 kg compared with baseline [74]. The Women's Intervention Nutrition Study (WINS) included the randomization of 2,437 women with a history of breast cancer to a low-fat diet versus a control diet [76]. After a median follow-up of 60 months, the intervention group had a significantly lower dietary fat intake ($p<0.0001$) and lower body weight of approximately 6 lb compared with the control group ($p=0.005$). There was a reported 9.6 and 12.4 % decrease in breast cancer relapse events in the dietary and control groups, respectively, representing a hazard ratio in the intervention versus the control group of 0.76 (95 % CI 0.60–0.98; $p=0.077$ for stratified log rank and $p=0.34$ for adjusted Cox model analysis) [76]. From 1993 to 2005, 40 US clinical centers participated in a randomized, controlled, primary prevention study in which 48,835 postmenopausal women without prior breast cancer history were randomly assigned to a dietary intervention promoting low fat (20 %) and increased fruits and vegetables (at least five servings daily) and increased grains (at least six servings daily) or to a comparison group that were asked not to alter their dietary intake [75]. Over an 8.1-year follow-up period, 0.42 % of the intervention group and 0.45 % women of the comparison group were diagnosed with breast cancer (7 % difference), representing a hazard ratio of 0.91 (95 % CI 0.83–1.01). At 6-year follow-up, the mean difference in body weight between the intervention and comparison groups was −0.8 kg ($p<0.001$) [75]. In addition to these reported cohort and randomized control trial studies, the review by Byers and Sedjo also identified several studies designed to examine changes in cancer-related hormonal biomarkers and proinflammatory agents following intentional weight loss [55]. The authors conclude:Because both cancer incidence and levels of circulating cancer biomarkers drop fairly rapidly following weight loss, intentional weight

loss may well lead to meaningful reductions in cancer risk with a short latency time [55].

An extensive and systematic review by Birks et al., published in 2012, examines the influence of weight loss upon cancer incidence and mortality [56]. Using PubMed and EMBASE, a systematic literature search was conducted for manuscripts that contained key terms such as "weight loss," "weight change," and "obesity" and were published between 1978 and April of 2011. From a total of 4,748 articles, 34 studies met that search criteria and were further analyzed. Of the 34 articles, the following categories were identified: surgical weight loss and cancer ($n=3$), intentional nonsurgical weight loss and cancer ($n=3$), any weight loss (i.e., intentionality not identified in the manuscript) and postmenopausal breast cancer ($n=10$), and any weight loss (i.e., intentionality not identified in the manuscript) and any cancer other than postmenopausal breast cancer ($n=6$ exploring all cancers and $n=12$ exploring other specific cancers) [56]. Studies identified by Birks et al. that were related to weight loss surgery will be discussed in the next section of this chapter. Of the nonsurgical weight loss surgical studies where weight loss intention was known ($n=3$), one of these studies [66] has been previously discussed. The other two reported articles were published by Williamson et al. and examined intentional weight loss and mortality in white women [77] and white men [29]. The white women-only study involved 43,457 overweight, never-smoking US participants (age range, 40–64 years) who self-reported weight, weight change information (i.e., how much weight (gain or loss), time interval and intentionality), and preexisting illnesses with specific reference to obesity-related illnesses. The vital status of participants was determined 12 years later [77]. For women who reported intentional weight losses of 1–19 lb and ≥20 lb and preexisting obesity-related illnesses, there was a significant reduction in cancer mortality risk, with an adjusted HR of 0.63 (95 % CI 0.43–0.93) and HR of 0.71 (95 % CI 0.52–0.97), respectively. Among women with intentional weight loss reported in these two weight loss ranges but without any preexisting illnesses, the cancer mortality risk varied from HR of 1.27 (95 % CI 0.98–1.65) for weight loss of 1–19 lb to HR of 0.84 (95 % CI 0.62–1.15) for weight loss ≥19 lb; neither was significant [77]. The men-only study of Williamson et al. reported no significant differences in cancer mortality risk associated with intentional weight loss [29]. Of the remaining studies reviewed by Birks et al. where weight loss intentionality was not known ($n=28$), the link between weight loss and cancer risk varied from inverse to null to positive associations [56]. As part of the discussion, Birks et al. reported:Although the literature reviewed compared cancer incidence between two equivalent groups of people (one of which achieved weight loss), only six studies (including the three [weight loss] surgery studies) investigated the effect of weight loss among specifically overweight or obese individuals. [Further] when intentional weight loss is achieved in those with excess weight, there is consistent evidence that the incidence of cancer is reduced. When intentionality is not known, results are less clear, although more than half of such studies analyzed here still demonstrate a significant inverse association between weight loss and cancer incidence [56].

Limited research has been conducted on the use of weight loss-specific pharmacological agents and subsequent cancer risk. Given the relationship between obesity and diabetes incidence and the associated pharmacological treatment of these disorders, additional studies are likely to provide additional insight related to cancer risk following the use of drug therapy that might "target the factors thought to play a role in the cancer risk-increasing mechanisms of obesity" such as metformin [9]. In a review/meta-analysis of metformin and cancer risk in diabetic patients (11 total studies), a 31 % reduction "in overall summary relative risk" was reported to be 0.69 (95 % CI 0.61–0.79) for patients who were reported to be taking metformin compared with other antidiabetic medications [78].

Studies have suggested that increased risk of cancer recurrence may be attributed to obesity [9, 79–82]. For example, for patients who were diagnosed with cancer, a BMI in the normal range was shown to be associated with more favorable outcomes for pre- and postmenopausal women [80]. A study by Joshu et al. reported that weight gain in the period of 5 years prior to and 1 year following a prostatectomy increased the risk of prostate cancer recurrence [9, 83]. As a result of these and other similar findings, whether or not to advise overweight or obese patients recently diagnosed with cancer to voluntarily lose weight or to avoid weight gain for reasons related to reducing risk for cancer progression or recurrence is an important consideration. Unfortunately, limited data exists regarding the influence of weight loss on cancer progression or recurrence.

Bariatric Surgery, Weight Loss, and Cancer Risk

While most of the large population cancer and weight loss studies previously cited in this report have included participants who are not necessarily overweight or obese, with little exception post-bariatric surgery patients are severely obese prior to their weight loss surgery. Most insurance companies require patients seeking bariatric surgery to have first engaged in nonsurgical weight reduction activity and have a BMI of ≥ 35 kg/m^2 but <40 kg/m^2 and at least two obesity-related risk factors or a BMI ≥ 40 kg/m^2 [10]. The adjustable gastric banding system (Allergan$^\copyright$) has also been approved as a surgical treatment option for patients whose BMI is ≥ 30 kg/m^2 and who have at least one preexisting obesity-related risk factor. Following these guidelines, treatment of severe obesity through bariatric surgery has gained greater favor over the past few decades, with an estimated 344,000 weight loss sur-

geries performed globally in 2008 [84, 85]. Because bariatric surgery is now recognized as the only successful treatment for substantial, long-term weight loss for most severely obese patients [86–88], and due to the fact that the prevalence of extreme obesity in the United States has increased at a greater rate than moderate obesity [2, 3], the popularity of weight loss surgery is likely to continue. These trends and the resulting increase in post-bariatric surgery patients provide an ideal patient population to study the association of meaningful and sustained weight loss on subsequent cancer incidence and, in some cases, cancer recurrence.

The longest ongoing prospective bariatric surgery study is the Swedish Obesity Subjects (SOS) study, with reported significant and sustained weight loss among surgical patients for a period of greater than 10 years when compared with matched severely obese control participants [89]. Further demonstration of significant, long-term weight loss (out to 6 years) following Roux-en-Y gastric bypass surgery has been reported in the prospective Utah Obesity Study [90]. To date, three randomized clinical trials have been published comparing diabetic patients with bariatric surgical procedures or intensive medical therapy [91–93]. Although the primary outcome for each of these trials related to improved diabetes status following bariatric surgery, these studies demonstrated the successful attainment of major weight loss. Dixon et al. randomized severely obese diabetic patients to an adjustable gastric banding group or to nonsurgical medical intervention, and after two years of intervention, the surgical patients had reduced their initial body weight by 20.7 % compared with a loss of 1.7 % in the nonsurgical group [93]. Schauer et al. reported a reduction in baseline weight at 1-year intervention of 27.5 % for gastric bypass patients, 24.7 % for sleeve patients, and 5.2 % for patients receiving an intensive lifestyle-based program only [92]. At 2 years post-intervention, patients participating in the study by Mingrone et al. achieved weight loss from baseline of 33.3 %, 33.8 %, and 4.7 % for gastric bypass, biliopancreatic diversion, and the intensive lifestyle therapy program, respectively [91]. To date, associations with weight loss and subsequent cancer incidence risk have not been reported for these three trials. Results from prospective and randomized control trial studies have clearly demonstrated that significant and sustained weight loss can be achieved through bariatric surgery. The question of whether or not this intentional weight loss can impact future cancer risk can now (and has recently been) be explored using the bariatric surgery model in a manner not previously undertaken in non-weight loss population groups due to weight loss sustainability limitations of interventions previously identified in this chapter.

Likely the first study demonstrating a possible link between post-bariatric surgery weight loss and cancer mortality risk was by MacDonald et al. who prospectively followed 154 type 2 diabetic patients who underwent gastric bypass surgery and 78 severely obese type 2 diabetic patients who did not have weight loss surgery and who were matched to the surgical patients by age, sex, and BMI [94]. The mean follow-up time was 9 years and 6.2 years for the surgical and nonsurgical groups, respectively. Although not significantly different between groups, the cancer mortality for the gastric bypass group was 0 % compared with 0.6 % cancer mortality for the nonsurgical group [94]. Since this initial paper, a number of studies have been published on the association of cancer mortality and cancer incidence risk with bariatric surgery, including review papers [25, 54–56, 84, 95–98] and prospective and retrospective studies [33, 89, 99–105].

As previously indicated, the Swedish Obesity Subjects study (SOS study) is a long-term study that has followed 2,010 patients who underwent bariatric surgery (71 % females) and 2037 severely obese participants who did not undergo weight loss surgery. Both groups were matched using multiple parameters. The study participants were followed at 25 surgical departments and 480 primary health care centers in Sweden and of the surgical group, 376 (18.7 %) underwent nonadjustable or adjustable gastric banding, 1,396 (68.1 %) had vertical banded gastroplasty, and 265 (13.2 %) Roux-en-Y gastric bypass procedures [106]. Study inclusion criteria included age between 37 and 60 years and a BMI of 34 kg/m^2 or more for men and 38 kg/m^2 for women. The initial SOS mortality study followed participants in both groups for an average of 10.9 years, and vital status was determined for all but three of the participants (follow-up rate of 99.9 %) [89].

As the SOS study is the only prospective investigation to report long-term changes in clinical variables and cancer incidence, a significant strength of this mortality study was the prospective tracking of weight. Maximum weight loss from baseline that occurred over the period of up to 15 years was 25 %, 16 %, and 14 %, respectively, for gastric bypass, vertical banded gastroplasty, and gastric banding, with an approximate ±2 % weight change among the control group [89]. The unadjusted overall total mortality HR in the surgery group when compared with the control group was 0.76 (95 % CI 0.59–0.99; $p=0.04$), and when adjusted for sex, age, and risk factors, the HR was similar at 0.71 ($p=0.01$). The SOS study reported a total of 129 deaths (6.3 %) among the control group and 101 deaths (5.0 %) in the surgical group. Interestingly, cancer was the most common cause of death over this mean 10-year period (48 deaths in the control groups compared with 29 deaths in the surgical groups), and myocardial infarction was the second leading cause of death (25 deaths among the control group and 13 deaths in the surgical group) [89].

As a follow-up study (mean follow-up of 10.9 years; range from 0 to 18.1 years) among SOS study participants, Sjöström et al., reported on the incidence of cancer [100]. The number of reported cancers among the post-bariatric surgery group was 117 compared with 169 cancers among the control group, representing an HR of 0.67 (95 % CI 0.53–0.85; $p=0.0009$). Because the SOS study consisted of primarily female participants, the female-only analysis showed the surgical group had a reported 79 cancers compared with 130 cancers in the control females, giving an HR value of 0.58 (95 % CI 0.44–0.77; $p=0.0001$). Unlike the cancer results of female-only participants, SOS reported that there were no effects related to bariatric surgery and subsequent cancer incidence in males (38 cancer cases among men in both the surgical and control groups) [100]. The lack of significant differences in cancer incidence between the male post-bariatric surgery patients and nonoperated comparison participants may have been influenced by the fewer numbers of male subjects. Exploration of possible variables associated with cancer incidence showed that the degree of weight loss or changes in energy intake among the SOS subjects participating in the bariatric surgery group were not significantly related to the reduction in cancer incidence [98]. However, sagittal trunk diameter (a substitute measure for intra-abdominal adiposity [100, 107]) was shown to contribute significantly to cancer incidence [100].

Christou et al. conducted an observational study (mean follow-up approximately 2.5 years; maximum of 5 years) of weight loss following bariatric surgery of 1,035 patients (65.6 % female; operated on between 1986 and 2002) in which bariatric surgical patients were compared with a comparison group of 5,746 age- and gender-matched severely obese patients. The comparison group was obtained from a large health care claims database (which included hospitalizations) using ICD codes that are commonly related to obesity [101]. The types of bariatric surgery included open Roux-en-Y gastric bypass (79.2 %), vertical banded gastroplasty (18.7 %) and laparoscopic Roux-en-Y gastric bypass (8 %) procedures. The mortality rate was reported as 0.68 % for the surgical group and 6.17 % for the control group [101].

As a follow-up to this initial cancer-focused study, Christou et al. published a study in which first-time physician/hospital visits were linked to eventual "all cancer diagnosis." The study population included 1,035 post-bariatric surgical patients (surgery performed between 1986 and 2002). Similar to Christou's earlier study, the age- and gender-matched morbidly obese group ($n=5,746$) of participants were identified using ICD codes for morbid obesity, who had not undergone bariatric surgery and whose data were part of a single-payer administrative database [102]. Any surgical or control participant found to have visited a physician or hospital for purposes that were related to cancer (diagnosis or treatment) within 6 months before their inclusion into the study was excluded from the analysis [54]. Analysis of the data after a maximum of 5 years follow-up showed the number of visits to the physician/hospital that led to a cancer-related diagnosis for the weight loss surgical group was 21 visits (2.0 %) compared with 487 visits (8.5 %) among the comparison group, with a relative risk of 0.22 (95 % CI 0.14–0.35; $p=0.001$) [102]. Reported relative risk for breast cancer was 0.17 (95 % CI 0.01–0.31; $p=0.001$), but menopausal status in relation to these cancers was not noted. The risk ratio for colorectal cancer between the two groups was 0.32 (95 % CI 0.08–1.31; $p=0.63$). This study did not report all-cause mortality between study groups [54].

Drawing upon post-gastric bypass patient data collected by surgeons of the Rocky Mountain Associated Physicians (Salt Lake City, UT) over two decades, Adams et al. conducted a retrospective cohort study of long-term mortality (from 1984 to 2002) [99]. The study included 7,925 post-Roux-en-Y gastric bypass patients matched to 7,925 severely obese comparison subjects who had applied for a Utah driver's license. Matching included age, sex, BMI, and the date of bariatric surgery with the year the comparison participant applied for their driver's license. The self-reported BMI of all driver's license applicants was corrected using gender-specific regression equations derived from a subset of 592 subjects using weight that had been clinically measured before bariatric surgery. To assure that none of the comparison group participants had previously undergone weight loss surgery, they were linked to the state hospitalization registry. If a comparison participant had ICD codes for bariatric surgery, they were excluded from the study analyses [99]. Names, date of birth, Social Security numbers, and state of birth of all patients and comparison group participants were submitted to the National Death Index for the purpose of obtaining mortality status and cause of death.

Total study follow-up was 18 years with a mean follow-up of 7.1 years. For all-cause deaths, there were 213 deaths among the surgical group and 321 deaths among the group (hazard ratio of 0.60, 95 % CI 0.45–0.67; $p<0.001$, after covariate adjustment). Prevalent cancers for the surgical and comparison groups were 1.67 % and 1.59 %, respectively, not significantly different ($p=0.71$). With specific reference to cancer deaths, the gastric bypass surgery group (31 deaths; 5.5 cancer deaths per 10,000 person years) was 60 % lower than the comparison group (73 deaths; 13.3 cancer deaths per 10,000 person years) ($P=0.001$). Any cancer deaths occurring within 5 years of baseline were eliminated from the analysis [99]. Unlike the SOS study, weight and other associated clinical data at the time of death were not obtainable, and as indicated, only self-reported baseline weight was available for the comparison group participants.

Adams et al. extended the mortality follow-up study to 24 years (mean, 12.5 years) and added cancer incidence data by linking all participant data to the Utah Cancer Registry (UCR) [33]. Cancer site (type), stage, date of diagnosis, vital status, and date of death were also obtained. Subjects included gastric bypass patients who were Utah residents (6,596 of a total 9,949 post-gastric bypass patients) and severely obese comparison participants ($n=9,442$) as identified through Utah driver's license applications. There were no differences between groups for baseline cancer prevalence. Results showed that 254 (3.1/1,000 person years) and 477 (4.3/1,000 person years) incident cancers were detected in the post-gastric bypass and comparison groups, respectively [33]. For all cancers

combined, the gastric bypass surgery group demonstrated a 24 % reduction in cancer incidence when compared with the comparison group (HR 0.76, 95 % CI 0.65–0.89; $p=0.0006$). Similar to other reported studies where women represent the greater percentage of bariatric surgical patients, in this study only 14 % and 17 % of the surgical and comparison participants, respectively, were men. The small number of male subjects may have influenced the finding of no significant group differences in incidence of all cancers when only males were compared. However, all incident cancers were significantly lower for females of the surgical group compared with comparison female-only group (HR 0.73, CI 0.62–0.87; $p=0.0004$). When cancers identified as "likely" to be obesity-related were grouped (esophageal adenocarcinomas, colorectal, pancreas, postmenopausal breast, corpus and uterus, kidney, non-Hodgkin lymphoma, leukemia, multiple myeloma, liver and gallbladder), incident risk for these obesity-related cancers was significantly lower in the surgery group compared with the comparison group (HR 0.62, 95 % CI 0.49–0.78), whereas the grouped "nonobesity"-related incident cancers were not significantly different between groups. Results from this study estimated that approximately 71 gastric bypass surgeries would be necessary to prevent one incident cancer [33].

When specific stratification of cancer by stage [108] at first diagnosed was performed, there were no stage differences between groups in the in situ (stage 0) and local (stage 1). However, the regional cancers (stages 2–5) were significantly lower in the surgical group compared with the comparison group (HR 0.61, 95 % CI 0.43–0.89; $p=0.009$). The distant cancers (stage 7) were also significantly lower in the surgical patients compared with comparison participants (HR 0.61, 95 % CI 0.39–0.96; $p=0.03$). Finally, the cancer case fatality rates were not significantly different between groups nor were the mean times to cancer detection [33]. As has been previously indicated, unlike the SOS study, this study only had baseline weight available, and no follow-up clinical data for surgical patients and comparison groups (other than incident cancer information) were obtained. Further discussion related to strengths and weaknesses of this study have been previously reviewed [33]. This study further surmised that:...regional and distant cancers that would have resulted without the surgery [gastric bypass] were detected in the in situ and local stages and in situ and local stage cancers that would have occurred without surgery were prevented or delayed beyond the end of the follow-up period [33].

A study by Östlund et al. addresses whether or not bariatric surgery reduces the postsurgical cancer risk to the risk of the general population [103]. Östlund et al. analyzed the incidence of obesity-related cancers among 13,123 post-bariatric surgical patients operated on in Sweden over a 26 years period (1980–2006). Cancers were identified through the Swedish Cancer Registry, and follow-up after surgery included three different intervals: 1–4, 5–9, and ≥10 years, and the mean follow-up time was 9 years. Of the total post-bariatric surgery cohort, there were 296 obesity-related cancers identified. The number of obesity-related cancers were divided by the expected number of cancers (representing the risk at baseline and derived using the "entire background population in Sweden") to determine a standardized incidence ratio (SIR). The primary outcome for this study was the time trends for SIR.

There were no significant differences in the SIR for all obesity-related cancers combined (SIR 1.04, 95 % CI 0.93–1.17) with a p for trend of 0.40 for follow-up time [103]. However, when individual obesity-related cancers were reported, breast cancer did show a significant decrease in risk following bariatric surgery (SIR 0.55, 95 % CI 0.44–0.68) [103]. When analyzed individually, colorectal, endometrial, and kidney cancers demonstrated increased risks, with SIR values of 2.14 (95 % CI 1.33–3.22), 2.15 (95 % CI 1.62–2.81), and 2.68 (95 % CI 1.71–3.98), respectively [103]. The difference in comparison group selection between the Östlund et al. study and studies previously reviewed (i.e., using the general population versus severely obese-only subjects) presents the possibility that bariatric surgery may be associated with a reduction in obesity-related cancers when compared to nonoperated severely obese individuals, but this reduction in cancer risk, except possibly for breast cancer, may not drop to the cancer rates of the general population (whose average BMI is considerably lower than that of the severely obese and usually lower than post-bariatric surgery patients).

Reporting on the relationship of female cancers related to bariatric surgery, McCawley et al. identified women whose cancer had been diagnosed prior to their having bariatric surgery as well as women free of cancer before surgery but diagnosed with cancer following bariatric surgery [104]. Of a total of 1,482 women who underwent bariatric surgery, 34 (64.1 %) had been diagnosed prior to their surgery, with a mean interval between their cancer diagnosis and subsequent bariatric surgery of 9.9 years [104]. A total of 17 (32 %) of surgical women were diagnosed with cancer, on average, 4.2 years postsurgery [104]. Finally, one patient (1.9 %) had cancer discovered during the perioperative evaluation, and in one patient (1.9 %) the time of diagnosis was not known. McCawley et al. also included a control population of women ($n=3,495$) who were severely obese. Their study results indicated that the bariatric surgical group had fewer cancers (3.6 % versus 5.8 %; $p=0.002$) when compared with the severely obese comparison group [104]. However, the bariatric surgery women were significantly younger (41.7 versus 46.9 years; $p<0.001$) and had cancer diagnosed as a younger age (45.0 versus 56.8 years; $p<0.001$) when compared with the nonoperated group [104]. The most commonly diagnosed cancers in the bariatric surgical women were breast ($n=15$, 28.3 %), endometrial ($n=9$, 17 %), and cervical ($n=6$, 11.3 %) cancers [104]. Although the inclusion of women whose cancer was diag-

nosed well before their participation in bariatric surgery makes this study design rather unique, sorting out the long-term impact of bariatric surgery-related weight loss on cancer (or cancer recurrence) may be problematic.

Gagne et al. reported on a large case series ($n=1,566$; 1999–2008) of bariatric surgery patients with reference to cancer diagnosed prior to, during, or following their bariatric surgery [105]. They reported that of these patients, 36 (2.3 %), 4 (0.26 %), and 16 (0.9 %) of patients had diagnosed cancers before undergoing bariatric surgery evaluation, preoperatively, and postoperatively, respectively. In addition to this study by Gagne et al., there are multiple small case studies in the literature that report on malignancies discovered during workup for bariatric surgery, at the time of bariatric surgery, when bariatric revisional surgery is performed, and among bariatric surgical patients who at a later point in time after their bariatric surgery undergo surgery for an unrelated reason. The extent to which weight loss is related to these findings is not certain.

Concluding this section, mention is made of the increasing interest in measuring specific biomarkers in patients before and following bariatric surgery. For example, Sainsbury et al. collected mucosal biomarkers in bariatric patients ($n=26$) before and 6 months after surgery and compared with mucosal biomarkers of 21 age- and sex-matched normal weight participants [109]. They reported that the mucosal biomarkers, "accepted as indictors of future colorectal cancer risk," were found to be increased in the bariatric surgical patients at 6 months after surgery when compared with the normal weight comparison group [109]. As indicated, this study was only 6 months in duration. No doubt, longer follow-up studies with greater numbers of post-bariatric surgical patients will be conducted with the intent to follow cancer-related biomarkers. Currently, however, there are a limited number of cancer biomarkers that can be included in such studies.

Exploring Potential Mechanisms Associated with Bariatric Surgery and Subsequent Cancer Risk

Highlighted in Fig. 1 is a schematic by Ashrafian et al. that presents probable physiologic mechanisms that occur following bariatric surgery and that may result in a decrease in future cancer incidence [84].

These authors suggest that bariatric (or metabolic) surgery "interrupts" the postulated mechanistic pathways that are thought to promote both obesity and subsequent cancer. As review authors, we predict that during the next few years, there will be a significant escalation in research related to the potential mechanisms postulated by Ashrafian et al., leading to a clearer understanding of the relationship of voluntary weight loss and cancer risk.

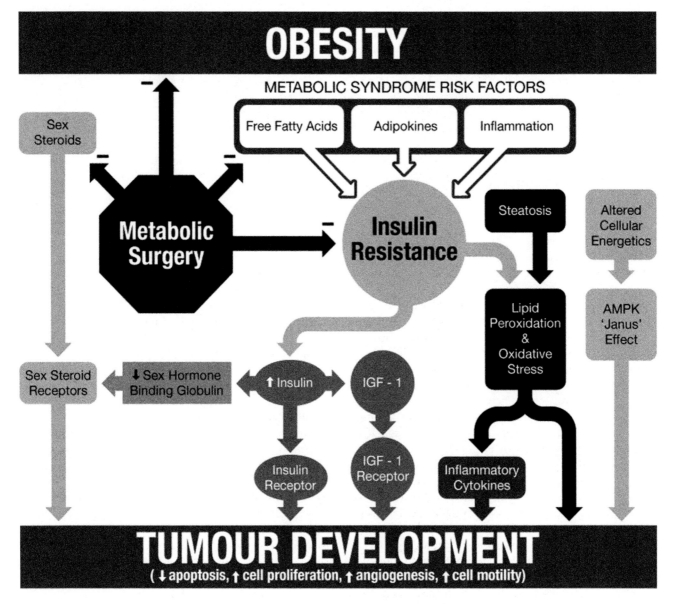

FIG. 1. Mechanisms of decreased cancer risk by metabolic surgery. IGF-1 = Insulin-like Growth Factor 1, AMPK = 5′ adenosine mono-phosphate-activated protein kinase. (Figure adapted from Ashrafian, et al. [84] and reprinted by permission).

Conclusion

The link between increased adiposity (i.e., obesity) and greater risk for cancer has been well established. However, due to the difficulty in achieving meaningful and sustained weight loss in large population studies, whether or not voluntary weight loss reduced the risk of cancer incidence and cancer recurrence is not entirely clear. The opportunity to study cancer risk following voluntary weight loss is possible when bariatric surgical patients are followed over time. Although limited in number, studies have demonstrated a reduction in cancer mortality among post-bariatric patients compared with severely obese, nonoperated controls. In addition, one prospective study (SOS study) and a few observational studies have shown a lower risk for cancer incidence among patients who have undergone bariatric surgery compared with nonoperated, severely obese comparison groups. One study has suggested that the risk for obesity-related cancers following bariatric surgery is not reduced below cancer rates of the background population. Further, reported reductions in obesity-related cancer risk have been limited to females, perhaps due to the greater percentage of women who undergo weight loss surgery when compared with men. With reference to the various types of bariatric surgical procedures, there is limited evidence of how these procedures might differ in relation to their potential for reducing subsequent cancer risk. There is an increasing consensus that intentional weight loss may lead to lower cancer incidence [56]. Finally, recent national and international guidelines that have recommended weight loss for individuals (if clinically indicated), for the purpose of reducing cancer incidence risk, appear to be supported by the few weight loss and cancer studies that have been published, including those related to bariatric surgery.

Acknowledgments We wish to thank Maureen Rice of the McMaster University Evidence-based Practice Center (MU-EPC), McMaster University, Hamilton, Ontario, for conducting a medical literature review. We also express appreciation to Kenneth Adams, Ph.D.; the late Eugenia Calle, Ph.D.; Paul Hopkins, M.D.; Richard Gress, M.S.; Nan Stroup, Ph.D.; Sherman Smith, M.D.; Steven Simper, M.D.; and Rodrick McKinlay, M.D.

T.D.A. receives partial funding through the *Huntsman Fellowship— Advancing Community Cancer Prevention*, Intermountain Research and Medical Foundation, Intermountain Healthcare Corporation, SLC, UT. T.D.A., S.C.H., and L.E.D. are supported by grant DK-55006 from the National Institutes of Health/the National Institute of Diabetes and Digestive and Kidney Diseases.

Review Questions and Answers

a. Question 1: Do pre-menopausal obese women have a greater risk for incidence of breast cancer compared to pre-menopausal normal weight women?

Answer 1: No, population-based research suggests that pre-menopausal obese women are at lower risk for developing breast cancer compared to pre-menopausal normal weight women. However, post-menopausal obese women are at a greater risk for breast cancer compared to post-menopausal normal weight women.

b. Question 2: What are considered to be the primary mechanistic links between obesity and specific cancer types?

Answer 2: Generally, three major categories have been identified as mechanisms associating obesity and obesity-related cancers. These include chronic inflammation, over-release of steroid-related hormones and tumor growth promotion (secondary to hyperinsulinemia.

c. Question 3: How strongly does the evidence support the recommendation that traditional weight loss reducesincident risk of cancer as well as cancer recurrence?

Answer 3: The evidence relating weight loss from traditional therapies (i.e. diet, physical activity and behavioral modification) and reduced cancer risk are limited primarily because of the difficulty achieving significant and sustained weight loss among overweight and obese population groups.

d. Question 4: What is the evidence for reduced cancer incidence and cancer mortality among patients who have had bariatric surgery compared to obese, non-bariatric surgical subjects?

Answer 4: Because patients who have undergone bariatric surgery generally lose a large amount of weight (i.e. greater than 20% of initial weight) and maintain significant weight loss for an extended period of time (i.e. years), these patients are ideal to study weight loss and subsequent cancer risk. There are multiple studies that have shown when bariatric cancer patients are compared to severely obese non-surgical subjects, the bariatric surgical patients demonstrate lower cancer mortality and cancer incidence when compared to severely obese non-operated controls.

References

1. Cowie CC, Rust KF, Ford ES, et al. Full accounting of diabetes and pre-diabetes in the U.S. population in 1988-1994 and 2005-2006. Diabetes Care. 2009;32(2):287–94.
2. Freedman DS, Khan LK, Serdula MK, Galuska DA, Dietz WH. Trends and correlates of class 3 obesity in the United States from 1990 through 2000. JAMA. 2002;288(14):1758–61.
3. Sturm R. Increases in clinically severe obesity in the United States, 1986-2000. Arch Intern Med. 2003;163(18):2146–8.
4. Fox CS, Coady S, Sorlie PD, et al. Increasing cardiovascular disease burden due to diabetes mellitus: the Framingham Heart Study. Circulation. 2007;115(12):1544–50.
5. Preis SR, Hwang SJ, Coady S, et al. Trends in all-cause and cardiovascular disease mortality among women and men with and without diabetes mellitus in the Framingham Heart Study, 1950 to 2005. Circulation. 2009;119(13):1728–35.
6. Olshansky SJ, Passaro DJ, Hershow RC, et al. A potential decline in life expectancy in the United States in the 21st century. N Engl J Med. 2005;352(11):1138–45.
7. Preston SH. Deadweight?–The influence of obesity on longevity. N Engl J Med. 2005;352(11):1135–7.
8. Food, Nutrition, Physical Activity, and the Prevention of Cancer: A Global Perspective. Washington, DC: AICR: World Cancer Research Fund/American Institute for Cancer Research;2007.
9. Patlak M, Nass SJ. The role of obesity in cancer survival and recurrence: Workshop summary. Washington, DC: Institute of Medicine of the National Academies; 2012.
10. National Institutes of Health (NHLBI). Clinical guidelines on the identification, evaluation, and treatment of overweight and obesity in adults: the evidence report. Obes Res. 1998;6(2):51S–209.
11. National Task Force on the Prevention and Treatment of Obesity. Overweight, obesity, and health risk. Arch Intern Med. 2000;160: 898–904.
12. Calle E. Obesity and cancer (Chapter 10). In: Hu F, editor. Obesity Epidemiolog. Oxford: Oxford University Press; 2008. p. 196–215.
13. Reeves G, Pirie K, Beral V, Green J, Spencer E, Bull D. Cancer incidence and mortality in relation to body mass index in the Million Woman Study: cohort study. Br Med J. 2007; 335:1134–9.
14. Calle EE, Rodriguez C, Walker-Thurmond K, Thun MJ. Overweight, obesity, and mortality from cancer in a prospectively studied cohort of U.S. adults. N Engl J Med. 2003;348(17): 1625–38.
15. Rapp K, Schroeder J, Klenk J, et al. Obesity and incidence of cancer: a large cohort study of over 145,000 adults in Austria. Br J Cancer. 2005;93(9):1062–7.
16. Samanic C, Chow WH, Gridley G, Jarvholm B, Fraumeni Jr JF. Relation of body mass index to cancer risk in 362,552 Swedish men. Cancer Causes Control. 2006;17(7):901–9.

17. Renehan A, Tyson M, Egger M, Heller R, Zwahlen M. Body-mass index and incidence of cancer: a systematic review and meta-analysis of prospective observational studies. Lancet. 2008;371(9612): 569–78.

18. Calle EE, Thun MJ. Obesity and cancer. Oncogene. 2004; 23(38):6365–78.

19. IARC. IRAC handbooks of cancer prevention weight control and physical activity. Lyon: International Agency for Research on Cancer; 2002.

20. Schouten LJ, Goldbohm RA, van den Brandt PA. Anthropometry, physical activity, and endometrial cancer risk: results from the Netherlands Cohort Study. J Natl Cancer Inst. 2004;96(21): 1635–8.

21. Rodriguez C, Freedland SJ, Deka A, et al. Body mass index, weight change, and risk of prostate cancer in the Cancer Prevention Study II Nutrition Cohort. Cancer Epidemiol Biomarkers Prev. 2007;16(1):63–9.

22. Xu WH, Xiang YB, Zheng W, et al. Weight history and risk of endometrial cancer among Chinese women. Int J Epidemiol. 2006;35(1):159–66.

23. Aune D, Greenwood DC, Chan DS, et al. Body mass index, abdominal fatness and pancreatic cancer risk: a systematic review and non-linear dose-response meta-analysis of prospective studies. Ann Oncol. 2012;23(4):843–52.

24. Calle EE. Obesity and cancer. BMJ. 2007;335(7630):1107–8.

25. Basen-Engquist K, Chang M. Obesity and cancer risk: recent review and evidence. Curr Oncol Rep. 2011;13(1):71–6.

26. Vainio H, Kaaks R, Bianchini F. Weight control and physical activity in cancer prevention: international evaluation of the evidence. Eur J Cancer Prev. 2002;11 Suppl 2:S94–100.

27. Anderson AS, Caswell S. Obesity management–an opportunity for cancer prevention. Surgeon. 2009;7(5):282–5.

28. Yaari S, Goldbourt U. Voluntary and involuntary weight loss: associations with long term mortality in 9,228 middle-aged and elderly men. Am J Epidemiol. 1998;148(6):546–55.

29. Williamson DF, Pamuk E, Thun M, Flanders D, Byers T, Heath C. Prospective study of intentional weight loss and mortality in overweight white men aged 40-64 years. Am J Epidemiol. 1999; 149(6):491–503.

30. Calle EE, Kaaks R. Overweight, obesity and cancer: epidemiological evidence and proposed mechanisms. Nat Rev Cancer. 2004;4(8):579–91.

31. Khandekar MJ, Cohen P, Spiegelman BM. Molecular mechanisms of cancer development in obesity. Nat Rev Cancer. 2011;11(12): 886–95.

32. Kolonin MG, editor. Adipose tissue and cancer. New York: Springer Science; 2013.

33. Adams TD, Stroup AM, Gress RE, et al. Cancer incidence and mortality after gastric bypass surgery. Obesity (Silver Spring). 2009;17(4):796–802.

34. Force USPST, Barton M. Screening for obesity in children and adolescents: US Preventive Services Task Force recommendation statement. Pediatrics. 2010;125(2):361–7.

35. Whitlock EP, O'Connor EA, Williams SB, Beil TL, Lutz KW. Effectiveness of weight management interventions in children: a targeted systematic review for the USPSTF. Pediatrics. 2010;125(2):e396–418.

36. USPSTF. Screening and interventions for obesity in adults: Summary of the evidence by the U.S. Preventive Services Task Force. 2010; http://www.uspreventiveservicestaskforce.org/3rduspstf/obesity/obessum2.htm

37. Wang Y, Beydoun MA. The obesity epidemic in the United States–gender, age, socioeconomic, racial/ethnic, and geographic characteristics: a systematic review and meta-regression analysis. Epidemiol Rev. 2007;29:6–28.

38. Ogden CL, Carroll MD, Curtin LR, Lamb MM, Flegal KM. Prevalence of high body mass index in US children and adolescents, 2007-2008. JAMA. 2010;303(3):242–9.

39. Ogden CL, Lamb MM, Carroll MD, Flegal KM. Obesity and socioeconomic status in children and adolescents: United States, 2005-2008. NCHS Data Brief. 2010;2010(51):1–8.

40. Reilly JJ, Methven E, McDowell ZC, et al. Health consequences of obesity. Arch Dis Child. 2003;88(9):748–52.

41. Must A, Spadano J, Coakley EH, Field AE, Colditz G, Dietz WH. The disease burden associated with overweight and obesity. JAMA. 1999;282(16):1523–9.

42. Thompson DR, Obarzanek E, Franko DL, et al. Childhood overweight and cardiovascular disease risk factors: the National Heart, Lung, and Blood Institute Growth and Health Study. J Pediatr. 2007;150(1):18–25.

43. Jasik CB, Lustig RH. Adolescent obesity and puberty: the "perfect storm". Ann N Y Acad Sci. 2008;1135:265–79.

44. Petridou E, Syrigou E, Toupadaki N, Zavitsanos X, Willett W, Trichopoulos D. Determinants of age at menarche as early life predictors of breast cancer risk. Int J Cancer. 1996; 68(2):193–8.

45. Titus-Ernstoff L, Longnecker MP, Newcomb PA, et al. Menstrual factors in relation to breast cancer risk. Cancer Epidemiol Biomarkers Prev. 1998;7(9):783–9.

46. Stoll BA. Western diet, early puberty, and breast cancer risk. Breast Cancer Res Treat. 1998;49(3):187–93.

47. Kushi LH, Doyle C, McCullough M, et al. American Cancer Society Guidelines on nutrition and physical activity for cancer prevention: reducing the risk of cancer with healthy food choices and physical activity. CA Cancer J Clin. 2012;62(1):30–67.

48. Boyle P, Autier P, Bartelink H, et al. European Code Against Cancer and scientific justification: third version (2003). Ann Oncol. 2003;14(7):973–1005.

49. Lichtenstein AH, Appel LJ, Brands M, et al. Diet and lifestyle recommendations revision 2006: a scientific statement from the American Heart Association Nutrition Committee. Circulation. 2006;114(1):82–96.

50. Bantle JP, Wylie-Rosett J, Albright AL, et al. Nutrition recommendations and interventions for diabetes: a position statement of the American Diabetes Association. Diabetes Care. 2008;31 Suppl 1:S61–78.

51. The 2010 Dietary Guidelines for Americans. Washington, DC: US Department of Agriculture and the US Department of Health and Human Services; 2010.

52. Physical Activity Guidelines for Americans. Washington, DC: US Department of Health and Human Services; 2008.

53. Wolin KY, Colditz GA. Can weight loss prevent cancer? Br J Cancer. 2008;99(7):995–9.

54. Adams TD, Hunt SC. Cancer and obesity: effect of bariatric surgery. World J Surg. 2009;33(10):2028–33.

55. Byers T, Sedjo RL. Does intentional weight loss reduce cancer risk? Diabetes Obes Metab. 2011;13(12):1063–72.

56. Birks S, Peeters A, Backholer K, O'Brien P, Brown W. A systematic review of the impact of weight loss on cancer incidence and mortality. Obes Rev. 2012;13(10):868–91.

57. Fisher BL, Schauer P. Medical and surgical options in the treatment of severe obesity. Am J Surg. 2002;184(6B):9S–16.

58. Knowler WC, Barrett-Conner E, Fowler SE. Diabetes Prevention Program Research Group: Reduction in the incidence of type 2 diabetes with lifestyle intervention or metformin. N Engl J Med. 2002;346(6):393–403.

59. Look ARG, Pi-Sunyer X, Blackburn G, et al. Reduction in weight and cardiovascular disease risk factors in individuals with type 2 diabetes: one-year results of the look AHEAD trial. Diabetes Care. 2007;30(6):1374–83.

60. Diabetes Prevention Program Research Group, Knowler WC, Fowler SE, et al. 10-Year follow-up of diabetes incidence and weight loss in the Diabetes Prevention Program Outcomes Study. Lancet. 2009;374(9702):1677–86.

61. Wadden TA, West DS, Neilberg RH, et al. One-year weight losses in the Look AHEAD study: Factors associated with success. Obesity. 2009;17(4):713–22.

62. Ryan DH, Espeland MA, Foster GD, et al. Look AHEAD (Action for Health in Diabetes): design and methods for a clinical trial of weight loss for the prevention of cardiovascular disease in type 2 diabetes. Control Clin Trials. 2003;24(5):610–28.

63. McTiernan A, Irwin M, Vongruenigen V. Weight, physical activity, diet, and prognosis in breast and gynecologic cancers. J Clin Oncol. 2010;28(26):4074–80.

64. Rapp K, Klenk J, Ulmer H, et al. Weight change and cancer risk in a cohort of more than 65,000 adults in Austria. Ann Oncol. 2008;19(4):641–8.

65. Ahn J, Schatzkin A, Lacey Jr JV, et al. Adiposity, adult weight change, and postmenopausal breast cancer risk. Arch Intern Med. 2007;167(19):2091–102.

66. Parker E, Folsom A. Intentional weight loss and incidence of obesity-related cancers: the Iowa Women's Health Study. Int J Obese Relat Metab Disord. 2003;27:1447–52.

67. Trentham-Dietz A, Nichols HB, Hampton JM, Newcomb PA. Weight change and risk of endometrial cancer. Int J Epidemiol. 2006;35(1):151–8.

68. Harvie M, Howell A, Vierkant RA, et al. Association of gain and loss of weight before and after menopause with risk of postmenopausal breast cancer in the Iowa Women's Health Study. Cancer Epidemiol Biomarkers Prev. 2005;14(3):656–61.

69. Adams KF, Schatzkin A, Harris TB, et al. Overweight, obesity, and mortality in a large prospective cohort of persons 50 to 71 years old. N Engl J Med. 2006;355(8):763–78.

70. Webb P. Commentary: weight gain, weight loss, and endometrial cancer. Int J Epidemiol. 2006;35(1):301–2.

71. Eliassen AH, Colditz GA, Rosner B, Willett WC, Hankinson SE. Adult weight change and risk of postmenopausal breast cancer. JAMA. 2006;296(2):193–201.

72. Radimer KL, Ballard-Barbash R, Miller JS, et al. Weight change and the risk of late-onset breast cancer in the original Framingham cohort. Nutr Cancer. 2004;49(1):7–13.

73. Eng SM, Gammon MD, Terry MB, et al. Body size changes in relation to postmenopausal breast cancer among women on Long Island, New York. Am J Epidemiol. 2005;162(3):229–37.

74. Pierce JP, Natarajan L, Caan BJ, et al. Influence of a diet very high in vegetables, fruit, and fiber and low in fat on prognosis following treatment for breast cancer: the Women's Healthy Eating and Living (WHEL) randomized trial. JAMA. 2007;298(3):289–98.

75. Prentice RL, Caan B, Chlebowski RT, et al. Low-fat dietary pattern and risk of invasive breast cancer: the Women's Health Initiative Randomized Controlled Dietary Modification Trial. JAMA. 2006;295(6):629–42.

76. Chlebowski RT, Blackburn GL, Thomson CA, et al. Dietary fat reduction and breast cancer outcome: interim efficacy results from the Women's Intervention Nutrition Study. J Natl Cancer Inst. 2006;98(24):1767–76.

77. Williamson DF, Pamuk E, Thun M, Flanders D, Byers T, Heath C. Prospective study of intentional weight loss and mortality in never-smoking overweight US white women aged 40-64 years. Am J Epidemiol. 1995;141(12):1128–41.

78. Decensi A, Puntoni M, Goodwin P, et al. Metformin and cancer risk in diabetic patients: a systematic review and meta-analysis. Cancer Prev Res (Phila). 2010;3(11):1451–61.

79. Ligibel J. Obesity and breast cancer. Oncology. 2011;25(11):994–1000.

80. Protani M, Coory M, Martin JH. Effect of obesity on survival of women with breast cancer: systematic review and meta-analysis. Breast Cancer Res Treat. 2010;123(3):627–35.

81. Hewitt M, Greenfield S, Stovall E. From cancer patient to cancer survivor: lost in the transition. Washington, DC: Institute of Medicine and National Research Council; 2005.

82. Demark-Wahnefried W, Campbell KL, Hayes SC. Weight management and its role in breast cancer rehabilitation. Cancer. 2012;118(8 Suppl):2277–87.

83. Joshu CE, Mondul AM, Menke A, et al. Weight gain is associated with an increased risk of prostate cancer recurrence after prostatectomy in the PSA era. Cancer Prev Res (Phila). 2011;4(4):544–51.

84. Ashrafian H, Ahmed K, Rowland SP, et al. Metabolic surgery and cancer: protective effects of bariatric procedures. Cancer. 2011;117(9):1788–99.

85. Buchwald H, Estok R, Fahrbach K, et al. Weight and type 2 diabetes after bariatric surgery: systematic review and meta-analysis. Am J Med. 2009;122(3):248–256e245.

86. Courcoulas AP. Progress in filling the gaps in bariatric surgery. JAMA. 2012;308(11):1160–1.

87. Flum DR, Belle SH, King WC, et al. Perioperative safety in the longitudinal assessment of bariatric surgery. N Engl J Med. 2009;361(5):445–54.

88. Kushner RF, Noble CA. Long-term outcome of bariatric surgery: an interim analysis. Mayo Clin Proc. 2006;81(10 Suppl):S46–51.

89. Sjostrom L, Narbro K, Sjostrom CD, et al. Effects of bariatric surgery on mortality in Swedish obese subjects. N Engl J Med. 2007;357(8):741–52.

90. Monti V, Carlson JJ, Hunt SC, Adams TD. Relationship of ghrelin and leptin hormones with body mass index and waist circumference in a random sample of adults. J Am Diet Assoc. 2006; 106(6):822–8.

91. Mingrone G, Panunzi S, De Gaetano A, et al. Bariatric surgery versus conventional medical therapy for type 2 diabetes. N Engl J Med. 2012;366(17):1577–85.

92. Schauer PR, Kashyap SR, Wolski K, et al. Bariatric surgery versus intensive medical therapy in obese patients with diabetes. N Engl J Med. 2012;366(17):1567–76.

93. Dixon JB, O'Brien PE, Playfair J, et al. Adjustable gastric banding and conventional therapy for type 2 diabetes: a randomized controlled trial. JAMA. 2008;299(3):316–23.

94. MacDonald Jr KG, Long SD, Swanson MS, et al. The gastric bypass operation reduces the progression and mortality of non-insulin-dependent diabetes mellitus. J Gastrointest Surg. 1997; 1(3):213–20.

95. Kaul A, Sharma J. Impact of bariatric surgery on comorbidities. Surg Clin North Am. 2011;91(6):1295-1312, ix.

96. Menendez P, Padilla D, Villarejo P, Menendez JM, Lora D. Does bariatric surgery decrease gastric cancer risk? Hepatogastroenterology. 2012;59(114):409–12.

97. De Roover A, Detry O, Desaive C, et al. Risk of upper gastrointestinal cancer after bariatric operations. Obes Surg. 2006;16(12): 1656–61.

98. Renehan AG. Bariatric surgery, weight reduction, and cancer prevention. Lancet Oncol. 2009;10(7):640–1.

99. Adams TD, Gress RE, Smith SC, et al. Long-term mortality after gastric bypass surgery. N Engl J Med. 2007;357(8):753–61.

100. Sjostrom L, Gummesson A, Sjostrom CD, et al. Effects of bariatric surgery on cancer incidence in obese patients in Sweden (Swedish Obese Subjects Study): a prospective, controlled intervention trial. Lancet Oncol. 2009;10(7):653–62.

101. Christou NV, Sampalis JS, Liberman M, et al. Surgery decreases long-term mortality, morbidity, and health care use in morbidly obese patients. Ann Surg. 2004;240(3):416–23.

102. Christou NV, Lieberman M, Sampalis F, Sampalis JS. Bariatric surgery reduces cancer risk in morbidly obese patients. Surg Obes Relat Dis. 2008;4(6):691–5.

103. Ostlund MP, Lu Y, Lagergren J. Risk of obesity-related cancer after obesity surgery in a population-based cohort study. Ann Surg. 2010;252(6):972–6.

104. McCawley GM, Ferriss JS, Geffel D, Northup CJ, Modesitt SC. Cancer in obese women: potential protective impact of bariatric surgery. J Am Coll Surg. 2009;208(6):1093–8.

105. Gagne DJ, Papasavas PK, Maalouf M, Urbandt JE, Caushaj PF. Obesity surgery and malignancy: our experience after 1500 cases. Surg Obes Relat Dis. 2009;5(2):160–4.

106. Sjostrom L. Surgical intervention as a strategy for treatment of obesity. Endocrine. 2000;13(2):213–30.

107. Sjostrom L, Lonn L, Chowdhury B. The sagittal diameter is a valid marker of visceral adipose tissue volume. In: Angel A, Anderson H, Bouchard C, Lau D, Leiter L, Medelson R, editors. Recent advances in obesity research VII. London: John Libbey; 1996. p. 309–19.

108. Johnson C, Adamo M. The SEER Program: coding and staging manual 2007. Bethesda: Surveillance Research Program, Cancer Statistics Branch, Division of Cancer Control and Population Sciences, National Institutes of Health; 2007. NIH Pub. No. 07-5581.

109. Sainsbury A, Goodlad RA, Perry SL, Pollard SG, Robins GG, Hull MA. Increased colorectal epithelial cell proliferation and crypt fission associated with obesity and roux-en-Y gastric bypass. Cancer Epidemiol Biomarkers Prev. 2008;17(6):1401–10.

51

Obstructive Sleep Apnea in Bariatric Surgery Patients

Christopher R. Daigle and Stacy A. Brethauer

Introduction

Obstructive sleep apnea (OSA) is a chronic disease that affects up to 24 % of North American adults and is characterized by partial or complete airway obstructions that occur during sleep [1]. Patients with OSA suffer from loud snoring, fragmented sleep, daytime somnolence, and cardiorespiratory sequelae (hypoxia) which may go undiagnosed for years. There is a strong link between obesity and OSA, with the typical patient being overweight with numerous comorbidities; thus, a keen understanding of the perioperative diagnosis and management of sleep apnea is paramount when caring for bariatric surgery patients. Sleep apnea is also one of the many comorbidities that improve or resolve after bariatric surgery [2]. This chapter will review the pathophysiology, clinical features, preoperative evaluation, perioperative management, and postoperative outcomes of OSA in patients undergoing bariatric surgery.

Epidemiology and Pathophysiology

The general prevalence of OSA with daytime somnolence has been reported in the range of 3–7 %, but there are numerous factors like gender, age, comorbid conditions, alcohol, smoking, and obesity that influence the prevalence of OSA [3–5]. The incidence of OSA in bariatric surgery patients is up to 30 times greater than in the general population, and studies have shown that underdiagnosis is commonplace among obese patients. In fact, sleep studies performed during the preoperative assessment for bariatric surgery have suggested an overall prevalence of 48–91 % [6–10].

As previously mentioned, OSA is characterized by periodic episodes of hypopnea (partial airway obstruction) or apnea (complete airway obstruction) during sleep that are a direct result of narrowing in the upper airway. These events, which typically lead to loud snoring and restlessness, prevent the patient from achieving restful sleep and typically lead to significant daytime somnolence. Furthermore, the resulting hypoxia can have severe cardiovascular consequences, with OSA being linked to hypertension, ischemic heart disease, arrhythmias, stroke, and sudden/premature death, among other conditions [11–14]. The mechanism of periodic apneic or hypopneic episodes is thought to be due to increased amounts of upper airway (pharyngeal and tongue) soft tissue which preclude the passage of air to the larynx and, ultimately, the lungs [15]. While this can be seen as an anatomical variance in nonobese patients, this phenomenon is certainly more prevalent in overweight populations.

There are many factors that contribute to the degree of collapse of the upper airway that is seen in patients with OSA, and it is worth noting that these changes in airway caliber may not be present during wakefulness. With the onset of sleep, there is a physiologic reduction in neural-mediated activation and tone of the upper airway muscles. The decrease in airway tone is actually more than what is seen for the respiratory muscles proper, and the negative intrathoracic and intra-airway pressures that are generated during inspiration are transmitted to the more pliable pharynx. This normal physiologic phenomenon may have no consequences for those with normal amounts of upper airway soft tissue but can cause significant airway narrowing in patients with bulky upper airway soft tissue [16]. It has been hypothesized that the improvements seen in OSA patients who lose weight by any means (including bariatric surgery) are at least partially a result of a decrease in upper airway tissue bulk [17]. It is also recognized that increased levels of inflammatory cytokines and decreased expression of anti-inflammatory regulators are present in obese subjects with OSA, but their role in the pathophysiology is still unknown [17, 18].

The consequences of periodic hypopneic and apneic events are numerous, and a complete review is perhaps beyond the scope of this chapter. However, it is important to note that the effects reach far beyond disturbances in sleep patterns. For instance, the brief desaturations that occur while sleeping lead to drops in oxyhemoglobin concentrations and a subsequent decrease in both heart rate and blood pressure. When the obstruction is relieved, there is a reflex

S.A. Brethauer et al. (eds.), *Minimally Invasive Bariatric Surgery*,
DOI 10.1007/978-1-4939-1637-5_51, © Springer Science+Business Media New York 2015

surge in sympathetic autonomic tone, which leads to tachycardia and hypertension and can predispose to cardiac arrhythmias [19]. Some subjects with OSA also demonstrate hypercapnia and chronic respiratory acidosis during wakefulness, known as the obesity hypoventilation syndrome. These patients usually also suffer from chronic obstructive pulmonary disease (COPD) and are thought to be at even higher risk than those with OSA alone [20].

The constellation of effects that OSA imparts on obese individuals is significant and certainly raises concerns when considering bariatric surgery on patients who suffer from it. The importance of thorough preoperative assessment and testing by a multidisciplinary team cannot be overstated as it can drastically affect outcomes in an already high-risk population.

Clinical Features

Unfortunately, many of the clinical symptoms of OSA are nonspecific, and this may lead to delayed diagnosis. Patients may be asymptomatic or experience symptoms at night, during wakefulness, or both. The classic presentation is loud snoring with periods of "snorting" that are usually witnessed by a partner, and this is typically accompanied by excessive daytime sleepiness and the need for naps. While less common, patients may give a history of conscious "gasping" or "choking" episodes while abruptly waking from sleep [21, 22]. Over a prolonged period of time, these symptoms can lead to frequent headaches, irritability, and depressed mood, all of which can negatively affect quality of life for the patient and those around them [23].

Diagnosis

The diagnosis of OSA is made by clinical history, physical examination, validated screening tools, and polysomnography (PSG). While the numerous screening tools available can be useful in establishing a diagnosis (Table 51.1) (Maintenance of Wakefulness Test, the Epworth Sleepiness Scale, the Berlin 60 questionnaire, and the STOP-BANG questionnaire), their sensitivities vary, and a more reliable

TABLE 1. STOP-BANG scoring tool

Do you **S**nore loudly?	Yes/no
Do you often feel **T**ired, sleepy, or fatigued during the day?	Yes/no
Has anyone **O**bserved you stop breathing?	Yes/no
Have you been diagnosed with high blood **P**ressure?	Yes/no
BMI>35?	Yes/no
Age>50?	Yes/no
Neck circumference>17″ (male), 16″ (female)?	Yes/no
Gender=male?	Yes/no
Three "Yes" responses place the patient in the category of suspected high risk of having OSA	

Modified from Frances Chung et al. A tool to screen patients for obstructive sleep apnea. Anesthesiology 2008; 108:812–21

diagnosis can be achieved by PSG [24]. For a PSG study, the patient is admitted overnight to a sleep study lab, and the number of apneic and hypopneic events per hour is quantified. To be defined as apnea during the study, there must be a complete cessation of upper airway flow; to be defined as a hypopneic event, there must be a 50–90 % decrease in flow and at least a 4 % decrease in oxygen saturation for over 10 s. From this data, an apnea-hypopnea index (AHI) is calculated and used to not only diagnose OSA but also to characterize the severity of disease [25].

Treatment

While surgical procedures aimed at increasing airway patency do exist, their efficacies vary and many are not validated in morbidly obese patients [26, 27]. For the purpose of this review, we will focus on the medical treatment of OSA.

Continuous positive airway pressure (CPAP) is currently the mainstay in treatment of both obese and nonobese OSA patients (Fig. 51.1). It delivers continuous airway pressure that keeps the upper airway open during sleep, and studies have shown that it improves OSA-related desaturation events, hypertension, and "sleepiness" in those with an established diagnosis of OSA. Conventional nasal CPAP masks can be difficult to tolerate for some patients, and compliance is a constant concern, but numerous types of masks exist, and some may be better tolerated than others. For patients with significant nasal dryness or obstruction, a CPAP facemask can be utilized to improve therapy [28–30]. While no clear consensus exists on the duration of CPAP therapy before considering surgery, the patient should be given ample time to adjust to the system before moving ahead with surgery [10].

Previously, there have been concerns regarding the postoperative use of CPAP and the risk of anastomotic leak after Roux-en-Y gastric bypass based on studies that reported increased complication rates in those using postoperative CPAP [31, 32]. Because of these concerns, some have suggested omitting positive airway pressure therapy in the immediate postoperative period to avoid adverse surgical events. The American Society for Metabolic and Bariatric Surgery (ASMBS) released their position statement in 2012 addressing this issue and concluded that there was no evidence that postoperative CPAP increased the risk of anastomotic leak and that the usage of CPAP immediately after bariatric surgery was appropriate if indicated for pulmonary concerns [10].

Postoperative Care of the Bariatric Patient with Sleep Apnea

The level of postoperative monitoring and care required will ultimately depend on numerous patient- (OSA severity, other comorbidities) and procedure-specific factors (type of surgery,

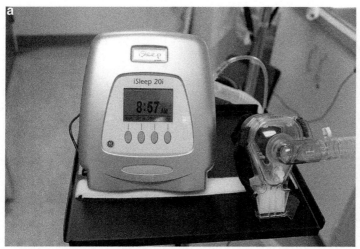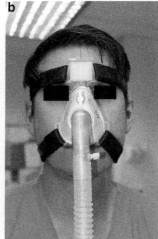

Fig. 1. (**a**) Continuous positive airway pressure (CPAP) device, with face mask (**b**). (GE Breas iSleep™ 20i self-adjusting CPAP; courtesy of GE Healthcare).

laparoscopic vs. open). Our patients are placed on continuous telemetry including pulse oximetry monitoring while on the surgical ward. Higher-risk patients such as those with severe OSA, numerous other comorbidities, superobesity, or advanced age may be better served with a brief ICU stay depending on the facility and airway expertise available at night. There are numerous published guidelines on the postoperative care of bariatric patients, and institutions vary regarding the protocols they incorporate into practice [33, 34]. The level of monitoring should be at the discretion of the surgeon in consultation with the medical consultants managing the patient. For instance, Grover et al. omitted intensive monitoring for their bariatric patients undergoing laparoscopic RYGB. Their cohort included over 200 patients with OSA, and they reported no increase in overall or pulmonary complications despite non-routine use of intensive monitoring [34]. There is consensus, however, that patients should continue their CPAP therapy postoperatively to avoid potential cardiopulmonary events in a patient already under considerable physiologic stress. Patients are encouraged to bring their own masks from home to ensure they have a properly fitting mask during their admission. It is also helpful to have experienced respiratory therapists who are comfortable with positive pressure therapy in morbidly obese patients. The surgeon and the multidisciplinary team should discuss the perioperative usage of CPAP at length with the patient prior to surgery.

Effect of Bariatric Surgery on Obstructive Sleep Apnea

Bariatric surgery is now considered to be the most effective way to achieve durable weight loss and has been shown to improve many obesity-related comorbidities like type 2 diabetes and metabolic syndrome [35–37]. Many studies have also shown that bariatric surgery is capable of improving or resolving OSA, which is not surprising given the fact that even modest weight loss can achieve some degree of improvement. Interestingly, many patients develop clinical improvement or resolution of symptoms of OSA after bariatric surgery, regardless of whether a normal BMI is achieved. In fact, 10–20 % weight loss has been associated with improvement of symptoms and a significant reduction in AHI [38]. It is important to note that not all causes of OSA are obesity related, and bariatric surgery may not improve symptoms of sleep apnea in all patients [39].

Marti-Valeri et al. reported prospective outcomes in 30 subjects who required CPAP (or BiPAP) therapy before RYGB surgery. At 1 year after RYGB, patients experienced significant weight loss and achieved a decrease in mean RDI assessed by PSG (63.6 ± 38.4 preoperatively, 17.4 ± 16.6 postoperatively; $p = 0.004$) [40]. Dixon and colleagues published their prospective randomized control trial assessing surgical (LAGB, $n = 30$) vs. conventional weight loss ($n = 30$) therapy for the treatment of OSA. At 2 years follow-up, the surgical cohort lost significantly more weight and achieved greater AHI reductions (reduction of 25.5 events/h vs. 14 events/h) than the conventional weight loss cohort [41]. Greenberg et al. performed a meta-analysis in 2009 looking at the effects of surgical weight loss on objective measures of OSA. Their analysis included 12 studies ($n = 342$ patients) that had polysomnography performed before and at least 3 months after bariatric surgery. The cohort achieved a 17.9 kg/m² reduction in BMI, which corresponded to a pooled cohort reduction of 38.2 hypopneic/apneic events per hour [2].

While many patients subjectively notice improvement in their sleep apnea after bariatric surgery and stop using their CPAP at home several months after surgery, we recommend that they continue to follow up with their pulmonologist to have their CPAP titrated down during the rapid weight loss phase. Patients should also undergo a repeat PSG 6–12 months after surgery to determine the need for further CPAP therapy.

Conclusion

Obstructive sleep apnea is prevalent in the morbidly obese, and bariatric surgeons must be aware of the history and symptoms suggestive of OSA, as well as the evaluation and management of these patients. A multidisciplinary approach involving the patient, surgeon, anesthetist, medical specialists, respiratory therapists, and support staff is paramount if these patients are to achieve therapeutic success. Metabolic surgery can offer these patients durable weight loss and improvement or remission of OSA.

References

1. Young T, Peppard PE, Gottlieb DJ. Epidemiology of obstructive sleep apnea: a population health perspective. Am J Respir Crit Care Med. 2002;165(9):1217–39.
2. Greenburg DL, Lettieri CJ, Eliasson AH. Effects of surgical weight loss on measures of obstructive sleep apnea: a meta-analysis. Am J Med. 2009;122(6):535–42.
3. Summers CL, Stradling JR, Baddeley RM. Treatment of sleep apnoea by vertical gastroplasty. Br J Surg. 1990;77(11):1271–2.
4. Bixler EO, Vgontzas AN, Lin HM, Ten Have T, Rein J, Vela-Bueno A, Kales A. Prevalence of sleep-disordered breathing in women: effects of gender. Am J Respir Crit Care Med. 2001;163:608–13.
5. Young T, Palta M, Dempsey J, Skatrud J, Weber S, Badr S. The occurrence of sleep-disordered breathing among middle-aged adults. N Engl J Med. 1993;328(17):1230–5.
6. Kyzer S, Charuzi I. Obstructive sleep apnea in the obese. World J Surg. 1998;22(9):998–1001.
7. Palla A, Digiorgio M, Carpene N, Rossi G, D'Amico I, Santini F, et al. Sleep apnea in morbidly obese patients: prevalence and clinical predictivity. Respiration. 2009;78(2):134–40.
8. Hallowell PT, Stellato TA, Schuster M, Graf K, Robinson A, Crouse C, et al. Potentially life-threatening sleep apnea is unrecognized without aggressive evaluation. Am J Surg. 2007;193(3):364–7.
9. Frey WC, Pilcher J. Obstructive sleep-related breathing disorders in patients evaluated for bariatric surgery. Obes Surg. 2003;13(5):676–83.
10. ASMBS position statement on peri-operative management of obstructive sleep apnea. 2012. www.asmbs.org
11. Somers VK, Dyken ME, Clary MP, Abboud FM. Sympathetic neural mechanisms in obstructive sleep apnea. J Clin Invest. 1995;96(4):1897–904.
12. Parra O, Arboix A, Bechich S, Garcia-Eroles L, Montserrat JM, Lopez JA, et al. Time course of sleep-related breathing disorders in first-ever stroke or transient ischemic attack. Am J Respir Crit Care Med. 2000;161(2 Pt 1):375–80.
13. Gami AS, Howard DE, Olson EJ, Somers VK. Day-night pattern of sudden death in obstructive sleep apnea. N Engl J Med. 2005;352(12):1206–14.
14. Mehra R, Benjamin EJ, Shahar E, Gottlieb DJ, Nawabit R, Kirchner HL, et al. Association of nocturnal arrhythmias with sleep-disordered breathing: the sleep heart health study. Am J Respir Crit Care Med. 2006;173(8):910–6.
15. Schwab RJ, Pasirstein M, Pierson R, Mackley A, Hachadoorian R, Arens R, et al. Identification of upper airway anatomic risk factors for obstructive sleep apnea with volumetric magnetic resonance imaging. Am J Respir Crit Care Med. 2003;168(5):522–30.
16. Kryger MH, Roth T, Dement WC. Principles and practices of sleep medicine. 3rd ed. Philadelphia: WB Saunders; 2000.
17. Vgontzas AN, Papanicolaou DA, Bixler EO, Hopper K, Lotsikas A, Lin HM, Kales A, Chrousos GP. Sleep apnea and daytime sleepiness and fatigue: relation to visceral obesity, insulin resistance, and hypercytokinemia. J Clin Endocrinol Metab. 2000;85(3):1151–8.
18. Sharma S, Malur A, Marshall I, Huizar I, Barna BP, Pories W, Dohm L, Kavuru MS, Thomassen MJ. Alveolar macrophage activation in obese patients with obstructive sleep apnea. Surgery. 2012;151(1):107–12.
19. Salah HA. Obstructive sleep apnea and cardiac arrhythmias. Ann Thorac Med. 2010;5(1):10–7.
20. Kessler R, Chaouat A, Schinkewitch P, et al. The obesity-hypoventilation syndrome revisited: a prospective study of 34 consecutive cases. Chest. 2001;120:369–76.
21. Sleep-related breathing disorders in adults: recommendations for syndrome definition and measurement techniques in clinical research. The Report of an American Academy of Sleep Medicine Task Force. Sleep. 1999;22:667–89.
22. Kimoff RJ, Cosio MG, McGregor M. Clinical features and treatment of obstructive sleep apnea. Can Med Assoc J. 1991;144:689–95.
23. Ohayon MM. The effects of breathing-related sleep disorders on mood disturbances in the general population. J Clin Psychiatry. 2003;64:1195–200. quiz, 1274–1276.
24. Abrishami A, Khajehdehi A, Chung F. A systematic review of screening questionnaires for obstructive sleep apnea. Can J Anaesth. 2010;57(5):423–38.
25. Norman D, Loredo JS. Obstructive sleep apnea in older adults. Clin Geriatr Med. 2008;24(1):151–65.
26. Holty JE, Guilleminault C. Surgical options for the treatment of obstructive sleep apnea. Med Clin North Am. 2010;94(3):479–515.
27. Khan A, Ramar K, Maddirala S, Friedman O, Pallanch JF, Olson EJ. Uvulopalatopharyngoplasty in the management of obstructive sleep apnea: the mayo clinic experience. Mayo Clin Proc. 2009;84(9):795–800.
28. Chai CL, Pathinathan A, Smith B. Continuous positive airway pressure delivery interfaces for obstructive sleep apnoea. Cochrane Database Syst Rev. 2006;18(4), CD005308.
29. Giles TL, Lasserson TJ, Smith BH, White J, Wright J, Cates CJ. Continuous positive airways pressure for obstructive sleep apnoea in adults. Cochrane Database Syst Rev. 2006;19(3), CD001106.
30. Rauscher H, Formanek D, Popp W, Zwick H. Self-reported vs measured compliance with nasal CPAP for obstructive sleep apnea. Chest. 1993;103(6):1675–80.
31. Perugini RA, Mason R, Czerniach DR, et al. Predictors of complication and suboptimal weight loss after laparoscopic Roux-en-Y gastric bypass: a series of 188 patients. Arch Surg. 2003;138:541–5. discussion 545–546.
32. Fernandez Jr AZ, DeMaria EJ, Tichansky DS, et al. Experience with over 3,000 open and laparoscopic bariatric procedures: multivariate analysis of factors related to leak and resultant mortality. Surg Endosc. 2004;18:193–7. Epub 2003 Dec 29.
33. Schumann R, Jones SB, Cooper B, Kelley SD, Bosch MV, Ortiz VE, et al. Update on best practice recommendations for anesthetic perioperative care and pain management in weight loss surgery, 2004-2007. Obesity (Silver Spring). 2009;17(5):889–94.
34. Grover BT, Priem DM, Mathiason MA, Kallies KJ, Thompson GP, Kothari SN. Intensive care unit stay not required for patients with obstructive sleep apnea after laparoscopic roux-en-Y gastric bypass. Surg Obes Relat Dis. 2010;6(2):165–70.

35. Schauer PR, Kashyap SR, Wolski K, Brethauer SA, Kirwan JP, Pothier CE, Thomas S, Abood B, Nissen SE, Bhatt DL. Bariatric surgery versus intensive medical therapy in obese patients with diabetes. N Engl J Med. 2012;366(17):1567–76.

36. Mingrone G, Panunzi S, De Gaetano A, Guidone C, Iaconelli A, Leccesi L, Nanni G, Pomp A, Castagneto M, Ghirlanda G, Rubino F. Bariatric surgery versus conventional medical therapy for type 2 diabetes. N Engl J Med. 2012;366(17):1577–85.

37. Aminian A, Daigle CR, Romero-Talamás H, Kashyap SR, Kirwan JP, Brethauer SA, Schauer PR. Risk prediction of complications of metabolic syndrome before and 6 years after gastric bypass. Surg Obes Relat Dis. In Press, Available online 29 January 2014.

38. Peppard PE, Young T, Palta M, Dempsey J, Skatrud J. Longitudinal study of moderate weight change and sleep-disordered breathing. JAMA. 2000;284(23):3015–21.

39. Lettieri CJ, Eliasson AH, Greenburg DL. Persistence of obstructive sleep apnea after surgical weight loss. J Clin Sleep Med. 2008; 4(4):333–8.

40. Marti-Valeri C, Sabate A, Masdevall C, Dalmau A. Improvement of associated respiratory problems in morbidly obese patients after open roux-en-Y gastric bypass. Obes Surg. 2007;17(8):1102–10.

41. Dixon JB, Schachter LM, O'Brien PE. Polysomnography before and after weight loss in obese patients with severe sleep apnea. Int J Obes (Lond). 2005;29(9):1048–54.

52

Ventral Hernias in the Bariatric Patient

Krzysztof J. Wikiel and George M. Eid

Introduction

Ventral hernia, a collective term for incisional, umbilical, and other anterior abdominal wall defects, is quite common in obese population. With almost 40 % of the population considered obese, and nearly two-thirds are overweight, today's general surgeons will encounter this disease process often. Management of these hernias, especially in the morbidly obese population, poses multiple dilemmas and challenges, and requires a careful and holistic approach to the patient.

Epidemiology, Etiology, and Risk Factors

Over one-third of adult the US population is now considered obese, and by some accounts, over six is considered morbidly obese [1, 2]. As prevalence of obesity and morbid obesity increases, general surgeons will encounter this and related disease processes quite often. The morbidly obese patient group is thought to be at a particularly high risk of development and progression of abdominal wall defects because of increased intra-abdominal pressure and poor wound healing potential. Additionally, comorbidites often associated with obesity, such as type 2 diabetes mellitus, sleep apnea, previous incisional hernias, obesity hypoventilation syndrome, and wound infections, can play a role in the development of hernias [3]. It is also important to mention that smoking is another important risk factor for development of incisional hernias as well as hernia recurrences, as smoking has been clearly associated with altered surgical wound healing [4].

Ventral hernias are more common in the older population, with mean age 51 [5] and a male-to-female ratio of 1.6:1. Umbilical hernias are also relatively common and will most likely occur in the fifth and sixth decades of life [5, 6]*. Primary hernias, like umbilical hernias, tend to be an acquired defect in over 90 % of adults [7]. About 8 % of these are recurrent, with omental incarceration in 30 %. The average size of the hernia defect in this population is 25.4 cm^2 with multiple defects in 5 % [8].

Incisional hernias complicate 3–13 % of laparotomies in the general surgical population [9]*. This number is much higher in the bariatric population; this was especially noted in the group of patients who have undergone open bariatric procedure [3]. As open bariatric surgery is falling out of favor, many hernias are now detected when patients undergo another procedure. Nassar et al. report a 12 % incidence of umbilical or periumbilical defects in patients undergoing laparoscopic cholecystectomy [10]. Eight percent of bariatric patients will have a ventral hernia discovered during their bariatric procedure and these may create additional treatment dilemmas [11].

Clinical Presentation

While most patients with a ventral hernia present with a bulge on the abdominal wall, this may not be the case in the morbidly obese patient where the diagnosis may present a challenge [12]. Occasionally, the obese patients may present for the first time with abdominal pain, nausea, or small bowel obstruction. It should be noted that due to patient body habitus, it may be difficult to feel the hernia defect due to a thick abdominal wall, and a computed tomography (CT) scan of the abdomen may be warranted [13]. Often, even large ventral hernias may go unnoticed, and the diagnosis is first made intraoperatively during other procedures.

Treatment

Appropriate management of obese patients with ventral hernias is a complex and controversial topic with lack of consensus among the surgical community on the ideal approach to treating this condition. Those controversies range from the

S.A. Brethauer et al. (eds.), *Minimally Invasive Bariatric Surgery*,
DOI 10.1007/978-1-4939-1637-5_52, © Springer Science+Business Media New York 2015

need for concomitant repair at the time of a bariatric procedure as opposed to a delayed treatment following weight loss to the appropriate approach to use in cases that violate the intestinal tract to appropriate mesh and procedure selection. With the understanding that the literature provides little guidance regarding the ideal method to address hernias in obese patients or in conjunction with bariatric surgery, we present the approach we utilize at our institution.

The question that needs to be immediately answered is whether the patient is symptomatic or asymptomatic. This could aid in the selection of method as well as timing of ventral hernia repair in this patient population. As a good proportion of these defects are noted during bariatric procedures, an important consideration is whether to place mesh into a clean-contaminated field encountered during bariatric procedures that violate the gastrointestinal tract, such as laparoscopic Roux-en-Y gastric bypass or laparoscopic sleeve gastrectomy, as opposed to performing a primary hernia repair. On the other hand deferring surgical repair may result in significant morbidity. In our experience, 36 % of patients whose hernia repair was deferred at the time of gastric bypass developed small bowel obstruction due to incarceration in the postoperative period. The time interval for this complication is an average of 63 days (range 10–150 days) from the bariatric procedure [8]. The risk of infecting a prosthetic mesh by contamination with enteric contents is also well documented, and the authors of this text do not recommend using these meshes if the defect repair is concomitant with a bariatric procedure which violates the gastrointestinal system.

The basis of our approach is the notion that all hernias are not created equal, and that every bariatric patient with an abdominal wall defect should be approached individually. Certain factors, such as the patient's past medical history, body mass index (BMI), body habitus, defect size and location, level of operative field contamination, and the presence or absence of symptoms, should always be taken into consideration while developing a surgical plan.

In our opinion, the most important factors to consider when planning a hernia repair are body habitus based on fat distribution (android versus gynecoid), BMI, hernia location, and reducibility. During the work-up, computer tomography is used for a precise evaluation of the defect size, contents, and abdominal wall thickness. The above criteria are then used to divide patients into favorable and unfavorable anatomy groups. If the defect is located centrally or in the upper half of the abdomen, it allows for easier accessibility and laparoscopic port placement; it is considered favorable. Lower abdominal defects are considered unfavorable. Android body habitus is considered unfavorable due to less compliant abdominal wall and intra-abdominal fat distribution causing increased technical difficulty, as opposed to favorable gynecoid fat distribution. Patients with abdominal wall thicker than 4 cm are placed in the unfavorable group, as thicker abdominal wall tends to cause greater torque on laparoscopic instruments, leading to increased surgical difficulty

of the hernia repair. Patients with a thinner abdominal wall were considered to have favorable anatomy. Hernia reducibility is considered a favorable feature, as incarcerated contents may be more difficult to reduce intraoperatively. Hernias of 8 cm or less in greatest diameter were also considered favorable, because they allow the surgeon to approximate the edges of the defect with primary sutures under reduced pneumoperitoneum. Finally, a BMI of 50 kg/m^2 or greater was considered unfavorable due to the elevated operative risks associated with super-obese patients [14].

Our algorithm divides the patients into four treatment subgroups (Fig. 1):

1. Symptomatic patients with favorable anatomy: Here we recommend that these patients undergo ventral hernia repair as an initial and separate procedure. This repair may be followed by bariatric procedure of choice at a later date. Generally this group qualifies for laparoscopic hernia repair which is described later in this text.

2. Asymptomatic patients with favorable anatomy: These patients are good candidates to undergo concomitant bariatric surgery and ventral hernia repair. We recommend that after performing laparoscopic bariatric procedure, the surgeon addresses the hernia defect. If possible abdominal wall is repaired primarily with the placement of nonabsorbable sutures using a suture-passing device through the abdominal wall and fascia to decrease rate of recurrence (Fig. 2, photo 1). The approximated defect was then reinforced using biologic mesh (Fig. 2, photo 2). The mesh was introduced through the abdomen via one of the port sites and secured in place with both sutures and circumferential tacks.

3. Symptomatic patients with unfavorable anatomy present the biggest challenge from surgical standpoint. In this population we recommend a medically supervised very low calorie diet for up to 12 weeks. Dietary supplements, including daily multivitamins as well as ursodiol treatment to prevent gallstone formation during rapid weight loss, should be given to these patients. This group requires careful monitoring with qualified medical staff to ensure no adverse health changes. Once appropriate weight loss is achieved these patients are candidates to undergo a hernia repair either with concomitant or deferred bariatric procedure.

4. Asymptomatic patients with unfavorable anatomy are best treated with bariatric surgery first, followed by a ventral hernia repair at a later date, only after significant weight loss had occurred. At our institution laparoscopic gastric bypass and sleeve gastrectomy are the preferred options, given the more likely early rapid weight loss. This would allow a timely repair of the abdominal wall hernia. Nevertheless, the decision for which procedure to perform should be made jointly by the patient and the surgeon after thorough discussion and counseling.

Next consideration is the choice of surgical modality. Ventral hernia repairs have evolved considerably over the

FIG. 1. Algorithm for ventral
hernia repair in the morbidly
obese patient.

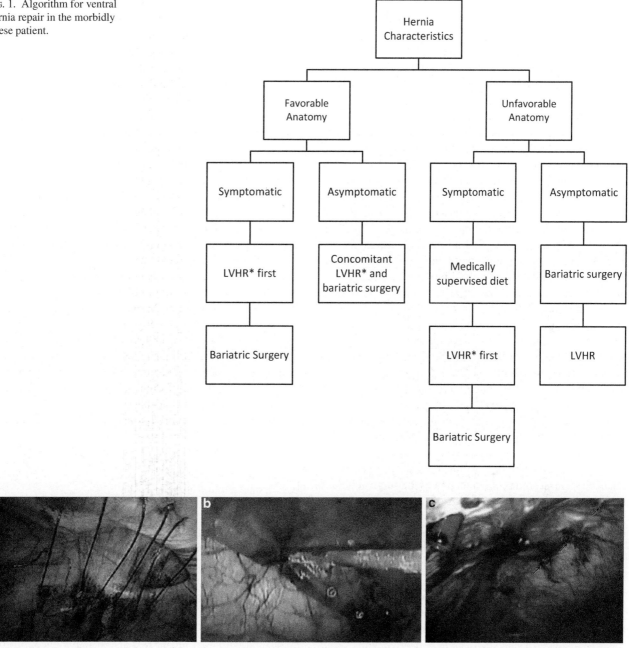

FIG. 2. Ventral hernia repair at time of bariatric surgery with follow-up laparoscopy 1 year later. (**a**) Suture repair of the hernia defect at the time of a laparoscopic Roux-en-Y gastric bypass (step #1). (**b**) Subsequent placement of biologic mesh as a reinforcement of the primary suture repair during a laparoscopic Roux-en-Y gastric bypass (step #2). (**c**) Anterior abdominal wall of the patient above who was undergoing an elective laparoscopic cholecystectomy at the 24-month time mark. Note the absence of the hernia defect and visible partially peritonized surgical tacks.

years. Traditional open primary suture repairs are falling out of favor especially in the obese population, as the reported recurrence rates have been over 50 % [15]. Open tension-free mesh repairs, including separation of components procedure, have considerably lower recurrence estimated at 20–30 %. Unfortunately, large abdominal incisions in the morbidly obese patients with wide tissue dissection and flap creation result in a fairly high incidence of postoperative morbidity and wound complications [15]. Nevertheless the latter still remains a good option in some patient groups and is still widely used.

Laparoscopic ventral hernia repair was first reported about 20 years ago. Application of this method in certain situations might be advantageous, as it is associated with fewer complications and faster recovery [15–17]. It appears that this advance in hernia repair might benefit the bariatric patient as well, just as recent studies have demonstrated an advantage of the laparoscopic approach over open bariatric surgery [18]. Similarly, shorter hospital stays, decreased pain, lower wound complications, lower recurrence rates, and quicker return to work are reported for laparoscopic ventral hernia repair patients [15–19].

The technique we have chosen to use in our patient population is based on the modified Rives-Stoppa technique. This involves reduction of the hernia and, under laparoscopic vision, outlining the hernia defect on anterior abdominal wall skin using a marker pen. A further outline adds an extra 4-cm overlay margin. An appropriate mesh, depending on the level of contamination during the case, is placed and then tailored to size using the outline on the abdominal wall. Nonabsorbable sutures are placed onto the corners of the mesh, which is then rolled up and introduced into the abdomen through a trocar. Using a Carter-Thomason device, the mesh is anchored into the desired position using the previously placed sutures. The mesh is further anchored with several rows of titanium helical tacks placed circumferentially at about 1-cm intervals. Through several small stab incisions, the mesh is secured in place using nonabsorbable sutures at 3-cm intervals along its circumference. This is also done with the Carter-Thomason device.

Weight loss surgery may be an important adjunct treatment in the management of ventral hernia. Unfortunately, laparoscopic gastric bypass as well as sleeve gastrectomy both require division of the gastrointestinal tract, which results in at least some contamination of the surgical field. In such cases, there is a general lack of acceptance within the surgical community of concomitant bariatric surgery and hernia repair with permanent mesh, due to risk of mesh infection. However, limited data has been reported demonstrating the feasibility of such an approach. A small trial in which ventral hernias were repaired with prosthetic dual meshes in conjunction with laparoscopic gastric bypass has been reported. No mesh infections and two recurrences were seen in this study [20]. While such data does exist, it is by no means considered a standard of care, as it only involves small series with lack of long-term follow-up. Mesh infection, necessitating subsequent mesh removal, is a very morbid and costly problem in an already high risk bariatric patient population, not to mention the high recurrence rates associated with mesh infections and the potential medical-legal implications. For those reasons, we do not favor this approach.

High recurrence rates have been encountered when bio-absorbable mesh is used as a bridge to close the hernia defect in a similar fashion to permanent mesh. Although initial data reported zero recurrence rates at short-term follow-up using this technique concomitantly with laparoscopic gastric bypass, unfortunately, majority of patients will present with a recurrence when followed for over 2 years. While some surgeons routinely use the above technique as a temporary fix with the main goal of avoiding bowel strangulation, clearly it cannot be considered a permanent repair. The reasoning behind this is that deferring repair of the defect carries a significant risk of bowel incarceration and possibly even strangulation, especially when the surgeon reduces an omental incarceration without addressing the underlying hernia [8]. Based on our experience, we believe that the use of bio-absorbable mesh with concomitant laparoscopic gastric bypass can only be effectively utilized as reinforcement for suture repair. On the other hand, concomitant bariatric surgery and hernia repair in patients with unfavorable hernia and body habitus characteristics as described above can be challenging and time consuming. Performing a bariatric procedure at the time of the hernia repair not only adds considerable operation time and risk, but also introduces contamination with subsequent risk for mesh infection as previously mentioned.

As mentioned above, it is not unusual to find incidental hernias during laparoscopy which have remained asymptomatic while performing bariatric surgery. Most of these defects, missed during preoperative work-up, are small and have greatest diameter less than 2 cm. These defects should be repaired primarily with the use of permanent sutures using a Carter-Thomason suture-passing device with simple or figure-of-eight stitches (Fig. 3). It is also important to mention that these small hernias need to be addressed as they are more likely to lead to potential bowel strangulation requiring emergent surgery with potential poor outcomes [5, 8].

Clinical Pearls

Hernias still present a therapeutic challenge in the morbidly obese and as the prevalence of obesity increases, so does the incidence of ventral hernias in the obese population. Those patients require a complex and thought-out approach, devised on a case-by-case basis. It is also important to make the morbidly obese patient aware of the potential intraoperative discovery of incidental hernias and the high risk of recurrence associated with their repair. It is also strongly encouraged to repair all incarcerated incisional hernias in the morbidly obese population, that required reduction to complete the bariatric procedure, because of the high risk of strangulating bowel obstruction in the postoperative period [8].

Concomitant hernia repair with bariatric procedure versus a staged approach should be based on patients' symptoms and the hernia characteristics. Our suggested algorithm has been helpful in our practice with the selection of timing, mesh, and type of repair. All decisions are made on individual case basis. In cases of concomitant repair, reinforcing defects that are >2 cm in diameter with biomaterial mesh as an underlay following primary repair may help reduce the incidence of hernia recurrences [5].

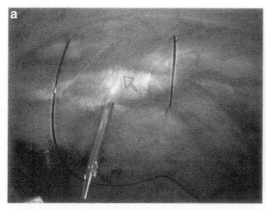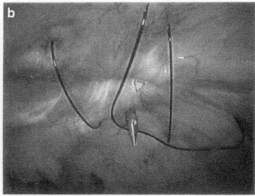

FIG. 3. (**a**) Sutures are placed across the fascial defect (*arrow*) with a Carter-Thomason device. (**b**) All sutures are tied once the pneumoperitoneum has been released.

Review Questions and Answers

Question 1

Bariatric patients are thought to be at increased risk of incisional hernia development because of:

(a) Increased Intra-abdominal pressure.
(b) Poor wound healing potential in the morbidly obese.
(c) Respiratory issues such as sleep apnea and obesity hypoventilation syndrome commonly seen in the morbidly obese population.
(d) Comorbidities such as diabetes mellitus.
(e) All of the above.

Answer: *E*. All of the mentioned answers are thought to play a role in increased risk of incisional hernia development in the obese patients.

Question 2

One of the major advantages of laparoscopic hernia repair in the bariatric population is:
(a) Better cosmetic outcome.
(b) Better visualization of the defect.
(c) Decreased risk of postoperative wound complications.
(d) All of the above.

Answer: *C*. Decreased risk of wound complications is considered one of the major advantages of laparoscopic over open repair.

Question 3

The best treatment option for an incidental periumbilical hernia encountered during a laparoscopic gastric bypass which contains omentum and with greatest diameter of 4 cm is:

(a) This defect will never need to be addressed and therefore should be left alone.
(b) This defect should be left alone for now and repaired at a later time with the use of permanent mesh.
(c) The omentum should be reduced to prevent incarceration, but the defect itself should be repaired at a later time.
(d) This defect should be repaired at the time of the bariatric surgery.

Answer: *D*. We suggest that the best treatment option for such defects is to perform the repair at the time of the initial bariatric surgery. This is done to prevent strangulation of bowel.

References

1. Sturm R, Hatton A. Morbid obesity rates continue to rise rapidly in the United States. Int J Obes (Lond). 2012;6:889–91.
2. Flegal KM, Carroll MD, Kit BK, Ogden CL. Prevalence of obesity and trends in distribution of body mass index among US adults 1999–2010. JAMA. 2012;307(5):491–7.
3. Sugerman HJ, Kellum Jr JM, Reines HD, DeMaria EJ, Newsome HH, Lowry JW. Greater risk of incisional hernia with morbidly obese than steroid-dependent patients and low recurrence with prefascial polypropylene mesh. Am J Surg. 1996;171:80–4.
4. Sorensen LT. Wound healing and infection in surgery: the pathophysiological impact of smoking, smoking cessation and nicotine replacement therapy. Ann Surg. 2012;255:1069–79.

5. Eid GM, et al. Laparoscopic repair of umbilical hernias in conjunction with other laparoscopic procedures. JSLS. 2006;10:63–5.

6. Harmel RP. Umbilical hernia. In: Nyhus LM, Condon RE, editors. Hernia. Philadelphia: Lippincott Williams & Wilkins; 1989. p. 347–52.

7. Morgan WW, White JJ, Stumbaugh S, Haller Jr JA. Prophylactic umbilical hernia repair in childhood to prevent adult incarceration. Surg Clin North Am. 1970;50:839–45.

8. Eid GM, et al. Repair of ventral hernias in morbidly obese patients undergoing laparoscopic gastric bypass should not be deferred. Surg Endosc. 2004;18:207–10.

9. Mudge M, Hughes LE. Incisional hernia: a 10 year prospective study of incidence and attitudes. Br J Surg. 1985;72:70–1.

10. Nassar AH, Ashkar KA, Rashed AA, Abdulmoneum MG. Laparoscopic cholecystectomy and the umbilicus. Br J Surg. 1997;84:630–3.

11. Datta T, Eid G, Nahmias N, Dallal RM. Management of ventral hernias during gastric bypass. Surg Obes Relat Dis. 2006;2(3):389–92.

12. Ianora AA, Midiri M, Vinci R, Rotondo A, Angelelli G. Abdominal wall hernias: imaging with spiral CT. Eur Radiol. 2000;10:914–9.

13. Rubio PA, Del Castillo H, Alvarez BA. Ventral hernia in a massively obese patient: diagnosis by computerized tomography. South Med J. 1988;81:1307–8.

14. Cottam D, Qureshi FG, Mattar SG, et al. Laparoscopic sleeve gastrectomy as an initial weight-loss procedure for high-risk patients with morbid obesity. Surg Endosc. 2006;20:859–63.

15. Heniford BT, Park A, Ramshaw BJ, Voeller G. Laparoscopic repair of ventral hernias: nine years' experience with 850 consecutive hernias. Ann Surg. 2003;238:391–9;discussion 9–400.

16. Novitsky YW, Cobb WS, Kercher KW, Matthews BD, Sing RF, Heniford BT. Laparoscopic ventral hernia repair in obese patients: a new standard of care. Arch Surg. 2006;141:57–61.

17. Birgisson G, Park AE, Mastrangelo Jr MJ, Witzke DB, Chu UB. Obesity and laparoscopic repair of ventral hernias. Surg Endosc. 2001;15:1419–22.

18. Hutter MM, Randall S, Khuri SF, Henderson WG, Abbott WM, Warshaw AL. Laparoscopic versus open gastric bypass for morbid obesity: a multicenter, prospective, risk-adjusted analysis from the National Surgical Quality Improvement Program. Ann Surg. 2006;243:657–62;discussion 62–6.

19. Park AE, Roth JS, Kavic SM. Abdominal wall hernia. Curr Probl Surg. 2006;43:326–75.

20. Schuster R, Curet MJ, Alami RS, Morton JM, Wren SM, Safadi BY. Concurrent gastric bypass and repair of anterior abdominal wall hernias. Obes Surg. 2006;16(9):1205–8.

53

Plastic Surgery Following Weight Loss

Dennis Hurwitz

Minimally invasive gastrointestinal bypass surgery for morbid obesity was successfully pioneered at the University of Pittsburgh Medical Center [1]. Soon dozens of women demanded a solution to their hanging skin and ptotic breasts and buttocks. I accepted the request by the surgeon director, Philip Schauer, to focus my plastic surgery skills on body contouring after massive weight loss. Speaking in lecture halls full of these patients, I learned of the disheartening changes in body contour with repulsive hanging skin and bizarre rolls of skin and fat. In the course of achieving extraordinary weight loss and alleviation of comorbidities, successful bariatric surgery creates these problems that diminish patients' quality of life. The Bariatric Center clinical staff in Pittsburgh and then throughout the country anticipate these issues and encourage completion of rehabilitation through skilled body contouring surgery.

In the late 1990s, many plastic surgeons agreed that skin redundancy of the trunk and thigh is best treated by a circumferential abdominoplasty and a lower body lift [2–8]. However, results vary, and there is no consensus on approach. The magnitude of the challenge for each patient was just being appreciated. The concept of multiple operations during a single operative session was introduced but by no means accepted. There are few reports that include body contouring surgery after massive weight loss. Those patients of the 1970s usually underwent the physiologically disruptive jejunal-ileal bypass and were poor candidates for prolonged body contouring surgery. Minimally invasive surgery with the Roux-en-Y gastrointestinal bypass delivered a much less traumatized and healthier patient. Consistent patterns of deformity were discovered, necessitating individualization and new combination of procedures. Hence, I was in a position to explore a variety of approaches, procedures, and patient intraoperative positioning. An innovative approach evolved that featured comprehensive and coordinated planning in one to three stages, termed the total body lift. Not only was loose skin to be removed but the body was to be sculpted by what was left behind and by autogenous flaps

for breast and buttock augmentation and suspension. These are extensive and complex operations over large portions of the body, requiring a team of operators, working in consort from 6 to 12 h under general anesthesia. Minor wound healing complications were common, but major morbidity was fortunately rare.

By diligent assessment of outcomes, feedback from numerous presentations and the work of others, I have tailored body contouring surgery to adequately treat the deformities and needs of the patient. A complete medical and nutritional evaluation with comprehensive consideration of the total body deformity is essential. The plan is based on the application of plastic surgical principles that incorporate artistry, efficiency, and tight closures, with minimal trauma to tissues (Table 1).

This chapter presents the patient profile, preoperative preparation, and operative planning. There is a summary of the operative technique, as well as selected case presentations. Advances since the first edition of this text will be highlighted. The principles of treatment are detailed, followed by an evaluation of the surgical outcomes. Over the past 12 years, this author has performed over 1,600 procedures on more than 500 patients after massive weight loss, pregnancy, or aging. These include singly or in combination abdominoplasty, lower body lift, upper body lift, medial thighplasty, brachioplasty, mastopexy, breast reduction, facelift, gynecomastia correction liposuction, and lipoaugmentation. The body mass index (BMI) ranged from 24 to 42. Due to the potential of a high rate of complications, we have treated few patients with morbid obesity [9].

Patient Profile

Obesity is a stigmatizing disorder, especially among women, which may explain why women predominate in seeking weight loss treatment [2]. The increased demand is due to word-of-mouth comments on the improved results and lower

S.A. Brethauer et al. (eds.), *Minimally Invasive Bariatric Surgery*,
DOI 10.1007/978-1-4939-1637-5_53, © Springer Science+Business Media New York 2015

TABLE 1. Plastic surgical principles

1. Analyze deformity and patient
2. Be efficient in design and execution
3. Excise excess as much as possible transversely
4. Position incisions favorably, and respect scars
5. Focus on the ultimate contour and tissue tension
6. Preserve healthy dermis and subcutaneous fascia
7. Remove fat from flaps gently and effectively
8. Make closure tight and secure
9. Minimize swelling, infection, phlebitis, and seroma
10. Analyze your experience

morbidity, supported by reports in scientific journals, the Internet, and the media [10]. Over 80 % of the patients in this series seeking body contouring after weight loss are women.

Most patients report to me that their laparoscopic bypass operation was brief, followed by easily controlled pain. Through four to six small incisions, their peritoneal cavity has been inflated to expose intestines for rerouting and/or partition over what has routinely become a 2-h session. They are discharged within days to return to work within a week. Those who are converted to open procedures due to technical considerations tend to have a slightly more prolonged post-operative course. Delayed wound healing and incisional hernia are common in the open group. Extensive scars and abdominal hernias are important considerations in abdominoplasty planning.

With small gastric pouches and a moderately long Roux-en-Y jejunal bypass (the length varies directly with the degree of obesity [11]), the patients shed pounds rapidly due to limited intake, reduced absorption, and early satiety. Many experience mild gastrointestinal dumping after minimal sugar or fat intake. Most become uninterested in food, which may be a hormonally mediated change. All are encouraged to maintain a small caloric multiple-meal diet and an active exercise program, in anticipation of increased gastrointestinal capacity over time. In general, patients lose weight because of reduced food intake and increased physical activity and not intestinal malabsorption. Many become champions of bariatric surgery and encourage others at a variety of organized support group meetings. Most have been introduced to the results of plastic surgery at these group meetings and individually through the bariatric nurse coordinators, who have personal experience. A referral program called Life after Bypass has been instituted at the University of Pittsburgh. Patients receive automatic appointments and an informative brochure about body contouring surgery, shortly after their bypass. Patients find their way to the Hurwitz Center for Plastic Surgery through Internet searches, word-of-mouth referrals, and national television programs featuring the total body lift (the author's signature procedure).

After a steady weight loss to about 70 % of their excess weight over 18 months, most regain about 20 % over the next few years [12]. Therefore, if a patient's weight loss reaches a plateau, waiting beyond 18 months before initiating body contouring surgery is counterproductive. Commonly, over the next year patients gain much of the weight removed during body contouring surgery. On the other hand, in some patients unanticipated further weight loss occurs, from 20 to 60 lb, because of partial gastrointestinal mechanical obstruction. This causes malnutrition reflected in low serum prealbumin fraction, anemia, and measurably low trace elements [13]. The nutritional deficiency may prolong what would otherwise be minor wound healing problems [14]. Additional weight loss results in new skin laxity, which will detract from what could have been an optimal outcome.

The patients who struggle with their layers of hanging skin and fat and have the courage to consider surgery present to plastic surgeons. When obese, their massive size presented an unappealing but recognizable shape. Hanging skin distorts the body shape and patient age and appearance, and it flaps around during vigorous activity. Skin beneath folds becomes moist, malodorous, and inflamed. Clothes fit poorly. Embarrassment of their hanging pannus, mons pubis, and inner thighs thwarts sexual intimacy. While many comprehend that plastic surgery is an anticipated part of their rehabilitation, they still may resent and even regret the bypass operation. The plastic surgeon's empathy is important, especially when asking the patient to accept the new risks and self-pay costs of body contouring surgery. If the patient has limited financial means, we offer national cosmetic surgery finance plans at reasonable rates for those with good credit.

With the ease of convalescence, effective weight loss, improved exercise habits, and encouragement from others who have gone before them, patients are accepting of the arduous body contouring procedures yet ahead. The opportune time to perform body contouring is when the patient has completed the catabolism and has reduced comorbidities. These include sleep apnea, hypertension, gastroesophageal reflux disease (GERD), cardiomyopathy, diabetes, leg edema, osteoarthritis, and mental depression. Because of their diseases and prolonged postoperative negative nitrogen balance (starvation), we avoid panniculectomy coincidental to the intestinal bypass. Moreover, the panniculectomy scar may preclude optimal subsequent surgical planning for definitive contour correction.

We find most patients understand the goals and limitations and the need for multiple stages and possible revisions. We impress upon them that optimal contour improvement entails a very tight closure with risk of suture line dehiscence. If that complication is unacceptable, then less pull will be made. While the scars are generally thin, they may be thickened and uneven. After revealing the common and serious risks of their operations, we offer a detailed consent form for each procedure. We have established a Web site (www.hurwitzcenter.com) that patients may visit before the first office appointment. They learn about the surgery, see results of operations on a variety of patients, and are cautioned about the risks. There is a detailed intake form, which is instructive to the patient and gathers important information for the surgeon. The Hurwitz Center for Plastic Surgery sends each patient who seeks a consultation a complimentary copy of a consumer directed book, *Total Body Lift: Reshaping the Breasts, Chest, Arms, Thighs, Hips, Back, Waist, Abdomen, and Knees After Weight Loss, Aging, and Pregnancies*, published by MDPublish, New York, New York, 2005. We attempt to exclude candidates suffering from chronic medical and psychiatric illnesses and those with unrealistic expectations.

Digital imaging is used during the second visit several weeks before the scheduled surgery. The patient's preoperative photographs are displayed. Electronic pens allow for drawing anticipated incision lines, indicating the direction of tissue tensions and final scar placement on multiple views of their images. Their new silhouette can be drawn, but no promises are made. Technique and outcomes vary according to the patient's basic body habitus. Oversized people, endomorphs, cannot be transformed into ectomorphs. During office follow-up, impatient and disappointed patients, as well as pleased patients, are graphically reminded of the extent of their original deformity by having a monitor with all possible images available within view of the examination room.

The surgeon considers the body shape (endomorph, mesomorph, or ectomorph), extent of deformity, size, sex, patient priorities, lifestyle, and tolerance for risk. Before embarking on such lengthy procedures, the surgeon and the support team and hospital should have experience working together on less extensive procedures. Three days of hospital care are essential. The larger the patient and the longer the procedure, the more likely are complications.

The Deformity

The massive weight loss patient has a deflated shape based on familial and gender-specific fat deposition and skin to fascia adherence. The most susceptible regions are the anterior neck, upper arms, breasts, lower back, flanks, abdomen, mons pubis, and thighs. In men there is a tendency to accumulate fat around the flanks, intra-abdominally, and the breasts. In women the fullness lies in the subcutaneous fat of the abdomen, hips, and thighs. Patterns of deformity are emerging that seem to be affected by the magnitude of initial BMI and change in BMI.

Redundant skin hangs over regions of fibrous adherence to deep fascia (Fig. 1). The skin of the trunk is densely adherent along the inframammary fold, down the upper midline to the linea alba, and in the groin. Adherence is variably dense across the rectus abdominis transverse tendinous inscriptions (more so in the male) and along one or two transverse levels across the anterolateral ribs, flanks, and back. Skin flaps undermined beyond adherences will readhere after the operation and have less tension on the skin, which explains why the epigastrium usually maintains an unwanted roll after an abdominoplasty.

Both anteriorly and posteriorly, there is medial to lateral staggered sweep of redundant tissue. Thigh skin is adherent below the anterior superior iliac spine, along the midlateral and midmedial regions and to a lesser extent along the entire posterior thigh. By the time the weight loss plateaus, the amount of fat within this redundant skin varies considerably. With massive weight loss, there are extensive layered folds or wrinkling. The skin is like an oversized suit and in no dimension, vertical or horizontal, is there normal skin tension. Unlike posttraumatic or congenital deformity surgery, there is no displaced normal tissue to relocate. All the skin is disordered and is treated accordingly.

Etiology of Skin Laxity

The etiology of skin laxity after rapid weight loss is inadequately understood. The subdermal to aponeurosis fibroelastic spans, overflowing with adipocytes in the obese, have fractured elastin fibers on microscopic study. The damaged elastin and collagen allow for no skin retraction after weight loss. With rapid weight loss, there is no way to prevent sagging of the abdominal skin, skin of the breasts and buttocks, and the inner portions of the arms and thighs. It is important to repair the abdomen with the best quality of skin, usually from the upper portions. Unfortunately, in massive and rapid weight loss patients, there is usually no quality skin. The problem is compounded in individuals over 55, who lose considerable skin elasticity without weight loss. Until we are able to reverse this complex disorder of subcutaneous disease, we are forced to excise the widest possible areas of skin and then close the skin flaps as tightly as possible.

Three factors contribute to postoperative skin laxity. First is the diseased skin collagen and elastin. Second, the farther the skin is from the line of closure, the less effective is the pull. I refer to this as the law of skin laxity. Otherwise stated, skin laxity is corrected closest to the line of closure and is progressively increased farther away. Third, the adherence of the skin to underlying fascia prevents tightening beyond the adherence. Surgical disruption of these customary and unique adherences mobilizes the flaps, but since perforating blood supply usually occurs there, flap vitality may be compromised.

As yet there are no proven means to improve skin and subcutaneous tissue elasticity. I am pleased with the applicability of Endermologie (LPG, Montreal, Canada), a computer-modulated differential vigorous massage and suction machine, to treat these patients. LPG claims that significant skin laxity can be reduced with about 20 twice-weekly treatment sessions. We have initiated treatments to improve our surgical results and substantiate this claim. We are convinced that if expertly performed, Endermologie hastens resolution of postoperative performed, Lipomassage® reduces swelling and induration. It softens most hypertrophic scars and reduces scar-related neuralgia. It is Food and Drug Administration (FDA) approved to temporarily

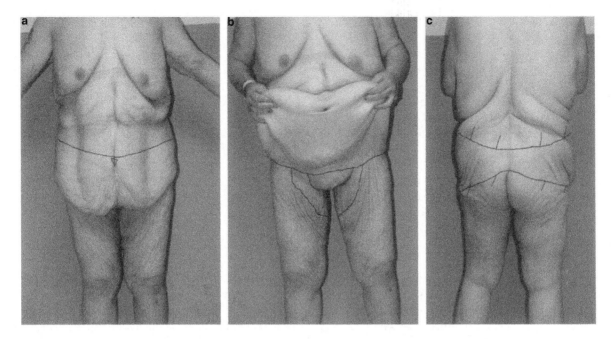

FIG. 1. Massive weight loss deformity varies according to the original fat distribution and pattern of skin adherence. (**a**) This 33-year-old, 203-lb woman lost 300 lb 2 years after Roux-en-Y gastrointestinal bypass. She has a large hanging pannus and considerable skin laxity in the mid-torso, hips, and medial thighs. The redundant skin and fat torso rolls cascade from midline to lateral. There is an anterior midline adherence along the linea alba and umbilicus, which is somewhat accentuated in the epigastrium by her vertical surgical scar. There are paramedian vertical folds reflective of the semilunar lines along the lateral rectus margins extending from the costal margins to the end of the hanging pannus. Beginning with the inframammary folds, there is an asymmetrical stairstep array of transverse skin adherences. Immediately superior to the costal margin, the skin is broadly adherent, more on the left than on the right side. Inferiorly, two transverse lines reflecting the tendinous inscriptions cross from lateral rectus border to the midline in the epigastrium and at the umbilicus. (**b**) On lifting the pannus, one sees the broad adherence along the iliac crests, across the suprapubic region, and diverting along each labial thigh junction. There is a progressive lateral flowing of rippled skin from upper medial thigh to the suprapatellar region. (c) Back folds begin inferior to the scapula. The left back has two oblique lines of back fascia adherence, while the right has a series of three. The last rolls overlap the pelvic rim. The firmly adherent central buttock fullness is framed laterally and inferiorly by numerous thin folds of lax skin. The posterior and lower lateral thigh skin below the lateral trochanter is broadly adherent to the fascia lata. The markings for a circumferential abdominoplasty, lower body lift, and medial thighplasty are drawn. Surgical lines for the first stage have been drawn while the patient reclines, pulls her pannus out of the way, and stands. The vertical lines ensure proper alignment for closure. The markings begin with the patient reclined and pulling up on her pannus. A 14-cm transverse line is centered about 8 cm above the labial commissure. With firm oblique upward pull on the pannus to the opposite costal margin, the incision line is continued across each groin and over the anterior superior iliac crests. The inferior incision continues across the hip with the patient in lateral decubitus and abducting the thigh. With all excisable skin drawn cephalad, the transverse line extends posteriorly to end immediately superior to the intergluteal fold. When the patient is standing, as seen here, the line dips inferiorly to the extent there is lateral thigh skin laxity. The anterior superior incision is along the umbilicus and is planned by pulling down the superior flap to the bikini line, because unraveling upper redundancy will be limited by costal margin skin adherences. The medial thighplasty has an inner line along the labial thigh groove extending to border the lateral mons pubis. The outer line is an estimate of skin removal, aided by the patient raising her leg while in the supine position. The posterior extension of the medial thighplasty overlies the ischial tuberosities and ends along the inferior gluteal folds.

improve cellulite. We find that minor contour deformities are smoothed by these treatments. There is experimental evidence in pigs that subcutaneous organized collagen can be produced by these treatments over a short period of time [15]. Clinical studies have failed to show a reliable improvement for contour deformity but show promising results for cellulite and as a helpful adjunct to ultrasonic and traditional liposuction [16–19]. The recent introduction of advanced electronic technology into the CELLU 8 promises to deliver on improved body contour sooner.

Panniculectomy

Many patients request plastic surgery referral from the bariatric nurses for a panniculectomy. They know that most insurance companies will reimburse when overhanging pannus is symptomatic. Our bariatric nurses explain that panniculectomy is inadequate to treat their myriad of abdominal skin redundancy problems. A panniculectomy is simply the removal of hanging panniculus by a long anterior transverse excision of skin and fat between the umbilicus and pubis.

There is no undermining of the superior flap or alteration or reconstruction of the umbilicus. It is often complemented with liposuction of surrounding, nonundermined bulging skin. It satisfies the medical indications by correcting the inflammatory sequelae of an overhanging pannus. This limited abdominoplasty is aesthetically adequate in the rare patient who has most of the deformity between the umbilicus and pubis. After an ill-advised panniculectomy, a subsequent abdominoplasty results in a much higher and less aesthetic lower abdominal scar.

Operative Planning and Care

Operative planning and sequencing is based on the deformity and patient priorities. The majority of patients are prepared for removal of excess tissue of the lower torso and thighs through a circumferential abdominoplasty and lower body lift. Unwanted redundancy distal to the mid-thighs requires long vertical medial excision of skin. Most patients accept this long scar, which usually heals favorably and is concealed by the thighs, in exchange for the distasteful skin redundancy. Many want the midback rolls and sagging breasts also corrected, which is usually performed more than 3 months later.

Upper and Total Body Lift

An upper body lift treats epigastric skin and midback folds and flattened, distorted breasts. Similarly, upper body lifts treat ptotic gynecomastia in continuity with back rolls. In women the upper body lift focuses on establishing a higher and firm inframammary fold. In men the fold should be obliterated. Abdomens that have defined midlevel skin adherence resulting in a two-tiered pannus (Fig. 43.1) will not have adequate correction of the epigastrium without an upper body lift. Due to abdominal flap blood supply concerns and the magnitude of the complex operation, a total body lift is usually staged with the lower body preceding the upper. The ideal scenario for a single-stage total body lift lasting up to 10 h are the correction of difficult gynecomastia back and abdomen, and taller female patients who want as much accomplished as possible in a single operative session. The single-staged TBL is controversial and is uncommonly performed. When it is, it should be limited to the most experienced operative teams, including a second experienced plastic surgeon, a physician assistant, and talented residents in plastic surgery training.

Each of the body contouring procedures takes 2–3 h. Unless medically contraindicated, cosmetic procedures were added to a medically necessary (insurance reimbursed) procedure. At Magee Women's Hospital, which is part of the University of Pittsburgh Medical Center, facility and anesthesia-related costs and hospital convalescence costs are considerably reduced this way.

Experienced anesthesiologists will be prepared for the position change and protection of the face and weight-bearing surfaces. A foam rubber mask with a cutout for the endotracheal tube has been our preferred approach (Gentle Touch™ 5" headrest pillow by Orthopedic Systems Inc., Union City, CA). Intravenous fluids are scaled down in consideration of the use of several liters of saline tumescent subcutaneous injections for liposuction. Intraoperative fluid and medical management are controlled by the anesthesia team. The need for colloid and blood replacement is discussed during the procedure. All patients are continuously monitored, which includes urine output. Hemoglobin concentration is optimized with iron and vitamin supplements, resorting to iron infusions if necessary. Erythropoietin may be taken a month before surgery, accepting an increased risk for thromboembolism. Larger patients pre-donate 1–3 units of blood for later transfusion. Or preferably, our anesthesiologist removes about 500 cm³ at the beginning of the case, replenishes the volume with saline and then administers the donated blood at the end of the case. In that way patients do not receive thrombogenic old banked blood. A liter of Hespan colloids helps resort both volume and oncotic pressure.

Intermittent leg pressure pumps are activated and intravenous antibiotics are given before the induction of general anesthesia. Additional risk factors for thrombophlebitis, a history of phlebitis, thromboembolism, lower extremity swelling, over 50, prolonged surgery, and obesity prompt the use of low-molecular-weight heparin.

Patients are hospitalized for about 3 days for fluids, electrolytes, and pain management. Also their movements are assisted to reduce excessive tension on tight suture lines.

In my patients, there have been rare medical complications or documented thrombophlebitis. Minor wound dehiscence, requiring bedside suture line closure, was allowed to heal in 52 patients. Minor skin necrosis occurred in ten patients. Skin loss requiring debridement and grafting occurred in one cigarette-smoking woman after an upper body lift. Multiple seroma aspiration was required in eight patients.

Summary of Operative Technique

Our basic operative technique has been reported elsewhere [18]. In essence, a circumferential abdominoplasty with a lower body lift removes a wide swath of skin and fat along the bikini line (Figs. 1, 2, 3, 4 and 5). The panniculectomy is a small portion of the procedure. This approach requires at least one turn of the patient. This procedure varies according to patterns of truncal skin adherence and the patient's BMI.

The full abdominoplasty features removal of all the redundant skin of the lower abdomen, central undermining to the xiphoid, and minimal lateral undermining of the superior flap. A running #2 PDO Quill® barbed suture (Angiotech, Vancouver, Canada) has replaced large braided permanent

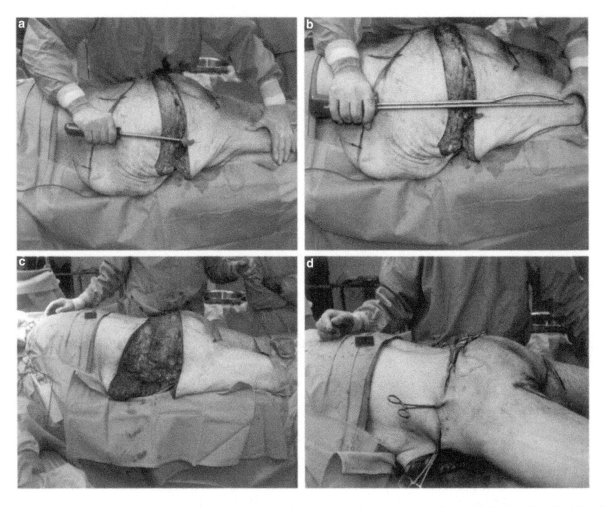

Fig. 2. The operation was started with the patient in the prone position. A scalpel cut was made for the inferior incision. (**a**) After direct undermining to just beyond the lateral trochanter, a long blunt underminer designed by Dr. Ted Lockwood is used. (**b**) Pushing against the fascia lata, the surgeon repeatedly thrusts the underminer down the lateral, posterior, and anterior thigh. When skin mobilization is complete, the thigh flap is pulled up to the proposed superior incision. If appropriate, the superior transverse incision is made. (**c**) Then the intervening island of skin and fat is excised, leaving behind the appropriate amount of large globular fat along the flank. The wound is very large. (**d**) To avoid persistent thigh skin laxity, the incision should be closed as tightly as possible. Several maneuvers assist in obtaining a secure closure. The thigh is fully abducted onto a padded utility table placed next to the operating room table. The wound margins are approximated with towel clips. Closely placed large braided permanent sutures are used to approximate the subcutaneous fascial system as the clips are replaced. Before the patient is turned for the abdominoplasty, the lateral triangular shape extensions of the medial thighplasties are excised and closed

suture to imbricate the central fascia from xiphoid to pubis. The operating table is flexed as the superior flap is approximated to the incision over the pubis and groins with lateral oblique tension. That tension narrows the waist and raises the anterolateral thighs. High central skin tension is created through the umbilicoplasty by deepithelializing three small flaps in the abdominal flap umbilical cutout and suturing them around the base of the isolated umbilicus. The lower body lift, performed with the patient in the prone position, incorporates extensive undermining distally along the hips and thighs followed by a very tight subcutaneous fascial closure with #2 PDO Quill, aided by full abduction of the leg

onto arm boards that swing the legs out from the operating room table. Liposuction is liberally used except through the distal central flap. A medial thighplasty frequently accompanies the lower body lift in massive weight loss patients. Smaller patients may have additional coincidental major procedures, such as mastopexies and brachioplasties.

Proper preoperative marking of the incisions plans for the removal of excess skin and estimates the closure tension, which affects the contour for the surrounding tissues and final location of the scars. Long abdominal scars must be respected, to avoid a narrow ischemic segment of skin between the incision and scar. The surgeon can either include

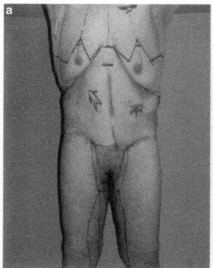 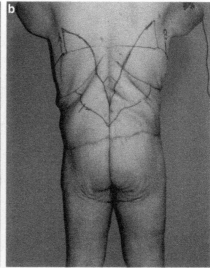

FIG. 3. (**a**, **b**) The result 4 months after the first stage is seen as well as the surgical markings for the upper body lift, mastopexy, and vertical thighplasty. (**a**) The wide vertical resect. of medial thigh skin was performed because of an inadequate correction from the high transverse medial thighplasty. A broad rim of skin is resected from the lower thorax to the inframammary fold. (**b**) The excision is continued around the back. Because of the severe skin redundancy, a broad oblique excision of skin crosses the transverse band. The operation was begun with the patient in the prone position. After the reverse abdominoplasty is done, a Wise pattern mastopexy completed the upper body lift. Then the medial thighplasty was performed.

the scar in the incision or leave enough space between the incision and scar to ensure adequate blood supply to the intervening skin. Because of the physical difficulties of marking the heavy hanging tissue while the patient is standing, many of the surgical lines are made with the patient reclined, and then reevaluated with the patient standing. Others have advocated a similar approach [4, 6].

Principles of Treatment

These multiple operations are lengthy, envelop large portions of a big body, and require position changes and high-tension closure of undermined and thinned flaps. Accordingly, we have listed the relevant plastic surgery principles for successful results with a low complication rate. The precise technique varies according to the deformity and surgeon preferences, but the principles are inviolate (Table 1).

The first principle is to analyze the patient and the deformity, which has been discussed. We need to emphasize that the farther from the suture line, the less effective is the pull. Therefore, following a bikini line closure, residual laxity is seen in the epigastrium, midlateral trunk, and distal thighs. This upper laxity can be treated secondarily through a reverse abdominoplasty, which we have developed into the upper body lift. The lower laxity is corrected by direct excisions along the medial and posterior thighs. Excessive intra-abdominal girth limits the aesthetic contour of even tight skin closures. This may be reduced by a month of preoperative

abdominal binding, several days of purging, and avoiding nitrous oxide anesthesia (gaseous distention) during abdominal wall plication. If obesity is the cause, then further weight loss is indicated.

Efficiency is the second principle. Inefficiency lengthens an already long operation, thereby increasing bleeding, medical and wound healing complications, surgeon fatigue, and costs. The surgeon should develop a consistent procedure so that the surgical assistants can anticipate the surgeon's needs. Unusual equipment or sutures should be requested ahead of time. With experience, preoperative assessment of the width of the resection becomes accurate (especially for the thinner patients) but does require nearly an hour of vigorous skin displacement while the patient lies, sits, and stands for the markings.

The most effective and efficient positioning and turning of the patient starts in the prone and ends in the supine positions, which includes the recent modification of placing the leg in abduction [19].

Prone followed by supine requires only one position change. The flap with the greatest movement is elevated first. The operation starts with the patient in the prone position, with the inferior incision of the lower body lift. Once suctioned and mobilized, the buttock and thigh flap is pulled superiorly and the anticipated superior incision line is confirmed and incised. The intervening low back and flank skin is removed as an island of skin and fat from side to side. Appropriate traction and countertraction permit rapid resection through a potentially bloody and vague plane of dissection.

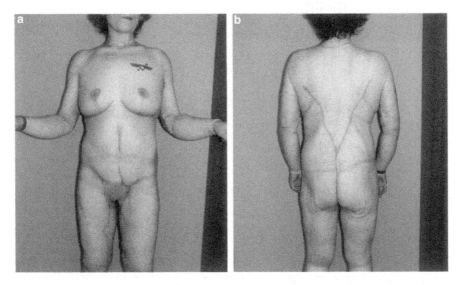

FIG. 4. (**a**, **b**) The result 6 months later than that shown in Fig. 3 is seen and immediately after bilateral brachioplasties [24]. The patient had a staged total body lift. Prior to her body contouring surgery, she weighed 210 lb and now she weighs 170 lb. (**a**) Her breasts are well shaped and symmetrical [25]. All redundant skin is removed and a natural hip and waist contour is established. (**b**) The thighs have a natural tapered contour. Most of her extensive back scars can be covered by underwear.

Care is taken to leave behind the ideal and symmetrical amount of fat along the flanks and hips. The central back closure is not tight; hence, it better tolerates the marked flexion needed for the abdominal closure later in the operation. Before the patient is turned, the posterior portion of the medial thighplasty is performed superficially along the inferior gluteal fold. Later the patient is turned and placed in the supine position onto a second operating room table and sterile sheets for the abdominoplasty. Experienced residents assist or perform portions of the procedure with both the attending and the residents suctioning fat or suturing simultaneously.

The third principle is to excise skin transversely. Skin redundancy is predominantly vertical, and crisscrossing with vertical excisions leaves compromised flap tips. Transverse scars are easily placed within underwear areas and are less likely to hypertrophy. Plan the trunk scar along the bikini line, which is easily covered and represents the greatest circumference of the female torso (Fig. 5). When the relatively narrow waist level excess skin is advanced over the iliac crests, much of the transverse excess is taken in.

Inverted superior anterior midline V excision is reserved for removal of widened and depressed surgical scars. A posterior V-shaped excision is limited to the midline buttock flap, to help rotate in excessively redundant lateral thigh skin. A broad vertical segment of midline back skin is invariably adherent, and therefore it is only excised as the end of a transversely oriented ellipse. Further exceptions to the rule of transverse excisions are the correction of severe gynecomastia and midback rolls, where obliquely and vertically oriented ellipses have been used.

Proper incision planning, the fourth principle, as discussed previously, leaves level scars along the bikini line. Most excisions are made with the patient reclining, but checked standing. Mid- and upper abdominal transverse scars are included in the excision, to avoid possible skin necrosis, whenever possible.

The fifth principle is to focus on the contour and tension of the tissue left behind, much as in a breast reduction. When great closure tension is present, some late thinning of the subcutaneous tissues can be anticipated, particularly in the lateral buttock region. Nevertheless, the central buttock assumes a more spherical shape over time. The inclusion of a deepithelialized upper buttock flap often fills out the flattened buttocks.

We follow the sixth principle, preservation of dermis and subcutaneous fascia, by preliminary infiltration along the anticipated incision of 100 of milliliters of lactated Ringer's solution with 1 mg of epinephrine and 40 cm^3 of 1 % Xylocaine per liter. This preparation minimizes bleeding and limits the use of electrocautery. The incision is slightly beveled along the dermis and perpendicularly through the fat and subcutaneous fascia, as the flaps are retracted from each other. The use of a vasoconstrictor follows the second principle, efficiency, requiring interruption to coagulate bleeders only after considerable tissue is incised.

The seventh principle is gentle fat removal, which is possible by liposuction with prior infiltration of Xylocaine and epinephrine. A brief run with an ultrasound probe reduces the vigor of the liposuction cannula stokes. Both the LySonix (Mentor Corporation, Santa Barbara California) and the VASER (Sound Surgical Technologies, Louisville, CO)

Fig. 5. This is a composite before and after photograph of a 34-year-old female corporate executive. After losing 170 lb, she weighed 160 lb. A single-stage operation was done, consisting of a circumferential abdominoplasty, a lower body lift, medial thighplasties, and 450-mL silicone gel smooth round implant partial subpectoral breast augmentations beneath concentric ring mastopexies. Her scars lie within brief underpants and inconspicuously around the areolas. While the thighs are still large, they have excellent contour with no redundant and sagging skin. Her larger, symmetrical, shapely, and soft breasts complement her full-sized hips and lateral thighs. Her sagging mons pubis has been raised and contoured with the lower central abdomen.

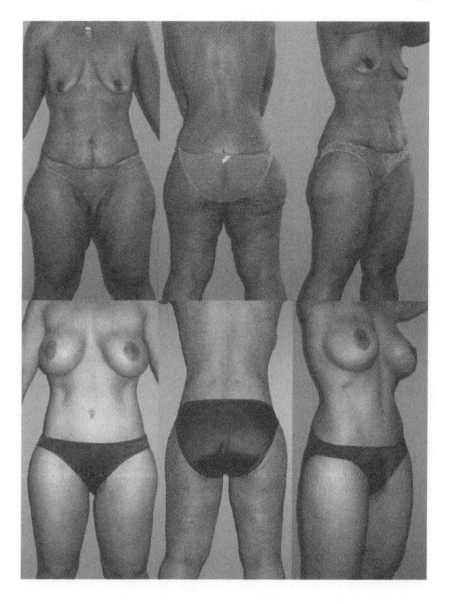

ultrasound systems are satisfactory. Bleeding rarely occurs, and if some blood is seen in the cannula, significant vessel damage of the flap is presumed and the liposuction is stopped. Flap edge direct resection of excess sub-Scarpal fat does not diminish overlying skin blood supply.

The eighth principle dictates a high-tension skin flap closure. After massive weight loss the trunk skin flaps are relatively inelastic. The flap vessels are large, a remnant of the prior obesity, which appears to increase blood flow, permitting greater undermining and tension on the flaps than one would generally consider safe. Correction of the lateral thigh saddlebag deformity has been improved by fully abducting the leg onto a side utility table while closing with the patient in the prone position (Fig. 2) [21]. Preliminary approximation with towel clips keeps the tension during closure of the wound minimal. Optimal abdominoplasty closure is achieved by flexing the trunk, approximating the wound edges with #2

PDO Quill large subcutaneous tissue bites followed by intradermal 3-0 Monoderm®. The reverse abdominoplasty, the central aspect of the upper body lift, is successful after establishing the new inframammary fold with high-tension advancement of the upper abdominal skin flap fixed about the ribs with running #2 PDO.

The ninth principle is that swelling, infection rate, phlebitis, and seroma are reduced by closing wounds as expeditiously as possible over long dwelling suction catheters. Elasticized garments with minimal pressure over the lower abdomen are comfortable and reassuring to the patient. Aside from some flap tacking sutures in the groins, we have not closed the dead space. Lower abdominal sub-Scarpa fascia lymphatics are preserved as much as possible. Seromas are a rare experience. Preoperative adipose preparation and postoperative Lipomassage™ speed recovery and improve results.

The tenth principle is that analyzing the aesthetic results and the patient outcomes a year or more postoperative is very instructive. Persistent heavy tissues, particularly of the thighs, lower the transverse scars and depress the contours. Review of standard photography is the best gauge of our efforts. We have developed a deformity and outcome grading scale, which we have applied to our results [19, 20]. Correction of deformity may not always equate with optimal aesthetic results, but it is an improvement. The best aesthetics leave the most unobtrusive symmetrical scars and gender-specific contours.

The Surgical Challenge

The ongoing presentation of many reasonably healthy, body-conscious weight loss patients has offered me a rare surgical opportunity and challenge. Complex planning based on clinical experience and artistic skills, followed by a physically demanding and tedious procedure, is rewarded by incredible body transformations. The metamorphosis is greeted with patient elation and gratitude. This is plastic surgery that melds reconstructive and cosmetic procedures for eagerly anticipating patients. Effective, reliable, and reduced risk procedures are evolving so that future contributions are available to the legion of surgeons who want to commit their talents to this needy population [21–23].

References

1. Schauer PR, Ikramuddin S, Gourash W, Ramanathan R, Luketich J. Outcomes after laparoscopic Roux-en-Y gastric bypass for morbid obesity. Ann Surg. 2000;4:515–29.
2. Lockwood TE. Lower body lift with superficial fascial system suspension. Plast Reconstr Surg. 1993;92:1112–22.
3. Lockwood TE. Lower body lift. Aesthet Surg J. 2001;21:355–60.
4. Hamra S. Circumferential body lift. Aesthet Surg J. 1999;19(3):244–51.
5. Pascal JF, Le Louarn C. Remodeling body lift with high lateral tension. Aesthetic Plast Surg. 2002;26:223–30.
6. Aly AS, Cram AE, Chao M, et al. Belt lipectomy for circumferential truncal excess: the University of Iowa experience. Plast Reconstr Surg. 2003;111:398–413.
7. Van Geertruyden JP, Vandeweyer E, de Fontanie S, et al. Circumferential torsoplasty. Br J Plast Surg. 1999;52:623–30.
8. Hunstad JP. Addressing difficult areas in body contouring with emphasis on combined tumescent and syringe techniques. Clin Plast Surg. 1996;23:57–80.
9. Matory Jr WE, O'Sullivan J, Fudem G, et al. Abdominal surgery in patients with severe morbid obesity. Plast Reconstr Surg. 1994;94:976–80.
10. Mitka M. Surgery for obesity, demand soars amid scientific, ethical questions. JAMA. 2003;289(14):1761.
11. Schauer PR, Ikramuddin I. Laparoscopic surgery for morbid obesity. Surg Clin North Am. 2001;81:1145–51.
12. Buchwald H. Overview of bariatric surgery. J Am Coll Surg. 2002;194:367–75.
13. Agha-Mohammadi S, Hurwitz DJ. Nutritional deficiency of post-bariatric body contouring patients: what every plastic surgeon should know. Plast Reconstr Surg. 2008;122(2):604–13.
14. Agha-Mohammadi S, Hurwitz DJ. Potential impacts of nutritional deficiency of post-bariatric patients on body contouring. Plast Reconstr Surg. 2008;122(6):1901–14.
15. Adcock D, Paulsen S, Davis S, Nanney L, Shack RB. Analysis of the cutaneous and systemic effects of Endermologie in the Porcine model. Aesthet Surg J. 1998;18:414–20.
16. Latrenta GS. Endermologie versus liposuction with external ultrasound assist. Aesthet Surg J. 1999;19:1110–4.
17. Ersek RA, Mann II GE, Salisbury S, Salisbury AV. Noninvasive mechanical body contouring: a preliminary clinical outcome study. Aesthetic Plast Surg. 1997;21:61–7.
18. Latrenta GS, Mick S. Endermologie after external ultrasound-assisted lipoplasty (EUAL) versus EUAL alone. Aesthet Surg J. 2001;21:128–36.
19. Dabb RW. A combined program of small-volume liposuction, Endermologie, and nutrition: a logical alternative. Aesthet Surg J. 1999;19:388–93.
20. Hurwitz DJ, Zewert TE. Body contouring after bariatric surgery. Oper Tech Plast Reconstr Surg. 2002;8(2):77–85.
21. Hurwitz DJ, Rubin JP, Risen M, Sejjadian A, Serieka S. Correcting the saddlebag deformity in the massive weight loss patient. Plast Reconstr Surg. 2004;114(5):1313–25.
22. Song AY, Jean RD, Hurwitz DJ, Fernstrom MH, Scott JA, Rubin JP. A classification of contour deformities after massive weight loss: the Pittsburgh Rating Scale. Plast Reconstr Surg. 2005;116(5):1535–44.
23. Hurwitz DJ. Single stage total body lift after massive weight loss. Ann Plast Surg. 2004;52(5):435–41.
24. Hurwitz DJ, Holland SW. The L brachioplasty: an innovative approach to correct excess tissue of the upper arm, axilla and lateral chest. Plast Reconstr Surg. 2006;117(2):403–11.
25. Hurwitz DJ, Agha-Mohammadi S. Post bariatric surgery breast reshaping: the spiral flap. Ann Plast Surg. 2006;56(5):481–6.

54

The Female Patient: Pregnancy and Gynecologic Issues in the Bariatric Surgery Patient

Karina A. McArthur, Giselle G. Hamad, and George M. Eid

Polycystic Ovary Syndrome and Morbid Obesity

Polycystic ovary syndrome (PCOS) was initially named Stein-Leventhal syndrome for the physicians who recognized in 1935 a clinical triad of hirsutism, amenorrhea, and obesity. Since then, the National Institutes of Health (NIH) has updated this definition to the Rotterdam consensus criteria requiring two of the three following clinical manifestations: menstrual irregularity, hyperandrogenism (clinical or biochemical), and polycystic ovaries on ultrasound [1]. Estimates of the prevalence of polycystic ovary syndrome (PCOS) have ranged between 4 and 18 % [2].

The etiology of PCOS remains largely unclear. It is currently thought to represent a complex interaction of genetics and environmental factors, including intrauterine factors that predispose an individual to having endocrine abnormalities including insulin resistance, hyperandrogenemia, and infertility. Recently several studies have been published implicating candidate genes from genome-wide association studies [3, 4]. This represents an exciting avenue for further elucidation of the etiology of PCOS. Obesity is also thought to influence the phenotype of PCOS strongly [5], potentially forming a part of a "vicious" cycle further contributing to androgen excess [6].

PCOS is primarily a disorder of ovary function, resulting in menstrual irregularities, infertility, and hyperandrogenism. Hyperandrogenism is manifested in a number of ways, including hirsutism and acne. There is also a strong prevalence of insulin resistance in the PCOS population, in both obese and lean women [7]. The relationship between hyperandrogenism and insulin resistance is not clearly defined. However, hyperandrogenism predisposes to central obesity, which itself correlates with insulin resistance [8]. As a result of these endocrinopathies, women with PCOS may be at risk for cardiovascular events and other end organ complications [9].

The prevalence of obesity in women with PCOS ranges from 30 to 80 % [6, 9]. The role that obesity plays in the pathophysiology of PCOS is controversial. Nevertheless, obesity undoubtedly exacerbates some of the features of PCOS, including insulin resistance [9]. The prevalence of obesity in US women aged 20 and older is 35.8 % in 2009–2010 [10]. Obesity is clearly associated with a number of comorbidities including cardiovascular disease, hypertension, diabetes mellitus, sleep apnea, osteoarthritis, dysfunctional uterine bleeding, and endometrial carcinoma. When compared to their nonobese PCOS counterparts or to obese women without PCOS, women with PCOS and obesity have an even higher risk of developing the comorbidities that overlap between the two conditions. In other words, the risks are additive [11].

PCOS treatment focuses on the clinical manifestation of the syndrome such as hyperandrogenemia and insulin resistance. Insulin-sensitizing agents are one of the mainstays of treatment of PCOS. Advocates of their use believe that high insulin levels trigger the cascade of endocrinopathies that lead to anovulation and hyperandrogenism. While some studies have shown an improvement in ovulation and pregnancy rates with the use of insulin-sensitizing agents, a recent meta-analysis did not show any improvement in live birth rates with the use of insulin-sensitizing agents in PCOS [12]. A potential explanation for the heterogeneity of the results of insulin-sensitizing agents in studies looking at PCOS and improvement of metabolic dysfunction is the broader Rotterdam consensus criteria, including many patients without metabolic dysfunction in the definition of PCOS [13]. Treatment with antiandrogens is generally effective for the amelioration of hirsutism and acne but does not produce an insulin-sensitizing effect. Similarly, oral contraceptives may improve menstrual cycle regularity and acne [14].

Currently, there is no ideal treatment for PCOS, as none of the treatments described can remedy all of the biochemical aberrations, signs, and symptoms of the disease. Instead,

S.A. Brethauer et al. (eds.), *Minimally Invasive Bariatric Surgery*,
DOI 10.1007/978-1-4939-1637-5_54, © Springer Science+Business Media New York 2015

most treatments tend to target only one or a few components of PCOS. Weight loss is the only treatment that improves many of the endocrine aspects of the disease in the obese PCOS patient. A recent Cochrane review [15] showed that lifestyle intervention reduces adiposity and improves hyperandrogenism and insulin resistance in women with PCOS. However, weight loss achieved by lifestyle intervention is generally modest (5–10 %) and is followed by a regain in weight in the majority of cases [16].

Surgical management of weight is, therefore, an attractive option for improving the symptomatology of PCOS. Although studies on this subject are limited, they appear to show a significant benefit of bariatric surgery in treating PCOS [6]. One retrospective study evaluated 24 patients with an established diagnosis of PCOS [17]. All patients were oligomenorrheic, 96 % had hirsutism, 20 % had acne, and 50 % had ovary cysts on ultrasound. All of the patients had resolution of their menstrual abnormalities and the five patients who wished to conceive postoperatively were able to do so without clomiphene.

Similarly, in another retrospective study of 20 patients with PCOS who underwent Roux-en-Y gastric bypass, 82 % of patients had improvement in menstrual cycle irregularity, and all six patients who desired pregnancy were able to achieve it, five without any additional intervention [18]. In regard to the effect of restrictive bariatric procedures on PCOS, a study of the Swedish adjustable gastric band showed improvement of symptoms in 48 % of the patients with PCOS [19]. While several small studies have shown promising results in PCOS treatment with bariatric surgery, further research is necessary to establish bariatric surgery as a standard therapy for PCOS.

Pregnancy After Bariatric Surgery

Because preoperative menstrual irregularities and infertility frequently improve following bariatric surgery, female patients of reproductive age may become more fertile [17, 20]. Patients should be advised that they are at increased risk of becoming pregnant following bariatric surgery. Given that micronutrient deficiencies can result in deleterious effects on the fetus, it is critical to discuss the importance of compliance with micronutrient supplementation.

Bariatric surgery is associated with improved perinatal outcomes. Obese pregnant women are at higher risk of a number of perinatal complications, including preeclampsia, gestational diabetes, hypertension, post-datism, meconium staining, and prolongation of labor [21–23]. In a review of 75 published articles, post-bariatric surgery mothers had lower rates of pregnancy-related complications than obese women without bariatric surgery [24]. A population-based study demonstrated a lower risk of macrosomia following bariatric surgery, but these patients were more likely to be anemic, hypertensive, and deliver small for gestational age infants [25].

Another population-based study over a 20-year period compared pregnancy outcomes after different types of bariatric surgeries, including laparoscopic adjustable gastric band (LAGB), vertical banded gastroplasty, silastic ring gastroplasty, and Roux-en-y gastric bypass (RYGB). Among the groups, there was no significant difference in low birth weight, macrosomia, low Apgar scores, or perinatal mortality [26].

Gestational diabetes confers an increased risk of cesarean delivery and macrosomia [27]. Following bariatric surgery, the rate of gestational diabetes decreases [28]. In a retrospective study of a private insurance claims database, women who underwent bariatric surgery were less likely to have gestational diabetes and cesarean section compared to those who delivered before having bariatric surgery [29].

Pregnancy Following Gastric Bypass

A common question among women of reproductive age who are potential candidates for bariatric surgery concerns the safety and optimal timing of subsequent childbearing. The period of rapid weight loss following RYGB was initially thought to be a vulnerable time period for a pregnancy. Traditionally, bariatric surgeons have counseled patients to avoid pregnancy for up to 24 months following RYGB because of the concern that rapid weight loss leads to adverse fetal outcomes. However, recent studies have challenged the notion that pregnancy should be avoided in the first 2 years after bariatric surgery. In a retrospective review comparing RYGB patients who became pregnant within 1 year of surgery with those who became pregnant after 1 year, there was no increase in malnutrition, adverse fetal outcomes, or complications in pregnancy in the women who became pregnant within 1 year after surgery [31]. These data suggest that recommending a delay in conceiving beyond 1 year after bariatric surgery is unnecessary.

One theoretical challenge in the management of this population is the possibility that the anatomy of the RYGB impairs absorption of oral contraceptives, which might lead to unintended pregnancy [31]. There are few pharmacokinetic studies in the literature to guide clinical practice and more clinical trials are needed.

Gastric bypass has been shown to reduce the rate of pregnancy-related complications. In an analysis of insurance claims data from bariatric surgery patients who had at least one pregnancy [32], mothers having prior bariatric surgery had lower rates of preeclampsia, eclampsia, and gestational hypertension compared to deliveries prior to bariatric surgery. The majority (81.5 %) had undergone RYGB surgery.

A small bowel obstruction is a potentially catastrophic complication following RYGB that may result in major morbidity and mortality for both mother and fetus [33–35]. The gravid uterus displaces the intestines cephalad and a closed-loop obstruction through an internal hernia defect may occur.

This may progress to infarction or perforation if not recognized promptly. A small bowel intussusception is another possible etiology of small bowel obstruction that can lead to bowel necrosis [35]. A pregnant post-RYGB patient who complains of abdominal pain may present with vague clinical complaints which make diagnosis difficult. Clinicians may be reluctant to submit pregnant patients for CT scanning because of the radiation exposure. In addition, imaging studies may fail to diagnose an internal hernia or even intestinal volvulus [36]. Therefore, in a pregnant post-GBP patient with unexplained abdominal pain, serious consideration should be given to exploratory laparotomy or diagnostic laparoscopy, as early surgical intervention is needed to avoid a delay in diagnosis [37].

Pregnancy Following Restrictive Procedures

A low rate of pregnancy-related complications has been noted among patients having restrictive procedures. Following LAGB, there is a lower risk of gestational diabetes, pregnancy-induced hypertension, preeclampsia, cesarean section, macrosomia, and low birth weight babies compared to pregnancies in obese mothers who did not undergo bariatric surgery [38].

An advantage of LAGB is that the restriction may be adjusted during pregnancy to decelerate weight loss or to relieve hyperemesis. Dixon and colleagues cite the adjustability of the gastric restriction of the LAGB as an ideal method to control the weight of pregnant bariatric patients [39]. Of 1,382 gastric band patients, 79 pregnancies were compared with the patients' previous pregnancies and with matched obese subjects and community outcomes data. Birth weights were comparable to the community birth weights. Gestational diabetes and pregnancy-induced hypertension were comparable to the community incidence and were less frequent compared to the obese cohort. Stillbirths, preterm deliveries, and abnormal birth weights were concordant with the community data.

Conceiving within a year after LAGB appears to be safe according to a retrospective study which demonstrated that bariatric surgery patients who became pregnant during the first postoperative year did not have a higher rate of perinatal complications compared to those who became pregnant more than 12 months postoperatively [26]. In this study, the majority of patients had undergone LAGB (61.5 %). These data suggest that it is safe to conceive within 1 year of bariatric surgery.

The timing of pregnancy after LAGB is related to the rate of revisional surgery [40]. Among LAGB patients who became pregnant following LAGB, excess weight loss was equivalent at 3 years compared to nonpregnant controls. The rates of revisions of the band, port, and tubing were equivalent between the two groups. However, the women who became pregnant sooner after LAGB and pregnancy had a higher rate of band revisions.

Pregnancy Following Biliopancreatic Diversion

There are few studies in the literature evaluating pregnancy outcomes in BPD patients. One study with 18-year follow-up has addressed pregnancy following biliopancreatic diversion (BPD) [41]; 239 pregnancies occurred in 1,136 women who had previously undergone BPD. Thirty-five women experienced improvement in fertility following BPD. Eighty-five percent delivered at term and 28 % were small for gestational age. Total parenteral nutrition was required in 21 %. Two birth malformations were observed and three fetal deaths occurred.

In another study of pregnancy in BPD patients, a survey of 783 women showed an improvement in fertility in 47 % of patients who were unable to conceive preoperatively [28]. Although fetal macrosomia improved after the BPD, the miscarriage rate remained elevated at 26 %. The authors supported delaying pregnancy until weight stabilization.

The most recent study of pregnancy outcomes after BPD retrospectively evaluated ten BPD patients who previously had type 2 diabetes mellitus which resolved after BPD [42]. None of the mothers developed gestational diabetes and none of the infants had macrosomia.

Nutritional Issues

Several essential micronutrients are malabsorbed in GBP patients [43]. Therefore, compliance with vitamin and mineral supplementation is of utmost importance in pregnant patients following gastric bypass surgery. Deficiencies in vitamin A, iron, calcium, vitamin D, vitamin B12, thiamine, and folate have all been described. Thiamine deficiency may lead to Wernicke's encephalopathy, which may have devastating neurologic consequences.

The post-GBP reduction in calcium absorption may lead to a decrease in bone density which potentially places a female patient at risk for osteoporotic fractures [44]. Longer-term follow-up of 3 years reveals that the reduction in bone density continues [45].

Premenopausal women are at risk of iron deficiency anemia because of menstrual losses. Following GBP, these women are even more predisposed to iron deficiency. Gastric acid is required for release of iron and cobalamin from food. Iron is maximally absorbed in the duodenum, while cobalamin is absorbed in the terminal ileum. Following gastric bypass, the parietal cells in the distal stomach are bypassed, thereby reducing gastric acidity and subsequent absorption of iron and cobalamin. Therefore, daily iron supplementation is mandatory in GBP patients. Prenatal vitamins or multivitamin supplements containing iron are generally inadequate to meet the needs of the GBP patient; a separate iron supplement is required.

In the setting of folate deficiency, neural tube defects may occur after GBP and may result in devastating fetal abnormalities [46]. Therefore, patients must be counseled about the importance of folic acid supplementation, especially as an increasing number of adolescent and childbearing-aged females undergo bariatric surgery.

Urinary Stress Incontinence and Obesity

Obesity is a risk factor for urinary stress incontinence [47]. It has been postulated that the increased intra-abdominal pressure due to obesity increases the intravesical pressure until it overcomes the maximal urethral closing pressure [48]. Neurogenic mechanisms for urinary stress incontinence in the obese have also been proposed [49].

Weight loss appears to be an essential element in sustained improvement in stress incontinence. The effect of nonsurgical weight reduction resulting in weight loss of ≥ 5 % had a ≥ 50 % reduction in incontinence frequency compared to only 25 % of women with <5 % weight loss ($p < .03$) [50]. Similarly, a recent randomized controlled trial demonstrated that a weight loss of 8.0 % resulted in a self-reported decrease in incontinence episodes in 47 % of patients in the intervention group, compared to 28 % in the control group that had 1.6 % of weight loss ($p = 0.01$) [51].

There has been increasing support in the literature citing the improvement of stress incontinence after bariatric surgery. One prospective study demonstrated that urinary incontinence resolved in 64 % and improved in 92 % at 1 year after gastric bypass [52]. Whitcomb et al. found that the overall prevalence of stress urinary incontinence decreased from 32 % at baseline to 15 % at 6 months ($p = 0.006$) [53].

The impact of obesity on the surgical treatment of urinary stress incontinence has been investigated in a modest number of studies. The literature looking at results of traditional surgical treatment such a Burch colposuspension in obese patients is mixed. However, there is an increasing consensus that cure rates and complication rates after tension-free vaginal tape repair are similar between obese and nonobese patients [49].

Conclusion

Obesity and PCOS are closely related; surgically-induced weight loss improves menstrual irregularities, hirsutism, and infertility. Postoperative bariatric patients are at increased risk of becoming pregnant. During pregnancy, compliance with vitamin supplementation is of utmost importance. Pregnancy outcomes are improved following bariatric surgery. If possible, close prenatal surveillance should be established with an obstetrician with experience in high-risk pregnancies. Elevated BMI is a risk factor for urinary stress incontinence, which improves with surgically-induced weight loss.

Review Questions and Answers

Question 1

What combination of characteristics does not meet the requirement for the diagnosis of PCOS according to the Rotterdam criteria?

(a) Obesity and polycystic ovaries on ultrasound
(b) Hyperandrogenism and menstrual irregularity
(c) Menstrual irregularity and polycystic ovaries on ultrasound
(d) Hyperandrogenism and polycystic ovaries on ultrasound

Answer: A

The Rotterdam consensus criteria requires two of the three following clinical manifestations: menstrual irregularity, hyperandrogenism (clinical or biochemical), and polycystic ovaries on ultrasound. Although obesity exacerbates many of the clinical abnormalities of PCOS, it is not a required component of the diagnosis.

Question 2

A 24-year-old G2P1 woman is 32 weeks pregnant and presents with dehydration, nausea, vomiting, and left upper quadrant abdominal pain. She underwent a gastric bypass 2 years ago and has lost 150 lb. Physical exam reveals tachycardia of 110, blood pressure of 90/50, and a gravid abdomen with left upper quadrant tenderness without peritonitis. White blood cell count is 11.0. CT scan reveals distended bowel loops and swirling of the small bowel mesentery. What is the next step in diagnosis and treatment?

(a) Insertion of nasogastric tube
(b) Upper endoscopy
(c) Serial abdominal exams
(d) Surgical exploration

Answer: D

Internal hernia is a devastating complication in a gastric bypass patient, possibly resulting in necrosis of the bowel, perforation, peritonitis, and short gut. Pregnancy complicates the diagnosis of internal hernia due to a gravid uterus displacing intra-abdominal contents. Clinicians may be reluctant to subject the fetus to ionizing radiation, making diagnosis challenging. In a patient with high suspicion of internal hernia, there should be no delay in intervening surgically.

Question 3

A 35-year-old female presents to a general obstetrician at 20 weeks of pregnancy for a first prenatal visit. She has had a gastric bypass 10 years ago and has not followed up for the last 5 years with the bariatric surgeon. She has not taken any nutritional supplements during this pregnancy. A routine CBC reveals anemia. The deficiency of what nutrient early in pregnancy could have predisposed this woman to deliver an infant with severe spinal cord abnormality?

(a) Cobalamin
(b) Iron
(c) Folate
(d) Calcium

Answer: C

This patient's anemia could potentially be multifactorial, with causes that include iron, folate, and cobalamin deficiency. However, folate deficiency can lead to neural tube defects. Many of these abnormalities occur early in pregnancy. Female bariatric patients of childbearing age should be counseled on the need for close monitoring of micronutrients starting early in their pregnancy.

References

1. Rotterdam ESHRE/ASRM-Sponsored PCOS consensus workshop group. Revised 2003 consensus on diagnostic criteria and long-term health risks related to polycystic ovary syndrome (PCOS). Hum Reprod. 2004;19(1):41–7.
2. Teede H, Deeks A, Moran L. Polycystic ovary syndrome: a complex condition with psychological, reproductive and metabolic manifestations that impacts on health across the lifespan. BMC Med. 2010;8:41.
3. Chen ZJ, Zhao H, He L, Shi Y, Qin Y, Li Z, et al. Genome-wide association study identifies susceptibility loci for polycystic ovary syndrome on chromosome 2p16.3, 2p21 and 9q33.3. Nat Genet. 2011;43(1):55–9.
4. Shi Y, Zhao H, Cao Y, Yang D, Li Z, Zhang B, et al. Genome-wide association study identifies eight new risk loci for polycystic ovary syndrome. Nat Genet. 2012;44(9):1020–5.
5. Pasquali R, Gambineri A, Pagotto U. The impact of obesity on reproduction in women with polycystic ovary syndrome. BJOG. 2006;113(10):1148–59.
6. Escobar-Morreale HF. Surgical management of metabolic dysfunction in PCOS. Steroids. 2012;77(4):312–6.
7. Randeva HS, Tan BK, Weickert MO, Lois K, Nestler JE, Sattar N, et al. Cardiometabolic aspects of the polycystic ovary syndrome. Endocr Rev. 2012;33(5):812–41.
8. Kahn BB, Flier JS. Obesity and insulin resistance. J Clin Invest. 2000;106(4):473–81.
9. Moran C, Arriaga M, Rodriguez G, Moran S. Obesity differentially affects phenotypes of polycystic ovary syndrome. Int J Endocrinol. 2012;2012:317241.
10. Ogden CL, Carroll MD, Kit BK, Flegal KM. Prevalence of obesity in the United States, 2009–2010. NCHS Data Brief. 2012;82:1–8.
11. Hoeger K. Obesity and weight loss in polycystic ovary syndrome. Obstet Gynecol Clin North Am. 2001;28(1):85–97; vi-vii.
12. Tang T, Lord JM, Norman RJ, Yasmin E, Balen AH. Insulin-sensitising drugs (metformin, rosiglitazone, pioglitazone, D-chiro-inositol) for women with polycystic ovary syndrome, oligo amenorrhoea and subfertility. Cochrane Database Syst Rev. 2012;5, CD003053.
13. Duleba AJ. Medical management of metabolic dysfunction in PCOS. Steroids. 2012;77(4):306–11.
14. Moghetti P, Toscano V. Treatment of hirsutism and acne in hyperandrogenism. Best Pract Res Clin Endocrinol Metab. 2006;20(2):221–34.
15. Moran LJ, Hutchison SK, Norman RJ, Teede HJ. Lifestyle changes in women with polycystic ovary syndrome. Cochrane Database Syst Rev. 2011;7, CD007506.
16. Yanovski SZ, Yanovski JA. Obesity. N Engl J Med. 2002;346(8):591–602.
17. Eid GM, Cottam DR, Velcu LM, Mattar SG, Korytkowski MT, Gosman G, et al. Effective treatment of polycystic ovarian syndrome with Roux-en-Y gastric bypass. Surg Obes Relat Dis. 2005;1(2):77–80.
18. Jamal M, Gunay Y, Capper A, Eid A, Heitshusen D, Samuel I. Roux-en-Y gastric bypass ameliorates polycystic ovary syndrome and dramatically improves conception rates: a 9-year analysis. Surg Obes Relat Dis. 2012;8(4):440–4.
19. Brancatisano A, Wahlroos S, Brancatisano R. Improvement in comorbid illness after placement of the Swedish Adjustable Gastric Band. Surg Obes Relat Dis. 2008;4(3 Suppl):S39–46.
20. Musella M, Milone M, Bellini M, Sosa Fernandez LM, Leongito M, Milone F. Effect of bariatric surgery on obesity-related infertility. Surg Obes Relat Dis. 2012;8(4):445–9.
21. Chu SY, Callaghan WM, Kim SY, Schmid CH, Lau J, England LJ, et al. Maternal obesity and risk of gestational diabetes mellitus. Diabetes Care. 2007;30(8):2070–6.
22. Stuebe AM, Landon MB, Lai Y, Spong CY, Carpenter MW, Ramin SM, et al. Maternal BMI, glucose tolerance, and adverse pregnancy outcomes. Am J Obstet Gynecol. 2012;207(1):62. e1–7.
23. Vahratian A, Zhang J, Troendle JF, Savitz DA, Siega-Riz AM. Maternal prepregnancy overweight and obesity and the pattern of labor progression in term nulliparous women. Obstet Gynecol. 2004;104(5 Pt 1):943–51.
24. Maggard MA, Yermilov I, Li Z, Maglione M, Newberry S, Suttorp M, et al. Pregnancy and fertility following bariatric surgery: a systematic review. JAMA. 2008;300(19):2286–96.
25. Belogolovkin V, Salihu HM, Weldeselasse H, Biroscak BJ, August EM, Mbah AK, et al. Impact of prior bariatric surgery on maternal and fetal outcomes among obese and non-obese mothers. Arch Gynecol Obstet. 2012;285(5):1211–8.
26. Sheiner E, Balaban E, Dreiher J, Levi I, Levy A. Pregnancy outcome in patients following different types of bariatric surgeries. Obes Surg. 2009;19(9):1286–92.
27. Marshall NE, Guild C, Cheng YW, Caughey AB, Halloran DR. Maternal superobesity and perinatal outcomes. Am J Obstet Gynecol. 2012;206(5):417. e1–6.
28. Lesko J, Peaceman A. Pregnancy outcomes in women after bariatric surgery compared with obese and morbidly obese controls. Obstet Gynecol. 2012;119(3):547–54.
29. Burke AE, Bennett WL, Jamshidi RM, Gilson MM, Clark JM, Segal JB, et al. Reduced incidence of gestational diabetes with bariatric surgery. J Am Coll Surg. 2010;211(2):169–75.
30. Dao T, Kuhn J, Ehmer D, Fisher T, McCarty T. Pregnancy outcomes after gastric-bypass surgery. Am J Surg. 2006;192(6):762–6.
31. Merhi ZO. Challenging oral contraception after weight loss by bariatric surgery. Gynecol Obstet Invest. 2007;64(2):100–2.
32. Bennett WL, Gilson MM, Jamshidi R, Burke AE, Segal JB, Steele KE, et al. Impact of bariatric surgery on hypertensive disorders in

pregnancy: retrospective analysis of insurance claims data. BMJ. 2010;340:c1662.

33. Gagne DJ, DeVoogd K, Rutkoski JD, Papasavas PK, Urbandt JE. Laparoscopic repair of internal hernia during pregnancy after Roux-en-Y gastric bypass. Surg Obes Relat Dis. 2010;6(1):88–92.

34. Loar 3rd PV, Sanchez-Ramos L, Kaunitz AM, Kerwin AJ, Diaz J. Maternal death caused by midgut volvulus after bariatric surgery. Am J Obstet Gynecol. 2005;193(5):1748–9.

35. Tohamy AE, Eid GM. Laparoscopic reduction of small bowel intussusception in a 33-week pregnant gastric bypass patient: surgical technique and review of literature. Surg Obes Relat Dis. 2009;5(1): 111–5.

36. Boland E, Thompson JS, Grant WJ, Botha J, Langnas AN, Mercer DF. Massive small bowel resection during pregnancy causing short bowel syndrome. Am Surg. 2011;77(12):1589–92.

37. Torres-Villalobos GM, Kellogg TA, Leslie DB, Antanavicius G, Andrade RS, Slusarek B, et al. Small bowel obstruction and internal hernias during pregnancy after gastric bypass surgery. Obes Surg. 2009;19(7):944–50.

38. Vrebosch L, Bel S, Vansant G, Guelinckx I, Devlieger R. Maternal and neonatal outcome after laparoscopic adjustable gastric banding: a systematic review. Obes Surg. 2012;22(10):1568–79.

39. Dixon JB, Dixon ME, O'Brien PE. Birth outcomes in obese women after laparoscopic adjustable gastric banding. Obstet Gynecol. 2005;106(5 Pt 1):965–72.

40. Haward RN, Brown WA, O'Brien PE. Does pregnancy increase the need for revisional surgery after laparoscopic adjustable gastric banding? Obes Surg. 2011;21(9):1362–9.

41. Friedman D, Cuneo S, Valenzano M, Marinari GM, Adami GF, Gianetta E, et al. Pregnancies in an 18-year follow-up after biliopancreatic diversion. Obes Surg. 1995;5(3):308–13.

42. Adami GF, Murelli F, Briatore L, Scopinaro N. Pregnancy in formerly type 2 diabetes obese women following biliopancreatic diversion for obesity. Obes Surg. 2008;18(9):1109–11.

43. Bal BS, Finelli FC, Koch TR. Origins of and recognition of micronutrient deficiencies after gastric bypass surgery. Curr Diab Rep. 2011;11(2):136–41.

44. Fleischer J, Stein EM, Bessler M, Della Badia M, Restuccia N, Olivero-Rivera L, et al. The decline in hip bone density after gastric bypass surgery is associated with extent of weight loss. J Clin Endocrinol Metab. 2008;93(10):3735–40.

45. Vilarrasa N, San Jose P, Garcia I, Gomez-Vaquero C, Miras PM, de Gordejuela AG, et al. Evaluation of bone mineral density loss in morbidly obese women after gastric bypass: 3-year follow-up. Obes Surg. 2011;21(4):465–72.

46. Moliterno JA, DiLuna ML, Sood S, Roberts KE, Duncan CC. Gastric bypass: a risk factor for neural tube defects? Case report. J Neurosurg Pediatr. 2008;1(5):406–9.

47. Hunskaar S. A systematic review of overweight and obesity as risk factors and targets for clinical intervention for urinary incontinence in women. Neurourol Urodyn. 2008;27(8):749–57.

48. Kolbl H, Riss P. Obesity and stress urinary incontinence: significance of indices of relative weight. Urol Int. 1988;43(1):7–10.

49. Greer WJ, Richter HE, Bartolucci AA, Burgio KL. Obesity and pelvic floor disorders: a systematic review. Obstet Gynecol. 2008;112(2 Pt 1):341–9.

50. Subak LL, Johnson C, Whitcomb E, Boban D, Saxton J, Brown JS. Does weight loss improve incontinence in moderately obese women? Int Urogynecol J Pelvic Floor Dysfunct. 2002;13(1):40–3.

51. Subak LL, Wing R, West DS, Franklin F, Vittinghoff E, Creasman JM, et al. Weight loss to treat urinary incontinence in overweight and obese women. N Engl J Med. 2009;360(5):481–90.

52. Laungani RG, Seleno N, Carlin AM. Effect of laparoscopic gastric bypass surgery on urinary incontinence in morbidly obese women. Surg Obes Relat Dis. 2009;5(3):334–8.

53. Whitcomb EL, Horgan S, Donohue MC, Lukacz ES. Impact of surgically induced weight loss on pelvic floor disorders. Int Urogynecol J. 2012;23(8):1111–6.

55

Medicolegal Issues: The Pitfalls and Pratfalls of the Bariatric Surgery Practice

Kathleen M. McCauley

Historical Perspective

There was an explosion in the number of medical malpractice lawsuits filed in the early part of this century, and general surgeons experienced the effects of this boom in and out of the operating room. While medical negligence lawsuits have been recognized for over two centuries, the modern-day impact of this type of litigation in the United States has been simmering for decades. With litigation reaching crisis proportions in the mid-1980s and again in the last decade, medical risk management has become an integral part of every surgical practice [8].

The legal theory behind medical malpractice claims originates in English jurisprudence dating back to the eighteenth century; however, lawsuits alleging medical malpractice were filed sparingly in the United States until the middle of the nineteenth century [9]. By 1850, medical malpractice litigation as we know it today was entrenched in the American legal landscape. Historians have attributed the precipitous increase in professional negligence actions in the United States to the cultural decline in fatalist philosophical thought and the marked increase in religious perfectionism, both concepts having grown out of the Christian revivals of the 1820s and 1830s [10]. The increase in the number of suits filed in later decades of the nineteenth century has been attributed to the birth of what has been called "marketplace professionalism" [11]. The concept of marketplace professionalism, unique to the United States during this stage in the country's development, illustrates the most dramatic American divergence from traditional European models of professional evolution [11]. Historically, the learned professions of Western Europe were granted authority by the ruling class. In the United States, however, this sanction was not embraced by American society and became most evident in the 1830s when concepts of social status, economic class, monopoly, and elitism garnered great public criticism [11]. The professions, including law and medicine, were thrust into the marketplace to fend for themselves in an environment of Darwinian competition. Consequently, the medical profession expanded to include those who were trained and untrained, alternative, and traditional, with little quality control. At the same time, lawyers found themselves in an equally hostile culture of competition, and medical malpractice became an area of growth for the legal profession [11].

The result of this fight for professional survival was an unprecedented increase in the number of medical malpractice suits filed in the United States. Between 1840 and 1860, the number of lawsuits alleging medical negligence grew by 950 % [11]. Although medical malpractice litigation exploded onto the scene in the middle of the nineteenth century as a result of a cultural shift, the phenomenon has perpetuated in response to both scientific innovation and the call for professional regulation. Historically, with every new era of medical innovation or expansion came an increase in claims for negligence. Once the innovation became passé, the wave of litigation abated but it never fell back to zero [12].

Despite the recognition that medicine is not perfection and physicians are fallible, our culture demanded a standard by which mistakes could be measured. Accordingly, the mid-nineteenth century saw the advent of various professional organizations, including the American Medical Association. As a result of this self-regulation, unqualified physicians were identified and driven from the profession. However, the impact on those who remained was the creation of uniform standards by which medical professionals would be judged. In the wake of these new licensing requirements and standards of care, the profession was exposed to more litigation as lawyers now judged physicians by the profession's own standards [12].

Finally, the introduction of professional liability insurance in the late nineteenth century proved to be both a champion and an enemy of the physician. Insurance virtually erased risk to the financial survival of the individual practitioner, but at the same time it guaranteed resources to the malpractice plaintiff [13]. As a result, the introduction of insurance to the profession effectively guaranteed the survival of medical malpractice litigation into the twentieth century and beyond [13]. Today, medical malpractice litigation is pervasive. One economic study by the Joint Economic Committee of the US Congress suggests that the current state of the medical malpractice litigation system has had a negative impact on the access to and the cost of professional liability insurance, the quality of health care, and the cost of and access to health care in this country [14]. While the future of the current medical liability system in the United States is unknown, the prudent bariatric surgeon must be able to identify potential risks associated with litigation and how best to avoid it.

Medical Negligence Litigation and Recent Trends

Despite having preconceived ideas of how they will be perceived, physicians should be reassured to learn that juries usually "get it right." Over 30 years of data show us that outcomes in medical malpractice litigation are remarkably consistent with the quality of care provided to a patient as critiqued by physician peers [15]. In general, physicians win 80–90 % of those cases where other physicians conclude there is weak evidence of medical negligence, 70 % of the borderline cases, and 50 % of cases where other physicians believe that the plaintiff should prevail [15]. In fact, one study suggested that favorable physician outcomes in the face of no documented evidence of negligence have improved and that the perception of a broken American tort system is misplaced [16].

After the litigation crises of the mid-1980s and early 2000s, a 2006 study by Aon, a global provider of risk management and insurance and reinsurance brokerage, revealed that claims against hospitals and physicians began to stabilize. In its seventh annual Hospital Professional Liability and Physician Liability Benchmark Analysis, Aon attributed the decrease in frequency and increase in severity to claims management, tort reform, and patient safety and quality assurance efforts [17]. This stabilization in frequency of claims remained true for several years until the economy took a turn for the worse [18]. A new study suggests that by the end of 2012, claim severity for hospitals and physicians nationwide had increased by 2.5 % with claim frequency increasing by 1 %. In its 2012 Benchmark study, Aon and the American Society for Healthcare Risk Management concluded that we should expect to see a sharp increase in medical malpractice claims and warn that loss rates for both hospitals and physicians are projected to grow by 3.5 % by 2013 [19].

Medical Negligence Litigation and the Bariatric Surgeon

What is medical malpractice? How does a plaintiff prove medical malpractice? Why the surge in medical malpractice claims involving bariatric surgery? Why do people sue their physician? What is the impact of a medical malpractice lawsuit on the physician's career? What is the impact on the physician's job satisfaction and personal happiness? These are the questions that cause the medical profession angst, despair, and insomnia. For some, the topic inspires only ire and frustration.

The word *malpractice* has been defined as "any professional misconduct, unreasonable lack of skill or fidelity in the profession or fiduciary duties, evil practice or illegal or immoral conduct" [20]. The term *medical malpractice* is derived from the Latin *mala praxis*—bad practice—and was first applied to the profession of medicine by Sir William Blackstone in 1768 [21]. To prevail in a medical negligence suit, the plaintiff must prove by the greater weight of the evidence all four elements of the cause of action. That is, to prove a prima facie case of medical negligence, the plaintiff must establish:

1. A duty to the patient
2. A breach of that duty or standard of care
3. A compensable injury
4. Proximate causation to the injury or damages [22, 23]

Once the physician–patient relationship is established, the physician owes his or her patient the duty of due care. "Due care" is defined as the care required of a reasonably prudent physician in the same field of practice under the same or similar circumstances [24]. In most cases, the duty of due care—or the standard of care—must be proved through expert testimony. Likewise, any alleged breach of the standard of care and proximate causation must be proved through the introduction of expert testimony. The plaintiff often uses documents such as medical records, medical literature, and demonstrative aids such as models, charts, medical chronologies, and diagrams at trial as well.

Physicians are sued for myriad reasons, from the sublime to the ridiculous. That said, most suits for malpractice allege the following:

- Failure to communicate or miscommunication
- Failure to diagnose
- Failure to treat
- Failure to document appropriately
- Failure to perform a procedure appropriately
- Failure to get appropriate consultations
- Inappropriate orders or delegation of duties
- Breach of confidentiality
- Failure to admit a patient to the hospital or premature discharge
- Failure to order appropriate diagnostic tests or studies
- Misinterpreted diagnostic tests or studies
- Bad outcomes and unreasonable expectations
- Complications and failure to timely address recognized complications
- Inadequate informed consent or no informed consent
- Failure to follow up or patient abandonment

In recent years, there has been a focus on finding data to support why plaintiffs choose to sue healthcare practitioners.

One recent survey reveals that the number of years in practice dictates the likelihood of being named in litigation. A 2011 survey sent out by the ASMBS Patient Safety Committee determined that the probability of reporting at least one lawsuit independently increased with the number of years a surgeon was in practice [25]. Another study revealed that only about 5 % of physicians are sued annually but that 42.2 % of physicians have had medical malpractice claims filed against them during their career [26]. Pediatricians and psychiatrists were sued least often with their colleagues in surgery and obstetrics/gynecology having higher frequency data [26]. That said, a subsequent American Medical Association study revealed that 55 % of all cases filed against physicians are dismissed, with less than 5 % of cases making it to trial [27]. Of those cases tried to a judge or jury, 79.6 % of cases resulted in verdicts in favor of the physician [27]. The study involved claims closed between 2002 and 2005 and outcomes varied across specialties, with medicine-based specialties enjoying the highest rate of dismissal (61.5 %) and pathologists suffering the lowest (36.5 %) [27].

So why do surgeons get sued? Anecdotally, we know that bad clinical outcomes are at the heart of most litigation. The data shows that those bad clinical outcomes can be tied to injury to adjacent organ or anatomic structure. In a 2008 survey of 91 lawsuits against general surgeons, 30 % of those suits involved iatrogenic injury to adjacent structures, 37 % of which involved nerve injury [28]. However, patients and their families also sue because they are angry, offended, or grieving. As well, experience tells us that plaintiffs often use the litigation process to apportion blame, shift accountability, manage guilt or grief, and seek closure.

Bariatric surgeons see claims of malpractice for similar reasons, although weight-loss procedures and morbidly obese patients are unique in the medical litigation mise-en-scéne. Cases against bariatric surgeons include many of those claims delineated above but also may include the following allegations:

- Inexperience of the operator
- Inadequate facilities or equipment for the bariatric patient
- Failure to monitor or inadequate postoperative monitoring
- Failure to diagnose or to timely diagnose a lethal complication
- Inadequate preoperative workup or substandard patient selection
- Contraindications to surgery, including history of gallstones or cholecystitis
- Poor follow-up support after surgery
- Unrecognized or unaddressed psychiatric issues
- Misguided motivation for surgery

Today, the lion's share of litigation involving weight-loss procedures concentrates on allegations of negligence during the postoperative period, immediate postoperative inpatient care, and follow-up once the patient is discharged to home [29]. Specifically, postoperative leaks and delayed diagnosis of recognized complications of the procedure are the most common cause for a subsequent medical negligence claim [30]. Regardless of the theory of liability against the bariatric surgeon, the suits continue to be filed across the nation.

Informed Consent

Informed consent is a process, not a piece of paper. It is a common misconception that one proves informed consent with a signed "consent for treatment" form. To the contrary, the signed consent form is merely one piece of evidence that the attending physician completed the informed consent process. The doctrine of informed consent is based on the premise that people have a right to decide what happens to their own bodies and minds. It is based on the concept of autonomy—a concept firmly grounded in philosophy, not law. Autonomy—or self-determination—embraces the notion that people have the right to choose the course of their own medical treatment in accordance with their own values, mores, religious beliefs, and life goals. The principle is also grounded on the premise that no other person, institution, or other entity should be permitted to intervene to overrule an individual's wishes, whether or not those wishes are "right," as long as the decision does not negatively affect another individual [31]. That choice, however, must be based on information regarding diagnosis, prognosis, risks, and benefits of the procedure or course of therapy, as well as the consequences of refusing treatment.

The doctrine of informed consent is composed of two discrete components: permission and knowledge. A patient is entitled to give express permission for any touching by another and that permission is to be based on information that is deemed to be important by the patient's physician. That is, it is incumbent on the medical practitioner to impart all information necessary for the patient to make a well-reasoned, educated choice regarding treatment. Informed consent is of paramount importance when dealing with elective procedures, as consent is implied in the case of an emergency. As bariatric surgery is a high-risk elective procedure by its very nature, the informed consent process must be well planned and well executed.

Causes of action involving issues of informed consent fall into two categories: the tort of battery (no consent) or negligence (inadequate consent). Battery—or unauthorized touching—occurs when the physician fails to obtain informed consent or if the touching exceeds the scope of the informed consent. Negligent informed consent is consent that is based on inadequate information. In most jurisdictions, informed consent is based on the "reasonable" man standard; that is, consent is informed when it is based on the information that a reasonably prudent surgeon would convey to his or her patient during the informed consent process. Suits alleging negligent informed consent usually require expert testimony on the subject; cases alleging battery do not.

Generally, the informed consent process should include the following:

1. A discussion in laymen terms regarding the description of the surgical procedure to be performed
2. A discussion of the significant risks and benefits of the procedure to be performed
3. A discussion of the alternatives to the proposed surgical procedure
4. A discussion of the consequences of the procedure being declined by the patient
5. Documentation of the informed consent process *and* the actual consent, including a signed consent form, a note in the physician's progress notes, in the patient's clinic chart, and in the operative report

It is important to be sensitive to false or unrealistic expectations in the patient population and to dispel any misconceptions about the procedures of anticipated outcome. It is reasonable to assume that any representation about obesity surgery made on a Web site, in promotional materials, or in informational pamphlets or videotapes will be relied upon by patients and their families. Surgeons should be wary of making promises and predictions.

Documentation

The most credible piece of evidence in litigation is medical record documentation. Accordingly, the medical record must be complete, concise, accurate, legible, timely, and authentic. While this may seem a daunting task, physicians may be asked to interpret or rely upon a medical record several years after the provided care and treatment to a patient. In the busy practice, particularly one in the academic milieu, it is of paramount importance to maintain an accurate and comprehensive medical record.

Why document in the medical record? Is the documentation strictly used to defend the surgeon who finds himself embroiled in litigation? No. The medical record memorializes care and treatment contemporaneously in an effort to promote continuity of care, accurate communication among the care team members, and data for retrospective review and analysis and to defend surgeons who find themselves embroiled in litigation.

Accurate and complete documentation may prove to be the most important tool in the management of the bariatric patient. In this highly specialized practice of surgery, both the pre- and postsurgical phases of treatment require effective communication among various disciplines (i.e., medicine, surgery, nutrition, psychology, and occupational and physical therapy) and adequate data to provide comprehensive, timely, and safe treatment to this unique patient population. In general, effective inpatient documentation describes in an objective manner all noteworthy data regarding a patient's presentation, history and physical,

recommendations for treatment, actual ongoing care and treatment, and follow-up. It is important to include the most current information available, which will ensure that the patient's chart will be the most reliable resource for ongoing patient care and the best evidence that appropriate and timely care was provided. As the medical record is the primary conduit for continuing care and communication among a patient's care providers, it should include all pertinent clinical information, including the physician's assessment and reaction to laboratory reports, radiology, and other studies. Surgeons often fail to include their rationale for clinical decisions, including data to support the differential diagnosis; however, this information is critical. Physicians should be sure to document a differential diagnosis when the facts permit a reasonable inference that something other than the primary diagnosis may be valid. It is far more difficult to allege that a surgeon failed to consider all of the options when faced with clinically pertinent data if it is documented in the medical record, especially in an area of medicine where potential complications are many, are potentially lethal, and often occur quickly.

Regardless of the procedure, the operative note should be dictated expeditiously—ideally on the same day—and should include all findings and complications encountered and the related management of those findings. Operative notes dictated weeks or months after the procedure are a "red flag" in litigation, particularly in situations where complications were encountered by the surgical team. Despite the routine nature of some surgical procedures, the prudent surgeon should avoid using "boilerplate" language, rather endeavoring to personalize the operative note to the individual patient. Furthermore, all dictation should be reviewed, corrected, and signed promptly and include the results of the sponge and instrument counts. Likewise, postoperative orders should be legible and signed by the operating surgeon, and follow-up and discharge instructions should be signed by the patient or his or her responsible party.

In the bariatric clinic setting, it is important to document all preoperative patient encounters, referrals, and consultations. Preoperative screening should be comprehensive and noted in the patient's chart, as well as all relevant discussions with the patient and family and any consultants. All consultation reports should be contained in the record, as well as preoperative laboratory results, radiology, and other screening exams pertinent to the bariatric patient headed for surgery. When documenting the informed consent process, include the risks, benefits, and alternatives discussed, as well as whether additional information was provided to the patient and family (e.g., videotape, brochure, pamphlets, referral to support groups, or other forms of patient education). In most cases, the informed consent process for bariatric procedures is lengthy, is candid, and may be included in the patient screening mechanism. That being said, it should be well documented to protect the care team from claims alleging inadequate consent after a bad outcome.

Postoperative follow-up is arguably the most important phase in caring for the bariatric patient. Accordingly, the surgeon or professional staff should document clearly all follow-up instructions, appointments, referrals, prescriptions and refills, and the plan of care going forward. As the medical record is used as a communication tool and for documentation of continuing care, it is critical that all telephone communications are entered in the chart, as well as missed, canceled, and rescheduled appointments. Above all, document and include all correspondence related to the physician's decision to terminate the physician–patient relationship or when the patient informs the physician that the physician's services are no longer necessary.

Do's of Effective Charting

- Do use precise, concise, specific language.
- Do use objective, factual statements.
- Do document a patient's verbatim statements.
- Do date and time each entry in the medical record.
- Do make sure the patient's name appears on the page before writing.
- Do draw diagonal lines through all blank space after an entry.
- Do document adverse reactions to medications or therapy.
- Do "red flag" all allergies.
- Do ensure that all procedure notes and chart entries are timely and accurate.
- Do be sure to read a medical record entry before cosigning.
- Do include time and specific action in all discharge instructions.
- Do include all pertinent communications with residents, attending physicians, nursing staff, and consults.
- Do include an addendum or late entry if necessary.
- Do include the words "addendum" or "late entry"; time and date the note.

Don'ts of Effective Charting

- Do not alter the medical record… ever. This is a criminal act.
- Do not obliterate errors or remove pages from the chart.
- Do not use personal abbreviations, initials, or ditto marks.
- Do not include derogatory or discriminatory remarks.
- Do not document conflicts with other physicians or nursing staff.
- Do not use subjective statements about prior treatment or poor outcomes.
- Do not include a late entry after an adverse event.
- Do not include non-patient care information.
- Do not perpetuate incorrect information.
- Do not write any finger-pointing or self-serving statements.
- Do not alter existing documentation or withhold portions of the chart once a claim has been made or after the record has been copied.

- Do not use phrases that imply a risk.
- Do not include incident reports, quality assurance information, or documents involving the legal process in the patient chart… ever.

While the patient chart is first and foremost a medical document, it is also a legal document. It is the best defense to any claim of medical malpractice and should reflect the attention to detail required of the prudent bariatric surgeon.

Confidentiality

Since the Clinton Administration, patient privacy and medical record confidentiality have garnered much public and political attention. Congress passed the Health Insurance Portability and Accountability Act (HIPAA), historically known as the Kassebaum-Kennedy Law, in 1996 [32]. Its primary purpose was to improve continuity and portability in the delivery of health care while preserving the privacy of certain sensitive health information [32]. Furthermore, it seeks to "combat waste, fraud and abuse in health insurance and health care delivery… [and] simplify the administration of health insurance" [32]. In an effort to carry out these purposes in the age of technology, HIPAA targets three areas of the healthcare industry: (1) insurance portability, (2) fraud enforcement, and (3) administrative simplification [33]. It is the administrative simplification section of HIPAA that concentrates on patient privacy and that is of most interest to healthcare professionals and their staff [34].

The privacy regulations (Privacy Rule) of HIPAA are designed to provide patients a process by which to maintain the confidential nature of certain protected health information (PHI). The final Privacy Rule was published in December 2000, to be effective in April 2001 [35]. It applies to specific "covered" entities including health plans, healthcare clearinghouses, and healthcare providers who transmit health information in electronic form related to a transaction covered by the federal regulations [36]. The final modifications to the Privacy Rule were published in August 2002 [37], and the previously specified entities were required to comply with the Privacy Rule by April 14, 2003 [38].

The Privacy Rule protects individually identifiable health information (the PHI) that is maintained or transmitted by a covered entity, whether oral or written [39]. Individually identifiable health information includes even the most basic demographic information collected from an individual patient [39]. It also includes any information created by or received by a health plan, a patient's employer, a healthcare clearinghouse, or a healthcare provider that relates to past, present, or future physical or mental health condition of an individual [39]. Further, the Privacy Rule relates to information regarding the past, present, or future payment for health care by the individual, if the information identifies the individual patient [39].

The Privacy Rule does not prohibit disclosure of PHI; rather, it requires that the information be disclosed only in accordance with the provisions of HIPAA [40]. That is, when a covered entity discloses PHI or when it is requesting protected information from another covered entity, it must make reasonable efforts to limit the transmission of protected information to the minimum disclosure necessary to meet the requirements of the request [40]. However, the Privacy Rule requirement does not apply to the release of PHI in the following scenarios:

1. Requests from or disclosure to a healthcare provider for the purpose of medical treatment
2. Release of PHI to the patient himself
3. Disclosure of PHI to the US Department of Health and Human Services
4. Disclosures or requests required by law
5. Release of or request for information in accordance with the Privacy Rule [41]

The Privacy Rule requires that a covered entity not disclose or use PHI without an authorization, unless the disclosure is contemplated by the regulations [42]. For an authorization to be valid under HIPAA, it must include the following:

1. A description of the information to be disclosed
2. Identification of the persons or class of persons authorized to use or disclose the PHI
3. Identification of the persons or class of persons to whom disclosure will be made
4. A description of the purpose of the use of disclosure
5. An expiration date certain or precipitating event
6. The individual's signature and date
7. A description of the authority of the signatory to act on behalf of the individual, if signed by a personal representative [43]

The authorization for disclosure under HIPAA must also include the following:

1. A statement that the individual may revoke authorization and instructions regarding how to do so.
2. A statement that medical treatment, payment, enrollment in a plan, or eligibility for benefits may not be predicated on obtaining the authorization from the individual if such a condition is prohibited by the Privacy Rule. To the degree it is not prohibited, the authorization must include a statement about the consequences of not authorizing use and/or disclosure.
3. A statement about the likelihood that the recipient will disclose the PHI [43].

Patient authorization is *not* required for disclosure in accordance with public health activities; reporting victims of abuse, neglect, or domestic violence; health oversight activities; judicial and administrative proceedings; or law enforcement purposes (i.e., pursuant to court order or subpoena) [44].

As one would expect, patients are granted rights to their own PHI under HIPAA's Privacy Rule. Specifically, patients may request certain restrictions be placed on the disclosure of their PHI [45], the right to review and copy their PHI [46], the right to amend their PHI [47], the right to receive a copy of the HIPAA notice from the covered entity [48], and the right to receive an accounting of disclosures of PHI [49].

It is important to note that any provision of the HIPAA Privacy Rule that is contrary to individual state law preempts that provision of state law [50]. That being said, federal law will not preempt state law if the state law is promulgated to prevent fraud and abuse related to payment for medical services; to ensure state regulation of the insurance industry and healthcare plans; to report on the delivery of health care and related costs; to serve a compelling need related to public health, safety, or welfare; or to regulate controlled substances [51]. Furthermore, HIPAA will not preempt the state law if the state law is more restrictive than the federal statute [51]. It is extremely important for physicians to be aware of their state's confidentiality statutes that control when and how private health information may be disclosed.

Under the American Recovery and Reinvestment Act of 2009, the federal government included a set of provisions titled the Health Information Technology for Economic and Clinical Health Act (HITECH) that advance the use of technology in health care. The Act encourages physicians and hospitals to purchase and incorporate electronic medical record systems (the Act calls them electronic health records (EHR)) into their practice before the end of 2015. The goal of the Act is to improve quality of care and to control escalating costs associated with the delivery of health care in the United States. In an effort to facilitate and ease the transition from paper-based medical records to EMR, the Act includes incentive payments to qualifying professionals and hospitals.

The Centers for Medicare & Medicaid Services (CMS) administers the Medicare and Medicaid EHR incentive payments to eligible physicians, hospitals, and critical access hospitals [52] as they "adopt, implement, upgrade, or demonstrate meaningful use" of EMR technology. An estimate of $27 billion has been set aside to accomplish the Act's goals and specifically to assist in the implementation of the EMR, with roughly $17 billion going toward incentives. The incentive payments are available to hospitals and physicians when they adopt certified EMR and the numbers are significant. In recent years—and in large part due to these incentives— EMRs are being adopted, implemented, and used by hospitals and surgeons in increasing numbers. The process has not been seamless for most and the transition has been, and will continue to be, fraught with complications and unintended consequences. Nevertheless, the EMR is here to stay.

Along with the implementation of this technology in the office, clinic, and hospital setting comes new requirements for maintaining confidentiality. The HIPAA/HITECH Final Rule was published by the Department of Health and Human

Services, Office for Civil Rights (OCR) on January 25, 2013 [53]. The effective date is March 26, 2013, and compliance is required by September 23, 2013. The HITECH Act required that certain aspects of HIPAA be modified, including the August 24, 2009, interim final rule on Breach Notification for Unsecured Protected Health Information; the October 7, 2009, proposed rule modifying the HIPAA Privacy Rule as required by the Genetic Information Nondiscrimination Act (GINA); the October 30, 2009, interim final rule adopting changes to the HIPAA Enforcement Rule; and the July 14, 2010, proposed modifications to the HIPAA Privacy, Security, and Enforcement Rules [54].

It is important to be aware that the new rules include (1) the redefinition of "business associate" under HIPAA; (2) the broader liability application to business associates and their agents and subcontractors; (3) changes to the breach standards; (4) prohibitions regarding the sale of PHI without authorization; (5) new rules related to fundraising, marketing, immunization information to schools, and the disclosure of deceased patients' PHI; (6) broader individual access to electronic PHI; and (7) penalties associated with violations of these and other provisions of HIPAA. For purposes of this chapter, we will only discuss the changes to patient access to electronic PHI.

As with the original Privacy Rule, patients have the right to access their own health information. Under the HITECH Act, Congress gave patients the right to electronic *copies* of PHI in EHR; however, in the new rule, OCR expanded this right to include all electronic designated record sets (DRS). Accordingly, if an individual requests an electronic copy of PHI that is maintained electronically in more than one DRS, the provider must produce it in the electronic form and format requested, if it is readily reproducible. If it is not readily reproducible in the requested form or format, it must be produced in a readable electronic form and format as agreed upon by the parties. If the individual declines to accept any format that is readily reproducible by the provider, then the provider may produce a hard copy. There is no requirement that the provider scans paper copies. Finally, providers must comply with individuals' requests that their PHI be sent directly to another person if that request is in writing, is signed by the individual, and clearly identifies the designated person to whom the PHI should be sent.

The provider, at his or her discretion, may accept verbal requests for PHI or require written, signed authorizations. You have 30 days to provide access to a patient's PHI, and a 30-day extension may apply in situations where a hard copy or electronic PHI must be retrieved from off-site storage or where other time constraints make the extension necessary. Nonetheless, the provider must apprise the individual of any delay in making the PHI available if not within the 30-day period and provide a date when the information may be reasonably expected. If not otherwise provided by state law, the final rule permits providers to charge reasonable cost-based fees for complying with a request for PHI. This fee may include actual labor costs for copying PHI in paper or electronic form, actual costs for technical staff to create and copy electronic files, and costs for postage and supplies.

There is no requirement that a provider use portable devices brought by patients or other individuals (i.e., flash drives), as these pose a security risk. A provider may send PHI in an encrypted email; however, they must first advise the individual that there is some level of risk associated with email and that the PHI may be accessed and read by a third party [55].

With continued attention to patient privacy, surgeons and their professional staff have become increasingly more sensitive to the requirements of HIPAA and the HITECH Act; however, the principles behind the law have been part and parcel of good medicine for centuries. The concept of patient privacy is based on the principles of fidelity and confidentiality; two ideals articulated in the Oath of Hippocrates and the Prayer of Maimonides. Accordingly, the ethics of HIPAA and the requirements to keep private that information imparted to the surgeon for purposes of treatment shall remain tantamount to the prudent practice of medicine.

Risk Management and Prevention

Physicians in modern American society cannot control whether or not they are sued; they can, however, control how they defend themselves. The best defense in litigation amounts to the best practices of the profession.

The Physician

While an excellent education is imperative to the practice of surgery, experience is the keystone to a successful bariatric surgery practice. Because obesity surgery has been in the media spotlight in recent years, dozens of surgeons have broadened their practices by adding weight-loss procedures. By the surgical community's own admission, the procedures generate revenue and the practice area has proven to be lucrative. It has also provided hope and recovery to a large portion of the population for whom other weight-loss programs have proven to be a miserable failure. It saves lives. However, a fact that must not be ignored is that bariatric surgery is extraordinarily dangerous at the hand of the inexperienced or under-experienced surgeon. Obesity surgery was not included in the general surgery residency training as a matter of course until recent years and is not widely available even today. Accordingly, many surgeons learn the procedures in weekend classes and mini-fellowships. This training, while provided by the professional community's finest bariatric surgeons, is inadequate to arm the general practitioner with the skills and experience necessary to maintain a safe surgical weight-loss practice.

Continued Assessment of Outcomes

It is recommended that the local facility review the surgeon's outcome data within 6 months of initiation of a new program and after the surgeon's first 50 procedures (performed independently) as well as at regular intervals thereafter, to confirm patient safety. In addition, the surgeon should continue to meet Global Credentialing Requirements for bariatric surgery at the time of reappointment. Documentation of continuing medical education related to bariatric surgery is also strongly recommended.

In addition to the ASMBS, the American College of Surgeons (ACS) and the Society of American Gastrointestinal and Endoscopic Surgeons (SAGES) have crafted guidelines and resources for credentialing bariatric surgeons. Further, the Metabolic and Bariatric Accreditation and Quality Improvement Program (MBSAQIP) is a national program that maintains a data registry and provides guidance and standards for quality improvement for bariatric surgery. It is important for physicians to be aware of these recommendations even if the hospital at which they seek privileges has not adopted the ASMBS or other guidelines, as the recommendations were crafted and endorsed by the leaders in bariatric surgery. It is noteworthy that literature published in 2010 suggests that these credentialing initiatives for training and practice are justified in light of improved clinical outcomes for bariatric patients [56]. In the current litigation climate where the experience of the operator increasingly has been called into question, expertise may be the best defense to such allegations at trial.

As discussed earlier in the chapter, the physician's best line of defense in litigation is documentation. The physician should be concise, clear, and complete, as malpractice litigation is often won or lost on the content and quality of the medical record. The documentation the physician creates today may be used years later in litigation; therefore, good record keeping should be an integral part of the bariatric surgeon's daily routine. Because meticulous medical records constitute the very best evidence at trial, this aspect of malpractice litigation remains in the exclusive control of the practitioner: Document, document, document… and document well.

Patients and their families sue for a variety of reasons, some that are within the control of the surgeon and some that are not. The most important human relationship in bariatric surgery exists between the patient and the surgeon, not between the surgeon and his or her attorney. Accordingly, surgeons should treat the physician–patient relationship with as much care as they treat the actual patient. This interpersonal relationship is becoming more important in the increasingly more hostile healthcare environment. Patients who are treated with compassion and respect are less likely to resolve their feelings or disagreements in court. Physicians must give the patient their time and their undivided attention.

While bad outcomes are not always preventable, it has been suggested that physicians who apologize for bad outcomes are less likely to be the subject of a malpractice claim. Because anger is often the driving force in a lawsuit, contrition and honesty have been shown to dispel anger long before litigation is ever contemplated [57]. Good communication between physician and patient has been linked to a decrease in physician shopping, noncompliance, and malpractice claims as well [58]. Not only have communication and honesty been shown to positively impact the physician–patient relationship, but the manner in which the information is communicated may dictate the likelihood of a lawsuit resulting from a bad outcome [59].

The Facility

With the unprecedented growth in obesity surgery programs nationwide, more and more hospitals are providing the surgical venue, but without the appropriate facilities and equipment for the bariatric patient population. The key to a successful and safe surgical weight-loss program is strategic planning for this unique population, adequate spending to retrofit or build the appropriate facilities, and appropriate staffing and staff education.

While bariatric procedures are elective, they are not cosmetic surgery. Because bariatric patients are often very ill and require complex care, hospitals and staff must be prepared and equipped to manage their preoperative, perioperative, and postoperative courses. Accordingly, facilities should be equipped with appropriately sized surgical instruments, blood pressure cuffs, endotracheal and nasogastric tubes, and adequate imaging equipment including computed tomography and magnetic resonance imaging. Further, surgical weight-loss patients require specialty beds, chairs, and intensive care unit facilities.

Outpatient facilities should include large examination tables and enough chairs to accommodate patients and their families. It is important to be aware of the needs of this patient population and to respect their unique perspective. Every detail should be taken into consideration down to the magazines available in the waiting room.

In 2000, the American College of Surgeons published recommendations for facilities caring for the morbidly obese [60]. These comprehensive guidelines provide facilities with recommendations for equipping and managing a safe and appropriate venue for weight-loss surgery and for the even more important follow-up period.

Staff education is as important as having the appropriate equipment. As the bariatric surgeon cannot be at the bedside 24 h a day, well-trained staff must be the eyes and ears of the surgical team. Precious time is lost when postoperative complications manifest if the condition is not diagnosed and treated immediately. Accordingly, nursing staff must be attuned to the special needs of the bariatric population and must be quick to recognize and react to pertinent clinical information. The best solution is to have a devoted bariatric service and floor of the facility. When such a solution is unavailable, specialized training and education of hospital medical-surgical staff is the best defense to allegations of missed postoperative complications and negligent nursing care.

The Program

Bariatric surgeons treat the most complex patient population in the general surgery community—the morbidly obese. Bariatric surgical candidates often have multiple and varied comorbidities, which make the care and treatment of these special patients challenging. Patients who meet the criteria for weight-loss surgery present with myriad health problems, including asthma and sleep apnea, gout, heart disease, stroke, diabetes, gallbladder disease, hypertension, hypercholesterolemia, osteoarthritis, and a higher incidence of cancer. As a result, many of these patients have low reserves and a profoundly compromised ability to recover from the many complications associated with surgical weight-loss procedures. A comprehensive preoperative screening process, detailed informed consent discussions, and an appropriate and a well-supported long-term follow-up program are of paramount importance to the successful bariatric practice.

The safest and most successful bariatric surgery programs are built on an interdisciplinary approach to health care. This interdisciplinary approach contemplates the special needs of the morbidly obese and the health concerns with which they present. A successful program includes a comprehensive introduction to weight-loss surgery, patient/family education, and sensitivity to the patients served.

The program should include a thorough preoperative workup and a well-documented informed consent process based on the interdisciplinary approach. Morbidly obese patients come with myriad diagnoses, which require attention and management throughout the patient's journey from surgery to follow-up. Therefore, preoperative and postoperative care should include consultations with various subspecialties of internal medicine (including cardiology, endocrinology, pulmonology, etc.), psychiatry, nutrition, and physical and occupational therapy. The program should include a process for choosing the appropriate weight-loss procedure for the individual patient, based on the patient's diagnoses, risk factors, and other needs. This decision should be well documented, including the thought process employed by the surgeon in formulating the patient's plan of care.

The prudent program should also include long-term follow-up with appropriate specialists, support staff, and a mechanism to ensure the continuity of care. Patients who are provided quality care and treatment in a friendly and respectful environment, by compassionate and patient practitioners, are likely to be happy and healthier. Likewise, a deliberate program designed to care for the morbidly obese protects the surgical professional from allegations involving poor planning, inadequate facilities, inappropriate equipment, and inadequately trained staff.

Conclusion

It is safe to expect that the bariatric surgical community will continue to thrive as the demand for weight-loss surgery continues. As we move toward the future of bariatric medicine, it is important to recognize the risks of practicing in this exciting and rewarding field. With education, conscientious bariatric surgeons can avoid many of the legal pitfalls, despite the fact that it is impossible to insulate your practice from lawsuits. Nevertheless, prudent practices, complete medical record documentation, appropriate informed consent, and a healthy physician–patient relationship will provide the best defense for surgeons who find themselves exposed to the litigation process.

Review Questions and Answers

1. What must the plaintiff prove in order to prevail in a medical malpractice lawsuit?
   A. Duty
   B. Breach
   C. Proximate causation/damages
   D. All of the above

   Answer: D

2. What organizations do not provide guidance for credentialing bariatric surgeons?
   A. ASMBS
   B. ACS
   C. SSAT
   D. SAGES

   Answer: C

3. Q: True or false: After an increase in litigation in the early 2000s, there was a decrease in frequency of filing medical malpractice lawsuits until 2012.

   Answer: True

References

1. Mathias JM. Increase in bariatric surgery brings a surge in legal cases. OR Manager 2002;18(2).
2. Kowalczyk L. Gastric bypass risk is linked to inexperience. Boston Globe 2004 Jan 4.
3. Alt SJ. Market memo: liability insurance premiums on bariatric surgery soar. Health Care Strategic Manag. 2004;22(1):1.
4. Rice B. How high now? Med Econ. 2004;81:57–9.
5. Twiddy D. Associated Press 2004 Aug 26.

6. Nguyen NT, Masoomi H, Magno CP, Nguyen XT, Laugenour K, Lane J. Trends in use of bariatric surgery, 2003–2008. J Am Coll Surg. 2011;213(2):261. doi:10.1016/j.jamcollsurg.2011.04.030.

7. Livingston EH. The Incidence of bariatric surgery has plateaued in the United States. Am J Surg. 2010;200(3):378–85. doi:10.1016/j.amjsurg.2009.11.007 [Epub 2010 Apr 20].

8. For a more extensive discussion about the current medical malpractice crisis in the United States, see Studdert DM, Mello MM, Brennan TA, Medical malpractice. N Engl J Med. 2003;348(23):2281, corrected in N Engl J Med. 2003;349(10):1010; and Mello MM, Studdert DM, Brennan TA. The new medical malpractice crisis. N Engl J Med. 2004;350(3):283.

9. Mohr JC. American medical malpractice litigation in historical perspective. JAMA. 2000;283(13):1731.

10. Mohr JC. American medical malpractice litigation in historical perspective. JAMA. 2000;283(13):1732.

11. Mohr JC. American medical malpractice litigation in historical perspective. JAMA. 2000;283(13), citing Mohr JC. Doctors and the law: medical jurisprudence in nineteenth-century America. New York: Oxford University Press; 1993.

12. Mohr JC. American medical malpractice litigation in historical perspective. JAMA. 2000;283(13):1734.

13. Mohr JC. American medical malpractice litigation in historical perspective. JAMA. 2000;283(13):1735.

14. Miller D. Liability for medical malpractice: issues and evidence. Joint Economic Committee, U.S. Congress, Vice Chair Jim Saxton (R-NJ), May 2003. www.house.gov. Accessed 6 Sept 2004.

15. Peters PG. Twenty years of evidence on the outcomes of malpractice claims. Clin Orthop Relat Res. 2009;467:352–7.

16. Studdert DM, Mello MM, Gawande AA, Gandhi TK, Kachalia A, Yoon C, Puopolo AL, Brennan TA. Claims, errors, and compensation payments in medical malpractice litigation. N Engl J Med. 2006;354:2024–33. doi:10.1056/NEJMsa054479.

17. Aon Seventh Annual Hospital Professional Liability and Physician Liability Benchmark Analysis. 2006. www.aon.com/hpl_study.

18. See Aon Hospital Professional Liability and Physician Professional Liability Benchmark Analysis 2007–2010. www.aon.com/hpl_study; Zurich 2010 Claims Benchmarking Perspective. 2010;16(3). www.zurichna.com/internet/zna/SiteCollectionDocuments/en/Products/healthcare/HC_Perspectives_newsletter_Fall.pdf.

19. Aon 2012 Hospital Professional Liability and Physician Liability Benchmark Analysis. 2012. www.aon.com/hpl_study.

20. Black's Law Dictionary, citing Mathews v. Walker, 34 Ohio App.2d 128,296 N.E.ed 569, 571.

21. Mohr JC. American medical malpractice litigation in historical perspective. JAMA 2000;283(13):1731, citing Blackstone W. Commentaries on the Laws of England, vol. 3. Oxford, England: Clarendon Press, 1768:122.

22. See, generally, Fiscina S et al. Medical liability. Eagan, MN: West Group; 2004:209. West Publishing; 1991.

23. It is important to note that the law of torts is customarily controlled by the individual states. Accordingly, medical negligence case law may vary from jurisdiction to jurisdiction, although it is based on the more general common law.

24. Pike v. Honsinger, 155 N.Y. 201, 49 N.E. 760 (1898).

25. Dallal R. Survey: long surgical career raises likelihood of lawsuit. Clinical Endocrinology News Digital Network 2012 Jul 12.

26. American Medical Association Policy Research Perspectives. Carol K. Kane, Medical Liability Claim Frequency: A 2007–2008 Snapshot of Physicians. AMA Economic and Health Policy Research, 2010 Aug.

27. Outcomes of medical malpractice litigation against US physicians. Arch Intern Med. 2012;172(11):892–94.

28. van Heerden JA, Farley DR. Why do surgeons get sued? Common causes revealed. Contemp Surg. 2008;64(6):284–5.

29. Misreading Obesity Surgery Risk. www.rmf.harvard.edu. Accessed 7 Aug 2004.

30. Cottam D, Lord J, Dallal RM, Wolfe B, Higa K, McCauley K, Schauer P. Medicolegal analysis of 100 malpractice claims against bariatric surgeons. Surg Obes Relat Dis. 2007;3(1):60–6; discussion 66–7 [Epub 2006 Dec 27].

31. Furrow BR et al. Bioethics: health care law and ethics. 3rd ed. St. Paul: West.

32. Pub. L. No. 104–191,110 Stat. 1936 (1996) (codified in portions of 29 U.S.C., 42 U.S.C., and 18 U.S.C.).

33. For a more comprehensive discussion of the administrative simplification process, see Perrow et al. The Health Insurance Portability and Accountability Act: An Overview of Administrative Simplification, XIV J. Civ. L. 231 (2002).

34. 42 U.S.C. § 1320d et seq (2002).

35. Standards for Privacy of Individually Identifiable Health Information. 65 Fed. Reg. 82462 (December 28 2000).

36. Standards for Privacy of Individually Identifiable Health Information. 45 C.F.R. § 164.502 (2001).

37. Standards for Privacy of Individually Identifiable Health Information. 67 Fed. Reg. 53181 (August 14, 2002).

38. 42 U.S.C. § 1320d-3 (2002). Small health plans must have complied by April 14, 2004. Ibid.

39. 45 C.F.R. § 164.501 (2001).

40. 45 C.F.R. § 164.502 (2001).

41. 45 C.F.R. § 164.506.

42. 45 C.F.R. § 164.508 (2001).

43. 45 C.F.R. § 164.

44. 45 C.F. R. § 164.512 (2001).

45. 45 C.F.R. § 164.522 (2001).

46. 45 C.F.R. § 164.524 (2001).

47. 45 C.F.R § 164.526 (2001).

48. 45 C.F.R § 164.520 (2001).

49. 45 C.F.R. § 164.528 (2001).

50. 42 U.S.C. § 1320d-7 (2002). "Contrary to state law" is defined as impossible to comport with both state and federal law or that the state law is a major obstacle to the implementation to the Privacy Rule. 45 C.F.R. § 160.203 (2001).

51. 45 C.F.R. § 160.203(a) (2001).

52. Critical access hospitals (CAH) are small facilities (25 beds or less) located in geographically remote areas that provide acute care services to the community. To be designated as a CAH by CMS, a hospital must be located in a rural area, provide 24-hour emergency services; have an average length of stay for its patients of 96 hours or less; be located more than 35 miles (or more than 15 miles in areas with mountainous terrain) from the nearest hospital or be designated by its state as a "necessary provider."

53. 78 Fed. Reg. 5566 (Jan. 25, 2013).

54. HIPAA Administrative Simplification Regulations are found at 45 C.F.R. Parts 160, 162, and 164. To learn about the Rulemaking History of the HIPAA Enforcement Rule, see 42 C.F.R. Part 160, subparts C, D, and E.

55. 42 CFR §164.524.

56. Kohn GP, Galanko JA, Overby DW, Farrell TM. High case volumes and surgical fellowships are associated with improved outcomes for bariatric surgery patients: a justification of current credentialing initiatives for practice and training. J Am Coll Surg. 2010;210(6):909–18.

57. Zimmerman R. Doctors' new tool to fight lawsuits: saying "I'm sorry." The Wall Street Journal 2004 May 18.

58. Levinson W, Roter DL, Mullooly JP, Dull VT, Frankel RM. Physician–patient communication: the relationship with malpractice claims among primary care physicians and surgeons. JAMA. 1997;277:553–9.

59. Ambady N, LaPlante D, Nguyen T, Rosenthal R, Chaumeton N, Levinson W. Surgeon's tone of voice: a clue to malpractice history. Surgery. 2002;132:5–9.

60. Bariatric surgery: American College of Surgeons recommendations for facilities performing bariatric surgery. Bull Am Coll Surg. 2000;85(9).

Index

S.A. Brethauer et al. (eds.), *Minimally Invasive Bariatric Surgery*,
DOI 10.1007/978-1-4939-1637-5, © Springer Science+Business Media New York 2015